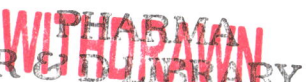

GASTROINTESTINAL PROBLEMS IN THE INFANT *Second Edition*

By JOYCE GRYBOSKI, M.D.

Professor of Pediatrics
Yale University
New Haven, Connecticut

and W. ALLAN WALKER, M.D.

Professor of Pediatrics
Harvard Medical School;
Chief, Pediatric Gastrointestinal and Nutrition Unit
Massachusetts General Hospital
Boston, Massachusetts

1983   W.B. Saunders Company

Philadelphia • London • Toronto

Mexico City • Rio de Janeiro • Sydney • Tokyo

W. B. Saunders Company: West Washington Square
Philadelphia, PA   19105

1 St. Anne's Road
Eastbourne, East Sussex BN21 3UN, England

1 Goldthorne Avenue
Toronto, Ontario M8Z 5T9, Canada

Apartado 26370 — Cedro 512
Mexico 4, D.F., Mexico

Rua Coronel Cabrita, 8
Sao Cristovao Caixa Postal 21176
Rio de Janeiro, Brazil

9 Waltham Street
Artarmon, N.S.W. 2064, Australia

Ichibancho, Central Bldg., 22-1 Ichibancho
Chiyoda-Ku, Tokyo 102, Japan

Library of Congress Cataloging in Publication Data

Gryboski, Joyce.

Gastrointestinal problems in the infant.

1. Pediatric gastroenterology.   I. Walker, W. Allan.
II. Title. [DNLM: 1. Gastrointestinal diseases — In
infancy and childhood. WS 310 G894g]

RJ446.G78 1983	618.9′23	81-48621
ISBN 0–7216–4329–9		AACR2

Listed here is the latest translated edition of this
book together with the language of the translation
and the publisher.

Italian (*1st Edition*) — Edizioni Medico Scientifiche,
Torino, Italy

Gastrointestinal Problems in the Infant   ISBN   0-7216-4329-9

Last digit is the print number: 9   8   7   6   5   4   3   2   1

To my family, without whose
continued love and caring this text
would not have been accomplished.

JOYCE GRYBOSKI

To the loving memory of my parents,
Allan and Cecelia Walker,
whose efforts and encouragement
were instrumental in my entering
the field of medicine.

ALLAN WALKER

Contributors

JOEL M. ANDRES, M.D.
Associate Professor
University of Florida College of Medicine
Department of Pediatrics
Division of Gastroenterology
Gainesville, Florida

STANLEY A. COHEN, M.D.
Clinical Assistant Professor
Medical College of Georgia;
Director, Gastroenterology, Nutrition and Pediatric Research
Scottish Rite Hospital for Children
Atlanta, Georgia

KRISTY MARIE HENDRICKS, M.S., R.D.
Research Dietitian
Pediatric Gastrointestinal and Nutrition Unit
Massachusetts General Hospital
Boston, Massachusetts

RONALD ELLIS KLEINMAN, M.D.
Assistant Professor of Pediatrics
Harvard Medical School;
Assistant in Pediatrics
Gastrointestinal and Nutrition Unit
Massachusetts General Hospital
Boston, Massachusetts

ALAN M. LAKE, M.D.
Assistant Professor of Pediatrics
The Johns Hopkins University School of Medicine;
Division of Pediatric Gastroenterology and Nutrition
The Johns Hopkins Hospital
Baltimore, Maryland

SUSAN H. LARAMEE, M.S., R.D.
Instructor
MGH Institute of Health Professions;
Department of Dietetics
Massachusetts General Hospital
Boston, Massachusetts

REBECCA NILOFF, M.D., C.M.
Clinical Fellow in Pediatrics
Harvard Medical School;
Fellow in Pediatric Gastroenterology and Nutrition, Children's Service
Massachusetts General Hospital
Boston, Massachusetts

Preface

In this second edition of the textbook, we have revised the format to allow readers more convenience in addressing gastrointestinal problems that develop during infancy. The textbook is divided into three major parts. The *first* deals with an approach to the evaluation of common gastrointestinal signs and symptoms presenting in infants. In these chapters we attempt to differentiate between developmental, self-limiting problems, such as neonatal jaundice and regurgitation, and potentially life-threatening conditions that must be identified and managed with expedience.

In the *second* part, we have provided an approach to managing the more complicated gastrointestinal problems that result in failure to thrive. This section provides a practical guide to parenteral and enteral nutritional support, which is based on the editors' experience over the decade. In many instances, the consequences of the gastrointestinal disorders are more dangerous to the young infant than the actual problems. Nutritional support to prevent damage to the developing brain or secondary infections due to inadequate host defenses ultimately may be more beneficial to the young infant than an aggressive approach to establishing the primary diagnosis. In fact, in many instances, such as with intractable diarrhea of infancy, the primary basis for the insult is never completely established, and nutritional support represents the most important approach to the problem.

In the *third* part, specific gastrointestinal problems unique to or also encountered in infancy are described. These conditions, as in the first edition, are presented according to location within the gastrointestinal tract. A considerable effort has been made to deal primarily and comprehensively with the most common disorders encountered and yet be as complete as possible. Extensive attempts to update the expanding literature in this area have been made, and chapters are referenced with the most recent articles appearing in the medical literature.

Finally, an expanded appendix has been provided to facilitate the access of practicing physicians to important objective data for interpreting diagnostic tests and for managing patients with specific problems.

As with the first edition of this textbook, the editors have tried to be as complete as possible in providing the most recent information on gastrointestinal problems in infants. However, the tenet of this edition is also clinical and directly primarily toward house officers, practicing pediatricians, and gastroenterologists. We have attempted to answer questions that we ourselves have asked. We are hopeful that this expanded edition will provide an appropriate reference text to be kept in your office for perusal when you encounter a young infant with symptoms or signs relevant to the gastro-intestinal tract. Much of what is written comes from our own collective experience in diagnosing and managing infants in our own practices of pediatric gastroenterology. We hope that it is of benefit to you in your practice.

JOYCE GRYBOSKI

ALLAN WALKER

Acknowledgments

We wish to thank all the individuals who contributed to the quality of this edition. This includes Dr. Ronald Kleinman, who contributed to Part II, on Nutritional Support of the Newborn with Gastrointestinal Problems; Dr. Rebecca Niloff, who contributed to the section on Pancreatic Disease States; Dr. Stanley Cohen, who contributed in Part I on Chronic Diarrhea and in Part III on Infectious and Miscellaneous Causes of Diarrhea; Dr. Alan Lake, who made major contributions to the chapter on Inherited and Metabolic Disorders; Dr. Joel Andres, who contributed to Symptoms of Liver Dysfunction in Part I and Diseases of the Liver in Part III; and Ms. Susan Laramee and Ms. Kristy Hendricks, who diligently prepared much of the Appendix material for this edition.

Finally, we would like to express our gratitude to the Saunders staff: Mary Cowell, Associate Medical Editor, with whom we worked closely and Bill Preston of the Production Department for both his patience and his skill.

Contents

to the mother is all that is required. If symptoms progress, gastroesophageal reflux must be suspected and investigated.

ABDOMINAL MASS

The time of development of an abdominal mass does not establish whether it is malignant or benign in nature. The consistency is more helpful, for masses that are soft more often represent an abscess or a cystic lesion than a tumor. As noted in Table 1–2, the location of the mass may be a clue to its diagnosis. Although each of the gastrointestinal lesions will be discussed in appropriate sections of the text, it is timely in this section to review the diagnostic techniques in current use.

A flat film of the abdomen is of value in determining a large intra- or extraluminal lesion of the gastrointestinal tract. Localized air-fluid levels or distention of a viscus suggest intrinsic obstruction, whereas displaced loops of bowel suggest an extrinsic mass. The presence of abnormal calcification suggests a teratoma. Liver, spleen, and kidney size may be evaluated from this film.

Ultrasonography is a rapid technique for determining consistency of an intra-abdominal mass and will easily differentiate fluid-filled from solid lesions.[8b] In the upper quadrants it will reveal the texture, consistency, and size of the solid organs, such as pancreas, liver, spleen, and kidneys, and ascertain the size of the external bile ducts and gallbladder (Figs. 1–1 and 1–2).[8b, 37]

Further studies, such as intravenous pyelography and radiologic examination of the gastrointestinal tract, are performed as indicated.

Table 1–2 Abdominal Mass in Infancy

Left upper quadrant	Splenomegaly
	Enlarged kidney
	Wilms' tumor
	Neuroblastoma
	Gastric distention
	Gastric duplication
	Gastric hematoma
	Gastric teratoma
	Pancreatic pseudocyst
	Enlarged left lobe of liver
	Volvulus of small bowel
Right upper quadrant	Hepatomegaly
	Hydropic gallbladder
	Choledochal cyst
	Mesenteric cyst
	Neuroblastoma
	Enlarged kidney
Epigastrium	Left lobe of liver
	Choledochal cyst
	Gastric tumor
	Gastric or duodenal duplication
	Pancreatic pseudocyst
Left lower quadrant	Fecal impaction
	Ovarian tumor or cyst
	Appendiceal abscess and malrotation of colon
Right lower quadrant	Appendiceal abscess
	Lymphangiomatous cyst
	Mesenteric cyst
	Ovarian cyst or tumor
Suprapubic or midabdominal	Fecal impaction
	Omphalomesenteric abnormalities
	Sacral teratoma
	Anterior meningocele
	Distended bladder
	Ectopic kidney

GASEOUSNESS

The usual cause of increased belching or passage of flatus is air-swallowing due to excessive sucking of a nipple with poor flow. Crying, improper feeding techniques, and poor burping are additional factors in accumulation of gastrointestinal air.

Disaccharide intolerances, particularly lactose intolerance, may cause significant gas production within the colon, but in infants are usually accompanied by diarrhea. A simple examination of the stool pH will determine the presence or absence of sugar malabsorption.

The most effective diagnostic tool is observation of the infant during feeding and burping. Silicone-containing preparations are occasionally given to diffuse the air bubbles but are generally not required.

PAIN

Pain is a difficult symptom to interpret in the infant. Normal periods of irritability may represent pain to the insecure or inexperienced mother, and in such instances, observation and examination of the infant

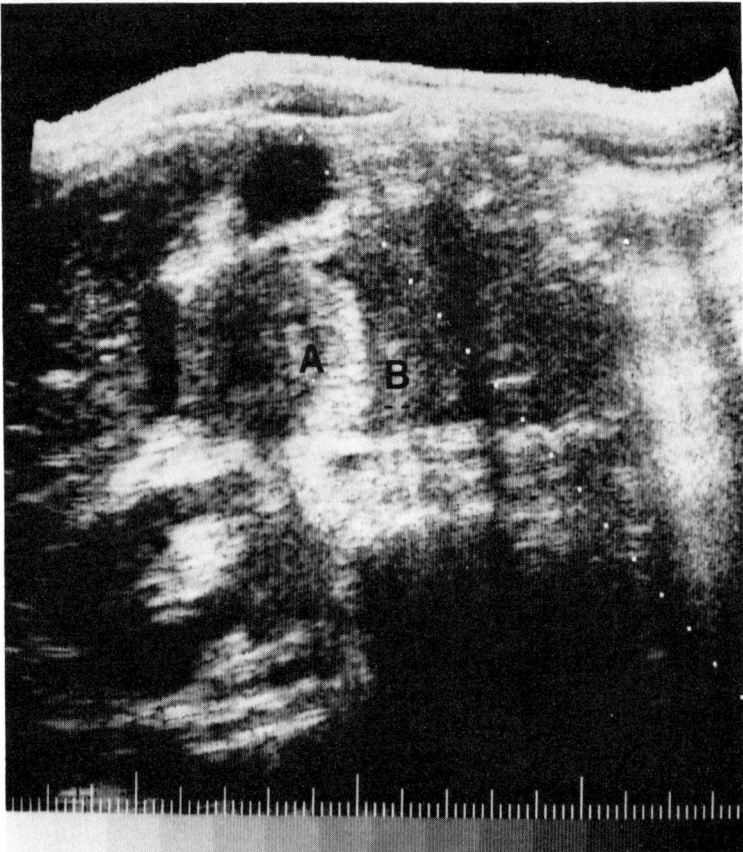

Figure 1–1 Ultrasonographic cross section of abdomen showing duodenal hematoma (*A*) and edematous pancreas (*B*). Skin surface (top) is shown for orientation.

during an attack of pain are crucial to the diagnosis. Some characteristic patterns, may, however, be discerned from a careful history. A cry after a brief period of staring may represent a seizure. The infant with esophageal pain arches his back in an effort to propel a nutrient bolus through an irritated or partially obstructed esophagus and is usually without symptoms between feedings. The pain of pancreatitis and peritonitis is of such severity that the infant lies quite still, has grunting respirations, and resists any efforts to examine his abdomen or to move him.

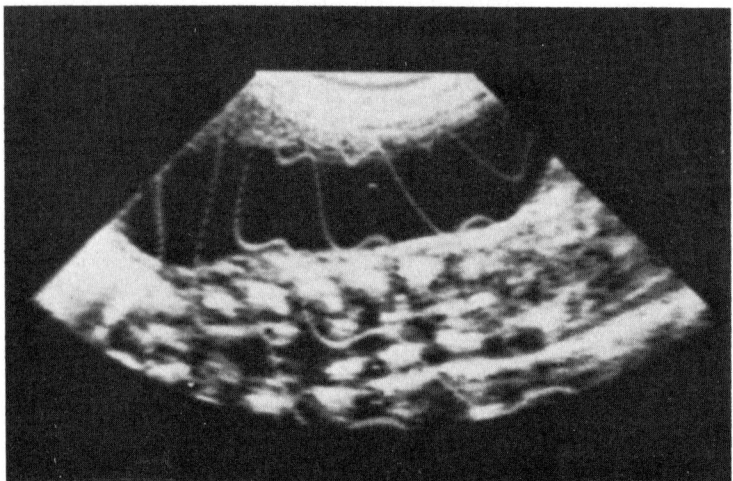

Figure 1–2 Suggested ultrasound study of 800-gm one-month-old infant with hepatomegaly and right lower quadrant mass. The view is such that orientation shows upper abdomen (left) and lower abdomen (right). Mottled opaque material (upper left) represents liver and the large lucent area, an enlarged gallbladder.

Table 1–3 Causes of Abdominal Pain
in Infants and Children

Lactose intolerance
Constipation
Milk allergy
Pancreatitis
Peptic ulcer disease
Esophagitis
Inflammatory bowel disease
Gastroenteritis
Duplication cysts
Meckel's diverticulum
Porphyria
Giardiasis
Psychogenic problems
Errors of rotation of the intestine
Ectopic pancreas
Annular pancreas
Spinal cord tumor

Intermittent, acute, or colicky pain may indicate intestinal obstruction or acute gastroenteritis . In the former, stools decrease, whereas in the latter, diarrhea predominates. If the pain persists in a wave-like pattern and is associated with vomiting or decreased stooling, the infant should be evaluated for intestinal obstruction. A sudden loss of consciousness or the passage of currant-jelly stools suggests intussusception. Postprandial discomfort and abdominal distention that seem to be relieved by the passage of flatus suggest disaccharide intolerance.

The causes of abdominal pain are listed in Table 1–3. Depending upon the study and the interests of the investigator,[27] one may identify the more common causes as lactose intolerance,[5, 35a] peptic ulcer disease,[29] pancreatitis,[11] constipation,[16] or a psychosomatic condition.[3] The individual disorders are discussed separately in the text.

Psychosomatic aspects of abdominal pain are less frequent in the infant and toddler than in older children. Apley notes, however, that the "gut is a psychosomatic target organ, and often the main one"[3] throughout childhood years; constipation, colic, and "irritable colon" are found to be more frequent manifestations of psychosomatic symptomatology in children under three years than is abdominal pain. After studying well over 100 children with recurrent abdominal pain, considered to be functional,

Stone and Barbero[35] found a high incidence of prenatal and perinatal problems as well as abdominal complaints in other family members. In long-term follow-up, there is a 2 per cent or less incidence of actual intestinal disease.[34] Often, however, one tends to term pain "functional" when a cause cannot be identified. We have seen a teratoma of the lumbar spine and others have reported an astrocytoma of the thoracic cord[8a] in children with entirely negative gastrointestinal evaluations. Each, significantly, had unexplained and persistent scoliosis.

COLIC

Colic is a symptom complex of presumed gastrointestinal etiology that is characterized by unexplained crying or screeching. It is associated with abdominal pain and some inability to pass gas.[8, 23]

Incidence. The incidence varies directly with the criteria used for diagnosis, for these are largely subjective. Approximately 11 per cent of full-term and low birth weight infants have been estimated to suffer from colic, but in a few studies, incidences range as high as 23 to 40 per cent. Caucasians are most often affected, but there seems to be no predilection for either sex.[2, 16]

Etiology. A multitude of factors have been implicated in the quest for the etiology of this disorder. Originally, the most popular theories included family tensions, central nervous system immaturity, allergies, and the position in the family as first-born child. Later, rather extensive studies have discovered no correlation with home environment, finding most mothers to be well educated, intelligent, stable, and cheerful.[32] Indeed, colicky infants at one year appear to be more active and inquisitive than their noncolicky peers. The majority of infants have, however, proved to be first-born and, as symptoms continued over several weeks, did generate conflict in many homes as well as concerns about parental inadequacy. Postulations of soft neurologic damage or central nervous system immaturity cannot be entirely dismissed, for we have seen several such infants grow into hyperactive youngsters.

Milk protein allergy remains a consideration in the diagnosis of colic, for it may be a presenting symptom in some infants before the onset of diarrhea. In recent years, colic in breast-fed infants has been related to the passage of cow's milk protein through breast milk.[20, 25] Nursing mothers are often instructed to drink 1 to 1½ quarts of milk per day, and colic is often relieved by simply decreasing or eliminating milk protein in the diet.

Lactose intolerance, which results in the accumulation of a large volume of colonic gas, may cause abdominal distress prior to the passage of large quantities of explosive stool. Similarly, *high lactulose concentrations* in commercial canned formulas may cause increased colonic gas, for lactulose is a synthetic carbohydrate formed from lactose and is not hydrolyzed by mammalian small intestinal mucosa.

Alprostadil (prostaglandin E_1) is used often in the neonate for the treatment of congenital cardiac defects and may cause intestinal colic and diarrhea.[32a]

Health food–additive colic is a more recently encountered form of the disorder. In this age of physical fitness and emphasis upon organic foods, we occasionally encounter an infant whose mother is supplementing his formula with natural sugars, yeast, pancreatic enzymes, and minerals.

Certain anatomic disorders may cause symptoms resembling those of colic. *Gastroesophageal reflux* may rarely cause repeated episodes of crying, fussing, and difficulty in feeding in infants without apparent regurgitation. *Anal stenosis or anal membrane* was a diagnosis made in five infants referred during the last two years for the evaluation of colic. Examination revealed a slightly anterior location of the anus in four infants and an incomplete anal membrane in the fifth. Anal stenosis was noted in rectal examination of four infants. Excision of the membrane or dilatation of the rectum was curative. *Urinary tract* obstruction, particularly in the ureteropelvic region, and even uncomplicated urinary tract infections have caused symptoms of colic in infants.[14]

Immunoglobulin abnormalities, such as transient IgA or IgG deficiency, have been associated with colic that is accompanied by or followed by chronic diarrhea. In such instances, a hypoallergenic formula will result in cessation of colic.

Feeding problems caused by inadequate nipple size or by leaving an infant with a propped bottle result in excessive air swallowing and the accumulation of large quantities of gastric and intestinal gas.

Pathophysiology. The gastrointestinal tract in true colic is hypermotile, with the stools being either loose or hard and containing mucus. There are increased nonpropulsive contractions in the rectum.

Symptoms. Typically, the onset of colic is at three weeks of age, although the condition may develop any time during the first three months of life. If the symptoms are rather mild and occur for the most part in late afternoon and early evening, the term "paroxysmal fussing" is often used. Brazelton,[6] in a classic study of crying in infancy, noted that the six-week infant had a maximal fussy period between 6 and 8 P.M. and that infants with colic had exaggerated fussiness that progressed until approximately six weeks of age and lasted for a period of four hours or longer for the next two weeks.

In its more obvious form, the attack is sudden in onset, with the infant becoming flushed and the abdomen distended. He cries constantly, often shrieking, and flexes his legs to his abdomen. The attack may last for several hours and is frequently terminated with the passage of stool and flatus. Symptoms improve spontaneously between 10 and 12 weeks, explaining the often-designated term "three months' colic."

Diagnosis. The diagnosis is often based upon a "typical history." However, a complete physical examination, urinalysis, determination of stool pH, and examination of the stool for milk precipitins are probably warranted in most infants. Observation of the infant's behavior and positioning during and after feedings is as essential as the physical examination, for feeding in the supine position and poor burping techniques are often major factors in air-swallowing.

Treatment. Folklore remedies are legion, ranging from fennel tea to a few drops of brandy. Many pediatricians begin therapy with antihistamines and, when these prove ineffective, move on to antispasmodics or sedatives, continuing any regime that seems effective. Results with most are often no better than with placebo.[31] Illingworth[23, 24] has found methyscopolamine to be therapeutic, but this has not been confirmed by other experiences. White has noted the most beneficial therapy to be thickened feedings.[36] The old remedies of walking, rocking, or laying the infant over the mother's lap on a warm heating pad offer some degree of solace. Most important in treatment is reassurance to the parents that they or their relationships with their baby are not the cause of his distress.

Prognosis. A number of children seen later for treatment of allergies do have a history of infantile colic. Similarly, Davidson and Wasserman[12] have noted a high incidence of colic and familial constipation or diarrhea in their series of children with the "irritable bowel syndrome."

DISORDERS OF STOOLING

In order to determine the abnormal, one must be aware of the normal frequency of stools. The majority of infants pass their first stool within 36 hours of birth.[9] Retention of stool beyond that period is considered to be abnormal and suggests Hirschsprung's disease, meconium plug, neonatal small left colon syndrome, or low intestinal obstruction.

CONSTIPATION

Constipation is a term describing the consistency of the stool rather than its frequency. Hard, firm, or pellet-like stools indicate constipation, whether they are passed several times a day or once a week. Indeed, infrequent stools are not unusual in the breast-fed infant. In babies, the gastrocolic reflex is most pronounced and the stools are typically passed during or just after feeding. With increasing age and variation in diet, stools become more firm and fewer. The transit time in infants of three to five days is 3 to 13 hours, but by 45 days this increases to longer than ten hours in breast-fed infants but remains less than ten hours in formula-fed ones.[18] Stool frequency, weight, and water content are noted in Table 1–4, showing that although stool frequency decreases and weight increases with age, there is actually little variation in water content of stools passed by infants one week to one year of age. By three years, most children have learned voluntary control and can withhold their movements until they reach the potty chair or toilet.

Etiology. Physiologic constipation is a major cause of this disorder and may well be familial, since one or both parents will have a history of constipation as a child or young adult. It is likely that this is due to an exaggerated water-absorptive mechanism in the colon. Symptoms often become quite marked when the infant is given regular milk containing 4 per cent lactose after taking infant formula containing 7 to 7.5 per cent sugar.

Sensory or motor impairment can cause abnormalities in defecation and result in fecal retention.[19] Those conditions often responsible are spina bifida and myelodysplasia, Hirschsprung's disease, Chagas' disease, neurofibromatosis of the colon, immaturity of the ganglion cells as in prematurity, porphyria, the lipoidoses, and hypothyroidism. A Hirschsprung-like disease due to atrophic myositis of the colon has

Table 1–4   Stool Frequency and Weight in Normal Infants

	1 WEEK	8–28 DAYS	1–12 MONTHS	13–24 MONTHS
No. stools/24 hours	4	2.2	1.8	1.7
Weight	4.3 gm	11 gm	17 gm	35 gm
Water content	72%	73%	75%	73.8%

been reported in Bantu children. One metabolic disorder that has received little attention as a cause of constipation is idiopathic hypercalcemia, or Williams' disease. Anatomic lesions such as anal stenosis or ectopic anus may cause constipation as well as colic symptoms.[21, 26]

The most common cause of constipation, however, is anal fissure, which results from the passage of hard stool and is associated with such pain that it leads to withholding. A vicious cycle is established, for as the fecal bolus remains in the rectum, it becomes even firmer. Rarely, fecal impaction leads to gastrointestinal bleeding from local ulceration or to partial intestinal obstruction. Intermittent or paradoxical diarrhea is frequent in the chronically constipated child and results from the overflow of soft material around the impacted bolus. With increasing colonic distention, the sensation of a distended rectum, needed to initiate defecation, disappears.

In older infants, improper or traumatic toilet training can be the origin of chronic constipation. The use of infant seats that attach over the adult toilet are to be condemned. They not only are frightening, they also are physiologically inappropriate, for they provide no means for the child to brace his feet, a position necessary for adequate abdominal muscle contraction.

Pathophysiology. Physiologically, in constipation due to irritable bowel there is a predominance of contractions that are increased in both number and amplitude.[1, 13] Davidson, in 1956, described a nonpropulsive pattern of colonic motility in normal children and an increased propulsive activity in diarrheal states. He noted that mecholyl caused a relaxation of the phasic activity of the distal colon. In 50 per cent of children with Hirschsprung's disease, this relaxation occurred only in normally innervated distal colons but was absent from the aganglionic segment. Davidson further described three children with "achalasia of the distal rectal segment" who had normal ganglion cells.[14]

Since it is imperative to differentiate Hirschsprung's disease, particularly the short-segment form, from physiologic constipation, considerable research has been done on anorectal function.[33] Internal sphincter relaxation has been demonstrated in most term infants and in some premature ones, the youngest being 34 weeks' gestational age. The sphincter response depends upon postnatal age as well as upon the actual presence of ganglion cells and develops with daily age. Increased anal canal pressure and decreased sensitivity of the internal sphincter relaxation have been noted as early as the first day of life. Cyclic rhythmic contractions in the anal canal, often seen in those infants with Hirschsprung's disease, have been, for some, a normal finding in the neonate.[10]

Meunier et al.[30] studied a variety of rectal responses in constipated children. The rectoanal inhibitory reflex threshold (internal sphincter relaxation in response to transient rectal distention) was increased in 6.2 per cent of constipated children. Anal hypertony was present in 46 per cent and decreased rectal sensitivity to distention, in 68 per cent. Abnormally large amounts of air may be required to fill the rectal balloon in order to initiate internal sphincter relaxation in extremely constipated children. If this is not recognized, Hirschsprung's disease may be erroneously diagnosed. A low mean resting tone of the anus, thought by some to represent a weak internal sphincter, may simply be a result of chronic impaction, since the pressure normalizes after treatment.[29a]

Symptoms. The truly constipated infant has a history of fretfulness, poor appetite, intermittent abdominal pain, and distention. Weight gain may be impaired. Frequently the child has been treated for one or more urinary tract infections. The stools are pellet-like and hard or massive in size. Older infants sometimes perform what Davidson[12] has termed the "duty dance," in which they tighten their gluteal muscles and wiggle in a dance-like motion in order to withhold stool. This may be misinterpreted by the parent as an episode of acute abdominal pain.

Diarrhea or partial intestinal obstruction may be the initial symptom, indicating the need for a rectal examination as an integral part of every physical examination. Stool is palpable above the pubis and in the left colon. In some, the entire colon, filled with firm masses of stool, is palpable. The abdomen is often distended and tympanitic to percussion. Rectal examination reveals hard stool within the ampulla. Rarely, if the patient is examined after a movement, the ampulla may be empty, a finding typical of Hirschsprung's disease.

Differential Diagnosis. Metabolic and physiologic disorders must be evaluated by physical findings and laboratory studies. Ectopic anus and anal membrane must be ruled out. Thyroid studies and analyses of serum carotene, calcium and phosphorus rule out the common metabolic disorders and celiac disease, which may present with constipation. Of these, celiac disease has been most often found by our group.

Diagnosis. The history and physical examination will often confirm the diagnosis of physiologic constipation, other family members and even a partner twin having constipation.[4] If rectal examination confirms the presence of hard stool in the ampulla, Hirschsprung's disease is unlikely, although the short-segment form cannot be eliminated. Barium enema is usually of no assistance, for it reveals only a dilated, redundant colon, and its use in the infant is not warranted. If there is anything atypical in the history, anorectal manometry is the most fruitful diagnostic tool in differentiating functional constipation from Hirschsprung's disease.

Treatment. The young infant is most easily treated by increasing the carbohydrate content of his diet, using Karo syrup, dextrins, maltose, or sucrose. If a large fecal impaction is present, this is best relieved by a mineral oil retention enema, followed by a normal saline or Fleet pediatric enema (3 ml/kg). Rarely, phosphate enemas cause problems owing to their high osmolarity and tendency to decrease serum calcium. They should therefore be used with caution or not at all in those infants suspected of having Hirschsprung's disease. In older children, addition of fiber to the diet in the form of bran cereals and breads and fresh fruits and vegetables will soften and provide increased bulk to the stools. Of course,

adequate fluid intake is essential for all age groups.

If dietary means are not sufficient, mineral oil, 3 to 5 ml/per kg/per day, will, after several days, soften the stools. The initial dose may be adjusted upward if necessary to guarantee several large, loose stools each day to ensure emptying of the colon. The dosage is gradually adjusted downward until the child is passing one large, soft stool per day. Staining of oil or the passage of small quantities of oily stool usually denotes inadequate mineral oil dosages. Several weeks to months of therapy may be required before the child is confident that stooling is without pain and until the sensation for defecation has returned. Lactulose, a nonabsorbable sugar, is also an effective stool softener and bypasses the staining problems of oil. A dosage for children, however, is not yet established.

Proper toilet training is essential to establishing patterns of defecation and should imply a happy, rewarding experience for both parent and child. Training is best not initiated before two years of age and only at a time when the child is responsive. He should be placed in the potty chair at a time when he is most likely to stool and for no longer than ten minutes. If this is not successful, attempts to train should be discontinued for several weeks. Training is facilitated by the use of training pants and clothing that the child may remove easily.

DIARRHEA

Diarrhea describes the consistency rather than the frequency of stools and implies an increased water content. Stools therefore may vary from soft and mushy to liquid. Occasionally, a central core of stool is surrounded in the diaper by a large water ring. The patient's history is extremely important, for what might seem to be a single episode of diarrhea is actually an acute manifestation of a more chronic disorder, such as food allergy, celiac disease, sugar intolerance, or cystic fibrosis. An infectious etiology is most likely if other members of the household are or have been ill. A family history of gastrointestinal disease in infancy suggests gastrointestinal protein allergy, celiac disease, or cystic fibrosis. The stools of infants with malabsorption are characteristically pale, large, bulky, and foul-smelling, sometimes containing visible oil droplets. Stools associated with disaccharide intolerance tend to be frothy and explosive, with a sour or vinegar-like odor. Those of infants with milk or soy protein allergies are soft to liquid, are often explosive, and contain mucus and occasional streaks of blood. Fine sand-like particles or pea-sized pellets resembling cottage cheese represent milk curds. Visible fruit or vegetable particles indicate rapid transit rather than any specific intolerance to these foods. Green, watery, "starvation" stools are passed by infants deprived of oral bulk for several days and are often seen in those with acute diarrhea who are taking electrolyte solutions. The causes and treatment of diarrhea are discussed in detail in Chapter Five.

REFERENCES

1. Almy, T.: Constipation in gastrointestinal disease. *In* Sleisenger, M., and Fordtran, J. (eds.): Gastrointestinal Disease. Philadelphia, W. B. Saunders Company, 1978.
2. Anders, T. F., and Weinstein, P.: Sleep and its disorders in infants and children. Pediatrics 50:317, 1972.
3. Apley, J.: Psychosomatic aspects of gastrointestinal problems. Clin. Gastroenterol. 6:311, 1977.
4. Backwin, H., and Davidson, M.: Constipation in twins. Am. J. Dis. Child. 121:179, 1971.
4a. Barlow, C. F.: Headaches and brain tumors. Am. J. Dis. Child. 126:99, 1982.
5. Barr, R. G., Levine, M. D., and Watkins, J.: Recurrent abdominal pain of childhood due to lactose intolerance. N. Engl. J. Med. 300:1449, 1979.
6. Boulton, T. J. V., and Rowley, M. P.: Nutritional studies during early childhood. III. Incidental observations of temperament, habits and experiences of ill health. Aust. Paediatr. J. 15:87, 1979.
7. Brazelton, T. B.: Crying in infancy. Pediatrics 29:579, 1962.
8. Breslow, L.: A clinical approach to infantile colic: a review of 90 cases. J. Pediatr. 50:196, 1957.
8a. Bucke, E., and Bodensteiner, J.: Thoracic cord tumor appearing as recurrent abdominal pain. Am. J. Dis. Child. 135:574, 1981.
8b. Cantu, T., Leopold, G., and Wolf, D. A.: Ultrasound in antenatal diagnosis of anomalies. Ann. Surg. 194:353, 1981.
9. Clark, D. A.: Time of first void and first stool in 500 newborns. Pediatrics 60:457, 1977.
10. Cohen, M., Duffner, P., and Lacey, D.: Neurologic aspects of swallowing, vomiting and defecation. *In* Lebenthal, E. (ed.): Textbook of Gastroenterology and Nutrition in Infancy. New York, Raven Press, 1981.
11. Cox, K. L., Ament, M., Sample, W., Sarti, D., O'Donnell, M., and Byrne, W.: The ultrasonic and biochemical diagnosis of pancreatitis in children. J. Pediatr. 96:407, 1980.
12. Davidson, M.: Irritable colon in children. *In* Sleisenger, M., and Fordtran, J. (eds.): Gastrointestinal Disease. Philadelphia, W. B. Saunders Company, 1978.
13. Davidson, M., and Bauer, C.: Studies of colonic motility in children. IV. Achalasia of the distal rectal segment despite presence of ganglia in the myenteric plexus of this area. Pediatrics 21:746, 1958.
14. Davidson, M., Sleisenger, M. H., Almy, T., and Levine, S. Z.: Studies of distal colonic motility in children. I. non-propulsive patterns in normal children. Pediatrics 17:820, 1956.
15. Davidson, M., and Wasserman, R.: The irritable colon of childhood. J. Pediatr. 69:1027, 1966.
16. Dimson, S. B.: Transit time related to clinical findings in children with recurrent abdominal pain. Pediatrics 47:666, 1971.
17. Du, J. N. H.: Colic as the sole symptom of urinary tract infection in infants. Can. Med. Assoc. J. 115:334, 1976.
18. Fomon, S. J.: Infant Nutrition. Philadelphia, W. B. Saunders Company, 1974.
19. Gryboski, J. D.: Gastrointestinal Problems in the Infant. Ed. 1. Philadelphia, W. B. Saunders Company, 1975.
20. Harris, M. J., Petts, V., and Penny, R.: Cow's milk allergy as a cause of infantile colic. Aust. Paediatr. J. 13:276, 1977.
21. Hendren, W. H.: Constipation caused by anterior location of the anus and its surgical correction. J. Pediatr. Surg. 13:505, 1978.
22. Holmes, C. A.: Infantile colic. Clin. Pediatr. 8:566, 1969.
22a. Honig, P., and Charney, E.: Children with brain tumor headaches. Am. J. Dis. Child. 136:120, 1982.
23. Illingworth, R. S.: Three months' colic. Arch. Dis. Child. 29:165, 1954.
24. Illingworth, R. S.: Three months' colic. Treatment by methylscopolamine nitrate. Acta Paediatr. Scand. 44:203, 1955.
25. Jakobsson, I., and Lindberg, T.: Cow's milk as a cause of infantile colic in breast fed infants. Lancet 2:437, 1978.
26. Leape, L., and Ramenofsky, M.: Anterior ectopic anus: a common cause of constipation in children. J. Pediatr. Surg. 23:627, 1978.
27. Lebenthal, E.: Recurrent abdominal pain in childhood. Am. J. Dis. Child. 134:347, 1980.
28. Lemoh, J. N., and Brooke, O. G.: Frequency and weight of normal stools in infancy. Arch. Dis. Child. 54:719, 1979.
29. Liebman, W.: Recurrent abdominal pain in children. Clin. Pediatr. 17:149, 1978.
29a. Loening-Baucke, V., and Younoszai, M. K.: Abnormal anal sphincter response in chronically constipated children. J. Pediatr. 100:213, 1982.
30. Meunier, P., Marechal, J. M., and deBeaujeau, M. J.: Rectoanal pressures and rectal sensitivity

studies in chronic childhood constipation. Gastroenterology 77:330, 1979.

31. O'Donovan, J. C., and Bradstock, A. S., Jr.: The failure of conventional drug therapy in the management of infantile colic. Am. J. Dis. Child. *133*:999, 1979.

32. Paradise, J. J.: Maternal and other factors in the etiology of infant colic: report of a prospective study of 146 infants. JAMA *197*:123, 1966.

32a. Sankaran, K., Conly, J., Boyle, C., and Tyrrell, M.: Intestinal colic and diarrhea as side effects of intravenous Alprostadil administration. Am. J. Dis. Child. *135*:664, 1981.

33. Siegel, M., and Lebenthal, E.: Development of gastrointestinal motility and gastric emptying during the fetal and neonatal periods. *In* Lebenthal, E. (ed.): Textbook of Gastroenterology and Nutrition in Infancy. New York, Raven Press, 1981.

34. Stickler, G., and Marltl, D. B.: Recurrent abdominal pain. Am. J. Dis. Child. *133*:486, 1979.

35. Stone, R. T., and Barbero, G.: Recurrent abdominal pain in childhood. Pediatrics *45*:732, 1970.

35a. Wald, A., Chandra, R., Fisher, S., Gartner, J. C., and Zitelli, B.: Lactose malabsorption in recurrent abdominal pain of childhood. J. Pediatr. *100*:65, 1982.

36. White, P. J.: Management of infantile colic. Am. J. Dis. Child. *133*:995, 1979.

37. Wilson, D. A.: Ultrasound screening for abdominal masses in the neonatal period. Am. J. Dis. Child. *126*:147, 1982.

Chapter Two

SUCK AND SWALLOW

The mechanisms of suck and swallow develop during prenatal life,[1] and the sucking response is elicited *in utero* as early as 18 weeks' gestation.[1] The presence of lanugo hairs and epidermal debris in meconium indicates that they have been swallowed *in utero*. Studies using radioactive materials also document fetal swallowing;[6] most of chromium-51–labeled maternal red blood cells injected into the amniotic sac disappear, and only a negligible number enter the maternal circulation. More than half the labeled cells have disappeared from the amniotic fluid in women delivered 23 to 29 hours after such an injection, and more

than 40 per cent of the cells are recovered from their infants' stools. Studies using iodine-131–labeled albumin yield like results and indicate a rate of fetal swallowing of 5 ml per kg per hour; those using colloidal gold suspended in normal saline show the fetus to swallow an average of 198 ml per day (range, 87 to 287 ml per day), with no difference in results of normal mothers and those with oligo- or polyhydramnios. The near-term fetus swallows, on the average, 500 ml of amniotic fluid per day. The amount of amniotic fluid remains constant because fetal urination in late pregnancy equals the amount of fluid swallowed. Fetal

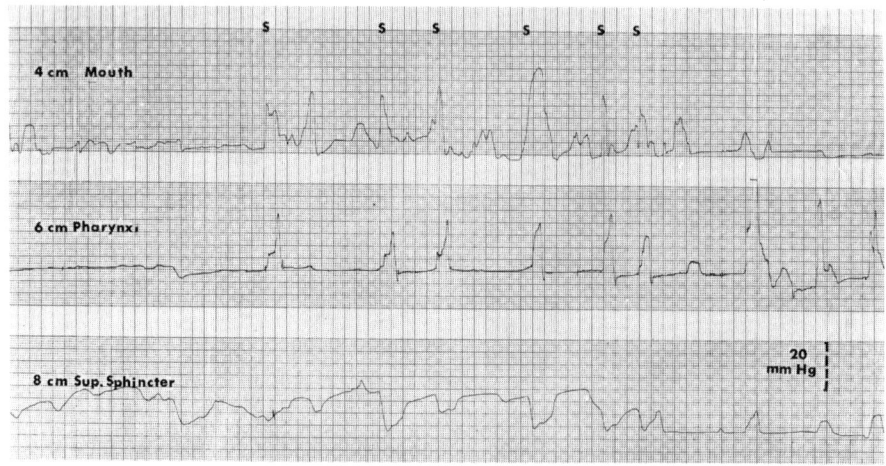

Figure 2–1 This tracing from an 1800-gm infant one day old shows considerable mouthing of the nipple in the 4-cm record but no regular suck pattern. At 6 cm, pharyngeal pressure peaks represent the pharyngeal contraction of deglutition. At 8 cm, the superior esophageal sphincter relaxes with deglutition.

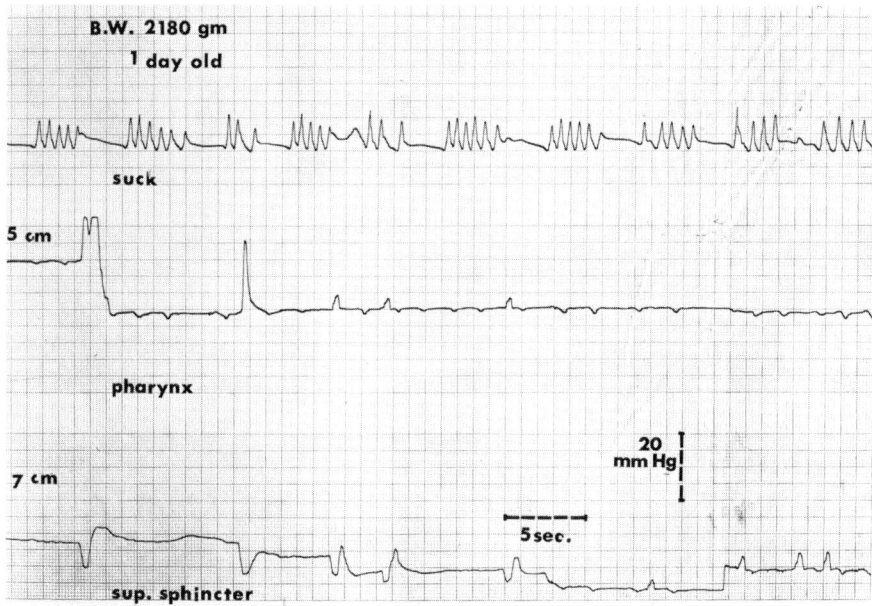

Figure 2–2   Tracing from a one-day-old premature infant of birth weight 2180 gm. A fairly immature suck pattern is represented by sucking bursts of 3 to 6 sucks per burst. Pharyngeal contraction (at 5 cm) appears at the end of or after each burst, and the superior sphincter (7 cm) relaxes.

urine output averages 24.1 (10 to 35) ml per hour. Failure to ingest amniotic fluid occurs in anencephalic fetuses and in those with upper gastrointestinal obstruction and is likely a causative factor for the polyhydramnios associated with these conditions.[39, 59] Conversely, renal abnormalities and genitourinary obstruction in which urination is diminished are associated with oligohydramnios.

The responses of suck and swallow mature most rapidly after several feeding experiences, when the infant is making his first contacts with the environment.[19, 42, 47-50, 62]

SUCK

Individual infants differ in their behavior and likewise in their sucking responses. In general, however, full-term infants demonstrate a transient "immature suck pattern" during their first feeding attempts (Figs. 2–1 to 2–3).[34-36] This is characterized by short bursts of three to five sucks that are preceded or followed by swallows. Within 24 to 48 hours they increase the number of sucks to between 10 and 30 in each burst and often swallow during a sucking burst. This we term the "mature sucking pattern" (Figs.

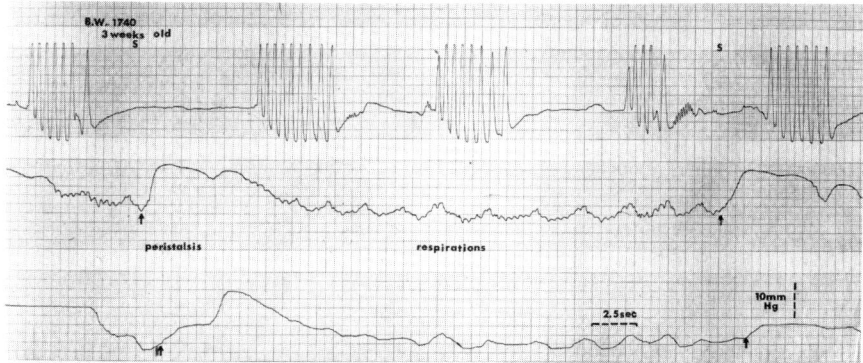

Figure 2–3   Tracing from a premature infant of 1740 gm birth weight taken at three weeks of age. Sucking bursts of six to eight sucks are represented with regular respirations noted in lead 2.

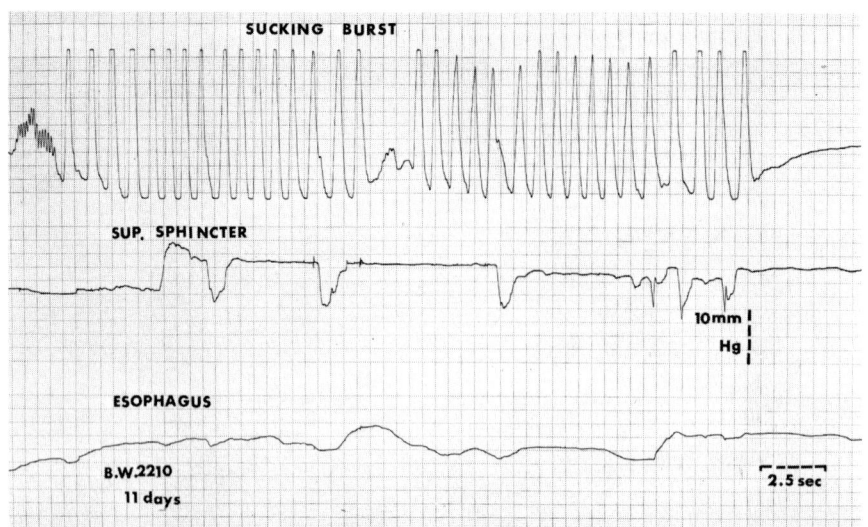

Figure 2–4 Studies in an 11-day-old premature infant of birth weight 2210 gm. A burst represents 16 or more sucks, and the superior sphincter relaxes with swallows during the continuous burst. Small esophageal pressure responses representing peristalsis follow some, but not all, swallows.

2–4 and 2–5). During this transition period the non-nutritive sucking rate increases from one to one and a half or two per second.[34-36] The nutritive sucking rate is approximately one per second but may vary in accordance with the ease of nipple flow. Sucking is affected by a number of factors: Infants suck milk more effectively than sugar-water formula; the rate is slowed by a rigid nipple; and the normal development of a sucking pattern can be depressed for up to four days if the mother has received obstetric sedation.[46-49]

In the premature infant, the development of the sucking response depends largely upon birth weight and degree of maturity.[35] Larger premature infants have a stronger and more effective suck than smaller ones. In those of birth weight between 1700 and 1790 gm, a mature suck pattern develops by the time they reach 1900 gm. An early sucking rate of one per second increases to two per second as infants attain the mature pattern. A mature suck develops at two to four weeks in infants of 1800 to 1890 gm birth weight, at one to two weeks in those of 1900 to 2100 gm, and by the fifth day of life in those of over 2100 gm.

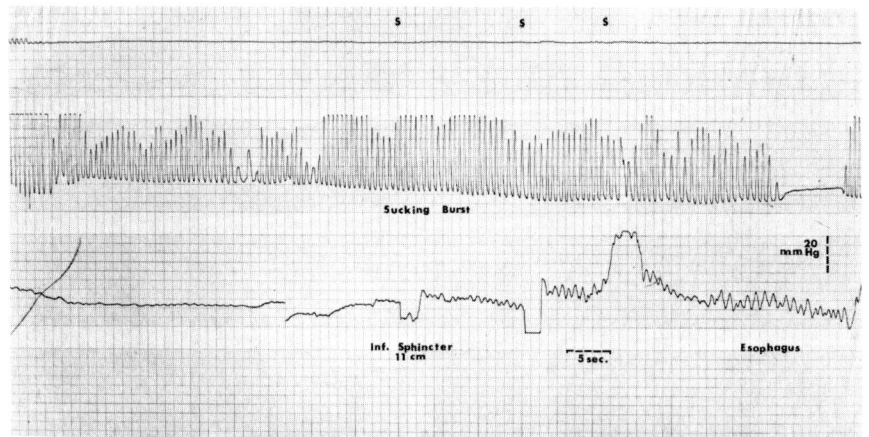

Figure 2–5 Tracing from a mature term infant one week old. Sucking bursts are maintained with swallows represented by relaxation of the inferior sphincter.

Negative intraoral sucking pressures vary from a low of 15 mm Hg to a high of 110 mm Hg, with the lowest pressures in the low birth weight infants. Sucking pressure is more consistent for the individual infant than is the rate of suck.[47, 48, 50]

SWALLOW

The oropharynx performs the function of bringing the nutrient bolus into the mouth and propelling it backward to the pharynx, where, once it reaches the superior esophageal sphincter, its transport becomes automatic or a matter of reflex.

The act of swallowing is divided into three phases.[3, 4, 7, 11, 17, 67]

1. The first phase is concerned with delivery of nutrient into the mouth. The pressures of the lips and jaws upon the nipple combined with negative intraoral pressure brings a flow of liquid into the mouth, where it collects between the tongue and the hard and soft palates. The soft palate and dorsum of the tongue form a seal that prevents the bolus from entering the pharynx. The mouth is separated from the respiratory tract, and the infant can breathe during this process. In some young infants, however, a bit of the bolus collects between the tongue, epiglottis, and soft palate.

2. In the second phase, the tongue, with a roller-like motion, separates from the soft palate and carries the bolus back into the pharynx. The soft palate moves up and backward to close the palatopharyngeal isthmus, and the tongue moves back to contact the pharyngeal wall. These closures occur behind the bolus and, assisted by peristaltic action of the pharynx, force air from the pharynx and the bolus into the upper esophagus. The hyoid bone and larynx move up and forward, the epiglottis closes, and, for the moment, breathing is inhibited.

3. In the last phase, the normally closed superior esophageal sphincter relaxes, the cricoid cartilage moves forward, and the sphincter contracts to begin the peristaltic transport of the bolus through the esophagus.[11] The pharynx and tongue separate, the epiglottis rises, and air flow into the trachea is re-established.

Until the infant is at least three months old, solids placed in his mouth will be forced by the tongue up against the palate and will be either swallowed or forced back out through the mouth. As he matures, solids are recognized, selectively transferred to the back of the pharynx, and swallowed.[17]

The coordination of suck and swallow is mediated through a number of oropharyngeal nerves.[29, 32] The motor supply of the lips is derived from the seventh cranial nerve, and sensation is carried through the trigeminal nerve. The maxillary division of the trigeminal sends branches to the upper teeth and alveoli, the hard and soft palate (except the posterior end), and the uvula. A mandibular division contains sensory branches to the tongue, lower cheek and lip, oral floor, auriculotemporal area, lower teeth, and alveolar process, and motor branches to the mylohyoid and anterior belly of the digastrics. The tenth cranial nerve, the vagus, supplies motor endowment to the palate and superior and middle pharyngeal constrictors. A branch from the fifth cranial nerve supplies the tensor veli palatini. Sensation of the palate and uvula is through the ninth cranial nerve and branches of the fifth. The sensory and motor supplies of the pharynx and fauces are therefore primarily from the ninth and tenth cranial nerves. The motor supply of the tongue is primarily from the twelfth cranial nerve, and sensation and taste are mediated through the seventh and ninth nerves.[15, 69]

ABNORMALITIES IN SUCK AND SWALLOW

Disorders contributing to difficulties in suck and swallow are listed in Table 2–1 and discussed below.

ABSENT OR DIMINISHED SUCK

Central nervous system damage due to perinatal anoxia or hyperbilirubinemia may

Table 2–1 Causes of Difficulties with Suck and Swallow

ABSENT OR DIMINISHED SUCK	MECHANICAL PROBLEMS WITH SUCK	DIFFICULTY IN SWALLOWING	
Anoxia	Ankyloglossia superior syndrome	High lesions— aspiration with swallowing or nasal regurgitation of formula	Low lesions— associated with aspiration after feeding or pain during feeding
Kernicterus	Fusion of gums	Cleft palate	Esophageal motor dysfunction
Trisomies 13–15, 21	Macroglossia	Choanal atresia	Familial dysautonomia
Amyotonia congenita syndrome	Aglossia	Pharyngeal tumors	Achalasia
Prader-Willi syndrome	Ankylosis of the temporomandibular joint	Pharyngeal cysts	Chalasia
Werdnig-Hoffmann disease	Cleft lip	Tracheoesophageal fistula	Post vagotomy
Myasthenia gravis	Tumors	Laryngotracheo-esophageal cleft	Congenital lesions of the esophagus
Congenital muscular dystrophy		Infectious diseases of the pharynx	Vascular compression
Bulbar palsy		Micrognathia	Duplication cyst
		Pharyngeal diverticulum	Esophageal stenosis or web
		Pharyngeal perforation	Acquired lesions of the esophagus—
		Myotonic dystrophy	Leukemic infiltrate
		Palatal paralysis	Caustic burns
		Bulbar paralysis	Peptic esophagitis
		Transient palatal or pharyngeal dysfunction	Esophageal stricture
		Laryngeal nerve paralysis	Infection
		Cricopharyngeal dysfunction or achalasia	
		Post tracheotomy	

cause a disordered or diminished sucking response. This alone may be the first manifestation of central nervous system disease.[68, 73]

Chromosomal disorders such as trisomy 13–15 and trisomy 21 may be associated with abnormal sucking responses.[73]

Neuromuscular disorders of the amyotonia congenita syndrome may present with diminished sucking ability. This syndrome encompasses a number of disease states characterized by hypotonia, flaccidity, and poor or absent suck. Included in the differential diagnosis of infantile amyotonia are toxoplasmosis, metachromatic leukodystrophy, atonic diplegia, kernicterus, Werdnig-Hoffmann disease, infantile polyneuritis, myasthenia gravis, and the congenital myopathies.[16, 18, 21, 33, 41]

The Prader-Willi syndrome is accompanied by absent or abnormal suck.[30, 75]

Cleft lip, with or without cleft palate, occurs in about 1 in 1000 births. These clefts are related to maternal age, with an incidence of 0.37 per 100,000 live births to mothers under 23 years and 1.41 per 100,000 live births to mothers over 37 years. In one quarter of the cases the defect is bilateral. Of the unilateral clefts, 70 per cent are on the left and 30 per cent are on the right (Figs. 2–6 and 2–7). Cleft lip is twice as frequent in males as in females and is more common in relatives of affected persons.

There is a concordance rate of 40 per cent in monozygotic twins and of only 5 per cent in dizygotic twins. The defect is believed to be of either an autosomal recessive or a conditioned dominance inheritance, with sex limitation to males. The risk to future siblings is 5 per cent if a sibling or parent is affected but rises to 15 per cent if both a sibling and a parent are affected. About 10

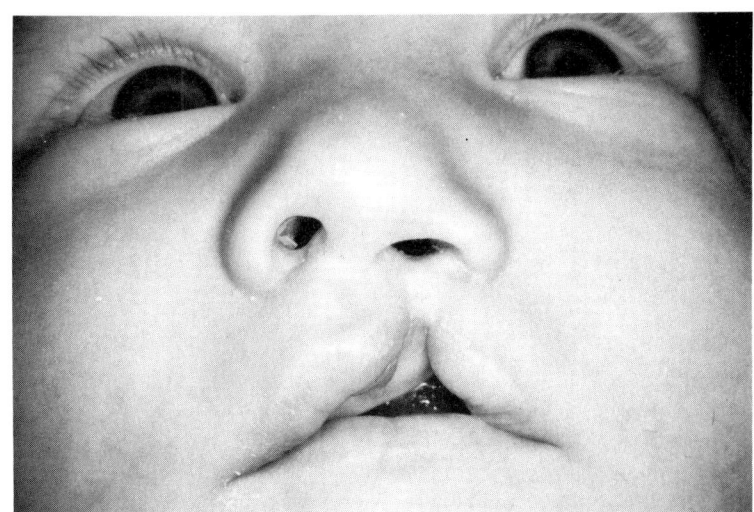

Figure 2–6 Unilateral cleft of the lip. (Courtesy of Howard Smith, M.D.)

per cent of these infants have mental retardation, 10 per cent have congenital heart disease, and 3 per cent have digital anomalies.[32]

Most of the median clefts of the lip are truly bilateral clefts with aplasia or hypoplasia of the philtrum. This type of cleft may be associated with bifid nose and ocular hypertelorism. Polydactyly of the hands and feet is an occasional finding.

The sucking difficulties caused by cleft lip are due to the infant's inability to grasp and enclose the nipple completely. This does not permit development of sufficient intraoral pressure for delivery of the nutrient from the nipple. The swallowing mechanism is not impaired in these infants. Surgical correction, with the establishment of excellent symmetry, may be accomplished as soon as the child has regained his birth weight.[28]

DIFFICULTIES IN INTRODUCING FOOD INTO THE MOUTH

Ankyloglossia superior syndrome is a rare constellation of congenital defects, the major one of which, and the source of its name, is a dense fibrous adhesion between the tongue and the roof of the mouth.[71] This immobilizes the tongue and prevents manipulation of the nipple by the tongue for the development of adequate intraoral pressure. Associated defects are almost always limited to the extremities as amputations or

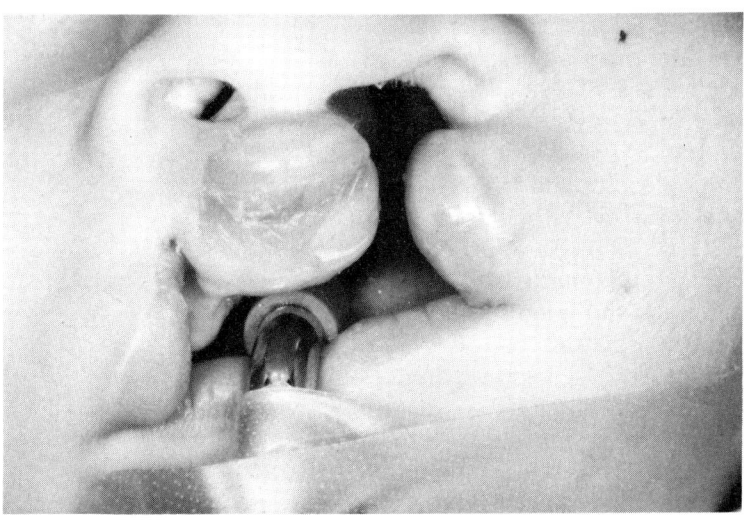

Figure 2–7 Bilateral cleft lip and palate. The right cleft is less extensive than the left, which involves the nostril. (Courtesy of Howard Smith, M.D.)

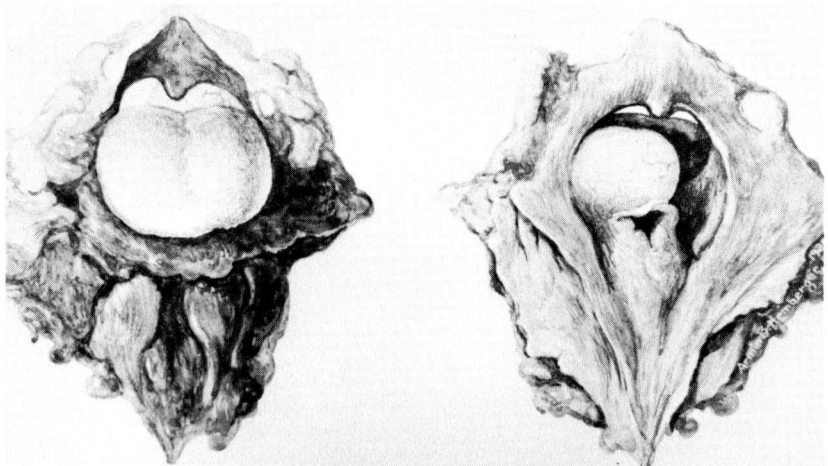

Figure 2–8 Anterior and posterior views of a pharyngeal cyst. Posteriorly, the cyst compresses the posterior aspect of the tongue. (Illustration by A. Hemberger. Yale University School of Medicine Collection.)

syndactyly of the fingers or toes. Rarely, cleft palate and sixth or seventh nerve palsy are associated. The etiology is not known, but developmentally the disturbance takes place between the eighth and twelfth weeks *in utero.* In at least one case reported, good function was restored after blunt dissection to separate the tongue from the palate.

Fusion of the gums is another rare congenital defect and is usually unaccompanied by other congenital anomalies. Surgical resolution of the problem is relatively easy.

Macroglossia may be of minor degree and cause little, if any, difficulty. This form is encountered in infants with Down's syndrome, in cretins, and in those with Pompe's disease. Less often it occurs with trisomy 21, acrocephalosyndactyly (Apert's syndrome), craniofacial dysostosis, Crouzon's disease, Hurler's syndrome, mandibulofacial dysostosis (Treacher Collins syndrome), or Beckwith's syndrome (giantism, omphalocele, and symptomatic hypoglycemia with or without other congenital defects).[32] In none of these is it of much clinical importance.[51]

Rarely, the tongue is so large that it protrudes from the mouth and overfills the buccal cavity, making it impossible for the newborn to suck. Two disorders may be responsible: muscular hypertrophy and lymphangioma. Diagnosis must be made by biopsy. If enlargement is due to muscular overgrowth, watchful waiting, with assisted feeding by gavage or syringe, is indicated. The tongue can be expected to shrink slowly over the next few weeks or months. If lymphangioma is discovered, staged operations are called for.

Aglossia-adactylia syndrome consists of absence of the tongue and failure of digital development. The face is sharp and narrow

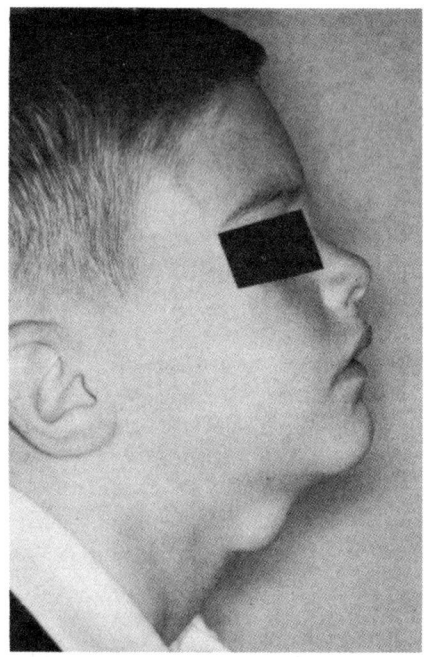

Figure 2–9 Lateral view of a thyroglossal cyst. (Courtesy of Howard Smith, M.D.)

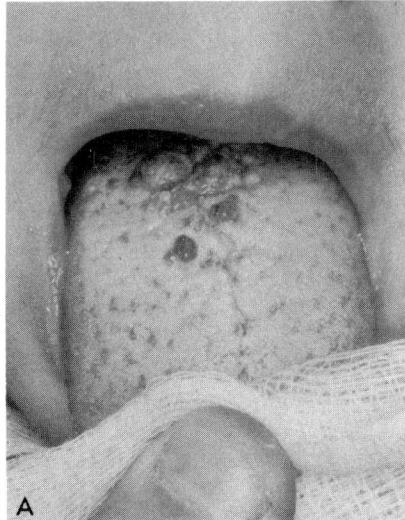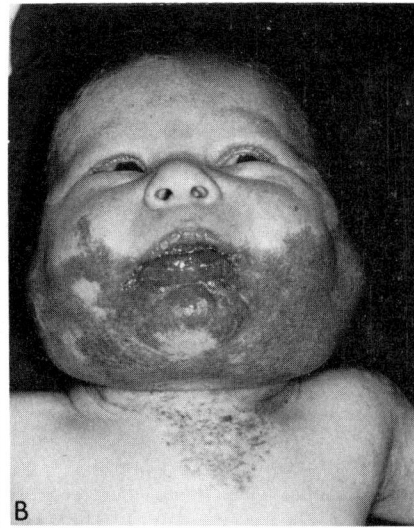

Figure 2-10 A, Hemangioma of the tongue. The cherry red nubbin is typical of the lesion. B, Extensive hemangioma of the face and neck, with macroglossia. (Courtesy of Howard Smith, M.D.)

with a receding bird-like chin. The tongue may appear as only a small nubbin in the posterior mouth, and the sublingual ridges are enlarged. Cleft palate and bony fusion of the jaws may be associated.[32]

Ankylosis or hypoplasia of the temporomandibular joint is a rare congenital anomaly in which the infant is unable to open his jaw. Obviously, sucking motions are affected and limited. Malocclusion is a late complication. Condylectomy is an effective treatment.

Some tumors or cysts that arise in the mouth or pharynx can impede the entrance of food. Reported examples of tumors of great size include epulis, epignathus, dermoid cysts, duplication cysts, teratomas, and thyroglossal duct cysts.[44] Those of lesser size are hemangiomas, lymphangiectasias (hygroma), and ectopic thyroid (Figs. 2-8 to 2-13).[12, 31a, 46, 51, 51a, 56, 61a]

Tongue-tie must be mentioned, although it is hardly ever significant in the newborn. Normally, the frenulum that binds the tongue to the floor of the mouth is short and not very elastic. The infant does not require a great deal of tongue extension, and he can usually feed and suck without difficulty.

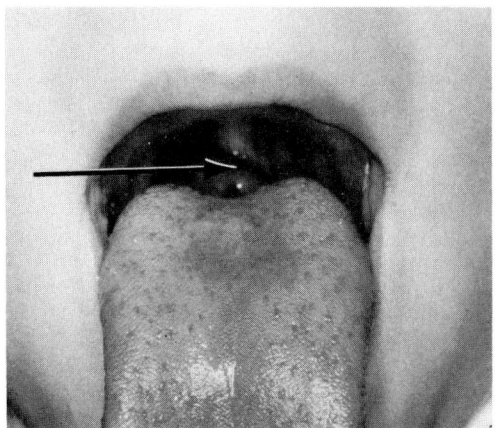

Figure 2-11 Lingual thyroid causing difficulties in approximation of the tongue and posterior pharynx. Denoted by the arrow, it appears as a mass of red-brown tissue. (Courtesy of Howard Smith, M.D.)

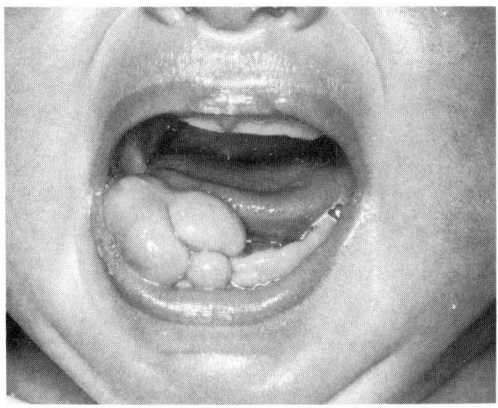

Figure 2-12 Myeloblastoma and a rare benign tumor arising probably from perineural fibroblasts. If submucosal, as in this child, hyperplasia of the overlying epithelium is marked. (Courtesy of Howard Smith, M.D.)

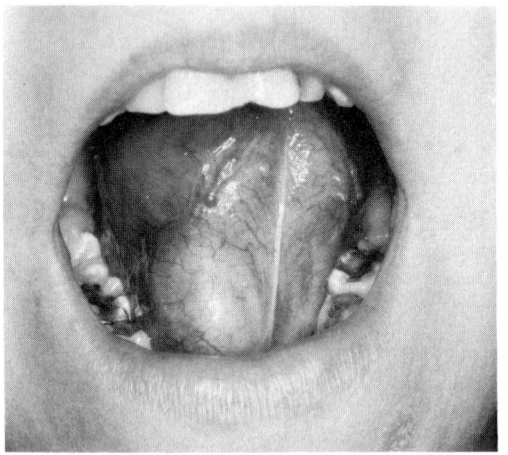

Figure 2–13 Dermoid cyst arising from the floor of the mouth and displacing the tongue. (Courtesy of Howard Smith, M.D.)

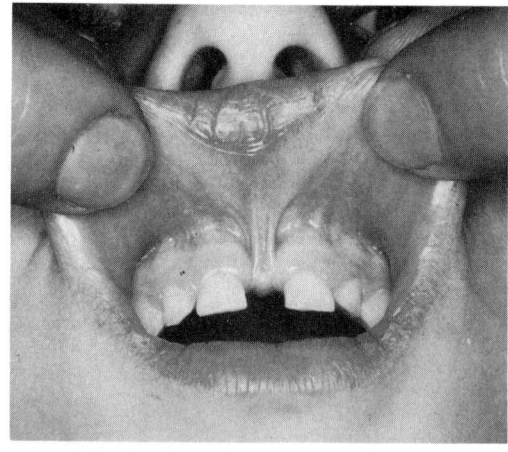

Figure 2–15 Superior labial frenulum associated with spacing between the front teeth. (Courtesy of Howard Smith, M.D.)

The frenulum will lengthen and should not be cut. In rare cases, it interferes with protrusion of the tongue in later years and should be severed (Fig. 2–14).[71]

A large labial frenulum may be associated with spacing between the front teeth but is not significant in causing any impairment in eating or in speech (Fig. 2–15).

DIFFICULTIES IN SWALLOWING BECAUSE OF ABNORMAL CONNECTIONS BETWEEN FOOD PASSAGE AND AIRWAY

Laryngotracheoesophageal cleft is discussed in Chapter Three. Tracheoesophageal fistula is discussed in Chapter Three.

Cleft Palate

Isolated cleft palate is inherited as a simple dominant trait with sex limitation to females.[32] Its incidence is about 1 in 2500 live births. If the parents are normal and one sibling is affected, the risk for another child is 2 per cent; if one parent is affected, the risk rises to 7 per cent; and if one parent and a sibling are affected, the risk increases to 15 per cent. Associated anomalies are 30 times more frequent than in the general population. The clefts may be small and submucous or extensive and associated with considerable nasal regurgitation and choking during feeding (Figs. 2–16 and 2–17). In the most severe cases, double clefts extend from the soft palate through the cleft lips on either side of the nose. Feeding problems

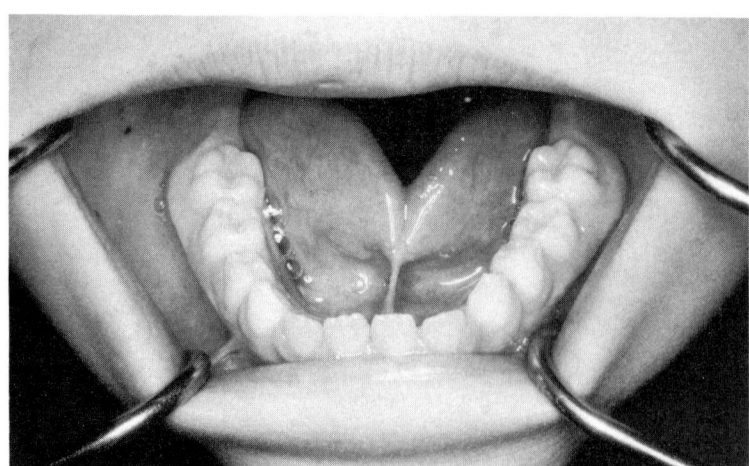

Figure 2–14 Tongue-tie. Note the degree of traction upon the tongue as the child attempts to elevate. (Courtesy of Howard Smith, M.D.)

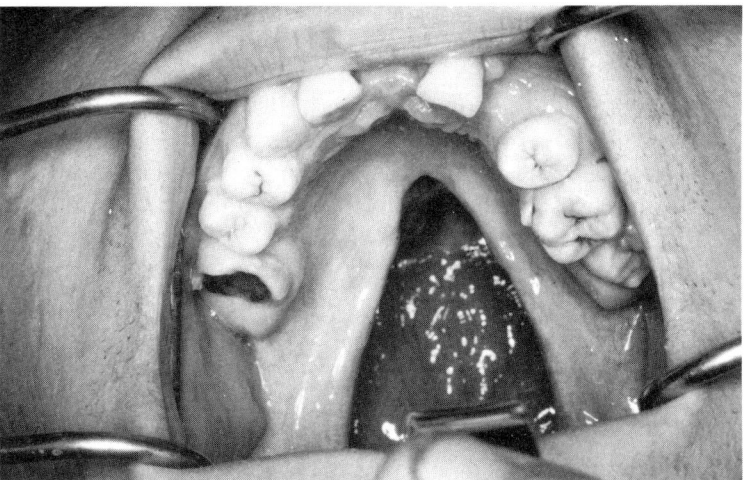

Figure 2–16 A complete cleft palate permits free flow of liquid and oral contents into the nasopharynx. (Courtesy of Howard Smith, M.D.)

are greatest in those with associated anomalies and require the most gentle techniques, using syringe, dropper, or even gavage. Surgical repair is undertaken when the child is between one and two years of age, but problems in speech and dental alignment require years of corrective procedures.[72]

Cleft palate is associated with mental retardation, congenital heart disease, the Pierre Robin syndrome, and Larsen's syndrome (cleft palate, flattened facies, and congenital dislocations).[32] Another association worthy of mention is cleft lip and palate, popliteal pterygium, hypoplasia or agenesis of the digits, and genital anomalies.

DIFFICULTIES IN SWALLOWING

Choanal Atresia

Choanal atresia consists of a membranous or bony obstruction of one or both choanae.[38, 40, 64] It is caused by failure of rupture of the embryonic bucconasal membrane (Fig. 2–18). The mode of inheritance is not well understood, but there seems to be a familial tendency. Associated anomalies of the cardiovascular, ophthalmic, and gastrointestinal systems or the facial skeleton occur in 10 to 50 per cent of infants, and the disorder has been described in the Treacher Collins, Apert, and Down syndromes.[57a] Unilateral choanal atresia is not a great problem and causes symptoms later in life only when the

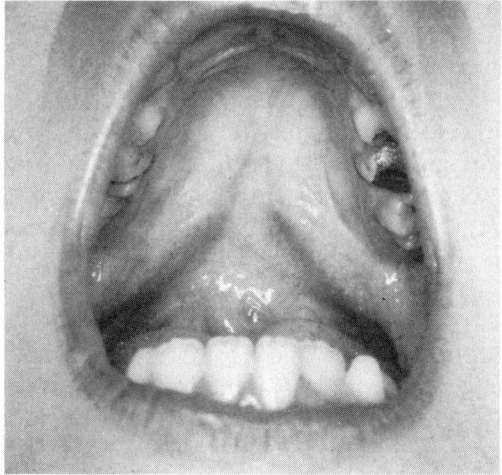

Figure 2–17 A submucous cleft palate is visualized as an elevated ridge in the palate and is best diagnosed by palpation. (Courtesy of Howard Smith, M.D.)

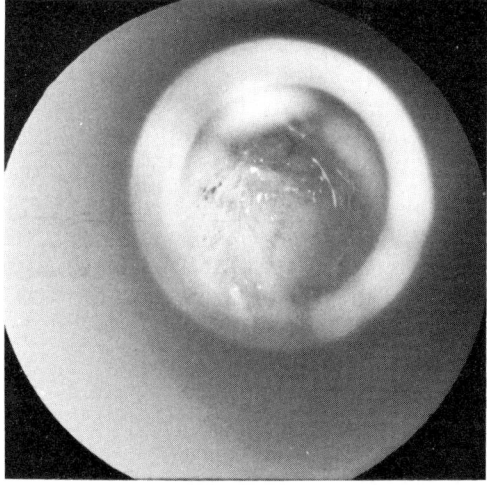

Figure 2–18 Choanal atesia. The imperforate membrane is visualized through the nostril. (Courtesy of Howard Smith, M.D.)

other nasal choana is obstructed. In this unilateral form, the right side is more often involved than the left.

Polyhydramnios is present in half the mothers. Bilateral involvement is as common as unilateral and is more common in girls than in boys. Infants with the bilateral type have symptoms early. Some are limp and unable to breathe at birth; others breathe initially but experience difficulty within the first few hours, and some attempt mouth breathing but cannot breathe during feedings. Breathing improves with crying, but as the infant quiets, breathing is impossible, and the more he struggles for air, the tighter his lips close. The respiratory problem is severe, for the young infant has not learned to breathe through his mouth. The diagnosis is made by listening over the nares with a stethoscope — there are no breath sounds. A catheter cannot be passed through the nose. Methylene blue instilled into a nostril does not appear in the nasopharynx and posterior pharynx if the nares is not patent. Similar results are obtained with radiographic studies using Lipiodol.

In either type of choanal atresia — membranous or bony — placement of an endotracheal airway is lifesaving until the child's condition is stable and the type of defect has been identified.[40] True membranous obstruction (10 to 15 per cent of cases) is treated by perforation of the membrane and introduction of a rubber catheter through it, with the catheter left in place for a few days. Bony obstruction (85 to 90 per cent of cases) should not be repaired until the infant is 12 to 18 months old; in this case, the use of an oral airway and gavage feedings is necessary until the infant learns to breathe through his mouth. A progression is made through dropper to bottle feedings. Surgical treatment of the bony deformity consists of the creation of choanal windows through a transpalatal approach.

Pierre Robin Syndrome

This syndrome consists of micrognathia, glossoptosis, and cleft palate. In a number of cases there is a family history either of the syndrome or of cleft palate and lip.[20] The

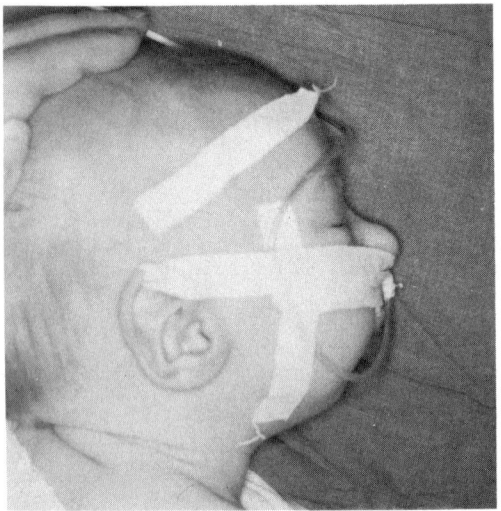

Figure 2–19   The infant with Pierre Robin syndrome requires prone positioning. The characteristic micrognathia is evident. (Courtesy of Howard Smith, M.D.)

condition is more common in infants born to older mothers. Intrauterine insult during the fourth to fifth month of gestation is considered the cause. Congenital heart disease is present in more than 15 per cent of those affected, and 20 per cent are mentally retarded. Eye anomalies such as esotropia, congenital cataracts and glaucoma, microphthalmia, and retinal detachment may be present, as may deafness and low-set ears. The mortality in this syndrome is reported to be between 20 and 65 per cent, but in many of the cases other anomalies were responsible for death.

Feeding problems are caused by inadequate tongue control. These infants must be fed slowly with a syringe or even by gavage. The problem is compounded by the cleft palate, and the tongue may even become impacted in the cleft. The respiratory problems are the most significant, for the small jaw does not support the musculature of the tongue. The tongue falls backward and downward (glossoptosis) and obstructs the epiglottis, causing cyanosis and respiratory distress. Immediate relief is provided by anterior traction of the tongue with a clamp. In general, if the infant can maintain the airway while sleeping in the prone position, surgery will not be necessary. The mild cases show marked improvement in symptoms within six weeks. More severe cases are treated by the Douglas operation — suturing of the tongue to the lower lip — or by the creation of tongue-lip adhesions. These are temporizing procedures, for during the first few months the jaw grows less rapidly than the tongue. They therefore may be abandoned when the baby is about six months of age. Jaw growth reaches adequate dimensions by the fourth to sixth year.

Micrognathia

This is a frequent finding in arthrogryposis, in the bird-headed dwarf syndrome of Seckel, trisomy 18, the triploidy syndrome, Turner's syndrome, and lateral facial clefts. It is associated also with renal agenesis, mandibulofacial dysostosis, Ullrich-Feichtiger syndrome (micrognathia, polydactyly, and genital anomalies), Möbius syndrome (congenital oculofacial paralysis), and progeria. The micrognathia is usually not severe, but the problems of glossoptosis already described may be apparent in early infancy.

Neuromuscular Disorders[38a, 69a]

Familial Dysautonomia. Familial dysautonomia is a disease of autonomic dysfunction in which there are swallowing difficulties due to esophageal motor dysfunction. It is discussed in detail in Chapter Eleven.

Werdnig-Hoffmann Disease. Werdnig-Hoffmann disease is the most serious of the amyotonias and the one in which differential diagnosis is most important. There is a familial incidence and probably a recessive type of inheritance. A history of diminished fetal movements can usually be elicited, and the infant may be hypotonic or areflexic at birth or shortly thereafter. Degenerative lower motor neuron disease progresses and is associated with severe muscle wasting. Motor neurons are lost in a caudocephalad progression that eventually involves the cranial nerve motor nuclei. Fibrillations of the tongue appear, the ability to suck is lost, swallowing becomes difficult, and respiratory paralysis eventually develops.

Benign Congenital Hypotonia. This is also important in the differential diagnosis of the amyotonias, for this disease is not progressive. It too may be familial. Although usually the mother has felt fetal movements *in utero*, the infant is hypotonic at birth. The joints are hypermobile, the suck is poor, and there is difficulty in swallowing. There is some evidence of deep tendon reflexes. Respiratory distress may be present early and may be associated with sternal and intercostal retractions, but the disease does not progress further. Motor development is delayed because of poor muscle tone, and only half these infants ever achieve adequate muscle function.

Myasthenia Gravis. This disease may appear in the neonate in one of two types.[5, 53, 63] Neonatal transient myasthenia gravis occurs in 10 to 15 per cent of infants born to myasthenic mothers and is now recognized as an immunologic disease. Maternal antiacetylcholine antibodies that cross the placenta bind to acetylcholine receptor protein at the myoneuronal junction.[22] Arthrogryposis may result from decreased fetal movement. If decreased movements are noted *in utero*, maternal plasmapheresis may be appropriate.[5, 23]

Within the first hours or days of life, symptoms of generalized weakness, poor Moro response, poor suck, voiceless cry, flat facial expression, dysphagia, and respiratory weakness develop. Aspiration and respiratory failure may follow. The course of this disease lasts from several hours to seven weeks and is followed by complete recovery. In most cases, symptoms are mild and need no treatment. If required, edrophonium chloride (Tensilon), 0.1 ml intramuscularly or subcutaneously, produces complete, temporary relief of symptoms. Therapy with neostigmine (neostigmine methylsulfate), in an initial dose of 0.1 mg given 10 to 20 minutes before feeding, is continued as long as the infant presents signs of weakness. As he improves, the medication may be given through a nasogastric tube and tapered as tolerated.

Neonatal persistent myasthenia gravis occurs in 1 per cent of all patients with myasthenia and appears in infants of unaffected mothers. There may be affected relatives, however. Millichap and Dodge[53] classify this condition as distinct from the juvenile type. The symptoms these infants have at birth are milder than those of the transient form, but they persist. Rest and anticholinesterase medication provide some relief of the ptosis, ophthalmoplegia, and generalized weakness, but the course is protracted and relatively resistant to therapy.

Juvenile myasthenia gravis, with the onset of symptoms occurring after the age of one year, is the most common form encountered in childhood. Inheritance is of the recessive type. The disease is more common in girls than in boys. Ptosis, unilateral or bilateral, is the most common presenting sign. Weakness of the extremities occurs in many patients. Respiratory difficulty develops in at least 40 per cent of patients and may be so severe as to require respiratory assistance. These children must be treated with medication; thymectomy is not recommended until later in life.

The defect in this disease may be one of several: defect of acetylcholine resynthesis, reduced acetylcholine release and end-plate acetylcholinesterase deficiency, or a defect of membrane ion channels normally induced by acetylcholine release.[5] The differential diagnosis includes all of the disorders of the amyotonia congenita syndrome, and administration of edrophonium chloride (Tensilon) or neostigmine, with the ensuing relief of weakness, is diagnostic.

Myotonic Dystrophy of Early Onset. This disorder is inherited as an autosomal dominant trait.[21, 57b, 70, 74] The myopathy, which appears in early infancy, consists of hypotonia, facial diplegia, and delayed motor development. A low birth weight is often noted, and feeding problems, particularly swallowing difficulties, may develop early. Some infants may require gavage feedings for the first few months of life. Sucking ability is less involved. The muscles primarily affected are those of the face, tongue, and pharynx, and weakness of the jaw muscles permits sagging of the mandible and drooling. Ocular myopathy with ptosis may be striking. In the early-onset group there is weakness of the proximal and truncal muscles, whereas children who acquire the disease after the

age of five have distal muscular weakness. In the latter group, too, achalasia of the superior esophageal sphincter may be found.

Congenital Muscular Dystrophy. This disorder, considered to be of autosomal recessive inheritance, is thought to run its course during intrauterine life, with little progression afterward. It is characterized by contractures, which may be congenital or may develop postnatally, severe hypotonia and weakness, and diminished tendon reflexes. The weakness characteristically involves the arm, leg, facial, extraocular, and oropharyngeal muscles, and the infant may be unable to suck and swallow, so that gavage feeding is required. About half the patients die by the age of 13 from intercurrent respiratory infection.[75]

Bulbar Palsy. In the infant, bulbar palsy is most commonly supranuclear. If it is confined to the bulbar muscles, the infant sucks poorly and has difficulty chewing and swallowing solid foods when they are introduced into the diet. Drooling is a prominent symptom.[33] Speech is delayed and dysarthric. Diagnostically, the jaw jerk is exaggerated. Usually, however, a picture of generalized cerebral palsy and spasticity is present or develops within several weeks of birth.[18, 33, 65]

Less common is the lower motor neuron type, in which suck is poor and there is nasal regurgitation of formula. Delayed speech and nasal dysarthria follow. As in supranuclear lesions, there may be generalized motor involvement, but the paralysis is flaccid. Flaccid bulbar paralysis associated with facial diplegia constitutes the syndrome of Möbius.[25] Nasopharyngeal reflux has led to neonatal apnea.[58a]

Transient Palatal or Pharyngeal Muscle Dysfunction. This disorder has been reported in premature infants and in those with cerebral palsy.[2, 27, 51, 52, 54] It is characterized by choking during feeding and dribbling of formula. Constrictor paralysis and a flaccid soft palate are noted in cineradiographic studies. Swallowing improves after several weeks as compensatory tongue movements develop. Aspiration is a danger during the first two months of life, and tube feeding or gastrostomy may be necessary.

Facial immobility develops later in some infants, as do dysarthria and nasal intonation of the voice. Results of cricopharyngeal and esophageal motility studies are normal. Infants with extremely mild symptoms may show marked improvement in their ability to feed within two weeks. Myographic studies have not demonstrated this disorder to be a denervating process.

Selective Laryngeal Nerve Paralysis. Selective paralysis of the superior laryngeal nerve in the neonate has been reported. It is likely caused by intrauterine posture with the face turned away from the midline before the head has flexed, so that the superior laryngeal nerve is compressed between the thyroid cartilage and the hyoid bone. Affected infants prefer to lie with the head turned and may have unilateral facial weakness or paralysis. Dysphagia and diminished esophageal motility are noted. Recovery is spontaneous and occurs by the first birthday.[14]

Isolated Palatal Paralysis. Paralysis involving the tenth cranial nerve has been reported in three cases.[57] It is apparent shortly after birth and causes nasal regurgitation of formula during feeding. Later, speech is hypernasal and unintelligible. In one infant the palate was foreshortened, but in the other two it was of normal length (Fig. 2–20). In all three infants the uvula was in the midline. This tenth nerve palsy prevents closure of the velopharyngeal space during phonation and deglutition. Surgical suturing of the soft palate to the posterior pharynx or the use of prosthetic devices to elevate the palate is required to prevent regurgitation and ensure normal phonation.

Cricopharyngeal Dysfunction. *Achalasia* of the cricopharyngeus or superior esophageal sphincter is often not recognized[38a, 52, 55, 66] and may occur in Down's syndrome.[31] It is characterized by intermittent, recurrent difficulties of swallowing.[69a] As in typical achalasia, which involves the lower esophageal sphincter, there is failure of the sphincter to relax with swallowing. The diagnosis is suggested by cineradiography and confirmed by manometric studies. Over the years, increased pressure develops in the upper esophagus and pharynx and leads to the development of posterior pharyngeal diverticulum. This type of achalasia and small diverticula as well are relieved by Heller-type myotomy.

Cricopharyngeal incoordination of infancy has recently been described. It resembles cricopharyngeal achalasia and is far more serious than the transient palatal and pharyngeal incoordinations.[7, 13] The disorder is present at birth, and although no anatomic obstruction exists, there is failure of a bolus to pass the cricopharyngeus and the superior esophageal sphincter. Sucking is normal, but the baby soon begins to resist feeding because of choking and aspiration. These infants have, in addition, small jaws that open poorly. The diagnosis is made after cineradiographic study of the swallowing mechanism, in which it can be seen that the bolus is propelled to the posterior pharynx, where it meets vigorous propulsive movements and undergoes retropulsion back into the mouth. In one infant who died, there was marked dilation of the pharynx above the area of obstruction and hypertrophy of the pharyngeal constrictors. Aganglionosis of the proximal third, but not of the distal third, of the esophagus was noted. Aspiration is a constant fear in such infants and is the life-threatening manifestation of this disorder. Infants who have survived have been spoon-fed until they were four to six months old, at which time they were considered well. This disorder must be differentiated from tracheoesophageal fistula and laryngotracheoesophageal cleft. The latter also may be associated with an

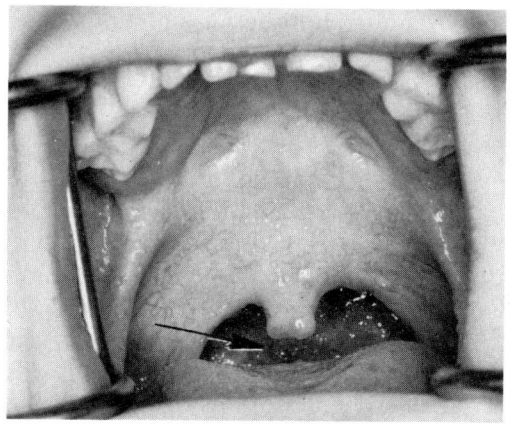

Figure 2–20 Left palatal paralysis. (Courtesy of Howard Smith, M.D.)

underdeveloped lower jaw, but the cleft can be detected by digital examination of the posterior pharynx. An attempt to pass a nasogastric tube may permit identification of a blind esophageal pouch. Cineradiography is the most useful diagnostic tool.

The Prader-Willi syndrome consists of obesity, growth and psychomotor retardation, cryptorchidism, and hypotonia. There may be abnormal or absent sucking responses in the neonatal period.[30, 76] Amyotonia and difficulties in swallowing are accompanying symptoms. These feeding difficulties generally improve when the infant reaches the age of two to six months.

Acquired Difficulties in Swallowing

Pharyngeal Diverticulum. Pharyngeal diverticulum has been discussed previously under disorders of the superior esophageal sphincter. It usually develops from increased pharyngeal pressure secondary to cricopharyngeal dysfunction. It has been associated with hiatus hernia.

Perforation of the Pharynx. Perforation of the pharynx after catheter aspiration of pharyngeal secretions may mimic the symptoms of esophageal atresia with coughing, choking with feeding, and cyanosis. The examiner is unable to pass a nasogastric tube beyond the pharynx.[24] Spasm of the cricopharyngeus caused by the perforation is persistent, and contrast material may be prevented from entering the esophagus. If the contrast material is diverted into the tract formed by the perforation, an erroneous diagnosis of tracheoesophageal fistula may be made, but the distance between the trachea and the fistulous tract is greater than in esophageal atresia and the tract is elongated and irregular. Direct surgical repair of the perforation has been done, but conservative management with cervical drainage and establishment of a feeding gastrostomy is probably adequate therapy.

Swallowing Dysfunction after Tracheostomy. This develops occasionally and may resemble bulbar paralysis, although there is no neurologic deficit.[26] Three possible explanations are (1) desensitization of the larynx by diversion of the normal air current; (2) fixation of the larynx and prevention of its elevation, a function necessary for coordinated swallowing; and (3) least likely, compression of the esophagus by tracheotomy tube cuff.

Esophageal Erosions. Erosions caused by recurrent vomiting, cerebral damage, or viral disorders may produce dysphagia.

Leukemic Infiltrate. Leukemic infiltrate in the lower third of the esophagus will cause difficulty in swallowing.

Postvagotomy Dysphagia. This occurs after any type of vagotomy[37] and is reported to have an incidence of greater than 30 per cent after selective proximal vagotomy. In the majority of cases it disappears within two weeks to three months.

Infectious Diseases. Streptococcal pharyngitis is a common cause of oropharyngeal dysphagia, but it responds rapidly to appropriate antibiotic therapy. Herpetic stomatitis is a common oral lesion that may persist for up to ten days. Good mouth hygiene is essential to prevent secondary bacterial infection. Maalox has proved helpful in coating the oral lesions and facilitating feeding. Moniliasis of the oropharynx, or oral thrush, is characterized by white, cheese-like plaques on the mucous membranes and tongue. It may be painful enough to interfere with feeding and swallowing. Oral nystatin in a dose of 100,000 to 200,000 units every six hours is curative within several days. Oral moniliasis may extend to the esophagus and cause dysphagia and aspiration, and in infants so affected there is a hazard of monilial pneumonitis.

Less common infectious diseases, but those with more serious consequences, include tetanus, diphtheria, infectious mononucleosis, botulism, poliomyelitis, aphthous stomatitis, and Stevens-Johnson syndrome. Tetanus is a rare disease in the United States but is common in underdeveloped countries.[58] Tetanus neonatorum results from passage of infection through the umbilical cord, and sucking difficulty due to trismus is one of its first signs. Other characteristic symptoms are tonic rigidity, nasal voice, and regurgitation of fluids through the nose when swallowing is attempted. The mortality rate may be as high as 95 per cent in the neonate. Antitoxin neutralizes the circulating toxin, and penicillin or tetracycline is useful. Additional supportive therapy may include use of a sedative and, perhaps, muscle relaxants. Tracheotomy may be necessary for control of laryngospasm and handling of secretions. Botulism is being recognized with increasing frequency and has been implicated as a factor in the sudden infant death syndrome.[43] The symptoms are rather nonspecific and include weakness, hypotonia, and absent gag reflex.[8, 60]

Diphtheria still occurs in nonimmunized populations. Its gastrointestinal import lies in the diphtheritic membrane that may form in the pharynx and extend over the tonsils and into the larynx, causing dysphagia and sometimes upper airway obstruction. The diphtheria endotoxin produces cranial and peripheral nerve damage, evident during the second to tenth week of the disease. Palatal paralysis is the most common of these neurologic manifestations and appears earliest, toward the end of the first week or during the second week of the disease. It is signaled by nasal voice tone and regurgitation of ingested fluids through the nose. Antitoxin affects the circulating, but not the tissue-bound, toxin. Antibiotics such as penicillin or erythromycin may be useful.

Infectious mononucleosis, although uncommon in infants, may mimic diphtheria. A pharyngeal membrane may develop and extend into the trachea.

The poliomyelitis virus is highly selective in its invasion of the central nervous system, choosing the brainstem, the precentral gyrus of the cerebral cortex, the roof nuclei of the cerebellum, the cerebral cortex, and the anterior horn cells of the spinal cord.[45]

Several different patterns of denervation are responsible for the dysphagia developing after poliomyelitis.[10] Few symptoms result from unilateral involvement of muscles. In the presence of unilateral palatopharyngeus weakness, there may be compensation by the contralateral palatopharyngeus and the pharyngeal constrictors to form an adequate palatopharyngeal partition. Two factors are important in occlusion of the retrooral area during swallowing: firm apposition of the tongue and palate, and lateral approximation of the palate against the tongue by the palatopharyngeus muscles. If motor function is impaired at this site, the bolus must be delivered posteriorly by upward tilt of the patient's head. If intrinsic musculature of the pharynx is affected, there is extension of the head with anterior displacement of the mandible. Impairment of the suspensory musculature of the pharynx leads to anterior displacement of the hyoid and larynx during swallowing. Weakness of the constrictor muscles of the pharynx causes incomplete swallowing and pooling of secretions, resulting in a "bubbling" type of speech. Palatal paralysis causes nasal regurgitation of a portion of the bolus. The most difficult type of paralysis is that of persistent closure of the cricopharyngeus, resembling achalasia.

Aphthous stomatitis associated with recurrent ulcerations of the eyes and genitalia carries the name Behçet's syndrome. The cause is not known, although a viral or allergic etiology is the most attractive hypothesis. Although this disease most commonly occurs in males during or after adolescence, we have seen it in one toddler. Recurrent conjunctivitis may precede by years other ocular lesions such as keratitis, uveitis, or retinitis. The genital ulcerations may involve the perianal areas as well and may begin as pustular lesions that break down to ulcerations. The oral ulcers occur in crops anywhere in the mouth. The base of the ulcer has a yellow or gray exudate, and the rather sharp margin is surrounded by a red halo. There may be a significant amount of tissue loss on the tongue periphery. Involvement of the pharynx and esophagus may follow, causing esophageal as well as oral dysphagia. There may be associated arthralgia, erythema nodosum, and meningeal signs as well as immunoglobulin A deficiency. These patients show a characteristic erythematous reaction when given an intracutaneous injection of saline.

Stevens-Johnson syndrome consists of mucocutaneous lesions involving the mouth, conjunctivae, and genitalia. A vesicular eruption may be noted on the extremities. Most cases are idiopathic, although there may be a history of allergy or drug sensitivity. The syndrome is most common in young adults, but it may develop in older infants. The cutaneous lesion is annular and may be maculopapular or vesiculobullous. It is especially apparent on the dorsa of the hands and feet. The oral lesions begin as small plaques that form bullae or vesicles, which then rupture to form erosions covered with exudate or pseudomembrane. There is crust formation on the lips. Bronchopneumonia and ulceration of the esophagus and colon have been noted in some cases with extensive involvement.

REFERENCES

1. Abramovich, D. R., Garden, H., Jandial, L., and Page, K. R.: Fetal swallowing and voiding in relation to hydramnios. Obstet. Gynecol., 54:15, 1979.
2. Ardran, G. M., Benson, P. F., Butler, N. R., Ellis, H. L. and McKendrick, T.: Congenital dysphagia resulting from dysfunction of the pharyngeal muscle. Dev. Med. Child. Neurol. 7:157, 1965.
3. Ardran, G. M., Kemp, F. H., and Lind, J. A.: Cineradiographic study of bottle feeding. Br. J. Radiol. 31:11, 1958.
4. Ardran, G. M., Kemp, F. H., and Lind, J. A.: Cineradiographic study of bottle feeding. Br. J. Radiol. 31:156, 1958.
5. Barlow, C.: Neonatal myasthenia gravis. Am. J. Dis. Child. 135:209, 1981.
6. Becker, R. F., Windle, W. F., Barth, E. E., and Schulz, M. D.: Fetal swallowing, gastrointestinal activity and defecation in amnio. Surg. Gynecol. Obstet. 70:603, 1940.
7. Benson, P. F.: Transient dysphagia due to muscular incoordination. Proc. R. Soc. Med. 55:237, 1962.
8. Berg, B. O.: Syndrome of infantile botulism. Pediatrics 59:321, 1977.
9. Bosma, J. F.: Deglutition: pharyngeal stage. Physiol. Rev. 37:275, 1957.
10. Bosma, J. F.: Studies of the pharynx. I. Poliomyelitic disabilities of the upper pharynx. Pediatrics 19:881, 1957.
11. Bosma, J. F., and Lind, J.: Roentgenologic observations of motions of upper airway associated with the establishment of respiration in the newborn infant. Acta Paediatr. 49 (Suppl. 123):18, 1960.
12. Brown, S., Kerr, R., and Wilson, R.: Intra-oral duplication cyst. J. Pediatr. Surg. 13:95, 1978.
13. Carre, I. J., and Astley, R.: The gastroesophageal junction in infancy. Thorax 13:159, 1958.
14. Chapple, C. C.: A duosyndrome of the laryngeal nerve. Am. J. Dis. Child. 91:14, 1956.
15. Chrispin, A. R., and Friedland, G. W.: A radiologic study of the neural control of oesophageal vestibular function. Thorax 21:422, 1966.
16. Cohen, S.: Motor disorders of the esophagus. N. Engl. J. Med. 301:184, 1979.
17. Colley, J. R. T., and Creamer, B.: Suckling and swallowing infants. Br. Med. J. 2:422, 1968.
18. Collis, E.: Some differential characteristics of cerebral motor defects in infancy. Arch. Dis. Child. 29:113, 1954.
19. Crump, E. P., Gore, P. M., and Horton, C.: The sucking behavior in premature infants. Hum. Biol. 30:128, 1958.
20. Dennison, W. M.: The Pierre Robin syndrome. Pediatrics 36:336, 1965.
21. Dodge, P. R., Gamstorp, I., Byers, R. K., and Russell, P.: Myotonic dystrophy in infancy and childhood. Pediatrics 35:3, 1965.
22. Donaldson, J. O., Penn, A., Lisak, R., Abransky, O., Brenner, T., and Schothand, D.: Antiacetylcholine receptor antibody in neonatal myasthenia gravis. Am. J. Dis. Child. 135:222, 1981.
23. Drackman, D. B.: Myasthenia gravis. N. Engl. J. Med. 298:136, 186, 1978.
24. Ducharme, J. C., Bertrand, R., and Debie, J.: Perforation of the pharynx in the newborn: a condition mimicking esophageal atresia. Can. Med. Assoc. J. 104:785, 1971.
25. Evans, P. R.: Nuclear agenesis: Mobius' syndrome, congenital facial diplegia syndrome. Arch. Dis. Child. 30:237, 1955.
26. Feldman, S. A., Deal, C. W., and Urquhart, W.: Disturbance of swallowing after tracheostomy. Lancet 1:954, 1966.
27. Frank, M. N., and Gatewood, O. M. B.: Transient pharyngeal incoordination in the neonate. Am. J. Dis. Child. 111:178, 1966.
28. Friede, H., Lilja, J., and Johanson, B.: Lip-nose morphology and symmetry in unilateral cleft lip and palate patients following a two-stage lip closure. Scand. J. Plast. Reconstr. Surg. 14:55, 1980.
29. Friedland, G. W., Melcher, D. H., Berridge, F. R., and Gresham, G. A.: Debatable points in the anatomy of the lower esophagus. Thorax 21:487, 1966.
30. Gabilan, J. C., and Royer, P.: Prader-Wabhardt-Willi syndrome: study of 11 cases. Arch. Fr. Pediatr. 25:121, 1968.
31. Gelfand, M., Dysphagia due to esophageal motility disorder in Down's syndrome. Gastroenterology 80:1154, 1981.
31a. Gellis, S., and Pierce, S.: Enteric duplication cyst of the tongue. Am. J. Dis. Child. 134:985, 1980.
32. Gorlin, R. J., and Pindborg, J. J.: Syndromes of the Head and Neck. New York, McGraw-Hill Book Company, 1964.
33. Graham, P. J.: Congenital flaccid bulbar palsy. Br. Med. J. 2:26, 1964.
34. Gryboski, J. D.: The swallowing mechanism of the neonate. Esophageal and gastric motility. Pediatrics 35:445, 1965.
35. Gryboski, J. D.: Suck and swallow in the premature infant. Pediatrics 43:96, 1969.
36. Gryboski, J. D., Thayer, W. R., and Spiro, H. M.: Esophageal motility in infants and children. Pediatrics 31:382, 1963.
37. Guelrud, M., Gomez, G., Simon, C., Zambrano, V., Plaza, J., and Toledano, A.: Postelective vagotomy dysplagia. Gastroenterology 80:1165, 1971.
38. Hall, B. D.: Choanal atresia and multiple congenital anomalies. J. Pediatr. 95:395, 1979.
38a. Hellemans, J., Peleman, S. W., and van Trappen, G.: Pharyngoesophageal swallowing disorders and the pharyngoesophageal sphincter. Med. Clin. North Am. 65:1149, 1981.

39. Hooker, D.: Fetal reflexes and instinctual processes. Psychosom. Med. *4*:199, 1942.

40. Hough, J. V. D.: The mechanism of asphyxia in bilateral choanal atresia. South. Med. J. *48*:588, 1955.

41. Illingworth, R. S.: Sucking and swllowing difficulties in infancy: diagnostic problems of dysphagia. Arch. Dis. Child. *44*:655, 1969.

42. Johnson, H. D., and Laws, J. W.: The cardia in swallowing, eructation and vomiting. Lancet *2*:1268, 1966.

43. Johnson, R. O., Clay, S., and Arnon, S.: Diagnosis and management of infant botulism. Am. J. Dis. Child. *133*:586, 1979.

44. Jover, P., Lassaletta, L., and Tovar, J.: Nasopharyngeal teratoma. Ann. Chir. Inf. *13*:95, 1972.

45. Kaplan, S.: Paralysis of deglutition, a postpoliomyelitis complication treated by section of the cricopharyngeus muscle. Ann. Surg. *133*:572, 1951.

46. Koop, C. E., and Moschakis, E. A.: Capillary lymphangioma of the tongue complicated by glossitis. Pediatrics *27*:800, 1961.

47. Kron, R. E., Ipsen, J., and Goodard, K.: Consistent individual differences in nutritive sucking behavior in the human newborn. Psychosom. Med. *30*:151, 1968.

48. Kron, R. E., Stein, M., and Goodard, K.: A method of measuring sucking behavior in newborn infants. Psychosom. Med. *25*:181, 1963.

49. Kron, R. E., Stein, M., and Goddard, K.: Newborn sucking behavior affected by obstetric sedation. Pediatrics *37*:1012, 1966.

50. Kron, R. E., Stein, M., Goddard, K., and Phoenix, M.: Effects of nutrient upon the sucking behavior of newborn infants. Psychosom. Med. *29*:24, 1967.

51. Logan, W. J., and Bosma, J. F.: Oral and pharyngeal dysphagia in infancy. Pediatr. Clin. North Am. *14*:47, 1967.

52. Macaulay, J. C.: Neuromuscular incoordination of swallowing in the newborn. Lancet *260*:1208, 1951.

52a. McCook, T. A., and Felman, A. H.: Retropharyngeal masses in infants and young children. Am. J. Dis. Child. *133*:41, 1979.

53. Millichap, J. G., and Dodge, P.: Diagnosis and treatment of myasthenia gravis in infancy, childhood and adolescence. Neurology *10*:1007, 1960.

54. Morgan, J.: Neuromuscular incoordination of swallowing in the newborn. J. Laryngol. Otol. *70*:294, 1956.

55. Murray, J. P.: Neuromuscular and functional disorders of the pharynx. J. Fac. Radiol. *9*:135, 1958.

56. Newstedt, J. R., and Shirkey, H. C.: Teratoma of the thyroid region. Am. J. Dis. Child. *107*:88, 1964.

57. Olmsted, R. W., Halfond, M. M., and Kirkpatrick, J. A.: Isolated palatal paralysis. J. Pediatr. *56*:795, 1960.

57a. Pagon, R., Graham, J., Zonana, J., and Yong, S.: Coloboma, congenital heart disease and choanal atresia with multiple anomalies: CHARGE association. J. Pediatr. *99*:223, 1981.

57b. Pearse, R. G., and Howeler, C.: Neonatal form of dystrophica myotonica. Arch. Dis. Child. *54*:331, 1979.

58. Pinheiro, D.: Tetanus of the newborn infant. Pediatrics *34*:32, 1964.

58a. Plaxico, D. T., and Loughlin, G. M.: Nasopharyngeal reflux and neonatal apnea. Am. J. Dis. Child. *135*:793, 1981.

59. Pritchard, J. A.: Deglutition by normal and anencephalic fetuses. Obstet. Gynecol. *25*:289, 1965.

60. Prolin, R. A., and Brown, L.: Infant botulism. Pediatr. Clin. North Am. *26*:345, 1979.

61. Seaman, W. B.: Functional disorders of the pharyngoesophageal junction. Radiol. Clin. North Am. *7*:113, 1969.

61a. Shah, B. L., Vasan, U., and Raye, J. R.: Teratoma of the tonsil in a premature infant. Am. J. Dis. Child. *133*:79, 1979.

62. Strawczinski, H., Bec, I. T., McKenna, R. D., and Nickerson, G. H.: The behavior of the lower esophageal sphincter in infants and its relationship to gastroesophageal regurgitation. J. Pediatr. *64*:17, 1964.

63. Teng, P., and Osserman, K. E.: Studies in myasthenia gravis: neonatal and juvenile types. J. Mt. Sinai Hosp. *23*:711, 1956.

64. Trail, M., Creely, J., and Landrum, C.: Congenital choanal atresia. South. Med. J. *66*:460, 1973.

65. Upjohn, C.: Multiple congenital nerve palsy. Proc. R. Soc. Med. *50*:333, 1957.

66. Utian, H. L., and Thomas, G.: Cricopharyngeal incoordination in infancy. Pediatrics *43*:402, 1969.

67. Vantrappen, G., and Hellemans, J.: Studies on the normal deglutition complex. Am. J. Dig. Dis. *12*:255, 1967.

68. Volpe, J.: Neurology of the Newborn. Philadelphia, W. B. Saunders Company, 1981.

69. Waller, S. L., Misiewicz, J. J., Anthony, P. P., and Gummer, J. W. P.: In vitro pharmacologic and histopathologic studies on the human cardiac sphincteric muscle from achalasic and control patients. Am. J. Dig. Dis. *16*:566, 1971.

69a. Waters, P. F., and Demeester, T. R.: Foregut motor disorders and their surgical management. Med. Clin. North Am. *65*:1235, 1981.

70. Watters, G. V., and Williams, T. W.: Early onset myotonic dystrophy. Clinical and laboratory findings in five families and review of the literature. Arch. Neurol. *17*:137, 1967.

71. Wilson, R. A., Kilman, M. R., and Hardyment, A. F.: Ankyloglossia superior (palatoglossal adhesion in the newborn infant). Pediatrics *31*:1051, 1963.

72. Witzel, M. A., Clarke, J., Lindsay, W., and Thomson, H.: Comparison of results of pushback or Langenbeck repair of isolated cleft of the hard and soft palate. Plast. Reconstr. Surg. *64*:347, 1979.

73. Wolff, P. H.: The serial organization of sucking in the young infant. Pediatrics *42*:943, 1968.

74. Zellweger, H., and Ionasecu, V.: Early onset of myotonic dystrophy in infants. Am. J. Dis. Child. *125*:601, 1973.

75. Zellweger, H., McCormick, W. F., and Mergner, W.: Severe congenital muscular dystrophy. Am. J. Dis. Child. *114*:591, 1967.

76. Zellweger, H., and Schneider, H. J.: Syndrome of hypotonia-hypomentia-hypogonadism-obesity or Prader-Willi syndrome. Am. J. Dis. Child. *115*:588, 1968.

Chapter Three

GASTROESOPHAGEAL REFLUX

No subject has been more controversial during the last five years than that of gastroesophageal reflux (GER). Originally, reflux was attributed to hiatus hernia or chalasia and was readily explained as being due to a poorly functioning lower esophageal sphincter (LES) (Table 3–1).[7, 29] It is now recognized, however, that GER may occur in the presence of low, normal, or even hypertensive sphincters and that various pathophysiologic mechanisms contribute to its genesis. It must therefore be considered a symptom complex, rather than a single disease state. Regardless of etiology, the complications are the same, with severe reflux causing failure to thrive or recurrent pneumonitis and esophagitis leading to gastrointestinal blood loss, pain, and stricture formation.[1, 21, 27a]

Reflux is best defined as the flow of gastric contents into the esophagus and is usually accompanied by regurgitation. It may vary in intensity, however, and cannot always be differentiated from vomiting.

Physiologic reflux and chalasia exist in the normal neonate, for up to 38 per cent of healthy infants regurgitate during the first five days of life and have radiologic evidence of chalasia.[20] The LES pressure in our studies is normally low during the first week or so in the term infant and for the first few weeks in the premature infant. Sphincter pressure gradually increases with age after the first week until at several months the LES is quite competent.[3, 20] Some infants demonstrate a prolongation of this period of physiologic chalasia and may have episodes of reflux lasting for several

Table 3–1 Manometric Data in Normal Infants and Those with Gastroesophageal Reflux

AGE	LOWER ESOPHAGEAL SPHINCTER *mm Hg Pressure*		UPPER ESOPHAGEAL SPHINCTER *mm Hg Pressure*	
	Control	*Reflux*	*Control*	*Reflux*
2–6 wk				
rapid pull	av. 46.3	av. 48	10–90	10–80
slow pull	20–30	4–48		
6 wk–1 yr				
rapid pull	av. 43.3	28–55	20–110	10–80
slow pull	20–35	5–45		
1–3 yr				
rapid pull	av. 30.6	10–40	20–110	15–85
slow pull	22–36	6–34		

months. They reflux only small quantities of formula and grow well, as symptoms decrease by six months and abate by one year.[20]

Recently, with the use of newer techniques, the evidence has been controversial, with some investigators noting a normal LES pressure at birth and others, the same developmental pattern observed by us. There seems to be no correlation between sphincter pressure and serum gastric levels in the neonate.[34a]

Pathophysiology of Reflux

The LES is not a readily identifiable muscular sphincter but exists as a region of increased resting pressure in the lower esophagus that forms a positive pressure gradient between the stomach and the body of the esophagus. The establishment and maintenance of resting sphincter pressure have been related to neuronal, hormonal, and muscular determinants. Each plays a role, with myogenic mechanisms alone, or those excited by postganglionic neurotransmitters, probably being the most significant. Acetylcholine, released by the vagus nerves, is also of considerable importance in maintaining LES pressures. Although intestinal hormones probably exert some effect upon sphincter pressure, the role of endogenous gastrin is questionable. Exogenous pentagastrin, however, does increase LES pressure.

A number of anatomic factors contribute to LES effectiveness: the acute gastroesophageal angle (which in the neonate is not fully established); compression of the sphincter area by sling and diaphragmatic fibers; pinchcock action of the diaphragm; and location of the LES below the diaphragm.[12, 34b] Again, developmental factors are operant, for the LES of most neonates lies at or above the diaphragm, and only later, with growth, does it move into the abdomen.[20] This phenomenon may not only affect LES pressure adversely but may also cause confusion in establishing a diagnosis of hiatus hernia in the young infant.

Esophageal manometric studies by Euler and Ament in 1977 showed that their infants with reflux had consistently lower LES pressures than did controls, whose average pressure was 21.5 mm Hg. Those who responded to medical therapy had pressures averaging 19.5 mm Hg, whereas those who failed to respond and required surgery had pressures averaging 12.7 mm Hg.[13] Johnson et al.[27] evaluated 55 infants and children who required surgical treatment for reflux and found LES pressures to vary from 2 to 25 mm Hg, with a mean of 8.3 mm Hg. Forty-seven of their patients had hiatus hernia. Other workers consistently substantiated low basal LES pressures in infants with GER,[20, 24, 34, 41] but in 1979 Herbst et al.[24] reported that infants with recurrent pneumonia and reflux had largely normal or even increased LES pressures. Certainly, other factors are operant, for we recognize now that the infants with severe reflux, disordered peristalsis, failure to thrive, or recurrent pneumonitis have often normal or hypertensive LES pressures and, in addition, have markedly delayed gastric emptying without evidence of antral spasm or pylorospasm. This observation implies that either the motility disorder is a primary one affecting stomach as well as esophagus or the gastric motor disorder is primary and causes reflux severe enough to lead to secondary disruption of esophageal motility.[26]

Increased intragastric pressure in itself will contribute to GER.[12] A normal degree of postprandial reflux exists in infants and adults. However, this may be exaggerated and pathologic when other factors increase intragastric pressure in a more sustained fashion. Excessive coughing, exercising, and constrictive body casts or braces are identified factors in causing GER and even esophagitis. Other intrinsic gastric disorders that promote reflux are antral spasm, pylorospasm, and perhaps the entity described as short-segment pyloric stenosis, in which there is resistance to gastric emptying. The upper gastrointestinal bleeding seen in some infants with pyloric stenosis is usually considered to be from mucosal erosions due to gastric stasis but has actually been shown to be caused by esophagitis.

Reflux has been identified in several conditions associated with mental retardation.[61]

Sondheimer and Vorris have reported significant reflux in severely retarded patients, most of whom were spastic and with scoliosis; few, however, developed stricture of the esophagus. We have noted reflux with pneumonitis or stricture as well as disordered motility in several patients with Down's syndrome.

Serious complications result from GER. Infants with inadequate caloric intake show signs of weight loss and eventually become severely malnourished if untreated.

The relationship between recurrent pneumonia or chronic pulmonary disease and GER has been recognized for years, but asthma has only recently been added to the group of related respiratory diseases.[2a, 16, 35] Some, but not all, asthmatic patients have improved after institution of medical or surgical antireflux therapy.[30] Those with the highest index of suspicion for GER are asthmatics with recurrent pneumonias. The pneumonia, as suggested by Winter and Grand,[43] may be due to actual aspiration of refluxed contents, to bronchospasm resulting from autonomic reflexes between the esophagus and the bronchial smooth muscle, or to hypersensitivity to refluxed antigen (i.e., milk or soy). A hypothesis that we entertain is that an autonomic reflex during the acute asthmatic attack causes hypotonia or decreased motor activity of the upper gastrointestinal tract that predisposes to GER. Antiasthmatic medications, such as theophylline, act to lower the LES pressure and may directly contribute to GER. However, abnormalities in LES function and demonstrable reflux are evident even in asthmatic patients who are not taking medication.

The "near-miss" sudden infant death syndrome characterized by cyanosis and apnea has, in some instances, been attributed to GER and to disordered or immature pharyngoesophageal coordination.[23] In support of these findings, it has been shown experimentally that chemosensitive reflexes initiated by fluid in the larynx will suppress respiration.[21]

In all instances of respiratory disease one must consider the role of secretions, for in adults it is well recognized that salivary secretions promote swallowing and aid in acid clearance from the esophagus.[12] Salivation is stimulated by eating but ceases during sleep — a time when pathologic reflux often takes place. Continued acid reflux has resulted in fibrosis of the epiglottis and even in inflammatory change in the larynx.

Esophagitis is caused by the reflux of gastric contents, alone or in combination with bile, and is usually associated with delayed clearance of material from the esophagus. Although hydrochloric acid below pH 2 denatures protein, the major damage from gastric contents is due to pepsin. This enzyme, active below pH 3.2, actually causes protein digestion. Bile has a corrosive effect and potentiates the damage caused by acid. Bile acids increase the permeability of the mucosa and promote back-diffusion of the hydrogen ion — a process similar to that observed in bile gastritis. The presence of proteolytic enzymes in refluxed bile further increases mucosal insult.

The resultant esophagitis causes spasm, pain, blood loss, and even upper gastrointestinal hemorrhage. More unusual complications are enteric protein loss and digital clubbing. If untreated, the lesion may progress to esophageal stricture.

Symptoms

Although a mother may state that her baby has been a spitter from the time of birth, these infants more typically have only minimal spitting during the first few weeks of life. Postprandial regurgitation becomes more problematic between four and eight weeks as the volume of the feeds increases. With more persistent GER, the infants become irritable, uncomfortable, and, often, inconsolable. Feeding periods are fraught with fussing, arching, and refusal to feed. Sleep may be interrupted by crying as if in pain.

Rarely, an infant will present with symptoms more typical of colic and little in the way of actual regurgitation.[15] In others, failure to thrive or recurrent episodes of pneumonia are the major complaints. Herbst[22] describes a separate group of infants with respiratory symptoms, delayed gastric emptying, and chronic diarrhea. We have seen a similar group with immunoglobulin A or G deficiency.

Anemia is the sole symptom in a few patients, and its origin, esophagitis, is suspected only after occult blood is found in the stool and a search for its source is instituted. Hematemesis is an unusual manifestation in the very young infant, but it does occur in those beyond six months of age.

Esophageal spasm causing dysphagia for solids may occur in the absence of radiologic obstruction and may precipitate apnea or cyanosis. Dysphagia from stricture is more usual and has a more gradual progression of symptoms.

Differential Diagnosis

These symptoms may be differentiated by history from disorders of outlet obstruction, in which regurgitation is intermingled with forceful vomiting. Those infants typically ingest only a few ounces and demand frequent feedings. Attempts to increase intake add to the volume and force of the vomitus. A mother may mention that colored medications or foods return several hours after their ingestion.

Infants with intractable vomiting should be evaluated for immunologic, neurologic, and metabolic disease, with particular emphasis placed on screening for hyperammonemia. A screen for renal disease includes BUN and creatinine analysis and urinalysis with evidence that the infant can concentrate his urine. Renal tubular acidosis, hydronephrosis, and urinary tract infection may cause persistent vomiting.

Diagnosis

The diagnosis is suggested by history and by careful observation of the infant during and after feeding. In all instances, the stool should be examined for occult blood, the presence of which suggests esophagitis. Radiologic examination of the chest and gastrointestinal tract should be performed initially to rule out pneumonitis and lesions of the esophagus or stomach, to describe the esophageal mucosa for irregularity or ulceration, and to note the integrity of the swallowing mechanisms.[39] Conclusive data are obtained by manometry, by intraluminal pH testing, and, if indicated, by gastric emptying studies and endoscopy.

Radiologic Examination. Radiologic examination of the upper gastrointestinal tract is the least accurate means of detecting GER, with the percentage of positive studies ranging from 45 to 95 per cent at different centers. In the "water siphon test," which employs fluoroscopy of the lower esophagus, the infant swallows water after the stomach has been filled with barium. This test is claimed to be more sensitive than the standard studies. Video tape or cinefluoroscopy should be employed in patients with neurologic or pulmonary disease to determine abnormalities in swallowing and to identify any aspiration of contrast material during deglutition. Mega-aero-esophagus may be a radiologic clue to the presence of reflux.[39a]

Esophageal Motility. Manometric techniques provide a permanent record of peristaltic amplitude and progression as well as sphincter location, pressures, and function. The studies are best performed using constantly perfused triple-lumen tubes with openings at 2-cm intervals. Those using single-lumen, rapid pull-through techniques yield pressures nearly twice those of standard measurements (31 to 58 vs. 10 to 32 mm Hg) and supply no other meaningful information. Even in the most careful studies it must be noted that there is temporal variation of LES pressure of up to 6 mm Hg (Table 3–1).

Acid Reflux Tests. These are the most sensitive means of detecting GER in both infant and adult. Although they detect the presence of acid and record the duration of time that it remains within the esophagus, they do not measure its quantity, nor do they discern alkaline reflux. Reflux is considered to be present when the intraesophageal measurements fall below pH 4.

Tuttle Test. This technique was the first used to measure intraluminal pH in infants and was performed after the introduction of 0.1 N HCl into the stomach.[8, 14] After the nasogastric tube was withdrawn, the esophagus was cleared of acid and the pH probe positioned 13 per cent of the esophageal distance above the LES. Spontaneous and induced reflux were measured over the next two hours. Christie found that only 55 per cent of children under two years of age who experienced vomiting and regurgitation had positive test results, but other workers, using abdominal compression, reported up to 96 per cent correlation. Obviously, the test was not recording the most physiologic conditions.

Yale pH Testing. A more physiologic approach consists of monitoring intraesophageal pH of the infant who has been fasted for four hours and who then has been fed. The probe is placed as described for the Tuttle test, and recordings are obtained for one hour with the infant in a semi-upright position in the infant seat. Forty ml per kg of apple juice (pH 4) are given by mouth, and monitoring is continued for two hours (Fig. 3–1). The number of refluxes and reflux time per hour are calculated on the basis of time the intraesophageal pH remained below 4. Those infants with mild reflux show a post-

prandial reflux time of 16.2 per cent, whereas those with failure to thrive or pulmonary disease and more severe symptoms have acid within the esophagus 38.4 to 49.5 per cent of the time (Table 3–2). The longest reflux periods in those with mild disease are less than eight and usually less than three minutes, but those with severe disease refluxed in 8 minutes and even up to 30-minute intervals.

Extended pH Monitoring. In the adult, these studies have identified three specific groups of patients:[31] (1) those who refluxed only after meals, (2) those who refluxed at night while supine, and (3) those who refluxed both day and night. Complications of reflux were greatest in the last group and absent in the first. The rate of acid clearance is undoubtedly a major factor in the development of esophagitis, for a similar study in young children showed that 38 control children under two years of age had some reflux after meals, but 14 symptomatic ones between 16 days and 25 months of age had more frequent and longer periods of reflux.[15, 25, 36] Sondheimer[36] established criteria for 18-hour monitoring using per cent

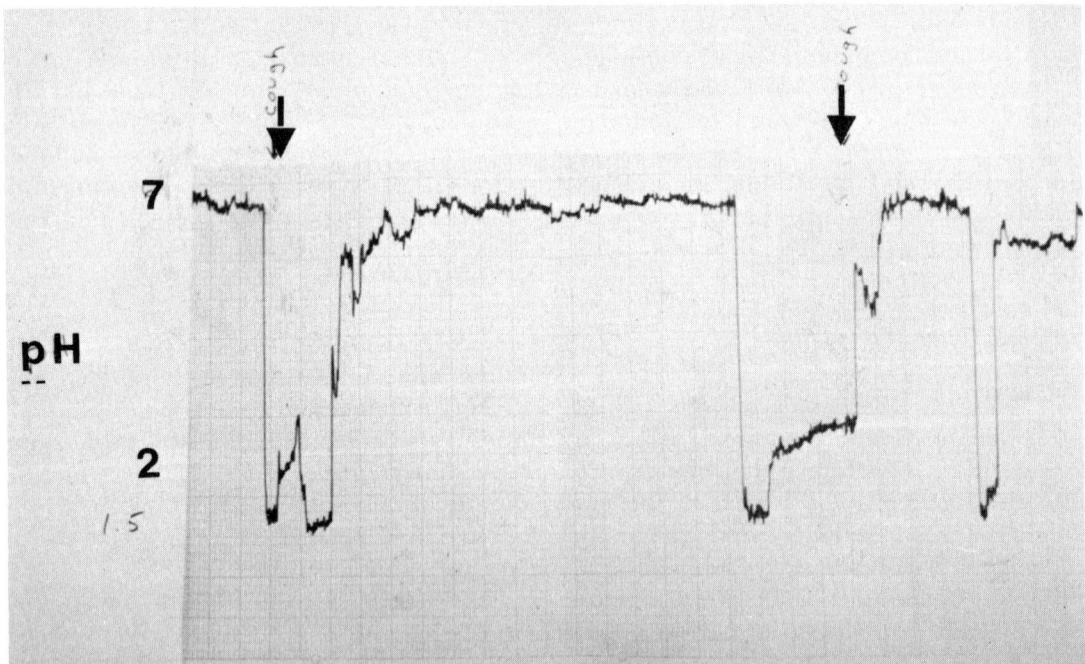

Figure 3–1 pH Probe showing normal esophageal pH 7 falling to 1.8 in infant during reflux. Arrows show coughs shortly after episode of reflux.

Table 3–2 Profiles of Infants with Gastroesophageal Reflux

Group	No.	% RT° 1 Hr	% RT° 2 Hr	Min. Longest Reflux	No. FTT	No. Pulm. Dis.	1 Hr % Gastric Emptying	Ampl. Wave Dist. Esophagus mm Hg	LESP mm Hg
Mild reflux	20	21.8	11.7	5.2	1	0	41.9 (35–55)	50.2	22.8
Severe reflux	25	53.5	37.2	16.5	14	9	21.6 (5–30)	28.7	19.1

°RT = reflux time.

time in which the pH was less than 4; the control value was 1.6 per cent and the value in children with reflux was 42 per cent. The frequency of reflux episodes per hour was 1.4 in controls and 6.1 in those with reflux.

Although one- to 2-hour postprandial monitoring is quite accurate, GER may be missed in a few infants. Those with negative or indeterminate postprandial testing and positive history should have pH monitoring extended over 24 hours.[15]

Isotope Scanning for GER. [99m]Technetium sulfur colloid is introduced into the stomach, and scintillations are counted over both stomach and thorax in 1- to 30-second intervals.[11, 18] A reflux index (RI) is calculated as

RI =

$$\frac{\text{no. counts esophagus / 1 to 30 sec. interval}}{\text{no. counts initially over stomach}}$$

This method has not proved very sensitive in infants, although it is helpful in identifying pulmonary aspiration of isotope. A computerized technique has been adapted to measure esophageal clearance of ingested isotope.

Gastric Emptying Studies. These studies provide information about gastric emptying as well as esophageal reflux. After a three-hour fast, the infant is given a meal consisting of 4 ounces of standard milk formula, to which 100 μc of [99m]technetium sulfur colloid are added. All infants are placed supine within three minutes of initiating ingestion and are maintained so for 60 minutes. Imaging of the upper gastrointestinal tract is performed using a gamma counter and dedicated computer. Emptying (E) is expressed as

$$E = \frac{CT^0 \text{ initial count in stomach} - CT^t \text{ count rate after correction for decay} \times 100}{CT^0}$$

Normal stomachs empty 44.3 per cent or more in one hour, whereas those of infants with severe reflux empty only 5 to 21.3 per cent (Figs. 3–2 and 3–3).

Endoscopy. This procedure is usually reserved for infants who fail to respond to conventional therapy. In combination with biopsy, it is highly accurate (92 to 96 per cent) in establishing the diagnosis of esophagitis. Since the mucosa may at times appear entirely normal, biopsy is essential. Extensive esophagitis is obvious as a red, friable mucosa, which may be covered with patchy exudate. Histologic examination of the biopsy specimen will show polymorphonuclear and eosinophilic infiltrate, elongation of the papillae (with rete peg length greater than 60 to 65 per cent of epithelial thickness), and thickening of the basal zone.[32] Transformation of squamous epithelium from normal to columnar represents Barrett's esophagus, a response to inflammation that carries a premalignant connotation.

Other. The string test uses methylene blue stain from material refluxed from the stomach.[9, 19] Although this may indicate reflux, other techniques provide more essential information.

A, GASTRIC EMPTYING < 10% AT 1 HOUR

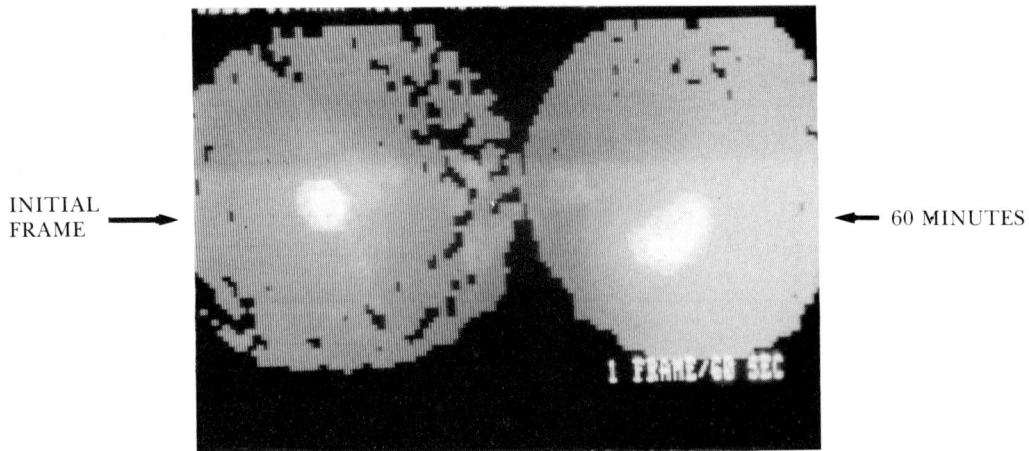

INITIAL FRAME ⟶   ⟵ 60 MINUTES

B, GASTRIC EMPTYING 35% AT 1 HOUR

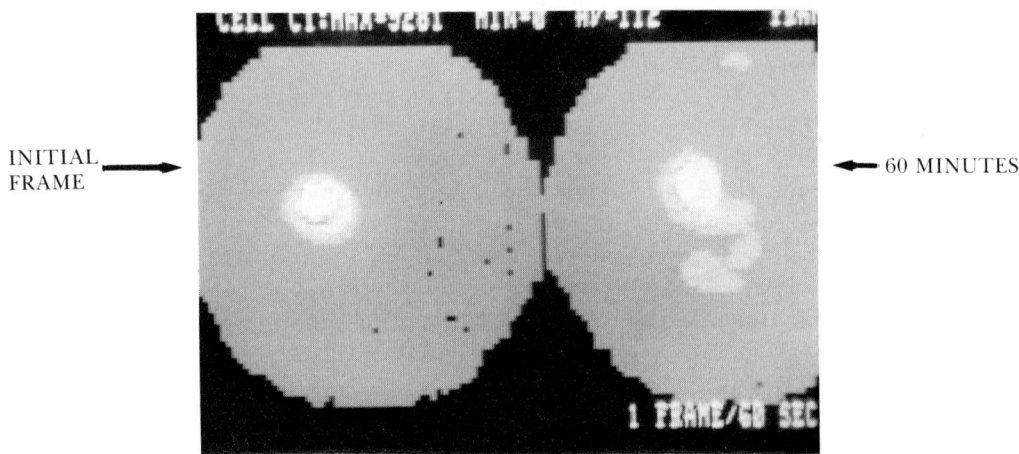

INITIAL FRAME ⟶   ⟵ 60 MINUTES

Figure 3–2   Scintiscan of normal (*A*) and abnormal (*B*) gastric emptying showing residual counts in stomach at end of one hour.

Treatment

The goals of therapy are to decrease episodes of GER and to coat the esophagus with a neutral material.

Position seems to have an effect upon GER, and most infants respond to constant elevation at a 30 to 45 degree angle. Maintaining the child in a semi-erect position for only an hour or so after feeding is ineffective. An infant seat is adequate during awake periods, and for sleep the crib mattress head is elevated. The prone position is more effective than the supine one.[33]

Feeding. Acid juices or fruits are contraindicated during the period of therapy, for these decrease LES pressure[40] and cause further irritation of the esophagus.[32a] Small, frequent feedings are given, and formula may be thickened by the addition of cereal. There is no documentation that the latter measure is effective, although mothers do report that it seems to decrease the volume that is regurgitated. Mothers are cautioned that a change in symptoms may not be obvious before two weeks. If, at that time, reflux is unchanged, antacids are added to the regimen in a dosage of ½ to 1 teaspoon given 15 to 30 minutes after meals. If there is evidence of bile reflux, an aluminum hydroxide antacid should be used for its ability to bind bile acids.

Cimetidine, 30 to 40 mg per kg per day in four divided doses, may be added if symptoms persist.[42] This functions to decrease gastric acid production through its H2 receptor antagonism. It has proved symptomatically effective in the treatment of GER in adults, but there are no controlled studies of its value in infants.[17a]

Bethanechol (urecholine), 8.7 mg per m^3 per day in three divided doses, has relieved symptoms and promoted weight gain in one group of infants with GER. It may, however, be associated with side effects such as diarrhea and agitation.

New drugs of the dopamine antagonist class are available (metoclopramide) or in limited investigational use (domperidone). Their action is central, rather than local, to promote increased peristaltic pressures and to increase gastric emptying. In proper dosage, they may be excellent agents to carry a child through the recovery period and should be considered in those patients with the more serious complications of GER. Side effects such as oculogyric crisis or rigidity seem to be less with domperidone than with metoclopramide, but they may develop in young infants with a relatively permeable blood-brain barrier. They should not be used in infants less than six months old or in cases of gastric outlet dysfunction.

Rarely, when regurgitation persists despite medical therapy, transpyloric feeds or surgical intervention are indicated. Surgery is indicated early in those with stricture or with serious episodes of apnea or pneumonitis.[27b] At least eight weeks of medical therapy should be attempted in other infants before surgical correction of GER is

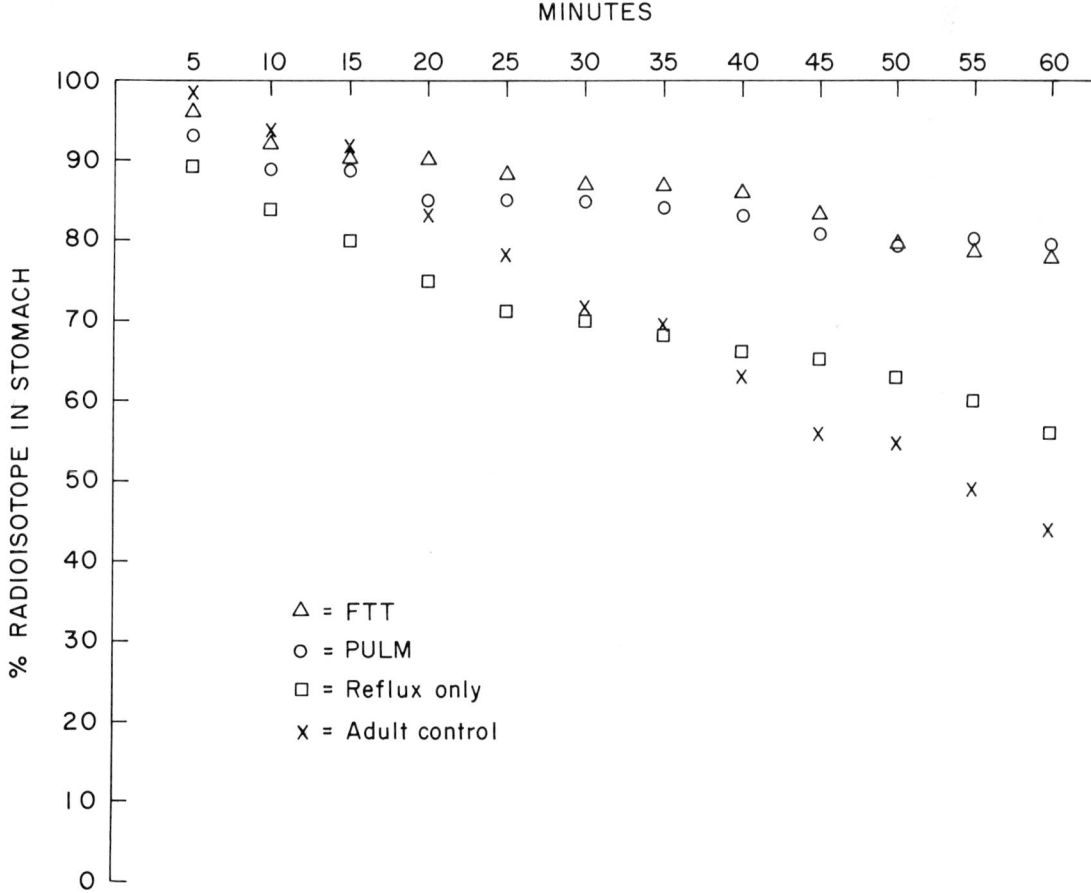

Figure 3–3 Per cent of gastric emptying with time in infants with mild reflux, failure to thrive, and recurrent pneumonitis, compared with normal adult controls.

undertaken. The Nissen fundoplication, which entails wrapping the fundus about the distal esophagus, is an often-used repair. Some surgeons are comfortable using a more simple gastropexy, while others use modifications of the two procedures.[1a, 2, 10, 17, 27, 28, 30] The Nissen procedure, however, leads to inability to belch or vomit and may promote a gastric bloat syndrome. It should be used with caution in infants with delayed gastric emptying. Children who have evidence of aspiration during swallowing do present postoperative complications and may not clear their pneumonitis. Feeding gastrostomy may be required for several months. A few continue to aspirate secretions; continuous drip through the gastrostomy, rather than bolus feeds, seems to decrease oral secretions and promote pulmonary clearing.

Prognosis

The prognosis for cure varies directly with the presence or absence of neurologic disease. Two thirds to four fifths of otherwise normal infants with GER respond to medical therapy and, once cured, experience no further problems. Now that sophisticated diagnostic techniques are available, those at risk for esophagitis and its complications (i.e., disordered peristalsis and/or delayed gastric emptying) may be identified early and aggressive medical management initiated. Pulmonary disease is cured or markedly improved in 85 to 95 per cent of infants after medical or surgical treatment.

Infants with neurologic disease are handicapped because of poor mobility, spasticity, and scoliosis — all of which tend to affect the normal anatomic relationships of the LES and diaphragm. Medical therapy is less successful, and there is an increased incidence of those requiring surgical intervention.[38] Complications after plication include esophageal perforation, gastric bloat syndrome, and herniated plication. Less often seen are intestinal obstruction, infection, gastric leak, esophageal stricture, and ulceration.[1a, 2, 5, 5a, 38] Although the complication rate after surgery was 59 per cent in retarded patients operated on for reflux,

in a 14-month follow-up study by Byrne et al.,[5a] none had recurrent vomiting.

REFERENCES

1. Arasu, T., Wyllie, R., Fitzgerald, J., Franken, E., Siddiqui, A., Lehman, G., Eigen, H., and Grosfeld, J.: Gastroesophageal reflux in infants and children. J. Pediatr. 96:789, 1980.
1a. Ashcraft, K., Holder, T., and Amoury, R.: Treatment of gastroesophageal reflux in children by Thal fundoplication. J. Thorac. Cardiovasc. Surg. 82:706, 1981.
2. Berlatzky, Y., Cohen, O., Freund, H., and Schiller, M.: Surgical treatment of gastroesophageal reflux with esophageal stricture in infancy and childhood. Am. J. Surg. 143:205, 1982.
2a. Berquist, W., Rachelefsky, G., Kadden, M., Siegel, S., Katz, R., Fonkalsrud, E., and Ament, M.: Gastroesophageal reflux, associated recurrent pneumonia, and chronic asthma in children. Pediatrics 68:29, 1981.
3. Boix-Ochoa, J., and Canals, J.: Maturation of the lower esophagus. J. Pediatr. Surg. 11:749, 1976.
4. Boix-Ochoa, J., Lafuente, J. M., and Gil-vernet, J. M.: Twenty four hour esophageal pH monitoring in gastroesophageal reflux. J. Pediatr. Surg. 15:74, 1980.
5. Bremner, C. G.: Gastric ulceration after a fundoplication operation for gastroesophageal reflux. Surg. Gynecol. Obstet. 148:62, 1979.
5a. Byrne, W., Euler, A., Ashcraft, E., Nash, D., Seibert, J., and Golladay, E. S.: Gastroesophageal reflux in the severely retarded who vomit: criteria for and results of surgery in twenty-two patients. Surgery 91:95, 1982.
6. Cadman, D., Richards, J., and Feldman, W.: Gastroesophageal reflux in severely retarded children. Dev. Med. Child Neurol. 20:95, 1978.
7. Carre, I. J.: Postural treatment of children with partial thoracic stomach. Arch. Dis. Child. 37:569, 1960.
8. Christie, D. L.: The acid reflux test for gastroesophageal reflux. J. Pediatr. 94:78, 1979.
9. Christie, D. L.: Methylene blue test for gastroesophageal reflux. Lancet 2:474, 1978.
10. Christie, D. L., Mack, D., Parker, A., Hall, D., and Cahill, J.: Use of intraoperative esophageal manometrics in surgical treatment of gastroesophageal reflux in pediatric patients. J. Pediatr. Surg. 23:648, 1978.
11. Christie, D. L., and Rudd, T. G.: Radionuclide test for gastroesophageal reflux (GER) in children. Pediatr. Res. 12:432, 1978.
12. Dodds, W. J., Hogan, W. J., Helm, J. F., and Dent, J.: Pathogenesis of reflux esophagitis. Gastroenterology 81:376, 1981.
13. Euler, A. R., and Ament, M.: Value of esophageal manometric studies in the gastroesophageal reflux of infancy. Pediatrics 59:58, 1977.
14. Euler, A., and Ament, M. E.: Detection of gastroesophageal reflux by Tuttle test. Pediatrics 60:65, 1977.
15. Euler, A., and Byrne, W.: Twenty four hour esophageal intraluminal pH probe testing a com-

parative analysis. Gastroenterology *80*:957, 1981.

16. Euler, A. R., Byrne, W. J., Ament, M., Fonkalsrud, E., Strobel, C., Siegel, S., Katz, R., and Rachelefsky, G.: Recurrent pulmonary disease in children: a complication of gastroesophageal reflux. Pediatrics *63*:47, 1979.

17. Euler, A., Fonkalsrud, E., and Ament, M. E.: Effect of Nissen fundoplication on lower esophageal sphincter pressure in children with gastroesophageal reflux. Gastroenterology *72*:260, 1977.

17a. Fiasse, R., Hanin, C., Lepot, A., Descamps, C., Lamy, F., and Dive, C.: Controlled trial of cimetidine in reflux esophagitis. Dig. Dis. Sci. *25*:750, 1980.

18. Fisher, R. S., Malmud, L. S., Roberts, G. S., et al.: Gastroesophageal (GE) scintiscanning to detect and quantitate GE reflux. Gastroenterology *70*:30, 1976.

19. Girardi, G., Vial, L., Fritis, E., et al.: Diagnosis of gastroesophageal reflux in infants and children by methylene blue test. Lancet *1*:1236, 1978.

20. Gryboski, J. D., Thayer, W. R., and Spiro, H. M.: Esophageal motility in infants and children. Pediatrics *31*:382, 1963.

21. Harned, H., Myraele, J., and Ferreiro, J.: Respiratory suppression and swallowing from introduction of fluids into the laryngeal region of the lamb. Pediatr. Res. *12*:1003, 1978.

22. Herbst, J.: Gastroesophageal reflux. J. Pediatr. *98*:859, 1981.

23. Herbst, J., Book, L. S., and Bray, P.: Gastroesophageal reflux in the "near miss" sudden infant death syndrome. J. Pediatr. *92*:73, 1978.

24. Herbst, J., Book, L., Johnson, D., and Jolley, S.: The lower esophageal sphincter in gastroesophageal reflux in children. J. Clin. Gastroenterol. *1*:119, 1979.

25. Hill, J. L., Pelligrini, C. A., Burrington, J. D., et al.: Technique experience with 24 hour esophageal pH monitoring in children. J. Pediatr. Surg. *12*:877, 1978.

26. Hillemeier, C., Lange, R., Seashore, J., McCallum, R., and Gryboski, J. D.: Delayed gastric emptying in infants with gastroesophageal reflux. J. Pediatr. *98*:190, 1981.

27. Johnson, D., Herbst, J., Oliveros, M., and Stewart, D.: Evaluation of gastroesophageal reflux surgery in children. Pediatrics *59*:62, 1977.

27a. Johnson, D., and Jolley, S. G.: Gastroesophageal reflux in infants and children. Surg. Clin. North Am. *61*:1125, 1981.

27b. Johnson, L. F.: New concepts in the study and treatment of gastroesophageal reflux disease. Med. Clin. North Am. *65*:1195, 1981.

28. Jolley, S., Herbst, J., and Johnson, D.: Surgery in children with gastroesophageal reflux and respiratory symptoms. J. Pediatr. *96*:194, 1980.

29. Kim, S. H., and Donahoe, P.: Gastroesophageal reflux and hiatus hernia in children: Experience with 70 cases. J. Pediatr. Surg. *15*:443, 1980.

30. Leape, L. L., and Ramenovsky, M. L.: Surgical treatment of gastroesophageal reflux in children. Am. J. Dis. Child. *134*:935, 1980.

31. Little, A., DeMeester, T., Kirchner, P., O'Sullivan, G., and Skinner, D.: Pathogenesis of esophagitis in patients with gastroesophageal reflux. Surgery *88*:101, 1980.

32. Livestone, E., Sheahan, D., and Behar, J.: Studies of esophageal epithelial cell proliferation in patients with reflux esophagitis. Gastroenterology *73*:1315, 1977.

32a. Lloyd, D. A., and Borda, I. T.: Food-induced heartburn: Effect of osmolality. Gastroenterology *80*:740, 1981.

33. Meyers, W. F., Herbst, J., and Jollan, S. G.: Superior efficacy of the prone and elevated position in treatment of post-prandial gastroesophageal reflux. Pediatr. Res. *15*:541, 1981.

34. Moroz, S., Espinoza, J., Cumming, W., and Diamant, N.: Lower esophageal sphincter function in children with and without gastroesophageal reflux. Gastroenterology *71*:236, 1976.

34a. Moroz, S., and Beiko, P.: Relationship between lower esophageal sphincter pressure and serum gastrin concentration in the newborn infant. J. Pediatr. *99*:725, 1981.

34b. O'Sullivan, G., De Meester, T., Joelsson, B., Smith, R., Blough, R., Johnson, L., and Skinner, D.: Interaction of lower esophageal sphincter pressure and length of sphincter in the abdomen as determinants of gastroesophageal competence. Am. J. Surg. *143*: 40, 1982.

35. Shapiro, G., and Christie, D. L.: Gastroesophageal reflux in steroid dependent asthmatic youths. Pediatrics *63*:207, 1979.

36. Sondheimer, J.: Continuous monitoring of distal esophageal pH: a diagnostic test for gastroesophageal reflux in infants. J. Pediatr. *96*: 804, 1980.

37. Sondheimer, J., and Vorris, B.: Gastroesophageal reflux among severely retarded children. J. Pediatr. *94*:710, 1979.

38. Sondheimer, J., Wilkinson, J., and Dudgeon, D. L.: Medical versus surgical management of gastroesophageal reflux in the severely mentally retarded. Pediatr. Res. *15*:547, 1981.

39. Stillman, A., Larter, W., Goldman, D.: Longitudinal esophageal bands associated with esophageal aperistalsis. Gastroenterology *74*:592, 1978.

39a. Swischuk, L., Hayden, C. K., and van Caillie, B. D.: Mega-aeroesophagus in children: a sign of gastroesophageal reflux. Radiology *141*:73, 1981.

40. Wallen, L., Boesby, S., and Madsen, T.: The effect of HCL infusion in the lower part of the oesophagus on the pharyngoesophageal sphincter pressure in normal subjects. Scand. J. Gastroenterol. *13*:82, 1978.

41. Werlin, S., Dodds, W., Hogan, W., and Wendorfer, R.: Mechanisms of gastroesophageal reflux in children. J. Pediatr. *97*:244, 1980.

42. Wesdorp, E., Bartelsman, J., Pape, K., et al.: Oral cimetidine in reflux esophagitis: a double blind controlled trial. Gastroenterology *74*:821, 1978.

43. Winter, H., and Grand, R. J.: Gastroesophageal reflux. Pediatrics *68*:134, 1981.

Chapter Four

MALNUTRITION AND FAILURE TO THRIVE

FAILURE TO THRIVE

Failure to thrive accounts for 1 to 5 per cent of all pediatric hospital admissions.[3, 9, 10, 26] It has been defined as weight below the third percentile for age or, more realistically, as two standard deviations below the expected average height and weight. Critical attention to height and weight at each office visit may enable early identification of the child who shows a fall-off from his standard height and weight percentiles. Half of children with failure to thrive are diagnosed by six months of age,[35, 39a, 56, 57] and, in the series of Shaheen et al.,[60] 54.3 per cent of those with systemic disease and 79.5 per cent of those with nonorganic disease were less than two years of age at the time of presentation (Table 4–1).

Table 4–1 Causes of Failure to Thrive

Organic	18–85%	
Gastrointestinal		12–19%
Neurologic		4–18%
Genitourinary		0–5%
Endocrine		1–5%
Cardiac		1–31%
Other		5–29%
Environmental	15–55%	
No cause	12–32%	
(short stature)		

Children with nonorganic failure to thrive may have feeding difficulties such as choking, spitting, or refusal to feed; many develop constipation. Since these symptoms are also associated with true gastrointestinal disease, their etiology must be investigated. In various series of children hospitalized for this problem, organic causes have been identified in 18 to 85 per cent (Table 4–1); in infants with organic disease, disordered family constellations and psychologic problems in the mother are identified in 15 to 40 per cent. Organic and psychologic factors may therefore exist side by side, contributing equally to the infant's disease.[11, 40, 46, 47, 47a, 47b, 49, 53, 59, 60, 62]

Although not consistently proven, families of children with nonorganic failure to thrive seem to be disorganized, to have more financial and emotional stresses, and to have an increased incidence of single parents.[27] Many mothers have come from deprived home situations and are themselves depressed, with feelings of inadequacy. They are unable to interact in a healthy, developing relationship with their children. The child with a physical problem or one who is difficult or demanding increases the inadequacies of such a parent. Feeding problems develop and result in hypocaloric intake[68] or the actual withholding of food.[47]

The normal term infant loses weight for

two to three days, and the premature infant loses weight for up to ten days after birth. Weight gain then progresses at extremely rapid rates until the age of two years. Gain in weight averages 0.5 to 1.0 kg per month for the first six months, 1.0 to 3.0 kg per month for the second six months, and 0.2 kg per month between the ages of one and two years. Linear growth averages 125 to 130 cm per year between six months and one year and 112 cm per year between one and two years. The head circumference increases by an average of 5 cm during the first three months and by 6 cm over the next nine months. Infant weight should double by five months, triple by one year, and increase fivefold by two years. During this most rapid period of growth there are concomitant changes in body composition, with total protein increasing from 12.5 to 18 per cent, fat increasing from 12.5 to 18 per cent, and carbohydrate decreasing from 1 to 0.7 per cent by two years; water content decreases from 73 to 60 per cent.

Malnutrition during this period carries a significant threat to long-term development, for it decreases cell size within the body and brain, increases body water, and decreases body fat and protein.[71] Catch-up growth is dependent upon continued cellular division and is depressed once this ceases.

Different types of growth failure may be recognized in the infant. *Intrauterine growth retardation* is identified in the neonate weighing less than the tenth percentile for gestational age.[28, 53a, 66a] Several intrauterine growth curves are available, the most commonly used being from Denver. The prognosis varies with the degree of retardation: (1) Infants of low birth weight who have normal length and head circumferences suffer from an insult late in gestation and have evidence of decreased subcutaneous tissue. They respond in time to adequate nutrition by relatively normal growth and developmental progress. (2) Those with low weight and height but normal head circumference may have slow to normal catch-up growth but normal intellectual development. (3) Infants born with retarded height, weight, and head development have endured an insult of long duration as the result

of early viral infection or placental insufficiency and fare poorly, remaining small, with 92 per cent below the fiftieth percentile and 35 per cent below the third percentile at ten years. Intellectual development is delayed or markedly abnormal in those whose head circumference continues at or falls below the tenth percentile.[7, 70]

Intrauterine growth retardation is due to maternal malnutrition, particularly of protein, excessive maternal smoking or alcohol consumption, maternal diabetes, chromosomal abnormalities, anomalies, placental insufficiency, twinning, or intrauterine viral infection.[7, 14, 42]

Decreased linear growth in excess of weight suggests hypothyroidism, various types of dwarfism, or the mucopolysaccharidoses. Such children appear more small than thin.

Weight decrease in excess of height occurs as a result of inadequate nutrition. This may result from increased energy expenditure as in cardiac disease, decreased caloric intake, or impaired gastrointestinal absorption, often with zinc malabsorption.[17] This pattern may be noted in the neonatal period or may develop during the first few years of life. Although celiac disease may present in an infant several months of age, it typically has its onset between 10 and 18 months, with a progressive fall-off from established percentile lines, first in weight and then in height (Fig. 4–1). Children placed on severely restricted diets may either mistakenly be given inadequate calories or may simply refuse to eat the new diet.[62a]

Emotional deprivation, sometimes termed "psychogenic dwarfism,"[58] is a symmetric growth retardation that develops during the first few months or years of life in children subjected to a lack of interaction and maternal affection. It may occur in any economic or social class. Functional hypopituitarism is documented by low growth hormone levels, which return to normal or near-normal after the child is removed from his environment. Parental withholding of food is an additional factor in some cases. Although weight gain and acceleration of growth velocity are marked during the recovery period, some children have

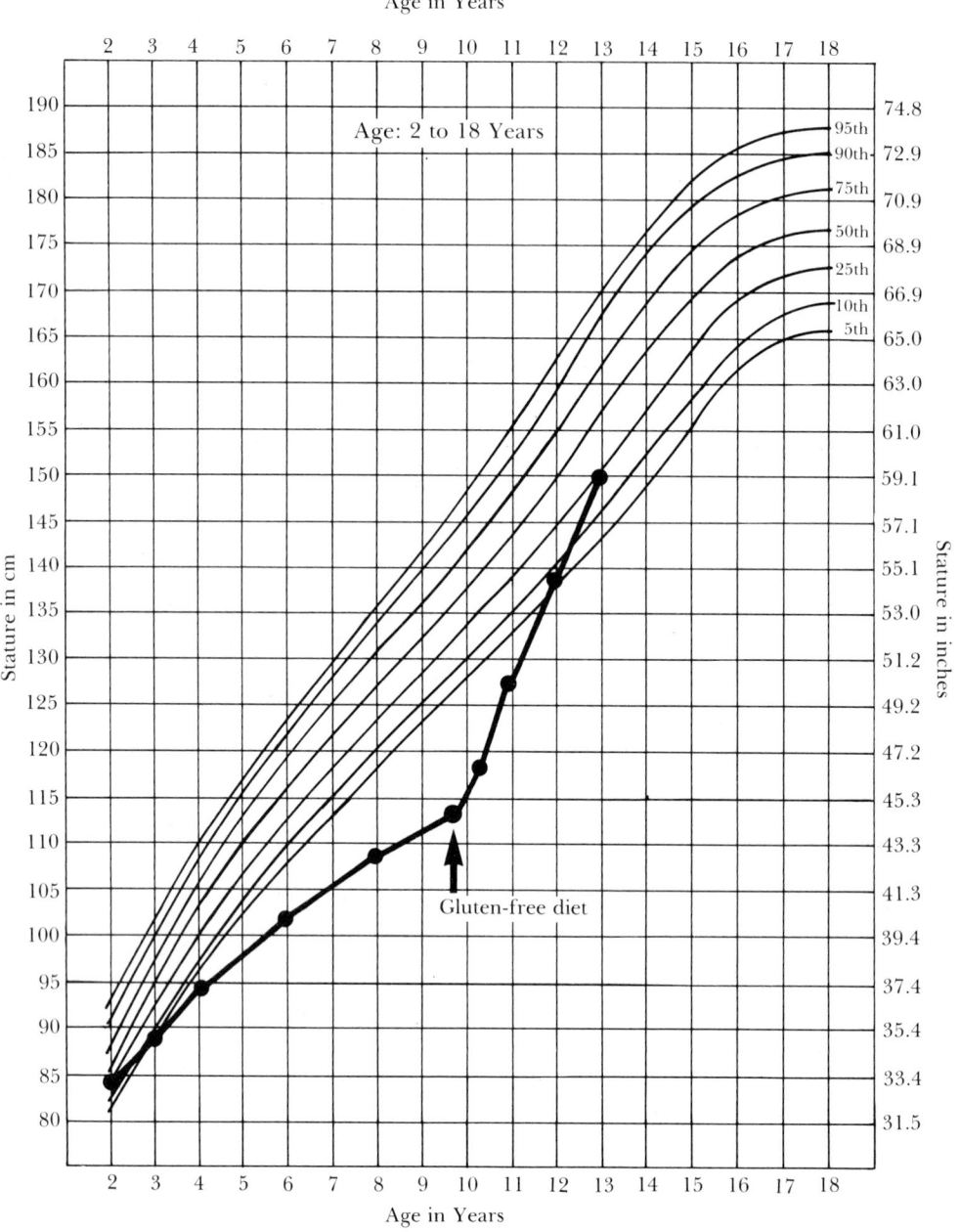

Growth Chart

Boys

Stature for Age

Figure 4–1 Growth chart of patient with celiac disease showing gradual decrease in velocity of linear growth from four years of age, with rapid increase of growth velocity after introduction of gluten-free diet.

impaired growth and intellectual development.[23, 24, 31, 36]

Constitutional short stature, represented by the infant or child who grows consistently along or below the lower percentiles,

reflects his genetic endowment. Small stature is usually present in one or more family members.

The preliminary screening tests for failure to thrive are listed in Table 4–2. Endo-

Table 4-2 Evaluation of Failure to Thrive

I. Careful history and physical examination
   Developmental examination
   CBC and urinalysis (test for ability to concentrate urine)
   Stool examination for blood, pH, reducing substances, fat
   Calorie count
   Feeding trial

II. Bone age, chest film, ECG (if indicated)
    BUN, creatinine
    Electrolytes, calcium, phosphorus
    Urine culture and genetic screen
    Carotene, folate, thyroid studies

crine testing for somatomedin and growth hormone profiles may be included if other organic diseases are not present. It is obvious, however, that organic disease may coexist with parental disarray, and both must be evaluated for the total care of the patient.

MALNUTRITION

The early recognition of malnutrition is possible in this country, where pediatric care is readily available. World estimates indicate that approximately 500 million preschool children suffer from mild to moderate protein-calorie malnutriton. This, with associated infections, is the major killer of infants and young children and the major cause of growth and developmental retardation. In third world countries, infant growth and development are normal during the first five months but become severely retarded between 18 and 24 months. Although the children continue to grow, their activity is limited and they never attain normal height or weight for their age. Malnutrition takes its greatest toll upon growth between weaning and the end of the second year. The diet in underdeveloped nations, which relies heavily upon cereals as a protein source, fails to provide a balanced amino acid intake for children. Protein-calorie malnutrition exists in the United States owing to inadequate intake in some instances and to fad or vegetarian diets in others.[20, 22, 43, 61, 64] Intestinal malabsorption is a less common cause.

Pathology and Pathophysiology. As the protein and caloric intakes decrease, the body attempts to maintain normal plasma protein levels by depleting the supply of protein in muscle and liver. It is only after 50 per cent of the protein store has been utilized that the plasma level begins to fall. This is nature's way of preserving the integrity of the life-supporting tissues: heart, brain, and lungs. A decrease in total body mass is reflected in wasting of the arms, legs, and gluteal musculature, but not all the tissue loss is apparent since extracellular fluid tends to be retained as body solids diminish.[20, 69] The ratio of noncollagen to collagen protein decreases. Only after weight loss is evident does linear growth cease. Essential amino acids, particularly taurine, are decreased.

Severe and prolonged malnutrition in infancy affects head circumference and brain growth.[4, 48] Particularly related to protein malnutrition, one of the most serious sequelae is irreversible central nervous system injury. Normally, the number of brain cells increases until the sixth month, and myelin synthesis, most rapid around the time of birth, continues until two years of age. In the brains of infants who die of marasmus during the first year of life, there is little evidence of cell division and the DNA content of the brain is decreased or normal. In general, the earlier the onset of malnutrition, the more severe the degree of permanent injury, owing to reduced brain weight and decreased cell number. A later onset of malnutrition causes a decrease in cell size rather than number. Malnutrition from birth has been associated with defective myelinization, abnormal dendritic growth of Purkinje cells, and reduced pyramidal cell volume. When adequate nutrition is offered, there is rapid brain growth, often associated with separation of sutures; brain scans show growth with obliteration of subarachnoid spaces and decreases in ventricular size. Certainly, malnutrition, particularly in small for gestational age infants who are born prematurely, is associated with an increased incidence of cerebral palsy and intellectual problems. Evidence is now accumulating that malnutrition with onset after six months of age may even be harmful to later intellectual development.[55]

Malnutrition begets malabsorption. The absence of adequate dietary intake leads to decreased gastrin production and atrophy of dependent tissues, i.e., stomach, duodenum, and colon. Achlorhydria is not unusual. The intestine and pancreas are most susceptible to protein depletion because of their high daily protein turnover (9 to 16 gm per day in the adult). There are varying degrees of intestinal atrophy and submucosal hemorrhage. Ten to 60 per cent of children with kwashiorkor have a small bowel mucosa resembling that of celiac disease: The intestinal wall is thin and the mucosa atrophic, showing decreased cell numbers and DNA content.[5, 15, 16, 50, 67] Changes are most marked in the proximal small bowel. The enterocytes are decreased in size, with the mucosa appearing cuboidal; crypt depth is increased; cell production and migration up the crypts are decreased; round cells infiltrate the lamina propria, and fat bodies are present within the absorptive cells. Electron microscopy shows disorganization of the brush border, collagen filament deposition, autophagosomes, and a dense granular deposition beneath the basal lamellae.[25] Changes in marasmus have been reported by some to be more severe and by others to be less severe than in kwashiorkor. The mucosal abnormalities may persist for a year or more after refeeding.

With flattening of the intestinal mucosa, cholecystokinin production by the duodenum is decreased.[44] Since this enzyme is trophic for the pancreas, its depletion further augments pancreatic insufficiency. Pathologically, patients with protein malnutrition show atrophy of acinar cells, decreased zymogen granules, vacuolization of cells, fibrosis, and dilatation of the pancreatic ducts. Mitochondria, endoplasmic reticulum, and cytoplasmic bodies are decreased. Clinically, the insufficiency is primarily acinar in type, with trypsin and lipase and, later, amylase being decreased. Volume and bicarbonate responses are usually normal. The defect is more marked in those with maramus than those with kwashiorkor and may persist for weeks to years after adequate intake is restored.[6, 23]

Secondary to the mucosal and brush border abnormalities in the small intestine are deficiencies of disaccharidases,[1, 12, 13] dipeptidases,[38] dipeptide hydrolase,[29] and alkaline phosphatase. Lactose deficiency is of major clinical import, although sucrose and even monosaccharide transport may be impaired in severely malnourished infants. Not only are peptides and carbohydrates poorly absorbed, but the resultant increased transit in itself may cause a mild generalized malabsorption. Changes are more severe in marasmus.

Steatorrhea results from these as well as other defects. Intraluminal micellar solubilization of triglycerides and fatty acids is deficient, probably as a result of both impaired bile acid absorption and deconjugation of bile acids by bacterial overgrowth.[52] Bacterial overgrowth itself is harmful to sugar absorption. Iron,[51] vitamin B_{12},[2] and folic acid absorption are impaired.

The liver is enlarged and fatty, and there is decreased synthesis of low-density lipoproteins. Beta-lipoprotein, cholesterol, and triglycerides are decreased, but alpha-lipoprotein and phosphatidylcholine remain normal. Children with kwashiorkor, unlike those with marasmus, have an abnormal glucose tolerance test, probably owing to decreased insulin production. Caloric expenditures are decreased, somatomedin levels are low, and growth hormone response to arginine is increased.[39] Thyroxine levels are often in the high normal range.[54] Aldosterone levels are normal in marasmus but increased in kwashiorkor.[8]

Poor resistance to infection is associated with depression of the thymolymphatic system and cell-mediated immunity.[18, 19, 30, 45, 65, 66] The skin window inflammatory response is normal in infants with marasmus but abnormal in those with kwashiorkor. Immunoglobulins G and M are normal, but immunoglobulin A is often increased. The immunologic abnormalities are compiled in Table 4–3.

Types of Malnutrition. There are no exact criteria for the determination of the various forms of chronic malnutrition, and, indeed, they may overlap.[36] Marasmus has been defined as a body weight below the expected fiftieth percentile weight[37] for age

Table 4–3   Immunologic Abnormalities
in Malnutrition

HUMORAL IMMUNITY	
Serum IgG, IgA, IgM	Normal or increased
Serum IgE	Increased
Antibody production	Normal or decreased
Secretory IgA	Decreased
CELLULAR IMMUNITY	
Thymus and lymphatic tissue	Decreased
T cell function	Decreased
Lymphocyte transformation	Decreased
Delayed hypersensitivity	Decreased
Inflammatory response	Decreased
COMPLEMENT	Decreased

and wasting of the muscles and subcutaneous fat. It represents both protein and calorie deficiency and is now termed (PCM (protein-calorie malnutrition) (Table 4–4). Kwashiorkor, or edematous PCM, indicates primarily protein deficiency. Marasmic kwashiorkor includes hepatomegaly, pitting edema, low serum proteins, and hair changes. There are intermediate cases in which there is marasmus with hair changes but without hepatomegaly or edema. (Kwashiorkor means "red body" and describes the change in hair color to red or white produced by protein malnutrition.)

Symptoms. The first signs of malnutrition are a falling-off of weight gain, followed by an arrest in linear growth. If malnutrition occurs early in the child's life, head growth is arrested. Dental development is not impaired. Signs of protein deficiency of kwashiorkor or marasmic kwashiorkor are pitting edema, as tested by firm pressure over the anterior tibia for at least three seconds; light, dry, brittle hair that can be plucked out easily without pain, and even alopecia; and, eventually, ascites. The infants are uninterested, apathetic, and appear acutely ill. Vitamin deficiencies are manifest as angular stomatitis or fissuring at the corners of the mouth, follicular keratosis or goosepimple type of skin, and friable red gums. There are areas of depigmentation of the skin or brawny pigmentation with ulceration and scaling. The abdomen is distended, and the infants have a great deal of gas along with diarrheal stools (Fig. 4–2). Because of edema, the extreme degree of malnutrition may not be obvious at first.

The marasmic child is small, thin, chronically ill, and wasted. His temperature is below normal.

Diagnosis. The full-blown clinical picture is unmistakable (Fig. 4–2). Radiologic examination of the long bones and wrists shows retardation of bone age and, if appropriate deficiencies are severe, rickets or scurvy. Examination of the gastrointestinal tract reveals some mildly dilated small bowel loops and flocculation of barium. Fat

Table 4–4   Clinical and Laboratory Findings in Malnutrition

	MARASMUS	KWASHIORKOR
Weight loss	+++	++
Edema	−	+++
Depigmentation	−	+++
Hair changes	−+	++
Vitamin deficiencies	+++	++
Small intestine	Villous atrophy	Villous atrophy
Pancreatic enzymes	Decreased	Decreased
Laboratory values		
Serum albumin	Normal to slightly decreased	Decreased
Lipase	Normal or decreased	Decreased
Amylase	Normal or decreased	Decreased
Esterase	Slightly decreased	Decreased
Triglycerides	Normal	Normal
Cholesterol	Normal	Decreased
Fatty acids	Increased	Increased

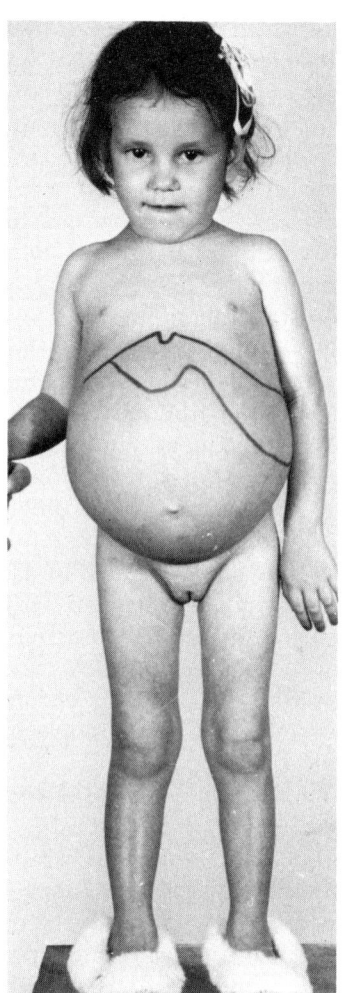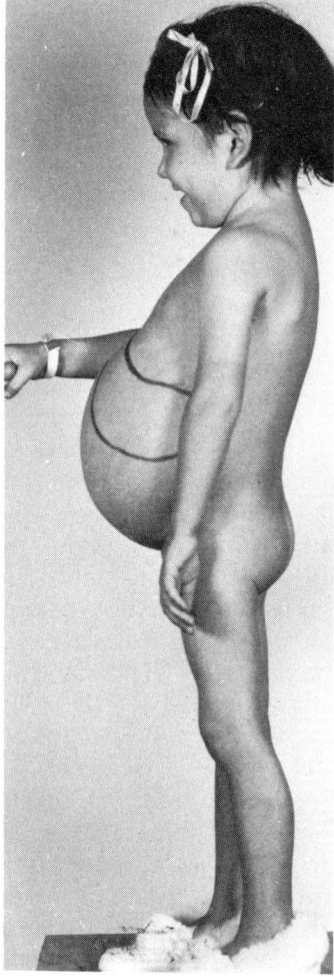

Figure 4–2 This five-year-old girl presented with diarrhea. Protein malnutrition is reflected in her sparse, coarse hair, pitting edema of the legs, and marked abdominal distention. The liver enlargement is due to fatty infiltration. Note the wasting of the extremities and gluteal musculature.

excretion is increased in quantitative stool examination, and trypsin is often absent. There is significant anemia, with a hemoglobin of as little as 6 gm per dl. Serum potassium and magnesium levels are depressed, but the sodium is either low or elevated. The serum albumin and prealbumin values are depressed and are probably the best indicators of early protein deficiency. The rate of albumin synthesis is decreased, as is the rate of its catabolism, as the body attempts to maintain a constant circulating albumin mass. Prealbumin is a sensitive index of protein status.[41] Liver function is usually normal, but as fatty infiltration of the liver increases mild abnormalities may be seen. Alkaline phosphatase is depressed, but in those with fatty liver it may be elevated. The creatinine-height ratio, representing the 24-hour creatinine

excretion of the subject as compared with that of a normal child of the same height, should be approximately 1.0. In malnourished children with edema the ratio is 0.25 to 0.75, and in those with no edema it is 0.35 to 0.85.

Treatment. Severely malnourished infants require intravenous therapy and electrolyte regulation. Pulmonary edema can be a complication during early hydration, and for this reason some recommend giving no more than 100 ml per kg per day during the first day. Others advocate up to 200 ml per kg per day.[33] Since the infant has increased intracellular fluid, he may lose weight during the first few days of therapy. Lactose intolerance is present in most infants tested, but milk is usually tolerated and remains the accepted nutriment; 2 to 4 gm per kg per day and up to 6 to 9 gm per kg per day of milk protein are given.[63] Recently, a formula of protein hydrolysate, medium-chain triglyceride, and glucose has been used successfully in depleted infants and seems a logical first-stage feeding.[32] If a large caloric load precipitates diarrhea, the load should be reduced and then increased gradually. Pancreatic enzyme supplementation is of benefit if the level of pancreatic enzymes is depressed. Rapid increase in caloric intake may provoke acute pancreatitis, and amylase and lipase should be monitored, particularly in the child who complains of abdominal pain.[40]

Complications. Because of the combination of achlorhydria, protein malnutrition, and impaired immunologic defenses, these children are particularly susceptible to bacterial and parasitic infections, which further compound their symptomatology. During the early recovery period the most common complications are heart or liver failure, pancreatitis,[34] hypoglycemia, and worsening of the diarrhea. An encephalopathy sometimes follows refeeding of high-protein diets to children with kwashiorkor, but the mechanism for this is poorly understood. The central nervous system sequelae have been noted earlier.

Prognosis. Even with our increasingly sophisticated knowledge of nutrition, enzymes, and fluid and electrolyte balance, the mortality rates in severe malnutrition remain between 30 and 50 per cent. Intercurrent infections are 50 times more frequent in these patients than in normal children. After weight gain has begun, it increases rapidly in velocity and approaches normal after several months. Linear growth, however, may remain delayed even three years after treatment and may never reach normal percentiles. If the onset of malnutrition occurs after infancy, there seem to be no serious sequelae. Obviously, the best therapy is prevention, with adequate prenatal care and supervision of infantile feedings.

REFERENCES

1. Adams, J. L., and Leichter, J.: Effect of protein-deficient diets with various amounts of carbohydrates on intestinal disaccharidase activity in the rat. J. Nutr. 103:1716, 1973.
2. Alvarado, J., Vargas, W., Dias, N., and Viteri, F. E.: Vitamin B_{12} absorption in protein-calorie malnourished children and during recovery: influence of protein and of diarrhea. Am. J. Clin. Nutr. 26:595, 1973.
3. Ambuel, J. B., and Harris, B.: Failure to thrive. Ohio Med. J. 59:997, 1963.
4. Babson, S. G., and Henderson, N. B.: Fetal undergrowth: relation of head growth to later intellectual performance. Pediatrics 53:890, 1974.
5. Barzebat, G. O., Bowie, M. D., Kashula, R. O. C., and Hansen, J. D. L.: Studies on the small intestinal mucosa of children with protein calorie malnutrition. S. Afr. Med. J. 41:1031, 1967.
6. Barzebat, G. O., and Hansen, J. D. L.: The exocrine pancreas and protein-calorie malnutrition. Pediatrics 42:77, 1968.
7. Beck, F. J., and van der Berg, B. J.: The relationship of the rate of intrauterine growth of low birth weight infants to later growth. J. Pediatr. 86:504, 1975.
8. Beitins, I., Graham, G., Kowarski, A., and Migeon, C.: Adrenal function in normal infants and in marasmus and kwashiorkor. J. Pediatr. 84:444, 1973.
9. Berwick, D. M.: Non-organic failure to thrive. Pediatr. Rev. 1:265, 1980.
10. Blackburn, G. L., and Thornton, P. A.: The nutritional assessment of the hospitalized patient. Med. Clin. North Am. 63:1103, 1979.
11. Boulton, T. J. C., and Rowley, M. P.: Nutritional studies during early childhood. Aust. Pediatr. J. 15:87, 1979.
12. Bowie, M. D., Barzebat, B. O., and Hansen, J. D. L.: Carbohydrate absorption in malnourished children. Am. J. Clin. Nutr. 20:89, 1967.
13. Bowie, M. D., Brinkman, G. L., and Hansen, J. D. L.: Acquired disaccharide intolerance in malnutrition. J. Trop. Pediatr. 66:1083, 1965.
14. Brasel, J., and Winick, M.: Maternal nutrition and prenatal growth. Arch. Dis. Child. 47:479, 1972.
15. Brunser, O.: Effects of malnutrition on intestinal structure and function in children. Clin. Gastroenterol. 6:341, 1977.
16. Brunser, O., Castillo, C., and Araza, M.: Fine structure of the small intestinal mucosa in infantile marasmic malnutrition. Gastroenterology 70:495, 1976.
17. Castro-Magana, M., Collipp, P., Chen, S., Cheruvansky, T., and Maddaiah, T.: Zinc nutritional status, adrogens and growth retardation. Am. J. Dis. Child. 135:322, 1981.
18. Chandra, R. K.: Lymphocyte subpopulations in human malnutrition: cytotoxic and suppressor cells. Pediatrics 59:423, 1977.
19. Chandra, R. K.: Immunocompetence in undernutrition. J. Pediatr. 81:1194, 1972.
20. Cheek, D. B., Hill, D. E., Cordano, A., and Graham, G. G.: Malnutrition in infancy and changes in muscle and adipose tissue before and after rehabilitation. Pediatr. Res. 4:135, 1979.
21. Coello-Raminez, P., and Lifshitz, F.: Enteric microflora and carbohydrate intolerance in infants with diarrhea. Pediatrics 49:233, 1972.

22. Dahlman, N., and Petersin, K.: Influence of environmental conditions during infancy upon final body stature. Pediatr. Res. *11*:695, 1977.

23. Danus, O., Urbina, A., Valenzuela, I., and Solimano, C.: The effect of refeeding upon pancreatic function in marasmic infants. J. Pediatr. 77:334, 1970.

24. Davis, R. D., Apley, J., Fill, G., and Grimaldi, C.: Diet and retarded growth. Br. Med. J. 2:539, 1978.

25. Duque, E., Lotero, H., Bolanos, O., and Mayoral, L. G.: Enteropathy in adult protein malnutrition: ultrastructural findings. Am. J. Clin. Nutr. 28:914, 1975.

26. English, P. C.: Failure to thrive without organic reason. Pediatr. Ann. 7:774, 1978.

27. Fitchoff, J., Whitten, C. F., and Pettit, M. C.: A psychiatric study of mothers of infants with growth failure secondary to maternal deprivation. J. Pediatr. 79:209, 1971.

28. Fitzharding, P. M., and Steven, R. M.: The small for dates infant. Pediatrics 49:671, 1972.

29. Gjessing, E. C., Villaneuva, D., Duquem, E., Bolanos, O., and Mayoral, L. G.: Dipeptide hydrolase activity of the intestinal mucosa from protein malnourished adult patients and controls. Am. J. Clin. Nutr. 30:1044, 1977.

30. Gleason, R., and Roodman, D.: Reversible T cell depression in malnourished infants. J. Pediatr. 90:1032, 1976.

31. Graham, G., and Adrianzen, B.: Late "catch up" growth after severe infantile malnutrition. Johns Hopkins Med. J. *131*:204, 1972.

32. Graham, G., Baertl, J., Cordano, A., and Morales, E.: Lactose free medium chain triglyceride formula in severe malnutrition. Am. J. Dis. Child. *126*:330, 1973.

33. Graham, G. G., Cordano, A., Blizzard, R. M., and Cheek, D.: Infantile malnutrition: changes in body composition during rehabilitation. Pediatr. Res. 3:579, 1969.

34. Gryboski, J. D., Hillemeier, C., Kocoshis, S., Anyan, W., and Seashore, J.: Refeeding pancreatitis in malnourished children. J. Pediatr. 97:441, 1980.

35. Hannaway, P. J.: Failure to thrive. A study of 100 infants and children. Clin. Pediatr. 9:96, 1970.

36. Hatch, T.: Effects of protein-calorie malnutrition on the digestive and absorptive capacities of infants. *In* Lebenthal, E. (ed.): Textbook of Gastroenterology and Nutrition in Infancy. New York, Raven Press, 1981, p. 767.

37. Hathaway, M. L.: Heights and weights of children in the U.S. USDA Home Econ. Res. Dept. #2. Washington, D.C., U.S. Government Printing Office, 1957.

38. Hazuria, R. S., Sarin, G. S., Srivastava, P. N., Misra, R. C., Bhatt, I. N., and Chuttani, H. K.: Intestinal dipeptidases in primary malnutrition. Am. J. Clin. Nutr. 27:760, 1974.

39. Hintz, R., Suskind, R., Amatayakul, K., and Thanangkul, B.: Somatomedin and growth hormone in protein-calorie malnutrition. J. Pediatr. 92:153, 1978.

39a. Homer, C., and Ludwig, S.: Categorization of etiology of failure to thrive. Am. J. Dis. Child. *135*:848, 1981.

40. Hufton, I. W., and Oates, R. K.: Non-organic failure to thrive: a long term follow-up. Pediatrics 59:73, 1977.

41. Ingenbleek, Y., DeVisscher, M., and DeNayer, P.: Measurement of prealbumin as index of protein-calorie malnutrition. Lancet 2:106, 1972.

42. Jackson, R. L.: Maternal and infant nutrition and health in later life. Nutr. Rev. 37:33, 1979.

43. John, T. J., Blanovitch, J., Lightner, E. S., Seiber, O. F., Corrigan, J. J., ahd Hansen, R.: Kwashiorkor not associated with poverty. J. Pediatr. 90:730, 1977.

44. Johnson, L. R., Copeland, E. M., and Dudreck, S. J.: Structural and hormonal alterations in gastrointestinal tract of parenterally fed rats. Gastroenterology 68:1177, 1975.

45. Katz, M., and Stiehm, E. R.: Host defenses in malnutrition. Pediatrics 59:490, 1977.

46. Kerr, M. A., Bogues, J. L., and Kerr, D. S.: Psychosocial functioning of mothers of malnourished children. Pediatrics 62:778, 1978.

47. Kreiger, I.: Food restriction as a form of child abuse in 10 cases of psychosocial deprivation dwarfism. Clin. Pediatr. *13*:127, 1974.

47a. Kristiansson, B., and Fallstrom, S. P.: Infants with low rate of weight gain. I. A study of organic factors and growth patterns. Acta Paediatr. 70:655, 1981.

47b. Kristiansson, B., and Fallstrom, S. P.: Infants with low rate of weight gain. II. A study of environmental factors. Acta Paediatr. 70:663, 1981.

48. Lacey, D., Cohen, M., and Duffner, P.: Malnutrition and the central nervous system: structural and functional consequences. *In* Lebenthal, E. (ed.): Textbook of Gastroenterology and Nutrition in Infancy. New York, Raven Press, 1981, p. 779.

49. Leonard, M., Rhymes, J. P., and Solnit, A.: Failure to thrive infants — a family problem. Am. J. Dis. Child. *111*:600, 1966.

50. Lifshitz, F., Teichberg, S., and Wapnir, R. A.: Malnutrition and the intestine. *In* Tsang, R., and Nichols, B., Jr. (eds.): Nutrition and Child Health: Perspectives for the 1980s. New York, Alan Liss, Inc., 1981.

51. Massa, E., MacLean, W., and de Romana, G.: Iron absorption in protein-calorie malnutrition. J. Pediatr. 93:1045, 1978.

52. Mata, L. J., Jiminez, F., and Cordon, M.: Gastrointestinal flora of children with protein-calorie malnutrition. Am. J. Clin. Nutr. 25:1118, 1972.

53. McArthur, R. G., and Fagan, J. E.: An approach to solving problems of growth retardation in the child and teenager. Can. Med. Assoc. J. *116*:1012, 1977.

53a. Miller, H. C.: Intrauterine growth retardation. Am. J. Dis. Child. *135*:944, 1981.

54. Parra, A., Garza, C., Garza, Y., Saravia, J., Hazelwood, C., and Nichols, B.: Changes in growth hormone, insulin and thyroxine values, and in energy metabolism of marasmic infants. J. Pediatr. 82:133, 1972.

55. Pereira, S. M., Sundararaj, R., and Bergum, A.: Physical growth and neurointegrative performance of survivors of protein energy malnutrition. Br. J. Nutr. 42:165, 1979.

56. Pollitt, E.: Failure to thrive: socioeconomic, dietary intake and mother-child interaction data. Fed. Proc. *34*:1593, 1975.

57. Pollitt, E., and Eichter, A.: Behavioral disturbances among failure to thrive children. Am. J. Dis. Child. *130*:124, 1976.

58. Powell, G. K., Brasel, J., and Blizzard, R. M.: Emotional deprivation and growth retardation simulating idiopathic hypopituitarism. N. Engl. J. Med. *296*:1271, 1967.

59. Riley, R. L., Landwirth, J., Kaplan, S., and Collipp, P. J.: Failure to thrive: an analysis of 83 cases. Calif. Med. *108*:32, 1968.

60. Shaheen, E., Alexander, D., and Truskowsky, M.: Failure to thrive: a retrospective profile. Clin. Pediatr. 7:255, 1968.

61. Shull, M. W., Reed, R. B., Valadian, I., Palombo, R., Thorne, H., and Dwyer, J.: Velocities of growth in vegetarian preschool children. Pediatrics *60*:410, 1977.

62. Sills, R. H.: Failure to thrive: the role of clinical and laboratory evaluation. Am. J. Dis. Child. *132*:967, 1978.

62a. Sinatra, F. R., and Merritt, R. J.: Iatrogenic kwashiorkor in infants. Am. J. Dis. Child. *135*:12, 1981.

63. Spady, D. W., Payne, R., Picou, D., and Waterlow, J. C.: Energy balance during recovery from malnutrition. Am. J. Clin. Nutr. *20*:1073, 1976.

64. Suskind, R. M.: Characteristics and causation of protein-calorie malnutrition in the infant and preschool child. *In* Greene, L. S. (ed.): Malnutrition, Behavior and Social Organization. New York, Academic-Press, 1977, p. 1.

65. Suskind, R. M., and Partington, M.: Effects of postnatal malnutrition on the development of the immune response. *In* Lebenthal, E. (ed.): Textbook of Gastroenterology and Nutrition in Infancy. New York, Raven Press, 1981, p. 791.

66. Vitale, J. J.: Impact of nutrition on immune function in nutrition and disease. Columbus, Ohio, Ross Laboratories, 1979.

66a. Voght, H., Haneberg, B., Finne, P. H., and Stensberg, A.: Clinical assessment of gestational age in the newborn infant. Acta Paediatr. *70*: 669, 1981.

67. Waterlow, J. C., Cravioto, J., and Stephen, J. M. L.: Protein malnutrition in man. Adv. Protein Chem. *15*:131, 1960.

68. Whittan, C. F., Perrit, M. G., and Fischoff, J.: Evidence that growth failure from maternal deprivation is secondary to undereating. JAMA *209*:1675, 1969.

69. Widdowson, E. M., and Dickerson, J. W.: Chemical composition of the body. *In* Comar, C. L., and Bonner, F. (eds.): Mineral Metabolism. Vol. II. New York, Academic Press, 1962, p. 1.

70. Wingard, J., and Schoen, E. J.: Factors influencing length at birth and height at 5 years. Pediatrics *53*:737, 1974.

71. Winick, M., and Rosso, P.: The effect of severe early malnutrition on cellular growth of human brain. Pediatr. Res. 3:181, 1969.

Chapter Five

PATHOPHYSIOLOGIC APPROACH TO ACUTE AND CHRONIC DIARRHEA

Diarrhea is one of the most common and easily recognized symptoms in pediatric gastroenterology and is generally considered a failure of the intestinal tract to conserve water and electrolytes.[4] It has been defined as fecal evacuations causing water losses exceeding 5 to 10 ml/kg/day.[5a, 5b]

Normally, the intestine functions as an efficient and sensitive regulator of extracellular fluid. Absorption and secretion take place concurrently throughout the bowel, resulting in a constant, bidirectional flux of predominantly isotonic fluid. The diet contributes only a small portion of the total intraluminal fluid content, the major contributor being secretions from the stomach and intestines as chyme and succus entericus (Table 5–1). The largest quantity of water and electrolytes is reabsorbed in the jejunum; however, although distal segments absorb less fluid per unit surface area, these sites contribute more to the ultimate absorption of total intraluminal contents and are therefore important to control of the final stool volume.

The end result of this process is that only 100 ml of water per m^2 of body surface area are excreted daily in the feces. Compared

Table 5–1 Approximate Volumes of Fluid Entering and Leaving the Human Intestinal Tract Daily (Per 1.73 m^2 Body Surface Area)*

	LITERS INTO LUMEN		LITERS REABSORBED	APPROXIMATE "EFFICIENCY"
Diet	2	Jejunum	4–5/9	50%
Saliva	1			
Gastric	2	Ileum	3–4/4–5	75%
Bile	1			
Pancreatic	2	Colon	1–2/1–2	>90%
Small intestine	1			
TOTAL	9		TOTAL 8–9	

*From Phillips, S.: Viewpoints on Digestive Disease 7:51, 1975. Used by permission.

with the net amount secreted each day, this volume represents a net filtration of 98 to 99 per cent and may result in a loss of greater than 200 ml of fecal water per m^2 per day, representing a difference of 2 per cent in the total fluid flux. With such a small margin of error in H$_2$O and electrolyte control, one can understand the ease with which diarrhea can be provoked by a variety of stimuli.

PATHOGENESIS

The excretion of excess fecal water, characterized clinically by an increase in frequency and/or loss of consistency in the stool, can be understood pathophysiologically as a reduced net absorption of fluid from the intestinal lumen into the extracellular and intravascular compartments.[14, 22] With the bidirectional flux, either an increased intraluminal fluid that exceeds the intestine's reabsorptive capacity or an increase in the actual secretion of fluid into the intraluminal space can contribute to the excessive volume of fluid manifest as diarrhea (Table 5–2).

MECHANISMS

DECREASED ABSORPTIVE CAPACITY

The intestine is normally well adapted to the absorption of fluid, electrolytes, and nutrients. Full-thickness mucosal folds, the valvulae conniventes, triple the surface area available in the small intestine. Finger-like villi extend along these folds, producing an additional tenfold increase in absorptive surface. The highly specialized epithelial cells on the villi contain numerous microvilli, where absorption actually occurs (Fig. 5–1). The composite 600-fold increase in luminal area over the simple cylinder results in an absorptive surface of approximately 2,000,000 square centimeters in the small intestine of an average adult (which is roughly the size of a single tennis court).

Any significant decrease in the surface area available can result in diarrhea. This

Table 5–2   Causes of Diarrhea

DECREASED ABSORPTIVE CAPACITY
Rapid intestinal transit
    Massive intestinal resection ("short gut")
    Hyperthyroidism
    Chronic nonspecific diarrhea (irritable colon
      of childhood)
Decreased Absorptive Surface
    Virus
    Shigella
    Amoeba
    Giardia
    Strongyloides
    Celiac syndrome
    Protein-calorie malnutrition
    Food allergy (?)
Vascular compromise (?)
    Ischemia
    Malrotation, volvulus

OVERWHELMED ABSORPTIVE CAPACITY
Osmotic
    Disaccharide deficiency
    Monosaccharide malabsorption
    Dietary diarrhea
    Laxative abuse
Secretory diarrhea
    Cyclic AMP stimulation
      Cholera
      Toxigenic *E. coli*
      Verner-Morrison syndrome
      Bacterial overgrowth
      Malabsorption
      Ileal resection
      Laxative abuse (anthraquinones)
      Antibiotic-associated diarrhea
    Prostaglandin stimulation
      Salmonella
      Campylobacter
      Enteroinvasive *E. coli*
      Inflammatory bowel disease (?)
    Congenital chloridorrhea

UNCERTAIN
    Hirschsprung's enterocolitis
    Immune deficiency states

could occur with a loss in length of the bowel or a reduction in the surface itself. Surgical correction of various congenital and acquired abnormalities often requires resection leading to a short bowel syndrome. Although compensatory hyperplasia of the mucosa provides adaptation with some increased nutrient absorption per centimeter of remaining gut, fatal diarrhea and steatorrhea can still result, particularly if the terminal ileum or the ileocecal valve or both are removed (Fig. 5–2).

The destruction of mucosa by infectious agents such as *Shigella* can produce a hem-

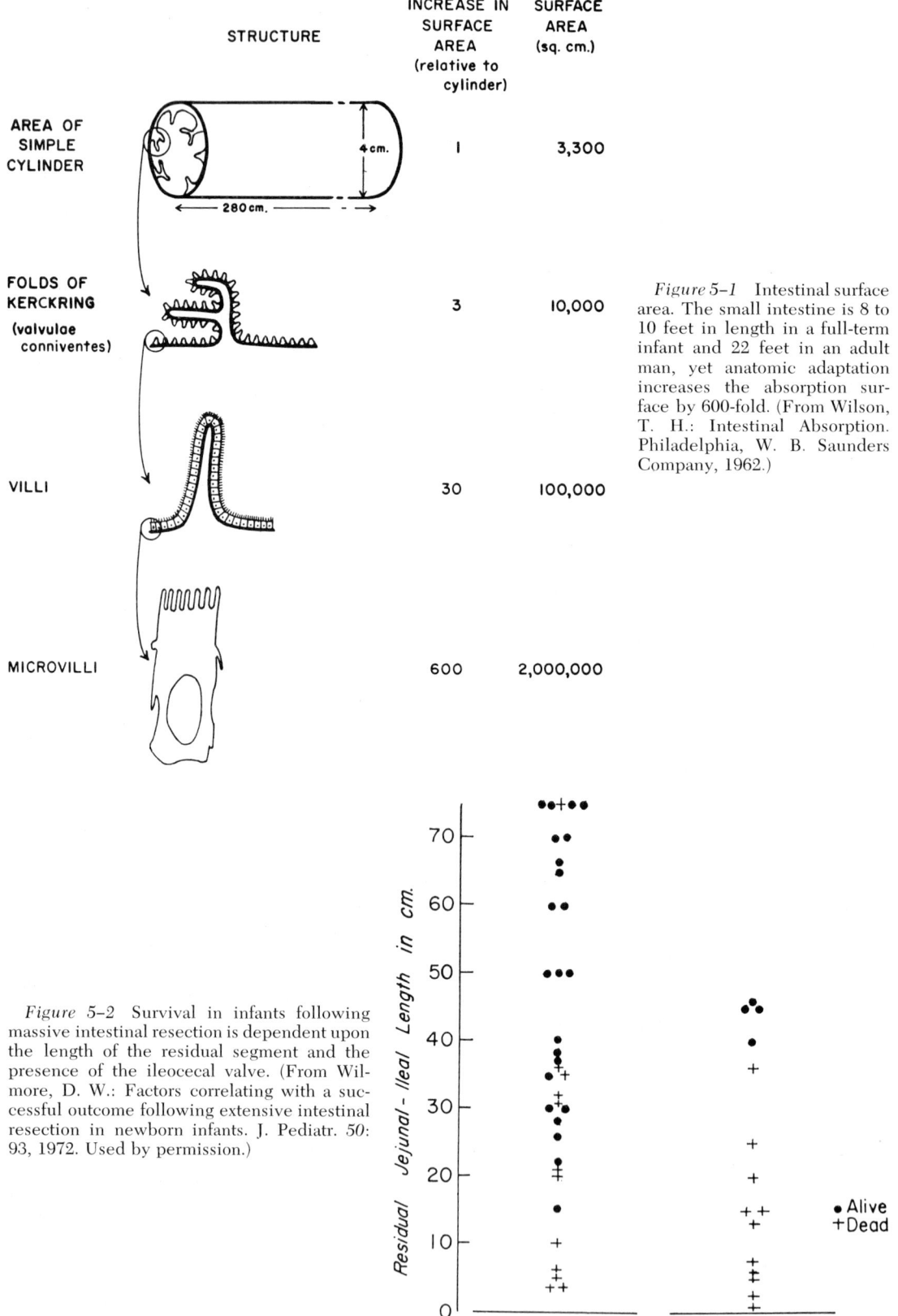

Figure 5–1 Intestinal surface area. The small intestine is 8 to 10 feet in length in a full-term infant and 22 feet in an adult man, yet anatomic adaptation increases the absorption surface by 600-fold. (From Wilson, T. H.: Intestinal Absorption. Philadelphia, W. B. Saunders Company, 1962.)

Figure 5–2 Survival in infants following massive intestinal resection is dependent upon the length of the residual segment and the presence of the ileocecal valve. (From Wilmore, D. W.: Factors correlating with a successful outcome following extensive intestinal resection in newborn infants. J. Pediatr. 50: 93, 1972. Used by permission.)

orrhagic and exudative diarrhea acutely. A virus invading histologically normal mucosa may damage microvilli and also reduce available surface area.[21] The flattening of villi in celiac syndrome, food allergies, and kwashiorkor results in steatorrhea and diarrhea, since the surface area available for the absorption of fluid and nutrients is diminished.[1, 17, 18] Involvement of the terminal ileum impairs bile acid and vitamin B_{12} absorption. Bile acids, which reach the colon, stimulate cyclic AMP and increase the diarrheal state.[5a, 5b]

A rapid intestinal transit limits exposure of nutrients to the mucosal surface, so that states with more rapid peristalsis, such as hyperthyroidism, often have diarrhea as a primary or secondary manifestation. *Giardia*, despite microscopic evidence of transmucosal penetration, has been postulated to cause diarrhea by preventing nutrients from reaching the villous surface, or by competing for those nutrients, thereby blocking their access to the mucosa for absorption.

OVERWHELMED ABSORPTIVE CAPACITY

Only two sources exist for excess intestinal fluids: (1) those orally ingested, and (2) those secreted by the gastrointestinal tract itself.

Osmotic Diarrhea

Osmotic diarrhea often occurs when poorly absorbed water-soluble substrates obligate luminal fluid retention in order to maintain intraluminal isotonicity. Polyvalent ions, such as Mg^{++} and $PO_4^=$, and carbohydrates, such as lactulose, have been used therapeutically to promote catharsis based on their osmotic effect.

Several disease states originate from the same factors. Sorbitol used as an artificial sweetener in dietetic candies has caused diarrhea, but osmotic diarrhea most frequently results from carbohydrate malabsorption. Monosaccharides are usually well absorbed by passive diffusion or active transport coupled with a sodium ion. Disaccharides require enzymatic hydrolysis

into monosaccharides at the cell-lumen interface prior to their absorption. If the appropriate enzymes are insufficient owing to congenital deficiency or mucosal abnormalities of the intestine, the nonabsorbed disaccharide (with lactose as the prototype) contributes an osmotic load causing fluid retention, which may result in diarrhea. However, the absorptive capacity of the intestine can often reabsorb most of the additional fluid load, making diarrhea a less prominent feature than abdominal distention. It is important to remember that amylase is deficient in infants until three to four months of age. Therefore, starches and complex carbohydrates are not well tolerated until that time and may also provoke diarrhea.

Secretory Diarrhea

Cholera has classically produced the most fulminant watery stools and has been the prototype of secretory diarrhea. The pathogenesis of the diseases in this category has been clarified by the demonstration that cholera toxin alone reproduces these symptoms and provokes parallel changes in mucosal adenylcyclase activity and cyclic AMP concentration.[5] Fecal sodium losses in secretory diarrhea exceed 50 mEq/L/day.

Cyclic AMP stimulates processes such as Na^+-K^+ ATPase activity, resulting in active intestinal secretion of fluid and electrolytes (Fig. 5–3). The cyclic AMP mechanism appears to be the final common pathway in a number of secretory diarrheal states. The toxins of *Escherichia coli* and *Clostridium perfringens* as well as *Vibrio cholerae* increase adenyl cyclase activity.[5] Vasoactive intestinal polypeptide, elaborated by the pancreas in the Verner-Morrison syndrome, similarly increases adenyl cyclase activity to provoke a watery diarrhea referred to as pancreatic cholera.

Malabsorbed bile salts and fatty acids can be deconjugated and hydroxylated, respectively, by bacteria and then may stimulate the same mechanism.[2, 8] The diarrhea can be prevented by removing the excess acids with anion exchange resins, such as cholestyramine, or Pepto-Bismol.

Prostaglandins can also induce secretion by the adenyl cyclase pathway but may act

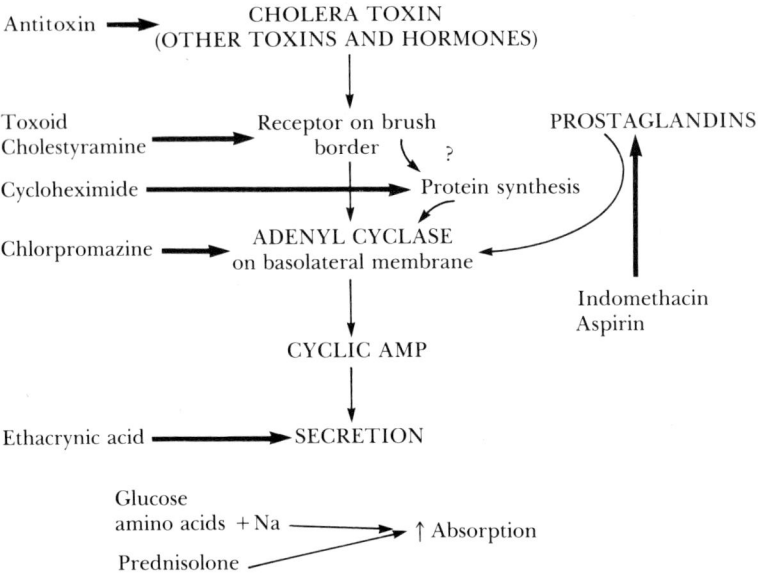

Figure 5-3. Secretory diarrhea appears to be mediated by the action of cyclic AMP on the sodium-potassium pump, resulting in net solute secretion. This can be stimulated or inhibited by numerous factors. (Modified from Turnberg, L. A.: Intestinal transport of salt and water. Clin. Sci. Mol. Med. *54*:343, 1978.)

by a separate mechanism. They have been implicated in the symptoms of salmonella enteritis, inflammatory bowel disease, and pancreatic tumors. Indomethacin and aspirin are among the nonsteroidal anti-inflammatory agents that appear to inhibit prostaglandin activity and may be useful in promoting water and electrolyte absorption during diarrheal illness.

In our own experience, a secretory diarrhea has been observed in several children under the age of two years with severe hypogammaglobulinemia. Biopsy has shown subtotal to total villous atrophy and invasion of the mucosa and lamina propria by bacteria. In such instances, oral antibiotic therapy has led to marked decrease in fluid volume of the stools and to regeneration of the villi within several weeks. Although the mechanism by which immunoglobulin deficiencies may cause chronic diarrhea in infancy is not well understood, it has been established that approximately 20 per cent of infants with chronic diarrhea have deficiencies of one or more of the immunoglobulins, i.e., IgA or IgG. These deficiencies are usually transient, and immunoglobulins return to normal values by 12 to 18 months of age. It is postulated that certainly in the absence of immunoglobulin A, there is a toxic macromolecular penetra-

tion of the gut and enhanced bacterial penetration in some instances.

The central roles of cyclic AMP and adenyl cyclase in secretory diarrhea may be manageable by therapeutic measures. Chlorpromazine and cycloheximide have been effective in the laboratory to inhibit the secretion induced by this mechanism, but they have seldom been utilized in human subjects. The recognition that the cyclic AMP and adenylate cyclase mechanism does not interfere with coupled sodium-glucose absorption has already proved to be of therapeutic significance. Rehydration has been utilized internationally in the treatment of cholera-like diarrhea by taking advantage of oral glucose/saline solutions, which promote salt and water absorption.

CLINICAL ILLNESS

Diarrheal illness may be ascribed, on occasion, to a combination of pathophysiologic mechanisms.[11] An intestine with decreased absorptive capacity will not only suffer loss of ability to absorb fluid and nutrients but will also retain osmotically active substances within the lumen, which may obligate additional fluid to the intestine. This will, of course, contribute to increased diarrheal fluid because of a limited ability for compensatory absorption within the colon. A common example of this phenomenon is viral gastroenteritis. The jejunal villus is invaded and may be destroyed; moreover, the mucosal disaccharidases may be diminished as well. Thus, an osmotic diarrhea secondary to lactose intolerance may be superimposed upon the diarrhea caused by decreased absorptive capacity.

The diarrheal states can be complicated further by secondary malabsorption and increased crypt cell turnover of epithelial cells.[1, 10] Infections can frequently produce these combinations of events. Enterotoxic organisms that disrupt the normal mucosa will also disrupt the normal absorptive processes and cause a decrease in the surface available for absorption of other nutrients as well as fluid and electrolytes. The organisms present are sufficient to create an infection and may also compete for metabolites with the host. Moreover, the infectious agents could also metabolize bile acids sufficiently to render them ineffective in facilitating absorption of fats. The fats themselves may be hydroxylated, thereby decreasing absorption. Together, the hydroxylated bile acids and fatty acids may stimulate cyclic AMP–associated intestinal secretion.

The noninfectious diarrheal states have less effect, but they too may influence the patient's nutritional status by impairing the absorption of water-soluble nutrients, e.g., folic acid.

With diarrheal illnesses that are not quickly reversed, these nutritional effects could result in a deteriorating spiral of malnutrition and malabsorption. This can be seen most clearly in the infant who develops intractable diarrhea. Chronic or intractable diarrhea is that which persists for more than three weeks. The initial cause of the diarrhea becomes less important than the sequelae that result (Fig. 5–4). The diarrhea is accompanied by decreased absorption. An infant with relatively little nutritional reserve who is maintained for extended periods on fluids to provide adequate hydration, but on few or no calories, develops severe malnutrition. The malnutrition results in decreasing mucosal and pancreatic function, thus further diminishing nutrient digestion and absorption. Unless this process is reversed and adequate protein and caloric substrates provided, the infant's immune status becomes impaired and infection results. The infection increases the infant's nutrient requirements and may be the cause of his death.

Such events have been prevented largely by aggressive, early attention to diarrheal illnesses and their sequelae. The require-

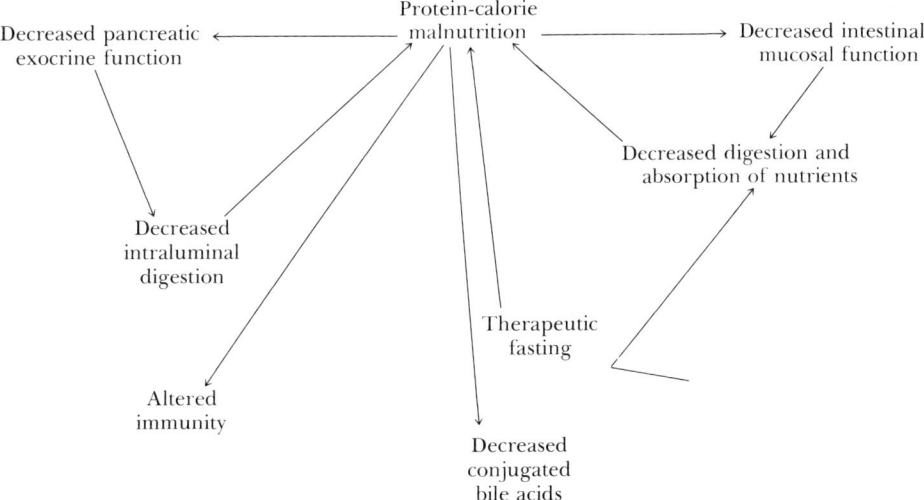

Figure 5–4 The cycle of chronic diarrhea and protein-calorie malnutrition can result in the syndrome of intractable diarrhea of infancy if it is not corrected early. (Modified from Sunshine, P., Sinatra, F. R., and Mitchell, C. H.: Intractable diarrhea of infancy. Clin. Gastroenterol. 6:445, 1977.)

ments for each clinical condition will be discussed individually in Part III.

DIFFERENTIAL DIAGNOSIS AND EVALUATION

The evaluation of diarrhea is largely dependent upon its character (severity and duration) and any associated finding, such as weight loss or weakness secondary to electrolyte abnormalities.

History

The first, and possibly most important, step is to determine whether diarrhea is in fact present. This entails a careful and complete history about the usual and the supposedly abnormal stool patterns. Stool consistency, frequency, and the presence of blood or mucus need to be recognized. Floating stools denote the admixture of flatus and stool but should be noted. Variability in these findings rules out secretory diarrhea and most infectious etiologies and may suggest dietary indiscretions. These historical findings are best confirmed by inspection and analysis of the diarrheal stool, as described below.

Further historical data will be most helpful. The onset and progression of the illness, weight changes, response to treatment, medications taken, and any other associated symptoms or other recent diarrheal episodes should be noted, as should such episodes in family members and schoolmates. Both acute and chronic diarrheal illnesses may follow travel exposures to *E. coli* or viral "traveler's diarrhea," which often affect individuals before they leave the country where they were infected. However, organisms such as *Giardia* may be acquired well before symptoms are apparent.

In young infants, the relationship of diarrhea to dietary factors may not be recognized by the parents. A careful nutritional history, best performed by a trained nutritionist, is important and should focus on total caloric and fluid intake and the percentage of intake from protein, fat, and carbohydrates. Many patients will present to the pediatric gastroenterologist on diets restricting milk and/or wheat intake. These restrictions often complicate the evaluation. Lactase insufficiency cannot be dismissed as a diagnostic possibility unless lactose, and not just milk, has been completely eliminated from the diet. Gluten restriction may result in celiac syndrome that is partially treated, making the patient difficult to diagnose.

Physical Examination

The physical examination usually will not enlighten one as to the character or cause of the diarrhea itself but may aid in evaluating secondary manifestations, such as dehydration and malnutrition. The acutely ill patient may demonstrate clinical signs of dehydration at various levels, which will help determine the fluid and electrolyte replacement required (Table 5–3).

Laboratory Studies

Laboratory investigations need to be considered in terms of cost effectiveness and benefit to the patient. For example, the patient with vomiting and diarrhea of one day's duration rarely requires any tests (unless those symptoms are prodigious and the patient is dehydrated), whereas the persistence of diarrhea for several days necessitates obtaining at least a stool culture and blood count. The continuation of these symptoms (even intermittently) for several weeks suggests that further, more extensive studies are in order. Thus, *duration* and *severity* of the symptoms usually dictate the primary guidelines for investigation.

The initial evaluation should attempt to assess the patient's clinical status as well as determine diagnosis. In the acutely ill patient, hydration and biochemical parameters should be evaluated with serum electrolytes, calcium, urea nitrogen, creatinine, proteins, pH (venous is adequate), hematocrit, and urine specific gravity.

Infections are the most common cause of acute diarrhea.[8, 11] A white blood cell count and differential blood count are useful in indicating leukocytosis, classic *Shigella* in-

Table 5–3 Physical Findings

SIGN	POSSIBLE SIGNIFICANCE IN DIARRHEAL DISEASE
Rapid pulse	*Shigella* infection (classic)
With normal temperature	
Blood pressure	Dehydration
Falls with sitting	
Dry mucous membranes	
Abrupt weight loss, decreased urine	
Decreased skin turgor	Dehydration, hypertonic
Decreased subcutaneous tissue	Marasmus
Edema	Hypoproteinemia
Glossitis, cheilosis	Iron or B-vitamin deficiency
Peripheral neuritis	B_{12} or other B-vitamin deficiency
Bone pain or fractures	Osteoporosis (hypoproteinemia)
	Osteomalacia (decreased calcium or vitamin D)
Tetany, paresthesias	Hypocalcemia, hypomagnesemia
Weakness/muscle cramps	Anemia, hypokalemia, hyponatremia
Abdominal distention	Carbohydrate intolerance
Hyperkeratosis	Vitamin A malabsorption
Night blindness	Vitamin A malabsorption
Bleeding disorders	Vitamin K malabsorption

fection, and the presence of large numbers of eosinophils indicative of parasites or food allergy. The erythrocyte sedimentation rate may be elevated in the bacterial enteritides as well as in inflammatory bowel disorders, but it should be normal in viral illnesses. Thrombocytosis is common in inflammatory bowel disease (the platelets acting much like an acute-phase reactant), but it is not a prominent finding in infections unless they are overwhelming.

Examination of the stool yields the most useful analysis, confirms the historical report of diarrhea, and may yield much information.[11] Visual inspection identifies the presence of blood or mucus and determines whether the consistency is watery, raising the possibility of a secretory process. Small amounts of fecal material (preferably mucus) may be placed on slides. Qualitative testing should include methylene blue staining for the presence of leukocytes, which is helpful in the diagnosis of invasive or inflammatory states (50 to 75 per cent accuracy).[15] Sudan staining will identify fat droplets quantitatively and will indicate the need for quantitative fecal fat determination in individuals with chronic diarrhea. Nitrazene paper can be used to obtain the stool pH. A pH of less than 6 implicates carbohydrate malabsorption as contributing to the diarrhea. Stool guaiac analysis should be performed to identify any occult blood loss.

In any patient investigated for diarrhea, several stool specimens should be sent for bacterial culture and for morphologic examination for ova and parasites. The number of specimens sent for study increases the accuracy of the test. For *Giardia*, one specimen alone will detect only 40 per cent of the cases, whereas three specimens will yield results of 60 to 95 per cent accuracy. These specimens should be sent fresh, since most parasites do not survive well in cold or dried specimens. The exception is coccidium, which must undergo prolonged incubation at room temperature before it can be identified. A Gram stain is of little value unless there is an overwhelming predominance of staphylococci.

Stool weight is often neglected, yet this provides a quantitative measure of volume and intestinal efficiency. North Americans and Europeans on routine diets usually excrete less than 0.1 liter of stool water per kilogram of body weight each day. A stool weight of greater than 150 to 200 mg per m^2 per day of watery stool verifies the presence of diarrhea. Quantitative stool fat can be determined using the same specimen. Stool analysis will be addressed in more detail in Chapter 14 on malabsorption; however, several points should be recognized. Fecal fat quantitation is valid only when considered in relation to the amount and type of fat ingested. The coefficient of absorption is an index of the amount of fat absorbed (grams ingested minus grams excreted) divided by the grams of fat ingested. In order for this to be an accurate measure, the patient must have an adequate fat intake preceding and during the stool collection period. If an infant is receiving a formula or supplements containing medium-chain triglycerides, special extraction techniques must be performed in order to detect medium- as well as long-chain fats.

Another extremely useful indicator of physiologic function is the measurement of mouth-to-anus transit time. Roy, Silverman, and Cozzetto have obtained a normal value of 25.4 ± 7.6 hours on patients six months to three years old.[19] More rapid transit suggests an increased intestinal motility, as in patients with chronic nonspecific diarrhea syndrome prior to treatment. The test is best performed by adding a small (10 ml) slurry of activated charcoal to the noon or evening meal and then observing for its passage. An acceptable alternative is the use of raisins or corn kernels in young patients capable of swallowing but unable to digest the exterior coating of these substances.

In order to categorize liquid diarrhea as either secretory or osmotic, a clinical period during which oral feedings are withheld can suggest the manner in which the patient is to be evaluated further. In patients continuing to have diarrhea despite fasting, stool osmolality and electrolytes should be determined. A secretory process is indicated by elevated sodium and potassium (Na^+ and K^+) in the stools. If the stool osmolality exceeds the electrolyte content of the stool, $(Na + K) \times 2$, then the etiology of an osmotic diarrhea should be sought. An infant with watery diarrhea and no response to fasting should also have a stool chloride analysis to rule out the slight possibility of congenital chloridorrhea.

There is controversy as to the efficacy of radiologic studies in this clinical setting. Abdominal flat plates may demonstrate gaseous distention indicative of obstruction or colitis and, on rare occasions, may depict a tumor elaborating hormones causing the diarrhea (e.g., a calcified ganglioneuroma). When tumors are suspected in secretory states, levels of specific hormones (VMA, catecholamines, vasoactive intestinal polypeptide, gastric inhibitory polypeptide, and pancreatic polypeptide) should be obtained.

Barium studies (upper gastrointestinal series with small bowel follow-through and barium enemas) are often ordered but are rarely helpful. Patients with malabsorption or diarrhea or both demonstrate little that can be differentiated from normal. Patients with chronic or bloody diarrhea should be investigated with fluoroscopic barium studies, particularly if other features (mucus, decreased growth, weight loss, or elevated sedimentation rate) are present to suggest inflammatory disease. However, routine patients with chronic diarrhea should not be automatically subjected to these studies.

Specialized Laboratory Tests. Sigmoidoscopy and rectal biopsy should be performed in any patient with bloody diarrhea or chronic diarrhea in which an inflammatory or infectious etiology is suspected. A biopsy of the rectal folds is recommended even in the event of a normal sigmoidoscopy, since biopsies diagnostic of Crohn's disease have been obtained frequently in this circumstance. A rectal biopsy (and, if possible, manometry) should be performed in infants suspected of having Hirschsprung's colitis, since approximately 25 per cent of infants with this disorder present with diarrhea. The absence of ganglia in infants of normal gestational maturity is indicative of this entity.

Jejunal biopsy may be necessary to confirm the diagnosis of allergic (eosinophilic) enteritis but is otherwise reserved for evaluation of patients with diarrhea who are suspected of having malabsorption, i.e., weight loss.

The need for obtaining intestinal disaccharidase levels can now be circumvented by a less invasive analysis of breath hydrogen after a lactose load or by measurement of isotopically labeled carbon dioxide. These tests are based on the fact that malabsorbed carbohydrate is hydrolyzed by co-

Ionic bacteria to gaseous products (H_2 or CO_2) that are excreted in constant proportion by the lungs. Various substrates can be tested by utilizing different carbohydrate loads. The breath analysis method is a more accurate reflection of intraluminal events than serum collection for glucose, which measures absorption and not malabsorption. It is also simpler than the biopsy approach, which is invasive and may miss the affected area.

TREATMENT

The initial therapy for diarrhea is largely independent of its cause. If a child is dehydrated, deficits must be replaced and ongoing losses must be met. If the child's fluid requirements are being administered to adequately, dietary measures and pharmacologic agents may be useful, even while the results of the diagnostic evaluation are awaited.

Fluid Therapy

The treatment of acute diarrhea with parenteral fluids is a standard part of the pediatrician's armamentarium and needs no further review here.[3] The principles of replacing deficits and ongoing losses, determined by the degree of hydration (i.e., per cent of body weight lost) and tonicity (hypo-, iso-, or hypertonic) encountered, still apply.

Recent data have continued to prove the efficacy of oral rehydration fluids developed during the 1940's. However, so many formulae have been espoused subsequently that confusion reigns — losing the more optimal solutions among the others. Part of this confusion stems from a difference of opinion regarding the optimal sodium concentration for the fluids. The concerns focus on infants and toddlers, those most prone to develop dehydration and hypernatremia. Their large surface area to weight ratio, increased metabolic rate, and relatively decreased renal filtration of sodium predispose to hypernatremia. This may be exacerbated, or even precipitated, by inappro-

priate milk feeding early in the infant's course. The high salt content of bouillon or boiled skim milk, in particular, and the acidosis induced by lactose intolerance, further increase the infant's loss of extracellular water and retention of sodium.

Hypernatremia, then, prompted the use of hypotonic (Na 30 to 60 mEq/L) solutions for correction of extracellular and intracellular water depletion. However, some clinicians feel that this correction requires an overly long period (24 to 48 hours) and that a slightly increased sodium concentration (75 to 100 mEq/L) would result in more rapid repair. Whether more patients are now becoming hyponatremic is currently under study.

The use of glucose in the solutions is less controversial. Glucose as well as galactose and some amino acids is absorbed in tandem with sodium in the jejunum. This coupled transport appears maximal at a 1:1 molecular ratio within a range of 60/40 mM of glucose per liter. Chloride appears to be preferred over other anions for this process. Bicarbonate may enhance sodium absorption separately. Substituting sucrose for glucose is less effective utilizing the same fluid volume.

Thus, each liter of oral rehydration fluids should contain 75 to 100 mEq Na, and 75 to 100 mM glucose, with chloride in high proportion (50 to 75 mEq) and bicarbonate making up the remainder of anions. Potassium should be added (20 to 30 mEq) because of an increased loss in both the urine (secondary to aldosterone effect) and the stools. Approximately 1 liter per day should be administered to infants, but it should not be used beyond a 24-hour period without monitoring of serum electrolytes. In infants and young children, every second to third bottle should contain an equal volume of free water or breast milk (low in osmolality) in order to decrease the child's total electrolyte consumption.

Commercially available solutions, such as Gatorade and Jell-O, have little to offer infants, as they have inadequate sodium and an overly generous glucose concentration and osmolality.[23] This, then requires the private manufacture of appropriate solutions. The dangers inherent in that method can be minimized by utilizing the WHO standard pediatric formula or by having a hospital pharmacy prepare the powder or already diluted solution.

Dietary Therapy

The only nutritional measure that is consistently followed in acute diarrheal states is the avoidance of lactose products. Loss of the β-glucosidase from villous cells diminishes the capacity to absorb lactose. Those patients with true secretory diarrhea not injuring epithelial cell structures probably do not require this restriction. The problem, however, is when to restore lactose-containing products to the diet. Individual variability and the extent of the destructive infection will dictate the time sequence. Perhaps the best measure is to perform repeated breath hydrogen analyses following lactose loads or simply lactose-product ingestion. Lacking availability of this tool, intermittent clinical trials should indicate whether lactose will be tolerated.

In rare situations, intestinal sucrose will be decreased as well. This requires the use of more elemental formulae containing glucose or its polymers (e.g., corn syrup derivatives). Those few children unable to absorb monosaccharides will require immediate intervention with parenteral alimentation.

Prolonged milk restriction may be necessary if lactose intolerance is present; however, other liquids or foods that contain fat should be included in the diet of youngsters with prolonged diarrhea. As evident in chronic nonspecific diarrhea, gastric emptying and the gastrocolic reflex are increased by high-carbohydrate liquids and may be modified by the inclusion of alternative sources of fat (either in soy formulae or in other foods). In diarrheal states, the more frequent the feedings, the more frequent the stools. Wheat restriction is of no benefit except in patients with true celiac disease. Such restrictions prior to referral and diagnosis may actually impede identification of this condition.

Aside from these measures, empiricism and our own training and experience have directed the use of other dietary programs. Bananas, rice cereal, applesauce, and toast (the "BRAT" diet) are often recommended as foods that can be eaten without harm during the course of gastroenteritis. The foods are bland. Bananas supposedly contain kaolin, and applesauce (when the skins are used in processing) contains pectin. However, controversy exists over whether ripe or green bananas contain pectin, for, as will be discussed under pharmacotherapy, kaolin plus pectin may not be beneficial at all. Lactobacillus has little effect and may be a gastric irritant.[13]

Pharmacotherapy

Medications have been employed for specific prophylactic and symptomatic abatement in diarrhea — depending on the severity, etiology, and chronicity of the illness (in that order).[16] The philosophy of benign observation with adequate fluid replacement is still the overwhelming choice of most physicians, especially in acute diarrheal illnesses. However, if the process is particularly severe or chronic, or if it affects one's own children, other therapeutic maneuvers are sought more readily.

Adsorbents. Cholestyramine is clearly the prototype. The resin exchanges its chloride for anions of other acidic compounds. Thus, it binds bile acids and enteric toxins. It binds other drugs as well, such as digitalis and antibiotics. Because of the affinity of cholestyramine for bile acids, patients unable to synthesize adequate replacement could deplete their bile salt pool and develop steatorrhea. The other complications that can occasionally result are hyperchloremic acidosis, diminished absorption of fat-soluble vitamins, and, from inadequate dilution, small bowel obstruction. Therefore, cholestyramine should be administered (in its usual dose of 4 gm two to four times per day) with a beverage between meals and well in advance of medication. Many children are averse to taking cholestyramine because of its taste. It should be contained in the first ounce of formula, fluid, or applesauce to assure its complete consumption. Honey may help to mask its flavor.

Colestipol hydrochloride, another resin, may be equally effective and better tolerated. Amphojel is another anionic exchanger but requires large volumes (150 mg [5 ml]/kg/day). Pepto-Bismol binds both toxins and bile acids and in a dosage of $1/2$ tsp four times daily is often remarkably effective in aborting diarrhea.[20a]

The combination of kaolin and pectin, often given in the form of the popular product Kaopectate, has been considered an adsorbent since the 1930's. Recent studies have demonstrated a lack of effect, however, and in animal studies, fecal electrolyte and fat losses actually increased. At this time, its use cannot be recommended.

Antiperistaltics. Opiates and synthetic alkaloids have been recommended in the past because of their alteration of smooth muscle contractibility, inhibiting fecal expulsion. This has been a major concern to pediatricians, because children could still secrete diarrheal fluid into the lumen unbeknownst to parent or physician. This third-space loss might go unrecognized and could contribute to a more significant illness. Furthermore, use of these agents may prolong the illness by interfering with propulsion, which may also be considered as a defense mechanism that enhances the removal of the bacteria and viruses that infect the gastrointestinal tract. In addition, the atropine present in Lomotil (along with diphenoxylate) is insufficient to alter diarrhea without significant side effects but is sufficient to result in both morbidity and mortality when ingested by those under two years of age.

The introduction of an apparently less toxic alternative, loperamide (Imodium), and the recent recognition that both the opiates and loperamide inhibit choleratoxin-induced small intestinal secretion have demonstrated a need for re-evaluation of these products.[12]

At present, drops of tincture of opium (an equivalent of 10 mg morphine/ml) or paregoric (2 mg morphine/5 ml) can be carefully titrated to provide symptomatic relief in chronic secretory diarrheas, when cholestyramine or prostaglandin inhibitors are ineffective. Thus, only when severe cramping accompanies an acute diarrheal illness should symptomatic relief be considered, since use of therapeutic agents may delay elimination of the offending infective organism.

The pediatric dosage for loperamide has not been established. The usual recommendation for adults is 4 mg initially and 2 mg thereafter as necessary, with a daily maximum of 16 mg. The medication should be reduced or eliminated upon normalization of the stool pattern.

The use of prostaglandin antagonists or steroids to inhibit intestinal secretions remains experimental at present. Salicylates, however, have been shown to decrease fluid losses.[1a] They should be restricted to secretory diarrheas (e.g., intractable diarrhea of infancy), when other modalities have been unsuccessful and clinical deterioration is apparent.

Antimicrobials. Since the demonstration by Aserkoff and Bennett that antibiotics do not shorten the duration of salmonella gastroenteritis, and that they actually prolong the carrier state, the role of antimicrobials has been controversial.

The basic tenet is that mild, transient illnesses do not require antibiotic therapy, which should be utilized only for severe or systemic bacterial infection. Some authors recommend the use of antibiotics for prolonged diarrheal illness associated with organisms that are potentially enteropathogenic. However, dietary modifications may yield the same result.

Parasitic infections appear to require therapy in order to eradicate the organism and resolve the illness. Because of the difficulty in diagnosing giardiasis in the past, some authors are empirically treating their patients with metronidazole. The evidence suggests, however, that an adequate number of specimens examined should render an accurate diagnosis.

Antimicrobials are now shown to be effective for prophylaxis against traveler's diarrhea (from a wide variety of pathogens). The question is whether these agents (e.g., doxycycline) should be used. The use of antibiotics promotes widespread bacterial resistance and may interfere with normal enteral

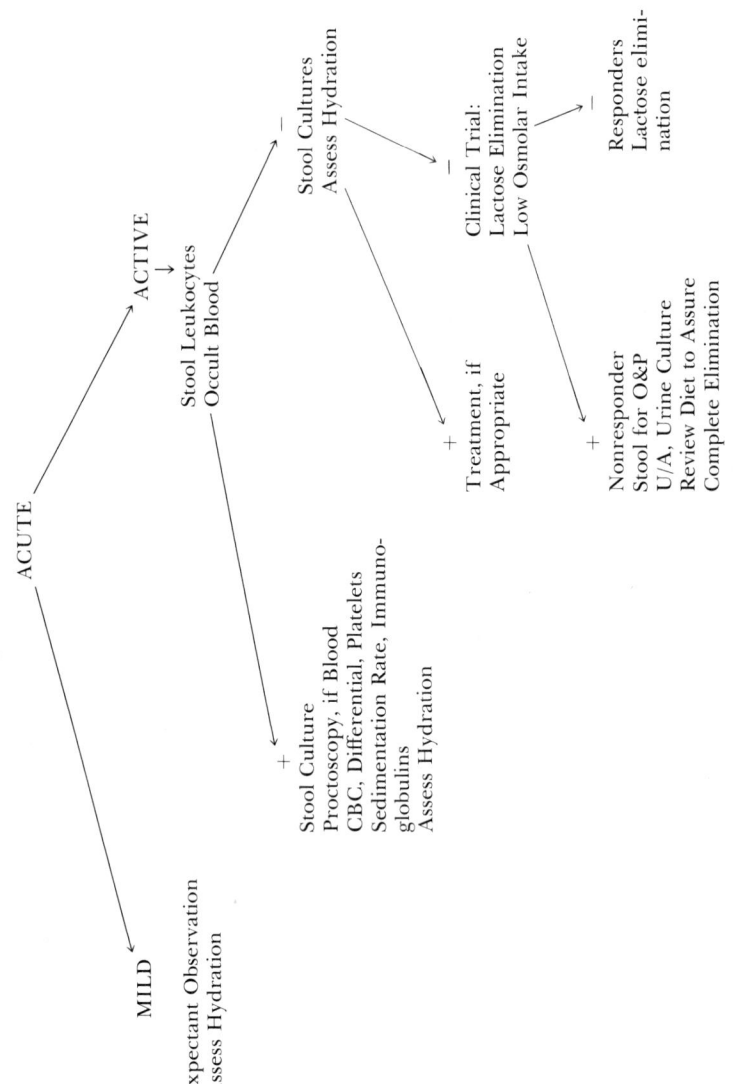

Figure 5–5 Algorithmic evaluation of diarrhea.

Illustration continued on opposite page

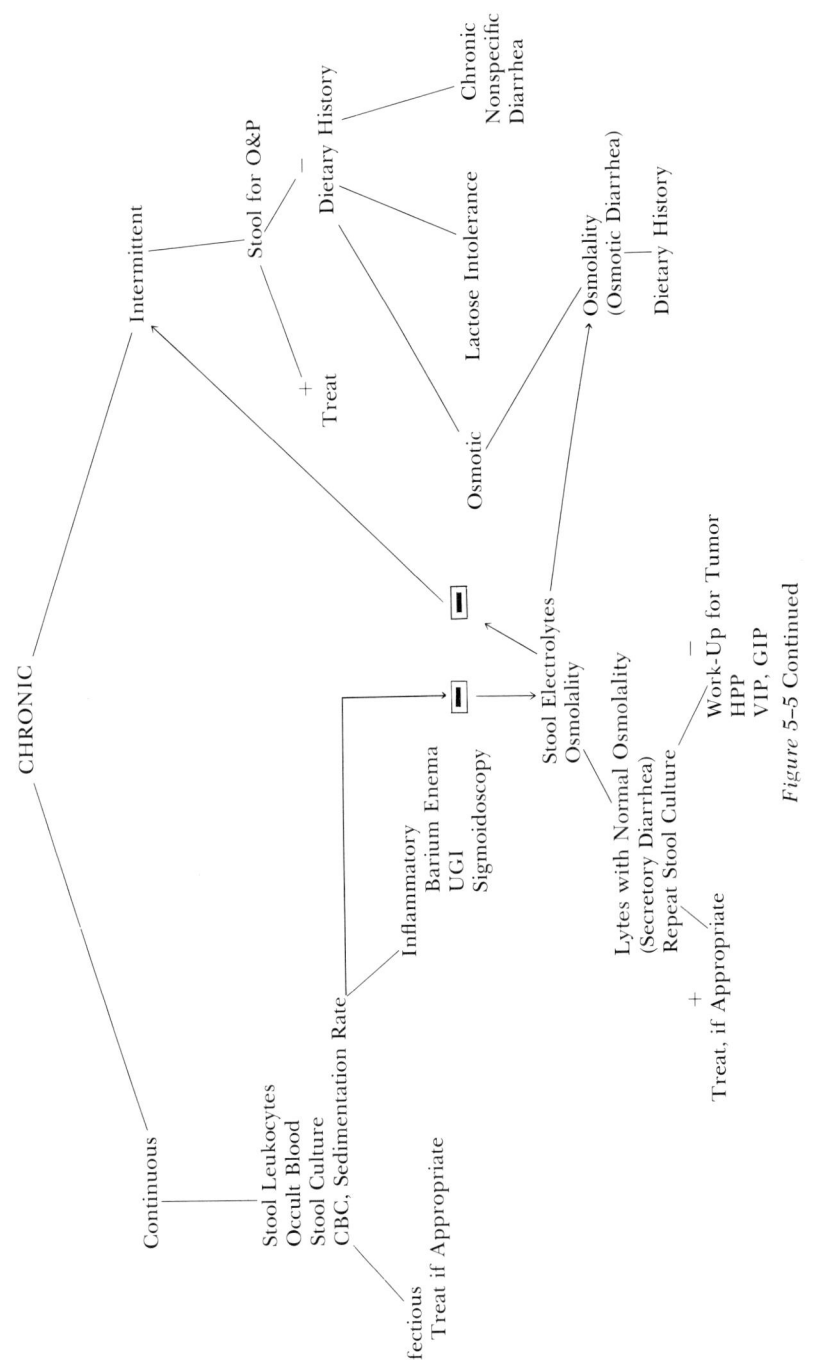

Figure 5-5 Continued

metabolism of bile acids and enzymes. The other problem is that of rebound. Despite the short-term protection afforded by doxycycline, one week after administration ceases, a small number of those protected go on to develop the illness. A long-term goal is the development of vaccines and agents such as bismuth subsalicylate (to decrease intestinal secretion). Until then, doxycycline prophylaxis (100 mg q.d.) should be considered for (nonpregnant) adults and older children who will be traveling for short periods to endemic areas, particularly those areas where good hygienic practices are not possible.

CONCLUSIONS AND SUMMARY

Thus, the patient with acute or chronic diarrhea should be evaluated in a systematic way, as in an algorithm (Fig. 5–5), that includes etiologic and physiologic parameters. Once the patient's illness is categorized, tests for specific etiologies can be performed. Differential diagnoses must be considered and ruled out by appropriate cultures and/or serologic studies. Laxative abuse should be evaluated in the analysis of the stool and urine.

Patients with diarrhea accompanied by hypoproteinemia and edema should be assessed for protein-losing enteropathy. Those with steatorrhea instead of or as well as chronic diarrhea should be considered as having malabsorption primarily (although patients with acute diarrhea may have fat and nitrogen losses accompanying their acute infection). The evaluation of these patients is considered in the chapter on malabsorptive states.

REFERENCES

1. Ament, M. E.: Malabsorption syndromes in infancy and childhood. J. Pediatr. 81:685, 867, 1972.
1a. Burke, V., Gracey, M., Suharyono, E., and Sunoto, T.: Reduction by aspirin of intestinal fluid loss in acute childhood gastroenteritis. Lancet 1:1329, 1980.
2. Donaldson, R. M.: Normal bacterial populations of the intestine and their relation to intestinal

function. N. Engl. J. Med., 270:938, 994, 1050, 1964.
3. Finberg, L.: The role of oral electrolyte-glucose solutions in hydration for children — international and domestic aspects. J. Pediatr. 96:51, 1980.
4. Gall, D. G., and Hamilton, J. R.: Chronic diarrhea in childhood: A new look at an old problem. Pediatr. Clin. North Am. 21:1001, 1974.
5. Grady, G. F., and Keusch, G. T.: Pathogenesis of bacterial diarrheas. N. Engl. J. Med. 285:831, 891, 1971.
5a. Gryboski, J.: Chronic diarrhea. Curr. Probl. Pediatr. 9:5, 1979.
5b. Gryboski, J., and Hillemeier, A. C.: Chronic Diarrhea in Children. Kalamazoo, Mich., Upjohn Company, 1982.
6. Hirschhorn, N.: The treatment of acute diarrhea in children: An historical and physiological perspective. Am. J. Clin. Nutr. 33:637, 1980.
7. Keusch, G. T.: Ecological control of the bacterial diarrheas: A scientific strategy. Am. J. Clin. Nutr. 31:2208, 1978.
8. Lifschitz, F.: The enteric flora in childhood disease — diarrhea. Am. J. Clin. Nutr. 30:1811, 1977.
9. Lloyd-Still, J. D.: Chronic diarrhea of childhood with the misuse of elimination diets. J. Pediatr. 95:10, 1979.
10. MacLean, W. E., Klein, G. L., deRomana, G. L., Massa, E., and Graham, G. G.: Transient steatorrhea following episodes of mild diarrhea in early infancy. J. Pediatr. 92:562, 1978.
11. Nelson, J. D., and Haltalin, K. C.: Accuracy of diagnosis of bacterial diarrheal disease by clinical features. J. Pediatr. 78:519, 1971.
12. Netchvolodoff, C. V., and Hargrove, M. D.: Recent advances in the treatment of diarrhea. Arch. Intern. Med. 139:813, 1979.
13. Pearce, J. L., and Hamilton, J. R.: Controlled trial of orally administered lactobacilli in acute infantile diarrhea. J Pediatr. 84:261, 1974.
14. Phillips, S. F.: Diarrhea: A current view of the pathophysiology. Gastroenterology 63:495, 1972.
15. Pickering, L. K., DuPont, H. L., Olarte, J., Conklin, R., and Ericsson, C.: Fecal leukocytes in enteric infections. Am. J. Clin. Pathol. 68:562, 1977.
16. Pietrusko, R. G.: Pharmacotherapy of diarrhea. Am. J. Hosp. Pharm. 36:757, 1979.
17. Poley, J. R.: Chronic diarrhea in infants and children. South. Med. J. 66:1035, 1049, 1133, 1973.
18. Rosenberg, I. H., Solomons, N. W., and Schneider, R. F.: Malabsorption associated with diarrhea and intestinal infections. Am. J. Clin. Nutr. 30:1248, 1977.
19. Roy, C., Silverman, A., and Cozzetto, F. (eds.): Pediatric Clinical Gastroenterology. St. Louis, C. V. Mosby Company, 1975. p. 450.
20. Sack, R. B., Froehlich, J. L., Zulich, A. W., Sidi Hidi, D., Kapikian, A. Z., Orskov, F., Orskov, I., and Greenberg, H. B.: Prophylactic doxycycline for traveler's diarrhea: Results of a prospective double-blind study of Peace Corps volunteers in Morocco. Gastroenterology 76:1368, 1979.

20a. Steinhoff, M., Douglas, R. G., Jr., Greenberg, H., and Callahan, D.: Bismuth subsalicylate therapy of viral gastroenteritis. Gastroenterology 78:1495, 1980.

21. Torres-Pinado, R., Rivera, C., and Rodriquez, A.: Intestinal absorptive defects associated with enteric infections in infants. Ann. N.Y. Acad. Sci. 176:284, 1971.

22. Turnberg, L. A.: Intestinal transport of salt and water. Clin. Sci. Mol. Med. 54:337, 1978.

23. Wendland, B. E., and Arbus, G. S.: Oral fluid therapy: sodium and potassium content and osmolality of some commercial "clear" soups, juices and beverages. Can. Med. Assoc. J. 121:564, 1979.

Chapter Six

DEVELOPMENT AND EVALUATION
OF LIVER FUNCTION

INTRODUCTION

Numerous conditions affect the liver during the period of infancy. Hepatic diseases described in older children and adults do not necessarily present in a similar manner in infancy, and the prognosis may be considerably different. This may be related, in part, to a unique pathologic response (e.g., active fibroblastic proliferation and early bile stasis) of the infant liver to a variety of insults, perhaps because of structural and functional changes that occur during maturation. Before a discussion of diseases and conditions that primarily affect the liver of infants, this chapter will be devoted to a review of (1) morphologic and biochemical development of the liver, which will help explain clinical manifestations of hepatic disease states in infancy, especially hepatomegaly and jaundice, and (2) current liver function tests and their practical application in infants.

LIVER DEVELOPMENT AND STRUCTURE

Hepatobiliary Development

Morphogenesis begins during the third week of gestation with the liver primordium as a ventral outgrowth from the foregut endoderm, which is destined to become duodenum (Fig. 6–1 A).[2] This hepatic outgrowth enlarges and buds off cords of epithelial cells that become the liver parenchyma (hepatic plate). The hepatocytes are closely aligned to sinusoidal endothelial cells and phagocytic cells known as Kupffer cells. The origin of the Kupffer cells is not settled; however, they may be derived from mononuclear cells of the blood and either proliferate locally or are continuously recruited from circulating monocytes.[49] The larger intrahepatic biliary ducts arise from liver cords that interact with mesenchymal tissue.[4] The origin of small bile ductules is uncertain, but it is well established that the bile canaliculus develops from specialized hepatocyte plasma membranes.[53] At five weeks' gestation, the extrahepatic biliary tree is a solid cord of epithelial cells that elongates and recanalizes to become the common bile duct, the hepatic duct, and possibly the larger intrahepatic bile ducts.[3] The gallbladder and cystic duct separate from the duodenum by elongation of the common bile duct. Biliary tract development is completed by ten weeks of gestation; arrest in development because of an intrauterine insult (e.g., infection) may presumably occur at this critical stage and contribute to anomalies such as biliary atresia.

Development of the liver is associated

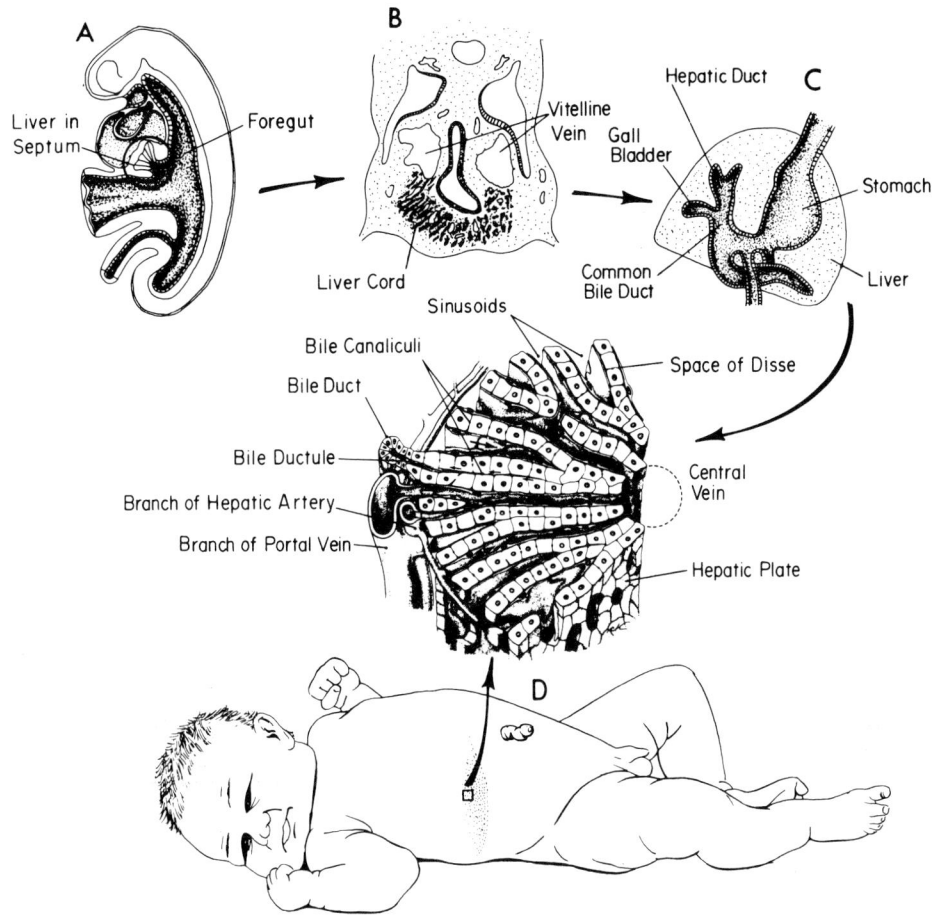

Figure 6–1 Comparative developmental changes of liver and biliary tract. *A*, Hemisection of 3.5-week embryo showing ventral outgrowth of hepatic diverticulum from foregut endoderm. *B*, Transverse section of 4-week embryo showing budding epithelial (liver) cords between the two vitelline veins. *C*, Hemisection of 7.5-week embryo with near-final recanalization of extra-hepatic biliary tract. *D*, Neonate, with representation of three-dimensional section of "classic" hepatic lobule showing radial distribution of hepatic plates and sinusoids. Arrows indicate flow of blood and bile in opposite directions. (From Andres, J. M., Mathis, R. K., and Walker, W. A.: Liver disease in infants. I. Developmental hepatology and mechanisms of liver dysfunction. J. Pediatr. 90:686, 1977.)

with drastic changes in the primordial vitelline and umbilical veins; Figure 6–1 *B* illustrates the development of the hepatic venous system throughout intrauterine existence.[28] The vitelline veins give rise to the portal and hepatic veins. At five weeks of gestation the umbilical veins extend branches into the liver; this change enables blood to be diverted to the heart by a more direct route through the hepatic sinusoids. By the eighth week of embryogenesis, however, *only* the distal left umbilical vein remains to supply the liver with oxygenated blood from the maternal circulation. Also, some of the hepatic sinusoids coalesce to

form the ductus venosus, which continues as a direct channel from the umbilical vein to the hepatic vein, giving no vascular tributaries to the liver substance. In this way, oxygenated blood is carried directly to the fetal heart. Fetal blood flow through the hepatic artery, which arises from the celiac artery, is small compared with that through the umbilical and portal veins.[3] At birth, however, umbilical vessels are obliterated, and blood flow to the liver abruptly shifts from well-oxygenated venous blood to less well oxygenated portal venous blood. This adaptive response may lead to significant liver dysfunction in early postnatal life, especially with neonatal distress, when the ductus venosus may remain open and cause blood to be diverted away from the liver sinusoids.

Liver Morphology

The liver of infants is relatively large, constituting approximately 5 per cent of body weight,[28, 54] and is made up of four incompletely separated lobes. Conventionally, the liver is divided into right and left lobes, which do not coincide with intrahepatic branching of blood vessels and biliary ducts. A Riedel's lobe is a tongue-like downward projection of the right lobe. Each lobe contains structural units known as hepatic lobules (Fig. 6–1), roughly hexagonal pieces of tissue with anastomosing plates of parenchymal cells, not single strands of liver cords, in addition to a system of blood sinusoids and perisinusoidal spaces. By two years, the majority of two-cell–thick plates have become one cell in thickness, which presumably improves the movement of materials through the hepatocyte. The lobule comprises a histologic unit with a central vein (smallest subdivision of the hepatic vein) and sinusoids extending toward the periphery, where portal triads (containing branches of hepatic artery, portal vein, and interlobular bile duct) are encountered. Blood from branches of the hepatic artery and portal vein flows toward the central vein through the sinusoids, in the opposite direction to bile. Bile produced by hepatic cells is secreted into the bile canaliculi located between parenchymal cells, and flow is toward biliary ductules located near the lobule periphery, in interlobular bile ducts in the portal tract, to hepatic ducts that unite in the porta hepatis to form the common hepatic duct. Lymph is formed in the perisinusoidal space and flows in the same direction as bile to lymphatic vessels of the portal tract, which are found adjacent to branches of the hepatic artery. Lymph vessels are also associated with hepatic veins and are found in the liver capsule. Toxins and products of local inflammation may be excreted into hepatic lymph, and studies of experimental bile duct obstruction have suggested that liver lymphatics are a potential excretory pathway for bile.[16]

EVALUATION OF THE PATIENT

HISTORY

The history is invaluable in approaching the question of whether the disease is acute or chronic. Dark urine often precedes jaundice, and this and yellow sclerae are often the only evidence to date the onset of disease. Anorexia, fatigue, and failure to thrive are often the only clues to chronic disease. Increasing prominence of the abdomen may be due to hepatomegaly or ascites, the latter often being accompanied by edema. The sudden appearance of an inguinal or umbilical hernia should alert the physician to check for ascites. Since many disorders are inherited, careful questioning for a family history of liver disease is imperative, as is a history of consanguinity within the family.[42]

CLINICAL ASSESSMENT OF THE LIVER

The infant liver is unique in that it is a large organ relative to body size during the first two years of life. It is normally palpable 2 cm below the right costal margin, just lateral to the rectus muscle.[9, 51] The liver should not be felt to the left of the midline. Palpation of the lower liver margin is unreliable for the evaluation of liver size until the position of its upper border is determined in the right midclavicular line by percussion. Determination of liver span by percussion only is not usually considered reliable in infants, however. Lawson et al.[31] measured liver span in 350 infants and children by percussion of upper and lower borders in the midclavicular line and found span to be related to age in a curvilinear fashion. Spans ranged from 1.9 cm at one week to 6 to 7 cm at 20 years of age. Determinations of vertical liver span in normal children may provide a guideline for estimating liver size in children less than two years of age; some consider a span greater than 7 cm an indication for further evaluation.[58] Abnormalities of structures adjacent to the liver can influence apparent liver size; for example, an emphysematous lung and gas in the hepatic flexure of the colon may obscure hepatic dullness, and hyperinflation with subsequent depression of the diaphragm displaces the liver downward, allowing the lower edge to be more easily palpated.

The consistency and character of the liver surface and the palpable edge may aid in determining the nature of the underlying liver disorder. The edge is normally sharp but soft and nontender. A large liver due to congestive heart failure has a rounded, smooth edge with a firm consistency; the cirrhotic liver is hard and has an irregular surface and edge. Auscultation is valuable in detecting the increased hepatic arterial flow (bruit) of primary liver tumors, metastatic disease, hemangiomas, or arteriovenous fistulas.

A complete abdominal examination of the infant with suspected hepatomegaly should include examination of the spleen. Until two years of age, the spleen is normally palpated 2 cm below the costal margin, but after two years it is no longer palpable. Large spleens can go undetected if palpation is not carefully performed by starting at the level of the left superior iliac crest with movement cephalad to the costal margin. Midabdominal venous hums may be heard in infants with splenomegaly and portal hypertension, and abdominal distention suggests ascites, especially in the infant with a prominent abdominal venous pattern and peripheral edema.

Hepatomegaly

Mechanisms. Physiologic enlargement of the liver during infancy is accounted for, in part, by increased, labile connective tissue,[20] which may initially result from the hypoxic stress associated with umbilical vessel obliteration at birth. Other normal mechanisms underlying early liver enlargement in the infant include active hematopoietic function (which declines after the first few postpartum weeks as the liver assumes a more central role in metabolism, such as increased protein synthesis necessary for rapid somatic growth) and increased amounts of liver glycogen. Numerous pathophysiologic mechanisms also account for hepatomegaly associated with hepatic disease states and include sinusoidal congestion, Kupffer cell hyperplasia, cellular infiltration, glycogen, and lipid storage, fatty infiltration, and intrinsic tumors (Table 6–1).[2, 51] Sinusoidal and other vascular spaces can rapidly expand with increased venous pressure associated with right heart failure or hepatic vein thrombosis (Budd-Chiari syndrome). Early postnatal changes in blood flow may accentuate the hepatic congestion[35] and contribute to mild elevation in serum transaminase levels, altered bilirubin metabolism, and depressed drug detoxification.

Kupffer cells constitute about 10 per cent of the total cell mass of the liver and are the largest component of the mononuclear phagocytic system of the body.[45] Pathologic processes in the liver profoundly affect Kupffer cell function and structure; a proliferative hyperplastic Kupffer cell response results in hepatomegaly, especially in septicemia, acute hepatitis, or any cellular inflammatory response to hepatocellular destruction. Because of the strategic relationship of Kupffer cells to the portal circulation within hepatic sinusoids, their hyperfunction is also associated with absorption of toxic agents and various drugs, since they actively phagocytize microbial pathogens, soluble protein, and particulate matter.

Polymorphonuclear leukocyte and monocyte inflammatory responses occur in acute and chronic liver disease. Also, hepatocellular infiltrative diseases, such as leukemia or histiocytosis, lead to an increase in liver mass, especially prominent in portal tract and periportal areas. Tumor infiltration may be diffuse but usually results in focal or asymmetric hepatomegaly. Storage of substances (e.g., glycogen) within hepatocytes or Kupffer cells produces enlargement of the liver. Hepatocyte fat accumulation can occur in protein malnutrition[46] because of

Table 6–1 Mechanisms of Hepatomegaly and Associated Clinical Conditions

MECHANISMS	CONDITIONS

Cellular infiltration and Kupffer cell hyperplasia	Infectious liver disease
	    Bacterial sepsis, hepatic abscess
	    Viral infection (e.g., HBV, HAV, CMV, rubella)
	    Parasitic infection (e.g., toxoplasmosis)
	Chemical liver injury
	"Benign" hepatomegaly

Sinusoidal congestion	Congestive heart failure Pericardial tamponade Budd-Chiari syndrome (hepatic vein thrombosis)

Tumor infiltration	Leukemia
	Lymphoma
	Histiocytosis
	Metastatic tumors
	    Neuroblastoma
	    Wilms' tumor

Cellular storage	Glycogen storage disease
	Lipid storage disease
	    Niemann-Pick
	    Gaucher's
	α_1-Antitrypsin deficiency

Fat accumulation	Malnutrition (kwashiorkor)
	Total parenteral nutrition
	Metabolic liver disease
	    Galactosemia
	    Hereditary fructose intolerance
	    Tyrosinemia
	Reye's syndrome
	Cystic fibrosis

Liver tumors	Hepatoblastoma
	Hepatoma
	Benign hepatic tumors
	    Hemangioma
	    Focal nodular hyperplasia

(From Walker, W. A., and Mathis, R. E.: Hepatomegaly: An approach to differential diagnosis. Pediatr. Clin. North Am. 22:929, 1975.)

inadequate synthesis of lipoproteins and consequent decrease in pinocytotic transport of lipid from the hepatocyte. Abnormal concentrations of hepatic fat (steatosis) also occur in infants receiving total parenteral nutrition and in specific disease states such as Reye syndrome, cystic fibrosis, and hepatotoxin-induced liver dysfunction, which will be discussed in Chapter Fourteen. Infants with choledochal cysts may present with apparent hepatomegaly. "Benign" hepatomegaly is common in nonspecific viral infections and is secondary to Kupffer cell hyperplasia and portal inflammatory cell infiltration.

Splenomegaly Associated with Hepatomegaly. Splenomegaly suggests portal hypertension associated with advanced liver disease (e.g., cirrhosis), cellular infiltrative or storage disease (e.g., Gaucher or Niemann-Pick disease), and reticuloendothelial cell hyperplasia. Infants with overt evidence of hepatitis have hepatosplenomegaly early in life; however, splenic enlargement may be the first manifestation of previously undiagnosed progressive liver disease.

LIVER FUNCTION: DEVELOPMENT AND CLINICAL MANIFESTATIONS

The fetal liver is primarily a hematopoietic organ. By late gestation, erythropoiesis commences in the bone marrow and hema-

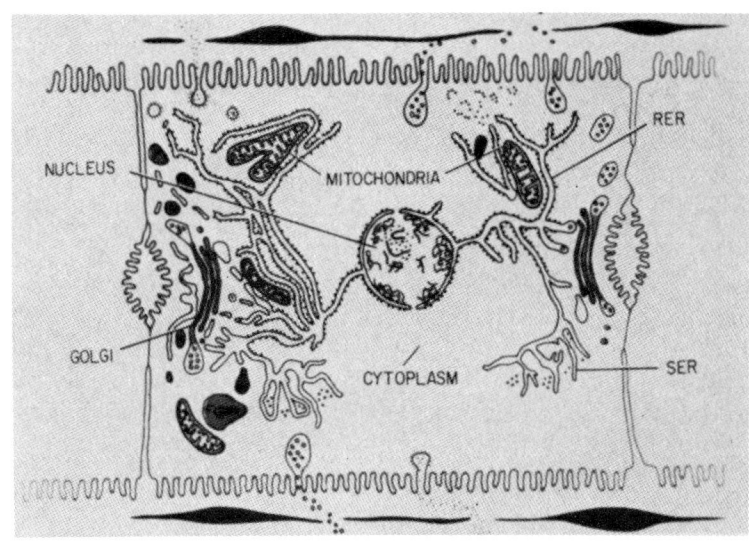

Figure 6–2 Diagram of functional hepatocyte with important subcellular structures. RER, rough endoplasmic reticulum; SER, smooth endoplasmic reticulum. (From Andres, J. M., Mathis, R. K., and Walker, W. A.: Liver disease in infants. I. Developmental hepatology and mechanisms of liver dysfunction. J. Pediatr. 90:686, 1977.)

topoiesis decreases as the infant liver assumes its vital role in metabolism, previously controlled by the maternal liver *in utero*.[15] These important metabolic processes, all developing at different rates during gestation, include bilirubin and bile acid conjugation and secretion, bile acid synthesis, glucose homeostasis, protein synthesis, detoxification of drugs, and development of infant reticuloendothelial function and host defense. Important aspects of developmental liver function will be discussed and then related to manifestations of liver disease, especially jaundice and cholestasis. A diagrammatic representation of the functional hepatocyte is shown in Figure 6–2 in order to facilitate a better understanding of this section.

Bilirubin Metabolism

The fetal liver is unable to completely conjugate bilirubin, and the unconjugated molecule is readily metabolized by the maternal liver.[33] Furthermore, decreased bilirubin glucuronyl transferase and increased beta-glucuronidase enzymes are present in fetal liver and intestine, respectively. The latter enzyme hydrolyzes conjugated bilirubin, allowing for rapid clearance by the placenta of the unconjugated molecule, and thus represents an important fetal protective mechanism. At birth, however, the neonatal liver must handle the total bilirubin load despite bilirubin metabolizing enzymes that are functionally immature.

A complete understanding of the various steps in bilirubin formation and excretion is necessary when jaundice is considered as a manifestation of liver disease in the infant[34b] (Fig. 6–3). Bilirubin is derived from hemoglobin after senescent red blood cells are taken up by the reticuloendothelial system,[17] and heme is converted to biliverdin by the microsomal enzyme heme oxygenase

Figure 6–3 Reactions necessary for bilirubin conjugation.

$$
\begin{array}{c}
\text{GLUCOSE + ATP} \\
\Updownarrow \text{ hexokinase} \\
\text{GLUCOSE-6-PHOSPHATE} \\
\Updownarrow \text{ phosphoglucomutase} \\
\text{GLUCOSE-1-PHOSPHATE} \\
\text{URIDINE TRIPHOSPHATE PP} \Updownarrow \\
\text{URIDINE DIPHOSPHATE GLUCOSE} \\
\Updownarrow \\
\begin{array}{l}
\text{2 NAD} \\
\text{2 NADH + 2H}^+
\end{array} \\
\text{URIDINE DIPHOSPHATE GLUCURONIC ACID} \\
\begin{array}{l}
\text{BILIRUBIN} \\
\text{UDP}
\end{array} \quad \downarrow \text{ glucuronyl transferase} \\
\text{BILIRUBIN GLUCURONIDE}
\end{array}
$$

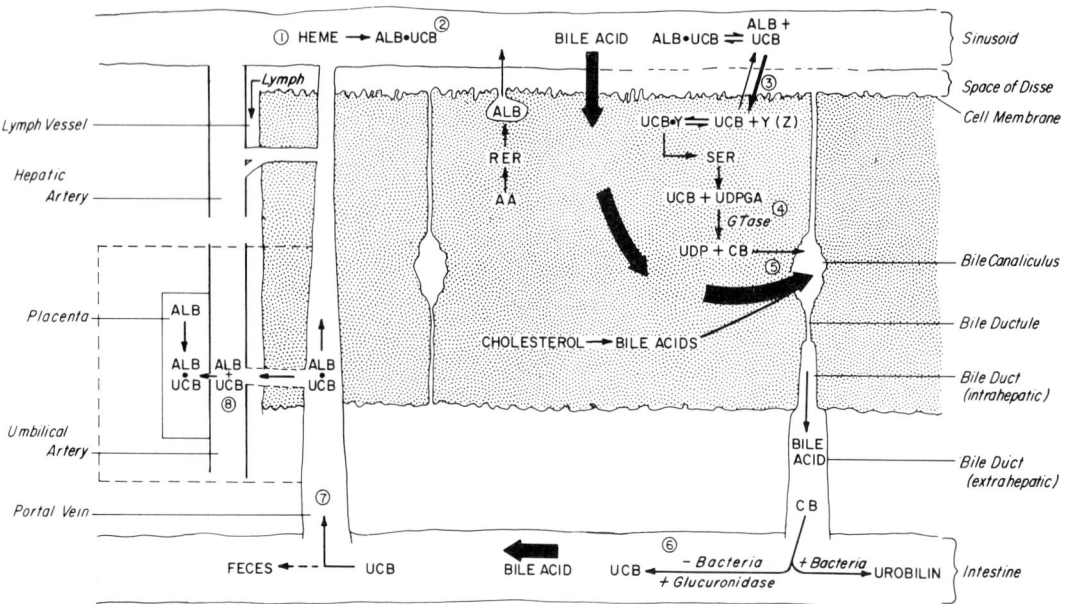

Figure 6–4 Representation of functional hepatocyte with important anatomic relationships and vital hepatic processes — that is, bilirubin metabolism, bile acid production, enterohepatic circulation, and albumin production with cellular secretion. The numbers 1 through 8 refer to steps of bilirubin metabolism. AA, amino acids; ALB, albumin; CB, conjugated bilirubin; GTase, glucuronyl transferase; RER and SER, rough and smooth endoplasmic reticulum; UCB, unconjugated bilirubin; UDP, uridine diphosphate; UDPGA, uridine diphosphoglucuronic acid. (From Andres, J. M., Mathis, R. K., and Walker, W. A.: Liver disease in infants. I. Developmental hepatology and mechanisms of liver dysfunction. J. Pediatr. *90*:686, 1977.)

and the cytochrome enzymes.[47] Biliverdin is subsequently reduced to bilirubin. Increased catabolism of fetal hemoglobin contributes a further bilirubin load to the neonatal liver. The newly formed unconjugated bilirubin becomes tightly bound to plasma albumin (Fig. 6–4) and is then transported to and taken up by the hepatocyte after dissociation from albumin at the hepatocyte plasma membrane. Within the cytoplasm, proteins Y (ligandin) and Z bind bilirubin and other organic anions.[17] The major cytoplasmic protein Y is probably diminished in fetal life and early infancy,[34] which contributes to decreased transportation of bilirubin to the smooth endoplasmic reticulum for conjugation and consequent water solubilization necessary for movement into bile. Conjugation requires uridine diphosphate (UDP) glucuronic acid in the presence of glucuronyl transferase, a microsomal enzyme that takes several days after birth to reach mature levels.[6, 17] UDP glucuronic acid is dependent on glucose and the enzyme UDPG dehydrogenase, both of which may be diminished at birth, especially in premature infants. The glucuron-

ide conjugates are rapidly secreted at the bile canaliculus into the bile and subsequently into the small intestine; immaturity of this secreting process *or* damage of the canalicular membrane undoubtedly contributes to elevated serum bilirubin values.

Colonic bacterial flora reduce conjugated bilirubin to urobilinogen, which is further reduced to urobilin and excreted in the feces. Urobilinogen can be reabsorbed, and small quantities normally escape into the systemic circulation and appear in the urine. However, in the fetus and newborn infant there is an absence of intestinal bacteria[37] and the meconium/feces of the newborn infant contains beta-glucuronidase, which deconjugates bilirubin.[5] Enterohepatic recirculation of deconjugated bilirubin occurs because this molecule can be rapidly reabsorbed across the intestinal microvillus membrane or excreted in the feces; placental clearance of the reabsorbed bilirubin occurs *in utero.*

Jaundice. Jaundice is the most common presenting manifestation of hepatic dysfunction or physiologic immaturity of the liver in infants.[34a] The clinical conditions associated with this important physical finding will be discussed in Chapter Fourteen. It is a yellow discoloration of skin, sclera, and other tissues caused by the accumulation of conjugated and/or unconjugated bilirubin. After maturation of the blood-brain barrier, *unconjugated bilirubin* in the serum of infants is of no pathologic significance. It may be "physiologic" and is noted in approximately 15 per cent of normal newborn infants.[23] Neonatal unconjugated hyperbilirubinemia, however, is potentially hazardous because of deposition of free bilirubin in neuronal tissues (kernicterus) with associated brain damage, especially in premature infants.[18] Jaundice is noted in the older infant when the total serum bilirubin concentration is approximately 2.5 mg per dl; in contrast, the neonate is not obviously jaundiced until the bilirubin concentration is about 7 mg per dl.[7, 8] Because the unconjugated bilirubin molecule is not secreted into bile, urobilinogen does not appear in the intestine or subsequently in the urine. Persistent, unconjugated hyperbilirubinemia without hepatomegaly suggests either a problem with overproduction of bilirubin or an inherited or acquired disruption of bilirubin transport, uptake, or conjugation. It should be carefully distinguished from the more serious, always pathologic, liver dysfunction causing hepatomegaly and *conjugated hyperbilirubinemia*. Increased serum levels of conjugated bilirubin, therefore, represent an important indicator of disease, but the molecule is not known to be chemically harmful to body tissues, including the central nervous system.

A serum conjugated (direct) bilirubin of greater than 1.5 mg per dl should always be considered secondary to hepatocellular injury with regurgitation of conjugated bilirubin from the hepatocyte or canaliculus into the circulation.[36] For most forms of liver disease to be discussed, conjugated and unconjugated bilirubin values are elevated and the conjugated fraction predominates.

Bile Acid Metabolism

Bile acids are the principal organic anions synthesized by the liver, and secretion into bile is quantitatively much greater than for other organic ions, such as bilirubin, and occurs by a separate mechanism.[25] Infants have low intraluminal bile acid concentration, resulting in inefficient intestinal dietary fat absorption. Furthermore, bile acid synthesis and pool size are less in premature infants as compared with full-term infants.[52] By 14 to 16 weeks of gestation, bile acids can be found in the liver; the dihydroxy bile acid, chenodexoycholic acid, predominates in bile from 22 to 26 weeks' gestation and is conjugated with taurine. Cholate appears after 28 weeks and is the bile acid that predominates at birth.[38] Glycine conjugate is the more common conjugate in the mature liver of later infancy. The conjugated bile acids are secreted into bile and enter the small intestine for micellar formation and subsequent reabsorption. Retention of bile acids in the enterohepatic circulation may be quantitatively adequate in infancy; however, bile acids lost in the stool must be resynthesized from cholesterol, and there appears to be a negative feedback control of intestinal bile and liver bile acid synthesis. Ultimately, bile flow in the infant is dependent on synthesis and release of bile acid from the hepatocyte by an active transport process (bile acid–dependent component) and an independent ionic pump mechanism (bile acid–independent component).[24] In addition, bile ductules and/or ducts may be capable of organic anion secretion and resorption, probably regulated by secretin.[13] Disruption of the canalicular membrane, poor development of bile acid secretory mechanisms, and immature bile acid synthesis may account for the decreased bile flow (cholestasis) noted in many liver diseases of infancy.

Cholestasis. Cholestasis is impairment of bile excretion; physiologically, it can be defined as reduction in bile flow; morphologically, it is the presence of bile pigment in histologic sections of liver. Symptoms of cholestasis in infancy may include irritability, perhaps a manifestation of pruritus secondary to increased serum and tissue bile acids, but dermal excoriations and associated physical findings are necessary for a clinical diagnosis because estimation of serum bile acids is not a routine or generally available laboratory procedure. Cholestasis is often associated with conjugated hyperbilirubinemia; since bilirubin is a small component of bile, jaundice is an indirect indicator of cholestasis and the term "cholestatic jaundice" has appeared in the literature. It should be recognized, however, that some infants with cholestasis become anicteric,[26, 27] or the onset of their cholestatic disease may have been anicteric. Bile secretory failure also leads to a defect in excretion of lipids, with resultant hypercholesterolemia; the infant may develop xanthomas, although this is unusual prior to two years of age. The clinical manifestations of a decrease in intestinal bile acid concentration, which will be discussed separately with the specific liver diseases, include the problems of steatorrhea, osteomalacia, and hypoprothrombinemia.

Carbohydrate Metabolism

The liver plays a central role in maintaining blood glucose levels. Increased concentrations of glucose have been demonstrated in livers of distressed fetuses as early as 13 weeks of gestation,[19] and lipid synthesis from carbohydrates occurs in early gestation.[40] Liver glycogen deposition, which requires hepatocyte uptake of glucose from portal blood and synthetase enzymes, occurs just prior to term and represents another important fetal protective mechanism. Liver glycogen decreases after birth as glucose-6-phosphatase (glucose-6-phosphate → glucose) increases, suggesting that the newborn infant is completely capable of glycogen synthesis and degradation. Gluconeogenesis may assume more functional importance when carbohydrate homeostasis is disturbed, even during a time of mild hepatic insult.[14] Hypoglycemia occurs with all forms of infant liver disease, especially in the premature infant.

Protein Metabolism

Except for immunoglobulins, most of the serum proteins are synthesized by the rough endoplasmic reticulum of the hepatocytes. Synthesis can be detected as early as four weeks' gestation[22]; at this time, the embryonic liver can produce albumin, alpha-fetoprotein, alpha$_1$-antitrypsin, and other important macromolecules.[21] A rapid decline in fetoprotein concentration,[22] which occurs during late gestation, is accompanied by active synthesis of albumin, suggesting a reciprocal relationship during fetal development.[29, 43] Alpha-fetoprotein is elevated in hepatitis, in some hepatic tumors, and in regenerating liver.[1] It has been suggested that fetoprotein is the gestational counterpart of albumin[1] and that their amino acid sequence is similar.[41] After birth, albumin is the major serum protein, with a half-life in the circulation of 21 days. Maintenance of adequate serum albumin is dependent, in part, on normal hepatic function. The site or mode of albumin degradation is unknown, but excessive losses can occur with certain pathologic conditions of the gastrointestinal or urinary tract, although low albumin levels are commonly found in premature infants. The mean value for total serum proteins is lower in term neonates than in their mothers, averaging 6.16 gm per dl. Levels rise slowly after birth to adult levels of 6.92 gm per dl by one to two years. Albumin constitutes 50 to 60 per cent of the total protein in all age groups. Significant hypoalbuminemia is usually not associated with acute liver disease but is relatively common in patients with cirrhosis or other forms of chronic liver disease.[42]

Albumin may quantitatively be the most important of the serum proteins, but alpha and beta globulins, transferrin, ceruloplasmin, and the clotting factors are also made in the liver. Albumin is synthesized by the hepatocyte, but alpha and beta globulins are synthesized by both the hepatocyte and the intestinal mucosa. Since biliary obstruction results in increases in cholesterol, which is principally carried by the beta globulins, hyperbetaglobulinemia is a frequent accompaniment of obstructive liver disease. Beta globulins are decreased or absent in patients with Tangier disease and abetalipoproteinemia, inherited disorders of lipoprotein formation associated with fatty infiltration of the liver.

Serum alpha globulin levels rise in a number of chronic inflammatory diseases but fall sharply and occasionally are absent during the acute stages of liver disease, and one may follow the course of acute viral hepatitis by noting the reappearance of these proteins in the serum. Nearly 90 per cent of the alpha₁ globulins are alpha₁-antitrypsin, a deficiency of which is associated with either chronic pulmonary or liver disease. The finding of this protein on protein electrophoresis strips is a convenient and simple screening test for this deficiency.

It is not well understood why patients with chronic liver disease have marked increases in gamma globulins, since these are made by the reticuloendothelial system and not by the liver. Values occasionally reach 6 to 10 gm per dl. In contrast, patients with agammaglobulinemia have an increased susceptibility to develop chronic liver disease.

Four clotting factors — Christmas factor, factor VII, Stuart-Prower factor, and prothrombin — are synthesized by the liver only if vitamin K is present.[34a] Fibrinogen, stable factor, serum prothrombin conversion accelerator, proaccelerin, and labile factor are also synthesized solely by the liver. The prothrombin time is often employed to assess the extrinsic pathway of thrombin formation and the partial thromboplastin time to assess the intrinsic pathway. Abnormalities of the clotting factors are usually manifestations of chronic liver disease, although clotting factors may be abnormal in subacute hepatic necrosis.

Ammonia is produced in the gut from deamination of amino acids by intestinal bacteria and by the breakdown of urease-producing bacteria. In patients with alkalosis, the increased activity of renal glutaminase provides a significant contribution to the blood ammonia level. There is an excellent correlation between rising blood ammonia and the development of hepatic coma in patients with overwhelming liver disease. This is because the liver is no longer capable of utilizing ammonia to aminate keto acids. Elevated blood ammonia levels also occur when there is portosystemic shunting of blood, since the liver is no longer in the mainstream of ammonia absorbed from the intestine, or when there are deficiencies of the urea cycle enzymes. In addition to the absolute level of blood ammonia, the amount of un-ionized ammonium hydroxide plays a key role, since this and not the ammonium ion is capable of crossing the blood-brain barrier (brain cell membrane). Alkalosis increases the concentration of un-ionized ammonium hydroxide, and therefore blood pH measurements must be considered in addition to simple blood ammonia measurements for optimal treatment of hyperammonemic patients. The most frequent cause of alkalosis in patients with liver disease is hypokalemia due to injudicious use of diuretics.[42]

Lipid Metabolism

The liver plays a central role in lipid metabolism.[42] In the fasting state, all of the triglycerides and phospholipids present in the serum are synthesized within the liver. Most of the cholesterol derives from the liver, with the rest being synthesized by intestinal mucosa and skin. Whenever there is obstruction to bile flow, synthesis of phospholipids, especially lecithin, increases. When serum lecithin rises, there is an outpouring of cholesterol from the reticuloendothelial system and an increase in hepatic synthesis of cholesterol. As a result, both phospholipids and cholesterol are increased in biliary obstruction. Occasionally, serum triglycerides also increase, but the serum does not become turbid because of the detergent action of the phospholipids. Cholesterol elevations are highest in patients with drug hepatitis and primary biliary cirrhosis, often reaching levels over 1000 mg per dl. In mechanical obstruction, cholesterol rarely rises above 500 mg per dl. Levels between 300 and 400 mg per dl may be seen during the cholestatic phase of viral hepatitis. Except in infants with inherited hyperlipoproteinemia type II, cord cholesterol levels are less than 100 mg per dl, but adult levels between 150 and 200 mg per dl are attained during the first few weeks of life.

Serum cholesterol esters are manufactured in the serum from cholesterol and lecithin, with the reaction catalyzed by lec-

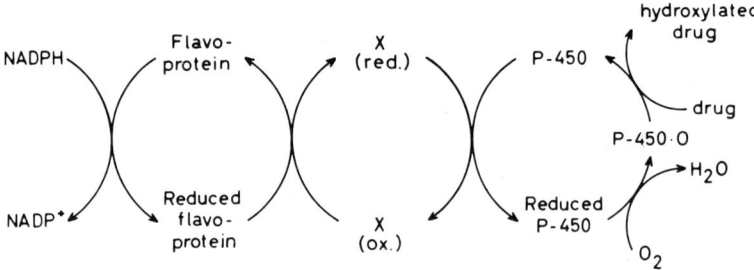

Figure 6–5 Drug-metabolizing enzyme system. Arrows represent oxidation/reduction reactions of the electron transport chain. Flavoprotein is the final oxidase in the system. Oxygen incorporation into drug is catalyzed by P-450, eventually yielding a hydroxylated metabolite. Maturation of the system is essential to extrauterine life when material detoxifying processes are no longer available. P-450·0, oxygen-activating component of system; NADPH, nicotinamide adenine dinucleotide phosphate (reduced); X, component of unknown structure. (From Andres, J. M., Mathis, R. K., and Walker, W. A.: Liver disease in infants. I. Developmental hepatology and mechanisms of liver dysfunction. J. Pediatr. *90*:686, 1977.)

ithin cholesterol acyl transferase (LCAT), which is manufactured by the liver. Liver disease therefore results in decreased esterification of cholesterol, and it has been shown that the percentage of cholesterol esters is inversely proportional to the level of serum bilirubin.

An abnormal lipoprotein appears to be reasonably specific for biliary obstruction. Termed lipoprotein X, this moiety migrates with the beta globulins on lipoprotein electrophoresis but is abnormal in having an increased content of phospholipid and free cholesterol. Forty per cent of its apoprotein is albumin. It disappears from the serum when obstruction is relieved or when hepatic decompensation develops.

Drug Metabolism

Oxidation and conjugation are the important drug metabolizing reactions of the mature liver; oxidation of a drug occurs at cytochrome P-450 (an oxidase), yielding a hydroxylated metabolite that is immediately conjugated with glucuronic acid,[12] sulfate, or certain amino acids (Fig. 6–5).[39] The water-soluble conjugated drug is more easily excreted into the bile, except in the fetus, where a functional immaturity of drug metabolism exists as another developmental protective mechanism; i.e., unconjugated lipid-soluble metabolites more readily pass across the placenta to be detoxified by the maternal liver. A drug-metabolizing enzyme system for the fetal liver has been noted at 14 to 25 weeks' gestation, but pre-mature infants[57] have a reduced ability to hydroxylate lipid-soluble substances[43] and therefore are more susceptible to drug toxicity. Inefficient drug metabolism occurs in young infants because of diminished microsomal enzymes at birth, a mechanism similar to the one responsible for delayed bilirubin excretion into bile.

Reticuloendothelial Function of the Liver

Kupffer cells constitute the greatest part of the mononuclear phagocyte system.[48] The function of these sinusoidal lining cells may be different from other phagocytic cells, especially with regard to the proposed role in controlling the immunogenicity of antigens in the general circulation. In the fetus the liver is an important hemopoietic organ, and Kupffer cells are probably derived from monocytes and bone marrow precursor cells present in the fetal sinusoids. Because of their strategic location and relationship to the portal blood flow, they are a protective filter, and endocytosis is their major cell function. Experimental studies have demonstrated that these phagocytic cells clear bacteria, viruses, and particulate matter from the circulation as well as participate in the uptake of antigens such as endotoxin. Immaturity of the Kupffer cell function may contribute to hepatic dysfunction in infants, especially since the intestine of the newborn has an increased permeability to antigens such as enzymes and various toxins.[50, 55] Also, transient depression of Kupffer cell phagocytosis occurs in protein-deficiency states and after exposure to various drugs (e.g., cyclophosphamide,[10] halothane, and pentobarbital[32]). It is becoming clear, therefore, that the liver is an important organ of host defense.

TESTS OF LIVER FUNCTION

Liver function tests are of limited value as far as the classification of hepatobiliary disease in infants is concerned, but liver function can be broadly divided into assessment categories to aid investigation of (1) hepato-

Table 6–2 Tests of Liver Function

FUNCTION BEING EXAMINED	TEST	MAJOR USE
Protein metabolism	Protein electrophoresis	
	Albumin	Decreased in cirrhosis; increased in dehydration and hamartoma
	Gamma globulin	Increased in chronic liver disease; occasionally absent in chronic hepatitis
	Beta globulin	Increased in biliary obstruction; decreased in abetalipoproteinemia and Tangier disease
	Alpha globulin	Decreased in acute liver disease and in α_1-antitrypsin deficiency; increased in some chronic inflammatory diseases
	Cephalin flocculation	3+ and 4+ positive with decreased albumin; increased γ globulin, viral hepatitis and cirrhosis; negative in drug hepatitis and fatty infiltration
	Prothrombin time	Abnormal in any severe liver disease and malabsorption of vitamin K
	Partial thromboplastin time	Abnormal in any severe liver disease
	Fibrinogen	Abnormal in any severe liver disease
	SGOT, SGPT, LDH	Abnormal in any acute hepatocyte damage
	Alkaline phosphatase	Increased in obstruction to bile flow, intrahepatic or extrahepatic
	Ammonia	Increased in liver failure and in portosystemic shunting of blood
Lipid metabolism	Cholesterol	Increased in obstruction to bile flow; decreased in abetalipoproteinemia and Tangier disease
	Cholesterol esters	Decreases in proportion to increasing bilirubin
	Phospholipids	Increased in obstruction to bile flow
	Triglycerides	Slightly increased in biliary obstruction; decreased in abetalipoproteinemia and Tangier disease
	Lipoprotein electrophoresis	Abnormal lipoprotein, LPX, in biliary obstruction migrating with β-lipoproteins
Carbohydrate metabolism	Blood sugar	Abnormal glucose tolerance test in all types of liver disease; hypoglycemia in hepatitis, acute yellow atrophy, and hepatoma
Drug metabolism	Bilirubin (unconjugated)	Increased in hemolysis, physiologic jaundice of newborn, any liver disease
	Bilirubin glucuronide	Increased in biliary obstruction, any liver disease
	Total bilirubin	May be increased in any liver disease
	BSP	Increased in any liver disease; falls faster than bilirubin when obstruction relieved

cellular injury, (2) abnormalities of bile secretion, and (3) disruption of hepatocyte metabolic function. These categories of tests will be reviewed and are cited in Table 6–2.

Tests for Hepatocellular Dysfunction

Aminotransferases. The aminotransferases (formerly called transaminases) are hepatocyte cytoplasmic enzymes and have little individual differential value. However, aspartate aminotransferase (glutamic-oxaloacetic transaminase, or SGOT) is also partially bound to cytoplasmic organelles, and therefore serum elevation may suggest more significant hepatocyte injury.[11] When the hepatocyte plasma membrane is damaged, it becomes permeable to cellular enzymes and their level increases in the serum; alanine aminotransferase (glutamic-pyruvic transaminase, or SGPT) is the better indicator of membrane "leakage"[44] because it is not organelle-bound and is more specific to the liver.[7] Both aminotransferases reflect the degree of hepatic damage. Serum levels greater than ten times the upper limit of normal favor acute hepatocellular injury, but moderate increases may be seen in infants with cholestatic or storage diseases. They have no predictive value, however, for the prognosis of the liver insult. A sharp fall in enzymes associated with clinical deterioration of the patient indicates liver decompensation and destruction.

Other Indices of Cell Injury. Lactic dehydrogenase (LDH) is a poor indicator of hepatocellular injury and is of no value in the detection of infant liver disease. Ornithine carbamyl transferase (OTC) and alcohol dehydrogenase (AD) are more specific to the liver than are aminotransferases, but their practical application is not justified because of difficulties in laboratory determinations. Glutamyl transpeptidase (GGTP) catalyzes the transfer of gamma glutamyl moieties from donor to other peptides and amino acids. Although present in hepatocytes and intrahepatic bile ducts, it is also present in other tissues. Wright and Christie report that levels of GGTP are lower in infants with neonatal hepatitis (mean 183 IU/L) than in those with biliary atresia (mean 760 IU/L).[56]

The SGOT is actually excellent for following the daily progress of liver integrity, since the half-life of the enzyme in the serum is between 18 and 21 hours.

The cephalin flocculation is positive when serum albumin levels fall or gamma globulin levels rise. The test has two specific uses: It is positive in over 95 per cent of patients with viral hepatitis but in only 20 per cent of those with drug hepatitis. It is also positive in the majority of patients with cirrhosis and not in those with fatty infiltration of the liver. (A positive test indicates 3 to 4+ flocculation.) The thymol turbidity test results are similar, but it should be noted that high serum triglycerides will precipitate thymol.

In the absence of vitamin K deficiency, an abnormal prothrombin time (not corrected by intramuscular vitamin K) indicates liver disease.

Tests for Abnormalities of Bile Secretion

Bilirubin. The metabolism of this organic anion has been discussed earlier: it constitutes only a small portion of bile, but conjugated (direct) bilirubin is an indicator of cholestasis because it is secreted across the hepatocanalicular membrane. Conjugated bilirubin is elevated in the absence of cholestasis only in the Dubin-Johnson or Rotor syndrome. Normally, conjugated bilirubin is less than 0.3 mg per dl in the serum, with total bilirubin levels normally measuring less than 1.0 mg per dl.

Bile Acids. Bile acids have been extensively studied in hepatobiliary disease using tedious and not generally available techniques such as gas-liquid chromatography. Therefore, the clinical assessment of bile acids has remained confusing. Recent development of specific radioimmunoassays has resulted in renewed interest in the use of bile acids as a reliable laboratory tool for measurement of hepatic excretory function. Increases in serum bile acids are usually determined to be conjugates of cholic and chenodeoxycholic acids, but contrary to earlier reports, the ratio of cholate/chenodeoxycholate or total serum bile acids does not precisely differentiate ductal from hepatocellular cholestasis.

Alkaline Phosphatase and Other Indices of Cholestasis. Hepatobiliary alkaline phosphatase is synthesized primarily by the bile canaliculi and bile duct epithelium and is located near the hepatocyte canalicular and sinusoidal membranes. In liver disease, its level is increased owing to inadequate bile flow subsequent to decreased bile excretion.[28a] The elevation is probably due to increased enzyme synthesis and regurgitation into the sinusoidal blood rather than leakage of the enzyme across the damaged plasma membrane. Isoenzyme activity, best determined by electrophoresis, is derived from liver, bone, intestine, and placenta. In the normal, actively growing infant, the serum alkaline phosphatase is generally two to three times that of the adult. This makes laboratory interpretation difficult, especially since alkaline phosphatase is commonly elevated in many infant liver diseases, including hepatitis, biliary atresia, and infiltrative liver disease. Congestion of the splanchnic bed, such as occurs in congestive heart failure, may result in increased alkaline phosphatase of intestinal origin.

Alkaline phosphatase levels should be compared to 5′-nucleotidase, a more specific liver enzyme, which is an alkaline phosphatase that catalyzes the hydrolysis of nucleotides such as adenosine-5′-phosphate.[57a] It appears to be specifically derived from liver and placenta. Determination of this enzyme is most useful when there is some doubt as to the origin of alkaline phosphatase. Increased levels are occasionally seen in malnourished infants with fatty infiltration of the liver. The enzyme is significantly increased in the presence of active bile duct proliferation and is most useful in the diagnosis of biliary obstruction in the growing child. Since the enzyme results from increased hepatic synthesis, a fall in its level during the course of unrelieved biliary obstruction usually indicates hepatocyte failure rather than clinical improvement. The levels are age-dependent, with those in infants under one month measuring less than 3 IU/L; in those between 1 and 11 months, 1.5 to 2 IU/L, and in those between one and five years, 1 IU/L. Some report 5′-nucleotidase levels to be inferior to gamma glutamyl transpeptidase (GGT) for the diagnosis of obstructive liver disease.[4a] *Leucine aminopeptidase* (LAP) is the least sensitive of the tests for cholestasis in infants and children.

[131]I-Rose Bengal Excretion. This is the most accurate test for determining bile excretion or degree of biliary obstruction.[43a] Rose bengal dye, handled like bilirubin by the hepatocyte, is rapidly taken up by the liver, excreted into the biliary system, and ultimately eliminated via the stool in normal infants. The test consists of the intravenous injection of radiolabeled rose bengal followed by a 72-hour collection of urine-free stool; radioactivity is measured in the stool specimen and expressed as a percentage of total injected dose. Complete biliary obstruction is suggested if the radiolabeled dye in the stool is less than 10 per cent; hence, the test is invaluable in differentiating biliary atresia (ductal cholestasis) from hepatocellular cholestasis. Because the rose bengal scan does not provide a quantitative analysis of biliary excretion, it is a less reliable test, and the diagnosis of patent bile ducts (e.g., extrahepatic biliary hypoplasia) could potentially be missed. This is especially important because hypoplasia regularly occurs with severe cellular cholestasis, a situation in which the hepatocyte canalicular membrane is damaged and secretion of conjugated rose bengal (with I-131) is markedly impaired.

Tests for Liver Metabolic Function

Bromsulphalein (BSP). Bilirubin and BSP dye are handled in a similar way by the hepatocyte except that BSP is conjugated with glutathione. The dye is given as an intravenous injection in a dose of 5 mg per kg body weight, and blood is obtained at 45 minutes to measure retention of the dye in the circulating blood; BSP retention is normally less than 8 per cent of the injected dose.[22a] This is one of the more sensitive tests of liver dysfunction, if other tests have proved to be normal in the infant with suspected liver disease. The test has some limitations, however, in that abnormal results are found in many nonhepatic disorders (e.g., congestive heart failure with decreased hepatic blood flow) and in infants with hypoalbuminemia. This procedure is time-consuming, but the newer BSP clearance test is technically simple and may provide a practical estimate of liver plasma flow and cellular excretory capacity (T_m, transport maximum) in complicated cases.

Liver Immunologic Tests

Immunologic reactivity is probably important in the pathogenesis of certain types of infant liver disease. For example, liver damage induced by hepatitis B virus may be an immunologic reaction against the B virus. Cytotoxicity of lymphocytes against specific liver antigens, rather than direct tissue damage by the hepatitis B virus has been suggested as the mechanism of injury, and immunoglobulin can be identified on the hepatocyte plasma membrane from patients with active liver disease.[36b, c] Non-organ-specific antibodies are detected in children with chronic liver disease, especially smooth muscle and antinuclear antibodies, which are present in more than 20 per cent of patients with chronic active hepatitis.[8a] The inflammatory response of the liver may be associated with elevated serum gamma globulins. Infants with acute hepatitis, however, usually have gamma globulin levels of less than 2.5 gm per dl, and serum levels greater than 3 gm per dl suggest the diagnosis of chronic hepatitis. Serum immunoglobulins vary considerably with age, but elevations of immunoglobulins A, G, and M are found in chronic liver disease of infancy and IgM may be raised in acute viral hepatitis. Furthermore, serum alpha-fetoprotein (AFP) levels greater than 40 μ per ml suggest the diagnosis of hepatitis in the young infant. The significance of AFP changes in the serum remains to be determined; however, this protein may contribute to the regulation of both cellular and humoral immune responses.[1b]

Radioisotope Scanning (Scintigraphy)

Several scintigraphic agents are available for localization of reticuloendothelial cells and leukocytes, for assessment of hepatocellular function, and for visualization of the biliary system. *Technetium (Tc-99) sulfur colloid* displays the distribution of functioning liver (spleen and bone marrow) reticuloendothelial cells and is currently favored for routine imaging of the liver.[1a] It reliably demonstrates masses in the liver greater than 1 cm as well as liver size and irregularity or displacement of the liver outline. Technetium scanning is useful in detecting focal liver lesions (e.g., abscess, cyst, tumor) and diffuse liver disease. Acute hepatocellular disease is suggested by a decrease in radionuclide uptake and an irregular pattern of isotope distribution. Reduced intensity of the hepatic image because of poor extraction of colloid by the liver, together with increased radionuclide uptake by spleen and bone marrow, is a characteristic scintigraphic feature of cirrhosis. *Gallium citrate (GA-67)* is another gamma-emitting radionuclide that is useful for localizing occult inflammatory masses when other clinical, radiologic, and radioisotopic procedures fail to detect an abnormality, especially in the febrile patient.[30a] The precise mechanism of hepatic uptake is unknown, but gallium may be associated with cytoplasmic lysosomes in leukocytes and macrophages. In addition to localization of abscesses, gallium scanning may help detect metastatic tumors and hepatic neoplasms. False negative scans occur in neutropenic patients, and normal accumulation of the radionuclide in the liver reticuloendothelial system could potentially delay detection of a subphrenic abscess. Newer agents, especially the [99m]*Tc-iminodiacetic acid* analogs (e.g., *p*-isopropyl-acetaniliodomino-diacetic acid, or PIPIDA), are organic anions that are taken up by the hepatocyte, conjugated, and excreted across the canalicular membrane.[39a, 45a] These agents rapidly clear from the blood, but their secretory mechanism, which is similar to that of rose bengal dye and bilirubin, is significantly disturbed by canalicular membrane damage and competitively inhibited by elevated serum bilirubin levels. In general, ^{99m}Tc-PIPIDA will demonstrate the common bile duct, gallbladder, and intestine if the serum bilirubin is less than 6 mg per dl; when the bilirubin level is greater than 6 mg per dl, the biliary system is poorly visualized and it is difficult to distinguish between bile duct obstruction and hepatocellular disease. In the normal infant, sequential demonstration of the liver, bile ducts, and small intestine occurs in approximately one hour.

Ultrasonic Scanning

Ultrasonography is complementary to scintigraphy and may confirm, or better characterize, radioisotope scan defects.[14a, 46a] Ultrasound yields high-frequency sound waves that are reflected back from tissues, and the transmitted oscilloscopic signals are finally imaged. This technique has proved useful in evaluating the parenchymal structure of the liver, including alterations in liver size and contour, and it is especially beneficial in differentiating fluid-filled lesions (e.g., cysts, abscesses) from focal lesions composed of solid tissue. Cystic lesions are more readily resolved (1 cm) than solid lesions (2 cm) and are more likely to be benign cysts or abscesses. Recent advances in sonography have improved its sensitivity, and minimal dilatation of the biliary tree can now be detected in adults. The normal or narrow bile ducts of infants are more difficult to display, but a choledochal cyst should be readily detected. Enlargement of the portal and splenic veins can also be demonstrated if there is significant increase in portal pressure. Diffuse hepatocellular changes cannot be distinguished from normal liver parenchyma, and tissue-transmitted sounds are similar for fat and interlobular collagen. Sonographic evidence of cirrhosis, however, includes diminution in liver size, dilatation of the portal venous system, and splenomegaly.

Computerized Axial Tomography (CAT) Scanning

Ultrasonic and CAT scanning have similar applications in clinical cross-sectional organ imaging. The CAT scan technique for liver evaluation gives superior image resolution of structural anomalies. However, because of the requirement for infant sedation, the potential hazard of ionizing radiation, and the high cost of the procedure, it is not regularly utilized unless other screening tests inconclusively define the liver abnormality.

Cholangiography

Intravenous cholangiography employing iodipamide (Cholegrafin) can be used to demonstrate the intrahepatic and extrahepatic biliary tree. However, the bile ducts are poorly visualized in infants because of their small caliber, especially if the serum bilirubin is greater than 6 mg per dl. Also, this method of investigation is not generally used in infants and children because the contrast agent can produce hypotension and renal damage when there is significant liver dysfunction. *Percutaneous transhepatic cholangiography* can now be performed with a fine-caliber (0.7-mm OD) Chiba needle, but there is little experience with this technique in infants who require anesthesia and respiratory control.[36a] After percutaneous hepatic puncture, contrast material is injected under fluoroscopic guidance. When bile ducts are entered, the contrast flows hepatofugally toward the main hepatic duct; dye in the duodenum excludes biliary obstruction. In adults, a high rate of bile duct opacification is reported. Small or normal ducts can be visualized in over 60 per cent of patients with jaundice due to intrahepatic disease and in 100 per cent of adult patients with dilated ducts secondary to obstruction. Transhepatic cholangiography is attended by certain risks, especially bile leakage and bleeding, which require prompt surgical intervention. Bacteremia is also a frequent complication; hence antibiotic prophylaxis is a routine recommendation. The introduction of contrast material by endoscopic cannulation of the papilla of Vater under direct vision (*endoscopic retrograde choledochopancreatography, or ERCP*) is another well-established technique in adults, but suitable fiberoptic instruments are not yet available for the evaluation of infants. Finally, when the accumulation of clinical and investigative data suggests complete biliary obstruction, *operative cholangiography* is essential for making a precise anatomic diagnosis.

Percutaneous Liver Biopsy

The percutaneous liver biopsy, utilizing a Menghini or Klatskin needle, has been established as a safe procedure in infants and children.[23a, 34c, 50a] Ultrasonic scanning prior to needle biopsy may be necessary to aid in accurately localizing a small liver or identifying focal lesions (e.g., cyst, abscess, angioma, tumor) that contraindicate close percutaneous biopsy. Other contraindications for this biopsy technique include coagulation abnormalities and the presence of ascites. In general, the liver biopsy is important for the accurate diagnosis and assessment of infants and children with persistent or recurrent direct hyperbilirubinemia, acute or chronic hepatomegaly, and chronic liver disease. Knowledge of the liver histology may serve as a guide to treatment and management and may aid in determining prognosis. In addition to light microscopy, comprehensive evaluation of the biopsy specimen may include electron microscopy for organelle pathology, histochemical and enzymatic analysis to facilitate the diagnosis of storage disease and enzyme deficiency, culture for detection of an infectious agent, and immunofluorescence studies for identification of specific antigens. Despite its obvious value, needle biopsy of the liver is associated with a significant risk. Complications such as intraperitoneal hemorrhage,

bile peritonitis, and pneumothorax are rare, however, as long as contraindications are carefully observed and the procedure is skillfully performed. When the percutaneous technique is unsafe, consideration should be given to an operative (open) or peritoneoscopic liver biopsy.

REFERENCES

1. Abelev, G. I.: AFP in oncogenesis and its association with malignant tumors. Adv. Cancer Res. *14*:295, 1971.
1a. Anderson, H., Pederson, L., Svendsen, K., Peters, N., Kilstrup, M., and Thayson, E.: The diagnostic value of liver scanning. Scand. J. Gastroenterol. 2:241, 1976.
1b. Andres, J. M., Lilly, J. R., Altman, R. P., Walker, W. A., and Alpert, E.: Alpha-1-fetoprotein in neonatal hepatobiliary disease. J. Pediatr. *91*:217, 1977.
2. Andres, J. M., Mathis, R. K., and Walker, W. A.: Liver disease in infants. I. Developmental hepatology and mechanisms of liver dysfunction. J. Pediatr. *90*:686, 1977.
3. Arey, L. B.: The digestive tube and associated glands. *In* Arey, L. B. (ed.): Developmental Anatomy. Ed. 7. Philadelphia, W. B. Saunders Company, 1974, pp. 245–262.
4. Bloom, W.: The embryogenesis of human bile capillaries and ducts. Am. J. Anat. *36*:451, 1926.
4a. Boone, D. J., Routh, J. I., and Schranta, R.: Gamma-glutamyl transpeptidase and 5′-nucleotidase: Comparison as diagnostic for hepatic disease. Am. J. Clin. Pathol. *61*:321, 1974.
5. Brodersen, R., and Hermann, L. S.: Intestinal reabsorption of unconjugated bilirubin: A possible contributing factor in neonatal jaundice. Lancet *1*:1242, 1963.
6. Brown, A. K., and Zuelzer, W. W.: Studies on the neonatal development of the glucuronide conjugation system. J. Clin. Invest. 37:332, 1958.
7. Burke, M. D.: Liver function. Hum. Pathol. 6:273, 1975.
8. Davidson, L. T., Marritt, K. K., and Weech, A. A.: Hyperbilirubinemia in the newborn. Am. J. Dis. Child. *61*:958, 1941.
8a. Dawkins, P. L., and Joska, R. A.: Immunoglobulin deposition in liver of patients with active chronic hepatitis and antibody against smooth muscle. Br. Med. J. 2:643, 1973.
9. Deligorgis, D., Yannakas, D., and Doxiadis, S.: Normal size of liver in infancy and childhood. Arch. Dis. Child. 48:790, 1973.
10. Deo, M. G., Bhan, I. L., and Ramalingaswami, V.: Influence of dietary protein deficiency on phagocytic activity of reticuloendothelial cells. J. Pathol. *109*:215, 1973.

11. Dumont, A. E.: Liver lymph. *In* Becker, F. F. (ed.): The Liver: Normal and Abnormal Functions: Part I. New York, Marcel Dekker, Inc., 1974, pp. 55–68.

12. Dutton, G. J.: The biosynthesis of glucuronides. *In* Dutton, G. J. (ed.): Glucuronic Acid. New York, Academic Press, 1966, p. 185.

13. Erlinger, S., and Dhumeaux, D.: Mechanisms and control of secretion of bile, water, and electrolytes. Gastroenterology 66:281, 1974.

14. Felig, P., Brown, W. V., Levine, R. A., and Klatskin, G.: Glucose homeostasis in viral hepatitis. N. Engl. J. Med. 283:1436, 1970.

14a. Ferrucci, J. T.: Body ultrasonography. N. Engl. J. Med. 300:590, 1979.

15. Finne, P. H., and Halvosen, S.: Regulation of erythropoiesis in the fetus and newborn. Arch. Dis. Child. 47:683, 1972.

16. Friedman, M., Beyers, S. O., and Omoto, C.: Some characteristics of hepatic lymph in the intact rat. Am. J. Physiol. *184*:11, 1956.

17. Gartner, L. M., and Arias, I. M.: Formation, transport, metabolism and excretion of bilirubin. N. Engl. J. Med. 280:1339, 1969.

18. Gartner, L. M., Snyder, R. N., Chabon, R. S., and Bernstein, J.: Kernicterus: High incidence in premature infants with low serum bilirubin concentration. Pediatrics 45:906, 1970.

19. Gennser, G., Lundquist, I., and Nilsson, E.: Glycogenolytic activity in the liver of the human fetus. Biol. Neonate *19*:1, 1971.

20. Ghosh, M. L., and Emery, J. L.: The connective tissue in livers of children. J. Clin. Pathol. 23:599, 1970.

21. Gitlin, D., and Biosucci, A.: Development of gamma G, gamma A, gamma M BIC, BIA, C'1 esterase inhibitor, ceruloplasmin, transferrin, hemopexin, haptoglobin, fibrinogen, plasminogen, alpha-1-antitrypsin, orosomucoid, B lipoprotein, alpha$_2$ macroglobulin and prealbumin in the conceptus. J. Clin. Invest. 48:1433, 1969.

22. Gitlin, D., Perricelli, A., and Gitlin, G. M.: Synthesis of alpha-fetoprotein by liver, yolk sac and gastrointestinal tract of the human conceptus. Cancer Res. 32:979, 1972.

22a. Hacki, W., Bircher, J., and Preisig, R.: A new look at plasma disappearance of sulfobromophthalein (BSP): Correlation with the BSP transport maximum and the hepatic plasma flow in man. J. Lab. Clin. Med. 88:1019, 1976.

23. Hardy, J. B., and Peeples, M. D.: Serum bilirubin levels in newborn infants. Distribution and association with neurological abnormalities during the first year of life. Johns Hopkins Med. J. *128*:265, 1971.

23a. Hong, R., Schubert, W. K.: Menghini needle biopsy and the liver. Am. J. Dis. Child. *100*:42, 1960.

24. Javitt, N. B.: The cholestatic syndrome. Am. J. Med. *51*:637, 1971.

25. Javitt, N. B.: Bile salts and liver disease in childhood. Postgrad. Med. J. *50*:354, 1974.

26. Javitt, N. B., Keating, J. P., Grand, R. J., and Harris, R. C.: Serum bile acid patterns in neonatal hepatitis and extrahepatic biliary atresia. J. Pediatr. *90*:736, 1977.

27. Javitt, N. B., Morrissey, K., and Siegel, E.: Cholestatic syndrome in infancy: Diagnostic value of serum bile acid pattern and response to cholestyramine. Pediatr. Res. 7:119, 1973.

28. Jones, A. L., and Mills, E. S.: The liver and gallbladder. *In* Greep, R. O., and Weiss, L. (eds.): Histology. Ed. 3. New York, McGraw Hill Book Company, 1974, pp. 599–644.

28a. Kaplan, M. M.: Alkaline phosphatase. Gastroenterology 62:452, 1972.

29. Kekomaki, M., Seppala, M., Einholm, C. C., Schwartz, A. L., and Raivio, K.: Perfusion of isolated human fetal liver: Synthesis and release of AFP and albumin. Int. J. Cancer 8:250, 1971.

30. Korman, M. G., Hofmann, A. F., and Summerskill, W. H. J.: Assessment of activity in chronic active liver disease. Serum bile acids compared with conventional tests and histology. N. Engl. J. Med. 290:1399, 1974.

30a. Kumar, B., Coleman, R. E., and Alderson, P. O.: Gallium citrate Ga-67 imaging in patients with suspected inflammatory processes. Arch. Surg. *110*:1237, 1975.

31. Lawson, E. E., Grand, R. J., Neff, R. K., and Cohen, L. F.: Clinical estimation of liver span in infants and children. Am. J. Dis. Child. *132*:474, 1978.

32. Lemperle, G., Herdter, F., and Gaspos, F.: The stimulating or depressing effect of various drugs on the phagocytic function of the RES. Adv. Exp. Med. Biol. *15*:87, 1971.

33. Lester, R., Behrmann, E., and Lucey, J. G.: Transfer of bilirubin C^{14} across monkey placenta. Pediatrics 32:416, 1963.

34. Levi, A., Gatmaitan, Z., and Arias, I. M.: Deficiency of hepatic organic anion-binding protein, impaired anion uptake by liver and "physiologic" jaundice in newborn monkeys. N. Engl. J. Med. 283:1136, 1970.

34a. Losowsky, M. S., Simmons, A. V., and Miloszewski, K.: Coagulation abnormalities in liver disease. Postgrad. Med. 53:147, 1973.

34b. Maisels, M. J.: Jaundice in the newborn. Pediatr. Rev. 3:305, 1982.

34c. Menghini, G., Lauro, G., and Caraceni, M.: Some innovations in the technic of the one-second needle biopsy of the liver. Am. J. Gastroenterol. *64*:175, 1975.

35. Meyer, W. W., and Lind, J.: Postnatal changes in portal circulation. Arch. Dis. Child. *41*:606, 1966.

36. Odell, G. B.: Neonatal jaundice. *In* Popper, H., and Schaffner, F. (eds.): Progress in Liver Disease. New York, Grune & Stratton, 1976, pp. 457–475.

36a. Okuda, K., Tanikawa, K., Emura, T., and Kuratami, S.: Nonsurgical percutaneous transhepatic cholangiography: Diagnostic significance in medical problems of the liver. Am. J. Dig. Dis. *19*:21, 1974.

36b. Paronetto, F.: Immunologic aspects of liver disease. Postgrad. Med. 53:156, 1973.

36c. Paronetto, F., Vernace, S. J., and Colombo, M.: Further studies on the cytotoxic activity of lymphocytes against liver cells in patients with chronic hepatitis. Gastroenterology 68:965, 1975.

37. Poland, R. O., and Odell, G. B.: Physiologic jaundice: The enterohepatic circulation of bilirubin. N. Engl. J. Med. *284*:1, 1971.

38. Poley, J. R., Dower, J. C., Owen, C. A., and Stickler, G. B.: Bile acids in infants and children. J. Lab. Clin. Med. *63*:838, 1964.

39. Remmer, H., and Bock, K. W.: The role of the liver in drug metabolism. *In* Schaffner, F., Sherlock, S., and Leevy, C. M. (eds.): The Liver and its Disease. New York, Intercontinental Medical Book Corporation, 1974, pp. 34–42.

39a. Riely, C. A., Caride, V. J., Lange, R. C., Gottschalk, A., and Klakskin, G.: The use of ^{99m}Tc-HIDA in evaluating pediatric liver disease. Gastroenterology *75*:983, 1978.

40. Roux, J., Grigorian, A., and Tokeda, Y.: In vitro 'lipid' metabolism in the developing human fetus. Nature *216*:819, 1967.

41. Royshahti, E., and Terry, W. D.: Alpha-fetoprotein and serum albumin show sequence homology. Nature *260*:804, 1976.

42. Scheig, R., and Gryboski, J. D.: The liver. *In* Gryboski, J.: Gastrointestinal Problems in the Infant. Philadelphia, W. B. Saunders Company, 1975, p. 311.

43. Sereni, F., Mandelli, M., Principi, N., Togoni, G., Pardi, G., and Morselli, P. L.: Induction of drug metabolizing enzyme activities in the human fetus and in the newborn infant. Enzyme *15*:318, 1973.

43a. Sharp, H. L., Krivit, W., and Lowman, J. T.: The diagnosis of complete extrahepatic obstruction by ^{131}I-rose bengal. J. Pediatr. *70*:46, 1967.

44. Skrede, S., Blomhoff, J. P., Elgjo, K., and Gjone, E.: Biochemical tests in the evaluation of liver function. Scand. J. Gastroenterol. *8*:37, 1973.

45. Souhami, R. I., and Bradfield, J. W. B.: The recovery of hepatic phagocytosis after blockage of Kupffer cells. J. Reticuloendothel. Soc. *16*:75, 1974.

45a. Sty, J. R., Babbitt, D. P., Boedecker, R. A., and Thompson, R. T.: ^{99m}Tc-PIPIDA biliary imaging in children. Clin. Nucl. Med. *4*:315, 1979.

46. Tandon, B. N., Ramanjan, R. A., and Tandon, H. D.: Liver injury in protein-calorie malnutrition. An electron microscopic study. Am. J. Clin. Nutr. *27*:550, 1974.

46a. Taylor, K. J. W., and Rosenfield, A. T.: Greyscale ultrasonography in the differential diagnosis of jaundice. Arch. Surg. *112*:820, 1977.

47. Tenhunen, R., Marver, H. S., and Schmid, R.: Microsomal heme oxygenase: Characterization of the enzyme. J. Biol. Chem. *244*:6388, 1969.

48. Thomas, H. C., Ryan, J., Benjamin, I. S., Blumgart, L. H., and MacSween, R. N. M.: The immune response in cirrhotic rats: the induction of tolerance to orally administered antigens. Gastroenterology *71*:114, 1976.

49. Van Furth, R., and Cohn, Z. A.: The origin and kinetics of mononuclear phagocytes. J. Exp. Med. *128*:415, 1968.

50. Walker, W. A., and Isselbacher, K. J.: Uptake and transport of macromolecules by the intestine: Possible role in clinical disorders. Gastroenterology *67*:531, 1974.

50a. Walker, W. A., Krivit, W., and Sharp, H. L.: Needle biopsy of the liver in infancy and childhood. Pediatrics *40*:946, 1967.

51. Walker, W. A., and Mathis, R. K.: Hepatomegaly: An approach to the differential diagnosis. Pediatr. Clin. North Am. *22*:929, 1975.

52. Watkins, J. B., Szczepanik, P., Gould, J. B., Klein, P., and Lester, R.: Bile salt metabolism in the human premature infant. Gastroenterology *69*:706, 1975.

53. Weibel, E., Straubl, W., Gnagi, H., and Hess, F.: Correlated morphometric and biochemical studies on the liver cell. J. Cell Biol. *42*:68, 1969.

54. Wilson, J. W., Groat, C. S., and Leduc, E. H.: Histogenesis of the liver. Ann. N.Y. Acad. Sci. *111*:8, 1963.

55. Wiznitzer, T., Better, N., and Rachlin, W.: In vivo detoxification of endotoxin by the reticuloendothelial system. J. Exp. Med. *112*:1157, 1960.

56. Wright, K., and Christie, D. L.: Use of γ-glutamyl transpeptidase in the diagnosis of biliary atresia. Am. J. Dis. Child. *135*:134, 1981.

57. Yaffe, S. J., Rane, A., Sjoqvist, F., Boreus, L. O., and Orrenius, S.: The presence of a monooxygenase system in human fetal liver microsomes. Life Sci. *9*:1189, 1970.

57a. Yeung, C. Y.: Serum 5′-nucleotidase in neonatal hepatitis and biliary atresia: Preliminary observations. Pediatrics *50*:812, 1972.

58. Younoszai, M. K., and Mueller, S.: Clinical assessment of liver size in normal children. Clin. Pediatr. *14*:378, 1975.

Chapter Seven

GASTROINTESTINAL BLEEDING

Significant gastrointestinal hemorrhage is one of the most serious emergencies in any age group, with blood losses from hematemesis being more severe than those from rectal bleeding.[114] Occasionally, blood swallowed by the infant during nursing by a mother with nipple fissures, or blood swallowed during a nosebleed, may be vomited to simulate upper gastrointestinal hemorrhage. A more unusual event in the older child is the vomiting of colored fruit-flavored drinks, which may simulate blood.

Upper gastrointestinal bleeding and hematemesis originate from lesions above the ligament of Treitz, with fresh blood appearing red and that which has remained in the stomach long enough to be converted to hematin appearing dark brown with the consistency of coffee grounds. Melena signifies dark, tarry stools that contain occult blood and denotes bleeding from the upper gastrointestinal tract or small bowel. However, infants with relatively rapid intestinal transit or any child with major bleeding in which blood exerts a laxative effect may pass bright red blood per rectum. Red-colored cereals and tomato skins may resemble flecks or spots of fresh blood in the stool, whereas dark chocolate, blueberries, grape juice, iron, and Pepto-Bismol give the stools a black appearance. Therefore, the importance of chemical testing of stools for blood cannot be overemphasized.

Lower gastrointestinal bleeding occurs from sites below the ligament of Treitz and usually from the distal small bowel and colon. Depending upon the site of the lesion and rapidity of transit it is signaled as either melena or hematochezia.

UPPER GASTROINTESTINAL BLEEDING

In the neonate the diagnostic considerations are largely influenced by the events of delivery. Hematemesis or melena within the first 24 hours of life is most often due to ingested maternal blood. Of 155 instances of neonatal bleeding, one third were due to ingested maternal blood. This is easily confirmed by the Apt test, which measures reduced fetal hemoglobin.[9] One part of gastric contents or stool is mixed with five to ten parts of water in a test tube, and these are centrifuged. The supernatant is separated, and to it is added 1 ml of 0.25 M (1 per cent) NaOH. After two to five minutes, adult hemoglobin produces a brown, and fetal hemoglobin a pink, color. If only a diaper is available for study, water and NaOH are added to it and the examination proceeds as above. Caution must be used in interpreting results when the specimen contains hematin (brown aspirate or black stools) or when the gastric acidity is 3.9 or less.[119a]

Hemorrhagic disease of the newborn is

Table 7–1 Causes of Upper
Gastrointestinal Bleeding

Esophagus	Varices
	Esophagitis
	Mallory-Weiss tear
	Duplication cyst
Stomach	Gastric erosions
	Ulcer
	Duplication cyst
	Tumor
	Hematoma
Duodenum	Duodenitis
	Duodenal erosions
	Ulcer
	Hemobilia
	Hematoma
Nonspecific	Swallowed maternal blood
	(neonate)
	Swallowed maternal blood from
	breast fissures
	Bleeding disorders
	Nosebleed

suggested by the presence of ecchymoses or petechiae or a history of aspirin,[53] anticonvulsant, or anticoagulant medication administered to the mother shortly before delivery. Stress ulcers (usually gastric) or gastric erosions are associated with anoxia, infection, or other perinatal insults and are the most frequent cause of true bleeding, as noted in Tables 7–1 and 7–2. Other lesions identified by endoscopy have been duodenal ulcer, tumor,[24] duodenitis, esophageal tear, and esophagitis (Table 7–2).[27, 30, 130, 131]

In the older infant, esophageal varices have contributed to the causes of upper gastrointestinal bleeding. Although it is unusual for varices to bleed before four to five years of age, they were associated in our patients with either intrauterine cytomegalovirus infection or portal vein thrombosis.

Diagnosis. The history is helpful in determining whether the bleed is intermittent or constant and whether the infant has had an associated illness or has been given medications associated with gastrointestinal irritation.[81] The family history should be studied for telangiectasias, ulcer disease, bleeding disorders, and gastrointestinal bleeding. Preceding feeding problems or vomiting indicate esophagitis or a Mallory-Weiss tear. The physical examination, although often unremarkable, may identify cutaneous lesions associated with gastrointestinal bleeding, such as hemangiomas or telangiectasia, or a gastric mass suggesting tumor. Hepatomegaly or splenomegaly indicates portal hypertension. Evidence of trauma should initiate a search for intestinal hematoma or hemobilia.

A positive nasogastric aspirate correlates well with a lesion above the ligament of Treitz; this should be the first diagnostic procedure in any type of gastrointestinal bleeding.[96a]

Before the advent of endoscopy, a lesion was not identified in one third to one half of older children and in even fewer infants with gastrointestinal bleeding. Superficial ulcerations and erosions are not visualized by conventional radiologic studies. Double-contrast techniques are now being refined to the point at which erosions can be demonstrated. These studies, however, are difficult to perform in the acutely ill child. Endoscopy may be performed even in the neonate by a trained endoscopist and is successful in identifying a lesion in 41 to 95 per cent of patients.[6, 7, 22, 25, 30, 31, 56, 59, 61, 91, 95, 165, 182] Failures to define a site of bleeding are due either to massive bleeding, which may obscure an ulcer crater, or to localization of the lesion below the site of visualization of the endoscope. Very small infants carry the risk of airway obstruction due to instrument compression of the trachea and are best examined under general anesthesia, during which an adequate airway is guaranteed. Older infants may be examined using sedation of 0.1 mg per kg of atropine, 0.05 to 1 mg per kg of Demerol, and 0.05 to 1 mg per kg of diazepam immediately before the procedure. The most frequently used endoscopes are the GIF P_1 with a shaft diameter of 7.2 mm and its P_2 modification with a diameter of 8.6 mm. Although larger, the P_2 unit may be used in most infants and has the advantage of four-way maneuverability, in contrast to its counterpart, which is bidirectional.

In older infants and children, bleeding from esophagitis has been related to known gastroesophageal reflux, to pyloric stenosis,[161] and to orthopedic procedures asso-

Table 7-2 Source of Upper Gastrointestinal Bleeding Determined by Endoscopy [6, 7, 25, 30, 61]

Age	Number of Patients	Duodenal Ulcer	Duodenitis	Gastric Ulcer	Gastric Erosions	Esophagitis	Esophageal Tear	Esophageal Varices
0–1 yr.	25	6	1	1	9	4		
1–2 yr.	17	1	2	4	3	2	1	2°

°One intrauterine CMV infection
One portal vein thrombosis

ciated with body casting. Half of the older children with esophageal varices bleed from other sites, as from gastric erosions or ulcer. Bleeding is often associated with aspirin ingestion (12 to 25 per cent), steroid therapy (12 per cent), or severe, life-threatening diseases, such as infection, respiratory distress, immune deficiency, central nervous system disease, or bleeding disorders (40 to 75 per cent).[30]

Angiography in the adult has been developed to the extent that it not only may identify the site of bleeding but also may be used therapeutically through arterial embolization using Gelfoam particles or balloon.[57, 72, 106, 129, 145]

Treatment.   The infant with hematemesis should be placed on his side to prevent aspiration, and bleeding studies should be performed immediately to determine any bleeding disorder. Rapid replacement of fluid volume is initiated with normal saline or lactate until colloid or blood is available. The stomach is aspirated and lavaged with ice water or saline, and constant nasogastric suction is applied. After hemostasis has been attained, antacids are administered in small amounts through the tube every half hour. Cold, constant-drip formula has been used successfully by us in the later treatment of some small infants, but care must be taken to intermittently aspirate the stomach to avoid fluid accumulation and vomiting. There are no controlled data to support the efficacy of cimetidine, a histamine receptor antagonist, in children with gastrointestinal bleeding. In adults it has proved effective in those with duodenal ulcer, but in controlled studies of patients with gastric ulcer it has seemed to increase the acute bleed. In adults who are critically ill or septic, cimetidine does not always decrease gastric acidity.

Patients with esophagitis are treated similarly but are placed in a moderately erect position, and the nasogastric tube is removed as soon as hemostasis is achieved. If there is evidence of bile reflux in the esophagus at the time of endoscopy, antacids of the aluminum hydroxide type are given because of their bile acid–binding proper-

ties. The treatment of esophageal varices is discussed in Chapter Eleven.

If bleeding persists or recurs, or if the initial blood loss is calculated to be greater than 85 ml per kg (the infant's total blood volume), immediate surgical intervention is indicated. Embolization has been employed in bleeding varices and in vascular malformations of the vessels supplying the duodenum.[43]

Prognosis.   Most infants and young children tolerate upper gastrointestinal bleeds fairly well. The first bleed from esophageal varices due to extrahepatic portal hypertension is usually not fatal, and that associated with intrahepatic disease is usually controlled by medical management. In 1964, Spencer[160] reported peptic ulceration in 54 infants, 65 per cent of whom expired. A 1969[8] review of gastrointestinal bleeding in 94 neonates failed to identify a lesion in 53 per cent, but all recovered. In our own experience during the last decade, only 3 per cent of infants and young children with upper gastrointestinal bleeding required surgical intervention. As in the series of Cox and Ament,[30] deaths were related to the underlying disease rather than to bleed.

RECTAL BLEEDING

The causes of rectal bleeding differ in the neonate from those of the older infant and child (Table 7–3). During the first few days of life, bleeding is most often due to swallowed maternal blood, confirmed by the Apt test, or to anal fissure, which is best identified by spreading the perineal skin to evert the anal canal. Less frequent are hemorrhagic diseases, intussusception, duplication cysts, Meckel's diverticulum, drug-induced colitis,[50] necrotizing enterocolitis, and gangrenous bowel.[26, 126, 152, 160, 162]

In the older infant and child, blood-streaking of the stool is often due to anal fissures or one of the enteric infections. Blood seen at the end of a stool may be caused by colonic or rectal polyps. Blood and mucus either mixed with stool or alone are often associated with infection, milk or

Table 7-3 Causes of Rectal Bleeding in Order of Frequency

Neonate	6 Weeks-1 Year	1-2 Years
Swallowed maternal blood	Anal fissure	Anal fissure
Anal fissure	Infection	Infection
Gangrenous bowel	Milk or soy allergy	Intussusception[71a]
Infection	Antibiotics	Polyp
Milk allergy	Intussusception	Lymphoid hyperplasia—colon[74]
Antibiotics	Lymphoid hyperplasia—colon	Meckel's diverticulum
Peptic ulcer	Gangrenous bowel	Milk allergy
Meckel's diverticulum[99]	Meckel's diverticulum	Antibiotics
Duplication cyst	Polyp	Hematoma
Intussusception	Hematoma	Arteriovenous malformation
Arteriovenous malformation	Duplication cyst	Colitis
Colitis of immune deficiency	Arteriovenous malformation	Tumor
Tumor	Peptic ulcer	Gastric heterotopia in ileum[25a]
Enterocolitis of Hirschsprung's disease	Foreign body	
	Tumor	
	Gastric heterotopia in ileum	

soy protein allergy, enterocolitis seen in infants with severe immune deficiency, and the hemolytic-uremic syndrome. Large quantities of blood are usually due to Meckel's diverticulum, duplication cyst, or intussusception. The bleeding of ileocolic intussusceptions produces stools that resemble currant jelly; Meckel's diverticulum typically produces alternating bright and dark blood.

There is normally a loss of minute quantities of blood from the gastrointestinal tract, measuring 0.5 to 1.0 ml per day in the adult and 0 to 0.4 ml per day in the infant. With the use of Cr-51 techniques, normal losses have measured as high as 3 ml per day. Approximately 5 ml of blood are required to produce a positive test for occult blood and 25 to 30 ml to produce a melanotic stool in the adult. Anyan and Clarkson,[8] using the orthotoluidine test, found a positive result in 14 per cent of infants examined at six days and in 33 per cent of those examined at six weeks. They postulated that the positive tests represented a milk-allergic reaction or a milk-related iron deficiency state. Woodruff et al.[185] noted guaiac positivity in 52 of 96 stools from infants 2 to 12 months old who were breast-fed or taking commercial infant formula. Foman et al.,[47a] using guaiac, reported 2.9 per cent positivity in stools from infants taking commercial formula and 9.6 per cent in stools from those taking whole cow's milk. Severe anemia and occult blood loss are associated with ingestion of large quantities of fresh cow's milk. Traces of blood are not unusual in stools from infants taking meats, and positive tests often revert to negative after elimination of meat from the diet.[184] In adults, significant meat intake causes 30 to 40 per cent of false positive test results. Of the commercial test materials, Fecatest has been shown to be less sensitive than benzidine and Hematest but more sensitive than Hemoccult I.[5] Since most tests depend upon the prior hemolysis of red blood cells, low-lying lesions may give a false negative test result. False positive findings may also be caused by banana, horseradish, turnips, and tomato skins.

Diagnosis. A description of the color, amount, and location of blood in or on the stool, or without stool, is essential. If blood is streaked along, or at the end of, the stool in an infant with diarrhea or constipation, the most likely cause of bleeding is an anal fissure. If the infant was and is entirely well, one must suspect a polyp. Gradually increasing diarrhea that becomes bloody denotes either infection or milk or soy protein allergy. The sudden onset of colicky pain, bleeding, and shock in a previously well infant suggests intussusception.

An abdominal mass may represent a du-

Table 7–4   Evaluation of Bleeding Disorders

UPPER GASTROINTESTINAL BLEEDING

1. Careful history for bleeding disorders, skin lesions, and aspirin or steroid ingestion
2. Bleeding studies
3. Treat—if no response, endoscopy
4. Upper gastrointestinal radiologic examination with air-contrast
5. If no identifiable lesion is discovered and bleeding has stopped, no further study
6. If bleeding persists or recurs, endoscopy

RECTAL BLEEDING

1. Careful history for bleeding disorders, skin lesions, and aspirin or steroid ingestion
2. Bleeding studies
3. Sigmoidoscopy
4. If no lesion identified:

Mild bleeding	*Severe*
Barium enema with air-contrast	Use Tc-labeled red cell study
Small bowel examination	to define site
Meckel's scan if above negative	Surgical exploration

plication cyst, intussusception, or, rarely, tumor. Emptiness of the right lower quadrant, on the other hand, is a typical finding in ileocolic intussusception. Palpation of the rectum may reveal a low-lying polyp or a pelvic mass of intussusception. Sigmoidoscopy will differentiate mucosal disease from bleeding lesions above the field of vision of the instrument and may define a sigmoid or rectal polyp. An aspirate of gastric contents must be examined for blood to rule out upper gastrointestinal hemorrhage as the origin of the rectal bleed. A plain film of the chest and abdomen may demonstrate large duplications, obstruction, or pneumoperitoneum. A barium enema will define an intussusception, abnormalities of rotation, or duplications. An air-contrast study is best for identification of polypoid lesions. Small bowel lesions, such as Meckel's diverticulum, vascular malformations, or polyps, are difficult to identify by radiologic means.

Isotope techniques using technetium-labeled red blood cells are helpful in identifying the site of a significant bleed, and in some instances arteriography is of value. The isotope techniques using T_c-99m sulfur colloid are certainly less complicated than, and considered by some superior to, angiography.[5a]

Treatment. The treatment consists of immediate replacement of fluid and blood and aspiration of the stomach. If there has been a history of chronic diarrhea or of prolonged use of antibiotics or milk-substitute formulas, intramuscular vitamin K is administered immediately after blood is obtained for cross matching, bleeding and clotting studies, and urea nitrogen and electrolyte determinations. Identified lesions are treated as discussed separately in the text.

The clinical evaluation for upper gastrointestinal and rectal bleeding is presented in Table 7–4.

HEMORRHAGIC DISORDERS

Gastrointestinal bleeding during the first two years of life often remains unexplained, even after extensive evaluation and surgical exploration. Fortunately, the majority of infants with negative findings at laparotomy have no further episodes of bleeding on subsequent evaluation. Patients with thrombocytopenia experience gastrointestinal mucosal bleeding only when the platelet count is reduced to several thousand or less.[148]

Children with hereditary coagulation factor deficiencies seldom bleed spontaneously unless an underlying lesion is present, although occasional cases with melena or hematemesis have been reported. The acquired coagulation disorder in the child with hepatic dysfunction is usually overshadowed by other manifestations of liver disease, leaving little problem in diagnosis. However, sudden, overwhelming hepatic failure has resulted in intestinal bleeding in the absence of jaundice or hepatomegaly.

A number of clinical entities must be considered in the child with unexplained gastrointestinal hemorrhage in whom no anatomic defect can be demonstrated. Some of these disorders are transient and are diagnosed only by the thorough and highly suspicious clinician.

Disseminated intravascular coagulation can present as massive gastrointestinal bleeding and may result from septicemia and endotoxic shock caused by enteric organisms, from bacterial, fungal, or viral infections, or from pancreatitis, giant hemangiomas, or malignancy.[76] This intravascular clotting is characteristically associated with decreased coagulation factors and increased plasma digestion products of fibrinogen and fibrin, although the exact mechanisms that initiate it are not fully understood. There is prolongation of the partial thromboplastin time owing to decrease of factors II, V, VII, VIII, and X and prolongation of the prothrombin time owing to decrease of factor VII. Platelet levels are usually low. Fibrin split products, as measured by the protamine sulfate dilution test or tanned red cell hemagglutination-inhibition assay, are increased. Unfortunately, in the early stages, clotting factors may be normal if their rate of production is equal to their rate of loss. Platelets are sometimes not reduced until the process has become well established. Kisker and Bush[76] therefore advocate measurement of circulating fibrin as a more sensitive indicator of active intravascular coagulation. Hemolytic anemia with fragmented erythrocytes may occur as a result of cellular mechanical destruction by fibrin strands.

Submucosal edema in the small and large bowel is seen in flat films of the abdomen, and radiologic examination with barium shows a characteristic deep thumbprint pattern. Once the diagnosis is established by the appropriate laboratory studies, heparinization is the treatment of choice. An initial dose of 50 units per kilogram is administered intravenously, and daily doses (given every six hours) are titrated to keep the clotting time greater than 20 minutes. In bacterial infections responding to antibiotic therapy, the clotting improves within 12 hours or so, but in viral infections the disease can persist for longer periods.

VITAMIN K DEFICIENCY

In 1935 Henrik Dam observed that a bleeding disease in chickens could be rapidly alleviated by feeding the birds a fat-soluble substance that he named vitamin K (Koagulation vitamin).[33] Vitamin K is now known to be a requirement for the hepatic biosynthesis of four coagulation factors, prothrombin (factor II), proconvertin (factor VII), plasma thromboplastin component (factor IX), and Stuart-Prower factor (factor X).[34]

Deficiency of vitamin K results in the most commonly acquired abnormality of the coagulation mechanism and is most frequently seen in the newborn period.[1-3] The term "hemorrhagic disease of the newborn" refers to a generalized, self-limited bleeding disorder resulting from a transient depression of the vitamin K–dependent clotting factors. At birth, the normal full-term infant has from 20 to 70 per cent of adult levels of these factors. The values are depressed even further in the premature infant and reach their nadir during the first two to three days of life. As little as $25 \mu g$ of vitamin K protects term infants from development of a prolonged prothrombin time. The response of the small premature infant is less predictable, probably because of hepatic immaturity. Since human milk has only one fourth the concentration of vitamin K of cow's milk, breast feeding has been implicated in hemorrhagic disease of the newborn.[32] It has been reported that bleeding episodes occurred twice as often in breast-fed infants receiving no supplementary vitamin K as in infants receiving cow's milk and no supplementary vitamin K. Synthetic formulas that alter enteric flora or have low concentrations of vitamin K have also been implicated.

Hemorrhage most commonly occurs on the second or third day of life. Hematemesis, melena, epistaxis, and profuse hemorrhage under the skin are the most common manifestations. There may be prolonged oozing from venipuncture sites or the umbilical cord. Death from exsanguination or central nervous system bleeding may occur.

Infants with hemorrhagic disease of the newborn respond dramatically to 1 mg of vitamin K, given either intramuscularly or intravenously, with a rise in clotting factors in three to four hours and correction of the prothrombin time in 24 hours. Under life-threatening circumstances, immediate correction can be achieved by the administration of 10 to 15 ml per kg of fresh plasma or one of the commerically prepared concentrates containing all of the vitamin K–dependent factors. This disorder can be effectively prevented by prophylactically treating all newborn infants with 0.5 to 1 mg of vitamin K parenterally as recommended by the American Academy of Pediatrics Committee on Nutrition.

Under certain circumstances, dietary vitamin K deficiency and hemorrhage have been reported in infants beyond the neonatal period. Bleeding has occurred in breast-fed infants who had not received prophylactic vitamin K and in infants with diarrhea being given antibiotics and special formulae with low concentrations of vitamin K. Observations in adults suggest that antibiotics play a minor role in causing vitamin K deficiency because significant vitamin K absorption from the colon does not occur. However, Aballi and coworkers[1] have demonstrated that vitamin K is readily absorbed from the colon of infants, suggesting that antibiotics may play an important role in causing a deficiency in the young child.

Hypoprothrombinemic bleeding has occurred in infants with significant fat malabsorption and occasionally has been the presenting symptom in children with cystic fibrosis during the first year of life. The American Academy of Pediatrics Committee on Nutritrion has recommended supplementing the diets of patients with fat malabsorption with 50 to 100 μg of water-soluble

vitamin K_1 each day, or giving 1 mg of vitamin K_1 parenterally once a month if oral feeding is impractical. It is also recommended that milk-substitute formulae contain 100 μg per liter of vitamin K_1 because these products are often used to treat conditions associated with malabsorption of this vitamin.

VON WILLEBRAND'S DISEASE

In 1926 Erik von Willebrand first described a familial hemorrhagic disorder in inhabitants of the Finnish Aland Islands.[176] Subsequent investigators have demonstrated low plasma factor VIII levels and abnormal platelet adhesiveness in patients with this disease. The disorder is inherited in an autosomal dominant manner, but, unlike other clotting disorders, the degree of the defect observed clinically or measured by laboratory tests varies considerably among affected members of the same family. Bleeding is mainly from the mucous membranes and gums and into the skin. Hemorrhage from the gastrointestinal tract occurs more commonly in this disorder than in other inherited hemorrhagic diseases and occasionally can be the presenting clinical symptom.

The response of the factor VIII levels of these patients to infusions of plasma or cryoprecipitate is unusual. There is an immediate increase in factor VIII activity, as occurs in patients with classic hemophilia, but this is followed by a continued increase due to the patient's own production of the coagulation factor for 20 to 30 hours. The factor that stimulates production of factor VIII in patients with von Willebrand's disease is also present in the plasma of persons with classic hemophilia.

The typical patient with von Willebrand's disease has a prolonged bleeding time, a level of factor VIII of less than 50 per cent, abnormal platelet adhesion to glass beads, and a family history of an autosomal dominant bleeding disorder. However, the laboratory abnormalities may vary from time to time in the same person, sometimes necessitating repeated testing and making the diagnosis difficult. Some investigators believe that the patient's factor VIII response to transfusion is the most important single criterion in establishing a diagnosis.

HEMOLYTIC UREMIC SYNDROME (HUS)

This syndrome exists in varying degrees of severity and is characterized by the triad of microangiopathic hemolytic anemia, thrombocytopenia, and renal failure. Ischemic colitis was not actually recognized as a major symptom until the early 1970's, 15 years after its original description. Indeed, the initial presenting symptom in young children may be rectal bleeding[170] in conjunction with an inappropriately low hematocrit and without evidence of renal disease.[39, 155, 158]

A milder form of the disease is reported from the Netherlands and California, areas where the disease has been endemic or epidemic. Patients are usually older (average of four years) and have a prodrome of diarrhea. Uremia is not a constant finding, and patients not oligemic tend to survive with total recovery. Even oligemic or anuric patients have an excellent outlook for recovery (94 to 99 per cent) if their disease does not persist beyond two weeks. Residual renal disease is likely (43 to 57 per cent) if oliguria or anemia is of longer than two weeks' duration. In families, twins are often affected and other members have the onset greater than one month apart.[41, 71]

In patients from Argentina and in sporadic cases in this country, the average age is one year, prodromal gastroenteritis is mild, and the number of patients who are oliguric or anuric for greater than 21 days is increased (29 per cent). The residual chronic renal failure rate is 21 to 24 per cent. When family members are affected, the onset of disease is more than one year apart.[75] Mortality rates in this familial form are as high as 68 per cent.[173, 175]

Incidence. Well over 1000 cases have been reported in the literature.

Etiology. The etiology is unknown. In Holland and the midwestern United States,

peak incidences are in May and June, whereas elsewhere in the United States and in Wales, cases cluster in late summer and autumn, suggesting a viral etiology. Simultaneous microangiopathic hemolytic anemia, thrombocytopenia, and acute nephropathy have been reported in a mother and child.[153]

Increased titers to coxsackievirus B, enterovirus, parainfluenza type 3, and varicella have been reported in one patient. The disease is related to shigellosis, and, recently, neuraminidase-producing microorganisms have been implicated.[151] Immunologic factors may play a role, for several reports have noted decreased B_1C globulin and total serum complement. Antigen-antibody complexes have been observed, and prostacyclin deficiency has been noted.[178] A familial form of the disease has been described in 41 families, affecting 83 siblings. Similar HLA typing has been observed in siblings with HUS and thrombotic thrombocytopenic purpura.[67]

Pathology. The disease is multisystemic, with vasculitis and microthrombi found in small vessels of kidney, lung, heart, gastrointestinal tract, pancreas, brain, and adrenal glands. Ischemia is evident in most organs examined. The kidneys show cortical necrosis as well as eosinophilic thrombi in glomerular capillary lumina and arterioles.[181]

Symptoms. There is often a mild to severe gastroenteritis or an upper respiratory infection lasting for several days to a week. In the form of disease presenting to the gastroenterologist, there is a sudden onset of vomiting, lower gastrointestinal bleeding, abdominal pain, or pallor. Oliguria dévelops in two thirds of patients; and nearly half have hepatomegaly. The hemoglobin may be as low as 5 gm per dl. Up to 50 per cent have seizures.[11] The children are pale, irritable, or lethargic, and the abdomen is diffusely tender to palpation with some rebound tenderness. Bowel sounds are variable. A few patients have rectal prolapse. The diarrhea usually abates with the onset of uremia.

Differential Diagnosis. The symptoms suggest bacterial or ulcerative colitis, or thrombotic thrombocytopenic purpura. The disproportionately low hemoglobin in the presence of a short-term colitis should suggest this disease.

Diagnosis. Immediate examination of a peripheral smear for microangiopathic red blood cell morphology (helmet cells and schistocytes) will support or rule out the diagnosis. The white blood cell count is increased, with a predominance of polymorphonuclear leukocytes. Although urinalyses are normal in the majority of patients, renal disease is not always evident early. The bilirubin may or may not be increased early, and the Coombs test is negative. Eighty per cent have platelet counts of less than 150,000 per cu mm. The blood urea nitrogen may not rise for several days. Sigmoidoscopy shows an actively bleeding, friable mucosa, and a few patients have a pseudomembrane. Barium enema shows typical thumbprinting of the colon, with irritability and spasm. Results of liver function tests, particularly the SGOT, are abnormal in the majority of patients, probably reflecting focal hepatitis. Barium enema shows edema of the bowel wall and, rarely, dilatation of the transverse colon.

Treatment. Treatment is in large part symptomatic, with blood and electrolyte replacement. Oliguria may initially be mistaken for dehydration. Early dialysis for renal failure decreases morbidity and mortality. The use of heparin is still controversial, as is the use of drugs such as aspirin and dipyridamole to inhibit abnormal platelet function.[110, 117] Colitic symptoms usually subside within a week. Nephrectomy and renal transplantation have been used for an infant with the familial syndrome.[121]

Complications. Immediate gastrointestinal complications are intussusception, segmental colonic gangrene,[142, 149] perforation, and toxic megacolon. The major late complication is ischemic stricture[142] in the splenic flexure or descending colon; another is cholelithiasis.[150, 174]

HENOCH-SCHÖNLEIN SYNDROME

Henoch-Schönlein syndrome is a common childhood disorder of unknown etiolo-

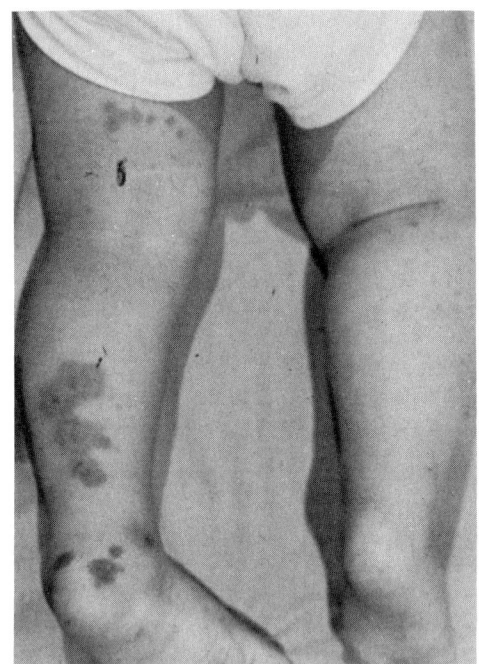

Figure 7–1 Henoch-Schönlein syndrome with urticarial skin lesions.

gy associated with a widespread vasculitis. There is often involvement of the gastrointestinal tract, kidneys, joints, and skin. The rash usually is urticarial initially (Fig. 7–1), followed by maculopapular lesions, often with ecchymoses and petechiae. The buttocks and lower extremities are most commonly involved. Lesions occasionally may be present on the upper extremities and face but seldom appear on the trunk. Edema of the periorbital area, scalp, and backs of the hands and feet is common and may be painful, especially in the younger patient.[138]

Periarticular pain and swelling without erythema occur in about two thirds of the children. The larger joints, particularly the knees, ankles, and elbows, are usually involved. The joint manifestations are transient and nonmigratory and leave no residual damage.

Evidence of renal disease with gross or microscopic hematuria and proteinuria is seen in approximately 40 per cent of patients. Although most children recover, renal dysfunction occasionally leads to oliguria, azotemia, and death. Biopsy specimens usually reveal a focal proliferative glomerulitis. Streptococcal antibody titers and B₁C globulin levels are no different from those of control subjects of the same age, as opposed to the elevated antibody titers and low B_1C globulin values found in patients with acute poststreptococcal glomerulonephritis. IgA-bearing lymphocytes in peripheral blood increase during the acute stage of the disease and return to normal as the activity subsides. In those who develop nephritis, the level remains increased.[84] Indeed, in certain family members, IgA lymphocytes are increased.

Gastrointestinal symptoms occur in about 70 per cent of patients.[93] The most distressing acute symptoms are colicky abdominal pain, vomiting, melena, and hematemesis. The abdominal pain may be severe enough to suggest an acute surgical problem, resulting in exploratory laparotomy. At surgery the bowel is edematous and hemorrhagic and grossly resembles that of acute regional enteritis. Massive gastrointestinal hemorrhage or intussusception may develop rapidly, sometimes with fatal outcome, necessitating careful observation of the child with visceral involvement. Malabsorption has been documented during the intestinal phase of the disease.[177]

Few radiologic studies of the gastrointestinal tract have been done in patients with Henoch-Shönlein syndrome. Dilatation, widely separated loops of bowel due to edematous intestinal walls, narrowing, loss of normal mucosal pattern, and filling defects appear in the small intestine. The roentgenographic studies revert to normal within a month. Similar radiographic changes may occur in the gastrointestinal tract in other bleeding disorders, such as intestinal lymphoma or regional enteritis.

Although the average duration of symptoms is about four weeks, they may last for as long as two years. Symptoms often recur after a period of apparent recovery. The disease in the child under two years of age is usually milder and accompanied by less severe renal and gastrointestinal involvement than is seen in the older patient.

Laboratory tests are of little use in establishing a diagnosis. There is usually a mild polymorphonuclear leukocytosis and an elevation of the erythrocyte sedimentation rate. Platelet counts, platelet function, and studies of the coagulation mechanism are normal. The diagnosis is based upon a characteristic clinical picture and is usually not difficult if the classic rash is present. It is important to realize that other manifestations of the syndrome may appear long before the occurrence of skin manifestations, and, rarely, a rash may never develop in a child who has all the other clinical findings of this disorder.

Corticosteroid treatment often gives prompt symptomatic relief of abdominal cramps, localized soft tissue edema, and joint swelling. It has been suggested that immediate steroid therapy be used in patients with gastrointestinal involvement in an effort to reduce the edematous areas of the bowel and possibly prevent intussusception and severe hemorrhage. These drugs have no effect on skin lesions, nor do they appear to influence the renal disease.

Evidence suggests that some form of anticoagulant therapy is indicated in all but the mild cases. Heparin and anti–platelet-aggregating agents such as aspirin do decrease acute morbidity and mortality. Streptokinase has reduced long-term proteinuria and hypertension.

VASCULAR LESIONS OF THE INTESTINE

Gastrointestinal telangiectasias or hemangiomas are relatively rare causes of gastrointestinal bleeding of infancy, although their cutaneous manifestations are not unusual.

ANEURYSMS

Aneurysms of the hepatic or gastroepiploic arteries have been associated with massive bleeding in infants.[62] The diagnosis of these extremely unusual lesions has been established by arteriography.

HEMANGIOMAS

Cutaneous hemangiomas in infants grow for several months before undergoing spontaneous regression. Such does not seem to be the case for intestinal lesions, which can bleed at any age.[4, 29]

Incidence. Intestinal hemangiomas are uncommon, and hemangiomatosis of the bowel accounts for only 2 to 12 per cent of all cases. Eight cases of diffuse neonatal hemangiomatosis were found in a review of the literature in 1970.[68]

Etiology. These congenital lesions originate in submucosal vascular plexuses as embryonic sequestrations of mesodermal tissue.

Pathology. The usual hemangioma is the cavernous one, which can be single or in a multiple of several hundred.[49, 104] Most often localized in the small bowel or rectum, they seldom involve other areas of the bowel. Small hemangiomas are often sessile, but some exist as small nodules or polyps and measure a few millimeters to several centimeters in size. Single lesions are often of the diffuse, expansive type. These hemangiomas extend from mucosa through serosa and are composed of dilated venous channels and poorly differentiated connective tissue stroma. Septa divide the larger venous sinuses. A few of the septa contain smooth muscle fibers. The channel walls are lined by flattened endothelial cells. The vascular supply derives from dilated mesenteric vessels that extend even to the root of the mesentery. One type of diffuse cavernous hemangioma encircles the circumference of the small bowel and may cause obstruction. Other lesions obstruct by sheer bulk, by intramural hemorrhage, or by causing intussusception.

Diffuse neonatal hemangiomatosis, by definition, involves three or more organ systems, including brain, lung, spleen, kidney, or heart as well as the intestines, and is lethal.

The capillary hemangioma grows as a nodule in the submucosa and eventually extends by stalk development into the intestinal lumen or by infiltration into the surrounding tissue. This lesion is characterized by endothelial hyperplasia, obliteration of vessels, and pericapsular fibrosis.

Symptoms. Bleeding in diffuse neonatal hemangiomatosis may be evidenced before birth as blood in the amniotic fluid and in the first voided urine, or by the rapid development of hydrocephalus. Seven of eight reported infants had extensive skin or mucous membrane hemangiomas. Respiratory distress, hepatomegaly, cardiac failure, gastrointestinal bleeding, and thrombocytopenia were other major manifestations of this generalized disease.[21]

In those with hemangiomas involving only the gastrointestinal tract, symptoms usually appear at any time between 2 months and 15 years. Nearly half have other hemangiomas or telangiectasias of the skin. Sudden gastrointestinal hemorrhage, unaccompanied by pain, is the usual mode of presentation. A few babies have a chronic hypochromic, microcytic anemia for months before the bleed, although a history of intermittent melena, listlessness, and cramping abdominal pain can usually be elicited by careful questioning. Very rarely, acute intussusception or intestinal obstruction is the first symptom of a hemanigoma.

Diagnosis. Similar symptoms may be produced by polyps or a Meckel's diverticulum. The diagnosis is a difficult one, for radiologic studies do not often demonstrate the lesions. An important clue of small, scattered calcifications throughout the small bowel is usually absent in infants. Characteristically, these calcifications involve a fairly long segment of bowel and show irregular, nodular filling defects that change in size during compression of the intestine. If they involve stomach, duodenum, or large bowel, they appear as polypoid filling defects. If a Meckel's scan and sigmoidoscopy show no lesions, visceral angiography may be required to demonstrate the dilated mesenteric vessels and dilated sinusoids.

Exploratory laparotomy is not always successful in localizing the lesions, but recent use of Doppler techniques has identified areas of increased blood flow and has proved invaluable in localizing these lesions.

Complications. Babies under one year of age are especially prone to develop thrombocytopenia and consumption coagulopathy with hypofibrinogenemia. This is particularly so in those with large lesions that sequester platelets. Intussusception, with the hemangioma serving as the lead point, is a complication in which bleeding is accompanied by acute, colicky abdominal pain.

Treatment. Some hemangiomas have undergone spontaneous remission or have resolved after steroid theapy.[48] If multiple lesions involve a localized area of bowel, or if one hemangioma is extensive, segmental excision of the bowel is indicated. Smaller lesions may be removed through serosal incisions.

Prognosis. Generalized neonatal hemangiomatosis is uniformly lethal, and affected infants have a life expectancy of only 71 days. Those with intestinal involvement alone have an excellent prognosis after excision of the lesion, although recurrent bleeding may develop if small lesions left behind increase in size.

OSLER-WEBER-RENDU DISEASE (HEREDITARY TELANGIECTASIA)

This disease, inherited as a dominant trait, can present in the neonate with cutaneous lesions. Telangiectatic tufts of dilated vessels appear on the skin and mucous membranes. Epistaxis is frequent during childhood, but gastrointestinal bleeding from gastric telangiectasias is a complication of later life and in 20 per cent of patients is associated with peptic ulcer disease. The radiologic diagnosis is extremely difficult, for the lesions sometimes have a foamy, reticular pattern. Endoscopy is the diagnostic tool of choice. Treatment is difficult; recently, coagulation by laser techniques has been employed.[101a]

THE BLUE RUBBER BLEB NEVUS SYNDROME

This oddly named syndrome derives its name from the appearance of the skin lesions, which look and feel like blue nipples, although they are actually cutaneous hemangiomas.[98, 102] The cutaneous lesions are present at birth and most often involve the upper limbs and trunk, although they may involve all extremities. Gastrointestinal hemangiomas are most common in the distal colon, small bowel, and stomach but occasionally may be seen throughout the gastrointestinal tract. Rarely, hemangiomas are found in other viscera, such as lungs, liver, spleen, deep subcutaneous tissue, and joints. Although the inheritance is not well defined, it has assumed an autosomal dominant form in several families. The major gastrointestinal symptom is chronic blood loss.

TURNER'S SYNDROME

Turner's syndrome has recently been shown to be associated with inflammatory bowel disease in greater than chance incidence. It is also associated with three different types of vascular abnormalities. This is of more than passing interest for the pediatrician, for hemorrhage occurs in 7 per cent of these patients.[144] The lesions are hemangiomas, telangiectases, or dilated and tortuous serosal vessels, which usually cause melena for several weeks to months before frank hemorrhage occurs. Although the bleeding is recurrent, it is usually self-limited. Sigmoidoscopy is helpful in diagnosing diffuse telangiectasia but does not permit visualization of hemangiomas. Angiography has been disappointing in localizing the lesions. Conservative treatment of gastrointestinal bleeding is the first line of therapy and usually suffices. If not, laparotomy and segmental resection of the involved region must be carried out. Recurrent bleeding episodes, however, are to be anticipated.

EHLERS-DANLOS SYNDROME

This syndrome is characterized by skin hyperelasticity, joint hypermobility, and a tendency to bruising and scarring. Because of tissue friability, passage of hard stools may rip anal skin to cause hemorrhage, or friability of the intestinal mucosa itself may contribute to hemorrhage.

THE VASCULAR INSUFFICIENCIES

Although vascular disease is extremely rare in infancy, it does occur in association with congenital vascular anomalies or after shock, sepsis, volvulus, or infection within the abdomen. An understanding of the anatomy of the intestinal vasculature is essential to delineate the extent of small bowel involvement. The superior mesenteric artery supplies the entire small bowel from just below the ligament of Treitz, the cecum, and the first few centimeters of ascending colon. Intestinal branches of the artery connect through a series of arcades from which small, straight vessels, the vasa recta, enter the intestine. Mesenteric veins return blood from the intestine to the portal vein. Arterial insufficiency involves the superior mesenteric artery more often than the inferior mesenteric because the former has a higher point of origin that runs almost parallel to the aorta, whereas that of the lower artery runs at a 45 degree angle. The patent foramen ovale or patent ductus arteriosus of the infant facilitates the transport of venous emboli into the arterial circulation.[166]

SMALL INTESTINAL INFARCTION

Intestinal infarction results from compromise of the arterial or venous circulation, or both, and each type accounts for approximately one third of the cases.

Etiology and Pathology. Arterial insufficiency results from embolization of the superior mesenteric artery in infants with congenital heart disease, polycythemia or trauma; from arteritis or extrinsic fibrous bands that compress the artery; or from narrowing of the artery itself.[108, 124] Intestinal necrosis has followed intra-arterial infusions and acute iron intoxication.[20, 79] Superior mesenteric artery insufficiency with eventual small bowel infarction has been related to a hepatic artery aneurysm and a vascular steal syndrome (Figs. 7–2 and 7–3).[62] Intestinal ischemia also follows any type of cardiovascular collapse that leads to splanchnic vasoconstriction, such as cardiac failure, shock, and gastroenteritis with septicemia, particularly from *Klebsiella, Proteus, Escherichia coli, Pseudomonas, Salmonella, Staphylococcus aureus,* and beta-hemolytic streptococcus.[47] Infection may be further complicated by a consump-

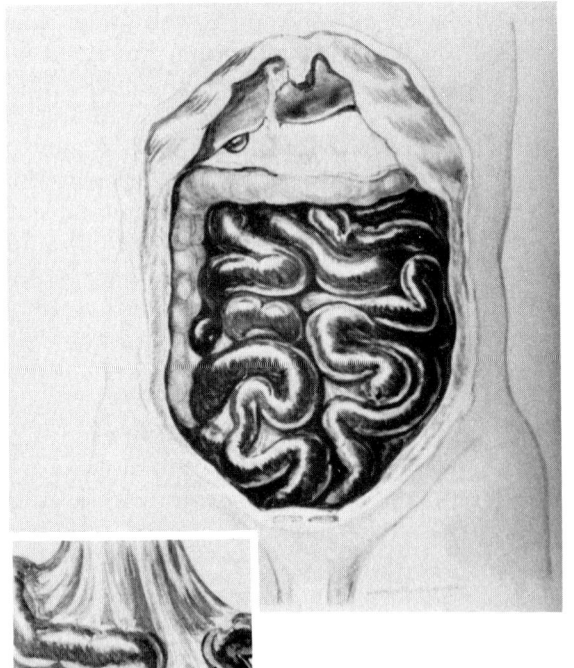

Figure 7–2 Artist's representation of superior mesenteric artery thrombosis, resulting in infarction of the small bowel from the ligament of Treitz to the mid–ascending colon. (Illustration by A. Hemberger, Yale University School of Medicine Collection.)

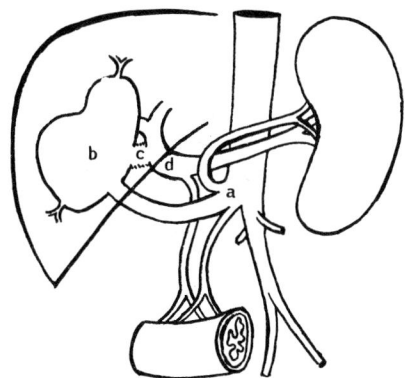

Figure 7–3 Diagrammatic representation of pathologic findings in a patient with hepatic artery aneurysm and superior mesenteric artery insufficiency. *a*, Common trunk from which the superior mesenteric and celiac arteries arise. *b*, Hepatic artery aneurysm. *c*, Intrahepatic arteriovenous communication. *d*, Portal vein. (From Gryboski, J. D., and Clemett, A.: Congenital hepatic artery aneurysm with superior mesenteric artery insufficiency. Pediatrics 39:344, 1967.)

tive coagulopathy. In such cases there is no evidence of vascular occlusion, although there is hemorrhagic necrosis of the bowel.

Segmental infarction of the small bowel has been reported in Thai children who have mesenteric adenitis.

Symptoms. Babies with small bowel infarction are usually ill for several days with diarrhea and vomiting before a paralytic ileus develops. The vomiting becomes constant and bilious, the abdomen distends, and the infant passes stools that contain large quantities of mucus and blood. In other cases, an apparently well infant becomes acutely ill with vomiting, abdominal distention, and diarrhea. The vomitus is clear at first but eventually contains bile and fecal material. The major symptom is acute, severe abdominal pain. The diagnosis is difficult because the abdominal findings are minimal early in the course of the disease and the child appears disproportionately ill, with fever, tachycardia, tachypnea, and hypotension. As tissue necrosis progresses and fluid pools in the bowel lumen, the baby becomes rapidly dehydrated. At this time, the abdomen is distended and tense, and bowel sounds are hypoactive or absent. Nearly one third of affected babies pass bright or dark blood in the stool, and one fifth have either diarrhea or constipation.

Diagnosis. It is difficult to differentiate this condition from sepsis, necrotizing enterocolitis, volvulus, or perforation with peritonitis. The leukocytosis is moderate to marked except in infants under one month old, in whom the white count can be normal or low. Clinically inorganic phosphates rise with intestinal ischemia as do base deficits and serum lactate. Three-way films of the abdomen show a paralytic ileus with air-fluid levels in the small bowel and cecum, edema of the valvulae, and thickening of the bowel wall. Barium examination of the small bowel (which should not be performed if peritonitis is suspected) shows separation of the loops and narrow, rather straight small bowel loops. Segmental spasm causes difficulty in filling the small bowel. Indentations resembling scallops or thumbprinting represent intramural hemorrhage. Radionuclide scanning with 99m Tc diphosphonate may be promising in the early diagnosis of intestinal infarction.[118] Use of Doppler ultrasound may also be helpful in determining the viability of ischemic intestine at the time of surgery.[28] An abnormal H_2 breath test has been shown to reflect intestinal ischemia.[120b]

Treatment. Supportive treatment includes nasogastric suction and replacement of electrolyte and fluid losses and perhaps low molecular weight dextran.[83] In patients with hypotension, isoproterenol not only affects the heart but also causes splanchnic vasodilatation. Early surgical reaction of segmental infarction is the ideal treatment, but if the infarction is extensive, a decompressing ileostomy is a palliative measure. Superior mesenteric artery embolectomy has been successful in one infant. In the future, prostaglandin therapy may be fruitful in providing vascular flow increases to relatively early ischemic bowel.

Prognosis. The prognosis is poor, and extensive infarctions carry a mortality rate of nearly 100 per cent.

INFARCTION OF THE LARGE BOWEL

This type of infarction is extremely rare because the branches of the inferior mesenteric artery rapidly develop collateral circulation through anastomoses of the marginal artery of Drummond with branches of the splenic or inferior hemorrhoidal arteries. The lesion, usually seen in elderly people or in young women taking oral contraceptives, is termed ischemic colitis and involves the distal transverse colon, cecum, and splenic flexure.

Symptoms. Diarrhea develops suddenly and is often associated with cramping abdominal pain. The stools contain blood and mucus. The abdomen is tender to palpation over the cecum and transverse colon.

Diagnosis. Sigmoidoscopy shows a normal rectal mucosa or proctitis, with fresh blood in the lumen of the rectum above the sigmoidoscope. Barium enema reveals the typical thumbprinting pattern in the colonic wall. Clinically and histologically, intestinal infarction cannot always be differentiated from ischemic colitis.

Treatment. In many cases, the colonic changes subside spontaneously over a period of several weeks, but in others, the ischemic segment must be resected.

CHRONIC SUPERIOR MESENTERIC ARTERY INSUFFICIENCY

Prolonged superior mesenteric artery insufficiency causes the "intestinal angina syndrome" of postprandial abdominal pain, disordered intestinal motility, anorexia, malabsorption, and weight loss.[40, 107]

Incidence. Sporadic cases have been reported in infants and children, but the disease is rare.

Pathology and Pathophysiology. This type of vascular insufficiency is caused by obstruction to the artery by bands, by the cruciate ligament, or by intimal thickening. The vascular lesion causes the development of arteriovenous shunts in the submucosa and muscularis of the small bowel, which deprive the more distal mucosal cells of adequate oxygen and blood. Secondary changes are enteric protein loss and impairment of mucosal enzyme systems and active transport mechanisms.[105] Jejunal biopsy shows a subtotal villous atrophy and plasma

cell infiltration of the lamina propria. The event that precipitates complete occlusion of the arterial flow is a sudden critical reduction of blood flow, such as might occur in anemia or dehyration.

Symptoms. Postprandial pain is characteristic of intestinal ischemia. Most patients have chronic diarrhea and malabsorption that leads to marked cachexia. The pain is of such severity that patients limit their intake of food. The physical findings are unremarkable, although in some cases a bruit is audible over the epigastrium. The history in one of our patients is described below.

Diagnosis. The quantitative fecal fat is elevated, and serum carotene, xylose absorption, and proteins are abnormal. Radiologic examination of the small bowel with barium shows dilatation of the small bowel, particularly in the mid- and distal jejunum, increased intraluminal fluid, and normal or delayed transit time. The mucosal folds may appear normal, thickened, or thin. Disordered peristalsis is evident by the appearance of intermittent small bowel intussusceptions. Arteriography will define the lesion.

Treatment. Division of a band is curative if the obstruction is extrinsic. Surgical approaches using endarterectomy or bypass are successful in adults but have limited use in small children and infants. Again, prostaglandin therapy, as yet experimental, may increase blood flow.

Prognosis. With relief of the obstruction, the small bowel function returns to normal within several months.

Case History. C.M. was a Caucasian male infant of birth weight 2980 gm (6 lb 3 oz). He was discharged at five days but was noted to scream and flex his knees or abdomen about 30 minutes after feeding. Stools numbered three to six per day and were watery. At seven weeks, bilateral inguinal hernias were repaired. A distended abdomen, hepatosplenomegaly, and hemoglobin of 6.7 gm per dl were noted. Diarrhea and pain continued until the infant was admitted to the hospital at nine weeks, dehydrated and lethargic. He weighed 2800 gm (5 lb 5 oz). There was a harsh grade II systolic murmur over the base of the heart and down the left sternal border. The abdomen was distended and tense. Liver and spleen were 4 cm below the costal margins. Bowel sounds were hyperactive. There was no bruit. During hospitalization, the serum protein levels fell from 5.9 to 3.8 gm per dl and he did not respond to any oral feedings. He became edematous at 14 weeks, passed gross blood per rectum, and was found at surgical exploration to have a purple, edematous small bowel. Postmortem examination revealed a large hepatic artery aneurysm, portal hypertension, and a superior mesenteric artery narrowed by intimal thickening. The heart was normal. It was concluded that increased hepatic artery flow caused a "steal" from the superior mesenteric circulation. Portal hypertension further compromised bowel perfusion.

MESENTERIC VENOUS OCCLUSION

Mesenteric venous occlusion in the infant is nearly as common as arterial occlusion, whereas in the adult it is less frequent.

Etiology. Superior mesenteric vein occlusion usually follows a septic intra-abdominal process, umbilical vein catheterization, or portal hypertension.

Pathology. The small bowel is thickened, reddened, and congested. There is enteric protein loss and serosanguineous ascites.

Symptoms. The symptoms can be acute, resembling those of intestinal infarction, or gradual, with abdominal pain and anorexia. In a few cases there is diarrhea. The physical examination shows abdominal distention and perhaps ascites. As the bowel becomes necrotic, there is fever, tachycardia, and vascular collapse, with signs of peritonitis and perforation.

Treatment. The treatment is the same as for arterial occlusion, including the use of supportive measures and operative resection of infarcted areas. If there is evidence of hypercoagulability, anticoagulant therapy may be of help.

Prognosis. The prognosis is related to the extent of bowel that is irrevocably damaged.

NECROTIZING ENTEROCOLITIS (NEC)

Over the past two decades, necrotizing enterocolitis has established itself as the major enteropathy of the neonate. Credit for the original description goes to Generish, who in 1891 reported an infant with perforation of the ileum. In 1944, von Willi described 62 patients, all fatalities, with "malignant enteritis."[109] Indeed, this disorder remains one of the most frequent causes of neonatal intestinal perforation.[45, 146a]

Incidence. Despite advances in neonatal care, the incidence of NEC has risen from an incidence of from 2.5 to 8 per cent a decade ago to an overall incidence of 10.1 per cent. Figures as high as 13.6 per cent to 80 per cent are reported in premature infants of less than 1500 gm birth weight who have survived long enough to feed. In one year, the Center for Disease Control investigated three nursery epidemics in three states. The disease is most common in the first six weeks of life and in premature babies of birth weight less than 2000 gm, who constitute 80 per cent of the total patients,[15-18] but it may occur in term and older infants.[76a, 100, 156]

Etiology. Over the years a number of factors have been incriminated in the etiology of NEC: septicemia, ingestion of infected amniotic fluid, hypoxia, exchange transfusion, lysozyme deficiency, and a Shwartzman-like phenomenon. Most affected infants have been premature or have suffered a perinatal insult such as hypoxia, respiratory distress, premature rupture of the membranes, or sepsis.[13] Touloukian[172] has proposed "ischemic gastroenterocolitis" as a more appropriate name for the disease, since gut ischemia is now considered to be the most important precipitating factor. Lloyd[95] first suggested that the fetus and premature infant have a "diving reflex" similar to that of the amphibious animals, in which blood is shunted away from the peripheral, mesenteric, and renal vascular beds in order to protect the delivery of oxygen to the brain. Experimental studies in asphyxiated piglets have shown first a reduction and then a rebound in gut perfusion. Although such vasoconstriction has not been demonstrated in the neonate, mucosal ischemia of the stomach, ileum, and colon has been produced in experimental animals. Electron microscopy has shown changes in the microcirculation before the development of mucosal lesions — changes similar to those of NEC. Hypoperfusion and hyperviscosity have also been implicated, but cardiac disease is not more prevalent in infants with NEC.

It has been repeatedly noted that NEC is extremely unusual in breast-fed infants, although it does rarely occur and has recently been reported in nine infants fed refrigerated breast milk.[77] The beneficial role of breast milk was evaluated by Santulli's group,[141] who subjected newborn rats to hypoxia or hypothermia: those fed artificial formula were predisposed to developing NEC, whereas those that were breast-fed remained well. The protective effect of breast milk is attributed to a variety of factors: a low pH, which inhibits the growth of coliform organisms and yeast and which enhances that of lactobacillus; increased lysozyme with its bactericidal properties; secretory IgA, which is not yet present in the infant intestine; bacteriostatic action of lactoferrin; and bactericidal action of lactoperoxidase, maternal macrophages, and T and B cells.[12, 85] NEC has been described in association with milk protein allergy.[122, 139]

Hyperosmolar formulae have also been implicated, not only for their osmolarity but also for their increased carbohydrate load.[89, 183] The incidence of NEC has increased in neonatal units where large feeding volumes or sudden increases in volume were given. Restricted feeding schedules have been associated with a low incidence of the disease, although isolated cases have been reported in infants fed by parenteral hyperalimentation.[44, 58]

The role of bacteria in the pathogenesis of NEC cannot be discounted, and some clusters of disease have been associated with isolation of *E. coli* strains 055 and 085, *Clostridium perfringens,* and *C. difficile* as well as *Klebsiella.*[46, 63, 78, 133, 159] Sporadic cases have been attributed to contaminated milk, enterovirus, *Salmonella, Clostridium butyricum,* and normal enteric flora. Even microbial toxins have been incriminated. Infants initially colonized with *Klebsiella pneumoniae* are three times more likely to develop NEC than are those colonized with other organisms. Clearly, the development of pneumatosis is dependent upon gas formation by bacteria. Recently, several epidemics of NEC in Paris have been associated with coronavirus.[25b] A definite relationship has been established between umbilical catheterization, mesenteric thromboembolism, and NEC.

Pathology. The right colon, cecum, appendix, and terminal ileum are most often affected, although the entire colon, small bowel, esophagus, and stomach may show evidence of the disease. Early microscopic findings consist of platelet-fibrin thrombi in the small arterioles of the muscular and submucosal layers, with little in the way of local tissue inflammatory reaction. Progression of disease is evident by mucosal ulceration, necrosis, and pseudomembrane formation. In the submucosa there is hemorrhage. The involved surfaces are dilated and the serosal surfaces covered with fibrin. Microscopically, the villi are broadened by dilated venules and capillaries, and the lamina propria is infiltrated by mononuclear cells and eosinophils. Mucosal hemorrhage is followed by epithelial slough, and large air-filled cysts are scattered through the submucosa and the serosal surfaces. The peripheral areas contain thrombi, evidence mucosal coagulation necrosis, and, again, show little inflammatory reaction. Mucosal injury decreases disaccharidase activity and glucose-galactose transport and leads to bacterial invasion of the mucosa.[92] Gastric aspirates from infants with NEC have shown an increase in gram-negative aerobes and a decrease in anaerobes.

Ileus results and leads to intestinal stasis and further bacterial proliferation. Intestinal perforation may occur within 24 hours or after several days in 33 to 80 per cent of infants. The perforations may be single or multiple and may appear days apart.

Septicemia, present in at least 50 per cent of the infants, is considered by some to be a prerequisite for the diagnosis. Certainly, pneumonia, otitis media, and meningitis are frequently encountered. Organisms recovered from the blood of infants with NEC are consistent among the series from which they are noted and include *Klebsiella, E.*

coli, *Proteus mirabilis*, *Pseudomonas*, *Staphylococcus aureus*, *S. epidermidis*, and *Salmonella*.

Healing begins as early as three days after onset, showing epithelialization, proliferation of fibroblasts, and granulation.

Symptoms. The triad of abdominal distention, vomiting, and blood in the stool typically heralds the development of NEC.[38, 141] Many infants have a history of prematurity, perinatal asphyxia, respiratory distress, umbilical catheterization, or exchange transfusion. The onset is usually after one or more days of feeding and between three and ten days of age. The course varies from a fulminant one, with intestinal necrosis within 12 to 24 hours, or a more chronic and benign one. Epidemic NEC typically affects larger infants with fewer neonatal insults and, although associated with higher temperature, has a lower mortality. Typically, the infant becomes suddenly ill with periods of apnea and abdominal distention. Vomiting is at first intermittent but later becomes continuous. Diarrhea is not common, but when it occurs, is watery and profuse. Because of large quantities of intraluminal secretions, dehydration is extreme. Some consider the presence of occult blood in the stool to be a more consistent finding than diarrhea. Gross rectal bleeding is not unusual.

The afflicted infants are sick and lethargic. Bowel sounds are at first hyperactive, and the distended abdomen is tender to percussion. A tense, silent abdomen indicates perforation. Ascites and/or crepitus of the abdominal wall signify extensive bowel necrosis and peritonitis. Some infants have few gastrointestinal symptoms and present either with sudden circulatory collapse or with signs of sepsis, such as apnea, lethargy, fluctuations in temperature, and hypotension.

A clinical classification for the severity of necrotizing enterocolitis has been proposed by Bell et al.[19]

Stage I. Suspected Disease
   a. History of factors producing perinatal stress
   b. Temperature instability, lethargy, apnea, bradycardia
   c. Gastrointestinal symptoms — poor feeding, increased pregavage residuals, emesis, occult blood in the stools, mild abdominal distention
   d. Radiologic evidence of mild ileus

Stage II. Definite Disease (treated medically)
   a. One or more of the historical features
   b. Signs and symptoms as above but with marked abdominal distention, persistent occult or gross bleeding
   c. Radiologic evidence of intestinal distention and ileus, separation of intestinal loops, "rigid bowel loops," pneumatosis intestinalis, portal vein gas

Stage III. Advanced Disease (requiring operative treatment)
   a. One or more of the historical features
   b. Signs and symptoms as above but with deteriorating vital signs, septic shock, gastrointestinal bleed
   c. Radiologic evidence of pneumoperitoneum

Differential Diagnosis. The disorder must be differentiated from intestinal malrotation and volvulus, Meckel's diverticulum, sepsis, and enterocolitis of Hirschsprung's disease (Table 7–5).

Diagnosis. Laboratory studies show either an elevated or a severely depressed white blood cell count with either leukocytosis or neutropenia. Thrombocytopenia and disseminated intravascular coagulation may ensue, and, in survivors, thrombocytopenia may persist for 7 to 31 days.[70] Serum proteins are often decreased through enteric losses. The diagnosis is established by radiologic examination (Figs. 7–4 and 7–5). Early studies often do not correlate well with the clinical stage of disease and show either generalized ileus or one dilated loop of bowel.[35, 112] Films repeated several hours later show an obstructive pattern, thickening of the bowel wall, pneumatosis intesti-

Table 7–5 Differential Diagnosis of Enteritis and Enterocolitis

	NECROTIZING ENTEROCOLITIS	PSEUDOMEMBRANOUS ENTEROCOLITIS	ILEAL ULCER	REGIONAL ENTERITIS
Past history	Neonatal anoxia Prematurity Exchange transfusion	Antibiotics Intussusception Hirschsprung's disease	None	None
Age of onset	First weeks	10 days to 1 year	Several months	Any age but usually older infants
Etiology	Vascular accident	Staphylococci or fungus in some Postoperative Above obstruction After antibiotics	None in infants Vitamin K in adults	None
Area involved	Terminal ileum Right colon	All colon ± Small bowel	Ileum	Ileum ± Right colon ± Jejunum
Symptoms				
Lethargy	++++	+	–	±
Distention	++++	++++	–	++
Diarrhea	++ to ++++	++++	–	++
Gross blood in stool	++	++	++	+ eventually
Diagnosis	Radiologic	Sigmoidoscopic	Laparotomy	Usually at laparotomy

nalis, ascites, free intraperitoneal air, or gas in the portal vein. Intestinal dilatation correlates best with disease activity and is present in half the infants with NEC. Persistently dilated loops suggest full wall necrosis.[180] Pneumoperitoneum occurs in 14 per cent; the presence of this or ascites indicates perforation. It may appear in the absence of pneumatosis. Pneumatosis intestinalis has been described in 25 to 88 per cent of cases, appearing first in the right lower quadrant as double rings or, in lateral views, as frames about involved bowel. Gas in the portal vein, although usually an ominous sign, does not in itself mandate laparotomy. Barium-contrast studies are utilized only in the barium enema to exclude Hirschsprung's disease or malrotation. Continuous sampling of peritoneal fluid to determine a dark brown color, or increase in white blood cells to indicate intestinal gangrene, is helpful in questionable cases.[123] Results of technetium scanning have been universally positive in infants with stage III disease.[143]

Complications. Perforation is the most common and urgent early complication, although thrombocytopenia and disseminated intravascular coagulation increase the risks of pulmonary, gastrointestinal, and intracranial hemorrhage. Oliguria and renal cortical necrosis may follow severe dehydration. Fluid and electrolyte complications are managed aggressively. Attention must be paid to nutrition, for not only are proteins lost through the bowel but the infants are deprived of caloric intake. Lymphoid hyperplasia may be seen in radiologic studies made during the recovery period.

Later complications, which may develop after several weeks to months, include small bowel or colonic strictures (30 per cent) and enterocysts, which may lead to intestinal obstruction or internal fistulas.[14, 94, 119] Many strictures resolve spontaneously.[171] Lactose intolerance may persist for months after

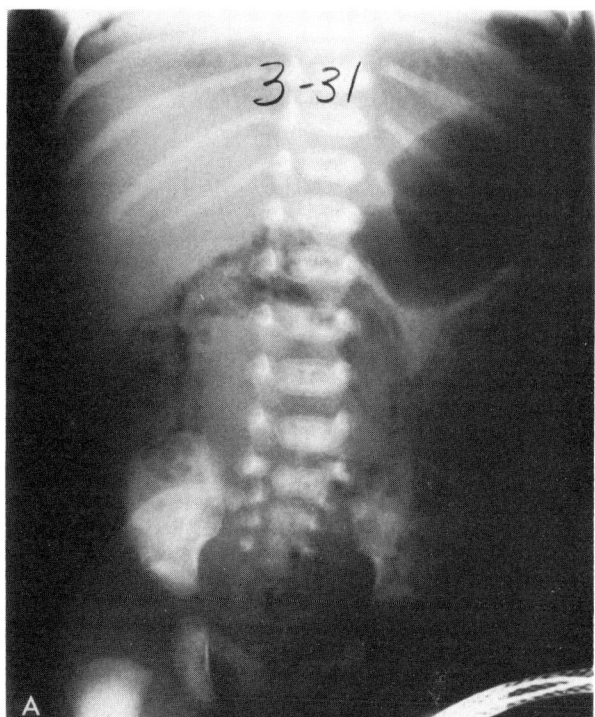

Figure 7–4 Necrotizing enterocolitis in an 1800-gm premature infant with tight pulmonic stenosis requiring a systemic artery to pulmonary artery anastomosis on the second day of life. The patient began vomiting during the following week and had progressive abdominal distention and grossly bloody stools. *A*, A chain of linear and small cystic lucencies, representing gas, is seen paralleling both walls of the entire colon. *B*, The linear and intramural gas is again seen on the lateral plain films, especially in the rectosigmoid area.

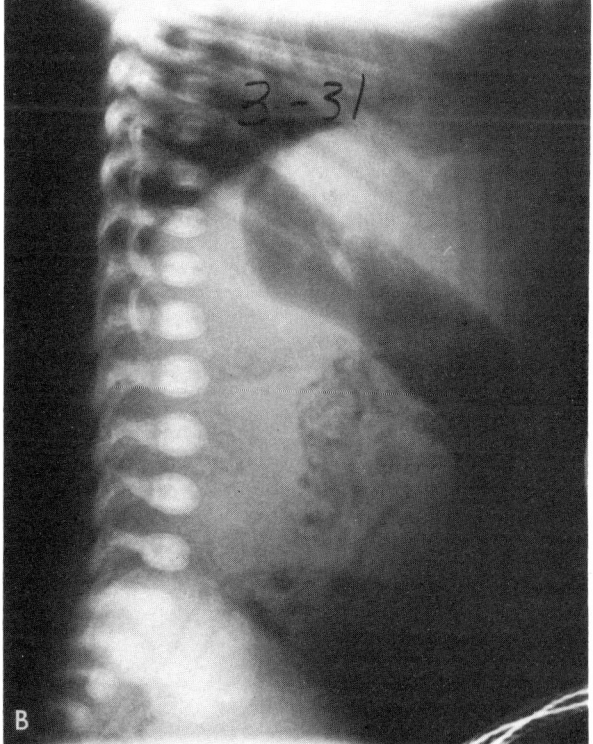

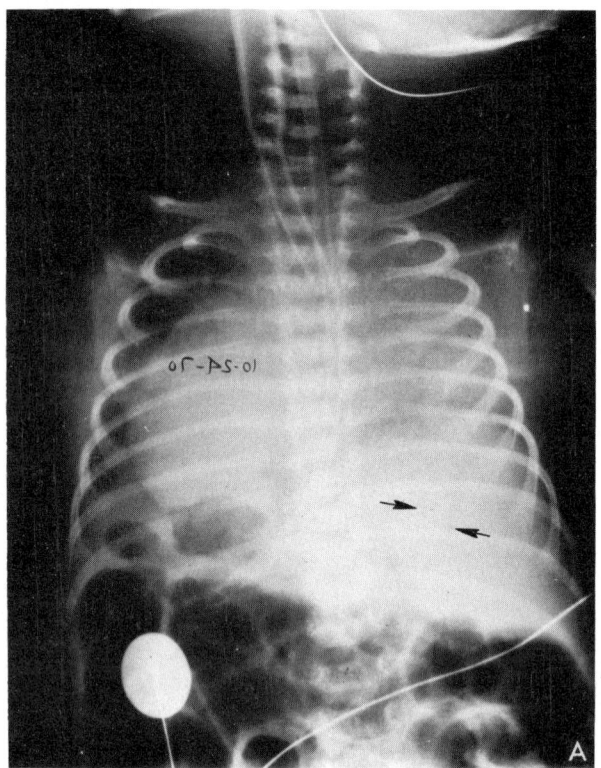

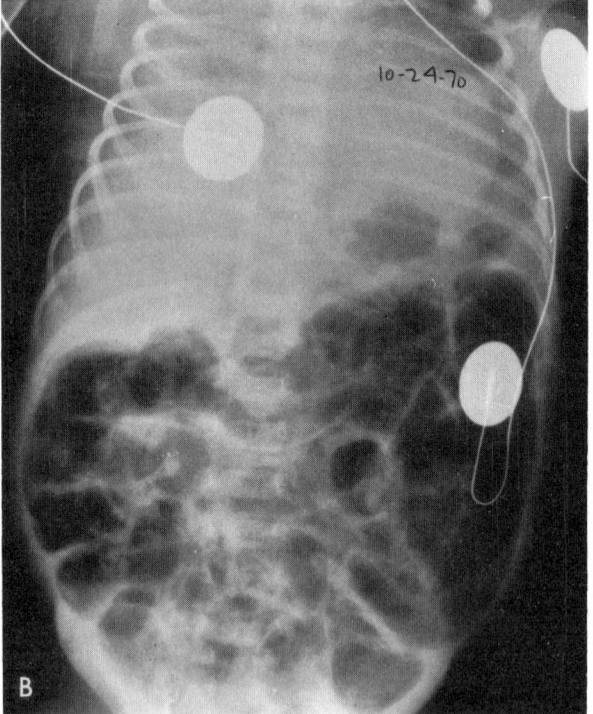

Figure 7–5 Premature newborn infant with pneumonia and progressive abdominal distention during the first week of life. Late in the course, blood was present in the stool. The infant died shortly after these studies and at autopsy was found to have extensive necrosis in the small bowel and colon. *A*, Diffuse gaseous distention of loops of bowel is seen throughout the abdomen. A linear lucency (*arrows*) represents dissection of gas into the wall of the bowel. *B*, A faint pattern of linear, branching lucencies is seen projected over the liver and is indicative of gas within the portal vein.

clinical recovery, and a hydrogen breath test should be performed to determine its severity.

Treatment. Oral feedings are withheld, and the infants are managed medically with continuous gastric suction, parenteral alimentation, and antibiotics appropriate for enteric organisms, i.e., ampicillin (150 to 200 mg/kg/24 h) and kanamycin (15 mg/kg/24 h) or clindamycin (30 mg/kg/24 h) and gentamicin (5 to 7.5 mg/kg/24 h). Early reports of the use of additional intragastric kanamycin (30 mg/kg/24 h) or gentamicin (10 to 15 mg/kg/24 h) noted the absence of perforation, but more recent controlled studies showed no difference between those who received the intragastric medications and those who did not.[42, 65] In fact, McCracken and Eitzman[103] do not believe that the aminoglycosides should be used routinely to prevent NEC because of the development of resistance and the growth of other potentially serious organisms such as clostridia. Changes in microflora are shown in Table 7–6. Low molecular weight dextran has been of some value, and half the infants so treated did not require surgery. Transcutaneous oxygen measurements (TcPo$_2$) have shown decreases in perfusion to herald intestinal necrosis and may be excellent indicators for early surgical intervention.[22]

Staging is important in the treatment program, for those in suspect stage I are treated with vigorous supportive measures; those in stage II are given parenteral and perhaps gavage antibiotics, and those in stage III are operated upon. Generally, if the disease progresses over 24 to 48 hours or if no improvement is noted, surgery is indicated. Kosloske et al.[82] use paracentesis findings, platelet count, and presence of clostridia as indications for surgery. O'Neill and Holcomb[116] feel that four hours is long enough to watch for improvement and believe that a decrease in platelet count by 150,000 m^3 or more is associated with gangrenous bowel. The surgical procedure often entails segmental resection and ileostomy with creation of a distal bowel fistula or Mikulicz double-fistula enterostomy. The fistula is closed after the infant has recovered.

Prognosis. The disease remits spontaneously in nearly 40 per cent of infants. NEC involving only the colon and without intestinal dilatation has a better prognosis than that involving the small bowel.[126] Even pneumatosis intestinalis, without associated dilatation, has a relatively benign course. The mortality is highest in those infants less than 1300 gm, those small for gestational age, or those with a rapid, fulminant course. Mortality rates in infants not operated upon until there are obvious signs of perforation

Table 7–6 Pre- and Post-Treatment Bacterial Isolates from Infants with NEC[18]

	YEAST	GRAM-NEGATIVE AEROBES	GRAM-POSITIVE AEROBES	GRAM-NEGATIVE ANAEROBES	GRAM-POSITIVE ANAEROBES
Gastric Juice					
Pre-Rx	0	14/22	16/22	0	0
Post-Rx					
48–72 hours	0	0/20	5/20	0	0
96–120 hours	1	2/25	5/15	0	0
Feces					
Pre-Rx	0	30/63	20/63	10/63	3/63
Post-Rx					
48–72 hours	2	18/46	17/46	6/46	3/46
Post-Rx					
96–120 hours	4	7/24	10/24	2/24	1/24

The majority of gram-negative aerobes are *Klebsiella pneumoniae* and *Escherichia coli*. The majority of gram-negative anaerobes are *Bacteroides* spp.

The majority of gram-positive aerobes are *Staphylococcus aureus* or *S. epidermidis*. The majority of gram-positive anaerobes are *Clostridium* spp.

Table 7–7 Gastrointestinal Polypoid Lesions

TYPE	INHERITANCE	PATHOLOGY	INVOLVEMENT	OTHER SYMPTOMS	PER CENT MALIGNANT
Familial polyposis	Dominant	Adenomatous	Colon (90–100%), stomach, rare in duodenum	—	85–90
Gardner's syndrome	Dominant	Adenomatous	Same	Osteomas, epidermal cysts, fibrous tumors, lipomas, adrenal and thyroid cancer	85–90
Turcot syndrome	Autosomal recessive	Adenomatous, villous	Colon	Medulloblastoma, glioblastoma, epidendyoma, thyroid cancer	85–90
Peutz-Jeghers syndrome	Dominant	Hamartoma of muscularis mucosae	Stomach, small bowel, colon	Buccal, facial pigmentation, clubbing	2–3 5 ovary
Juvenile polyp	Dominant or nonfamilial	Juvenile	Colon, rectum, sigmoid	—	Minimal
Diffuse juvenile polyposis	Dominant	Juvenile hamartoma	Stomach, small bowel, colon	Macrocephaly	Minimal
Cronkhite-Canada syndrome	?	Juvenile hamartoma	Stomach, small bowel, colon	Alopecia, nail dystrophy, hyperpigmentation of trunk and arms	Minimal
Cowden's disease[169] (multiple hamartoma syndrome)	? familial	Hamartoma	Colon, mouth, esophagus, stomach, small bowel	Multiple congenital anomalies, thyroid tumors, fibrocystic disease of breast	

approximate 70 per cent. Infants in stage II of the disease have an overall 85 per cent survival rate. The mortality rates for all infants with NEC now approximate 25 per cent, and, if corrected for later deaths from respiratory disease, fall to 15 per cent. Those patients with most severe neutropenia have a generally poor prognosis as do those with severe acidosis, hypertension, and shock.

In a long-term follow-up of 40 infants with NEC, only 19 were normal one to three years later, with six having moderate to severe neurologic impairment. Only four had gastrointestinal sequelae.[163]

POLYPS OF THE GASTROINTESTINAL TRACT

Infants and children may be affected by a variety of polypoid lesions of the gastrointestinal tract, most of which are benign but some of which are potentially malignant (Table 7–7).

A variety of lesions are associated with juvenile polyps.

JUVENILE POLYPS

The juvenile polyp is a benign lesion of the colon, which, once diagnosed, is best treated by watchful waiting, for such polyps cause few problems and tend to undergo spontaneous autoamputation.[168]

Incidence. Juvenile colonic polyps account for more than 90 per cent of the intestinal polypoid lesions in children, and two thirds of affected patients are males. In most cases there is no evidence of genetic transmission, but multiple familial juvenile polyposis has been reported in several sibships and in three to five consecutive generations of two families.[55, 59a]

Etiology. Some consider the polyps to result from chronic inflammation, but others consider them to be hamartomas, because they contain immature mesenchymal tissue.

Pathology. Eighty-five per cent of the polyps are solitary, and 90 per cent are located in the rectum or sigmoid (Fig. 7–6).[51] A few involve the ascending colon. Grossly, they appear as smooth, red or brown, round or ovoid, cyst-like projections

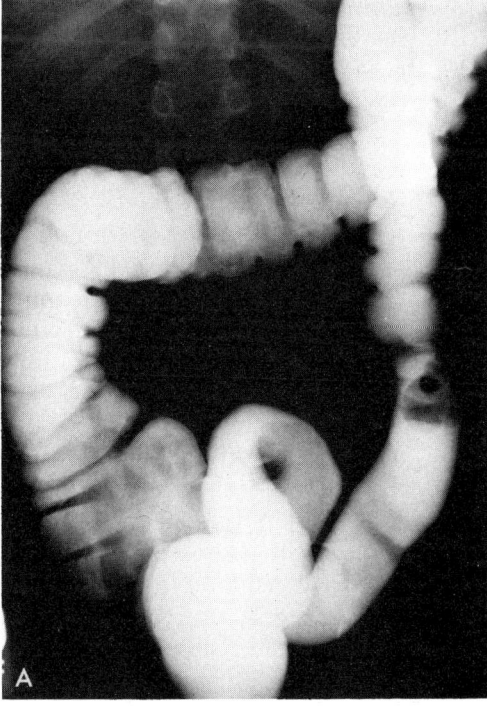
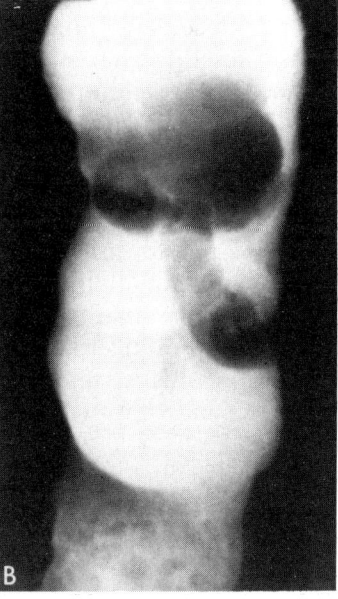

Figure 7–6 Juvenile polyp of the colon in a boy with bloody diarrhea. *A*, A single filling defect is seen in the mid–descending colon. *B*, Spot film of the area shows a typical polyp on a long stalk.

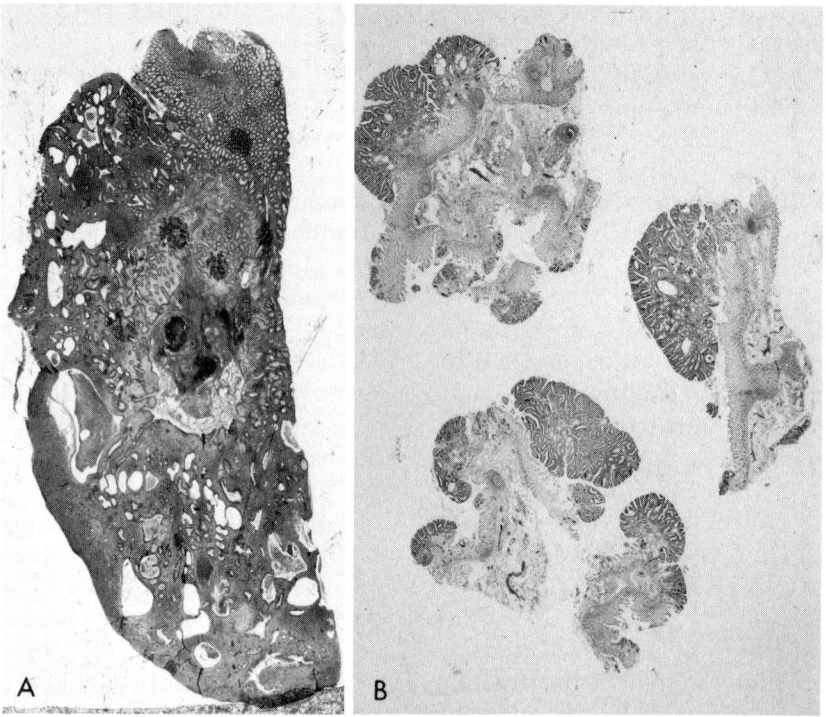

Figure 7-7   A, Typical biopsy from a juvenile polyp of the rectum. There is a great amount of stroma filled with granulation tissue and dilated lymphatics and capillaries. The surface is eroded. The overall pattern is one of disorganization. *B*, Adenomatous polyp of the colon in multiple sections. This polyp has a stalk and muscularis mucosa that are continuous with the lamina propria. The epithelium is that of the colon, and the glands are long and branched. The rather neat organization of the glands is in contrast to the wild appearance of the far more benign juvenile polyp. (Courtesy of D. Sheahan, M.D.)

into the intestinal lumen. The surface, covered with mucus, glistens but bleeds easily if wiped with a swab or scraped by the sigmoidoscope. Most of the polyps have a stalk containing muscularis mucosa, and only a few are sessile. The microscopic pattern is characteristic. The epithelium is continuous and composed of goblet cells except where it is interrupted by ulceration and granulation tissue. The glands are arborized, dilated, and cystic without any regular pattern. These too are lined by goblet cells, and their lumens are filled with debris and mucus. The stroma contains no smooth muscle and is filled with inflammatory cells — plasma cells, histocytes, polymorphonuclear cells, and eosinophils (Fig. 7–7A).

Symptoms. Most polyps produce symptoms by the age of ten years, with the majority presenting between three and six years. Rectal bleeding is invariably the presenting symptom, and it is not accompanied by pain. The blood is red and fresh or pink

and mixed with mucus. If the polyp lies in the right colon, dark blood is more prominent. Some patients note blood at the end of the stool and not in the first portion passed. Bleeding may accompany every stool or it may be intermittent, occurring one or more times a week or at monthly intervals. Intussusception is not common, but low-lying polyps tend to prolapse and can be a terrifying mode of presentation to a mother changing her baby's diaper. Older children may complain of recurrent, cramping lower abdominal pain.

Diagnosis. Polyps lying below the sigmoid flexure can be easily visualized through the sigmoidoscope in most cases. A small pink polyp can slide easily behind the wall of the sigmoidoscope, however, and require considerable manipulation before it is visualized. A barium enema and air-contrast study should be performed in all patients to detect other polyps higher in the colon (see Fig. 7–7). The true diagnosis of juvenile polyp is confirmed only after histologic examination, for the polyp may resemble follicular lymphoma.[52] A rare polyp may show both juvenile and adenomatous change.

Treatment. Once a polyp is identified as the cause of rectal bleeding, watchful waiting is the treatment of choice, for hemorrhage is not a problem. A yearly barium enema is performed to note the progress of the polyp and the presence or absence of others. If after one year the polyp remains and symptoms persist, elective polypectomy is performed, using colonoscopy if possible.[37]

Complications. Polyps are subject to volvulus and autoamputation and, rarely, serve as the lead point for intussusception. Intestinal lymphangiectasia has been associated with colonic polyps.[120]

Prognosis. Once removed, a simple juvenile polyp does not recur. In a family of 92, with 26 symptomatic and 19 diagnosed, 2 have developed colorectal carcinoma.[59a] Other families have noted deaths from colonic cancer, and a few from gastric, duodenal, or pancreatic carcinoma.

GENERALIZED JUVENILE GASTROINTESTINAL POLYPOSIS

This disease, otherwise termed fatal juvenile polyposis, follows a lethal course through early infancy.

Incidence. Fewer than 20 cases are known.[10, 125, 132, 135, 136, 157]

Etiology. These growths, like colonic juvenile polyps, are considered to be hamartomas. There is a dominant type of inheritance with variable age-dependent expressivity, for the symptoms appear earlier in each succesive generation.

Pathology. The polyps extend from the stomach through the small intestine, colon, and rectum, increasing in number from proximal to distal sites. All are typical juvenile polyps, sessile or on stalks, and measuring 0.3 to 3.5 cm in diameter. Their epithelial components vary according to the area from which they arise, with those from the stomach containing mucus-secreting cells; those from the small bowel, villous crypts with Paneth cells and Brunner's glands; and

those from the colon, colonic epithelium. Some exhibit adenomatous features.

Symptoms. Diarrhea beginning on the second or third day of life or during the first few weeks is the most common gastrointestinal symptom. In a number of babies, gastrointestinal disease is not suspected until chronic anemia and failure to thrive are found. A few present with prolapse of a polyp through the rectum, gastrointestinal hemorrhage, or intussusception. Any of the symptoms leading to the diagnosis are soon overshadowed by those of malnutrition and enteric protein loss. Diarrhea and gastrointestinal bleeding are more prominent with time, and hypoproteinemia leads to edema and ascites. The physical examination shows a cachectic infant who is anorectic, irritable, and critically ill. There is marked loss of subcutaneous fat and pallor of the mucous membranes.

Diagnosis. The diagnosis is suggested by a positive family history. Rectal prolapse of a polyp does not indicate diffuse disease, and further studies are required. Sigmoidoscopy shows numerous rectal and sigmoid polyps, and radiologic examination of the stomach, colon, and small bowel shows the extensive nature of the disease. Studies for enteric protein loss are of academic interest only.

Treatment. Rectal polyps are removed to prevent prolapse. The overall treatment is conservative, and the largest polyps are selectively removed through enterotomy. Fifty to 60 polyps can be removed during a single procedure. Parenteral hyperalimentation and albumin supplementation provide optimal nutrition before surgery, but the total gastrointestinal involvement precludes any long-term therapeutic optimism.

Prognosis. The disease carries a mortality rate of 100 per cent, with most babies dying before two years of age.

JUVENILE POLYPOSIS COLI

In this disorder, polyps are confined to the colon and are familial in nature.[80] Some relatives of these patients have colorectal carcinoma and others, adenomatous familial polyposis. Some children may have associated heart disease, hydrocephalus, malrotation of the gut, and hypertelorism.[115] The polyps may be segmental or diffuse and extend through the colon with age. One ten-year-old patient of ours with digital clubbing has had extension of his disease with development of adenomatous change. He also had lymphoid hyperplasia of the terminal ileum.

CRONKHITE-CANADA SYNDROME

This syndrome, described in approximately 50 adults, has been compared with fatal juvenile polyposis. It includes polyposis of the gastrointestinal tract, alopecia, nail atrophy, hyperpigmentation of the skin in an addisonian manner, malabsorption, hypoproteinemia and hypocalcemia, and hypokalemia and hypomagnesemia. The skin changes as brown macular lesions on face and extremities appear early enough in the disease to suggest that they are primary and not secondary in nature. The polyps are benign and of the juvenile type but cause severe diarrhea with electrolyte depletion and protein-losing enteropathy. They extend through the colon with lesser involvement of the stomach, the small bowel, and, rarely, the esophagus. Spontaneous remissions have occurred. Cowden's disease,[179] not reported in infants, is included in Table 7–7.

PEUTZ-JEGHERS SYNDROME

This disease consists of diffuse polyposis of the gastrointestinal tract associated with melanotic spots of the buccal mucosa, lips, and skin.

Incidence. The exact incidence is unknown, although the disease is well known in the medical literature.

Etiology. Inheritance is through a dominant gene of high penetrance, and the polyps are considered to be hamartomas of the muscularis mucosae.

Pathology. Although the small intestine is most often involved, the polyps actually extend from the stomach to the rectum.

They advance in segmental spurts with months to years of quiescent intervals. The new groups of polyps are separated from older ones by areas of normal bowel. These, like juvenile polyps, have a typical histologic appearance and contain all elements of intestinal mucosa. They develop about a fibromuscular stroma that arises from a smooth muscle mass in the muscularis mucosa. The glandular elements are well defined and contain Paneth, argentaffin, and goblet cells. Some polyps are so small as to be visible only microscopically, whereas others reach several centimeters in diameter. The polyps are subject to torsion with infarction and hemorrhage. A small number (2.3 to 12.6 per cent) undergo true malignant degeneration to adenocarcinoma. There is an increased incidence of the theca-cell ovarian and sex cord tumors in patients with this syndrome.

Symptoms. The typical mucosal pigmentation is the prerequisite for making this diagnosis. It varies from a blotchy, brown spotting in only a few areas to discrete, dark freckling involving the gums, palate, and face. In the skin at birth or early infancy there may be sharply demarcated, flat, dark brown macules grouped about the mouth, eyes, and nostrils. Other areas that are sometimes involved are fingers, palms, toes, forearms, and periumbilical region. All these lesions tend to fade somewhat at puberty. There may be digital clubbing and exostoses.

The polyps are not present at birth but develop with age. Some never cause symptoms, but others produce symptoms of large bowel or small bowel intussusception. Brief colicky bouts of pain occurring after feeding and appearing at intervals of weeks or months are typical complaints. The end of the attack of pain may be signaled by the passage of flatus. Colocolic intussusception with a polyp as a lead point has been reported in a four-month-old black infant. The majority of intussusceptions are transient, and gross bleeding is rare. Melena does occur in nearly one third of patients and causes a hypochromic, microcytic anemia. Rectal prolapse, accompanied by a polyp or not, is not unusual. Nasal polyps are also reported as well as those of the respiratory

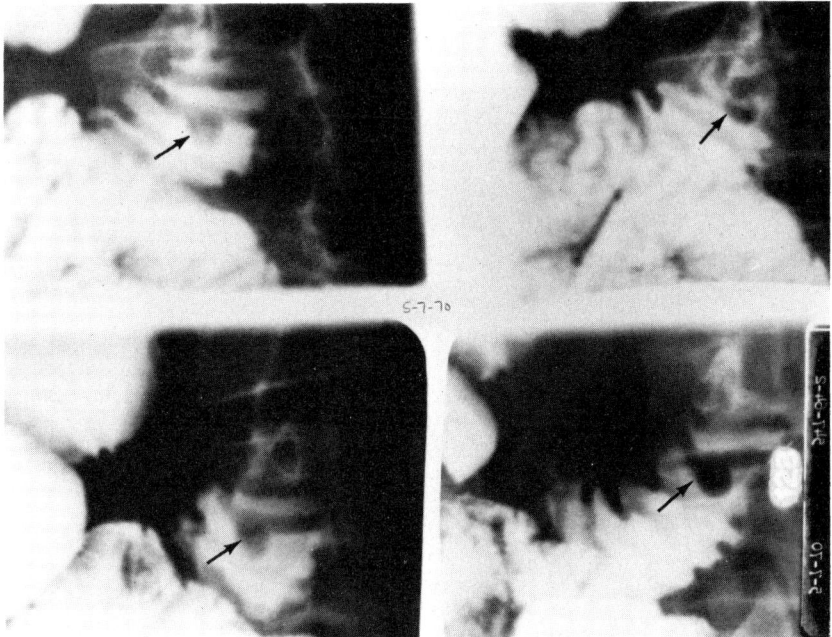

Figure 7–8 Peutz-Jeghers syndrome in a girl who had resection of a portion of small bowel at the age of five years for polyps. A series of spot films of the descending portion of the duodenum demonstrates a single polyp (*arrows*). Otherwise, the small bowel series was normal.

and urinary tracts. Clubbing of the fingers, congenital heart disease, and growth retardation are additional findings in this syndrome.

Diagnosis. All patients with the mucous membrane pigmentation have intestinal polyposis. Plain abdominal films taken in patients having pain show partial or complete intestinal obstruction or a soft tissue mass in a bowel loop, which represents the intussusception. Examination of the upper gastrointestinal tract and small bowel with barium shows solitary or multiple gastric polyps but does not always visualize small bowel polyps. A single jejunal polyp may be all that is shown (Fig. 7–8). Pedunculated small bowel polyps are seen more often during fluoroscopy. Barium enema shows 2 to 12 colonic polyps, which are often pedunculated, and differentiates this disease from familial polyposis, in which polyps carpet the entire colon.

Treatment. Asymptomatic polyps need not be treated, but those that cause obstruction or intussusception require resection.

Complications. As noted, gastric or duodenal carcinoma has developed, and tumors have metastasized, but this is extremely rare.[73] Females must be watched for the

development of ovarian tumors. Signs of an acute abdomen signal intussusception.[69]

Several syndromes are characterized by the familial adenomatous polyp lesions, perhaps representing both ends of a spectrum of the same genetic disorder.

FAMILIAL POLYPOSIS COLI

This inherited disease carries with it the formidable risk of carcinoma and, once recognized, must be treated by colectomy.[134] It has been called the most clearly defined precancerous lesion in medicine[36, 111] and must be distinguished from lymphoid hyperplasia.[86, 96, 128]

Incidence. It is estimated to occur once in every 8300 births and has a gene frequency of 1:16,000. The sexes are equally affected, but in 19 blacks reported, there was a female predominance. The condition has been reported in a four-month-old infant.

Etiology. The disease is transmitted as an autosomal dominant with some variation in gene penetrance.

Pathology. The polyps occur in greatest intensity in the sigmoid colon but extend through the entire colon and rectum in

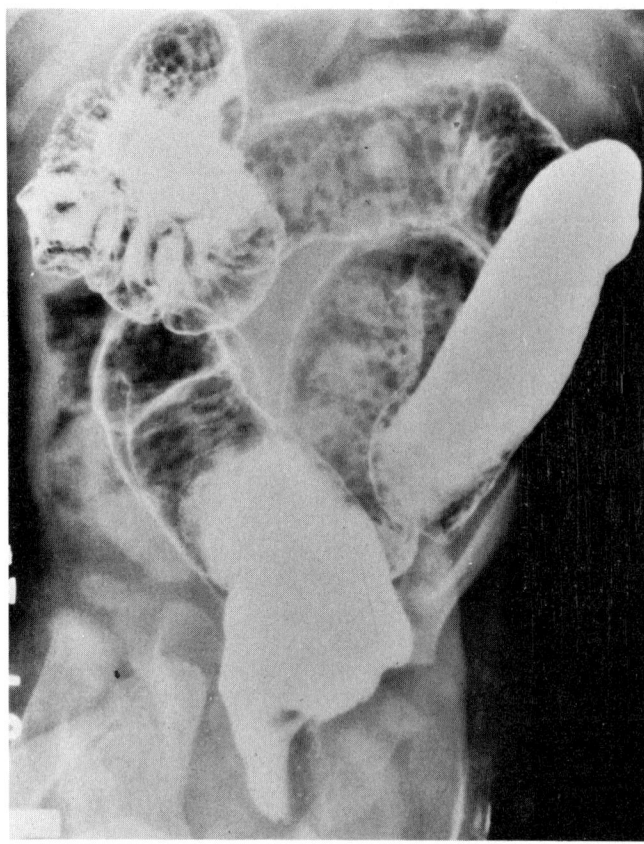

Figure 7–9 Familial polyposis of the colon in a baby girl who had one episode of bloody diarrhea in infancy. The contrast examination was done because of a history of polyposis in the mother. Small common nodular filling defects of varying size are seen throughout the colon.

numbers ranging from a few to thousands. Lesions beyond the colon are rare, but they do occasionally appear in the stomach and small intestine.[186] They originate as excrescences in the mucosa and progress to become sessile or pedunculated polyps. Many patients also have lymphoid hyperplasia of the terminal ileum and some have lymphoid polyps of the colon. Histologic examination shows changes that progress from the glandular proliferation to the development of a central core, as in the typical adult adenoma, in which there is branching of the glands and metaplastic epithelium (Fig. 7–9). Ten per cent of patients with familial polyposis have primary tumors of the thyroid or brain.

Symptoms. The onset of symptoms can be as early as the fourth month of life, although the disease is usually recognized in late childhood or adolescence. There may be no symptoms, or there may be diarrhea with the stool containing blood and mucus. Older children complain of recur-

rent cramping, abdominal pain, and weight loss. Intussusception and intestinal obstruction are not complications in early childhood but arise later and often in association with malignant change.

Diagnosis. Sigmoidoscopy shows numerous polyps in the rectum and sigmoid colon. The barium enema shows multiple polyps of varying size and configuration. Some are attached to the mucosa by a broad, flat base, and others by a narrow stalk. Larger polyps show superficial areas of ulceration. Not all the polyps are visualized when the colon is distended by barium, and the best films are obtained after partial evacuation of the contrast material, when one sees multiple rounded filling defects or ring-like shadows projecting into the lumen of the bowel. Air-contrast films are particularly helpful in demonstrating multiple polyps (Fig. 7–9).

Treatment. Until recently, the accepted treatment for this disease was proctocolectomy and ileostomy. Total colectomy with ileorectal anastomosis was later being performed, and spontaneous regression of the remaining rectal polyps has followed such procedures.[137] However, carcinoma has developed, and such a limited procedure cannot be recommended. A variation of the Soave procedure to include endorectal stripping and colectomy achieves ileoanal continuity.

Prognosis. In 5 per cent of untreated patients, carcinoma will develop in 5 years, and in 59 per cent it will develop within 23 years. Genetic counseling is imperative for the parents, for half the children born to an affected parent will have the disease. All siblings and relatives of affected patients should have sigmoidoscopic and radiologic examinations of the colon.

GARDNER'S SYNDROME

This variant of familial adenomatous polyposis of the colon includes subcutaneous tumors, epidermoid and sebaceous cysts, and bony tumors of the mandible, maxillae, and cranial bones.[113, 146, 147]

Incidence. More than 160 kindreds have been reported with Gardner's syndrome.[54] In a six-state study of familial polyposis, 72 families had Gardner's syndrome, 43 had familial polyposis, and 16 had Peutz-Jeghers syndrome. It is inherited in an autosomal dominant fashion and although twice as common in males as in females, does not appear to be sex-linked. It is estimated to occur once in 14,025 births. Some family members have only colonic lesions, and others, only soft tissue and bone lesions. Symptoms are more severe in blacks.[88]

The gene has a high a degree of penetrance, with 60 to 100 per cent of kindreds affected. Somatic cell culture of skin fibroblasts shows increased endoreplication with tetraploidy, a finding rare in normal individuals.[154]

Pathology. The pathologic changes in the colon and the malignant potential are the same as for familial polyposis coli. Skin lesions include epidermoid and sebaceous cysts, desmoid tumors (3.5 per cent), leiomyomas, lipomas, and neurofibromas. The desmoid tumors have a recurrence rate of 27 to 57 per cent but low malignancy. The epidermoid cysts are the most common and occur on the face and extremities. The normal trabecular bone of the mandible and maxillae is replaced by dense bone; involvement of the calvarium and long bones resembles osteosclerosis. Osteomas of the mandible may be extremely small. Dental abnormalities consist of absent or abnormal dentition. Mesenteric fibromatosis has been reported in several kindreds. Gastric polyps occur in at least 5 per cent, but some polyps are hyperplastic and not adenomatous. In the duodenum, the polyps are most often found in the second portion. In 12 per cent of patients, periampullary carcinoma may develop. Jejunal and ileal adenomas are rare, although a few polyps in these sites have become carcinomatous. Tumors in other organs include papillary carcinoma of the thyroid, adrenal adenoma, and sex cord tumors. Some patients also have lymphoid hyperplasia of the terminal ileum.

Symptoms. The disease has not yet been reported in infants, but one must realize that soft and hard tissue tumors appear early in life, years before intestinal polyps become apparent.[54, 167] Dentition is poor, and many teeth do not erupt. Some patients have supernumerary teeth. Gastrointestinal symptoms consist of cramping abdominal pain and mucoid or bloody diarrhea.

Diagnosis. The association of skin and bone tumors should spur investigation of the gastrointestinal tract in any patient in whom it is exhibited. Barium enema shows diffuse polyposis of the colon but to a lesser extent than that seen in familial polyposis.

Treatment. Total colectomy or ileorectal anastomosis is indicated for the same reasons as in familial polyposis. Surgery can be delayed until early adult life, however, because malignant transformation seems to occur later in this syndrome.

Prognosis. Although total colectomy removes the danger of colonic carcinoma, tumors in the ileum and primary tumors of the thyroid have developed in some patients.[64] Sarcomatous change has occurred in some bone lesions.

TURCOT SYNDROME

This syndrome consists of the association of adenomatous and, rarely, villous polyposis coli and malignant central nervous system tumors: glioblastoma, medulloblastoma, and ependymoma. Thyroid carcinoma has been found in one patient. The polyps may be adenomatous and villous and have all of the malignant potential of the other polyposis coli syndromes. The syndrome differs, however, in that inheritance seems to be in an autosomal recessive fashion.

REFERENCES

1. Aballi, A. J., Banus, V. L., De Lamerens, S., and Rozengvaig, S.: Coagulation studies in the newborn period. I. Alterations of thromboplastin generation and effects of vitamin K on full-term and premature infants. Am. J. Dis. Child. 94:594, 1957.
2. Aballi, A. J., and De Lamerens, S.: Coagulation changes in the neonatal period and early infancy. Pediatr. Clin. North Am. 9:785, 1962.
3. Aballi, A. J., Howard, C. E., and Triplett, R. F.: Absorption of vitamin K from the colon of the newborn infant. J. Pediatr. 68:305, 1966.
4. Abrahamson, J., and Shandling, B.: Intestinal hemangiomata in childhood and a syndrome for diagnosis. J. Pediatr. Surg. 8:487, 1973.
5. Adlercreutz, H., Liewendahl, K., and Virkola, P.: Evaluation of Fecatest, a new guaiac test for occult blood in feces. Clin. Chem. 24:756, 1978.
5a. Alavi, A., and Ring, E. J.: Localization of gastrointestinal bleeding— superiority of Tc-99m sulfur colloid compared with angiography. Am. J. Roentgenol. 137:741, 1981.
6. Ament, M. E., and Christie, D. L.: Upper gastrointestinal fiberoptic endoscopy in pediatric patients. Gastroenterology 72:1244, 1977.
7. Ament, M. E., Grans, S. L., and Christie, D. L.: Experience with esophagogastroduodenoscopy in diagnosis of 79 patients with hematemesis, melena or chronic abdominal pain. Gastroenterology 68:858, 1975.
8. Anyon, C. P., and Clarkson, K. G.: Occult gastrointestinal bleeding in the first 2 months of life. N. Z. Med. J. 70:315, 1969.
9. Apt, L., and Downey, W. S., Jr.: Melena neonatorum: the swallowed blood syndrome. A simple test for the differentiation of adult and fetal hemoglobin in bloody stools. J. Pediatr. 47:6, 1955.
10. Arbeter, A. M., Courtney, R. A., and Gaynor, M. F.: Diffuse gastrointestinal polyposis associated with chronic blood loss, hypoproteinemia and anasarca in an infant. J. Pediatr. 76:609, 1970.
11. Bale, J. F., Jr., Brasher, C., and Siegler, R. L.: CNS manifestations of the hemolytic uremic syndrome. Am. J. Dis. Child. 134:869, 1980.
12. Barlow, B., Santulli, T. V., and Herd, W.: An experimental study of necrotizing enterocolitis: the importance of breast milk. J. Pediatr. Surg. 9:587, 1974.
13. Barlow, B., and Santulli, T. V.: Importance of multiple episodes of hypoxia or cold stress on the development of enterocolitis in an animal model. Surgery 77:687, 1973.
14. Beardmore, H., Rodgers, B. M., and Outerbridge, E.: Necrotizing enterocolitis with the sequel of colonic atresia. Gastroenterology 74:914, 1978.
15. Bell, M., Kosloske, A., Benton, C., and Martin, L.: Neonatal necrotizing enterocolitis: prevention of perforation. J. Pediatr. Surg. 8:601, 1973.
16. Bell, R. S., Graham, C. B., and Stevenson, J. K.: Roentgenologic and clinical manifestations of neonatal necrotizing enterocolitis. Experience with 43 cases. Am. J. Roentgenol. Radium Ther. Nucl. Med. 112:123, 1971.
17. Bell, M., Shackelford, P., Feigin, R., Ternberg, J., and Brotherton, T.: Epidemiologic and bacteriologic evaluation of neonatal necrotizing enterocolitis. J. Pediatr. Surg., 14:1, 1979.
18. Bell, M., Shackelford, P., Feigin, R., Ternberg, J., and Brotherton, J.: Alterations in gastrointestinal microflora during antimicrobial therapy for necrotizing enterocolitis. Pediatrics 63:425, 1979.
19. Bell, M., Ternberg, J., Feigin, R., Keating, J., Marshall, R., Barton, L., and Brotherton, T.: Neonatal necrotizing enterocolitis: therapeutic decisions based upon clinical staging. Ann. Surg. 187:1, 1978.
20. Book, L. S., and Herbst, J.: Intra-arterial infusions and intestinal necrosis. Pediatrics 65:1145, 1980.
21. Brizel, H. E., and Giovanni, R.: Giant hemangioma with thrombocytopenia. Radioisotope demonstration of platelet sequestration. Blood 26:751, 1965.
22. Buntain, W., Conner, E., Enrico, J., and Cassady, G.: Transcutaneous oxygen (T_cPO_2) measurements as an aid to fluid therapy in necrotizing enterocolitis. J. Pediatr. Surg. 14:728, 1979.
23. Burdelski, M.: Endoscopy in pediatric gastroenterology. Eur. J. Pediatr. 1:33, 1978.
24. Cairo, M. S., Grosfeld, J., and Weetman, R.: Gastric teratoma: unusual cause for bleeding of the upper gastrointestinal tract in the newborn. Pediatrics 67:721, 1981.
25. Caledral, S., Rodesch, F., Peeters, J. P., and Cremer, M.: Fiber endoscopy of the gastrointestinal tract in children. Series of 100 examinations. Am. J. Dis. Child. 131:41, 1977.
25a. Chandrakamol, B.: Gastric heterotopia in the ileum causing hemorrhage. J. Pediatr. Surg. 13:484, 1980.
25b. Chany, C., Moscovici, O., Lebon, P., and Roussetis: Association of coronavirus infection with neonatal necrotizing enterocolitis. Pediatrics 69:209, 1982.

26. Chisholm, T., Spencer, B., and McParland, F.: Acute massive gastrointestinal hemorrhage. Pediatr. Clin. North Am. 9:201, 1962.

27. Collins, R. E. C.: Some problems of gastrointestinal bleeding in children. Arch. Dis. Child. 46:110, 1971.

28. Cooperman, M., Pace, W., Martin, E. W., et al.: Determination of viability of ischemic intestine by Doppler ultrasound. Surgery 83:705, 1978.

29. Copple, P., and Kingsbury, R.: Hemangiomas of the small bowel in children. J. Pediatr. 59:243, 1961.

30. Cox, K., and Ament, M. E.: Upper gastrointestinal bleeding in children and adolescents. Pediatrics 63:408, 1979.

31. Cremer, M., Peeters, J. P., Emonts, P., et al.: Fiberendoscopy in children: experience with newly designed fiberscopes. Endoscopy 6:186, 1974.

32. Dam, H., Glavind, J., Larsen, H., and Plum, P.: Investigations into the cause of physiological hypoprothrombinemia in newborn children. IV. The vitamin K content of woman's milk and cow's milk. Acta Med. Scand. 112:210, 1942.

33. Dam, H., and Schonheyder, F.: The antihaemorrhagic vitamin of the chick. Nature 135:652, 1935.

34. Dam, H., Schonheyder, F., and Tage-Hansen, E.: Studies on the mode of action of vitamin K. Biochem. J. 30:1075, 1936.

35. Daneman, A., Woodward, S., and de Silva, M.: The radiology of neonatal necrotizing enterocolitis. Pediatr. Radiol. 7:70, 1978.

36. Danes, B. S., and Krush, A. J.: The Gardner's syndrome: a family study in cell culture. J. Natl. Cancer Inst. 58:771, 1977.

37. Dawn, F., Zucker, P., and Boley, S.: Colonoscopic polypectomy in children. Am. J. Dis. Child. 131:566, 1977.

38. Denes, J., Gergely, K., Wohlmuth, G., and Leb, J.: Necrotizing enterocolitis of premature infants. Surgery 68:558, 1970.

39. Dolislager, D., and Tune, B.: The hemolytic uremic syndrome. Am. J. Dis. Child. 132:55, 1977.

40. Du Muth, W. E.: Mesenteric vascular occlusion in children. JAMA 179:130, 1962.

41. Edelstein, A. D., and Tuck, S.: Familial hemolytic uremic syndrome. Arch. Dis. Child. 255:6, 1979.

42. Egan, E. A., Mantilla, G. A,. Nelson, R. M., et al.: A prospective controlled trial of oral kanamycin prophylaxis for neonatal necrotizing enterocolitis. Pediatr. Res. 10:423, 1976.

43. Eggink, W. F., Perlberger, R. R., and van Urk, H.: Angiographic control of traumatic hemobilia by selective arterial embolization. Br. J. Surg. 64:635, 1977.

44. Eidelman, A., and Inwood, R. J.: Necrotizing enterocolitis and enteral feeding. Am. J. Dis. Child. 134:553, 1980.

45. Emmanuel, B., Zlotnik, P., and Raffensperger, J.: Perforation of the gastrointestinal tract in infancy and childhood. Surg. Gynecol. Obstet. 146:926, 1978.

46. Farmer, K., and Hassall, I. B.: An epidemic of E. coli 055: K 59 in a neonatal unit. N. Z. J. Med. 77:372, 1973.

47. Fines, J.: The intestinal circulation in shock. Gastroenterology 52:454, 1967.

47a. Foman, S., Ziegler, E., Nelson, S., and Edwards, B.: Cow milk feeding in infancy: gastrointestinal blood loss and iron nutritional status. J. Pediatr. 98:540, 1981.

48. Fost, N. C., and Esterly, N. B.: Successful treatment of juvenile hemangiomas with prednisone. J. Pediatr. 72:351, 1968.

49. Fowler, D., Fortin, D., Wood, W., et al.: Intestinal vascular malformations. Surgery 86:277, 1977.

50. Fox, V.: Gastrointestinal bleeding due to oral dicloxacillin therapy for osteomyelitis. Pediatrics 63:676, 1979.

51. Franklin, R., and McSwain, B.: Juvenile polyps of the colon and rectum. Ann. Surg. 175:887, 1972.

52. Frizzera, G., and Murphy, S. B.: Follicular lymphoma in childhood. A rare clinical pathological entity. Report of 8 cases from four cancer centers. Cancer 44:2218, 1979.

53. Fromm, D.: Salicylate and gastric mucosal damage. Pediatrics 62:938, 1978.

54. Gardner, E. J.: Follow-up study of a family group exhibiting dominant inheritance for a syndrome including intestinal polyps, osteomas, fibromas and epidermal cysts. Am. J. Hum. Genet. 14:376, 1962.

55. Gathright, J., and Cofer, T.: Familial incidence of juvenile polyposis coli. Surg. Gynecol. Obstet. 138:185, 1974.

56. Gleason, W. A., Tedesco, F. J., Keating, J. P., and Goldstein, P.: Fiberoptic gastrointestinal endoscopy in the infants and children. J. Pediatr. 85:810, 1914.

57. Goldblatt, M., Goldin, A. R., and Shaft, M. I.: Percutaneous embolization for the management of hepatic artery aneurysms. Gastroenterology 73:1142, 1977.

58. Goldman, H.: Feeding and necrotizing enterocolitis. Am. J. Dis. Child. 134:553, 1980.

59. Graham, D. Y., Klish, W. J., Ferry, G., and Sabel, J. S.: Value of fiberoptic gastrointestinal endoscopy in infants and children. South. Med. J. 71:558, 1978.

59a. Grotsky, H. W., Rickert, R. R., Smith, W. D., and Newsome, J. F.: Familial juvenile polyposis coli. Gastroenterology 82:494, 1982.

60. Gruenberg, J., and Mackman, S.: Multiple lymphoid polyps in familial polyposis. Ann. Surg. 175:552, 1972.

61. Gryboski, J. D.: The role of endoscopy in upper gastrointestinal bleeding in infants and children. Dig. Dis. 26:17S, 1981.

62. Gryboski, J. D., and Clemett, A.: Congenital hepatic artery aneurysm with superior mesenteric artery insufficiency: a steal syndrome. Pediatrics 39:44, 1967.

63. Guinan, M., Schaberg, D., Bruhn, F., Richardson, J., and Fox, W.: Epidemic occurrence of neonatal necrotizing enterocolitis. Am. J. Dis. Child. 133:574, 1979.

64. Hamilton, S. R., Bussey, H. J. R., Mendelsohn, G., Diamond, M. P., Pavides, G., Hutcheon, D., et al.: Ileal adenomas after colectomy in

nine patients with adenomatous polyposis coli Gardner's syndrome. Gastroenterology 77:1252, 1979.

65. Hansen, T., Ritter, D., Speer, M., Kenny, J., and Rudolph, A.: A randomized controlled study of oral gentamycin in the treatment of necrotizing enterocolitis. J. Pediatr. 97:836, 1980.

66. Headington, J. T.: Segmental infarcts of the small intestine and mesenteric adenitis in Thai children. Lancet 1:802, 1967.

67. Hellman, R. M., Jackson, D. V., and Bess, D. H.: Thrombotic thrombocytopenic purpura and hemolytic uremic syndrome in HLA identical siblings. Ann. Intern. Med. 93:282, 1980.

68. Holden, K. R., and Alexander, F.: Diffuse neonatal hemangiomatosis. Pediatrics 46:411, 1970.

69. Howell, J., Pringle, K., Kirschner, B., and Burrington, J.: Peutz-Jeghers polyp causing colocolic intussusception in infancy. J. Pediatr. Surg. 16:82, 1981.

70. Hutter, J. J., Hathaway, W., and Wayne, E. R.: Hematologic abnormalities in severe neonatal necrotizing enterocolitis. J. Pediatr. 88:1026, 1976.

71. Hymes, L., and Warshaw, B.: Hemolytic uremic syndrome in two siblings from a nonendemic area. Am. J. Dis. Child. 135:166, 1981.

71a. Janik, J. S., Cranford, J., and Ein, S. H.: The well nourished infant with intussusception. Am. J. Dis. Child. 135:600, 1981.

72. Janik, J., Culham, J. A. G., Filler, R., Shandling, B., and Stringel, G.: Balloon embolism of a bleeding gastroduodenal artery in a 1 year old child. Pediatrics 67:671, 1981.

73. Jones, T. R., and Nance, F.: Periampullary malignancy in Gardner's syndrome. Ann. Surg. 185:565, 1977.

74. Juda, J. Z., Belin, R. P., and Burke, J. A.: Lymphoid hyperplasia of the bowel and its surgical significance. J. Pediatr. Surg. 11:997, 1976.

75. Kaplan, B. S., Chesney, R. W., and Drummond, K. N.: Hemolytic uremic syndrome in families. N. Engl. J. Med. 292:1090, 1975.

76. Kisker, C. T., and Bush, R.: Circulating fibrin in meningococcemia. J. Pediatr. 82:787, 1973.

76a. Kleigman, R. M., and Fanaroff, A.: Neonatal necrotizing enterocolitis: a nine year experience. Am. J. Dis. Child. 135:603, 1981.

77. Kliegman, R., Pittard, W., and Fanaroff, A.: Necrotizing enterocolitis in neonates fed human milk. J. Pediatr. 95:450, 1979.

78. Kleigman, R. M., Fanaroff, A., Izani, R., and Speck, W.: Clostridia as pathogens in neonatal necrotizing enterocolitis. J. Pediatr. 95:287, 1979.

79. Knott, L., and Miller, R.: Acute iron intoxication with intestinal infarction. J. Pediatr. Surg. 23:720, 1978.

80. Knox, W. G., Miller, R. E., Begg, C. F., and Zintel, H. A.: Juvenile polyps of the colon: a clinicopathologic analysis of 75 polyps in 43 patients. Surgery 48:201, 1960.

81. Konturek, S., Piastucki, I., Brozozowski, T., Radecki, T., Dembinsakiec, A., Zmuda, A., and Gryglewski, R.: Role of prostaglandins in the formation of aspirin-induced gastric ulcers. Gastroenterology 80:4, 1981.

82. Kosloske, A. M., Papile, L. A., and Burstein, J.: Indications for operation in acute necrotizing enterocolitis of the neonate. Surgery 87:502, 1980.

83. Krasna, I., Becker, J. M., Schwartz, D., and Schneider, K.: Low molecular weight dextran and reexploration in the management of ischemic mid-gut volvulus. J. Pediatr. Surg. 13:480, 1978.

84. Kuno-Sakai, H., Sakai, H., Nomoto, Y., Takakura, I., and Kimura, M.: Increased IgA bearing peripheral blood lymphocytes in children with Henoch-Schoenlein purpura. Pediatrics 64:918, 1979.

85. Lake, A. M., and Walker, W. A.: Neonatal necrotizing enterocolitis: a disease of altered host defense. Clin. Gastroenterol. 6:463, 1977.

86. Laufer, I., and deSa, D.: Lymphoid follicular pattern: a normal feature of the pediatric colon. Am. J. Roentgenol. 130:51, 1978.

87. LeFevre, H. W., Jr., and Jacques, T. F.: Multiple polyposis in an infant of 4 months. Am. J. Surg. 81:90, 1951.

88. Letfall, L., Jr., Chung, E. B., Dewitty, R. L., Cornwell, E., and Blakey, T.: Familial polyposis coli in black patients. Ann. Surg. 186:324, 1977.

89. Lehmiller, D., and Kanto, W. P., Jr.: Relationships of mesenteric thromboembolism, oral feedings and necrotizing enterocolitis. J. Pediatr. 92:96, 1978.

90. Liebman, W. M.: Fiberoptic endoscopy of the gastrointestinal tract in infants and children. I. Upper endoscopy in 53 children. Am. J. Gastroenterol. 68:362, 1977.

91. Liebman, W. M., Thaler, M. M., and Bujanover, Y.: Endoscopic evaluation of upper gastrointestinal bleeding in the newborn. Am. J. Gastroenterol. 69:607, 1978.

92. Lifshitz, F., Liepner, R. A., and Pergolizzi, R.: Hypoxia effects on carbohydrate transport. Pediatr. Res. 10:356, 1976.

93. Lindenauer, S. M., and Tank, E. S.: Surgical aspects of Henoch-Schönlein's purpura. Surgery 59:982, 1966.

94. Lloyd, D. A., and Cwyes, S.: Intestinal stenosis and enterocyst formation as late complications of necrotizing enterocolitis. J. Pediatr. Surg. 8:479, 1973.

95. Lloyd, J. R.: The etiology of gastrointestinal perforations in the newborn. J. Pediatr. Surg. 4:77, 1969.

96. Louw, J. H.: Polypoid lesions of the large bowel in children with particular reference to benign lymphoid polyposis. J. Pediatr. Surg. 3:195, 1968.

96a. Luk, G., Bynum, T., and Hendrix, T.: Gastric aspiration in localization of gastrointestinal hemorrhage. JAMA 241:576, 1979.

97. Lux, G., Rosch, W., Phillip, J., et al.: Gastrointestinal fiberoptic endoscopy in pediatric patients and juveniles. Endoscopy 10:158, 1978.

98. Maier, C., and von Schulthess, F.: Blue rubber bleb nevus syndrome. Schioeiz. Med. Wscht. 100:878, 1870.

99. Maglinte, D., Jordan, L., van Hove, E., Chua, G., Brown, D., and Graffis, R.: Chronic gastrointestinal bleeding from Meckel's diverticulum: radiologic considerations. J. Clin. Gastroenterol. 3:47, 1981.

100. Malphus, E. W., Krishna, G. S., and Nichols, B. L.: Necrotizing enterocolitis and gastroenteritis in post neonatal term infants. Pediatr. Res. 15:539, 1981.

101. Matuchansky, C., Babin, P., Coutnot, S., et al.: Peutz-Jeghers syndrome with metastasizing carcinoma arising from a juvenile hamartoma. Gastroenterology 77:1311, 1979.

101a. Mayer, I. E., and Hersh, T.: Endoscopic diagnosis of hereditary hemorrhagic telangiectasia. J. Clin. Gastroenterol. 3:361, 1981.

102. McCauley, R. G., Leonidas, J., and Bartoshesky, L. E.: Blue rubber bleb nevus syndrome. Radiology 133:375, 1979.

103. McCracken, G., Jr., and Eitzman, D.: Necrotizing enterocolitis. Am. J. Dis. Child. 132:1167, 1978.

104. Mellish, R. W. P.: Multiple hemangiomas of the gastrointestinal tract in children. Am. J. Surg. 131:412, 1971.

105. Meyers, M., Kaplowitz, N., and Bloom, A.: Malabsorption secondary to intestinal ischemia. Am. J. Roentgenol. Radium Ther. Nucl. Med. 119:352, 1973.

106. Michael, J A., Brody, W. R., Walter, J., et al.: Transcatheter embolization of an esophageal artery for treatment of a bleeding esophageal ulcer. Radiology 134:246, 1980.

107. Miller, W. H., Maioriello, J. J., and Stein, D. B.: Mesenteric vascular occlusion in infancy and childhood. J. Pediatr. 59:567, 1961.

108. Ming, S., and Levitan, R.: Acute hemorrhagic necrosis of the gastrointestinal tract. N. Engl. J. Med. 263:59, 1960.

109. Mizrahi, A., Barlow, O., Berdon, W., Blanc, W., and Silverman, W. A.: Necrotizing enterocolitis in premature infants. J. Pediatr. 65:697, 1965.

110. Monnens, L., van Collenburg, J., deJong, M., Zoethout, H., and van Wieringer, P.: Treatment of the hemolytic uremic syndrome. Helv. Paediatr. Acta 33:321, 1978.

111. Murphy, E.: Hereditary polyposis coli. II. Genetic counseling. Johns Hopkins Med. J. 145:171, 1979.

112. Muta, A., and Rosengart, R.: Interobserver variability in the radiographic diagnosis of necrotizing enterocolitis. Pediatrics 60:68, 1980.

113. Naylor, E., and Lebenthal, E.: Gardner's syndrome. Recent developments in research and management. Dig. Dis. 25:945, 1980.

114. Northfield, T. C., and Smith, T.: Hematemesis as an index of blood loss. Lancet 1:990, 1971.

115. Onarau, L., Sahim, B., Temucin, G., and Gokoz, A.: Juvenile colonic polyposis associated with congenital heart disease. Dis. Col. Rectum 21:50, 1978.

116. O'Neill, J., and Holcomb, G.: Surgical experience with neonatal necrotizing enterocolitis. Ann. Surg. 189:613, 1979.

117. O'Regan, S., Chesney, R. W., Mongeau, J. G., and Robitaille, P.: Aspirin and dipyridamole therapy in the hemolytic uremic syndrome. J. Pediatr. 97:473, 1980.

118. Ortiz, V., Strakianakis, G., Haasi, G., and Boles, E. T., Jr.: The value of radionuclide scanning in early diagnosis of intestinal infarction. J. Pediatr. Surg. 13:616, 1978.

119. Paley, R. H., McCarten, K. M., and Cleveland, R. H.: Enterocolonic fistula as a late complication of necrotizing enterocolitis. Am. J. Roentgenol. 132:988, 1979.

119a. Parikh, N., Sebring, E., and Polesky, H.: Evaluation of bloody gastric fluid from newborn infants. J. Pediatr. 94:967, 1979.

120. Parsons, H. G., and Pincharz, P.: Intestinal lymphangiectasia and colonic polyps. Surgical intervention. J. Pediatr. Surg. 14:530, 1980.

120a. Pellerin, D., Harouchi, A., and Delmas, P.: Meckel's diverticulum: Review of 250 cases in children. Ann. Chia. Int. 17:157, 1976.

120b. Perman, J. A., Waters, L. A., Harrison, M. R., Yu, E. S., and Heldt, G. P.: Breath hydrogen reflects canine intestinal ischemia. Pediatr. Res. 15:1229, 1981.

121. Perret, B., Gaze, H., Zimmerman, A., et al.: Familial hemolytic uremic syndrome in an infant: nephrectomy and transplantation. Helv. Paediatr. Acta 34:167, 1979.

122. Pitt, J., Barlow, B., and Heird, W.: Protection against experimental necrotizing enterocolitis by maternal milk. I. Role of milk leukocytes. Pediatr. Res. 11:906, 1977.

123. Purker, T. W., and Hoy, G.: Technique for continuous sampling of peritoneal fluid for prediction of intestinal gangrene. J. Pediatr. Surg. 16:58, 1981.

124. Ratner, I. A., and Swenson, O.: Mesenteric vascular occlusion in infancy and childhood. N. Engl. J. Med. 263:1122, 1960.

125. Ravitch, M. M.: Polypoid adenomatosis of the entire gastrointestinal tract. Ann. Surg. 128:283, 1948.

126. Raffensperger, J. G., and Luck, S. R.: Gastrointestinal bleeding in children. Surg. Clin. North Am. 36:413, 1976.

127. Richmond, J. A., and Mikity, V.: Benign form of necrotizing enterocolitis. Am. J. Radiol. 123:301, 1975.

128. Riddlesberger, M., Jr., and Lebenthal, E.: Nodular colonic mucosa of childhood. Normal or pathologic? Gastroenterology 79:265, 1980.

129. Rosenkrantz, J. G., and Smiley, J. W.: Superior mesenteric arterial embolectomy in an infant. J. Pediatr. Surg. 1:70, 1966.

130. Ross, L.: Mallory-Weiss syndrome in a 10 month old infant. Am. J. Dis. Child. 133:1069, 1979.

131. Roth, D., and Cohen, H.: Hematemesis and melena in an infant. Am. J. Dis. Child. 134:995, 1980.

132. Ruymann, F. F.: Juvenile polyps with cachexia: report of an infant and comparison with Cronkhite-Canada syndrome in adults. Gastroenterology 57:431, 1969.

133. Ryder, R., Buxton, A., and Wachsmith, I.: Enterotoxigenic E. coli in necrotizing enterocolitis: lack of an association. J. Pediatr. 91:302, 1977.

134. Sachatello, C. R.: Familial polyposis of the colon: a four decade follow-up. Cancer 28:581, 1971.

135. Sachatello, C. R., Hahn, S., and Carrington, C.:

Juvenile gastrointestinal polyposis in a female infant. Surgery 75:107, 1974.

136. Sachatello, C. R., Pickren, J. W., and Grace, J. I., Jr.: Generalized juvenile gastrointestinal polyposis: an hereditary syndrome. Gastroenterology 58:699, 1970.

137. Safaie-Shirazi, S., and Soper, R.: Endorectal pull through procedure in the surgical treatment of familial polyposis. J. Pediatr. Surg. 8:711, 1973.

138. Sahn, D. J., and Schwartz, A.: Schönlein-Henoch syndrome. Pediatrics 49:614, 1972.

139. Sann, L., Senaneuch, C., and Bethenod, R.: Necrotizing enterocolitis and milk protein intolerance. Nouv. Presse Med. 8:4027, 1979.

140. Santos, M., Krush, A., and Cameron, J.: Three varieties of hereditary intestinal polyposis. Johns Hopkins Med. J. 145:196, 1979.

141. Santulli, T. V., Schullinger, J. N., and Heird, W. C: Acute necrotizing enterocolitis in infancy: a review of 64 cases. Pediatrics 55:36, 1975.

142. Sawaf, H., Sharp, M., Youn, K., et al.: Ischemic colitis and stricture after hemolytic uremic syndrome. Pediatrics 61:315, 1968.

143. Schick, J. B., Swanson, M. A., Cox, K. L., Smith, L. E., and Goetzman, B. W.: Technetium scan for necrotizing enterocolitis. Pediatr. Res. 15:546, 1981.

144. Schultz, L. S., Assimacopoulos, C. A., and Lillehei, R. C.: Turner's syndrome with associated gastrointestinal hemorrhage. Surgery 68:485, 1970.

145. Schuster, S. R., and Fellows, K. E.: Management of major hemoptysis in patients with cystic fibrosis. J. Pediatr. Surg. 12:889, 1977.

146. Schuchardt, W. A., and Ponsky, J. L.: Familial polyposis and Gardner's syndrome. Surg. Gynecol. Obstet. 148:97, 1979.

146a. Schullinger, J. N., Mollim, D. L., Vinocur, C. D., Santulli, T. V., and Driscoll, J. M., Jr.: Neonatal necrotizing enterocolitis. Am. J. Dis. Child. 135:612, 1981.

147. Schwabe, A., and Lewin, K.: Gastrointestinal polyposis syndromes. Viewpoints Dig. Dis. 12:1, 1980.

148. Schwartz, A.: Hematologic aspects of gastrointestinal disease. In Gryboski, J. D.: Gastrointestinal Problems in the Infant. Philadelphia, W. B. Saunders Company, 1975.

149. Schwartz, D., Becker, J., So, H., and Schneider, K.: Segmental colonic gangrene: a surgical emergency in the hemolytic uremic syndrome. Pediatrics 62:54, 1978.

150. Schweigofer, S., Primack, W. A., Slovis, T. L., Fleischmann, L. E., Slovis, T. L., and Higlet, D. W.: Cholelithiasis associated with the hemolytic uremic syndrome. Am. J. Dis. Child. 134:622, 1980.

151. Segr, R., Joller, P., Baerlocker, K., Keny, A., et al.: Hemolytic uremic syndrome associated with neuraminidase producing microorganisms. Helv. Paediatr. Acta 35:359, 1980.

152. Sherman, N. J., and Clatworthy, H. W., Jr.: Gastrointestinal bleeding in neonates. A study of 94 cases. Surgery 62:614, 1967.

153. Siegler, R. L., and Bond, R. E.: Simultaneous microangiopathic hemolytic anemia, thrombocytopenia and acute nephropathy in mother and child. Am. J. Dis. Child. 134:991, 1980.

154. Smith, W. G., and Kern, B. B.: The nature of the mutation in familial multiple polyposis. Dis. Colon Rectum 16:264, 1973.

155. Smith, C. D., Schuster, S., Gruppe, W., and Vawter, G.: Hemolytic uremic syndrome: a diagnostic and therapeutic dilemma for the surgeon. J. Pediatr. Surg. 13:597, 1980.

156. Solomon, A., Beck, J. M., and Dinner, M.: Necrotizing enterocolitis in older infants. S. Afr. Med. J. 46:395, 1972.

157. Soper, R. T., and Kent, T. H.: Fatal juvenile polyposis in infancy. Surgery 69:692, 1971.

158. Sorrenti, L., and Lewy, P.: The hemolytic uremic syndrome. Am. J. Dis. Child. 132:59, 1978.

159. Speer, M., Taber, L., Yow, M., and Rudolph, A. J.: Fulminant neonatal sepsis and necrotizing enterocolitis associated with a "nonenteropathogenic" strain of Escherichia coli. J. Pediatr. 89:91, 1976.

160. Spencer, R.: Gastrointestinal hemorrhage in infancy and childhood. 476 cases. Surgery 55:718, 1964.

161. Spitz, L., and Batcup, G.: Haematemesis in infantile hypertrophic pyloric stenosis: the source of the bleeding. Br. J. Surg. 66:827, 1979.

162. Stanley-Brown, E. G., and Stevenson, S.: Massive gastrointestinal hemorrhage in the newborn infant. Pediatrics 35:482, 1965.

163. Stevenson, D., Kerner, J., Malachowski, N., and Sunshine, P.: Late morbidity among survivors of necrotizing enterocolitis. Pediatrics 66:925, 1981.

164. Sturm, R., Staneck, J. L., Stauffer, L., and Neblett, W. W.: Neonatal necrotizing enterocolitis associated with penicillin-resistant toxigenic Clostridium butyricum. Pediatrics 66:928, 1980.

165. Tedesco, F. J., Goldstein, P. D., Gleason, W. A., Keating, J. P., et al.: Upper gastrointestinal endoscopy in the pediatric patient. Gastroenterology 70:492, 1976.

166. Texter, E. C.: Small intestinal blood flow. Am. J. Dig. Dis. 8:587, 1963.

167. Thomas, K. E., Watne, A. L., Johnson, J. G., Roth, E., and Zimmerman, B.: Natural history of Gardner's syndrome. Am. J. Surg. 11:218, 1968.

168. Toccalino, H., Gustavino, E., De Pinni, F., O'Donnell, J., and Williams, M.: Juvenile polyps of the rectum and colon. Acta Paediatr. Scand. 62:337, 1973.

169. Tyressen, H., and Doyle, R.: Cowden's disease (multiple hamartoma syndrome). Mayo Clin. Proc. 56:179, 1981.

170. Tochen, M., and Campbell, J.: Colitis in children with the hemolytic uremic syndrome. J. Pediatr. Surg. 12:213, 1977.

171. Tonkin, J. L. D., Bjelland, J. C., and Hunter, T. B.: Spontaneous resolution of colonic strictures caused by necrotizing enterocolitis. Am. J. Radiol. 130:1077, 1978.

172. Touloukian, R. J., Posh, J., and Spencer, R.: The pathogenesis of ischemic gastroenterocolitis of the neonate. Selective gut mucosal ischemia of asphyxiated neonatal piglets. J. Pediatr. Surg. 7:194, 1972.

173. Upadhyaya, K., Barwich, K., Fishaut, M., Kashgarian, M., and Siegel, N.: The importance of nonrenal involvement in the hemolytic uremic syndrome. Pediatrics 65:115, 1980.

174. van Stiegmann, G., and Lilly, J.: Surgical lesions of the colon in the hemolytic uremic syndrome. Surgery 85:357, 1979.

175. van Wieringen, P. M., Monueus, L. A., and Bakkeren, J.: Hemolytic uremic syndrome. Pediatrics 8:561, 1976.

176. von Willebrand, E. A.: Hereditar pseudohamofili. Finska Lak Sallsk Handl. 68:87, 1926.

177. Warter, J., Storck, D., Christmann, D., and Meyer, F.: Malabsorption syndrome during the initial phase of a case of severe Henoch-Schoenlein purpura. Nouv. Presse Med. 8:1245, 1979.

178. Webster, J., Ree, A. J., Lewis, P. J., and Hensby, C. N.: Prostacyclin deficiency in haemolytic uremic syndrome. Br. Med. J. 281:271, 1980.

179. Weinstods, J. V., and Kawanishi, H.: Gastrointestinal polyposis with orocutaneous hamartomas (Cowden's disease). Gastroenterology 74:890, 1978.

180. Wexler, H. A.: The persistent loop sign in neonatal necrotizing enterocolitis: a new indication for surgical intervention. Radiology 126:201, 1978.

181. Whittington, P., Freidman, A. L., and Chesney, R. W.: Gastrointestinal disease in the hemolytic uremic syndrome. Gastroenterology 76:128, 1979.

182. Willital, G.: Significance of pediatric endoscopy. Endoscopy 10:153, 1978.

183. Willis, D. M.: Hyperosmolarity of oral solutions contributing to necrotizing enterocolitis. Pediatrics 60:535, 1979.

184. Wilson, J. F., Lahey, M. E., and Huner, D. C.: Studies on iron metabolism. V. Further observations on cow's milk induced gastrointestinal bleeding. J. Pediatr. 84:335, 1974.

185. Woodruff, C. W., Wright, S. W., and Wright, R. P.: The role of fresh cow's milk in iron deficiency. Am. J. Dis. Child. 124:26, 1972.

186. Yao, T., Iida, M., Ohsata, K., Watanabe, H., and Omae, T.: Duodenal lesions in familial polyposis of the colon. Gastroenterology 73:1086, 1977.

Chapter Eight

INTESTINAL OBSTRUCTION

GASTROINTESTINAL OBSTRUCTION

Gastrointestinal obstruction occurs whenever there is interference with the flow of intraluminal contents through the digestive tract. One must differentiate the type of obstruction (mechanical or functional) and the site (gastric or small or large bowel).

Etiology. Some of the common causes of gastrointestinal obstruction in infancy are listed in Table 8–1. Those of functional origin include gastric atony, the more unusual disorders of motility such as aganglionosis, delayed maturation of ganglion cells, absence of intestinal musculature, and paralytic ileus. The last-named may result from hypokalemia, pneumonia (Fig. 8–1), respiratory distress, enterocolitis, cerebral trauma, mesenteric thrombosis, retroperitoneal hemorrhage, perforation, peritonitis, pancreatitis, shock, or surgery. Maternal medications or drugs such as heroin or ganglionic blocking agents can also produce temporary ileus. Although 83 per cent of infants with the congenital asplenia syndrome present with cardiorespiratory problems, 17 per cent present with intestinal obstruction due to malrotation or enteric duplications.[24b]

Pathogenesis. Mechanical obstruction of the stomach is dealt with in Chapter Twelve. When the small bowel is obstructed, the intestine proximal to the site of obstruction becomes distended by intestinal secretions, swallowed material, and air. As distention increases, the intestine loses its capacity to handle fluid and electrolytes, and as their intraluminal concentrations increase, so does their rate of secretion. Some question remains as to whether intraluminal fluid accumulation is due to increased secretion, decreased absorption, or both. Further fluid losses occur into the wall of affected bowel. Therefore, fluid losses, which are at first isotonic, become hypertonic.[34, 38] Vomiting further increases these losses, and the result is diminished plasma volume with severe dehydration, oliguria, azotemia, decreased cardiac output, tachycardia, and shock. Losses in colonic obstruction are less dramatic, but distention in the presence of a competent ileocecal valve carries the risk of cecal perforation. In the presence of stasis, intestinal flora proliferate.

Symptoms. Typical of gastrointestinal obstruction are pain that is periumbilical and colicky in nature, vomiting, abdominal distention, and some degree of obstipation. High intestinal obstruction, associated with lesions above the ligament of Treitz, is characterized by epigastric or upper abdominal distention with visible peristaltic waves traveling across the upper abdomen from left to right. The vomitus is clear and acid if the obstruction is gastric, clear and sometimes alkaline if it is above the ampulla of Vater, and bilious and alkaline if it is below the ampulla. In mid- and lower

Table 8–1 Causes of Intestinal Obstruction in Infancy

STOMACH	SMALL BOWEL	LARGE BOWEL
	Mechanical	
Pyloric stenosis	Atresia or stenosis	Imperforate anus
Prepyloric or antral diaphragm	Hypertrophic stenosis of the	Duplication
Pyloric gastric duplication cyst	duodenum	Atresia or stenosis
Volvulus of the stomach	Duplication cysts	
	Anular pancreas	
	Malrotation	
	Volvulus	
	Nonrotation with fibrous bands	
	Incarcerated hernia	
	Congenital adhesions or bands	
	Preduodenal portal vein	
	Meconium ileus	
	Acquired	
Foreign body	Intussusception	Drug-induced meconium ileus
Bezoar	Peritoneal adhesions	equivalent
	Mesenteric thrombosis	Meconium plug syndrome
	Necrotizing enterocolitis	Inspissated stool or milk
	Neuroma	syndrome
	Tumor	Fecalith
	Polyp	Toxic dilatation of the colon
	Foreign body	Intussusception
	Functional	
Gastric atony	Total aganglionosis of the colon	Hirschsprung's disease
	Absence of musculature	Neonatal small left colon
	Paralytic ileus	Hyperganglionosis
	Intestinal pseudo-obstruction	Microcolon, hypoperistalsis
		syndrome[2]
		Deficiency of argyrophil neurons
		of myenteric plexus[41]

intestinal obstruction, vomiting develops later than with high obstruction, and the vomitus often has a fecal odor. Failure to pass stool and gas occurs only after the bowel below the site of obstruction has been emptied. The bowel sounds may be normal, hypoactive, or hyperactive. Peristaltic rushes are not usual. The abdomen is tympanitic, and dilated loops of small bowel are visualized over the abdomen or palpated within it.

Partial small bowel obstruction is less typical and may present only as diarrhea or intermittent vomiting or both. Abdominal distention and colicky pain tend to subside and recur.

Diagnosis. Gastric aspiration is of diagnostic and therapeutic import. A large residual indicates high intestinal obstruction. Rectal examination will show whether the anus is patent. Films of the abdomen with the baby in decubitus, erect, and lateral positions will reveal typical patterns of obstruction: the massively dilated stomach of pyloric stenosis, the "double bubble" effect of duodenal obstruction, and the stepladder pattern of dilated small bowel loops in lower intestinal obstruction. The colon is distended proximal to a site of obstruction. Upright or lateral decubitus films show air-fluid levels throughout the small bowel. In paralytic ileus, both the small and the large bowel are dilated (Fig. 8–1).

If mechanical obstruction is suggested, barium studies, beginning with a barium enema, are performed to define the site of the lesion. Manometric studies show an increase in contractile pressures in the small bowel during early obstruction, which decrease as the obstruction persists.

Treatment. Medical therapy must begin the moment obstruction is suspected. The infant is given no food, is placed in a semi-upright position in an incubator or warm

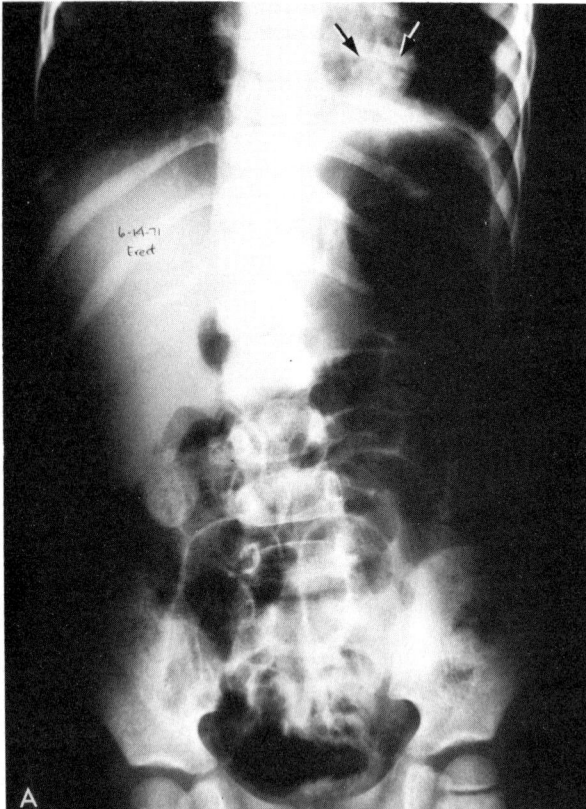

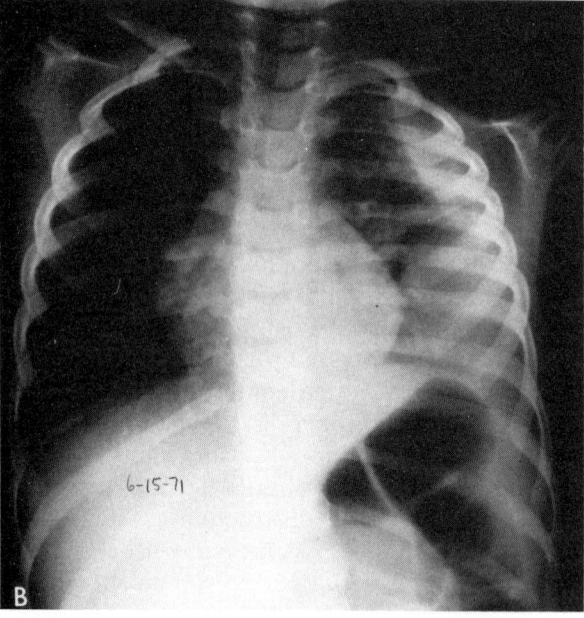

Figure 8–1 Acute abdomen secondary to basilar pneumonia. This young girl was brought into the emergency room with nausea, vomiting, and fever of 24 hours' duration. Diffuse abdominal guarding and absence of bowel sounds were found. There was no history of cough or sputum production. *A*, Initial plain film showed some mild and nonspecific dilation of bowel loops. A faint triangular area of density is seen just above the diaphragm partially hidden by the cardiac shadow (*arrows*); this represents a pneumonic infiltrate. There is an associated pleural effusion, which can be seen between the aerated lung and the lateral chest wall. *B*, Chest film one day later shows rather marked progression of the pneumonia and the effusion.

bassinet, and is given fluids intravenously. Hypovolemia is corrected by transfusion of whole blood, 10 ml per kg, or of plasma. The importance of correcting electrolyte imbalances and restoring good urinary flow cannot be overemphasized. Intermittent gastric suction not only places the bowel at rest but also prevents the accumulation of swallowed air and minimizes the opportunity for vomiting and aspiration of gastric contents. If sepsis is suspected, preoperative antibiotics are administered to provide effective coverage for enteric organisms. Surgical correction of recognized mechanical obstruction is the only definitive treatment.

Anatomic lesions causing obstruction are discussed in detail in later chapters under diseases of specific organs. Some of the more common lesions are described in the following pages.

INTUSSUSCEPTION

Although ileocolic intussusception is the type most frequently encountered, small bowel intussusceptions are less obvious but of more serious consequence.[10]

GASTRODUODENAL INTUSSUSCEPTION

Obstruction of the midportion of the stomach in a child should arouse immediate suspicion of gastroduodenal intussusception.

Incidence. Just over 60 cases have been reported in the literature, but only 3 were in children. Both sexes are affected equally in the adult group, but all of the children have been girls.

Etiology and Pathogenesis. All but one of the cases were associated with gastric tumors, and most of these were benign. A benign gastric polyp or, less often, an adenoma or leiomyoma serves as the lead point and is carried by peristalsis into the duodenum. Part of the gastric mucosa invaginates along with the polyp.

Symptoms. The symptoms are those of gastric obstruction. The youngest patient, a baby of 23 months, was always a poor eater and was fussy during the month prior to her illness. She had a three-day history of vague abdominal pain and vomiting, which increased until she could retain nothing and vomited even without eating. Each of the two older girls had a long history of recurrent epigastric pain and emesis. An inconstant mass was palpable in the epigastric or periumbilical area.

Diagnosis. Pyloric obstruction is differentiated by radiologic examination of the upper gastrointestinal tract. There is an abrupt cutoff of barium in the midportion of the stomach, narrowing of the body of the stomach, converging axial striations of the stomach and duodenum running parallel to the long axis of the organs, a central filling defect in the duodenum, and a coiled-spring appearance in the duodenum.

Treatment. Operative reduction of the intussusception and removal of the gastric polyp are performed as soon as the diagnosis is clear.

Complication. Perforation of the duodenum has followed this type of intussusception.

Prognosis. Complete recovery is the rule.

ILEOCECAL AND ENTEROENTERIC INTUSSUSCEPTION

Intussusception develops when a loop of bowel invaginates caudad in the direction of peristaltic flow. The type is dependent upon which part of the intestine, the intussusceptum, enters the intussuscipiens.

Incidence. Twice as common in boys as in girls, ileocolic intussusception is the most frequent cause of intestinal obstruction in infants, accounting for 80 to 90 per cent of all cases. Nearly three quarters of intussusceptions occur before the second year of life, with 70 per cent occurring in those under one year and 49 per cent occurring between the third and ninth months. The condition is rare in the neonatal period, but even intrauterine intussusception has been reported. Ein and Stephens reported 354 cases in a ten-year period.[10] Mollitt et al.[25] reviewed 119 cases of postoperative intussusception and found 86 per cent to involve small bowel, 8 per cent to be ileocecal, and 6 per cent to be cecocecal.

Etiology. No cause is identified in nearly 90 per cent of infants. This is in contrast to older children, in whom some etiologic factor, such as a polyp, is found in most cases. In many series a seasonal incidence is noted, with cases clustered in spring and fall. This is probably related to the high incidence at these times of enteric and respiratory infections, which cause reactive changes in the intestinal lymphoid tissue. There is considerable lymphatic tissue about the terminal ileum and ileocecal valve; it increases to its greatest size at one year and diminishes thereafter.

Infection with enlargement of this lymphoid tissue is considered causative in ileocecal intussusceptions, and rising titers of antibody to adenovirus have been noted in some infants with intussusception. Other etiologic factors are polyps, eosinophilic granuloma of the ileum, lymphoma, lymphosarcoma, duplication cysts, leukemic infiltration of the bowel, ectopic pancreas, hematoma, Henoch-Schönlein purpura, hemophilia, hypertrophied Peyer's patches, leiomyosarcoma, worms, foreign body, tumor, histoplasmosis of the appendix, and intestinal intubation.[14, 24, 43] Enteroenteric intussusceptions often follow intra-abdominal surgery and in some cases are caused by an inverted appendiceal stump or by ileal edema.

Pathology. Intussusception is categorized by the duration of symptoms and by the type of bowel involved in the invagination. It is acute if it is of less than one week's duration. In most cases the average duration is 34 hours. If symptoms have been present for one to two weeks, it is subacute. Chronic intussusception is that which persists for more than two weeks. The enteroenteric form entails invagination of small bowel into small bowel; the ileocecal or ileocolic, of ileum into cecum or colon; and the colocolic, of colon into colon. Transient small bowel intussusceptions occur in the normal infant and reduce spontaneously without causing symptoms. These are particularly frequent in children with celiac disease.

Intussusception is followed by edema and vascular compromise of the bowel and in time causes irreparable tissue necrosis with fever and elevation of the peripheral white blood cell count.

Three quarters of enteroenteric intussusceptions are associated with a specific organ lesion. The greater mobility of the small bowel reduces the dangers of infarction, but because of the longer duration of symptoms before diagnosis (average of seven days), there is an overall greater mortality and a higher small bowel resection rate. This type of intussusception has recently been reported as a complication of chemotherapy in children who are being treated for disseminated malignant disease.

Symptoms. Most of the intussusceptions of infancy are acute and of the ileocecal type (72 per cent). Of lower frequency are the enteroenteric (17 per cent) and the colocolic types (9 per cent). Colicky pain and vomiting characterize the low intestinal forms in more than 80 per cent of cases. The pain lasts for several minutes and occurs in 15- to 30-minute intervals. The infant screams, draws up his legs, and cannot be consoled. Between attacks he sleeps, only to awaken with a recurrence of pain. In 60 to 66 per cent of patients, blood is passed in the stool, which typically has the appearance of currant jelly. Others have blood-streaking of the stool, frank hemorrhage, or constipation. A few neonates have only painless rectal bleeding.

Rarely, the infant is perfectly well at one moment and lies ashen and unresponsive at the next. It is impressive that most patients with ileocolic intussusceptions are well nourished and, indeed, chubby babies.[17a]

The enteroenteric intussusceptions generally involve the ileum and are the most serious, because their symptoms are far less dramatic than those of the ileocecal type and their duration is much longer. There is no colic or rectal bleeding but only vomiting, which gradually increases in intensity and frequency. This lesion is to be suspected in any infant recovering from abdominal surgery and particularly in one who has had prolonged postoperative intestinal suction. The average age of onset is 17 months. Symptoms usually develop on the fourth to fifth postoperative day, although they can appear any time within the first month after surgery. The physical examination is not helpful, since small bowel intussusceptions are not usually palpable.

The baby with an acute ileocolic intussusception is toxic and dehydrated, is febrile, and has tachycardia. It is impossible to examine the abdomen during bouts of pain, but between attacks the abdomen is soft. A sausage-shaped mass is palpable in the right lower quadrant, along the ascending colon, or in the right upper quadrant. A right lower

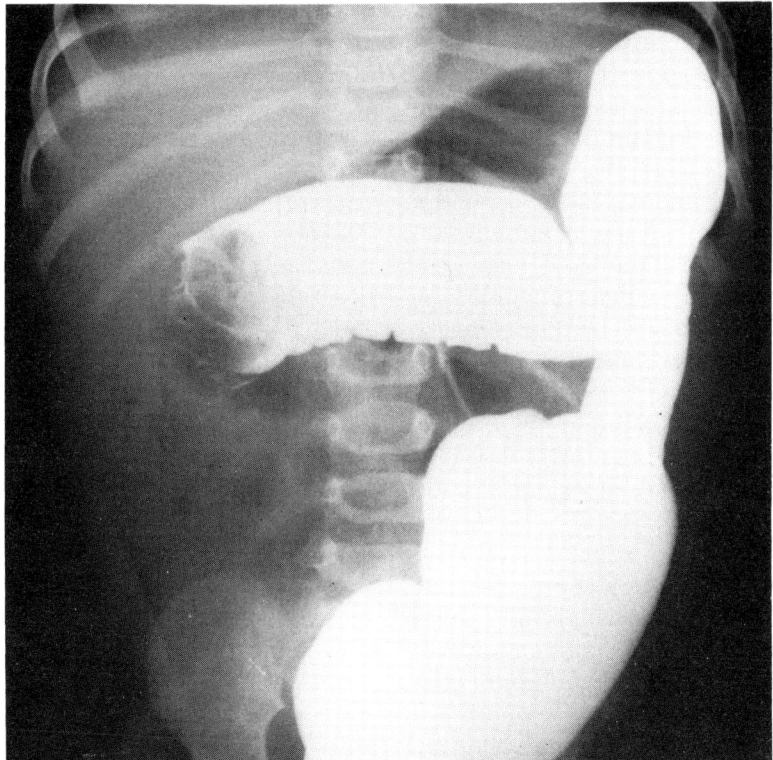

Figure 8–2 Intussusception in a five-month-old boy who had had intermittent sudden episodes of loud crying and apparent colic over 12 hours. A blood clot was found in the rectum at the time of initial examination. The barium enema demonstrates the intussuscipiens presenting as a mass near the hepatic flexure. This represents an ileocolic intussusception and was easily reduced by the barium enema. Surgery was not necessary.

quadrant mass is also palpable during rectal examination. If the intussusception has progressed into the transverse colon, it is palpable under the liver edge or it may be obscured by the liver. The absence of palpable bowel loops in the right lower quadrant (Dance's sign), is another diagnostic sign. Abdominal distention develops late, and the bowel sounds, which are hyperactive early, decrease as the vascular supply is compromised. The white blood count ranges between 10,000 and 18,000 cells per cubic millimeter. A rise to a level of 20,000 or more signifies gangrene of the bowel.

Plain films of the abdomen show dilated loops of small bowel with absence of air beyond the level of obstruction.[19] A soft tissue mass may be visualized at the site of obstruction. Although some feel that the diagnosis can be made by examination of the plain film, in one study such an examination by four skilled radiologists failed to confirm a correct diagnosis in more than half the cases. Barium enema is the diagnostic study of choice and should be performed in all infants who have had symptoms for less than 48 hours. With longer duration of symptoms there is increased danger of bowel necrosis and perforation. Not only will the study confirm the diagnosis, but it will reduce the intussusception in 80 per cent of cases. The barium flows into the colon until it ends at a cup-like cutoff (Fig. 8–2), and as it trickles between the intussusceptum and the intussuscipiens, it produces a coiled-spring or corkscrew pattern. Certain precautions must be taken during the procedure. A balloon-tipped catheter is inserted into the rectum, and the balloon is inflated and pulled against the levators. The barium canister must not be elevated more than 3 1/2 feet above the patient. Barium flow is stopped as the intussusception is met, and a gentle flow is resumed and continued for as long as the barium leaks ahead. If there is no change over five minutes, the enema is discontinued and the patient is taken to surgery. Manipulation of the abdomen in an effort to reduce the intussusception is contraindicated. Reduction is accomplished when the barium suddenly flows freely into the small bowel. Signs associated with successful reduction are the appearance of the cecum in the study, disappearance of the mass, passage of gas with the enema, and improvement in the clinical condition of the patient. Evacuation of charcoal in enema contents six hours after it is passed into stomach indicates that there is no residual obstruction. Glucagon has recently been used in reducing intussusception, but experience is still limited.[15]

Treatment. Surgical reduction is indicated if the intussusception is enteroenteric or if an ileocolic intussusception causes symptoms for more than 48 hours. Failure of the barium enema is an obvious indication for surgery.[45] One case has been reported in which the intussusception sloughed and the bowel underwent autoanastomosis.[27]

Prognosis. Idiopathic ileocolic intussusception of infancy carries a negligible mortality and recurs in only about 3 per cent of cases. Small bowel intussusceptions carry a higher mortality (7.6 per cent) as well as problems of segmental resection. Intussusceptions in older children do tend to recur if the causative lesion is not removed. Ileocolectomy is a rather drastic recommendation for recurrent idiopathic intussusception.

VOLVULUS

Volvulus is twisting of the bowel upon its own axis or the axis of its mesentery.

Etiology. Midgut volvulus is usually caused by abnormal re-entry of the bowel during its developmental return to the abdominal cavity. It is associated with faulty mesenteric attachments and is a frequent complication of errors of rotation.

Pathology. As the bowel undergoes volvulus, it rotates counterclockwise to any degree, so that the extent of intestinal obstruction and vascular compromise depends upon the degree of rotation. If it causes only obstruction, this is most common at the duodenojejunal junction and the duodenum above it is dilated. More advanced rotations cause strangulation with resulting tissue gangrene, perforation, peritonitis, and sepsis.

Symptoms. Symptoms develop in the neonatal period after the first few days of life and again after several months of age. The early symptoms of volvulus are those of intestinal obstruction, namely, abdominal distention and vomiting. The vomitus is at first gastric and later bilious or fecal in character. Obstipation or diarrhea may follow. Occasionally diarrhea is the only presenting symptom in an infant, and this can persist for days or weeks before the true diagnosis is recognized. Acute volvulus in infancy may even cause sudden gastrointestinal hemorrhage and shock as its first manifestation.

Recurrent volvulus later in infancy and in childhood mimics celiac disease when it causes chronic lymphatic obstruction, cyclic vomiting, or functional disease.

Diagnosis. This diagnosis is to be strongly suspected when intestinal obstruction or hemorrhage suddenly develops in a well infant. Intussusception, malrotation, and necrotizing enterocolitis must all be considered in the differential diagnosis. Perforation and bacterial peritonitis cannot be differentiated in infants with strangulation.

A flat film of the abdomen shows gastric and minimal to moderate duodenal dilatation. This is in contrast to the greatly dilated duodenum of intrinsic duodenal obstruction. In most cases of midgut volvulus, the obstruction is in the distal duodenum and there is scattered or no air in the distal small bowel. Occasionally, one or two greatly dilated small bowel loops are seen. The abdomen appears homogeneous. Less often, midgut volvulus is associated with jejunal or ileal obstruction. Although these obstructive findings are typical, they are not always present. Films of infants with complete volvulus may show only changes consistent with mild occlusive disease, such as intraperitoneal exudate and thickened bowel walls. A barium enema will show the position of the cecum.

Treatment. The volvulus must be reduced immediately, and any infarcted bowel should be resected.

Prognosis. Complete volvulus in the neonate is associated with an 80 per cent mortality, although in older infants it falls to between 10 and 20 per cent. Volvulus will recur in 5 per cent of cases.

MECONIUM ILEUS

Meconium ileus ranks third as a cause of neonatal intestinal obstruction, being exceeded in frequency only by intestinal atresia and malrotation. It must be stressed that although most cases are due to cystic fibrosis, a few are not.[37]

Incidence. The disease heralds the diagnosis of cystic fibrosis in 10 to 15 per cent of all infants with the condition. One third or more of the patients have affected siblings.[1] In a few series there is a slight preponderance of males over females, but in most the sexes are affected equally. The total reported incidence to date has been in Caucasian infants.

Etiology and Pathogenesis. The intestinal obstruction is caused by thick, abnormal meconium that resists passage beyond the terminal ileum.[9] Tar-like material fills the distal 10 to 30 cm of ileum, while the bowel proximal to it is dilated and its walls hypertrophied. The pancreatic changes are less severe in infants with cystic fibrosis and meconium ileus than in those without this complication. Intestinal changes, on the other hand, are more severe in those with cystic fibrosis, and masses of acidophilic secretions fill the lumens of Brunner's glands in the duodenum and the crypts of Lieberkühn in the colon. In two infants without cystic fibrosis, hypertrophied lymph nodules were noted in the ileal submucosa.

The abnormal meconium contains increased quantities of serum proteins, particularly albumin. The soluble proteins of meconium derive from intestinal secretions and ingested amniotic fluid. The quantity of albumin does not correlate with the presence or degree of clinical obstruction, for the mean percentage of albumin in normal meconium is 0.11; in that from babies with meconium ileus, 9.6; and in that from babies with cystic fibrosis without obstruction, 11.8. The tenaciousness of the meconium is due rather to an increase in the mucoprotein fraction and the formation of an insoluble calcium-glycoprotein compound in abnormal mucus (Table 8–2).

There is some question as to whether the

Table 8–2 Characteristics of Meconium in Normal Infants and Infants with Cystic Fibrosis[3, 29, 35, 39]

	NORMAL	CF
Water	74%	65%
Protein	8.5%	71.9%
Carbohydrate	4.6%	1.3%
Mucopolysaccharide	41.2%	8.8%
Mucoprotein	7.3%	15.1%
Globulins	0.6%	9.5%
Albumin	0.4%	22.2%
Enzymes		
Lactase mm/gm protein	0	5–22
Sucrase mm/gm protein	0	30–130
Maltase	0–95	55–240
Acid phosphatase mm × 60 mm/gm protein	0.2–0.9	0.1–0.7
Alkaline phosphatase	av. 5–35	30–148
Trypsin	>1:8	0
Metals	nl	↓

Adapted from Shwachman, H., and Antonowicz, I.: Studies on meconium. *In* Lebenthal, E. (ed.): Textbook of Gastroenterology and Nutrition in Infancy. New York, Raven Press, 1981.

complicating intestinal atresias in this disease are primary or secondary. Atresia may well result from intramural scarring and intraluminal obliteration after fetal volvulus, for a number of specimens with complete atresia show an extravasation of meconium and reaction to it within the intestinal wall at the site of the atresia. Specimens with partial atresia show obstruction from external cicatrization, mucosal ulceration, and a similar intramural reaction.

In most of the cases not associated with cystic fibrosis the etiology is unknown. Partial aplasia of the pancreas is one associated factor and an inspissated stool syndrome is consistent with some others.

Symptoms. One fifth of the babies are premature or have a history of maternal hydramnios. In most, abdominal distention develops during the first few days of life, although in some the abdomen is distended at birth. The infants do not pass meconium and begin to vomit when they are several hours to several days old. The vomitus is at first gastric in type, but later it becomes bilious. Depending upon the degree of pulmonary involvement, there are tachypnea, intercostal retractions, and grunting respirations. The distended abdomen shows patterns of dilated bowel loops that are doughy to palpation. Some of the loops contain scattered, firm, movable masses. Peristalsis is hyperactive. The rectal ampulla is empty, and sphincter tone is normal.

Meconium ileus therefore presents as low intestinal obstruction, but if it is complicated by volvulus, atresia, or perforation, as it is in one quarter of the cases, the symptoms resemble more closely those of upper gastrointestinal obstruction. A meconium ileus equivalent in older children is discussed under cystic fibrosis in Chapter Fifteen.

Diagnosis. Radiologic examination is diagnostic in 65 per cent of cases. The characteristic findings are air-fluid levels in the small bowel in 52 per cent; a sentinel loop in 45 per cent; atresia in 12 per cent; and intramural air and calcifications in 6 per cent (Figs. 8–3 to 8–5). The distended loops

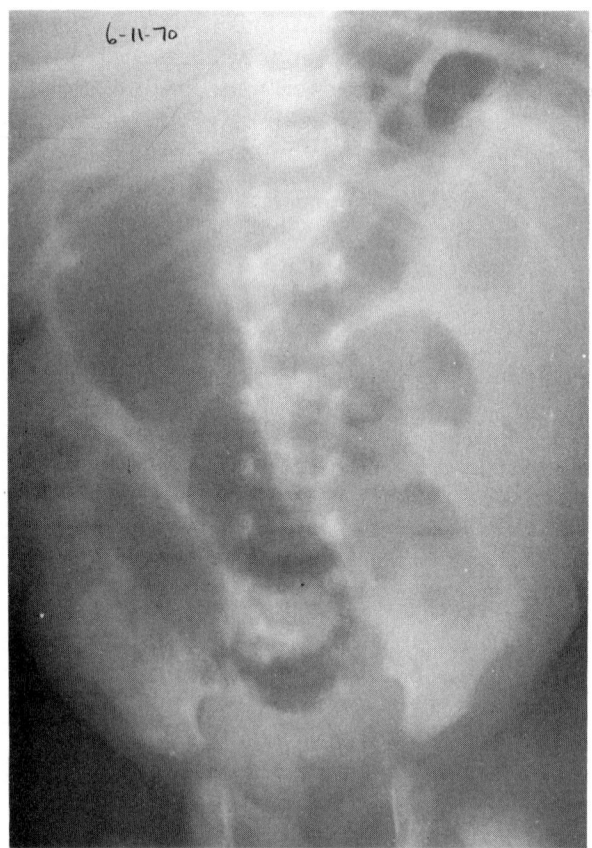

Figure 8–3 Meconium ileus in a four-day-old infant who had not passed any meconium. The KUB shows numerous dilated loops of bowel and a fairly characteristic mottled pattern of meconium and gas in the right lower quadrant. The clinical and radiologic impression was that this represented meconium ileus. The diagnosis was confirmed at surgery; the distal 10 to 12 cm of small bowel were obstructed with inspissated meconium. The meconium was disimpacted, but the obstruction recurred and repeat surgical disimpaction was necessary. The patient then made an uneventful recovery and is thought to have cystic fibrosis, although sweat test findings were equivocal.

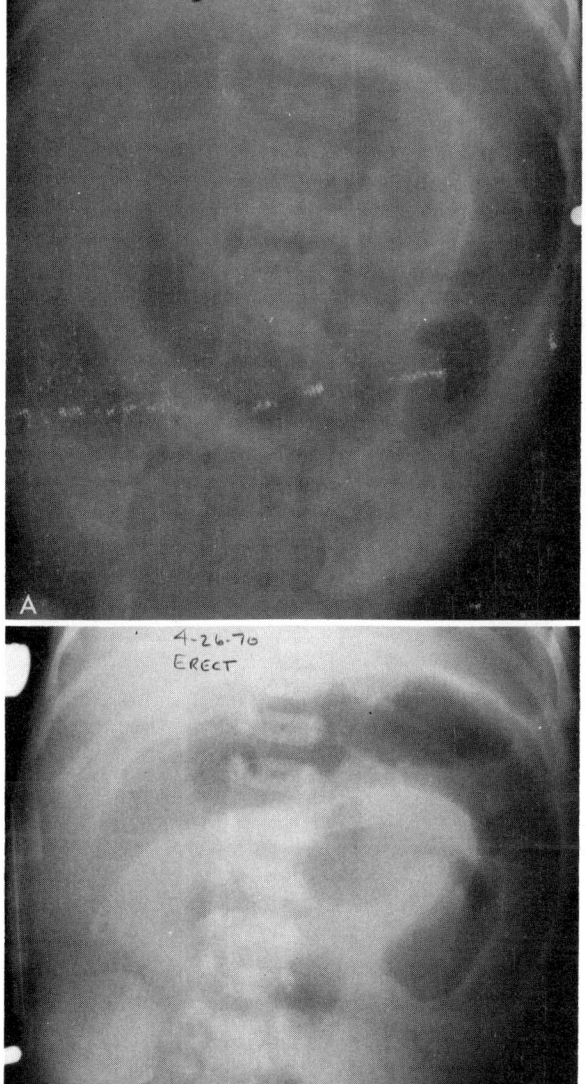

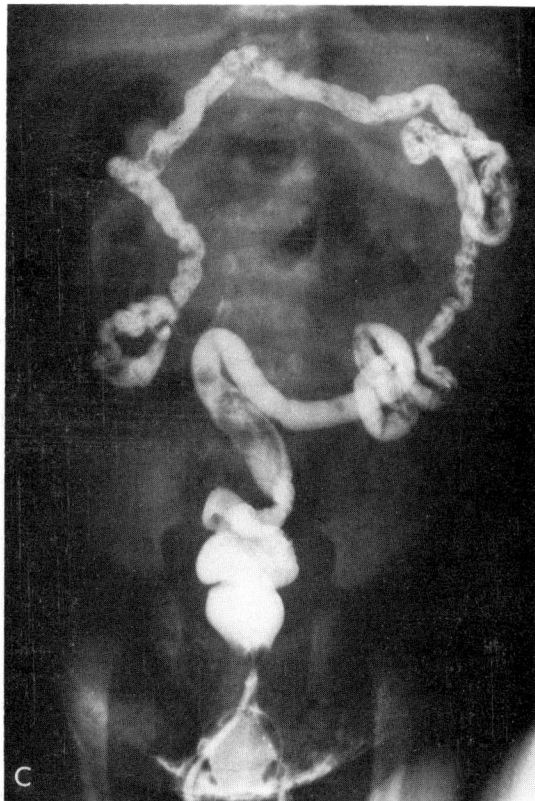

Figure 8–4 Meconium ileus in a neonate with progressive abdominal distention and failure to pass meconium during the first 24 hours of life. *A,* Supine film of the abdomen demonstrates several distended loops of bowel, but one cannot be certain from the plain film whether this is small bowel or colon or both. Mottled areas of lucency seen on both sides of the abdomen suggest the mixture of gas and meconium seen in meconium ileus. *B,* The distended bowel loops are again evident and several air-fluid levels can be seen on the left side. It is generally thought that the presence or absence of air-fluid levels cannot be used as a strong diagnostic point in consideration of meconium ileus. *C,* Barium enema shows that there is no obstruction at the colon level and that the large bowel is, in fact, abnormally small in caliber. This narrowed colon, or microcolon, suggests the presence of a long-standing obstructing lesion in the distal small bowel. The diagnosis of meconium ileus was confirmed at surgery, when impacted meconium was seen throughout the distal 10 cm of ileum. The inspissated meconium was surgically removed. The diagnosis of cystic fibrosis was made by a sweat test done somewhat later.

of bowel that contain air bubbles trapped in meconium have a "ground-glass" appearance. Barium enema shows an unused or "micro" colon. Bone films show abnormal metaphyseal bands in meconium peritonitis.[46]

The sweat test should be performed as soon as the diagnosis is suspected and is accurate in 90 per cent of infants. The major difficulty in this age group is to obtain sufficient quantities of sweat. Lactase in meconium is elevated.[3]

Treatment. Until recently, cases of simple meconium ileus were treated by surgi-

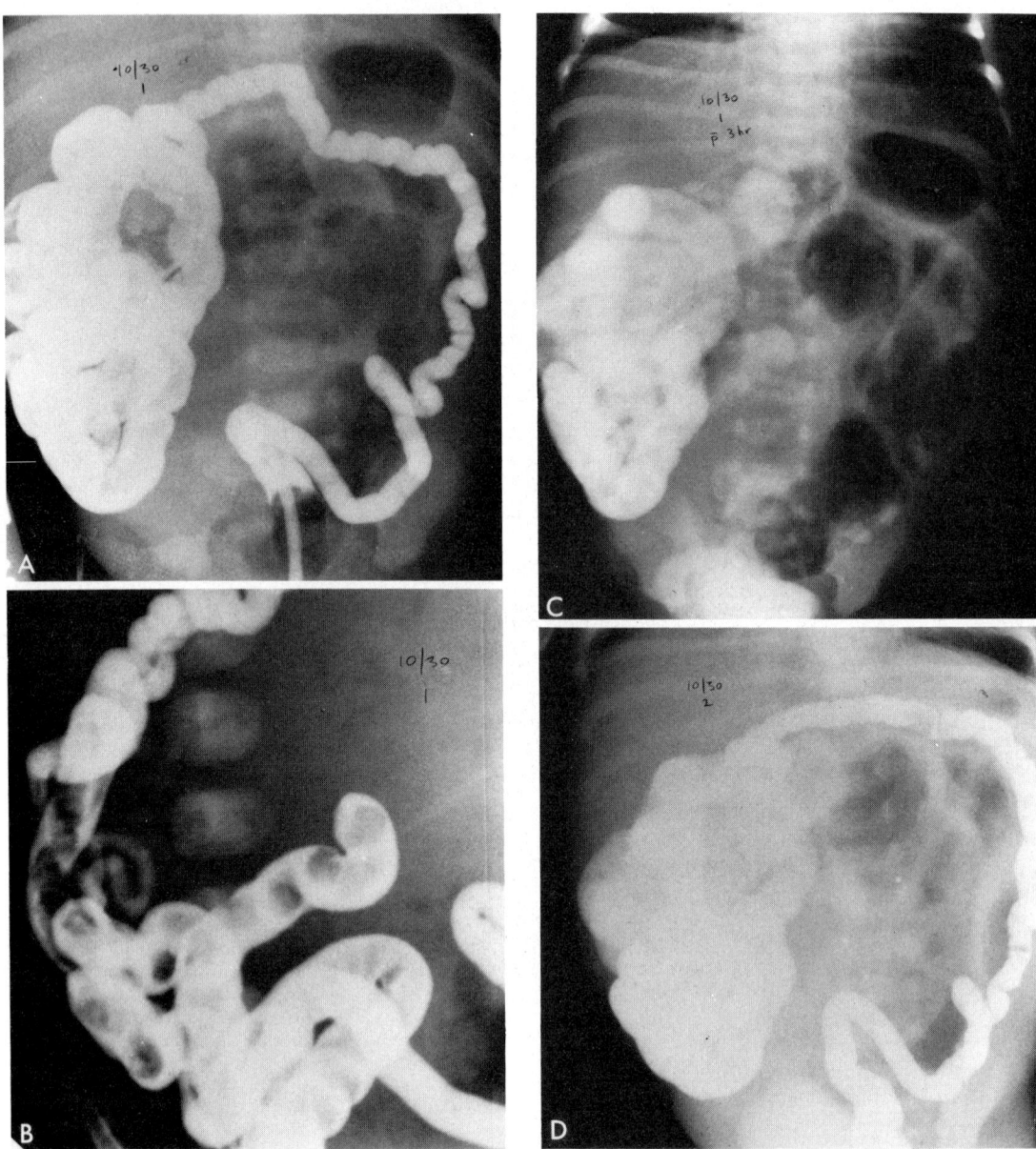

Figure 8–5   Relief of meconium ileus by multiple diatrizoate enemas in a neonate. There was progressive distention during the first day of life in this infant, and plain films of the abdomen demonstrated multiple dilated loops of bowel. *A*, Contrast study of the colon with a 50 per cent solution of diatrizoate demonstrates microcolon and moderately dilated small bowel loops. *B*, Spot film of the small bowel shows the pellets of meconium producing filling defects within the column of contrast medium. The contrast material was refluxed as far proximal in the small bowel as could be done easily.

C, Follow-up film done three hours later demonstrates some excretion of contrast medium through the urinary system. There is some dilution of the hypertonic contrast medium by fluid drawn from the circulating blood into the lumen of the small bowel. *D*, A repeat diatrizoate enema was performed as a therapeutic measure about five hours after the initial study and the fill-up films demonstrate somewhat more proximal filling of the small bowel than was evident in the first study. The infant began passing some small pellets of meconium over the next 12 hours.

Illustration continued on following page

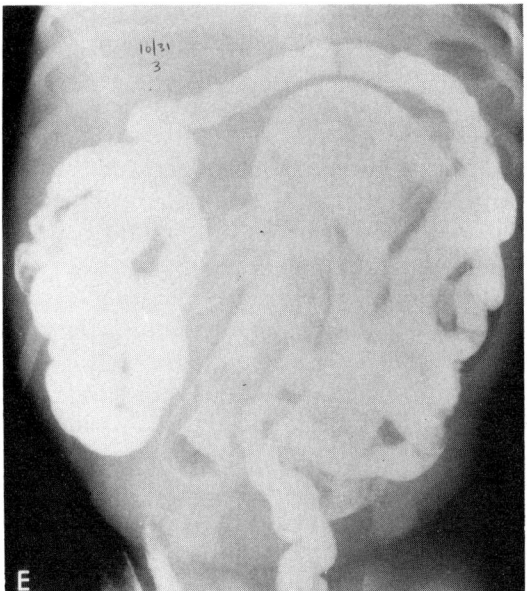

Figure 8–5 Continued. E, The third and final diatrizoate enema was performed about 20 hours after the initial examination, and in this study the contrast agent could be refluxed into some of the more dilated proximal loops of small bowel. Increasing amounts of meconium were passed in the ensuing 12 hours, and this was accompanied by decreasing abdominal distention. The stools were normal or near-normal after about the fifth day of life, at which time complete oral feeding was begun, and the infant was later discharged.

cal enterotomy and irrigation of the distal bowel segment with hydrogen peroxide or 4 per cent N-acetylcysteine.[16, 36] Hydrogen peroxide is no longer used for bowel irrigation, since it has been found to damage the bowel mucosa. Successful nonsurgical management now uses the Gastrografin enema performed under fluoroscopy until the dye is refluxed into the terminal ileum. The enema can be repeated in several hours. Meconium evacuation follows expulsion of the enema, and in most cases the obstruction is completely relieved. N-acetylcysteine enemas in 4 per cent concentration are also effective against simple meconium ileus, as the compound cleaves disulfide bonds in the mucoprotein molecules and decreases the tenaciousness of the abnormal meconium. Greater concentrations cause hyperemia and hemorrhage in the colonic mucosa and should not be used. If these methods are not successful, surgical intervention is required. In fact, these medical techniques are to be avoided in cases in which atresia, volvulus, or perforation is suspected. Some surgeons resect the dilated, hypertrophied proximal ileum and others do not, but all atretic or necrotic bowel must be removed. Feeding is resumed when peristalsis is well established. A readily absorbable formula, such as Pregestimil with its hydrolyzed protein, medium-chain triglyceride, and glucose composition, is used at first. Later feedings using more standard formulae and baby foods must all be supplemented with pancreatic enzymes.

Complications. Recurrent volvulus and intestinal obstruction are less frequent complications than in the past, but perforation with meconium and bacterial peritonitis still develop in about 40 per cent of the infants. In half the cases, perforation is due to gangrenous bowel and in the remainder, to atresia or volvulus. Hypoproteinemia is a particular problem but one that can be averted by the intramuscular injection of vitamin K.

Respiratory distress and pneumonia secondary to the primary disease must be treated accordingly with antibiotics and inhalation therapy. Prematurity itself carries the complications of kernicterus and the respiratory distress syndrome.

Intolerance to lactose and sucrose is not unusual and is a cause of persistent diarrhea. Treatment may be problematic, for necrotizing enterocolitis has followed Renografin treatment.[13]

Mortality and Prognosis. The overall mortality of the disease is between 50 and 67 per cent, but if it is complicated by peritonitis, it rises to 70 per cent. More than one third of these infants die of pulmonary complications during the first six months of life. The post-treatment pulmonary complications are fewer in those who are managed medically, but this group obviously has less severe disease at onset.

MECONIUM PLUG

The meconium plug syndrome is most often seen in premature, hypotonic, or brain-damaged infants.

Incidence. Meconium plugs are estimated to occur in about 1 per cent of neonates and are responsible for intestinal obstruction in 0.25 per cent. The incidence is greater in males than in females.

Etiology and Pathology. In addition to its relationship to prematurity and hypotonia, meconium plug has been attributed to hypomagnesemia,[40] respiratory distress, sepsis, hypothyroidism, and Hirschsprung's disease. Although Shwachman and Antonowicz[39] state that meconium plug is not a manifestation of cystic fibrosis, we have seen several infants presenting with meconium plug syndrome who later were diagnosed as having cystic fibrosis.[44] Rosenstein and Langbaum[28] described 12 of 37 infants with cystic fibrosis who had clinical features consistent with the syndrome and suggested that it was a milder form of meconium ileus. Premature infants rarely pass meconium *in utero*, whereas older infants do so in response to stress.[23]

The meconium plug differs from normal meconium in that it is firmer and has a normal or higher protein content. It contains no pancreatic enzymes because it is formed from mucus and secretions. Hypotonia and immature colonic expulsive mechanisms are contributory factors. The simple plug is gelatinous and yellow-white and usually is passed with the first stool. In some instances, there are multiple plugs, some as high as the ascending colon. If they are retained for more than 24 hours, they may cause intestinal obstruction.

Symptoms. Some infants are born to mothers who received magnesium sulfate for treatment of eclampsia. The infant passes no stool during the first 24 hours of life and develops signs of low intestinal obstruction, increasing abdominal distention, and vomiting. The vomitus is clear initially but later becomes bilious or even fecal. Bowel sounds are hyperactive. The anal canal is tight to rectal examination, and the firm plug may be distinguished at the tip of the examining finger.

Differential Diagnosis. Meconium ileus, ileal atresia, Hirschsprung's disease, and anal stenosis must be differentiated from simple meconium plug. A plain film of the abdomen shows low obstruction with multiple distended loops of small bowel or, occasionally, a presacral mass. A "soap bubble" effect in the colon is due to air mixed with meconium. The barium enema will outline the plug and the distended colon above it. There is no microcolon as in the atresias. Rarely, the plug is of such size that it extends into the terminal ileum.

Treatment. The rectal examination is often successful in dislodging the plug (Fig.

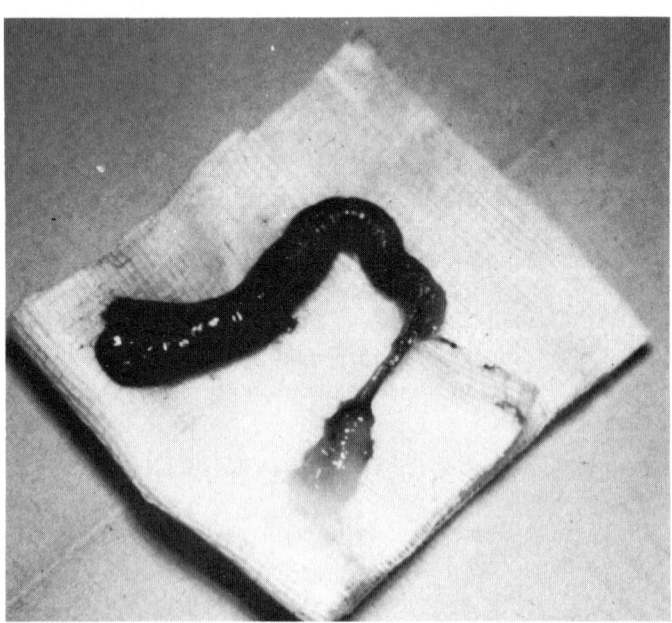

Figure 8–6 Meconium plug responsible for low intestinal obstruction.

8–6). Warm saline enemas, Gastrografin, enemas, or N-acetylcysteine enemas are the next procedures to be used and are nearly always successful. Hydrogen peroxide enemas are forbidden because of their proven hazard.

Prognosis. Once the plug is evacuated, most infants progress normally. If obstructive symptoms persist, additional plugs must be searched out and treated. If none is discovered, rectal manometry or biopsy should be undertaken to rule out Hirschsprung's disease and a sweat test should be performed. If the child is too small for an adequate test, the stool should be examined for trypsin. Our own recommendation is that a sweat test should be performed at some time on all infants with the meconium plug syndrome.

INSPISSATED STOOL SYNDROME FROM MILK (MILK CURD OBSTRUCTION)

The inspissated milk syndrome is reported in premature infants who have taken powdered milk or high-calorie formulae.[7, 26]

Incidence. In one center, 37 cases were noted in a 19-year period.[4]

Etiology and Pathology. The combination of high-calorie feeds and reduced intestinal motility in the premature infant leads to increased water absorption from the colon, causing hard milk curds that obstruct the colon, the ileocecal valve, and, at times, the terminal ileum. Etiologic factors are similar to those described for gastric bezoar. The curds contain increased fat and calcium, attributable perhaps to decreased bile acids.

Symptoms. A premature infant between 2 and 16 days of age becomes constipated and develops abdominal distention and vomiting. The vomitus eventually becomes bile-stained or fecal. Rope-like masses are palpable in the right lower quadrant, and pellets are felt through the remainder of the colon. There may be slight rectal bleeding, and symptoms may occasionally mimic those of necrotizing enterocolitis.

Diagnosis. This disorder must be differentiated from meconium ileus. Fortunately, the radiologic features are characteristic. Plain films show dense intraluminal masses in the colon and perhaps in the terminal ileum, all of which are surrounded by halos of air.[8] In the barium enema, the colon appears narrow and contains round, discrete, pellet-like filling defects.

Treatment. Gastrografin enema relieves the obstruction effectively.

MEDICALLY INDUCED COLONIC OBSTRUCTION

Several instances of colonic obstruction due to medications are worthy of mention.

Cholestyramine. This quaternary ammonium anion–exchange resin binds salts in the gastrointestinal tract to prevent their normal reabsorption. In children it is used for treatment of pruritus of biliary atresia, for bile salt diarrhea, for chronic diarrhea, and for type II hyperlipoproteinemia. Its usual complications are enhanced fecal excretion of fat and fat-soluble vitamins, nausea, flatulence, and constipation. The drug was first reported in 1969 to cause obstruction in a ten-month-old infant taking 3 mg per gm per day,[6] and in 1977, three more cases were noted.[21] The first infant required surgical removal of the resin from the ascending colon; the remaining infants recovered after discontinuation of the drug.

Antacid Obstruction. One of our own patients, a three-month-old infant taking an aluminum hydroxide gel antacid for treatment of a stress ulcer, developed abdominal distention and vomiting. A flat plate of the abdomen showed low intestinal obstruction with dilated, fluid-filled loops of small bowel. A putty-like mass was palpated in the right lower quadrant, and at laparotomy the ascending colon was filled with tenacious gel-like adherent material. Right hemicolectomy was performed, and the infant recovered. More recently, similar obstruction has been reported in a 12-year-old.[17]

Kaolin-Pectin Obstruction. Overzealous use of this product for treatment of diarrhea in a four-month-old infant has resulted in obstruction. The obstruction required laparotomy and removal of the mass blocking the right colon.

Kayexalate, a polystyrene sodium sulfonate, has also caused an obstructive bezoar in a neonate being treated for hyperkalemia.[24a]

CHRONIC INTESTINAL PSEUDO-OBSTRUCTION SYNDROME (CIPS)

Intestinal pseudo-obstruction is characterized by intermittent intestinal obstruction without identifiable lesions. It has also been termed hereditary hollow visceral myopathy, since stomach, esophagus, and bladder may be involved as well as the small and large intestine.[2, 30a, 42]

A similar syndrome may occur in systemic disorders such as scleroderma, myxedema, acute intermittent porphyria, or amyloidosis.

Incidence. In 1977, Byrne et al. reported CIPS in 11 children, 5 of whom were siblings.[5] In 1978 Faulk et al. reported a kindred of at least 18 members with visceral myopathy.[11, 12] Pseudo-obstruction has been reported in fewer than a dozen infants. Both sexes are affected in a pattern of autosomal dominant or sex-linked dominant inheritance with variable penetrance; consanguinity has been noted in several families.[12a]

Etiology and Pathophysiology. A variety of pathologic findings are reported and may represent separate diseases or stages of one disorder:[18, 31] (1) normal muscle and neuronal histology, a predominant finding in infants and children; (2) *progressive systemic sclerosis* (PSS) of the gastrointestinal tract, which may be associated with scleroderma. Smooth muscle is replaced by collagen in the absence of inflammatory reaction or vacuolar degeneration. Muscle width is normal or quite reduced, and the demarcation between normal and decreased muscle may be abrupt. The remaining muscle cells are normal. Smooth muscle fibrosis involves both circular and longitudinal muscle, while the myenteric plexus and neurons are normal. (3) Typical or *visceral myopathy* is vacuolar degeneration, which gives a honeycombed appearance to the muscle. The

vacuoles are empty or filled with debris of degenerating muscle cells and are bounded by collagen. Both or only the outer layer of muscle are involved, but myenteric plexus and neurons are normal. (4) Decreases in axon and neuron numbers are noted.

Abnormal small bowel mucosa as subtotal or patchy villous atrophy has been described and presumed secondary to bacterial overgrowth.[32, 33] Physiologically, the amplitude of peristalsis is decreased in the lower one third of the esophagus, and the lower esophageal sphincter pressure is decreased or above normal. Although the sphincter usually relaxes normally after deglutition, it is unresponsive to cholinergic stimulation. Peristalsis has been recorded from the stomach, and cholinergic mechanisms of the small intestine are probably intact. One adult patient was found to have no spontaneous electrical control activity in the jejunum. Prostaglandin E is elevated.[20, 22]

Symptoms. In children the onset of symptoms may occur at any time from the neonatal period to adolescence, with intermittent or continued abdominal distention being the major complaint. Vomiting, malnutrition, abdominal pain, diarrhea, or constipation is often associated. Attacks tend to increase in frequency and severity with age. The physical findings are limited to the abdomen, which, during an attack, is markedly distended and tense, with dilated loops of bowel easily palpated. Bowel sounds vary from absent to hyperactive. The course is most severe in infants born with evidence of obstruction.

Differential Diagnosis. Organic lesions causing obstruction must be ruled out as well as the systemic disorders such as scleroderma, myxedema, and porphyria. Duodenal intubation studies have documented the presence of bacterial overgrowth with coliforms and anaerobes. Biopsy of the small bowel has shown patchy villous atrophy with increased lymphocytes in the lamina propria. Rectal biopsies show normal rectal mucosa and a normal number of intact ganglion cells. Full-thickness surgical specimens of bowel contain normal smooth muscle and ganglion cells or changes noted earlier.

Radiologic examination shows dilated loops of bowel with air-fluid levels. Contrast studies show, in the colon, distention, redundancy, decreased haustral markings, and abnormal evacuation; and in the upper gastrointestinal tract, abnormal esophageal peristalsis, delayed gastric emptying, prolonged intestinal transit through a dilated duodenum, and segmentally dilated small bowel. In the small bowel there are abnormal to-and-fro propulsive movements. Intravenous pyelogram may be normal or may show a neurogenic bladder and hydronephrosis.

Treatment. Diverting surgical procedures are occasionally helpful but are not curative.[30] Nor have attempts at medical management using special diet agents to increase peristalsis or steroids been clinically successful. Oral broad-spectrum antibiotics to reduce bacterial overgrowth have reduced distention and pain. Parenteral hyperalimentation has been the only certain means of sustaining severely affected infants.

Other forms of motor-type obstruction may be due to abnormalities of circular musculature[16a] or of neurons.[22a]

REFERENCES

1. Allan, J. L., Robbie, M., Phelan, P. D., and Danks, D. M.: Familial occurrence of meconium ileus. Eur. J. Pediatr. 135:291, 1981.
2. Amoury, R. A., Fellows, R., Goodwin, C., Hall, R. T., Holder, T., and Ashcraft, K. W.: Megacystis-microcolon intestinal hypoperistalsis syndrome: Cause of intestinal obstruction in the newborn period. J. Pediatr. Surg. 12:1063, 1977.
3. Berry, H. K., Kellogg, F. W., Lichstein, S. R., and Ingberg, R. L.: Elevated meconium lactase activity. Am. J. Dis. Child. 134:930, 1980.
4. Berkowitz, G. P., Buntain, W., and Cassady, G.: Milk curd obstruction mimicking necrotizing enterocolitis. Am. J. Dis. Child. 134:1187, 1980.
5. Byrne, W. J., Cipel, L., Euler, A. R., et al.: Chronic idiopathic intestinal pseudo-obstruction syndrome in children. J. Pediatr. 90:585, 1977.
6. Cohen, M., Winslow, P., and Boley, S. J.: Intestinal obstruction associated with cholestyramine therapy. N. Engl. J. Med. 280:1285, 1969.
7. Cook, R. C. M., and Rickham, P. P.: Neonatal intestinal obstruction due to milk curds. J. Pediatr. Surg. 4:599, 1969.
8. Cremin, B. J., Smythe, P., and Cywes, M.: The radiologic appearance of the inspissated milk syndrome. Radiology 43:856, 1970.
9. Donnison, A. B., Schwachman, H., and Gross, R. E.: A review of 164 children with meconium ileus seen at the Children's Hospital Medical Center, Boston. Pediatrics 37:833, 1966.
10. Ein, S. H., and Stephens, C. A.: Intussusception: 354 cases in 10 years. J. Pediatr. Surg. 6:16, 1971.
11. Faulk, D., Anuras, S., Gardner, D., Mitros, F., Summers, R. W., and Christensen, J.: A familial visceral myopathy. Ann. Intern. Med. 89:600, 1978.
12. Faulk, D., Anuras, S., and Christensen, J.: Chronic intestinal pseudo-obstruction. Gastroenterology 74:922, 1978.
12a. Golladay, E. S., and Byrne, W. J.: Intestinal pseudoobstruction. Surg. Gynecol. Obstet. 153:257, 1981.
13. Grantmyre, E. B., Butler, G. J., and Gillis, D. A.: Necrotizing enterocolitis after Renografin 76 treatment of meconium ileus. Am. J. Roentgenol. 136:990, 1981.
14. Dudgeon, D. L., and Hays, D. M.: Intussusception complicating the treatment of malignancies in childhood. Arch. Surg. 105:52, 1972.
15. Haase, G., and Boles, T., Jr.: Glucagon in experimental intussusception. J. Pediatr. Surg. 14:664, 1979.
16. Harberg, F., Senekjan, E., and Pokorny, W.: Treatment of uncomplicated meconium ileus via T-tube ileostomy. J. Pediatr. Surg. 16:61, 1981.
16a. Humphry, A., Mancer, K., and Stephens, C.: Obstructive circular muscle defect in the small bowel of a one year old child. J. Pediatr. Surg., 15:197, 1980.
17. Hurley, R.: Bowel obstruction in a child during treatment with aluminum hydroxide gel. J. Pediatr. 92:592, 1978.
17a. Janik, J. S., Cranford, J., and Ein, S. H.: The well nourished infant with intussusception. Am. J. Dis. Child. 135:600, 1981.
18. Kapila, L., Haberkom, S., and Nixon, H. H.: Chronic adynamic bowel simulating Hirschsprung's. J. Pediatr. Surg. 10:885, 1975.
19. Lecine, M., Schwartz, S., Katz, I., Burke, H., and Rabinowitz, J.: Plain films in intussusception. Br. J. Radiol. 37:678, 1964.
20. Lewis, T. D., Daniel, E. E., Sarna, D., Waterfall, W. E., and Marzio, L.: Idiopathic pseudo-obstruction, report of a case with intraluminal studies of mechanical and electrical activity and response to drugs. Gastroenterology 74:107, 1978.
21. Lloyd-Still, J. D.: Cholestyramine therapy and intestinal obstruction. Pediatrics 59:626, 1977.
22. Luderer, J. R., Demers, L. M., Bonnem, E. M., et al.: Elevated prostaglandin E in idiopathic intestinal pseudo-obstruction. N. Engl. J. Med. 295:1179, 1976.
22a. Mathe, J. C., Khairallah, S., Phat Vuoung, N., Boccon-Gibod, L., Rey, A., and Costri, J.: Segmental dilatation of the ileum in a neonate. Nouv. Presse Med. 11:265, 1982.
23. Matthews, T. G., and Warshaw, J. B.: Relevance of gestational age distribution of meconium passage in utero. Pediatrics 64:30, 1979.
24. McGreevy, P., Doberneck, R., McLeay, J. M., and Miller, F.: Recurrent eosinophilic infiltrate of the ileum causing intussusception in a 2 year old child. Surgery 61:280, 1967.

24a. Menke, J., Stallworth, R., Binstadt, D., Strano, A., and Wallace, S.: Medication bezoar in a neonate. Am. J. Dis. Child. *136*:72, 1982.

24b. Mishalany, H., Mahnovski, V., and Woolley, M.: Congenital asplenia and anomalies of the gastrointestinal tract. Surgery *91*:38, 1982.

25. Mollitt, D. L., Ballantine, T. V., and Grosfield, J. L.: Postoperative intussusception in infancy and childhood: analysis of 119 cases. Surgery *86*:402, 1979.

26. Pochon, J. P., and Stauffer, U. G.: Milk curd obstruction. Helv. Paediatr. Acta *33*:25, 1978.

27. Rachelson, M., Jernigan, J. P., and Jackson, W.: Intussusception in the newborn infant with spontaneous expulsion of the intussusceptum. J. Pediatr. *47*:87, 1955.

28. Rosenstein, B., and Langbaum, T.: Incidence of meconium abnormalities in newborn infants with cystic fibrosis. Am. J. Dis. Child. *134*:72, 1980.

29. Rule, A. H., Baran, D. T., and Schwachman, H.: Quantitative determination of water-soluble proteins in meconium. Pediatrics *45*:847, 1970.

30. Sarna, S. K., Daniel, E. E., Waterfall, W. E., Lewis, T. D., and Marzia, L.: Postoperative gastrointestinal electric and mechanical activities in a patient with idiopathic intestinal pseudoobstruction. Gastroenterology *74*:112, 1978.

30a. Schuffler, M. D.: Chronic intestinal pseudo-obstruction syndromes. Med. Clin. North Am. *65*:1331, 1981.

31. Schuffler, M. D., and Beegle, R.: Progressive systemic sclerosis of the gastrointestinal tract and hereditary hollow visceral myopathy: two distinguishable disorders of intestinal smooth muscle. Gastroenterology *77*:662, 1979.

32. Schuffler, M. D., Kaplan, L., and Johnson, L.: Small intestinal mucosa in pseudoobstruction syndromes. Am. J. Dig. Dis. *23*:821, 1978.

33. Schuffler, M. D., Lowe, M. C., and Bill, A. H.: Studies of idiopathic intestinal pseudoobstruction I. Hereditary hollow visceral myopathy: clinical and pathological studies. Gastroenterology *73*:327, 1977.

34. Schwartz, S., and Storer, E.: Manifestations of gastrointestinal disease. *In* Schwartz, S. (ed.): Principles of Surgery. Ed. 3. New York, McGraw-Hill Book Company, 1979.

35. Sharp, H., Peller, J. Carey, H. B., Jr., and Krivit, W.: Primary and secondary bile acids in meconium. Pediatr. Res. *5*:274, 1971.

36. Shaw, A.: Safety of N-acetylcysteine in the treatment of meconium obstruction of the newborn. J. Pediatr. Surg. *4*:119, 1969.

37. Shigemoto, H., Endo, S., Isomoto, T., Sano, K., et al.: Neonatal meconium obstruction in ileum without mucoviscidosis. J. Pediatr. Surg. *13*:475, 1978.

38. Shields, R.: The absorption and secretion of fluid and electrolytes by the obstructed bowel. Br. Med. J. *52*:774, 1965.

39. Shwachman, H., and Antonowicz, I.: Studies on meconium. *In* Lebenthal, E. (ed.): Textbook of Gastroenterology and Nutrition in Infancy. New York, Raven Press, 1981.

40. Sokal, M. M., Koenigsberger, M. R., Rose, J. S., Berdon, W., and Santulli, T.: Neonatal hypermagnesemia and the meconium plug syndrome. N. Engl. J. Med. *286*:823, 1972.

41. Tanner, M. S., Smith, B., and Lloyd, J.: Functional intestinal obstruction due to deficiency of argyrophile neurons in the myenteric plexus (familial). Arch. Dis. Child. *51*:837, 1976.

42. Tanner, M. S., Smith, B., Lloyd, J.: Chronic idiopathic intestinal obstruction. J. Pediatr. *93*:169, 1978.

43. Touloukian, R. J., and DeLuca, F.: Unique aspects of small intestinal intussusception in infants and children: intussusceptions due to a metastatic malignant mesenchymoma and the indwelling long intestinal tube. Surgery *63*:346, 1968.

44. Townes, P. L., and Kopelman, A. E.: Meconium plug syndrome. Cystic fibrosis and exocrine pancreatic insufficiency. Am. J. Dis. Child. *132*:1043, 1978.

45. Wayne, E., Campbell, J., Burrington, J., and Davis, W.: Management of 344 children with intussusception. Radiology *107*:597, 1973.

46. Wolfson, J. J., and Engel, R.: Anticipating meconium peritonitis from metaphyseal bands. Radiology *92*:1055, 1979.

PART II / NUTRITIONAL SUPPORT FOR THE NEWBORN WITH GASTROINTESTINAL PROBLEMS

Chapter Nine

NUTRITIONAL ASSESSMENT AND ENTERAL FEEDING

Providing adequate nutritional support for infants with gastrointestinal disorders requires some knowledge of the digestive capability as well as the nutritional requirements of the growing infant. The ability to utilize nutrients presented enterically depends upon the maturity of the infant and on the particular limitations imposed by the gastrointestinal disorder. Requirements will also vary with the infant's age, metabolic demands, and method of feeding — i.e., parenteral nutrition versus enteric nutrition. In this section we will review the normal development of digestive functions and changes in nutrient requirements with age and relate this to the support of infants with gastrointestinal problems. The different techniques and formulas available for enteral alimentation will be discussed, as will the use of parenteral nutrition. Finally, nutritional support for infants with specific representative gastrointestinal disorders will be addressed.

DEVELOPMENT OF DIGESTIVE FUNCTIONS IN NORMAL INFANTS

Although the 16- to 17-week fetus is able to swallow amniotic fluid,[1] sustained coordinated deglutition with progressive peristaltic waves along the esophagus and competency of the lower esophageal sphincter are often absent or incompletely developed even in the full-term infant. By six weeks of age these muscular functions mature in the majority of infants, although a smaller group may require one to two years for lower esophageal sphincter tension to reach adult pressures.[2, 3] Further difficulties in retaining oral feedings may occur as a result of delayed gastric emptying, which often occurs in infants with respiratory distress syndrome.[4] Ganglion cells are present and distributed normally by 24 weeks' gestation, and small and large bowel motility do not appear to be affected by prematurity.[5] However, a number of medications, such as the neuromuscular blocking agents given to infants maintained on respirators, depress intestinal motility and may even paralyze the gut.

The absorption of nutrients depends upon an adequate surface area with developed absorptive sites composed of enterocytes lining the villus as well as active digestive enzymes. Surface area increases with advancing gestational age. A limited surface area does not appear to be of consequence in the healthy premature infant taking small amounts of enteric nutrients; however, further reduction in surface area, and hence absorptive sites, as a result of inflammation or surgical intervention may cripple the ability to nourish the infant enterally until compensatory hypertrophy of the small intestinal mucosa occurs. Newborn infants, whose small intestinal surface area is roughly three times their body length, can absorb only one seventh the glucose load per hour of a one-year-old.[6] Glucose absorption, which occurs by an energy-dependent mechanism, is surface area–related.[7]

More complex carbohydrates, such as disaccharides and starches, must be enzymatically hydrolyzed to simple sugars before they can be absorbed. Of the hydrolytic enzymes, only lactase and amylase are markedly low in activity in the premature infant.[8] Lactase begins to increase at 24 weeks of gestation, and highest levels are found at 38 to 40 weeks in the upper portion of the jejunum.[9] Lactase, sucrase, glucoamylase, and isomaltase are all located within the brush border of the enterocytes that line the villus. These enterocytes may be dam-

aged or destroyed following enteric infections or ischemic insults, which again will further limit the tolerance to a carbohydrate load. Exocrine pancreatic function may be severely limited even in the full-term infant.[10] Until one month of age, low levels of pancreatic amylase and lipase are found in duodenal fluid, with little increase occurring after stimulation by pancreozymin and secretin. Glucose polymers in the form of cornstarch hydrolysates appear to be well tolerated because they depend upon mucosal hydrolases for absorption.[11]

All infants absorb lipid inefficiently in comparison with adults. Lipid absorption begins with lipolysis by lipases from the sublingual glands and pancreas and, in breast-fed infants, with lipases in the breast milk. Lipase activity is augmented by the presence of bile salts secreted into the intestine. A minimal or critical bile acid concentration of 2 to 3 mM is necessary in the intestinal lumen to solubilize fats through the formation of micelles. Lipase activity is adequate in the newborn, but bile acid pools are diminished below the level necessary to maintain the critical intraluminal concentration.[12, 13] Animal studies suggest that the final phase of lipid absorption-uptake by mucosal cells and release of lipid bound to lipoproteins as chylomicrons may also be limited in the immature infant.[14] All of these limitations result in the loss of from 15 to 35 per cent of ingested fat in the newborn, depending on the type of fat ingested, with associated loss of fat-soluble nutrients such as vitamins A, D, and B.

Protein absorption, like lipid and carbohydrate absorption, is dependent on enzymatic activity both intraluminally and along the mucosal surface. Pepsin, which is present and active in the stomach in all premature infants and is maximally active between pH 1.8 and 3.4, does not function optimally in the markedly acidic milieu of the newborn's stomach, although this does not appear to prevent efficient protein digestion. Pancreatic peptidases and brush border peptidases are present with sufficient activity to allow protein digestion and absorption. That this digestive process is not as efficient as in the adult is clearly demonstrated by increased amounts of intact dietary proteins present in the serum of newborns when compared with that of adults.[15]

NUTRITIONAL REQUIREMENTS OF NEWBORN INFANTS

The question of whether nutrients should be supplied to prematurely born infants in amounts sufficient to achieve the same rate of growth as that occurring *in utero* has aroused considerable controversy.[16] This leaves open the question of what the optimal nutritional requirements are in this group. Even assuming that rapid growth is best, how to evaluate growth is itself controversial. Weight gain, gain in length, increase in brain growth as reflected in head circumference, and various serum protein values have been used to justify one set of requirements over another. With these controversies in mind, certain guidelines can be followed, with the awareness that requirements will continue to change as new data become available from clinical studies (see Recommended Dietary Allowances in Section 2 of Appendix).

Requirements of the various nutrients are interrelated, since one nutrient may influence the absorption or the metabolism of another. For example, feeding medium-chain triglycerides to premature infants appears to enhance fat absorption and allows a small reduction in the amount of dietary protein without diminishing the infant's rate of growth.[17] Similarly, nonabsorbable foodstuff, i.e., fiber, influences the availability of certain vitamins and trace minerals. Energy requirements to maintain intrauterine growth rates are approximately 120 to 130 kcal per kg per day by the end of the first week of life. Under certain circumstances, with unusual losses or high energy expenditures, this figure will be higher.

CARBOHYDRATE

Energy is supplied so that the carbohydrate furnishes approximately 55 per cent of the total calories. Lactose is the principal carbohydrate of mammalian milks, that of the sea lion being a notable exception. Using human milk as a standard, it has been the practice to supplement other mammalian milks with carbohydrate. Since the premature infant may not absorb lactose, other carbohydrates, mainly sucrose or glucose polymers, have been substituted in prepared formulae, with good infant growth as a result.[18] It is important to emphasize that, clinically, many premature infants tolerate lactose without developing an osmotic diarrhea. Furthermore, lactose enhances calcium absorption and the growth of *Lactobacillus bifidus*. This organism supplants gram-negative organisms and may help to protect the infant against potential enteric pathogens.[19]

FAT

Humans and horses consume the largest amount of carbohydrates in the perinatal period when compared with other mammals. There is often a reciprocal relationship between fat and carbohydrate in mammalian milks. Fat should supply approximately 40 to 50 per cent of calories in the diet of the human premature infant. The quality of the fat, in addition to the aforementioned limitations in the premature infant's ability to digest fat, influences absorption. Unsaturated fats are more readily solubilized and therefore more readily absorbed than saturated fats. The saturated fats present in breast milk are well absorbed because of the breast milk lipases, which are activated by bile salts in the intestine, and also because the saturated fatty acid, palmitic acid, is present in the beta position of the triglyceride molecule. In addition to supplying energy, the ingested fat must meet essential fatty acid requirements. Linoleic acid, 300 mg per 100 kcal, satisfies this requirement.

PROTEIN

No storage pool of protein or amino acids exists, as with fat and carbohydrates, to meet daily needs for growth. Premature infants show satisfactory growth on an intake of 2.2 to 5 gm per kg per day of protein with a biologic value equal to that of casein.[16] Other protein sources, such as soy, may be used but must be supplemented with amino acids and given in larger amounts to improve their biologic value.[20] Intakes below the recommended amounts lead to poor growth; intake above 5 gm per kg per day result in metabolic and central nervous system changes that may be deleterious to the infants. The quality of the protein is especially important to the premature infant, since several amino acids are essential at this time owing to immaturity of metabolic pathways that facilitate their formation from precursors. Histidine, tyrosine, cystine,[21] taurine,[22] and possibly carnitine[23] are included in this group, although premature infants fed on artificial formulae not supplemented with cystine or taurine do not demonstrate retarded growth. For the immature as well as the mature newborn, essential amino acids constitute 40 to 45 per cent of their total protein requirements. As the infant matures, this value declines, dropping to 19 per cent in the well-nourished adult. A major controversy today concerns the adequacy of pooled human milk to support growth in premature infants.[24] This milk is generally collected from donors well beyond parturition and therefore delivers less than 2.2 gm of protein per kg to the infant.[25, 26] Poorer rates of growth are seen in 28- to 32-weeks' gestation infants maintained on less than 1.5 gm of protein per kg when compared with infants on 2.2 to 3.0 gm of protein per kg.[27]

MINERALS

The newborn infant is limited in the ability to concentrate the urine to excrete a high solute load.[28] The main determinants of solute load in the diet include nitrogen, sodium, potassium, and chloride. When these are provided in excessive amounts, the result is hyperosmolarity with potential central nervous system damage. In contrast, however, sick preterm infants during the first week of life require 5 to 9 mEq Na per kg per day to balance the large natriuresis that occurs during this period.[29] Most of the body stores of minerals accrue during the latter half of the third trimester of pregnancy, so that immature preterm infants are particularly vulnerable to undermineralization of bone and poor growth if adequate calcium and phosphorus are not supplied. Recommended amounts between 300 and 500 mg per day for calcium with a calcium/phosphorus ratio of 2:1 have been shown to allow adequate bone mineralization with normal serum values.[30, 31] Diarrhea, one of the most common gastrointestinal problems of the newborn, results in both water and solute losses to the infant, often of 20 to 60 ml per kg with an osmolality of 150 osm per liter, which must be restored.

Of the trace minerals, the premature infant is at special risk for developing deficiencies of iron, copper, and zinc. Body stores of iron and copper are diminished in preterm infants, and, although zinc is not stored during late gestation, total body zinc increases at this time of rapid fetal growth.[32] The absence of copper and zinc from prepared formulae fed to premature infants has caused clinical deficiency states within the first six months of life. The deficiency states may be aggravated by gastrointestinal disease such as disaccharide intolerance, inflammatory bowel disease, or cystic fibrosis. Zinc absorption is markedly impaired in the presence of steatorrhea. Low iron stores also require replenishment, but supplementation of standard formulae or breast milk is not recommended until one to two months of age[33] to avoid the hemolytic anemia that can occur in the presence of vitamin E deficiency and high intakes of polyunsaturated fats.[34]

VITAMINS

Rickets has been reported in both breastfed[35] and formula-fed premature infants. In general, the infants have not taken sufficient quantities of the milk to receive 400

IU per day of vitamin D, or the milk has been deficient in the vitamin because of low maternal stores. Steatorrhea enhances loss of all the fat-soluble vitamins from the gastrointestinal tract, and therefore supplements of fat-soluble vitamins D and E are recommended. Folate and the water-soluble vitamins are often routinely administered as well, although there is no firm evidence to support this supplementation.

ASSESSMENT OF NUTRITIONAL STATUS

The clinical symptoms and evaluation of infants with gastrointestinal problems have been described in earlier chapters. The nutritional management of these infants depends not only on their particular disorder but also on their nutritional status at the time of presentation. Physical criteria and laboratory measurements of various serum substances, when compared with normal values derived from similar populations, allow us to judge the chronicity as well as the severity of nutritional deprivation. Unfortunately, these data for the most part have been derived from studies on normal infants greater than three months of age, making the nutritional assessment of the neonate more difficult. It is during this period that attention to nutritional status is most important. Energy stores of fat, protein, and carbohydrates are sufficient to support the starving immature infant for only a few days, compared with one month in the mature newborn and three months or more in the lean adult.

Physical Criteria

Regular increases in length occur with adequate nutrition, as reflected in the curves of the length for age in charts published by the National Center for Health Statistics (see Length Charts in Section 2 of the Appendix). Skeletal growth is less affected by acute changes in nutrition, and therefore a decreased length for age reflects chronic undernutrition. Infants should be measured in the supine position on a standardized length board. Head cir-cumference, which reflects the growth of both the skeleton and the brain, should be measured at the same points on the skull using a nonstretchable tape. When these measurements are made in a consistent manner on a single infant, the rate of growth can be evaluated accurately.[36] Soft tissues, such as muscle, adipose tissue, viscera, and body water, change more rapidly with acute deprivation. The weight for length measure assesses these tissues, although large and rapid changes in body water, which might occur with the rehydration of a premature infant, will obscure the nutritional status. Measurements of body fat can be calculated from skinfold thickness, using calipers in a standardized fashion. Total body protein can be estimated from measurements of midarm muscle circumference. Again, excess body water interferes with the interpretation of these measurements. A finding of two standard deviations below the fiftieth percentile is abnormal and requires intervention, as does failure to increase measurements at least along the fifth percentile.

Laboratory Measurements

A number of serum proteins have been used in children and adults as measures of nutritional status. None of these is well standardized in the premature infant before six months of age. Serum albumin has a half-life of 20 days, and so serum albumin values do not change as rapidly as do the values of some proteins with shorter half-lives, such as retinal-binding protein,[37] complement, and transferrin.[38] No standard values from large populations of newborns exist for these latter proteins. Values of albumin are also unreliable when there are unusual losses from the gastrointestinal tract or when albumin has been replaced with a parenteral transfusion. Deficiencies in immunologic capabilities are normal in the newborn and particularly so in the immature newborn. For this reason, skinfold testing with intradermal injections of various antigens is not useful. A total lymphocyte count of less than 1500 is always abnormal but is not specific for malnutrition and may occur with overwhelming infection. To summarize, we must rely on anthropometric values for the most part to evaluate nutritional status in the very young infant. Because nutritional reserves in this group of patients are extraordinarily limited, an adequate energy and nutrient intake must be accomplished as early as possible.

INFANTS WITH GASTROINTESTINAL DISORDERS

In infants with gastrointestinal problems, the failure to achieve adequate energy intake may develop for any number of reasons, some of which are listed in Table 9–1. Increased losses from the gastrointestinal tract may occur with recurrent emesis or protracted diarrhea. Because the young infant derives most of his nutrients from fluids, fluid restriction can be a major cause of caloric deprivation, especially in those with heart disease, renal failure, or chronic lung disease such as bronchopulmonary dysplasia. Digestion may be significantly impaired as a function of prematurity, reduced brush border enzyme activity, pancreatic insufficiency, or cholestatic hepatobiliary disease. The absorption of nutrients is primarily dependent on small intestinal surface area, which may be reduced by surgical resection, prolonged malnutrition, or chronic mucosal inflammation as encountered in gluten-, milk-, or soy protein–induced enteropathies, immunodeficiency states, or bacterial overgrowth. Energy requirements will also be increased by altered metabolism resulting from chronic inflammation, cardiopulmonary disease, or storage disease of glycogen or lipid.

The degree of impairment of absorption and digestion can be evaluated by fairly simple laboratory tests. The results of these tests, then, are useful in deciding whether to provide nutrition by the enteral route or to rely instead on parenteral nutrition. The absorption of D-xylose after a 5 gm oral dose is a measure of upper small bowel surface area in infants. A serum level that exceeds 25 gm at one or two hours after administration indicates adequate surface area.[39] The quantitative determination of fat excreted in stool collected over 72 hours with a daily intake of at least 25 mg/dl of long-chain fats gives information on mucosal integrity, pancreatic exocrine function, and sufficiency of bile acids. When both tests are normal for age, it is likely that the patient will tolerate some form of enteral nutrition.

Further tests done to define the type of diet that will be tolerated include specific carbohydrate tolerance tests, measuring the rise in serum glucose or increase in breath hydrogen after ingestion of 2 gm per kg of lactose, sucrose, or glucose. Increase in serum glucose of 20 mg per dl by two hours is normal. Direct tests of pancreatic function are difficult to perform in the small infant, since they involve intubation of the duodenum and are not standardized in premature infants. Newer tests, such as serum trypsin levels measured by radioimmunoassay[40] or the determination of metabolites of para-aminobenzoic acid (PABA) in urine following an oral dose of benzoyl-tyrosyl-PABA,[41] may improve our ability to detect pancreatic insufficiency in very young infants. Finally, biopsy of upper small bowel mucosa can confirm the diagnosis of a flattened villus lesion and, in certain cases, provide the etiology.

Table 9–1　Factors Limiting Energy Availability for Growth in Infancy

FACTOR	EXAMPLE
Caloric deprivation	Neglect, impaired suck/swallow
Fluid restriction	Cardiopulmonary failure
Impaired digestion	Pancreatic insufficiency
Impaired absorption (reduced surface area)	Celiac disease, malnutrition
Increased metabolism	Chronic inflammation
Impaired utilization	Storage diseases

SPECIALIZED ENTERAL FEEDING ALTERNATIVES

Composition of Formulae (See Section 3, Appendix)

Protein.　Commercially prepared formulae often attempt to mimic the protein composition of human milk, but casein is the standard against which alternative protein sources are compared. Although casein is an imperfect reference standard, it is accepted as such.[42] Modification of casein-based formulae to make them more like human milk includes enrichment with whey proteins such that the ratio of whey to casein is 60:40. This is in contrast to cow's milk, in which the ratio is 18:82. Formulae constituted in this way include SMA, PM 60/40, and Enfamil Premature. Other protein sources, such as vegetable protein, must be supplemented with amino acids to make them nutritionally adequate.

In infancy, recommended protein intake is expressed as percentage of total calories rather than as grams per kilogram per day, as cited earlier, owing to the tremendous variation in energy requirements for growth. With high-quality protein, protein intake should ideally be 8 per cent of total calories.[43] Higher levels do not further improve growth. Recent reports have documented higher amounts of protein and nonprotein nitrogen, sodium, and chloride in milk from mothers delivering preterm than was previously realized,[25] and persistence of these increased levels for at least several weeks. If the premature infant is able to tolerate the lactose load, this milk may provide adequate nutrition. As mentioned before, the adequacy of any human milk, especially of banked human milk which is usually pooled "mature" milk with only 6 per cent of calories as protein, remains under investigation for premature and malnourished infants. In neonates, protein toxicity has been documented with intakes exceeding 4 gm per kg per day. Acute manifestations of toxicity include CNS irritability, acidosis, and increased serum urea nitrogen.

Soy protein is a protein of lower quality owing to its reduced content of essential amino acids, especially methionine. The marketed soy formulae are thus methionine-enriched. Although soy protein formulae are adequate for normal infant nutrition,[44] they are not recommended for use in premature infants or in infants with cystic fibrosis.[45] A major indication for prolonged use of soy protein formulae is in infants raised by families adhering to vegetarian diets.

The casein hydrolysates are routinely amino acid–supplemented owing to loss of essential amino acids in hydrolysis. Recent studies have confirmed that dipeptides and oligopeptides are absorbed more efficiently than amino acids,[46] and the use of amino acid formulae in infancy has thus essentially ceased in favor of casein hydrolysates, except occasionally with milk protein intolerance.

Carbohydrates. The major carbohydrates in infant formulae have been disaccharides with lactose in the milk-based formulae and sucrose in the soy-based formulae. In an effort to reduce reliance on the more fragile brush border lactase and sucrase, manufacturers have turned to an alternative carbohydrate source, starch. This is primarily provided as tapioca, corn syrup solids, or the hydrolysis product of cornstarch, referred to as dextrins or glucose polymers. Digestion of starch requires amylase (pancreatic or mucosal glucoid-amylase) and maltase, a brush border disaccharidase. The only complete infant formulae that are lactose- and sucrose-free are Prosobee and Pregestimil.

Fat. The lipid content of infant formulae is generally a mixture of saturated and polyunsaturated long-chain fats. All of the standard formulae have been vitamin E–enriched owing to the polyunsaturated fat content. Infants with reduced lipolytic capacity may benefit from the use of medium-chain triglycerides (MCT), which have fewer than 12 carbon atoms. The medium-chain triglycerides do not require micellar solubilization for absorption and following absorption are transported via the portal vein rather than via the lymphatics. MCT-containing formulae are thus recommended for infants whose long-chain triglyceride (LCT) absorption is restricted as a result of prematurity, operative jejunal or ileal resection, mucosal inflammation, lymphangiectasia, pancreatic insufficiency, or cholestatic liver disease. None of the formulae provides fat exclusively as MCT, as the requirements for linoleic acid, an essential fatty acid that has 18 carbon atoms, would not be met.

Osmolality and Renal Solute Load. The osmolality of the formula may be a critical factor in gastric emptying and intestinal

Table 9–2   Electrolyte and Mineral Composition of Selected Infant Formulae

	MEQ/L					MG/L
	Na	*K*	*Cl*	*Ca*	*Phos*	*Fe*
Human milk	7	13	11	17	9	1.0
Cow's milk	24	35	29	60	54	0.5
Similac/Enfamil	12	19	15	26	23	1.4 or 12
SMA	7	14	10	22	16	12.7
PM 60/40	7	15	7	20	12	2.6
Similac LBW	16	26	24	36	33	3.0
Enfamil Premature	14	23	19	48	28	1.2
Isomil	13	18	15	35	29	12.0
Prosobee	18	19	12	40	31	12.7
Goat's milk	15	46	32	61	54	1.0
MBF	8	10	7	50	39	15.0
Probana	27	31	21	58	53	1.4
Nutramigen	14	17	13	32	28	12.0
Portagen	14	22	16	32	28	12.0
Pregestimil	14	18	16	32	28	12.0
CHO-free	16	23	15	42	25	8.5

transit, though the latter is usually of consequence only with intrajejunal feedings or short bowel syndrome. Impairment of gastric emptying does not appear to develop until osmolality exceeds 450 mOsm per kg H_2O.[47]

Renal solute load is rarely a factor in infants with normal renal function. When formulae are concentrated, however, the reduction in free water may become significant.

Electrolytes and Minerals. Table 9–2 lists the sodium, potassium, chloride, calcium, phosphorus, and iron content of the formulae. The values are those present when the formula is prepared at standard 30 or 24 calories per ounce, as noted previously. This table is included for reference rather than for extensive discussion. Routine iron supplementation is now recommened in infancy,[33] though the requirements may alternatively be met with cereals.

COMPLETE FORMULATIONS FOR INFANTS WITH GASTROINTESTINAL PROBLEMS
(See Section 3, Appendix)

Milk-Based Formulae

The nutritional, immunologic, and psychologic virtues of human breast milk have been repeatedly extolled.[48] We do encounter, however, limitations to the exclusive use of breast milk in infants with severe lactase deficiency, short bowel syndrome, hepatobiliary disease, and volume restriction secondary to congestive heart failure. Similac, Enfamil, SMA, PM 60/40, and related milk protein–based formulae share these limitations for use in infants with impaired digestive and absorptive capacity, as they contain lactose and long-chain fat. The advantages of milk-based formulae are low cost and ready availability (see Section 4, Appendix).

In an effort to meet some of the unique needs of premature infants, Similac LBW and Enfamil Premature have been introduced. When compared with breast milk, they are higher in protein (11 to 12 per cent of calories), vitamin D, and phosphorus. Since premature infants have reduced lactase, approximately 50 per cent of carbohydrate calories are derived from glucose polymer. Although lactose "intolerance" may manifest in neonates as osmotic diarrhea or acidosis or both, it appears that some lactose is essential for the development of normal colonic flora[19] and for maximal calcium uptake.[49] In light of the premature infant's well-documented reduction in jejunal micellar concentration, both formulae provide greater than 40 per cent of lipid calories as MCT. Widespread administration of these formulae has been restricted by the frequent constipation and scattered reports of lactobezoar formation associated with their use.[50]

Soy-Based Formulae

The soy-based formulae were introduced for use in infants who are "milk-intolerant." When this is secondary to isolated reductions in lactase, a soy formula will be tolerated well. Although soy formulae are extensively used in "allergic" children, recent studies suggest that soy protein is highly antigenic.[51] The major indication for soy formula is therefore in infants recovering from acute enteritis with acquired lactase deficiency or in those on vegetarian diets. Casein hydrolysate formulae are also lactose-free but are too expensive for routine use.

Goat's Milk

Goat's milk has also been heavily used in "cow's milk–sensitive" infants. Its value in diarrheal disease is limited, as its carbohydrate is lactose. Goat's milk is high in essential fatty acids and also has a higher MCT content than cow's milk. Although availability is restricted, it is an acceptable substitute for cow's milk, with several precautions. The high protein content precludes exclusive use in early infancy owing to acidosis. Routine folic acid supplementation of goat's milk is mandatory.

Casein Hydrolysates

Nutramigen. Nutramigen is the suitable formula for infants with milk or soy protein sensitivity with or without lactose intolerance. Protein is provided as casein hydrolysate. As sucrose provides 72 per cent of carbohydrate calories and all fat is long-chain, its utilization in severe malabsorption is restricted.

Portagen. Portagen is the only formula on the market providing the majority of fat as MCT. It is therefore the formula of choice in infants with severe steatorrhea as in pancreatic insufficiency, cholestatic liver disease, or severe malnutrition. Some sucrase activity is necessary, in as much as sucrose provides 25 per cent of carbohydrate calories. Until further studies are done, caseinate should not be considered "hypoallergenic."

Pregestimil. Pregestimil was reformulated in 1978 from an amino acid, dextrose, and MCT preparation of excessive osmolality to its present form. A major appeal is that it is lactose- and sucrose-free. Protein is provided as casein hydrolysate supplemented with cystine, tyrosine, and tryptophan. MCT provides 40 per cent of the lipid. This is therefore a suitable formula for infants recovering from severe diarrhea with attendant reductions in small bowel surface area and brush border enzymes.

Elemental and Modular Formulae

Amino acid formulations, as noted before, do not appear to offer any absorptive advantage over the supplemented casein hydrolysate formulae.[52] In addition, they are high-osmolar solutions, not specifically formulated for the newborn infant and therefore not optimal nutritional sources for this group. Modular formulae can be constructed for infants with nutritional requirements not met in standard formulae. The constituents of the diet can be varied in amounts and quality to suit most infants. Protein is usually supplied as casein (Casec) or soy, fat as corn oil or medium-chain triglycerides, and carbohydrate as glucose polymers.

FEEDING TECHNIQUES

When voluntary oral intake is inadequate or contraindicated, nutrients can be delivered directly into the stomach with small flexible orogastric or nasogastric catheters. When this method of feeding is necessary for several months or longer, a gastrostomy should be surgically constructed. The formula can be delivered either intermittently in bolus infusion or initially as a continuous infusion with progression to bolus infusions over several weeks or months. Disadvantages of bolus infusion include delayed gastric emptying secondary to volume and osmolality, risk of aspiration, bradycardia, and decreased ventilatory function.[53]

Continuous infusion using an infusion pump appears to reduce problems with gastric emptying and has the theoretical advantage of reducing substrate load to the mucosal and intraluminal digestive enzymes, thereby enhancing efficiency. Owing to concern for possible aspiration with intragastric infusion, no more than two hours' feeding should be in the chamber or syringe at any time. Aspirates are checked without prior cessation of the infusion. Although normal data of gastric aspirates in infancy are lacking, an aspirate in excess of the previous hour's feeding is considered significant. In special circumstances in which the risks of aspiration are particularly great, nutrients can be delivered continuously directly into the jejunum using a casein hydrolysate or elemental formula infused through a flexible transpyloric or jejunostomy tube.[54] A number of serious complications that may occur with this method of feeding include bacterial overgrowth, abdominal distention, and intestinal perforation.[55] In addition to the aforementioned complications, it may be difficult to pass the catheter through the pylorus. This is done either by leaving a length of catheter in the stomach and allowing it to pass with normal gastric motility over 24 hours or by placing the catheter through the pylorus under fluoroscopic guidance. In both cases, radiographic confirmation of placement is necessary, and care must be taken, by checking gastric aspirates, that the tube remains in the small bowel. All formulae are initially given in a concentration of 0.25 to 0.33 kcal per ml at 60 to 80 ml per kg per day.

Concentrations and volumes are increased daily until nutritional needs are met. With continuous intragastric feedings, an increase in osmolality seems to interfere less with gastric emptying than does a calorically equivalent increase in volume. With jejunal feedings, increases in volume may be tolerated better than increases in osmolality. Once the infant's volume limit has been reached, additional nutrients will have to be delivered by increasing the density of the formula. Increasing the concentration of the formula has the advantage of maintaining the distribution of calories derived from protein, carbohydrate, and fat.

The reduction in free water means that osmolality and renal solute load will increase. Initially, the caloric density is increased by concentrating the formula in a stepwise fashion to 1 kcal per ml. If this is not possible because of the sodium, solute, or protein load, and if further calorie increases are necessary, the formula is supplemented with carbohydrate and fat, diluting the protein intake to no less than 8 per cent of total calories. Fat (9 calories per gram) and carbohydrate (3 calories per gram) are usually added in equal caloric concentrations. Unless lipolysis is severely impaired, fat is added as long-chain corn oil to minimize the increase in osmolality. Carbohydrate is usually supplemented as glucose polymer (Polycose). Supplementation of protein is rarely indicated. While the infant's calorie and fluid intake is being increased, optimal intake can be achieved with supplemental parenteral nutrition.

Weaning from continuous infusion can be done by infusing a three-hour volume of formula in two hours with an hour without infusion, repeating this process over 24 to 48 hours, and then decreasing the three-hour infusion volume to one hour. It often requires a week or more to achieve bolus feedings after the infant has been fed continuously for a long period, and frequent reversions to continuous infusions are commonly necessary because of diarrhea or substrate intolerance.

Several medications have proved useful in managing the motility problems in young infants. Antispasmodics based on anticholinergic agents or opiates may be helpful to manage rapid transit times, as seen in the short bowel syndrome. Extreme care must be taken when using these agents not to produce an adynamic ileus, which can lead to sequestration of fluids in the intraluminal space or even perforation of the bowel. Paregoric and deodorized tincture of opium are two preparations commonly used for this purpose. Agents that enhance motility may be useful with delayed gastric emptying. Metoclopramide[56] and bethanechol increase gastric motility and are occasionally useful in the treatment of gastroesophageal reflux or in facilitating the placement of a transpyloric feeding tube.

REFERENCES

1. Pritchard, J. A.: Fetal swallowing and amniotic fluid volume. Obstet. Gynecol. 28:606, 1966.
2. Gryboski, J. D.: The swallowing mechanism of the neonate. Pediatrics 35:445, 1965.
3. Gryboski, T. D., Thayer, W. R., and Spiro, H. M.: Esophageal motility in infants and children. Pediatrics 31:382, 1963.
4. Yu, V. Y. H.: Effect of body position on gastric emptying in the neonate. Arch. Dis. Child. 50:500, 1975.
5. Aldridge, R. T., and Campbell, P. E.: Ganglion cell distribution in the normal rectum and anal canal. J. Pediatr. Surg. 34:475, 1968.
6. Younoszai, M. K.: Jejunal absorption of hexose in infants and children. J. Pediatr. 85:446, 1974.
7. Heyman, M., Desjeux, J. F., Grasset, E., et al.: Relationship between transport of D-xylose and other monosaccharides in jejunal mucosa of children. Gastroenterology 80(4):758, 1981.
8. Kien, C. L., Summers, J. E., Heimler, R., and Grausz, J. D.: Carbohydrate energy absorption in premature infants. Gastroenterology 78:52, 1979.
9. Antonowicz, I., Chang, S. K., and Grand, R. J.: Development and distribution of lysosomal enzymes and disaccharidases in human fetal intestine. Gastroenterology 51:481, 1966.
10. Lebenthal, E., and Lee, P. C.: Development of functional response in human exocrine pancreas. Pediatrics 66(4):556, 1980.
11. Russel, G., and Costalos, B.: Oral tolerance of Caloreen in babies. Arch. Dis. Child. 55:886, 1980.
12. Watkins, J. B.: Bile acid metabolism and fat absorption in newborn infants. Pediatr. Clin. North Am. 21:501, 1979.
13. Norman, A., Strandvih, B., and Ojama, O.: Bile acids and pancreatic enzymes during absorption in the newborn. Acta Paediatr. Scand. 61:571, 1972.
14. Holtzapple, P. G., Smith, G., and Koldovsky, O.: Uptake, activation and esterification of fatty acids in the small intestine of the suckling rat. Pediatr. Res. 9:786, 1975.
15. Robertson, D. M., Paganelli, R., Dinwiddie, R., and Levinski, R. J.: Milk antigen absorption in the premature and term neonate. Personal communication, 1982.
16. Barness, L.: Nutritional needs of low birth weight infants. Pediatrics 60:619, 1977.
17. Tantibhedhyangkul, P., and Haskin, S.: Medium-chain triglyceride feeding in premature infants: Effects on fat and nitrogen absorption. Pediatrics 55(3):359, 1975.
18. Fosbrook, A. S., and Whooton, B. A.: Added lactose and added sucrose cow's milk formula in nutrition of low birth weight babies. Arch. Dis. Child. 50:409, 1975.
19. Barbero, G. J., Runge, G., Fischer, D., Crawford, M. N., Torres, F. E., and Gyrogy, P.: Investigations on the bacterial flora, pH and sugar content in the intestine tract of infants. J. Pediatr. 40:152, 1952.
20. Fomon, S. J., Ziegler, E. A., Filer, L. J., Nelson, S. E., and Edwards, B. B.: Methionine fortification of a soy-protein formula fed to infant. Am. J. Clin. Nutr. 32:2460, 1979.
21. Sturman, J. A., Gaull, G., and Raiha, N. C.: Ab-

22. Gaull, G. E., Rassin, D. K., Räihä, N. C., et al.: Milk protein quantity and quality in low-birth-weight infants. III. Effects of sulfur amino acids in plasma and urine. J. Pediatr. 90:348, 1977.
23. Novak, M., Monhus, E. F., Chung, D., and Buch, M.: Carnitine in the perinatal metabolism of lipids. Pediatrics 67:95, 1981.
24. Fleischman, A. R., and Finberg, L.: Breast milk for term and preterm infants — optimal nutrition? Perinatology 3:397, 1979.
25. Atkinson, S. A., Bryan, M. H., and Anderson, G. H.: Human milk: Differences in nitrogen concentration in milk from mothers of term and preterm infants. J. Pediatr. 93(1):67, 1978.
26. Kleinman, R. E., Jacobson, L., Hormann, E., and Walker, W. A.: Protein values of milk samples from mothers without biologic pregnancies. J. Pediatr. 97(4):612, 1980.
27. Fomon, S. J., Ziegler, E., Gaull, G. E., Rassin, D. K., and Raiha, N. C.: Protein intake of premature infants. J. Pediatr. 90:504, 1977.
28. Edelmann, C. M., Barnett, H. L., and Troupkou, V.: Renal concentrating mechanisms in newborn infants. J. Clin. Invest. 39:1062, 1960.
29. Engelke, S. C., Bhavesh, S. L., Vasan, U., and Raye, J. R.: Sodium balance in very low birth weight infants. J. Pediatr. 93(5):837, 1978.
30. Committee on Nutrition, American Academy of Pediatrics: Calcium requirements in infancy and childhood. Pediatrics 62:826, 1978.
31. Tsang, R. C., Steichen, J. S., and Brown, D. R.: Perinatal calcium homeostasis: Neonatal hypocalcemia and bone demineralization. Clin. Perinatol. 4:385, 1977.
32. Sandstead, H. H., Vo-Khactu, K. P., and Solomons, J.: In Trace Elements in Human Health and Disease, Vol. 1. New York, Academic Press, 1976, p. 33.
33. Committee on Nutrition, American Academy of Pediatrics: Iron supplementation for infants. Pediatrics 58:765, 1976.
34. Williams, M. L., Shott, R. J., O'Neal, P. L., and Oski, F. A.: Role of dietary iron and fat on vitamin E deficiency anemia of infancy. N. Engl. J. Med. 292:887, 1975.
35. O'Connor, P.: Vitamin D–deficiency rickets in two breast-fed infants who were not receiving vitamin D supplementation. Clin. Pediatr. 16:361, 1977.
36. Usher, R., and McLean, F.: Intrauterine growth of live-born caucasian infants at sea level. J. Pediatr. 74:901, 1969.
37. Smith, F. R., Suskind, R., Thananakul, O., Lietzman, C., Goodman, D. S., and Olsen, R. D.: Plasma vitamin A retinol binding protein and prealbumin concentration in protein calorie malnutrition. Am. J. Clin. Nutr. 29:1089, 1976.
38. Smith, M. F., Moldawer, L. L., and Bistrian, B. R.: Transferrin as a measure of the efficiency of parenteral and enteral nutrition. J. Parent. Ent. Nutr. Vol. 1, 1977.
39. Buts, J. P., Morin, C. L., Roy, C. C., Weber, A., and Bonin, A.: One hour blood xylose tests. Reliable index of small bowel function. J. Pediatr. 90:729, 1978.
40. Toshes, P. D.: Serum trypsin as a test for chronic

pancreatitis. Gastroenterology 82:155, 1982.

41. Sacher, M., Korsa, A., and Shmerling, D. H.: PABA screening test for exocrine pancreatic function in infants and children. Arch. Dis. Child. 53:639, 1978.

42. Committee on Nutrition, American Academy of Pediatrics: Commentary on breast feeding and infant formulas including proposed standards for formulas. Pediatrics 57:278, 1976.

43. MacClean, W. G., and Graham, G. G.: The effects of level of protein intake in isoenergetic diets on energy utilization. Am. J. Clin. Nutr. 32:1381, 1979.

44. Fomon, S. J., Thomas, L. M., Filer, J. L., Anderson, T. A., and Bergmann, K. E.: Requirements for protein and essential amino acids in early infancy: Studies with a soy-isolate formula. Acta Paediatr. Scand. 62:33, 1973.

45. Lee, P., Roloff, D., and Howatt, W.: Hypoproteinemia and anemia in infants with cystic fibrosis, a presenting symptom complex often misdiagnosed. J.A.M.A. 228:585, 1974.

46. Matthews, D. M., and Adibi, S. A.: Peptide absorption. Gastroenterology 71:151, 1976.

47. Hunt, J. N., and Pathak, J. D.: The osmotic effects of some simple molecules and ions on gastric emptying. J. Physiol. 154:254, 1960.

48. Committee on Nutrition, American Academy of Pediatrics: Breast feeding. Pediatrics 62: 591, 1978.

49. Duncan, D. H.: The physiological effects of lactose. Nutr. Abst. Rev. 25:309, 1955.

50. Easenberg, A., Shaw, R. D., and Yousefzadeh, D.: Lactobezoar in the low birth weight infant. Pediatrics 63:692, 1979.

51. Eastham, E. J., Lichauco, T., Grady, M. I., and Walker, W. A.: Antigenicity of infant formulas: Role of immature intestine on protein permeability. J. Pediatr. 93:561, 1978.

52. Silk, D. B., and Fairclough, P.: Use of a peptide rather than free amino acid nitrogen source in chemically defined elemental diets. J. Parent. Ent. Nutr. Nov.–Dec. 1980, p. 548.

53. Patel, B. D., Dinwiddie, R., Kumar, S. P., et al.: The effects of feeding on arterial blood gases and lung mechanisms in newborn infants recovering from respiratory disease. J. Pediatr. 90:435, 1977.

54. Pereira, G. R., and Lemons, J. A.: Controlled study of transpyloric and intermittent gavage feeding in a small preterm infant. Pediatrics 67(1):68, 1981.

55. Penez-Rodriquez, J., Quero, J., and Frias, E. G.: Duodenal perforation in a neonate by a tube of silicone rubber during transpyloric feeding. J. Pediatr. 92:113, 1978.

56. Schluze-Delrieu, K.: Metoclopramide. Gastroenterology 77:768, 1979.

Chapter Ten

PARENTERAL NUTRITION

In spite of the wide variety of enteral formulations and techniques of enteral feeding available, several gastrointestinal problems arise in infants that preclude or severely limit the use of the intestine for nutritional support. Since 1944, when the first successful use of total parenteral nutrition in a malnourished infant was reported,[1] the use of total or supplemental parenteral nutrition has become a common practice. Premature infants with severe respiratory disease, congenital anomalies of the enteric canal, or inflammatory disease of intestinal mucosa (necrotizing enterocolitis) are frequent candidates for this form of nutritional support. Older infants with intractable diarrhea, severe malnutrition, or inflammatory bowel disease have been successfully rehabilitated with parenteral feedings as well. Extensive body surface burns, malignancies, and renal failure are examples of disorders outside the gastrointestinal tract in which parenteral support has been useful. Specific formulations and procedures are available for these latter situations and have been reviewed elsewhere.[2]

CATHETER PLACEMENT

Parenteral nutrition catheters can be placed in peripheral veins using standard peripheral intravenous catheters and isosmotic solutions. When higher osmolar solutions are employed, larger veins with a high blood flow volume must be used to avoid sclerosis and inflammation in the wall of the vein. The catheters, made either of flexible material such as Silastic or of stiffer polyethylene, are generally placed in the subclavian or internal jugular vein and advanced to the right atrium. The stiffer catheters can be introduced percutaneously into the subclavian vein, whereas the more flexible catheters must be placed by cutting down onto the vein or creating a subcutaneous tunnel into a superficial neck vein,[3] again advancing the catheter toward the right atrium. We prefer the surgical subclavian placement of Silastic catheters in the premature infant because of the lower incidence of vein perforation and thrombosis with these catheters.[4] On occasion, when jugular or subclavian sites have been unavailable, we have used the inferior epigastric vein as an alternative (Fig. 10–1).[5] Regardless of the site, radiographic confirmation of line placement is mandatory before the nutrition solutions are infused.

A number of complications that are directly related to the catheter itself may arise. Malposition of a central catheter outside the vein, with infusion of hypertonic solutions into the pleural or pericardial space,

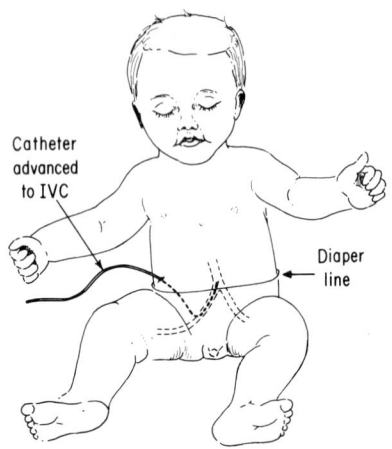

Figure 10–1 A Silastic catheter is threaded into the inferior epigastric vein and up the external iliac vein to a point just above the bifurcation of the inferior vena cava. The proximal catheter is tunneled subcutaneously upward to exit above the diaper line. With the catheter in situ, the baby can lie with the legs flexed or it can sit without angulating the catheter. (From Donahoe, P. K., et al.: J. Ped. Surg. *15*:737, 1980. Used by permission.)

may be life-threatening. A rapid fall in serum glucose or the acute onset of circulatory compromise should alert one to this complication. Hemorrhage, associated with erosion of central veins or of the wall of the right atrium, has also been reported. Pneumothorax and brachial plexus injuries are relatively common complications of percutaneous subclavian line insertion. Air embolus may occur if proper filters are not in place. Catheter emboli have resulted from rupture of Silastic catheters perfused under very high pressures or from the tips of polyethylene catheters sheared off when the catheter was pulled back through the hub of the needle used to insert it. Thrombophlebitis is seen in peripheral veins receiving hypertonic solutions. The most worrisome complication, however, is catheter sepsis, which may be life-threatening. Fever alone is not an indication for removal of a parenteral nutrition catheter. Other sources of infection should be searched for, and if none is found, removal of the catheter is then considered. Signs of sepsis in the neonate include lethargy, hyperbilirubinemia, temperature instability, and intolerance to previously tolerated glucose and lipid loads. Careful placement of the central catheter and strict adherence to established

guidelines for catheter care and maintenance markedly decrease the incidence of catheter-related complications.

COMPOSITION OF SOLUTIONS FOR INFANTS AND CHILDREN
(See Section 1, Appendix)

PROTEIN

Current solutions supply nitrogen requirements in the form of crystalline amino acids. Infants have demonstrated adequate growth with this source of nitrogen.[6, 7] Protein hydrolysate preparations no longer are commercially available. The various commercial amino acid preparations are available as concentrated solutions from 3.5 per cent to 10 per cent mixtures of crystalline amino acids, which can then be diluted to meet nutritional requirements of infants at different ages. None of the solutions available in the United States are qualitatively identical to the amino acid composition of breast milk, which has been used as the enteral standard formulation for optimal growth in healthy infants. None of the commercial solutions contain cystine, although separate packets of cystine are available to be added to the solutions. Cystine is an essential amino acid for premature infants, who have very low activity of hepatic cystathionase, which converts methionine to cystine.[8] Taurine, which is also formed from cystine, may be essential in this group of infants[9] and is absent from these solutions. Finally, none of the available solutions contain carnitine, which is required for the optimal oxidation of fatty acids in infants, for whom fat is a main source of energy.[10]

In spite of these recognized deficiencies, infants have tolerated and grown on the solutions available. Most of the metabolic complications related to protein in the solutions have developed when the infants received more than 4 gm per kg per day of protein. These problems included azotemia and acidosis. Our practice is to supply 2 to 3 gm per kg per day of protein, and we rarely encounter these complications. Hyperammonemia, associated with earlier solutions, is now also rarely seen owing to the increased amounts of arginine and decreased quantities of glycine in the formulations. Hyperchloremic metabolic acidosis was another problem noted with earlier crystalline amino acid solutions.[11] It has also been ameliorated by the substitution of acetate salts of lysine and sodium. Solutions containing high levels of branched-chain amino acids, or ketoanalogs of amino acids, have been used experimentally to treat the patients with severe hyperammonemia and those with hepatic failure. The use of these formulations has not been widespread in infants, for whom they are available only for research purposes.

CARBOHYDRATES

Glucose, fructose, galactose, sorbitol, glycerol, and alcohol have all been used as sources of carbohydrate calories in infant formulae. At present, almost all centers use glucose as the principal carbohydrate with the small amount of glycerol present in lipid solutions also contributing to carbohydrate calories. The other carbohydrate sources have fallen out of favor because they have no advantages over glucose and can produce serious complications in the premature infant. Tolerance to glucose infusion is variable in premature infants. We begin by infusing 5 mg per kg per minute and advance to 15 mg per kg per minute over a period of two days by increasing the concentration of glucose in the solution and keeping the volume of infusate constant at between 100 and 150 ml per kg per day, depending on the infant's fluid requirements (see the Pediatric Parenteral Nutrition Manual, Section 1 of the Appendix). In adult postsurgical patients, there appears to be no correlation between glucose clearance and the rate of oxidation of glucose.[12] That is, an increase in the glucose infusion rate from 4 mg per kg per minute to 7 mg per kg per minute is associated with an increased rate of glucose oxidation, but at higher infusion rates fat is synthesized from the glucose without any further increase in glucose oxidation or energy derived there-

from. Similar studies have not been completed in infants, but this suggests that higher glucose loads in the range of 20 to 30 mg per kg per minute may not be beneficial to infants and may contribute to the fatty infiltration of the liver seen with prolonged total parenteral nutrition. The increased production of CO_2 seen with high glucose loads may add a ventilatory burden to the compromised pulmonary functions in the premature neonate. The addition of insulin is difficult in the premature infant because of the unpredictable response to this hormone. Acute consequences of glucose intolerance are mainly hyperosmolarity of serum and osmotic diuresis, both of which can be avoided by careful serum monitoring.

LIPIDS

Lipid solutions are available as sources of energy and essential fatty acids. The two emulsions currently available in the United States have either soybean or safflower oil as the fat source, emulsified with egg phosphatides, and glycerol added to increase osmolarity. Essential fatty acid requirements can be met by infusing 0.5 gm per kg to 1.0 gm per kg per day.[13] Some controversy exists regarding the ability of fat to enhance nitrogen retention compared with glucose. Under conditions of starvation, fat and carbohydrates do appear to be equivalent in this regard after the first four days of parenteral feeding.[14] It is our policy, therefore, to use lipid as a calorie supplement to glucose infusions of 10 mg per kg per minute in small infants. Intravenous lipid is hydrolyzed to free fatty acids by lipoprotein lipase along the endothelial cells of blood vessels. The free fatty acids either are re-esterified and stored in adipose tissue or circulate, bound to albumin, and utilized as an immediate energy source. Premature infants of less than 32 weeks' gestation have decreased tolerance to intravenous lipid, although tolerance improves rapidly during the first week of life.[15] Small for gestational age infants,[16] septic infants, and infants with conditions requiring acute surgical intervention may develop hyperlipidemia at very low rates of lipid infusion and must be monitored continuously. There are no simple and reliable methods of determining lipid tolerance in the infant. Serum triglyceride and free fatty acid determinations cannot be done routinely. Our practice is to infuse up to 3 gm per kg per day over 20 hours and to check serum for lipemia just before restarting the infusion. Triglyceride levels are measured twice a week. If the serum triglyceride level is 150 mg per dl or the serum is lipemic, the infusions are held for 24 hours and then restarted at a lower amount and advanced over several days as tolerated. Lipemic serum also interferes with determination of serum bilirubin and calcium,[17, 18] and inaccurate values result unless the serum is centrifuged at high speed to remove the lipid.

Many potential adverse effects of lipid infusions have been reported; these are related to reticuloendothelial function, pulmonary function, albumin binding, and long-term effects of an elevated value of linoleic acid in serum and tissues. Intravenous lipid that is not cleared by lipoprotein lipase may deposit in lung[19] or reticuloendothelial tissues. Preterm infants have developed hypoxemia in the first week of life during lipid infusions, and fat globules have been demonstrated in alveolar macrophages both in animals and in premature infants who did not survive.

Anecdotally, some infants have proved difficult to wean from the respirator while on lipid infusion but improved sufficiently after termination of the lipid to discontinue assisted ventilation. Reticuloendothelial accumulation of lipid may alter immune function,[20] although there has been no clear *in vivo* evidence of this in human infants. Finally, hyperbilirubinemia is a common finding in premature infants but also may occur in newborn infants with liver disease. Free fatty acids compete with bilirubin for binding to albumin; with high serum concentrations of free fatty acids, bilirubin can be displaced from albumin-binding sites, increasing the risk of kernicterus in the small infant.[21] Because few laboratories have the capacity to measure serum free fatty acid levels, the American Academy of

Pediatrics Committee on Nutrition recommends that no more than 0.5 gm per kg per day of lipid be administered to infants with serum bilirubin concentrations of 8 to 10 mg per dl.[13]

MINERALS AND VITAMINS

Minerals must be supplied along with vitamins in all parenteral solutions. Metabolic complications have been described for excesses and deficiencies of all the nutrients. Although tract elements are present in varying amounts in different solutions, it has been our practice to add these to the commercial solutions, particularly for infants with severe diarrheal illness or enteric fistulas, in which losses are apt to be unusually high. In addition to standard multivitamin preparations, vitamin K, vitamin E, folate, and vitamin B_{12} are given either orally or by intramuscular injection to meet ongoing requirements.

GASTROINTESTINAL EFFECTS OF PARENTERAL NUTRITION

The single most problematic gastrointestinal complication of total parenteral nutrition is the development of liver disease, presenting clinically as hepatomegaly and jaundice and histologically as cholestasis, hepatocellular necrosis, and, in far advanced cases, cirrhosis or hepatic failure. First reported in 1971, liver disease is now recognized to occur in approximately one third of premature infants receiving total parenteral nutrition.[22] The etiology remains obscure. Toxic effects of the protein hydrolysates and lipid solutions have been proposed, although not corroborated on further study. Limited hepatic excretion function in premature infants has been demonstrated; this, combined with deficiencies in certain amino acids necessary for bile acid conjugation, such as taurine, may result in cholestasis. The appearance of liver disease, with elevations in transaminases, bilirubin, and alkaline phosphatase, usually occurs after two weeks of total parenteral nutrition and is often progressive, leading to portal fibrosis and, in a few infants, hepatic failure.[23] These infants are often compromised by a number of intercurrent illnesses, including sepsis and severe respiratory distress, and it has been difficult to separate these factors from the effects of parenteral nutrition on the development of hepatic dysfunction. Infants with surgical complications have a higher incidence of this problem than those with medical problems alone. But in both groups, there is no way to predict which infants will develop progressive liver disease, except that the longer the infusions are administered, the greater the risk of cholestasis.

Much less is known about the effects of chronic total parenteral nutrition on gastric, pancreatic, and small bowel functions. Studies in animals have documented pancreatic hyposecretion and intestinal mucosal atrophy, which are reversible upon resumption of enteric feeding.[24] The few studies made of human subjects suggest that a similar situation is present with decreased pancreatic excretion and parietal cell mass.[25] Intravenous amino acids do stimulate gastric acid secretion but much less so than amino acids placed into the stomach. Small bowel mucosal atrophy occurs as well. All of these findings revert to normal over eight to nine months following return to enteral nutrition. Although similar studies have not been done in premature infants, clinical experience suggests that, with time, enteric functions return to normal in these patients as well.

NUTRITION IN SPECIFIC GASTROINTESTINAL DISEASE STATES

Specific gastrointestinal disorders and their management are discussed in other chapters. For example, infants with milk or soy protein intolerance and gluten intolerance require diets free of the offending protein. Initially the formula should be a protein hydrolysate or amino acid and glucose polymer solution, with advancement to more complex formulae as the intestinal morphology returns to normal. With pancreatic insufficiency, supplemental pancreatic enzymes are necessary, although even with this supplementation together with antacid medication or enteric-coated capsules containing the enzymes, absorption of fat does not always return to normal. Whenever fat malabsorption is a prominent feature of the illness, vitamin requirements must be met by supplementing the formula with aqueous preparations of the fat-soluble vitamins, including vitamin E.

One gastrointestinal problem, however, that is often complicated by severe malnutrition is the short bowel syndrome. This can serve as an example for nutritional management of infants with severe gastrointestinal compromise.

The short bowel syndrome may be the result of a congenitally shortened bowel, or it may follow surgical resection of bowel either to correct a congenital malformation or to resect necrotic tissue, as with necrotizing enterocolitis. Infants with less than 50 cm of residual small bowel present at the extreme of absorptive limitation.

These infants will all initially require nutritional support by the parenteral route for several weeks. Our practice is to use the central route and to begin enteric feeding as soon as the viability of the residual bowel is confirmed. As the residual bowel has usually been ischemic, severe villous atrophy is assumed. Thus the initial feedings are with casein hydrolysate or elemental formulae. On day 1, the formula is prepared as 0.3 kcal per ml and delivered by continuous intragastric infusion at 10 kcal per kg per day. Calorie increases are made very slowly, and it is usually at least one month before 50 per cent of calories can be delivered enterically. At this point, the infant can be changed to peripheral parenteral nutrition as the enteric feedings are advanced. Lactose and solids are generally withheld for at least three months. Rapid intestinal transit may be managed with careful use of antimotility agents. Throughout the period of rehabilitation, care must be taken to meet the infant's requirements for vitamins, minerals, and trace elements either orally or intravenously in the face of continuing losses with diarrhea.

SUMMARY

Nutritional requirements of young infants, both premature and full-term, can be satisfied by recognizing the absorptive and digestive limitations present at this time. With gastrointestinal disease superimposed on an immature digestive system, these infants often require special support to maintain adequate growth. This support can be offered in the form of parenteral nutrition as well as with specialized feeding techniques and formulations. Continuous monitoring of the nutritional status is mandatory to assess the adequacy of nutritional support.

REFERENCES

1. Helfrick, F. W., and Abelson, M. M.: Intravenous feeding of complete diet in child; report of a case. Pediatrics 25:400, 1944.
2. Ghadimi, H.: Newly devised amino acid solutions for intravenous administration. *In* Ghadimi, H. (ed.): Total Parenteral Nutrition, Premises and Promises. New York, John Wiley & Sons, 1975, pp. 393–442.
3. Riordan, T. P.: Placement of central venous lines in the premature infant. J. Parent. Ent. Nutr. 3(5):301, 1979.
4. Pollack, P. F., Kadden, M., Byrne, W. J., Fonkalsrud, E. W., Ament, M. E.: 100 patient years' experience with the Broviac silastic catheter for central venous nutrition. J. Parent. Ent. Nutr. 5:1:32, 1981.
5. Donahoe, P. K., and Kim, S. H.: The inferior epigastric vein as an alternate site for central venous hyperalimentation. J. Pediatr. Surg. 15(6):737, 1980.
6. Shaw, J. C. L.: Parenteral nutrition in the management of the sick–low birthweight infants. Pediatr. Clin. North Am. 20:333, 1973.
7. Zlotkin, S. H., Bryan, M. H., and Anderson, G. H.: Intravenous nitrogen and energy intakes required to duplicate in utero nitrogen accretion in prematurely born human infants. J. Pediatr. 99(1):115, 1981.
8. Sturman, J. A., Gaull, G., and Raiha, N. C.: Absence of cystathionase in human fetal liver: Is cystine essential? Science 169:74, 1970.
9. Gaull, G. E., Rassin, D. K., Räihä, N. C., et al.: Milk protein quantity and quality in low-birth-weight infants. III. Effects of sulfur amino acids in plasma and urine. J. Pediatr. 90:348, 1977.
10. Schiff, D., Chan, G., Seccombe, D., and Hahn, P.: Plasma carnitine levels during intravenous feeding of the neonate. J. Pediatr. 95(6):1043, 1979.
11. Heird, W. D., Dell, R. B., Driscoll, J. M., Jr., and Winters, R.: Metabolic acidosis resulting from intravenous alimentation mixtures containing synthetic amino acids. N. Engl. J. Med. 287:943, 1972.
12. Wolfe, R. R., Allsop, J. R., and Burke, J. F.: Glucose metabolism in man: responses to intravenous glucose infusion. Metabolism 28:210, 1979.
13. Committee on Nutrition, American Academy of Pediatrics: Use of intravenous fat emulsions in pediatric patients. *In* Pediatric Nutrition Handbook, 1979, p. 312.
14. Jeejeebhoy, K. N., Anderson, G. H., Nakhodda, A. F., Greenberg, C. R., Sanderson, I., and Marliss, E. B.: Metabolic studies in total parenteral nutrition with lipid in man: Comparison with glucose. J. Clin. Invest. 57:125, 1976.
15. Pereira, G. R., Fox, W. W., Stanley, C. A., Baker, L., and Schwartz, J. G.: Decreased oxygenation and hyperlipemia during intravenous fat infusion in premature infants. Pediatrics 66(1):26, 1980.
16. Andrew, G., Chan, G., Schiff, D.: Lipid metabolism in the neonate. J. Pediatr. 88:2:273, 1976.
17. Giacoia, G., Krasner, J.: Interference of intravenous lipid emulsion with determination of calcium in serum. Am. J. Med. Technology 45(9):767, 1979.
18. Shennan, A. T., Cherian, A. G., Angel, A., Bryan, M. H.: The effect of intralipid on the estimation of serum bilirubin in the newborn infant. J. Pediatr. 88:2:285, 1976.
19. Barson, A. J., Chiswick, M. L., Doig, C. M.: Fat embolism in infancy after intravenous fat infusions. Arch. Dis. Child. 53:218, 1978.
20. DiLuzio, N. R., Blickens, D. A.: Influence of intravenously administered lipids on reticuloendothelial function. J. Reticuloendothelial Soc. 3:250, 1966.
21. Stasinski, R., and Shafrir, E.: Displacement of albumin-bound bilirubin by free fatty acids. Implications for neonatal hyperbilirubinemia. Clin. Chim. Acta 29:311, 1970.
22. Sondheimer, J. M., Bryan, G., Andrews, W., and Forstner, G. G.: Cholestatic tendencies in premature infants on and off parenteral nutrition. Pediatrics 62(6):984, 1978.
23. Cohen, M. I.: Changes in hepatic function in intravenous nutrition. *In* Winters, R. W., and Hasselmeyer, E. (eds.): Intravenous Nutrition in the High Risk Infant. New York, John Wiley & Sons, 1975, pp. 293–313.
24. Feldman, E. J., Dowling, R. H., McNaughton, J., and Peters, J. J.: Effects of oral and venous nutrition on intestinal adaptation after small bowel resection in the dog. Gastroenterology 70:712, 1976.
25. Kotler, D. P., and Levine, G. M.: Reversible gastric and pancreatic hyposecretion after long-term total parenteral nutrition. N. Engl. J. Med. 300(5):241, 1979.

PART III / GASTRO-INTESTINAL DISEASE STATES

Chapter Eleven

THE ESOPHAGUS

The esophagus in the newborn infant measures between 3 and 5½ inches in length from its functioning upper sphincter to its lower sphincter, and it extends through the posterior mediastinum. The diameter measures 4 to 6 mm.[63] It is fixed superiorly where the striated cricopharyngeus muscle joins the cricoid; inferiorly, it is somewhat fixed by the phrenoesophageal ligament as it passes through the diaphragmatic hiatus. The musculature of the esophagus is primarily smooth, although there is some mingling of striated muscle in the upper section. The lining is squamous epithelium, and there is serosal covering only at the insertion of the phrenoesophageal ligament. The arterial blood supply is from branches of the thoracic aorta, and the venous drainage is through three systems: superiorly, those vessels that drain into the superior vena cava; centrally, those that drain into the azygous system; and inferiorly, those that drain into the portal system through the gastric veins. The innervation of the organ is largely through the vagus and the sympathetic ganglia. Neural noncholin-ergic and nonadrenergic factors are also present, with evidence to suggest that VIP is the inhibitory neurotransmitter.

The esophagus develops from the embryonic foregut by the end of the first month of gestation. Anteriorly, the pharynx narrows and the tracheal bud arises. By the second month, the trachea and lung buds lie ventral to the short esophagus. During the next few weeks, the stomach moves from a position behind the heart into the abdomen and the esophagus grows in length. In children there is some correlation of esophageal length with height.[144] The lining epithelium, originally columnar, goes through a ciliated stage and finally attains its mature stratified squamous form. A few goblet cells in the proximal third provide mucus.

Since the major esophageal functions are to transport food from the mouth to the stomach and to provide an appropriate barrier against reflux of gastric contents, the manifestations of disease in this organ are either feeding difficulties or regurgitation. In young infants, problems in the initiation of swallowing indicate neurologic disorders

157

Table 11–1   Differential Diagnosis in Esophageal Disease

SYMPTOMS	DISEASE
Choking, cyanosis at onset of feeding	Tracheoesophageal fistula and atresia Laryngotracheoesophageal cleft Esophageal diverticulum Esophageal web or stenosis (high) Familial dysautonomia
Coughing, regurgitation after onset of and during feeding	Esophageal tumors Duplication cyst Vascular compression of esophagus Esophageal diverticulum Esophageal web or stenosis Tracheoesophageal fistula without atresia
Dysphagia	Esophageal stricture Achalasia Spasm Lower esophageal ring
Regurgitation after feeding	Esophageal stenosis Hiatus hernia Chalasia Achalasia Congenital short esophagus
Predominant symptoms of respiratory distress or pneumonia	Duplication cyst Diaphragmatic hernia Familial dysautonomia H-type fistula
Predominant symptoms of wheezing or stridor May or may not have dysphagia	Vascular compression Congenital diverticulum

or lesions of the oropharynx or the superior esophageal sphincter. Choking or cyanosis during feeding is due to aspiration because of swallowing incoordination, failure of closure of the epiglottis, laryngotracheoesophageal cleft, or tracheoesophageal fistula. Similar problems arising at the end of or after feeding suggest a lesion more distal in the esophagus, such as stenosis or hiatus hernia. Rumination is sometimes the only symptom of hiatus hernia in infancy.

The older infant who can talk often indicates the site of the lesion by his description of the symptoms. Pain or dysphagia produced by lesions in the body of the esophagus is located over the anterior chest or the back in the region of the lesion. Pain associated with involvement of the lower esophagus or inferior sphincter is referred to the suprasternal notch, the ears, or the jaws. Symptoms from the upper esophagus or superior sphincter are referred to the same areas. Major symptoms of esophageal disease are listed in Table 11–1.

PHYSIOLOGY OF THE ESOPHAGUS

Functionally, the esophagus is divided into three parts: the upper and lower sphincters and the body. The upper, or superior, esophageal sphincter, composed largely of the striated cricopharyngeus muscle and inferior pharyngeal constrictors, is a small segment (0.5 to 1.5 cm long in the infant) at the pharyngoesophageal junction.[54] Its resting pressure is higher than that of the body below it. The sphincter relaxes at the onset of swallowing and closes with a contraction well above its resting pressure. The striated muscle is innervated by special somatic motor fibers that probably arise from the central vagal nucleus and pass through the vagus. Basal pressures increase during distention or acidification of the esophageal lumen, but these changes do not occur in patients with chronic regurgitation.

Peristalsis in the smooth muscle body of

the esophagus follows relaxation of the sphincter within 0.3 to 0.4 second and extends down through the esophagus. The rate of peristalsis is 0.8 to 2 cm per second in very young infants and 0.8 to 4 cm in older ones. Innervation of the smooth muscle is through parasympathetic fibers of the esophageal plexuses, and it is believed that there is some sympathetic sensory innervation. Manometric tracings show the major peristaltic wave to be large and monophasic (see Fig. 2–4). Occasionally one notes a short negative wave that precedes the large one and coincides with deglutition. A short rise in esophageal baseline pressure sometimes precedes the peristaltic wave after a wet swallow. Another type of peristalsis, not related to swallowing and caused by material remaining in or refluxed into the esophagus, is termed secondary peristalsis. It may occur independently of vagal innervation. This is common in tracings from the esophagus of young infants and is undoubtedly related to the easy reflux of gastric contents noted so frequently in radiologic examinations.[11] Simultaneous or nonpropagative contractions constitute up to 20 per cent of the esophageal responses to deglutition in the young infant. They become less frequent after several months. The development of good propagative peristaltic waves in the infant esophagus coincides with maturation of the sucking pattern.[147]

The inferior esophageal sphincter, which functions to close the lumen at the gastroesophageal junction, is relatively incompetent in the normal neonate and in the premature infant.[25, 143] It measures 0.5 to 1 cm and in the majority of infants is located at or above the effective diaphragmatic hiatus.[24] Not only is sphincter tone poor during the first week of life, but the duration of sphincter relaxation is prolonged. Sphincter tone improves after the first week in the full-term infant and after several weeks in the premature one.[53, 54] The sphincter is of particular interest to the gastroenterologist, for in association with various disorders it may be either hypotensive or hypertensive. Drugs affect its tonus; methacholine (Mecholyl), bethanechol (Urecholine), acetyl-

choline, and histamine raise its pressure, and anticholinergics decrease it. Hormones act upon it too, with gastrin, pancreatic polypeptide, bombesin, serotonin, and prostaglandin F_2 increasing sphincter pressure and secretin and gastric inhibitory polypeptide decreasing it.[37] Selective destruction of vagal centers interferes with function of the sphincter, for the sphincter remains open in patients with vomiting due to central nervous system lesions. However, the fact that a lower sphincter, separated from the body of the esophagus, will still relax after deglutition suggests that there is an important central component in the neural pathways. Electromyographic studies show a continuous spiking activity in the basal LES that disappears before pressure is reduced by pharmacologic agents.

Radiologic investigation, particularly fluoroscopic or cinefluoroscopic examination, is especially helpful in documenting esophageal disease.[8, 71] Studies of the normal nursing infant show a smooth propulsion of the barium bolus through the pharynx and superior esophageal sphincter into the esophagus. In the infant, unlike the older child, esophageal stripping waves may not appear until after several swallows, when the esophagus is well distended with contrast material. The peristaltic contraction is seen to begin in the upper midesophagus and to continue smoothly to the cardia, where barium empties into the stomach. In oral and pharyngeal neuromuscular abnormalities there is gross incoordination of the swallowing mechanism and reflux of barium into the nasopharynx or aspiration into the larynx and trachea. The findings in abnormal communications between esophagus and trachea and in other disorders are discussed in detail later in this chapter.

CONGENITAL MALFORMATIONS OF THE ESOPHAGUS

ABSENCE OF THE ESOPHAGUS

Complete absence of the esophagus from the hypopharynx to the cardia has been reported. The condition is incompatible with life.

ESOPHAGEAL DUPLICATIONS

Duplication cysts of the esophagus present most commonly as expanding mediastinal masses.[104] These and bronchogenic cysts, classified as "foregut origin cysts,"[124] constitute about 16 per cent of the mediastinal masses of infancy and childhood.

Etiology. Although there have been a number of theories to explain the developmental defect causing duplications, only two are considered acceptable. The studies of Saunders[125] and others[51, 145] indicate that duplications arise from failure of separation of the notochord and the adjacent entodermal layer.[16, 125] The notochord plate between ectoderm and entoderm normally migrates dorsally and is pinched off from each side by mesodermal cells. If the notochord takes with it some entoderm, vertebral ossification may be incomplete, especially anteriorly. This postulate is supported by the frequent accompaniment of spina bifida or hemivertebrae and the more uncommon association of the Klippel-Feil syndrome with esophageal duplications. The second theory ascribes the defect to faulty recanalization of the intestinal tract. In the six- to seven-week embryo, the esophageal lumen is filled with proliferating epithelial cells in which vacuolization occurs to form a new lumen. An abnormally placed vacuole is presumed to be the origin of a duplication cyst.[56]

Pathology. The cysts are intramural or partially or completely separated from the esophagus. Although originally located in the posterior mediastinum, they extend to either hemithorax as they enlarge. The cyst walls contain one or more muscle layers and are lined by ciliated squamous or gastric epithelium. Clear, thick fluid fills the cyst. If the gastric mucosa is functional and if the cyst communicates with the esophagus, erosions and esophagitis appear at the site of communication. Noncommunicating cysts, unable to discharge their contents, enlarge and cause symptoms earlier than do communicating ones. Some cysts involve the entire esophagus, and others extend as long stalks through the diaphragm to attach to the pyloroduodenal area or even to the jejunum.

Symptoms. Since the cyst lies near the trachea as well as the esophagus, respiratory symptoms may be as prominent as gastrointestinal ones. Cyanosis and dyspnea are often present at birth, and, as the cyst enlarges, dysphagia and intermittent vomiting develop after several days or weeks. Recurrent pneumonia is the principal complaint in a few infants. Hemoptysis, hematemesis, or melena indicates esophagitis or digestion of the cyst wall. Some duplications of the cervical esophagus cause respiratory distress and stridor, but others present only as slowly enlarging, fluctuant, soft cervical masses.

Diagnosis. The demonstration of a mediastinal mass suggests bronchogenic cyst, neuroblastoma, thoracic abscess, or teratoma as well as a duplication cyst of the esophagus. Lesions in the neck must be differentiated from abscesses, cysts, and tumors (Fig. 11–1).[99]

Radiologic examination of the chest includes lateral and oblique views, for in the anteroposterior view the shadow of the lesion is difficult to separate from the cardiac opacity. In the oblique films the rounded shadow of the cyst becomes more prominent. A soft tissue mass is sharply defined in the posterior mediastinum, usually in the lower chest and most often on the right side. It may extend laterally well into the hemithorax, making its mediastinal origin difficult to appreciate (Fig. 11–1). Vertebral anomalies at the low cervical and upper thoracic levels are often associated with duplication cysts.

Barium swallow study demonstrates anterior displacement of the esophagus by an extrinsic or intramural mass. Less commonly, posterior mediastinal foregut cysts arise from small bowel, with extension through the diaphragm into the thorax.

Treatment. Surgical excision of the cyst results in complete relief of symptoms. Since duplications may be multiple, patients should be evaluated for other cysts, particularly of the small bowel or rectum.

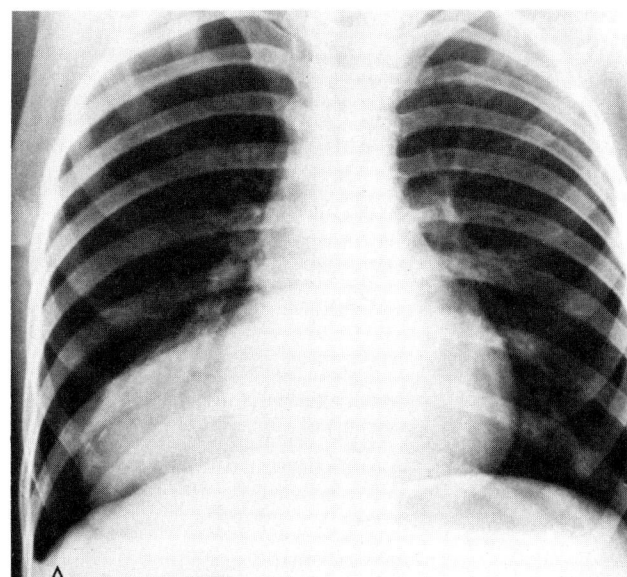

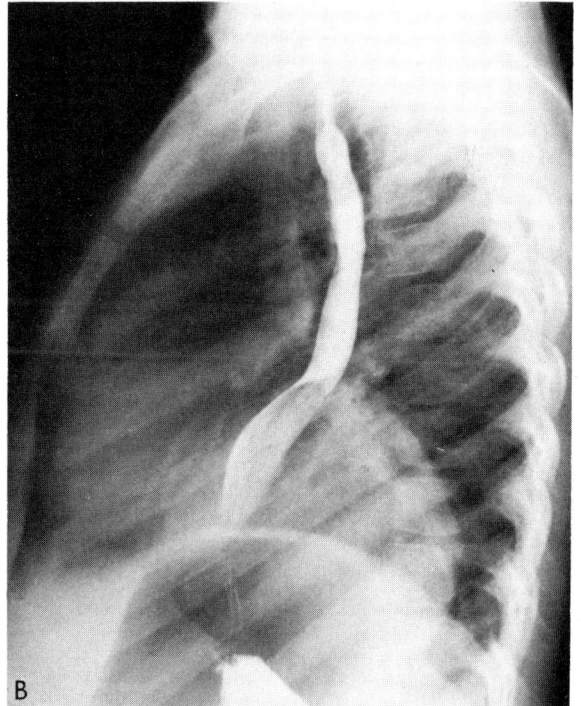

Figure 11–1 Five-year-old girl with poor feeding, frequent regurgitation, and a known chest mass since the age of nine months. Surgery performed after these studies confirmed the presence of a foregut cyst. The mass was surrounded by the outer muscle layer of the esophagus. *A*, Chest film demonstrates a large, sharply defined soft tissue mass in the right lower chest. No vertebral anomalies are present in this case. *B*, Lateral film during barium swallow shows distortion and displacement of the distal esophagus.

COMPRESSION OF THE ESOPHAGUS AND VASCULAR RINGS

Compression of the esophagus is most often produced by anomalous blood vessels, but mediastinal masses such as dermoids, anterior meningoceles, or duplication cysts can produce similar indentations or displacement of the esophagus.

Vascular Rings and Anomalies of the Aortic Arch

These vascular anomalies are considered significant if they cause compression of the esophagus or the trachea or both.[18, 41, 155]

Incidence. Several hundred cases have been reported in the literature. Undoubtedly, many more exist in which the defect has never produced significant symptoms.

Etiology. Anomalous vessels arise from faulty development of the aortic arch system while some arches are forming and others are regressing. The primitive basic pattern consists of a double aortic arch and a right and left ductus arteriosus. The descending aorta is in the midline. Normally, the right ductus and right aortic arch regress, so that at birth there are only a left aortic arch and a left ductus arteriosus, with deviation of the descending aorta.

Pathology. A double aortic arch is caused by failure of regression of either fourth arch. The posterior arch is the larger of the two. There are no symptoms if the space within the arch is adequate, but inadequate space results in compression of the trachea and esophagus. A right aortic arch in itself causes no symptoms, but when it is associated with a left ligamentum arteriosum or patent ductus arteriosus, it forms a vascular ring and causes symptoms identical to those of double aortic arch. Anomalous subclavian artery, also known as atresia lusoria, is the most common of the vascular anomalies. The right aortic arch is atretic, and the right subclavian artery arises as the fourth branch from the aorta. It passes upward and to the right of its normal position and lies either behind the esophagus or between it and the trachea. Very rarely does it pass in front of the trachea. It usually causes no symptoms, but in some infants it may compress the trachea or esophagus enough to produce respiratory symptoms or dysphagia. If there is an aberrant left subclavian artery arising as the fourth vessel from a right aortic arch, it passes upward and to the left.

Symptoms. Double aortic arch and right aortic arch with left ligamentum arteriosum cause the same symptoms. Tracheal compression is more severe than is esophageal compression. There is wheezing or stridor initiated or aggravated by feeding. Characteristically, hyperextension of the neck relieves the obstruction and flexion makes it worse. Recurrent pulmonary infections follow repeated aspiration. In most of these infants, symptoms appear before the fifth month, and in many they are present from birth.

Infants with an anomalous subclavian artery have esophageal difficulties. They hesitate in swallowing, take only small feedings, and show a preference for either liquid or solid foods.

Anomalous innominate, left carotid, and left pulmonary arteries produce obstructive respiratory, but not esophageal, symptoms.

Diagnosis. Vascular ring is a major consideration in the differential diagnosis of wheezing and dysphagia. Floppy epiglottis can be ruled out if symptoms are relieved when the infant is placed in the prone position. Visualization of the epiglottis confirms the diagnosis. Laryngeal stridor and laryngomalacia are ruled out by laryngoscopy.

Barium study of the esophagus demonstrates the indentations characteristic of each anomaly, usually at the level of the third or fourth thoracic vertebra. Posteroanterior and lateral films allow visualization of the trachea. Complete vascular rings cause an indentation of the anterior trachea above the carina and are best seen on lateral films. Barium swallow shows the posterior arch as an indentation of the dorsal margin of the esophagus at the same level or higher (Fig. 11–2). An aberrant left or right subclavian artery produces oblique pressure defects. An oval density between the trachea and the esophagus with anterior indentation of the esophagus suggests an aberrant left pulmonary artery.

In most of these vascular anomalies, angiography defines best the exact anatomy of the great vessels. Bronchoscopy permits determination of the degree of narrowing of the trachea above the carina but is hardly worth the discomfort it causes.

Treatment. The decision for surgery is based upon the severity of the clinical picture rather than upon the demonstration of the anomaly. Frequent pulmonary infections and severe feeding difficulties are the major indications for surgery. If symptoms are mild, surgery should be postponed until the infant is larger. This is particularly true for the infant with aortic ring, because the operative mortality is substantial. Surgery is followed by a high incidence of respiratory difficulty owing to persistence of the tracheal indentation; hence, elective tracheostomy at the time of correction is judicious.

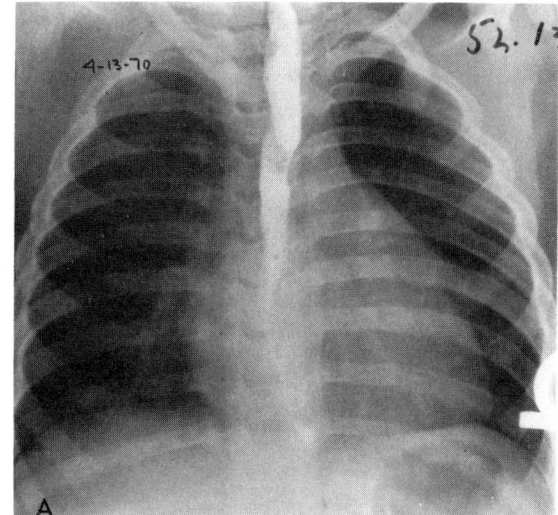

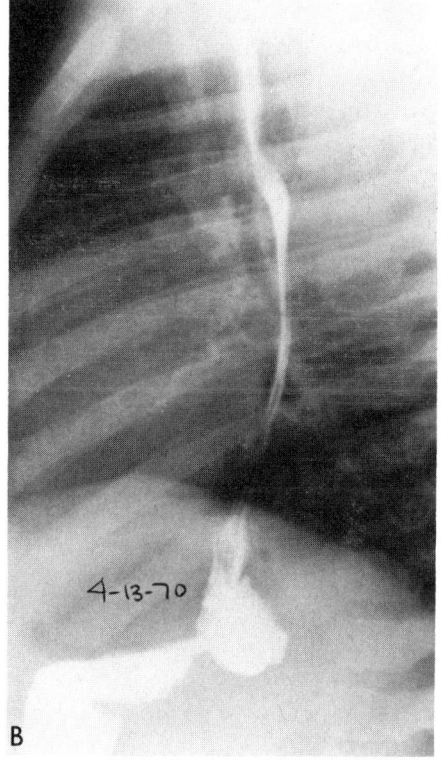

Figure 11–2 Three-year-old girl in whom a barium swallow cardiac series was taken because of a heart murmur. She was asymptomatic, but the findings are typical for aberrant right subclavian artery with left aortic arch, an incomplete vascular ring. *A*, Normal chest except for oblique defect across the esophagus at the level of the third and fourth thoracic vertebrae. The aortic arch is in normal position. *B*, There is a posterior impression on the esophagus without tracheal narrowing.

Prognosis. Surgical correction is generally curative except for the respiratory problems that may follow correction of the aortic ring.

CONGENITAL DIVERTICULUM OF THE ESOPHAGUS

This very rare anomaly is often asymptomatic for years until it is complicated by lodgment of a foreign body or development of an inflammatory process.[178] On the other hand, if it compresses the trachea or is associated with esophageal stenosis or fistula, as it is at times, symptoms are present at birth.

Pathology. This diverticulum arises from the upper third of the esophagus in the posterior midline just above the cricopharyngeal junction.[38] The neck of the diverticulum is either wide or narrow, and the sac, lined by squamous epithelium, contains all layers of the esophageal wall. If it attains a large enough size, it compresses both the esophagus and the trachea. A diverticulum has been associated with pyloric atresia.[103]

Symptoms. In infants with a large diverticulum, severe choking and regurgitation during the first feeding may resemble the signs of tracheoesophageal fistula. A smaller diverticulum can cause stridor, progressive dysphagia, and recurrent respiratory infections.

Diagnosis. On radiographic examination of the esophagus, with use of opaque material, a large diverticulum is seen arising from the upper esophagus.

Treatment. Removal of the diverticulum and closure of the esophagus should be done as soon as the diagnosis is established. Delay in the infant with symptoms only prolongs the period of feeding difficulty and increases the hazards of regurgitation and aspiration.

LARYNGOTRACHEOESOPHAGEAL CLEFT

This is an extremely rare and often fatal anomaly. As in other esophageal anomalies, there is an association with prematurity and maternal hydramnios. Some clefts are complicated further by tracheoesophageal fistula.

Etiology. Two processes are involved in the development of this anomaly: formation of the tracheoesophageal septum and dorsal closure of the cricoid cartilage.[23, 45, 70] The tracheoesophageal septum develops at the time the lung buds begin to grow from the lower end of the laryngotracheal groove. It grows in a caudocephalad direction and is complete to the level of the larynx at 33 gestational days. The cricoid cartilage is developed from the fifth or sixth branchial arch as two lateral centers of cartilage that fuse, first ventrally and then dorsally, during the third month of gestation. During this period the larynx has differentiated. Arrest in the advancement of the tracheoesophageal septum is followed by failure of dorsal

fusion of the cricoid cartilages and, thus, creation of the defect.

Pathology. There is no dorsal fusion of the cricoid cartilages, and the cleft extends down into the tracheoesophageal septum to the first few tracheal rings. The epiglottis fails to close over the glottis and appears shortened and rigid. Both these factors lead to aspiration, and malalignment of the arytenoids causes aberrations in phonation.

Symptoms. The symptoms are identical to those caused by tracheoesophageal fistula with esophageal atresia, type B — that is, with proximal fistula. Cyanosis is present at birth or develops with feeding. Excessive mucus accumulates in the oropharynx, with resultant choking, stridor, regurgitation during and after feedings, and bouts of apnea. The cry is feeble or hoarse. These infants often are subjected to repeated examinations for tracheosophageal fistula, but none is demonstrated. Tracheotomy is sometimes performed because of aspiration, and ingestion of formula or solids is followed by extrusion of these substances through the tracheostomy. Recurrent pneumonia and failure to gain weight and grow become apparent during the first month of life.

Routine examination of the oropharynx shows an epiglottis that is short and firm and does not fold over the glottis during respiration.

Diagnosis. Digital examination of the pharyngeal region provides a tentative diagnosis, for an examining finger passed into the throat moves freely between the trachea and the esophagus if the cleft is large. This procedure is of the utmost importance in any infant with the combined symptoms of choking and a hoarse, feeble cry. Endoscopy will demonstrate the lesion in most cases.

The defect is often overlooked in careful radiologic examinations, for the cricoid laminae tend to approximate one another and form a temporary closure of the defect. The chest film shows the tip of an endotracheal tube in the esophagus. Aspiration of barium during swallowing is often misinterpreted as spillage into the larynx due to neuromuscular incoordination, high tracheoesophageal fistula, or an H-type fistula. The esopha-

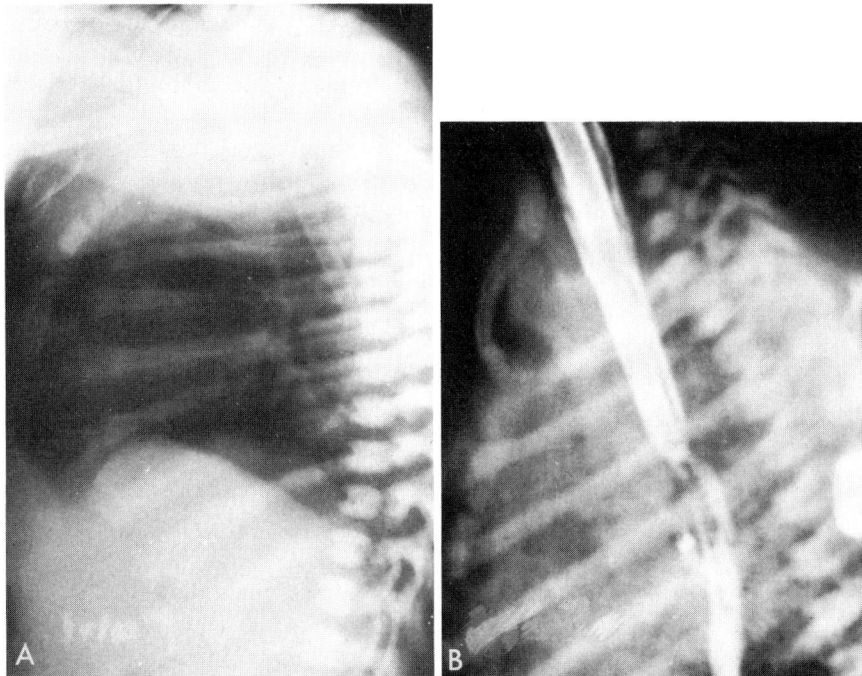

Figure 11–3 Neonate with tracheal agenesis and common tracheoesophageal canal. The infant died during the first hours of life. *A*, Lateral chest film. Despite the obvious malposition of the endotracheal tube, the infant's respiratory status was improved with the tube. *B*, Contrast study through the nasogastric tube outlines the tracheoesophagus. The anterior contrast material is at the junction of the mainstem bronchi, which communicate with the tracheoesophageal canal.

gus fills with air and empties in sequence with respiration. Extensive defects resemble a common tracheoesophagus, from which the main stem bronchi arise (Fig. 11–3).

Treatment. Satisfactory treatment consists of closure of the cleft. One patient we have followed for 17 years after repair has had no difficulties with phonation and has remained free of pneumonitis.

TRACHEOESOPHAGEAL FISTULA AND ESOPHAGEAL ATRESIA

These congenital anomalies are among the most serious surgical emergencies of the newborn period. The gravity of the situation is enhanced by the association of prematurity and other serious congenital anomalies.[67, 68, 139]

Incidence.[9] The reported incidence of these defects varies from 1 in 1000 to 1 in 4500 births. The figure most often cited is 1 in 3000 live births. A familial incidence is rare, but these anomalies have appeared in siblings. There is a history of maternal hydramnios in 16 per cent of such infants; seven cases of atresia and fistula in twins and two instances in parent and sibling have been reported.[77]

Embryology. During the fourth embryonic week, the trachea and bronchi develop from a bud of the foregut. Imperfect septal development between the trachea and the esophagus is considered the causative factor in tracheoesophageal fistula. In nearly all cases, the point of origin of the trachea is the region where the distal fistula occurs. The cause of atresia is not as well explained, although persistence of the obliterative stage of the esophageal lumen can result in abnormal septation of the foregut.[65] Some studies indicate that vascular anomalies at the level of the atretic area might be causative.[80] A reduced blood supply to the lower segment of the esophagus has been demonstrated in infants who died of esophageal atresia. Other investigators speculate that localized pressure on the developing esophagus by vascular anomalies or failure of complete closure of the laryngotracheal groove is a factor in causing atresia. Tracheomalacia, causing airway difficulty, has been associated with atresia and distal fistula.[36]

Foci of gastric epithelium are present in 34 per cent of upper esophageal pouches in infants with esophageal atresia,[42] as compared with 2.5 per cent in those with a normal esophagus. This finding places the development of the anomaly at a time before elongation of the esophagus takes place. Lipase activity is present in both the esophageal pouch and stomach, representing lingual and gastric lipases.[124a]

Pathology. The anomalies have been assigned types by the Surgical Section of the American Academy of Pediatrics: Type A (7.7 per cent of cases) is esophageal atresia without fistula; type B (0.8 per cent) is esophageal atresia with the tracheoesophageal fistula to the proximal segment; type C (86.5 per cent) is esophageal atresia with fistula to the distal segment (consistently, in all series, the most common form)[65b]; type D (0.7 per cent) is esophageal atresia with fistulas to both segments[47]; and type E (4.2 per cent) is tracheoesophageal fistula without atresia (Fig. 11–4). In 1978, 94 cases of atresia with double fistula were reported, and it was suggested the incidence of this type may be increasing to 5.3 per cent. Affected infants are larger and have fewer anomalies than other groups. Associated abnormalities have been reported in 52 per cent of infants with esophageal atresia, and 43 per cent of deaths were attributed to these anomalies. In more than 1000 patients reviewed by that group, congenital heart disease was present in 17 per cent, imperforate anus in 8 per cent, genitourinary anomalies in 10 per cent, and intestinal atresia in 3 per cent.[116] More than half the infants with associated cardiac anomalies weighed less than 2500 gm at birth.

A coincident congenital stricture distal to the site of the atresia is rare, with an incidence of 3 in 1000 cases of fistula or atresia. The stricture is at the junction of the middle and lower thirds of the esophagus. Several infants have also had foregut cysts.

When esophageal and duodenal atresia coexist, the type C lesion is the most common, and there is a wide variety of associated anomalies.[140a]

Symptoms. Infants with esophageal atresia swallow normally, but the secretions fill the esophageal sac and overflow into the oropharynx. Prior to feeding, one notes only excessive quantities of mucus in the mouth. If there is a distal fistula, crying forces air through it and into the stomach. Progressive distention of the abdomen leads to respiratory distress. Some of the air and gastric contents are forced back up the esophagus, through the fistula, and into the trachea, resulting in chemical pneumonitis. Upper esophageal contents also overflow into the trachea, causing atelectasis or bacterial pneumonia or both. In infants with a proximal fistula, saliva enters the airway directly and produces a more serious bacterial pneumonitis. In those with fistula but without atresia there is some airway contamination by oral contents, but regurgitated liquids seldom traverse the fistula (although air does); hence chemical pneumonitis is infrequent. A scaphoid abdomen indicates that there is no fistula or that it is proximal.

At birth the affected infant appears normal. Respiratory problems develop early, as there is difficulty in handling secretions. Pharyngeal suction is effective in removing the mucus and the infant seems well for a time, until he again becomes cyanotic, chokes, and has labored respirations. The first feeding suggests the diagnosis because the respiratory difficulties are aggravated and the food is regurgitated. Rales and rhonchi are present throughout the chest, and atelectasis becomes apparent. The infant must be given no further feedings until a diagnosis is established. The triad of excess mucus in the oropharynx, regurgitation of food, and respiratory distress indicates esophageal atresia until proved otherwise.

Diagnosis. A number 10 or 12 F-size catheter is passed through the nose. If it reaches the stomach, as determined by an acid pH of the aspirate, atresia is not present. If it meets an obstruction 10 to 13 cm distal to the nares, the diagnosis is nearly

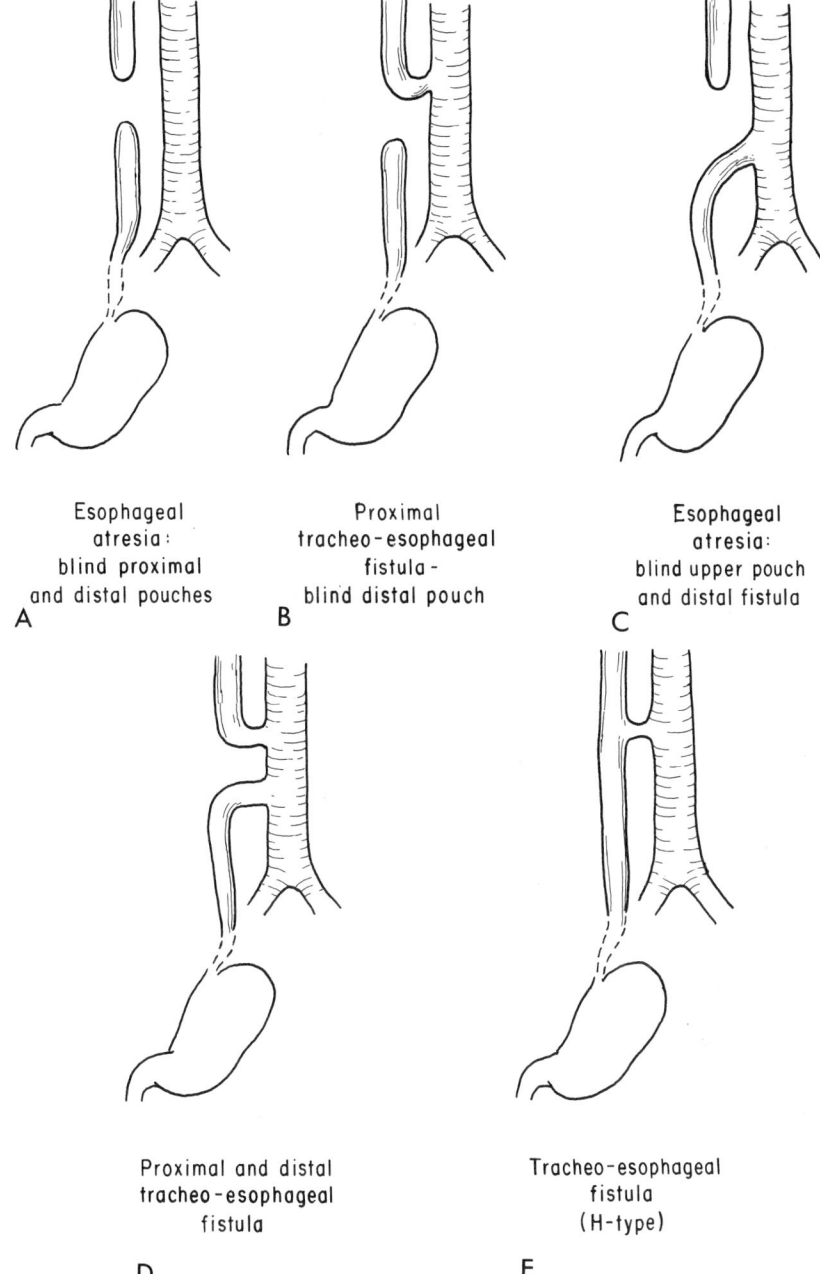

Esophageal
atresia:
blind proximal
and distal pouches
A

Proximal
tracheo-esophageal
fistula-
blind distal pouch
B

Esophageal
atresia:
blind upper pouch
and distal fistula
C

Proximal and distal
tracheo-esophageal
fistula
D

Tracheo-esophageal
fistula
(H-type)
E

Figure 11-4 Diagrammatic representation of the types of tracheal atresia and tracheoesophageal fistulas.

assured. A plain chest film demonstrates the position of the catheter and may show a dilated upper esophageal pouch that is filled with air (Figs. 11–5 and 11–6). Ventilation with 100 per cent oxygen will show increased gastric oxygen to 50 per cent or greater in infants with H-type fistula.[113] The presence of gas in the bowel indicates a

distal fistula; its absence, a proximal fistula or atresia without fistula. If there is any question about the nature of the esophageal obstruction or the presence of a fistula from the proximal pouch, a small amount of contrast material (usually less than 1 ml) is instilled under fluoroscopic control and removed through the tube after films have

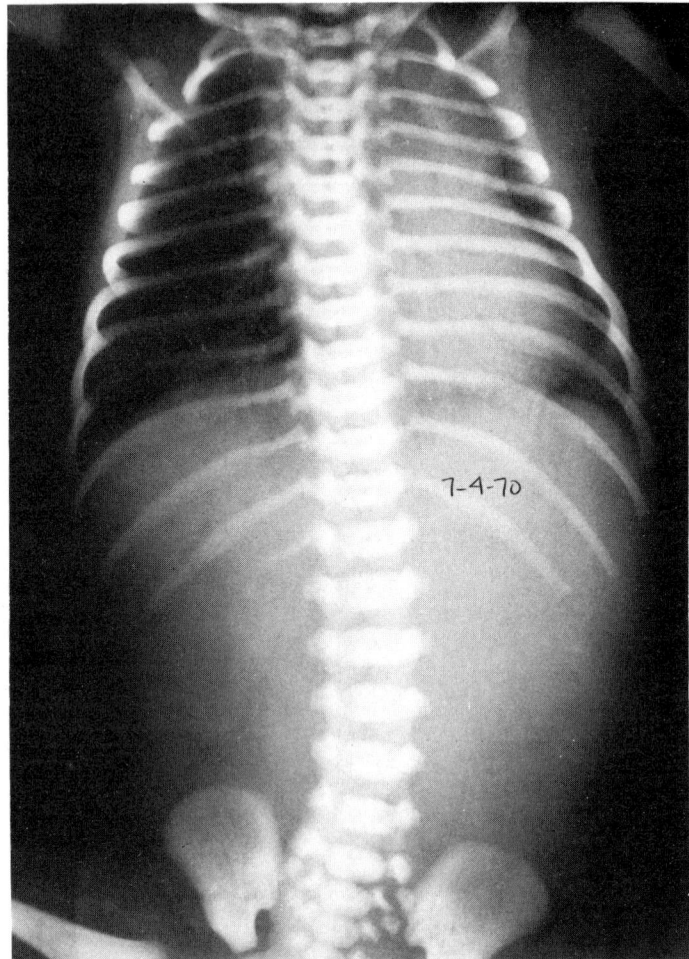

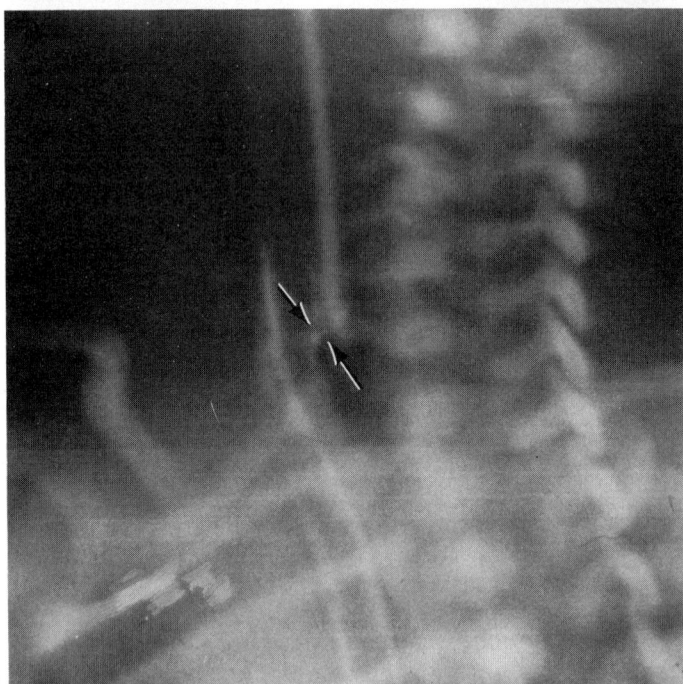

Figure 11–5 A, Atresia without fistula. Frontal film of chest and abdomen of a two-day-old infant, studied because of aspiration of feedings. Gas is absent from the stomach and intestine. *B,* Subsequent contrast study of the esophagus showed a blind upper pouch (arrows). The combination of such a clinical history and the absence of gas within the gastrointestinal tract in an otherwise vigorous, strong infant strongly suggests the diagnosis of esophageal atresia without distal tracheo-esophageal fistula.

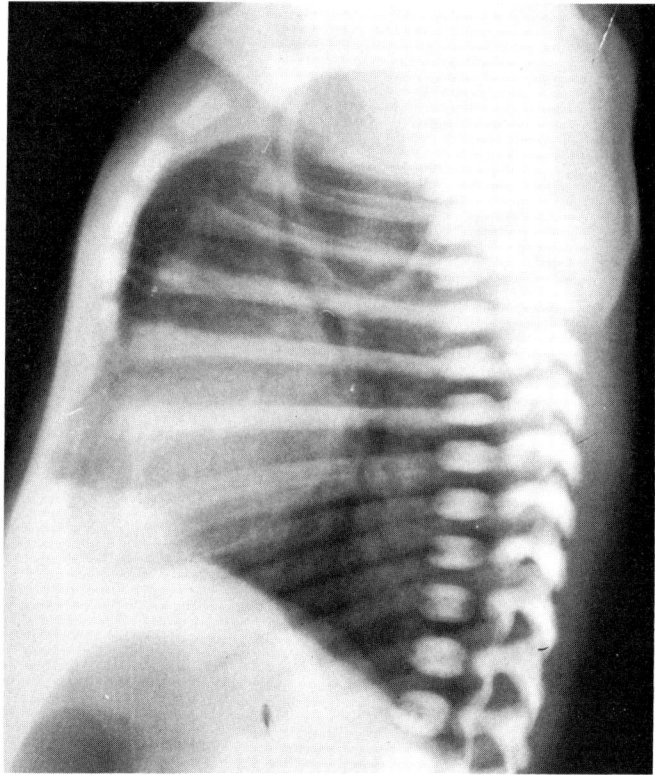

Figure 11–6 Atresia with distal fistula. Neonate with difficulty in handling secretions. The mother had polyhydramnios. The proximal esophageal pouch is markedly distended by air and compresses the trachea. Air within the stomach indicates a distal fistula.

been obtained. An oily contrast agent seems preferable, although barium mixtures are relatively nonirritating to the tracheobronchial tree. Water-soluble agents may be quite irritating and should not be used.

Treatment. Adequate preoperative management is imperative and must be aimed at controlling the pneumonitis[55] and attaining good nutritional status. Pneumonia is the cause of death in up to 75 per cent of infants with tracheoesophageal fistula; in such cases the normal cilitated tracheal and bronchial epithelium is replaced in whole or in part by squamous epithelium.[114] A debris-consolidation type of pneumonia has been reported in a number of mature infants with this anomaly.[115] The infant should be kept in an Isolette and given oxygen as needed. If the infant has a distal fistula, he should be maintained in a semi-Fowler position. Continuous suction of the proximal pouch is indicated, as is decompression gastrostomy to prevent reflux and to provide a pre- and postoperative portal for nourishment. Administration of antibiotics, usually penicillin and kanamycin, is started immediately, and the drug regimen is subsequently altered according to the culture reports. Intravenous fluids are given as required. Attaining the optimal conditions for surgery may take as little as 12 hours or as long as two weeks. Surgical correction should not be attempted until respiratory distress from pneumonitis or the respiratory distress syndrome has subsided.[67a]

Operative Treatment. The surgical treatment depends upon the size and condition of the infant.[13, 108a] The full-term infant weighing more than 2 kg without other anomalies or respiratory distress (type A) is a candidate for single-stage correction of the fistula and atresia. If pneumonia, respiratory distress, small size, or treatable anomalies (type B) are present, a gastrostomy should be performed and the primary repair delayed until the pneumonitis or respiratory distress syndrome has resolved. Those infants with severe cardiac disease may require deferment of surgery for four to eight weeks. End-to-end anastomosis with division of the fistula is a standard procedure but one that is followed by a high incidence

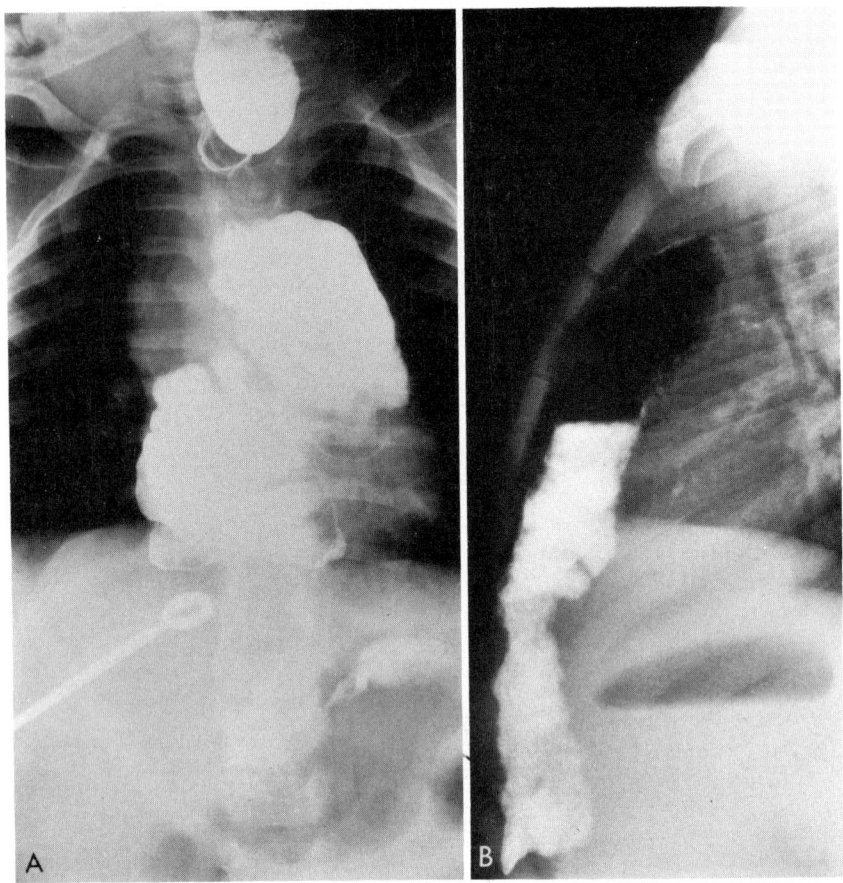

Figure 11-7 Surgical colon interposition done in a 14-month-old boy because of esophageal atresia with an atretic segment too long to allow primary anastomosis. Radiologic examination was performed several months after surgery because of symptoms of partial obstruction. *A*, Frontal projection shows the somewhat tortuous colon in the mid- and lower portions of the mediastinum. The dilated structure noted superiorly is the pre-anastomotic cervical esophagus. *B*, Lateral view with patient erect shows an air-fluid level in the mediastinal colon and poor drainage of barium into the stomach.

of postoperative stricture (up to 25 per cent) and longer duration before feeding (10.6 days). End-to-side anastomosis has a low incidence of stricture (7 to 9 per cent), and infants may feed two to three days after operation. Mortality rates for both techniques are similar.[111, 149]

If the infant is premature or is a poor candidate for surgery, a staged correction is appropriate, with gastrostomy and closure of the fistula first, followed in one to two months by esophageal anastomosis. The staged approach has reduced mortality from 61 to 11 per cent.[13] In these patients the length of the atresia can be evaluated by instillation of contrast material into the proximal esophageal pouch and the distal esophagus through the gastrostomy. If the

distance between the esophageal ends is too great for anastomosis without tension, a segment of colon is interposed (Fig. 11-7). Recent reports of stretching and elongation of the upper sac by bougienage and magnetic field indicate that this is an effective measure in avoiding tension at the suture line at the time of primary anastomosis.

Complications. An anastomotic leak sometimes develops between the second and seventh postoperative days and is due to incomplete approximation of the two segments, disruption of the suture line, or ischemic necrosis of the esophagus below the level of anastomosis. Contributing factors include tension at the suture line, devascularization, thinness of the esophageal wall, or infection at the suture line. Treatment consists of cervical esophagostomy, closure of the distal esophagus, and chest-tube drainage. Gastrostomy feedings are continued as long as reflux is not present.

Radiologic evidence of stricture is reported in up to 80 per cent of patients after repair of this anomaly. The area of repair normally appears narrowed for the first few weeks; this is attributed to tissue edema. True strictures become apparent at the anastomotic site after three weeks, when dysphagia and increasing pharyngeal secretions develop. The upper esophagus distends and sometimes causes stridor. Transient distention of the preanastomotic segment is seen during radiologic examination, when the infant feeds or cries, and can occur even when the anastomotic site is not narrowed enough to produce any holdup of barium. Depending upon their severity, the strictures are treated by dilation, local steroid injection, resection of the stricture with reanastomosis of the esophagus, or transplantation of colon or jejunum.

Recurrent tracheoesophageal fistula is to be suspected if the recovering infant begins to choke or cough or if he develops pneumonitis. Abdominal distention becomes extreme after crying, for air trapped in the fistula is diverted down the esophagus and into the stomach. This complication follows dilation of the esophagus above a previously unrecognized congenital or secondary stricture. Such fistulas are difficult to detect, but they will not close spontaneously and must be attacked surgically.[27]

Esophageal motility dysfunction occurs up to 19 years after repair. Most studies agree that there is diminished or absent motor activity below the area of repair.[86, 132, 158a] Some have described an aperistaltic spastic segment that responds to swallowing either by feeble, simultaneous, and often repetitive contractions or by no reaction at all. Sphincter function has been reported, however, as normal or reduced-pressure. Lind et al.[86] reported failure of the sphincter to relax with swallowing and described feeble contractions of the entire esophagus in response to swallowing. They suggested that this response is similar to the esophageal response to achalasia but that the sphincter

is unresponsive to bethanechol. Radiologic examinations show that the primary wave dissipates above the line of anastomosis, with antegrade and retrograde flow, or the "yo-yo" phenomenon, below. The cause of this motility disorder is not clear. Transection and resuturing of the esophagus are not followed by motor dysfunction. Destruction of esophageal branches of the vagus nerve, however, produces an aperistaltic segment without involvement of the inferior sphincter. This may be a congenital defect, or perhaps an iatrogenic one following mobilization of the atretic esophageal sac. Newer techniques of surgical anastomoses reduce the incidence of postoperative stricture and motor abnormalities.[57]

Hiatus hernia develops in a number of infants after repair of esophageal atresia. It is not certain whether this is an associated congenital defect or one that arises secondary to shortening of the esophagus from surgical manipulation.[109] Peptic esophagitis can result, and half of the patients require an antireflux procedure or treatment with cimetidine.[12a]

Recurrent pneumonitis and failure to thrive are seen in some infants late in the postoperative course. These conditions, which have been ascribed to sensitization to milk protein caused by repeated early aspiration of milk feedings, may represent a type of Heiner's syndrome, since milk precipitins are present in the serum.[59] Elimination of milk and milk products from the diet is often followed by an increase in growth rate and improvement or cure of pneumonitis.

Prognosis. A risk classification has been developed according to weight and presence or absence of pneumonia and congenital anomalies. Group A infants, that is, those weighing more than 2500 gm at birth and without pneumonia or anomalies, have a survival rate of 100 per cent. Group B infants, those of 1800 to 2500 gm birth weight and in good health, or full-term infants with moderately severe pulmonary disease or a non–life-threatening anomaly, have a survival rate of 57 to 65 per cent. Group C, the small, sick infants with associated severe anomalies, have a survival rate of only 6 per cent. A retropleural repair approach has decreased the overall mortality from 38 to 11 per cent. Survival in those with duodenal atresia approximates 33 per cent.

ESOPHAGEAL ATRESIA WITHOUT FISTULA

The symptoms of this lesion are similar to those of tracheoesophageal fistula, but there are fewer pulmonary problems.[82] Because there is no tracheal communication, there is no air in the stomach or in the lower gastrointestinal tract. The diagnosis is made as described previously for other types of esophageal atresia. Treatment entails cervical esophagostomy with feeding gastrostomy until the infant attains a large enough size (10 kg) for a definite anastomosis or, if necessary, a colon interposition. Small oral feedings should be offered so that the infant learns to suck and swallow.

TRACHEOESOPHAGEAL FISTULA WITHOUT ESOPHAGEAL ATRESIA

This anomaly, termed the H-type fistula, is rare and accounts for about 4.2 per cent of upper esophageal anomalies.[87] It occurs anywhere between the larynx and the carina, but its level is usually higher than that of fistula and atresia. Most fistulas are single, but three fistulas have been described in one patient. Esophagopulmonary fistula may occur.[22]

Symptoms. Choking and coughing follow the ingestion of fluids from the time of the first feeding. Cyanosis appears during feeding. The infant has less difficulty with thickened feedings, but there are recurrent bouts of pneumonitis, failure to gain weight, and even weight loss. Gastric distention is apparent after crying or coughing. Symptoms disappear during periods of gavage feeding but recur as soon as oral feedings are resumed.

Diagnosis. There is usually a delay in making the diagnosis because the fistula is often thread-like and difficult to visualize. Repeated esophagograms or cineradio-

graphic studies may be necessary, and image intensification should be used. Aspiration into the tracheobronchial tree is seen, but the fine fistulous tract is not always apparent. These fistulas are oblique, with the tracheal end situated higher than the esophageal end, so that contrast studies visualize the fistula only when the infant is in the prone or oblique position (Fig. 11–8). Satisfactory filling of the esophagus requires instillation of contrast material directly into the cervical esophagus through a nasogastric tube while spot films are made. The study is begun with oily contrast material; if no filling of the trachea is seen, it is our practice to switch to barium, which is less viscous and shows better detail. After the tube study, a cine-esophagogram is made while the infant drinks barium through a nipple until the esophagus and stomach are distended with barium. This allows exclusion of oropharyngeal swallowing dysfunction as the basis for aspiration and may, by showing abnormal esophageal motility, provide a clue to the presence of a fistula.

Treatment. Lesions at or above the level of the second thoracic vertebra are approached through the neck; those below that level are repaired through the thorax. After division of the fistula and closure of the esophagus and trachea, a flap of mediastinal tissue or pleura is interposed between the two organs.

CONGENITAL ESOPHAGEAL STENOSIS AND ESOPHAGEAL WEB

Both esophageal stenosis and esophageal web are forms of incomplete esophageal obstruction; they have common symptoms and derivation and are therefore discussed together.

Etiology. The defects are due to an error of maturation of the primitive foregut. There is resorption failure and faulty recanalization after the stages of proliferation and vacuolization. As with fistulas, in many cases the defect is located at the site of origin of the tracheal bud from the foregut.

Pathology. Congenital esophageal webs are mucosal lesions that form an incomplete

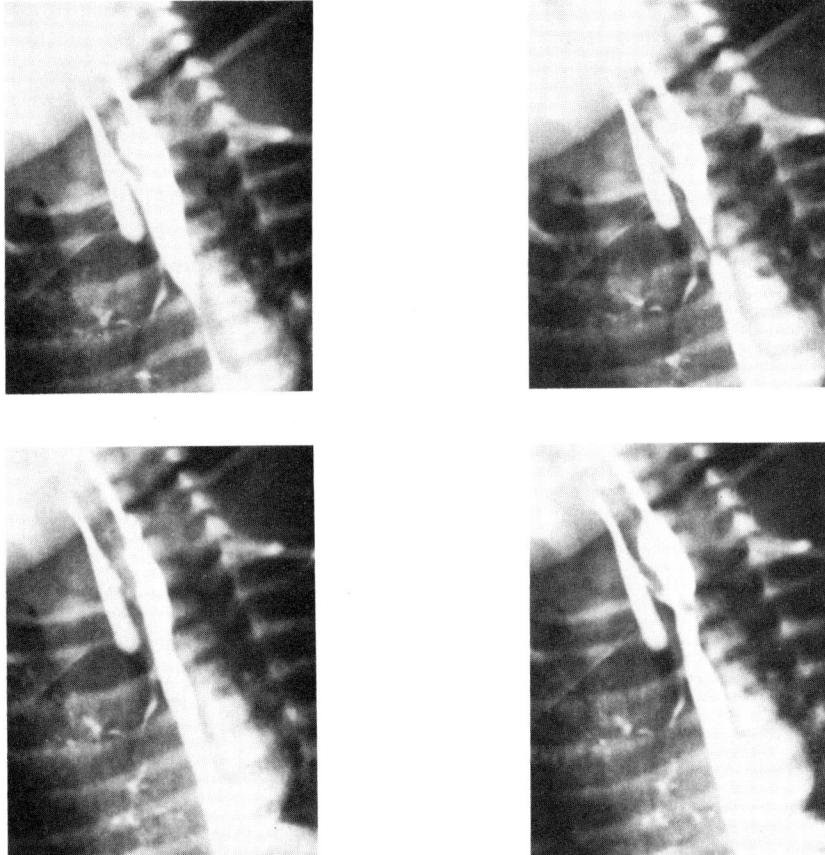

Figure 11–8 H-type fistula in a one-week-old infant with patchy pneumonic infiltrates, respiratory distress while feeding, and breath sounds audible over the stomach. A series of spot films taken during contrast examination of the esophagus demonstrates filling of the tracheoesophageal fistula and oily contrast material in the tracheobronchial tree.

mucosal diaphragm. The web is composed solely of squamous epithelium and does not include muscularis, and it is located in the cervical esophagus or at the junction of the lower and middle thirds. Stenoses are generally found between the middle and lower thirds of the esophagus, but some occur in the lower third. Only rarely are they found in the region of the cardia.

Symptoms. The symptoms vary with the position of the lesion. Infants with a cervical web have feeding difficulties during the first few days of life. Attempts to swallow are accompanied by choking. Symptoms of esophageal stenosis, on the other hand, do not become apparent until the second or third week of life, when vomiting begins, occurring during or at the end of feeding and increasing in frequency and amount until finally none of the food is retained. As

obstruction increases and the proximal esophagus becomes distended during feeding, pain causes the infant to arch his back, struggle, turn red, and cry. Arching and irritability can be so marked that the condition is mistaken for a neurologic disorder. After vomiting or regurgitation of esophageal content, the infant is comfortable and anxious to feed.

Rarely, the web or stenosis does not become apparent until solids are introduced into the diet and a preference for liquids becomes evident. Regurgitation is intermittent, and there are days when the infant is relatively free of symptoms. The regurgitated formula is never curdled or bile-stained. As regurgitation and dysphagia progress, the calorie intake is severely restricted, and failure to gain weight or actual weight loss is noted. Blood-streaking of the vomitus heralds the development of esophageal ulceration, and hematemesis indicates the more serious complication of esophageal tear or rupture.

Very rarely, impaction of solid food is the first sign of difficulty. We have seen impaction of a foreign body cause ulceration of the esophagus, tracheal compression, and death.

Diagnosis. Radiologic examination of the esophagus shows stenosis as a smooth, abrupt tapering (Fig. 11–9). The barium either trickles through the narrowed area or is propelled through in spurts. The esophagus below the area of stenosis is normal in caliber, but it is usually dilated above. It is not always possible to distinguish congenital stenosis from stricture caused by peptic esophagitis. Esophageal web is more difficult to delineate and is often visualized only in lateral views. There is a discrete narrowing that does not change caliber when the esophagus distends above and below it. During a barium swallow examination, it appears as a radiolucent intraluminal shelf or band only several millimeters in width (Fig. 11–10). More subtle degrees of narrowing require cinefluoroscopy in multiple projections to obtain satisfactory filling and delineation of the web.

Treatment. The treatment of choice is esophagoscopy and direct bougienage, for it accomplishes either fracture of the web or dilatation of the stenotic area. If it is unsuccessful, surgical excision of the web or retrograde dilatation of the stenosis through a gastrostomy is necessary. Retrograde dilatations will provide enough relief of a stenosis so that bougienage from above can be performed. One cannot overlook the fact that bougienage and dilatation are potentially hazardous procedures, and utmost care must be taken to avoid perforation.

Prognosis. The prognosis for both lesions is excellent if the original correction is satisfactory. Restricture of esophageal stenosis is not likely, and webs do not recur.

Case History. M.R. was a 45-day-old white male infant admitted because of difficult feeding, characterized by poor suck and irritability. He fed slowly and regurgitated frequently during the first week of life; thereafter he refused to suck. If urged with the nipple, he sucked feebly, turned red, arched his back, and screamed. The temperature and blood pressure were normal, the tongue was papillate, and he had a normal reaction to intradermal histamine. Neurologic examination showed hyperactive reflexes and increased muscle tonus. The cine-esophagogram showed narrowing of a 2 to 3 cm area at the cardioesophageal junction. The barium bolus hung above the region and trickled through in a

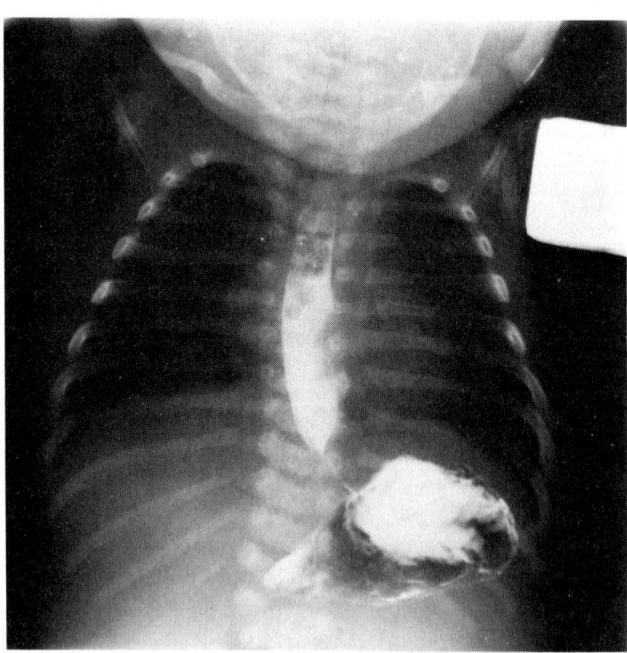

Figure 11–9 Esophageal stenosis in a six-week-old infant admitted for evaluation of vomiting and irritability with feeding. There is a delay of transit of barium from the stenotic area in the distal third of the esophagus and moderate dilation of the proximal esophagus.

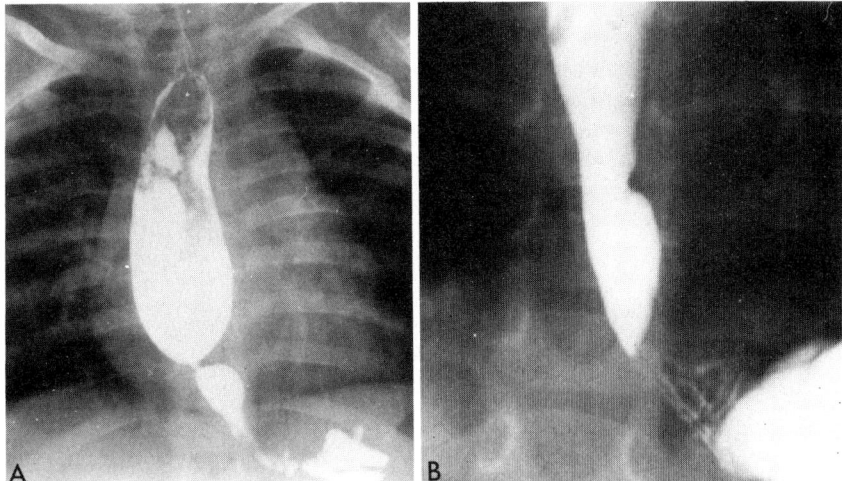

Figure 11–10 Esophageal web in a nine-month-old boy with a history of spitting since early infancy. *A*, Discrete narrowing in distal esophagus. The dilated proximal esophagus contains retained food and secretions as as well as barium. *B*, Films taken nine months and several dilatations later: Barium study shows minimal residual narrowing.

thin stream (see Fig. 11 –9). The esophagus above was dilated. Esophageal motility studies showed normal peristalsis in the body of the esophagus and a resting pressure in the region of the inferior sphincter of 15 mm Hg, two and one-half to three times normal for the age. Esophagoscopy was performed, and at bougienage a tight, narrowed area was encountered. The mucosa was normal. After dilatation with an 18F bougie and within 24 hours, he tolerated small amounts of formula. Within 48 hours he took regular feedings. At the time of five-year follow-up, he had remained free of dysphagia.

CONGENITAL DIAPHRAGMATIC HERNIAS

Congenital diaphragmatic hernias represent extrusion of abdominal contents through the diaphragm into the thoracic cavity. Stomach, liver, pancreas, kidney, and spleen are the organs most often herniated.[127, 140] Mortality is most directly related to hypoplastic lung tissue and is greatest in infants with bilateral hypoplasia.[4, 62]

INCIDENCE

These hernias occur in about 1 in 6000 live births and account for 5 in 10,000 admissions to children's hospitals. The most common type is posterolateral through the foramen of Bochdalek (83 per cent), and next is hiatus hernia (16 per cent). Retrosternal foramen of Morgagni defects account for most of the remaining 1 per cent. The perinatal mortality from these lesions is 1 in 2200 to 1 in 3500 live births.

Hernia of Bochdalek

These hernias present through a posterolateral defect of the diaphragm, in which there is no posterior diaphragmatic rim. The majority (85 to 90 per cent) are on the left side and occur in males. Despite advances in medical care, the overall mortality remains between 30 and 50 per cent.

Etiology.   The anomaly is caused either by defective closure of the pleuroperitoneal folds between the eighth and ninth weeks of gestation or by the early return of the abdominal viscera into the abdominal cavity. Diaphragm formation is completed by the ninth to tenth week of fetal life, the same period in which the gastrointestinal tract undergoes rotation. Since rotation is not completed until the twelfth week, viscera that herniate into the thorax remain malrotated.

Physiology.   Immaturity or hypoplasia of the lungs is a well-documented associated phenomenon, and pulmonary complications are the most common cause of death. Normal lung development with bronchial branching begins at four weeks and is completed by sixteen weeks; later development involves primarily alveolar growth. Lung buds therefore are in the early stages of development at the time of visceral herniation, and further maturation is inhibited. Pressure effects upon the developing lungs vary with the size of the hernia, being most severe in infants with the largest defects. The hypoplastic lungs contain fewer pulmonary vessels and increased muscle mass within the arterioles. The potential for lung growth and development remains, and growth continues after birth. These neonates have pulmonary hypertension (pressures from 44 to 88 mm Hg), shunting through the ductus arteriosus, and cardiomegaly.

Pathology. Since most of the hernias contain no sac, they are truly "false" hernias, and there is maldevelopment of all layers of the diaphragm. A sac covers the herniated contents in 10 to 20 per cent of cases and signifies that visceral migration occurred after the peritoneal lining was completed. If muscular elements are present, the defect is termed eventration of the diaphragm.[76] The organs that herniate are small intestine in 88 per cent, liver in 51 per cent, stomach in 60 per cent, colon in 56 per cent, spleen in 54 per cent, pancreas in 24 per cent, and kidney in 12 per cent. Malrotation of the intestine and associated congenital bands occur in 30 to 58 per cent of cases. Other associated anomalies are Meckel's diverticulum, omphalocele, patent ductus arteriosus, patent foramen ovale, coarctation of the aorta, and neurologic malformations (Figs. 11–11 and 11–12).

Symptoms. The severity of symptoms varies with the amount of viscera that has herniated into the chest. The onset of symptoms occurs at birth, after several days of life, or later in childhood. In the neonate with a large defect, there is cyanosis with respiratory distress from the time of delivery. After resuscitation, he grunts, gasps, and breathes irregularly. Direct administration of high concentrations of oxygen does little to alleviate the cyanosis. In some, symptoms of the respiratory distress syn-

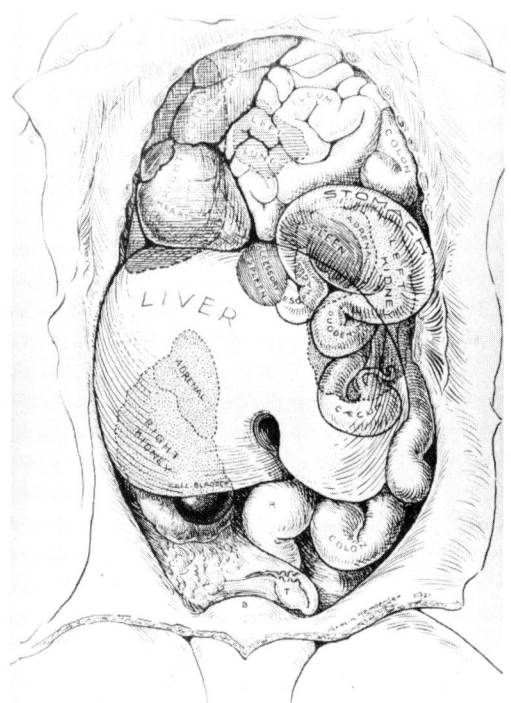

Figure 11–11 Post-mortem drawing of abdominal and thoracic contents of an infant who died of Bochdalek hernia: Stomach, intestine, and spleen are herniated into the left chest, displacing heart and lungs to the right. (Illustration by A. Hemberger, Yale University Art Collection.)

drome — tachypnea and substernal and intercostal retractions — predominate. Feeding attempts are futile, for the infants are too fatigued to suck. Those who develop symptoms before 72 hours are classified as the high-risk group, whereas those whose symptoms appear later and who have only mild respiratory or gastrointestinal complaints are considered to be low-risk patients.

Diagnosis. Breath sounds are diminished or absent over the involved side, and bowel sounds are sometimes heard in the thorax. The combination of flatness over one portion and tympany over another portion of the hemithorax is typical. The mediastinum and heart borders are shifted to the side opposite the lesion. Compression of the lung on the uninvolved side results in the changes of atelectasis: dullness to percussion, fine rales, and, perhaps, bronchial breath sounds. The abdomen is scaphoid. Radiologic examination of the chest shows gas-filled pockets or bowel loops in the

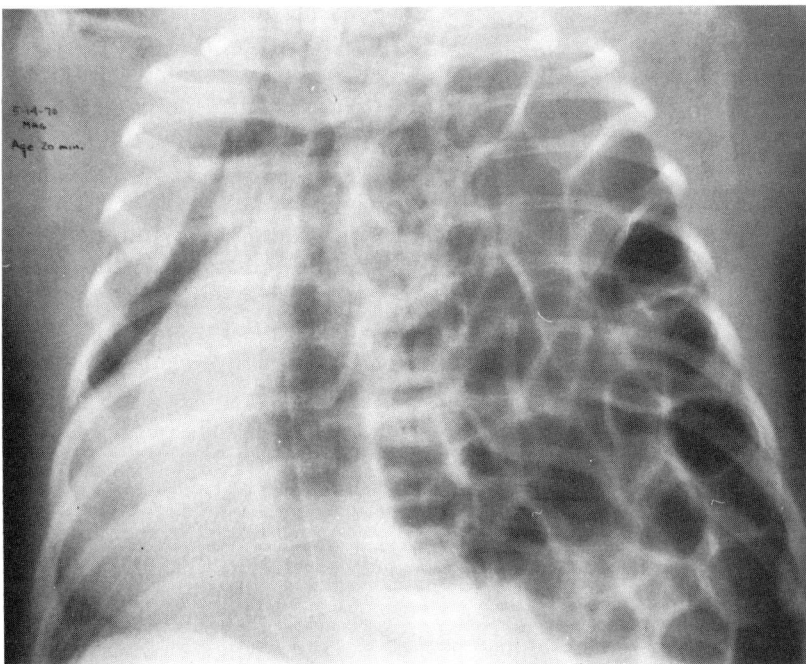

Figure 11–12   Congenital diaphragmatic hernia in a neonate who was cyanotic at birth. Ventilatory assistance aggravated respiratory distress by causing gaseous distention of stomach and small bowel loops in the chest.

thorax. A barium swallow is rarely necessary to define the involved viscera but should be carried out in doubtful cases, especially if the signs are on the right. Such an examination tends to increase respiratory distress because of distention of the intrathoracic stomach or bowel loops.

Treatment.   Delay in treatment of infants in the high-risk group only increases the mortality. Treatment is prompt laparotomy with reduction of the hernia and replacement of the viscera into the abdominal cavity. Exploration for and correction of associated congenital defects is imperative. Recently, cardiac catheterization, performed after surgery, is used as an indicator for pharmacologic therapy. Those with minimal pulmonary hypoplasia need no therapy, and those with bilateral hypoplasia are not benefited. It serves best for those with unilateral hypoplasia.[40a]

Complications.   Pneumothorax is a constant postoperative hazard. Another extremely serious complication stems from overlooking cystic enlargement of the hernia sac at surgery. The resulting symptoms are as severe as those that initiated the surgery. Tapping of the cyst contents is an emergency measure and must be followed by resection of the cyst. The hypoplastic lung does not always expand after repair,[31] and respiratory symptoms may persist for this reason. Persistent pulmonary hypertension is a serious complication.

A "honeymoon period" of improved pulmonary function may occur after surgery but is followed by deterioration and death.[22a] Such instances have been attributed to pulmonary vasospasm. Predictively, if the alveolar-arterial oxygen difference is greater than 500 mm Hg after surgery, the patient will probably die. A pH of less than 7.0 indicates a fatal outcome, whereas one greater than 7.2 is associated with survival.[122a] Measurements of ductal shunting have also been employed to determine the degree of pulmonary hypertension. Pharmacologic support with exogenous vasodilators, such as tolazoline, or endogenous ones, such as prostaglandins, to increase pulmonary circulation is under investigation.

Prognosis.   The mortality in high-risk infants is 50 to 70 per cent; that in the low-risk group is minimal. Operative mortality averages 30 per cent. Respiratory studies performed 6 to 12 years after surgery show normal functional residual capacity, residual volume, and total capacity, but reduced forced expiratory volume.

Parasternal Hernia of Morgagni

This hernia occurs most often on the right side, with herniation of the abdominal viscera through a triangular space bounded by fibers extending from the diaphragm to the xiphoid and ribs.[44]

Etiology. As the diaphragm develops between the eighth and tenth weeks of fetal life, the septum transversum forms beneath the heart and grows posteriorly to meet the dorsal mesentery of the foregut to form the central portion of the diaphragm. In this disorder, the retrosternal portion has failed to develop.

Pathology. The omentum and colon are the organs most frequently herniated, owing to their anterior position in the abdomen. The stomach and small intestine are sometimes involved. Associated anomalies are malrotation, congenital heart disease, and pectus carinatum. In several instances the hernia has extended into the pericardial sac.

Symptoms. These hernias, often asymptomatic, are discovered only by routine chest x-ray examination (Fig. 11–13). Some infants vomit intermittently or have repeated respiratory infections.

Diagnosis. The posteroanterior chest film shows a rounded shadow in the cardiophrenic angle and, on the lateral view, a rounded shadow in the anterior mediastinum. A barium enema is more effective in outlining the visceral contents of the hernia than is an upper gastrointestinal examination.

Treatment. Laparotomy and reduction of the hernia contents with repair of the defect are curative.

Hiatus Hernia

Persistent vomiting and failure to thrive are the major symptoms of infants with hiatus hernia.

Incidence. This hernia accounts for 16 to 20 per cent of the congenital diaphragmatic defects. It occurs more often and with greater severity in males than in females. It has been reported in twins, in siblings, and in children of an affected parent. We have

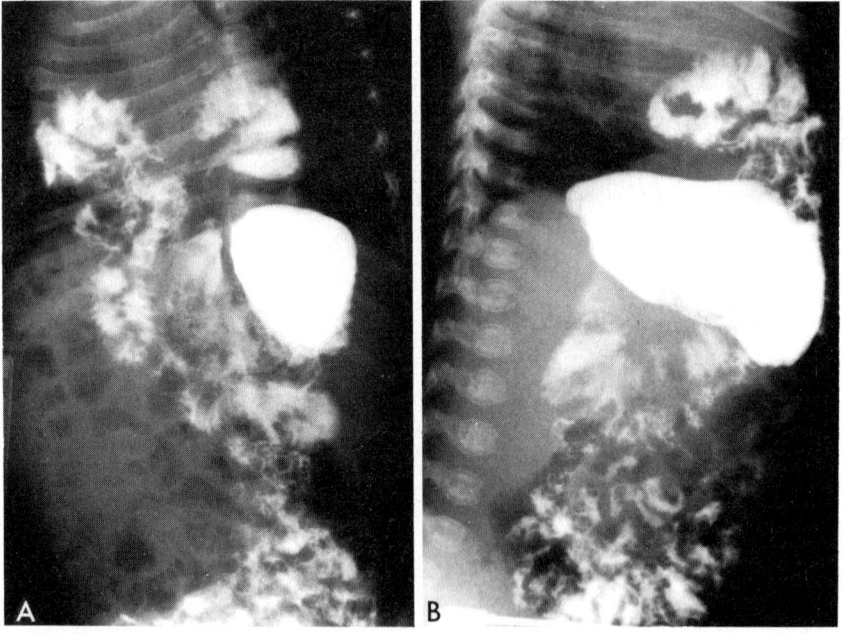

Figure 11–13　Foramen of Morgagni hernia in a male infant with omphalocele. The hernia and omphalocele were repaired, but films taken at three weeks show *(A)* recurrence of hernia in frontal projection with barium-filled duodenum and jejunum projected over the cardiac shadow. The anterior location of the diaphragm is demonstrated *(B)*.

noted these hernias to develop in children with neurologic diseases and scoliosis.

Etiology. Failure of complete elongation of the esophagus as the stomach moves into the abdomen during the fourth to seventh weeks of gestation leaves the esophagus somewhat short and the stomach incompletely descended into the abdomen. Some believe hiatus hernia develops after shortening of the esophagus from peptic esophagitis due to chalasia.[122]

Pathology. The hiatus is abnormally wide, and the muscle sling is often hypoplastic. A true hiatus hernia refers to a pouch of stomach that passes through the normal diaphragmatic hiatus into the chest.[83, 126] It is usually not contained in a peritoneal sac. The protective mechanisms about the inferior esophageal sphincter, such as fixation of the stomach, the muscle sling, and the angle of entry of the esophagus into the cardia, all are altered. The competency of the sphincter, which in the normal neonate is poor, is further impaired, so that it permits reflux of gastric contents into the esophagus. The degree of reflux is not related to the size of the hernia. The symptoms produced are due to peptic esophagitis and not to the hernia itself. Chronic reflux of gastric contents causes ulceration, bleeding fibrosis, stricture formation, and shortening of the esophagus.

Symptoms. Typically, the infant vomits from the time of birth, although in some cases the onset occurs only after several weeks or months. The vomiting takes place after feedings and may be projectile. The vomitus, which contains formula (changed or unchanged) and small quantities of mucus, is acid. The vomiting disappears for days at a time, only to recur. The infants are hungry and feed eagerly. Pain or dysphagia develops only after esophagitis or stricture formation has developed. Bleeding from esophagitis can be mild and go unnoticed until a severe anemia is found. The vomiting of blood-streaked mucus, gross blood, or coffee-ground material indicates severe esophagitis. Chronic pulmonary disease and even bronchiectasis follow repeated aspiration of gastric contents refluxed from the stomach during sleep.

Rumination has been linked with hiatus hernia[64] and in some cases is the only symptom. Such infants are characteristically alert and attentive, gathering what stimulation they may with their eyes and by oral manipulations. They suck and mouth their fingers until a point is reached when they regurgitate, chew, and reswallow the gastric contents.

Sandifer's syndrome consists of torsion spasms of the head and upper extremities associated with hiatus hernia.[58, 96, 150] It is believed that these abnormal postures (Fig. 11–14) are unconscious attempts by the child to reduce his hernia. There is an early history of recurrent or nocturnal vomiting, which subsides as the posturing pattern becomes dominant.

Moncrieff's syndrome includes hiatus hernia, sucrosuria, and mental retardation.[93] The syndrome is controversial, for some studies report small quantities of disaccharides in urine from normal populations and larger quantities in urine from mentally retarded populations. We have noted in our own patients an association with mental retardation and scoliosis.

Problems in pharyngeal swallowing arise in patients with pharyngeal pouch, cricopharyngeal dysfunction, and hiatus hernia.[136]

Pyloric stenosis is present in 3 to 10 per cent of infants with hiatus hernia. Other anomalies are jejunal stenosis, Down's syndrome, congenital heart disease, and the Klippel-Feil syndrome.

Complications. The two most serious complications of hiatus hernia are aspiration pneumonia and peptic esophagitis with stricture formation. The stricture, a localized ring or stenotic area extending half the length of the esophagus, occurred in about half the infants with hiatus hernia in one study. They had vomited from birth, and most had had one or more episodes of bleeding.

Diagnosis. Esophagoscopy will show the body of the esophagus to narrow distally with some friability and ulceration of the esophageal mucosa. As the narrowed area is passed, gastric mucosa is visualized in a saccular area that is above the diaphragm.

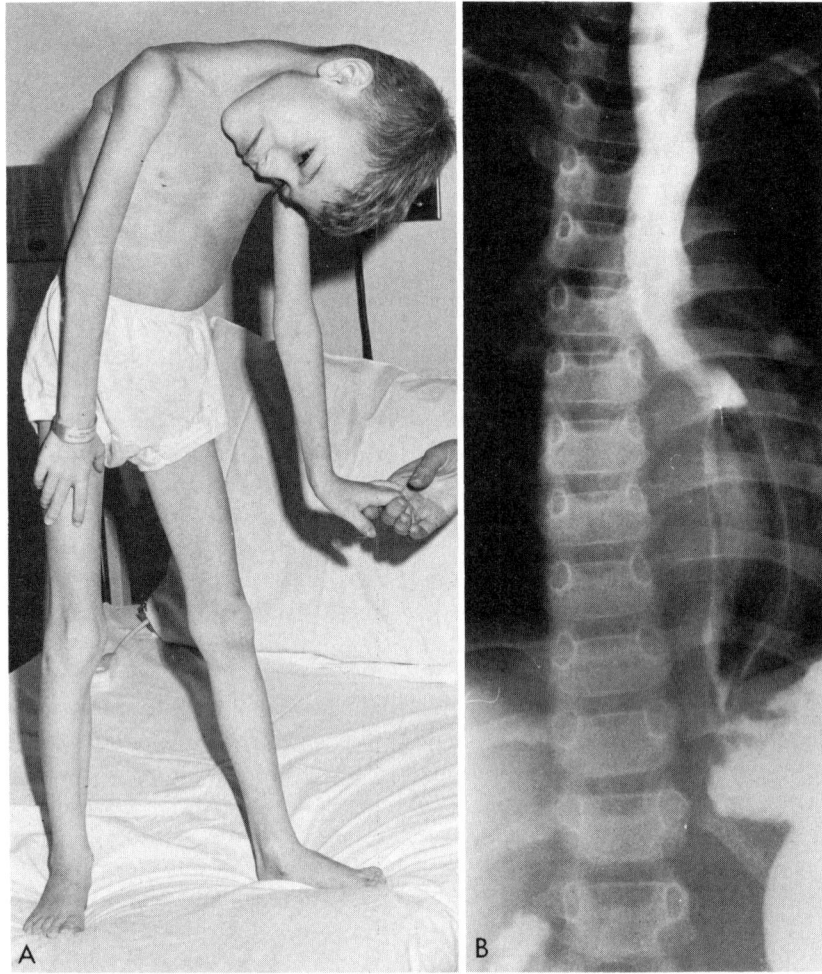

Figure 11–14   Eight-year-old boy with bizarre posturing. An initial chest film showed an air-fluid level in the
esophagus. The findings were consistent with Sandifer's syndrome. *A,* Unusual position of head and neck was a
position of comfort, although the child could voluntarily straighten both. *B,* Gastroesophageal reflux occurred
spontaneously during barium study of the esophagus. The motility was abnormal and stripping waves were
infrequent. (From Gellis, S. S., and Feingold, M.: Picture of the Month. Contributed by Siegel, N., Margolis, C.,
Long, J., and Spackman, T.: Am. J. Dis. Child. *121*:53, 1971. Copyright 1971, American Medical Association.)

The diagnosis is usually confirmed by radiologic techniques. A large hernia is noted as
an air-fluid level in the posterior mediastinum on a routine chest examination. Most
infant hernias containing 2 to 4 cm of stomach are visualized with contrast material as
gastric mucosal folds that extend uninter-
ruptedly from the stomach to above the
diaphragm (Fig. 11–15). Many of the smaller
hernias are very difficult to demonstrate,
and the Trendelenburg position should be
used in all studies.

It has been pointed out that some degree
of gastroesophageal reflux and transient prolapse of gastric mucosa above the diaphragmatic hiatus can be seen in normal
infants and that these radiologic findings
must be interpreted in the light of clinical
findings. Radiographic findings may not be
present if repeat studies are done weeks or
months later.

Esophageal motility studies in older infants will demonstrate that the inferior
esophageal sphincter lies above the point of
respiratory reversal at the diaphragm and
not within the intra-abdominal segment of
esophagus. Abnormalities of peristalsis may
be present and are attributable to esophagitis. These are usually represented by feeble
or nonpropulsive waves. It must be stressed

that in dissection of the gastroesophageal region of neonates, Botha[24] noted that the abdominal esophagus was nonexistent. In those a few months old, it measured several millimeters, and after several years its length was 5 to 15 mm. Similarly, in motility studies, the inferior esophageal sphincter is found to lie at or above the effective diaphragmatic hiatus in 80 per cent of neonates. Motility studies in infants with hiatus hernia are therefore difficult to interpret.

Treatment. The first line of treatment is medical and consists of maintaining the infant in an upright or semi-upright position during and after feeding. The commercial infant seat is ideal for this kind of positioning. If the infant must sleep in a crib, the head of the crib should be elevated on blocks and the infant placed prone. The use of pillows is unsuccessful because, by morning, most children are found curled up at the base of the pillow. Frequent, thickened feedings are offered, to coat the lumen of the esophagus and to counteract gastric acidity; thickened formula is more difficult to regurgitate. Older children are given antacids between feedings. Because of the recent studies showing lowering of inferior sphincter pressure by anticholinergics, we hesitate to use these drugs in patients with reflux. Some success has been achieved with agents that increase esophageal peristalsis.

The indications for surgical intervention are the appearance of blood in the vomitus, severe anemia with evidence of chronic blood loss, and stricture formation. Surgery is not always the definitive answer, for the condition recurs in at least one quarter of the patients. The results of the simple repair of gastropexy in children who do not have esophagitis at the time of operation are encouraging. The approach, the type of repair, and the decision as to whether or not to add vagotomy and pyloroplasty to the procedure are left to the individual surgeon. A small stricture can be treated by dilatations, but it is likely that it will recur. If the stricture is extensive, colon replacement is recommended.

Prognosis. The best medical results are achieved in infants in whom diagnosis is made and treatment is given before the third month; these patients become symptom-free within one year. Only half of those treated later improve significantly.[30] Seventy-five per cent of those who require surgery do well, whereas those who have esophageal stricture have the worst prognosis. Manometric studies after fundal plica-

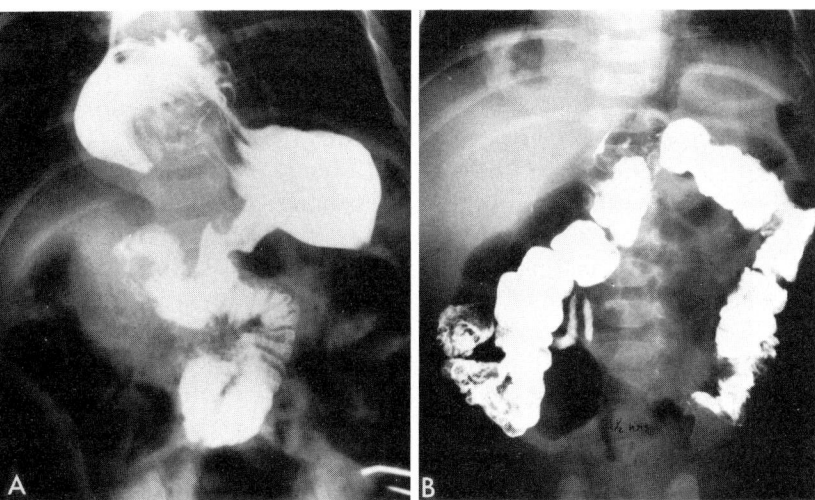

Figure 11–15 Congenital diaphragmatic defect and hiatus hernia in three-and-one-half-month-old infant who presented with vomiting and difficulty in swallowing. *A,* A large loculus of stomach lies above the hemidiaphragms and, owing to torsion, caused partial obstruction of barium flow into the distal stomach. The position of proximal small bowel loops in the midabdomen suggests an associated partial malrotation, *B,* Opacification of the colon demonstrates an inverted cecum, also indicating an abnormality of rotation and fixation. The thoracic portion of the stomach is seen as an air-containing structure.

tion procedures show an increase in length of the sphincter, but not always an increase in its basal pressure.

Paraesophageal Hernia

In this type of hernia, which is extremely rare in the infant, a small sac of peritoneum and part of the greater curvature of the stomach slide up through the hiatus beside a normally placed lower esophagus. The anatomy of the gastroesophageal junction is not disturbed, and there is no reflux. The esophagus is not shortened. These hernias are asymptomatic unless they become incarcerated or volvulus of the stomach is present. They can occur with a sliding hiatus hernia.

CONGENITAL SHORT ESOPHAGUS

Some consider congenital short esophagus to be a distinct entity, separate from that caused by peptic esophagitis and its resultant fibrosis. Not all agree, however. This discussion will present the disorder as it is seen by the former group.[29, 84]

Etiology. The cause is failure of elongation of the foregut.

Pathology. Included in the complex of congenital short esophagus is a portion of stomach within the thorax. Externally, the whole complex resembles esophagus, and it is not until esophagotomy is performed or the specimen is resected that the true lesion is ascertained. The intrathoracic stomach originates above the diaphragm and derives its blood supply from the aorta, not from the celiac axis as a herniated stomach would.[152] This segment is lined with mature, functioning gastric mucosa that contains parietal and chief cells. There may be areas of squamous metaplasia or of "intestinalization," i.e., areas of glands containing intestinal cells. The muscularis of the thoracic stomach consists of three muscle layers. There is no diaphragmatic defect. The short esophagus above is lined with stratified squamous epithelium and contains two muscle layers. There is no protective functioning inferior esophageal sphincter, and reflux of gastric contents leads to very severe esophagitis

and the development of esophageal stricture.

Symptoms. Vomiting may be associated with the first feeding experience, or progressive dysphagia and regurgitation of undigested food may develop gradually throughout infancy. Recurrent bouts of pneumonia or aspiration are a major complication.

Diagnosis. Radiologic examination of the esophagus will reveal the presence of gastric rugae above the diaphragm. Material injected into the stomach is immediately refluxed into the esophagus and even into the tracheobronchial tree. Lack of tonus or sphincter function is noted at the lower esophagus. Visalli has likened the reflux to fluid being sucked up through a straw.[152]

Treatment. Because of the severity of esophagitis and the propensity for stricture formation, esophageal resection with high esophagogastrostomy or colon transposition has been recommended.

BARRETT'S ESOPHAGUS

Barrett described a lower esophagus lined by columnar epithelium. It is extremely rare, and most cases have been seen in adults; a similar picture, however, has been reported in a six-year-old boy who had had dysphagia since the age of two years.[15, 89, 162] Barrett's esophagus is frequently associated with hiatus hernia or incompetency of the inferior esophageal sphincter.

Etiology. Some have considered this to be a congenital lesion, but it seems most likely to be acquired when columnar epithelium replaces squamous epithelium that has been destroyed by acid reflux. The new epithelium arises from the gastric or junctional epithelium. It has been suggested that islets of columnar epithelium in the esophagus are derived from superficial glands of the lamina propria that hypertrophy in response to reflux. This lesion often disappears after treatment.[87a]

Pathology. The lower esophagus is lined with columnar instead of squamous epithelium. This mucosa contains parietal cells, and there is evidence that it can produce acid. There is often hiatus hernia or chalasia of the inferior esophageal sphincter. Esophagitis develops above the mucosal squamocolumnar junction, and strictures of variable length[60] form at the squamocolumnar junction, which may be located at any point from just above the inferior esophageal sphincter to the level of the aortic arch. The columnar epithelium is not subject to esophagitis, although it sometimes contains a deep, solitary, inflammatory Barrett's ulcer.

Symptoms. The symptoms are long-standing and are related to the upper gastrointestinal tract. Regurgitation after feedings and nocturnal regurgitation of mucus are often the first complaints. Epigastric pain is difficult to ascertain in the infant, but abdominal pain is not relieved by food or by antacids. Dysphagia eventually develops and is more marked with solids than with liquids. If esophagitis or ulceration is significant, anemia or hematemesis complicates the condition.

Diagnosis. The diagnosis is suggested by the association of a mid-esophageal stricture and hiatus hernia or chalasia. Peristalsis is normal above and below the area of the stricture during radiologic examination. Esophagoscopy demonstrates the mucosal change, and biopsy shows the area of change to be columnar epithelium.

Treatment. The aim of treatment is prevention of reflux, as described for hiatus hernia. A medical regimen is adequate for many patients, but some require surgery to restore the competency of the inferior sphincter.

Prognosis. There is some evidence to indicate that persistence of Barrett's esophagus may predispose to the development of carcinoma.[89]

MOTOR DISTURBANCES OF THE ESOPHAGUS

FUNCTIONAL ESOPHAGEAL DISEASE

Achalasia

Achalasia is a motor abnormality of the esophagus characterized by failure of the lower esophageal sphincter to relax with swallowing.[10] The entire esophagus above the sphincter becomes progressively dilated and has little or no peristaltic activity. The resultant hypotonic organ is often termed megaesophagus. An identical clinical and physiologic picture occurs in Chagas' disease.[14, 79]

Incidence. The exact incidence is not known, but achalasia in infants and children accounts for only 4 to 5 per cent of all cases. Fewer than 100 pediatric cases have been reported. A hereditary factor is possible, for achalasia has occurred in six sets of siblings and has been reported in a father and son.[159]

Etiology. Although the true etiology is not known, the defect is considered to be neurogenic and the result of the congenital absence or degeneration of the ganglion cells of Auerbach's plexus. Since the myenteric plexus is established in a cephalo-caudal direction and is well developed by the twelfth week of gestation, it would be difficult to support the hypothesis of a congenital absence of ganglion cells in this area with normal development beneath it.[106, 107] Normal ganglion cells are found in esophageal tissue from young children with achalasia; from this, one may assume that degeneration of the ganglion cells follows prolonged dilation of the esophagus rather than precedes it. Experimentally, an achalasia-like disease has been produced by destruction of the caudate nucleus, section of the vagus nerves, selective destruction of the intramural ganglion cells, and prolonged cholinesterase inhibition. Achalasia sicca has been reported in a child with juvenile Sjögren's syndrome and gastric hyposecretion and in another child with autosomal deafness, short stature, vitiligo, and muscle wasting.[135]

Pathology and Pathophysiology. In older patients, microscopic examination of the esophagus reveals absence or diminution of the number of ganglion cells, most marked in the body of the esophagus and less so in the area of the lower esophageal sphincter. Smooth muscle cells appear normal by light microscopy but show cellular atrophy under electron microscopy. Electron microscopy also shows degenerative changes in the vagus and the dorsal motor nucleus of the vagus.

In vitro studies of achalasic muscle strips demonstrate a cholinergic innervation of both layers of the body of the esophagus and of the longitudinal layer of the inferior esophageal sphincter.[154] Excitatory and inhibitory adrenergic receptors are present in esophageal muscle, but the inhibitory receptors predominating in the longitudinal muscle are unresponsive to stimulation in the achalasic esophagus.

The obstruction in the esophagus is functional rather than mechanical because the inferior sphincter does not relax completely with deglutition. The increased sphincter pressure may decrease somewhat during swallowing but never reaches the level of gastric pressure.

Primary progressive peristalsis is absent, and there is no effective progression of a bolus through the esophagus. Simultaneous contractions are noted on manometric tracings, but they are weak and nonpropulsive. The esophagus empties when the weight of esophageal contents builds up enough hydrostatic force to overcome sphincter resistance. As the esophagus above the sphincter becomes more and more dilated, its walls become stretched and thin.

The esophagus is hypersensitive to methacholine (Mecholyl) given intramuscularly. Injection of this agent is followed by tonic contraction of the organ and chest pain. Manometric tracings show a sudden sustained increase in resting esophageal pressure in all of the esophageal leads (Fig. 11–16).[151] The sphincter is sensitive to gastrin, which causes a marked rise in its pressure. Gastric acidification, which suppresses endogenous gastrin formation, decreases the sphincter pressure. The LES contracts in response to cholecystokinin.[39]

Symptoms. The onset of symptoms is gradual. In children, most cases occur after the age of nine years, but occasionally a case is found in an infant. The youngest patient was a 900-gm, 14-day-old premature infant. Dysphagia, weight loss, regurgitation, and vomiting predominate. Pain is not a complaint. Dysphagia is experienced first with solids and later with liquids as well. Aspiration caused by nocturnal regurgitation of esophageal contents results in pneumonitis.[134] Indeed, recurrent pneumonitis is sometimes the major symptom.

Diagnosis. Chagas' disease is to be suspected if the patient lives in an endemic area. Infants with familial dysautonomia have similar esophageal problems, but other characteristics of the disease are evident. The diagnosis is usually made by radiologic studies. A huge dilated esophagus with little air in the stomach is seen in the chest x-ray. An esophagogram shows the dilated esophagus, which tapers to a smooth conical narrowing at the lower end (Fig. 11–17). Cineradiologic study is particularly helpful, for peristalsis is absent and barium passes through the lower sphincter in spurts. Intramuscular injection of Mecholyl causes forceful simultaneous contractions of the esophagus, as already described. Mecholyl should not be used routinely in radiologic examinations because of the danger of aspiration of the barium meal.

Treatment. In the small infant, temporary relief is provided by bougienage, and approximately 25 per cent are improved for some months. Pneumatic dilatation is dangerous in the young child owing to the danger of perforation[135a] and is not recommended in those under 9 years of age. Surgical treatment is the best therapy, with various techniques recommended. The Heller cardiomyotomy is the most widely used technique, although some prefer transabdominal esophagomyotomy, or the Wendel procedure, in which a vertical incision is made through all layers of the esophagus

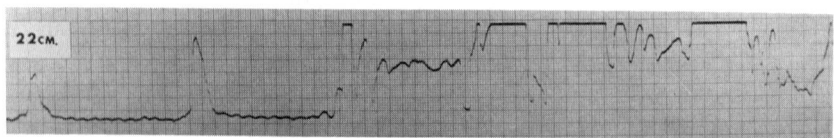

Figure 11–16   Positive methacholine test in achalasia. After injection of drug, there is an obvious rise in baseline esophageal pressure associated with multiple simultaneous esophageal contractions.

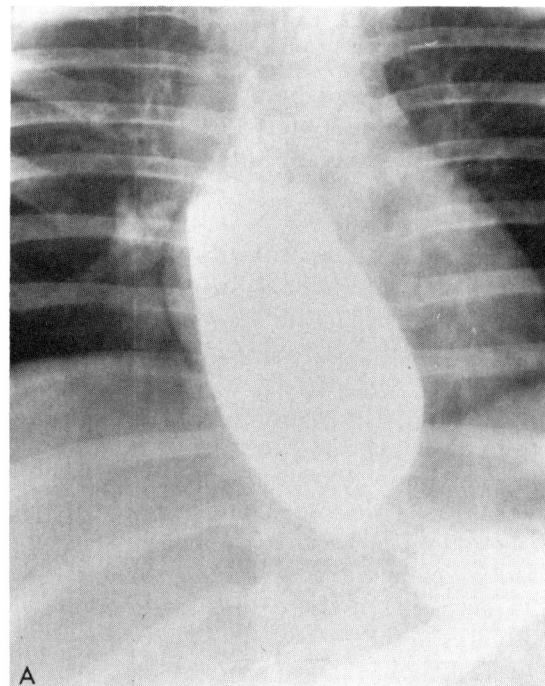

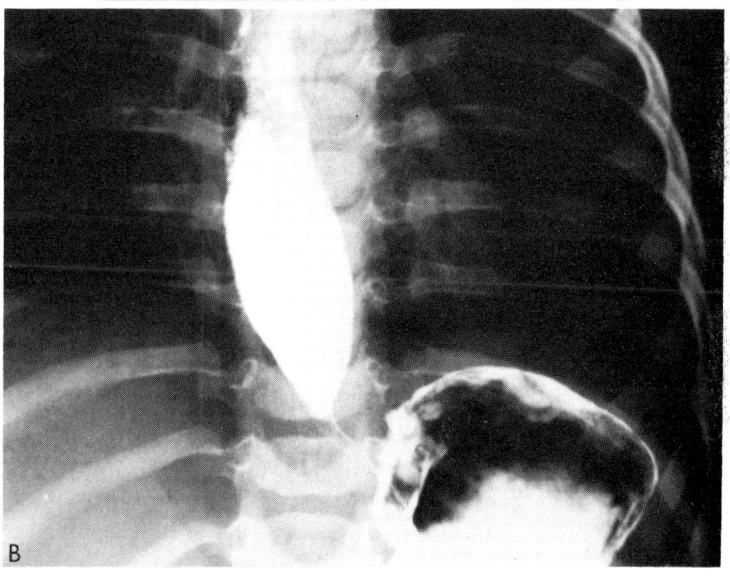

Figure 11–17 Nine-month-old infant with a history of poor feeding and regurgitation for six months. Barium swallow demonstrated a dilated esophagus with poor peristalsis. The distal esophagus tapers smoothly, and barium falls through intermittently. Films *A* and *B* were obtained at different intervals during the same study.

and cardia and closed transversely. This disturbs the anatomy of the esophagogastric junction and is associated with postoperative reflux esophagitis.[108] Simultaneous pyloromyotomy or vagotomy or both are added by some surgeons to ensure more rapid emptying of gastric contents.

Prognosis. The late results of mechanical dilatations in children are less satisfactory than those in adults, whereas surgical myotomy is usually followed by sustained improvement.[12] Recent studies in the pediatric literature, however, attest to the successes of pneumatic dilatation.[10, 26a] Although symptomatic cure is accomplished by either procedure and the resting pressure of the lower esophageal sphincter decreases, its abnormal response to deglutition remains. Surveillance of the patient is necessary throughout life, for the disease is associated with an increased incidence of carcinoma of the esophagus.

Esophageal Spasm

Esophageal spasm, also termed cardiospasm, is a motility disorder that involves the entire esophagus. Although a common disorder in the adult, it is rare in the infant and young child.

Etiology. The disorder is usually related to stress, rapid eating, or the drinking of very cold beverages. We have presumed that gastroesophageal reflux and esophagitis may be underlying factors in precipitating attacks.

Pathophysiology. The disorder is one of hypermotility, in which there are incoordinated, irregular contractions of the esophagus below the area of the aortic arch. Rarely, there is only intermittent constriction in the region of the lower sphincter. Sphincter function is normal, but there may be an associated hiatus hernia.[85]

Symptoms. Esophageal spasm causes intermittent dysphagia and severe substernal pain. Infants with spasm have choking spells after feeding.

Diagnosis. Radiologic examination may often be normal, and unless one persists by giving the patient barium-coated bread or marshmallows, spasm may not be elicited. Positive studies, however, show extensive areas of contraction alternating with dilated areas, giving the appearance of a corkscrew esophagus. Endoscopy is often unremarkable.

Treatment. Successful treatment has been achieved with atropine (1:1000 solution), given in dosage to the point of flushing, before each feeding. Spasm is occasionally dramatically relieved by the ingestion of a hot liquid. Esophageal dilatation is reserved for those who do not respond to medical therapy.

Prognosis. Spasm may be the first sign of developing achalasia and a persistence of symptoms should prompt further investigation for this disorder.

Lower Esophageal Ring (Schatzki Ring)

The lower esophageal ring is a cause of intermittent esophageal dysphagia in older children and adults, or it may be an incidental radiologic finding. It has also been termed contractile ring of the lower esophagus, or Schatzki ring. Recently, it has been described in a neonate.[78a]

Incidence. The frequency of rings in radiologic studies of adults has ranged from 0.2 to 14 per cent. Pathologic studies have yielded a frequency rate of 10 to 14 per cent, with males and females affected equally.

Etiology. Three theories for ring formation are presented: (1) plication, in which the ring represents redundant mucosa and the esophagus has shortened to form a hiatus hernia, (2) developmental, in which the ring represents a persistent congenital mucosal ridge, and (3) inflammatory, in which it is a manifestation of peptic esophagitis. The ring may also be a normal variant.

Pathology. Most mucosal rings lie at the squamocolumnar junction. The upper surface resembles esophageal mucosa and the undersurface, gastric mucosa. Microscopically, the ring contains esophageal mucosa on the proximal side and columnar epithelium on the distal side. The junction line may be even or irregular, at the margin or below it. The core of the mucosal ring contains fibrous tissue in varying amounts and plasma cells. The muscularis mucosa in the region of the ring may be normal or fragmented, with some muscle bundles extending into the lamina propria. Squamous epithelium has been described on both sides of the ring, but there is a question as to whether these lesions are actually rings or congenital webs. Rings are located proximal to the lower esophageal sphincter. Less frequently, another type of ring is noted. This is extremely firm, composed of hypertrophic muscle bundles separated by fibrous septa and chronic inflammatory cells, and covered by squamous epithelium.[48, 49] Most rings are associated with hiatus hernia.[40]

Symptoms. Many rings are diagnosed by chance and remain asymptomatic. In infancy and early childhood, rings may cause dysphagia after solids are introduced into the diet. In older adults, the typical presentation is one of intermittent dysphagia more marked for solids than for liquids, with steak as a particular offender. Symptoms vary with the diameter of the ring. Symptoms are often precipitated by stress, poor chewing of food, or rapid eating. Reflux symptoms are variable.

Differential Diagnosis. Rings must be differentiated from esophageal webs or diaphragms, strictures, and esophageal leiomyoma or neuroma.

Diagnosis. The history itself should suggest the diagnosis. Careful radiologic examination with maximal distention of the lower esophagus is definitive. Measures to increase intra-abdominal pressure aid in defining the ring and hiatus hernia. Barium-laden marshmallows or bread, or barium sulfate tablets, will often hold up at the site of obstruction and may be helpful in determining ring dimensions. In the past, rings were often missed by endoscopic examination with rigid instruments but now may be easily identified with the flexible fiberoptic ones. Typically, there is no or little evidence of esophagitis.

The muscular ring presents a different radiologic picture: a broad, smooth constriction in the lower esophagus well above the squamocolumnar junction.

Associated Lesions. As noted, most rings are associated with hiatus hernia. The converse does not hold, for rings are noted in only about 15 per cent of patients with hiatus hernia. Other associated lesions are gastric or duodenal ulcers, Zenker's diverticulum, achalasia, proximal esophageal webs, and iron deficiency anemia.

Clinical Course. Once diagnosed, most rings either remain unchanged or decrease in diameter.[50] Symptomatic cases often improve with no treatment. In a few patients, dysphagia may increase to the point at which no solids can be tolerated.

Treatment. Since symptoms are related to mucosal ring diameter, they can be minimized by careful chewing of food. Therapeutic dilatations by endoscope, bougienage, or Mosher bag have provided symptomatic relief, and one dilatation is usually curative. Treatment for muscular ring is identical.

Prognosis. Radiologic evidence of a ring persists despite treatment, and symptoms do tend to recur. Heartburn and esophagitis may follow treatment and are due to reflux. Surgical procedures include hiatus hernia repair, hernia repair with digital rupture, or partial excision of the ring.

ESOPHAGEAL MUSCULAR RING

Esophageal muscular ring has been described in the VACTERYL association, a syndrome of mesodermal malformations including vertebrae and rib anomalies, radial limb malformations, single umbilical artery, anal atresia, ventricular septal defect, and tracheoesophageal fistula.[65a]

Chalasia

Chalasia, or cardiochalasia, denotes relaxation or incompetence of the lower esophageal sphincter.

Incidence. In the very young infant this is considered a normal phenomenon, since in a study of 1100 normal infants, 38 per cent regurgitated during the first five days of life and had evidence of chalasia. In only a small percentage did reflux continue after the first week of life, however.

Etiology. The defect is most likely physiologic immaturity or delayed neuromuscular development of the inferior esophageal sphincter. A number of infants exhibit soft signs of central nervous system immaturity.

Pathophysiology. The lower esophageal sphincter is under both muscular and neurohumoral control, which must be balanced for well-coordinated sphincter function. During the first few days of life, the sphincter pressures approximate those of the stomach but rise to 2 to 6 mm Hg above gastric pressure by the end of the first week. Usually by one to two months the pressures approximate those of the normal childhood sphincter (Fig. 11–18). Botha's anatomic dissections demonstrated no abdominal segment of the esophagus in the neonate, and he proposed that chalasia represents a partial thoracic stomach with the cardia at or just above the diaphragm.[24]

In infants who regurgitate significantly after one month of age, esophageal motility

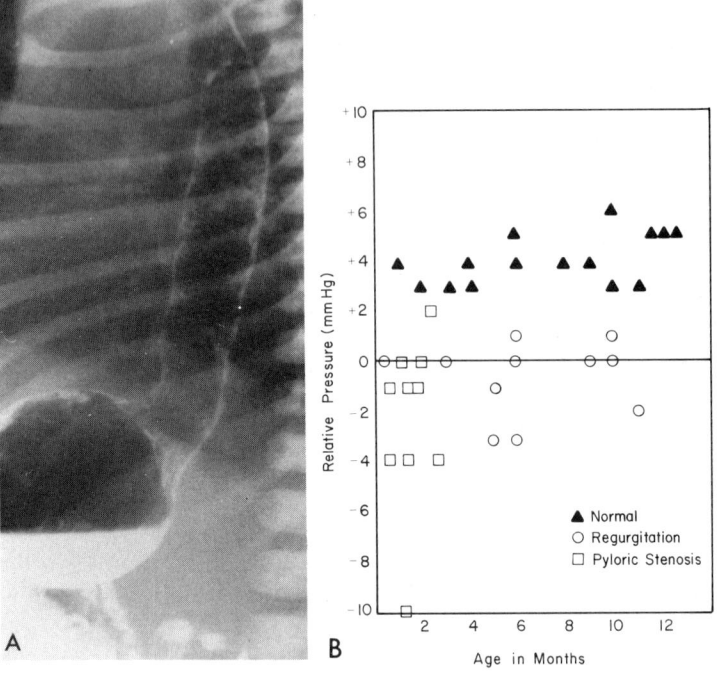

Figure 11–18 A, This premature infant had recurrent regurgitation and one episode of upper gastrointestinal bleeding during the first week of life. Barium study demonstrates a persistently open lower esophageal sphincter with free reflux of barium and gastric contents into the esophagus, findings typical for chalasia. B, Pressures of the lower esophageal sphincter in normal infants, in those with regurgitation, and in those with pyloric stenosis. The techniques used non-perfused water-filled catheters, yielding lower basal pressures. (From Gryboski, J. D., Thayer, W. R., Jr., and Spiro, H. M.: Esophageal motility in infants and children. Pediatrics 31:382, 1963. Used by permission.)

studies indicate the characteristics of chalasia. The sphincter relaxes normally after deglutition, but its resting pressure is lower than that of normal infants of the same age, measuring only a few mm Hg above intragastric pressure.

Symptoms. Regurgitation begins during the first week of life and occurs during and after feedings. Unchanged or curdled formula flows freely out of the mouth. Regurgitation is intermittent at first but increases in frequency until by several weeks it accompanies or follows every feeding. Many infants remain well nourished, and the regurgitation is more of a problem to the mother than to the child. It decreases in frequency and amount by the sixth month and ceases by the time the child is 12 to 18 months old. In others with the more severe form, caloric intake is inadequate and the child becomes malnourished. Recurrent pneumonia becomes a problem because of free reflux of gastric contents up the esophagus and into the trachea during sleep. As peptic esophagitis develops, there is some vomiting of blood-streaked material. Anemia and irritability are caused by chronic blood loss.

Diagnosis. A nasogastric tube passes into the stomach with ease. The diagnosis depends upon the demonstration of reflux of contrast material from the stomach into the esophagus. During inspiration, dye refluxes into the esophagus, and during expiration some is forced into the esophagus with the remainder passing into the stomach. Increased intra-abdominal pressure promotes reflux. The lower portion of the esophagus appears dilated (Fig. 11–18). More sensitive diagnostic procedures include pH monitoring and esophageal motility, as described in Chapter 3.

Complications. As in other obstructive esophageal disease, aspiration is a constant problem. Peptic esophagitis can reach such severity as to cause stricture, shortening of the esophagus, and the development of hiatus hernia.

Treatment. Reflux is decreased by maintenance of the infant in the semi-erect position at all times. The treatment is essentially the same as that for hiatus hernia and should be continued for three to six months. If small hiatus hernias are associated with this condition, they should be repaired. Small strictures respond to dilatations, but larger ones tend to recur and may require surgical correction.

Prognosis. The response to medical treatment in infants without significant esophagitis is extremely good, and regurgitation lessens within several days. The radiologic picture reverts to normal after a few weeks. Only a few infants with severe esophagitis require surgery for creation of a competent inferior sphincter.

Familial Dysautonomia

Sensory and motor dysfunction of the autonomic nervous system characterize familial dysautonomia, also known as the Riley-Day syndrome.

Incidence. An exact incidence is unknown, but the disease is rare.

Inheritance. Occurring exclusively in Eastern European families of Ashkenazi Jewish extraction, the disorder is inherited as an autosomal recessive trait.

Etiology. The disease is considered to represent an enzymatic defect in the metabolic pathway of catechol release.

Pathophysiology. Studies of the urinary metabolites of norepinephrine and its precursors show decreased excretion of vanillylmandelic acid (VMA) and increased excretion of homovanillic acid (HVA), a metabolite of dopamine and norepinephrine.[137] Dopamine-β-hydrolase (DBH) catalyzes the conversion of dopamine to norepinephrine and is found in the catecholamine-containing structures of sympathetic nerves and in the chromaffin granules of the adrenal medulla. DBH is detected in the blood and increases with stress, as do the catecholamines.[119] The blood content of the enzyme is low at birth and increases with age until it reaches adult levels by 11 or 12 years. Values at six months are 0 to 25 units; between six months and one year, a mean of 80 units; and between one and two years, a mean of 180 units per dl. The mean value of patients 11 to 24 years is 200 units per dl and of age-paired controls, 334 units per dl. One third of dysautonomic children under ten years of age have no measurable enzyme. Normal amounts of DBH were found in fathers of affected infants, but their mothers had low values.

There is a prolonged hypoglycemic response to insulin and an increased sensitivity to infused norepinephrine. Hypersensitivity to methacholine (Mecholyl) is demonstrated by constriction of the pupil after injection of this agent into the eye. The normal skin flare that develops after the intradermal injection of histamine is absent.

Esophageal function is affected, and there is dilation of the lower esophagus. Peristalsis is normal in the erect position but abnormal in the supine position. There is difficulty in the pharyngeal phase of deglutition because of delayed opening of the superior esophageal sphincter, but the lower esophageal sphincter is normal. This esophageal dysfunction is an important factor in the development of aspiration pneumonia.[87]

Symptoms. Swallowing difficulties are present from the first day of life, for there is a poorly coordinated suck and swallow reflex and secretions pool in the oropharynx.[110] Physical examination shows absence of deep tendon reflexes, postural hypotension, blotching of the skin, excessive perspiration, absence of tears, decreased pain and taste sensation, absence of circumvallate papillae of the tongue, episodic fever, and vomiting. As speech develops, there is dysarthria. In some children there is marked constipation and development of abdominal distention from a large, impacted colon.[52] Recurrent pneumonia is a major part of the history.

Diagnosis. The diagnostic considerations include neonatal cerebral trauma and achalasia, but as other symptoms evolve these conditions become less likely. Urinary catecholamine studies (reduced VMA and elevated HVA) and the responses to intraocular methacholine and intradermal histamine all corroborate the clinical diagnosis.

DBH measurements are not diagnostic because there is too much variation in normal values. A barium swallow study shows difficulty in swallowing and aspiration of barium into the trachea. There is cricopharyngeal spasm. The body of the esophagus is dilated and atonic.

Treatment. The only treatment is symptomatic. In some patients, parenteral neostigmine (Prostigmin) alleviates the swallowing difficulties. Sleeping in a semi-erect position prevents the aspiration of contents retained in the dilated esophagus. If recurrent pneumonitis is associated with the finding of milk precipitins in the serum, the elimination of milk and milk products from the diet sometimes improves the pulmonary status. Fundoplication or gastrostomy has been successful in patients with pneumonitis due to aspiration.[9a]

Prognosis. Many patients die in infancy, and those who mature to adulthood are plagued by postural hypotension, recurrent pneumonitis, taste disorders, periodic vomiting, and faulty coordination.

Dysautonomia-Like Disorders

Two female siblings of Sephardic Jewish origin with symptoms similar to those of the Riley-Day syndrome have been reported.[32, 128] They exhibited vomiting from infancy, dysarthria, hypotonia, labile blood pressure, postural hypotension, hypesthesia, blotching of the skin, abnormal temperature control, decreased lacrimation, constriction of the pupils with methacholine,

and psychomotor retardation. In addition, they had fixed, dilated pupils and irregular pupillary margins. The urinary VMA was normal, as were the sense of taste, response to insulin, and dermal reaction to histamine. One had a dilated, hypotonic esophagus.[138] We also have seen one Caucasian male infant with recurrent vomiting, severe motor retardation, blotching of the skin, hypesthesia, postural hypotension, abnormal reactions to histamine and intraocular methacholine, and a dilated, hypotonic esophagus.

ABNORMAL ESOPHAGEAL MOTILITY IN OTHER DISEASES

Abnormalities of esophageal persistalsis are described in a variety of neuromuscular disorders and collagen diseases as well as in diabetes mellitus. These are problematic in older children and adults but do not occur in the infant.[35] Abnormal motility may be an early sign of intestinal pseudo-obstruction.

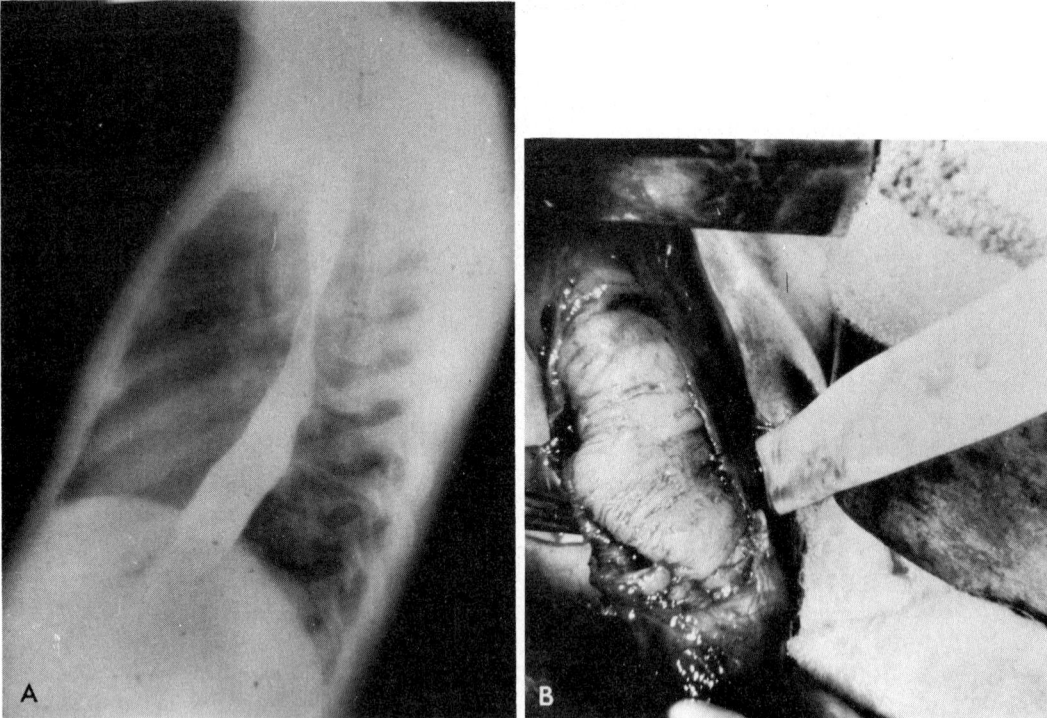

Figure 11–19 A, Lateral film of a five-year-old girl with a three-year history of dysphagia. Compression is evident in the middle third of the esophagus and the mucosal contour is abnormal below, suggesting a submucosal lesion. B, Surgical incision of the esophagus showing a pale, firm, diffuse leiomyoma, involving full thickness of muscle.

Illustration continued on opposite page

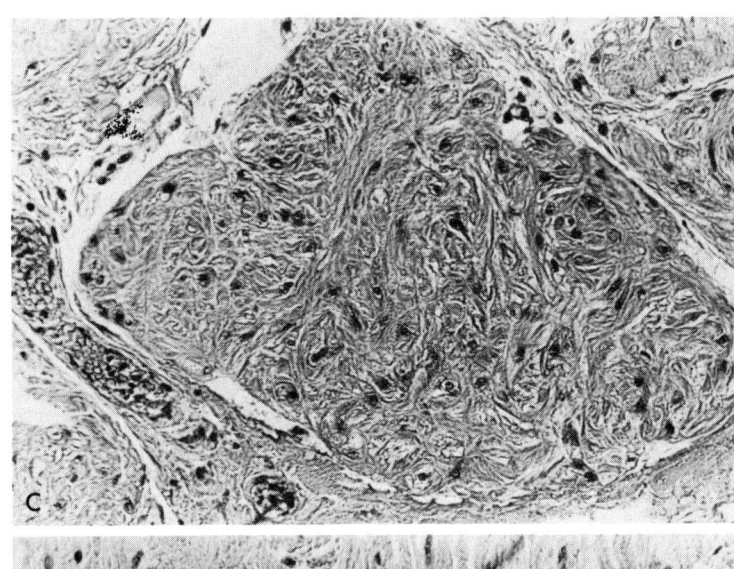

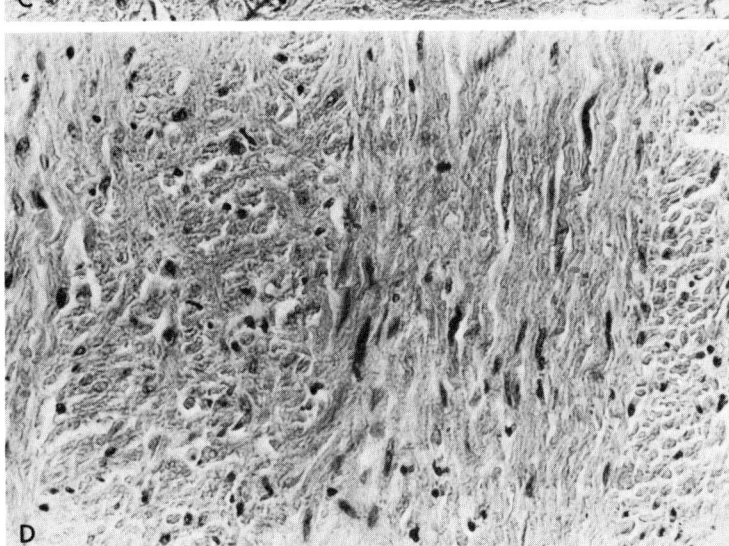

Figure 11–19 Continued C and D, Histology of benign leiomyoma. (Courtesy of Dr. A. Toole.)

Transient dysphagia sometimes follows vagotomy in the first few postoperative weeks. There is abnormal peristalsis in the lower third of the esophagus. Soft foods are taken without difficulty, and the symptoms subside within several weeks.

Longitudinal esophageal bands have been associated with esophageal aperistalsis.[142]

ACQUIRED DISEASES OF THE ESOPHAGUS

TUMORS OF THE ESOPHAGUS

Esophageal tumors are extremely rare in childhood, and, fortunately, most of them are benign.[148]

Pathology. The tumors are submucosal or polypoid. Most of the polypoid tumors are attached to the upper third of the esophagus and are neuromas, lipomas, polyps, hamartomas, or myxofibromas.[38] Submucosal neurofibromas are associated with von Recklinghausen's disease. Some even involve the thoracic vagus nerves.[100] Leiomyomas may be single, multiple, or diffuse (Fig. 11–19).[71]

Symptoms. There is a history of poor feeding, vomiting, and failure to gain weight from the first few weeks of age. In some infants the symptoms are present from the first day of life. As the tumors enlarge, the infants cough, wheeze, become dyspneic, and suffer recurrent pulmonary infections. Regurgitation of the tumor into the oropharynx is a frightening complication.

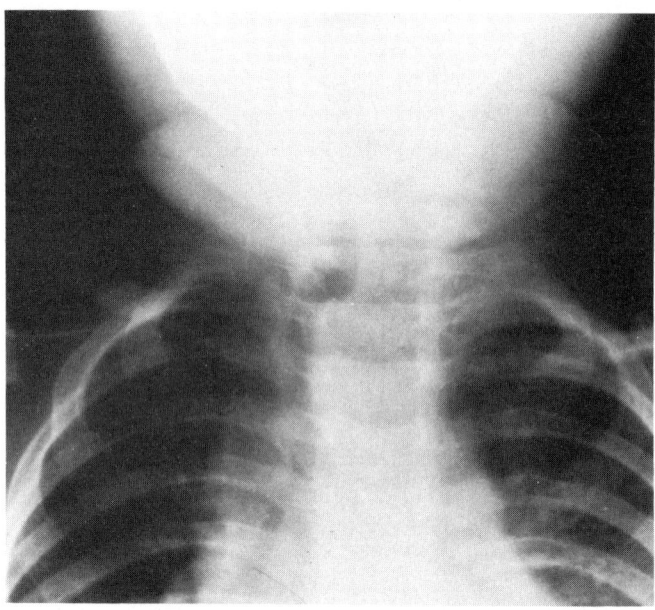

Figure 11–20 Six-month-old female infant with dysphagia due to neurofibroma of the posterior cervical esophagus: Note deviation of the trachea in plain film of the neck and chest.

Diagnosis. Cine-esophagography is particularly successful in demonstrating esophageal filling defects. Chest x-ray will show deviation of the trachea if the lesion is large enough (Fig. 11–20). Esophagoscopy further defines the characteristics of the lesion. Diffuse leiomyomas show thickening of the entire esophagus (Fig. 11–19).

Treatment. Surgical excision is the only treatment for these tumors. Local lesions are individually resectable, but diffuse leiomyoma requires excision of the esophageal muscle wall in its entirety.

EPIDERMOLYSIS BULLOSA DYSTROPHICA AND ESOPHAGEAL LESIONS

Epidermolysis bullosa exists in a variety of disease forms, which are divided into two major classifications: scarring and nonscarring. We are concerned here with the scarring type termed dermolytic bullous dermatosis.[1]

Inheritance. Two modes of transmission are encountered. The form with recessive inheritance is the more severe, whereas that with dominant inheritance affects the teeth and mucous membranes less severely.

Incidence. The incidence has been estimated at 1 in 300,000.

Etiology and Pathogenesis. The etiology is not known. Elastic tissue deficiency has been postulated, but this alone does not result in blistering. Allergy and thyroid, adrenal, and gonadal dysfunction have been suggested, but there is little supporting evidence for any of these causes. Collagenase activity in the skin of patients with epidermolysis bullosa dystrophica is increased.

Pathology. Trauma of even the most minimal sort causes separation of the epidermis from the dermis, with resultant blister formation (Fig. 11–21). The skin appears fine and crinkled. Hair is often lost. Blistering and recurrent skin infection result in scarring. Because of this the ears may be deformed, the hands may be involved with eventual contractures and loss of nails, and there may be fusion of the digits of the hands and feet. As in patients with second-degree burns, fluid loss, hypoproteinemia, and secondary infection all are problems. The disease affects all anatomic sites covered or lined by squamous epithelium. The teeth are dystrophic. Blisters appear at or shortly after birth. Involved areas of the gastrointestinal tract include the oropharynx, the esophagus, and the anus. Oral scarring leads to puckering of the lips and even to binding of the tongue. Anal lesions become easily infected and are associated with perirectal abscesses.

Symptoms. The infant with this characteristic skin disease shows increasing difficulty in swallowing, first of solids and later of liquids. These problems are not apparent early as long as soft nipples or puréed foods are used and provided that the infant does not injure his lips on a pacifier. As solids with roughage, such as toast, cookies, cold cereals, and hard uncooked vegetables, are added to the diet, they injure the oral and esophageal mucosa. Vesicles, bullae, edema, and ulcerations cause pain and spasm of the esophagus. Dysphagia on this basis is associated with pain and regurgitation during feedings. Later, as stricture formation develops in the esophagus, pain becomes less prominent and obstruction prevails. Food is swallowed with difficulty or not at all. There is considerable choking with attempts to eat, and most of the food or formula is regurgitated. Eventually, secretions are not swallowed, and the child sleeps in comfort only in the prone position.[70a]

Constipation becomes a problem as anal lesions progress. Because defecation causes pain, older infants withhold and become more constipated. Functional megacolon

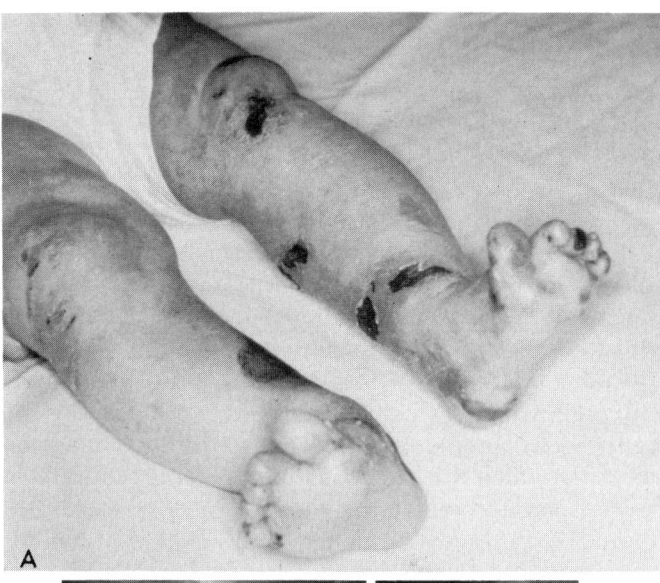

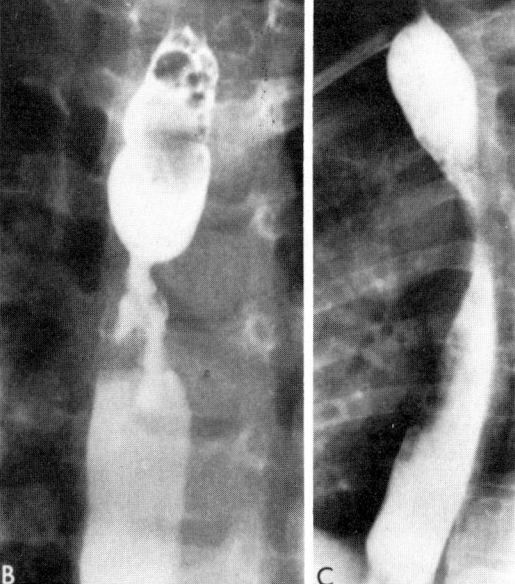

Figure 11–21 Three-year-old boy with long history of skin lesions of epidermolysis bullosa and history of increasing dysphagia of several months' duration. *A,* Typical skin lesions on the legs. Contact areas of legs and toes show ruptured bullae leaving denuded skin. (Courtesy of S. Hurwitz, M.D.) *B,* Barium swallow demonstrates long area of irregular stricture and ulceration within narrowed segment. *C,* Residual narrowing four years later after intermittent steroid therapy and several dilatations.

and even partial intestinal obstruction are complications of anal lesions.

Malnutrition, anemia, and hypoproteinemia related to inadequate protein-calorie intake and to protein and blood losses through the bullous lesion cause growth failure and delayed maturation.

Diagnosis. The appearance of the infant is diagnostic (Fig. 11–21A), and the diagnosis can be confirmed by skin biopsy. On barium swallow, edema and ulceration of the esophagus, with stricture in the middle or upper third of the esophagus extending over 3 to 5 cm, are seen (Fig. 11–21B). Esophageal web is often associated with esophageal disease and may preclude adequate filling of the esophagus.[66]

Treatment. In general, the blistering and denuding aspects of the disease are most common in infancy and early childhood.[102] Those who survive have less trouble as they advance in age. Supportive general measures are maintenance of an adequate intake in the form of high-protein liquid feedings, iron and vitamin supplementation, and treatment of the skin lesions with topical antibiotics to prevent secondary infection. We treat esophageal lesions with prednisone, 20 to 40 mg a day (up to 80 mg per day in older children) for three weeks, at which time improvement usually can be seen and the steroid dosage can be tapered very slowly. Dysphagia and bulla formation tend to recur when low dosage levels are reached. If there is no response to therapy at the end of three weeks, gentle dilatation with rubber bougies is attempted. This is done with extreme caution and in our patients has proved very effective. In some children, symptoms recur within a year or more but respond well to repeated dilatations. Colon transplantation has been successful in patients with extensive stricture.[43]

Case Report. R. B., a three-year-old Caucasian male with epidermolysis bullosa, entered the hospital with the chief complaint of inability to swallow. For three months before admission he had had difficulty in swallowing meats and had reduced his oral intake to soft solids, such as scrambled eggs, Jell-O, and hamburger. For the four weeks before admission he noted difficulty in swallowing liquids. At night he awoke choking and regurgitating mucus. Physical examina-

tion revealed a thin, irritable boy with the typical dystrophic changes of the hands and feet and absence of nails. His skin was covered by oozing, bleeding bullae. His mouth was puckered and scarred. Esophagography showed an esophageal stricture (Fig. 11–21B). After one week of therapy with prednisone, 60 mg a day, he could eat semi-solid foods. He was discharged, and steroid administration was continued for three months. He remained well until the age of five years, when the same complaints returned and another stricture was demonstrated. When a three-week regimen of steroids proved ineffective, bougienage was performed. Within 24 hours he was taking a soft diet. Now nine years old, the patient has had esophageal dilatation on two additional occasions. His height and weight are in the tenth percentile for his age.

ESOPHAGEAL WEB WITH DYSKERATOSIS CONGENITA SYNDROME

Esophageal web usually develops after the age of five years in children with dyskeratosis congenita, an extremely rare and often fatal disease consisting of hyperpigmentation, loss of nails, atrophic changes of the hands and feet, and leukokeratosis of the mucous membranes.[2]

Inheritance. This disease is inherited as an autosomal recessive, affecting males primarily and accompanied by a high incidence of parental consanguinity.

Pathology. The epidermis is atrophic and contains scattered areas of degenerating basal cells. Pigment is lost in the basal areas and accumulates in the dermal macrophages. Plaques of leukoplakia are present in the mucous membranes of the mouth and anus. The hematologic changes resemble those of Fanconi's anemia with varying degrees of bone marrow depression. The esophageal web is located in the cervical esophagus.

Symptoms. Skin pigmentary changes consist of linear streaks of light brown pigmentation that is darker in the areas of flexure. These changes are sometimes preceded by fine telangiectases most prominent over the face, neck, arms, and chest. Scattered throughout are areas of hypopigmentation. The palms and soles become hyperkeratotic and hyperhydrotic. Dystrophic nail changes progress to nail aplasia.

The teeth are poorly aligned and carious, the hair is sparse, and there is leukoplakia of the lips, mouth, conjunctivae, and anus as well as blepharitis and nasolacrimal obstruction. Some infants also have testicular hypoplasia, mental retardation, or hepatic cirrhosis. Esophageal involvement is indicated by intermittent dysphagia, which becomes continuous and is most marked with ingestion of solids (Fig. 11–22).

Diagnosis. The diagnosis is established by cine-esophagography, which reveals a discrete cervical web, by the typical skin lesions, and by bone marrow changes of aplastic anemia. A few patients have hyperglycinuria.

Treatment. There is no treatment for the disease. The web can be disrupted with an esophagoscope. Any oral or anal leukoplastic lesions should be resected.

Prognosis. Most patients die in the second or third decade as a result of pancytopenia or malignant transformation of the leukoplakia.

INFECTIOUS ESOPHAGITIS

Candidiasis

Candida albicans causes thrush in the mouth of the normal infant, but these lesions usually remain localized. In hypoparathyroidism, hypoadrenocorticism, and conditions in which the host resistance is abnormal, such as immunoglobulin deficiency, chronic illness, and long-term steroid, antibiotic, or immunosuppressive therapy, the fungus may assume the role of a virulent pathogen.[123, 131]

Pathology. When it is most extensively involved, the esophagus is lined with a yellow-white pseudomembrane. At earlier stages, one sees mound-like, grayish lesions with ulcerated centers. The typical fungal mycelia can be obtained from scraping either.

Symptoms. An infant with cutaneous or oral monilial infection in whom feeding problems or regurgitation develops is likely to have esophageal candidiasis.

Diagnosis. The isolation of *Candida* from the oropharynx is a prerequisite for the diagnosis. Radiologic studies of the esopha-

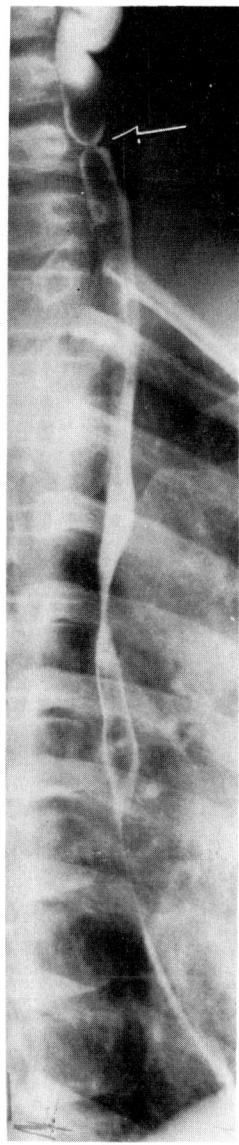

Figure 11–22 This 12-year-old boy had a long history of skin changes and mucosal ulcerations typical of dyskeratosis congenita. Barium swallow for evaluation of dysphagia demonstrated a discrete stricture of the cervical esophagus (*arrow*) and abnormal esophageal motility with infrequent stripping waves. (From Costello, M. J., and Buncke, C. M.: Dyskeratosis congenita. Arch. Dermatol. 72:123, 1956. Copyright 1956, American Medical Association.)

gus present varied findings. Early, there is irritability and spasm with an irregular and granular mucosal pattern. Later, the mucosa is shaggy, ulcerated, or edematous or has a cobblestoned appearance. (Fig. 11–23). A pseudomembrane with a double contour of barium is seen in the most severe cases.

Treatment. Oral nystatin, 100,000 to 200,000 units every six hours for one week,

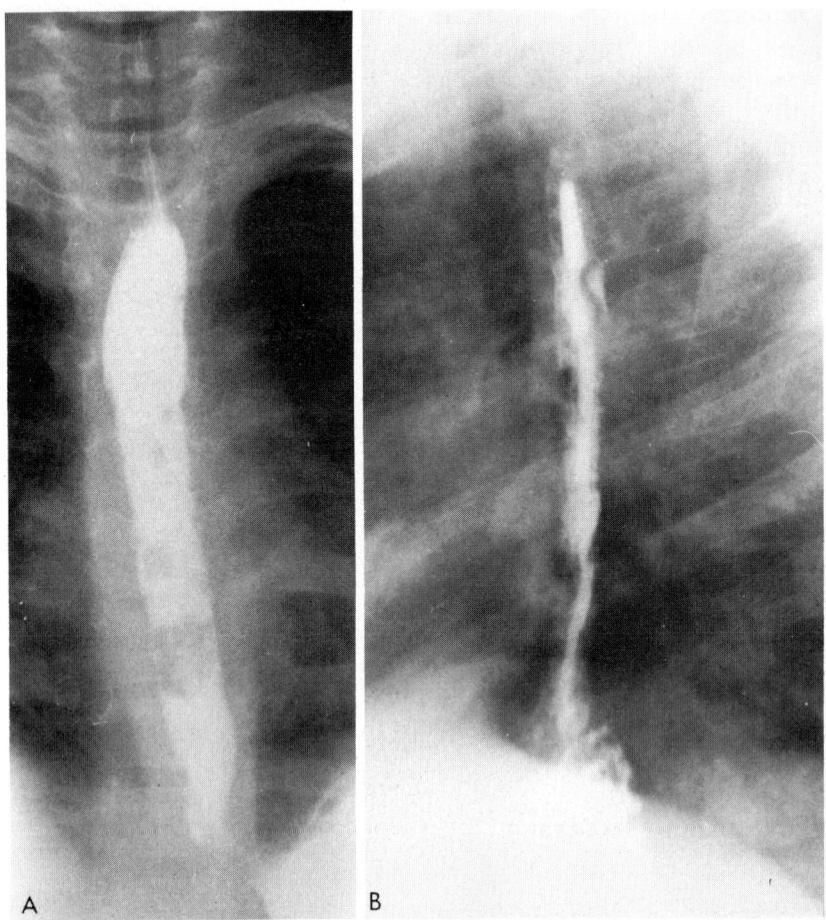

Figure 11–23   Three-year-old boy with acute lymphocytic leukemia who was being treated with steroids and antimetabolites and developed oral thrush and pain upon swallowing. *A,* Frontal view demonstrates irregularity of the esophageal wall associated with esophageal candidiasis. *B,* Lateral view showing severe marginal ulceration. The apparent extraluminal barium collection in the upper esophagus may represent a confluence of deep ulcers covered by a pseudomembrane.

is usually effective. Improvement is noted after two or three days of therapy. Amphotericin B, 0.25 to 1 mg per kg per day, given intravenously for a week, is reserved for refractory cases. Intravenous miconazole has also proved effective. Any underlying metabolic or immunologic disease requires correction.

Prognosis. In uncomplicated cases, healing is complete, but if the fungus has penetrated through the esophageal mucosa, healing is sometimes followed by scarring and stricture.

Meningococcemia

Meningococcemia has been followed by the development of esophageal stricture.

Dysphagia developed in a four-year-old boy four weeks after treatment of meningococcemia. At the time of diagnosis of the disease he had lesions of the conjunctivae and oropharynx as well as of the skin. At no time during treatment was a nasogastric tube passed. A stricture of the middle third of the esophagus was diagnosed and required two dilatations over a four-week period. The child had been free of all esophageal symptoms at a five-year follow-up visit.

Influenzal Viral Infection

This is sometimes associated with transient dysphagia and anterior chest pain accompanying swallowing. On radiologic examination the esophagus appears normal, and the dysphagia is self-limited and responds to treatment with antacids.

Herpes Infection

Generalized herpesvirus infection can cause esophageal ulceration; the ulcers do not often cause esophageal symptoms but may produce severe dysphagia in young children as well as upper gastrointestinal hemorrhage. The esophagus is the most common site of nongenital infection.[15a]

Chagas' Disease

Chagas' disease, caused by *Trypanosoma cruzi*, is endemic in South America, and congenital Chagas' disease has been described in nonendemic areas.[13] It causes a clinical picture resembling achalasia. The acute phase, with a mortality of 10 per cent, presents with fever, hepatomegaly, splenomegaly, cardiomegaly, and cardiac arrhythmias. The organism is identified in a peripheral blood smear. In the chronic phase, there is heart block and dilation of the hollow viscera, particularly the esophagus and colon. Less often, the duodenum, bladder, jejunum, and ureters are dilated. The parasite acts upon nerve and muscle, forming granulomas and cysts that rupture and release a toxin that destroys the ganglion cells. A complement-fixation test is diagnostic in the chronic phase. There is dilation of the esophagus with reduction in the number of ganglion cells. Some patients have acquired cell-mediated immunodepression.[146]

LEUKEMIC INFILTRATE OF THE ESOPHAGUS

As the survival of leukemic patients is prolonged, the incidence of gastrointestinal complications increases. Esophageal infiltrates are usually silent but occasionally cause symptoms of dysphagia and chest pain. Radiologic examination shows diffuse filling defects along the lower third of the esophagus. Radiation therapy to the area produces rapid relief of symptoms.

ANTIBIOTIC-INDUCED ULCERATION

Ulcerations of the esophagus have been attributed to both doxycycline and tetracycline.[42a, 159a]

ESOPHAGEAL ULCERATION AND CEREBRAL DISEASE

Localized or generalized lesions of the brain can produce peptic ulceration of the esophagus as well as of the stomach. The treatment is the same as that for peptic esophagitis.

TRAUMATIC ESOPHAGEAL LESIONS

Trauma from suction with a rigid tube or from a foreign body can cause ulceration or laceration of the esophagus.[20] Anterior laceration of the cervical esophagus has resulted from trauma of a laryngoscope blade. Many instances are associated with vigorous resuscitation of respiratory distress syndrome. Deep tears and perforation are associated with subcutaneous emphysema, pneumothorax and empyema, and mediastinitis (Figs. 11–24 and 11–25). Lesions predisposing to perforation are esophageal stricture, esophageal web, and achalasia. If the tear is high, antibiotic therapy and cervical drainage are effective therapy, but if it is lower, thoracotomy with closure of the tear and chest drainage is mandatory.[33]

Nasogastric intubation for as little as 24 hours can result in peptic esophagitis and stricture.

Vigorous resuscitation and aspiration of the pharynx and stomach of the newborn can perforate the cricopharyngeal wall and cause the formation of an esophageal pseudodiverticulum.[149a, 161] Perforation of the cricopharyngeal wall has followed breech delivery assisted by the obstetrician's finger in the infant's mouth. Traction diverticulum of the esophagus has been associated with a foregut cyst. The symptoms mimic those of tracheoesophageal fistula, with choking, cyanosis, and aspiration. The pseudodiverticulum may be small and confined to the

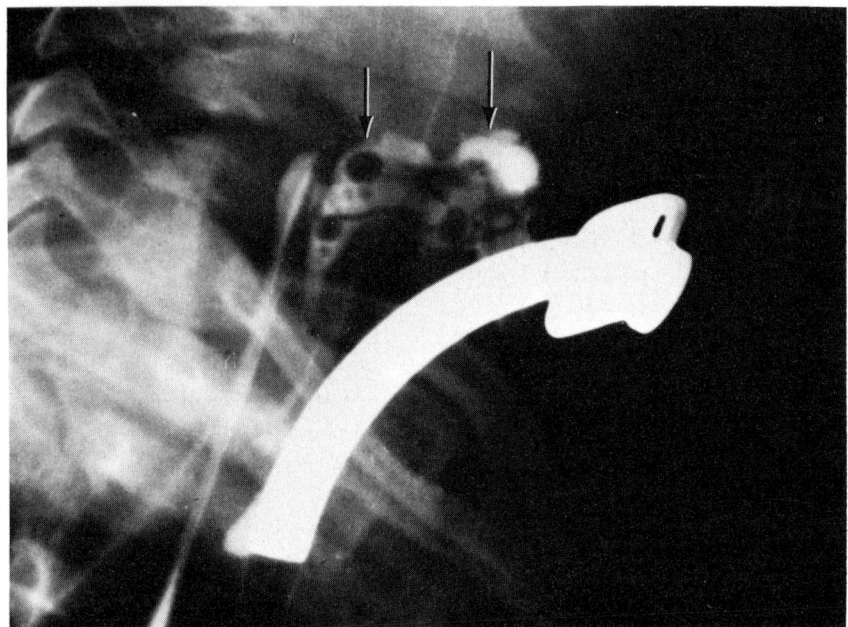

Figure 11–24 Laceration of the esophagus, which occurred at the time of emergency tracheostomy for croup. Lateral spot film of the neck during barium swallow shows extravasation of contrast material from the esophagus toward the anterior neck above the tracheostomy tube (*arrows*).

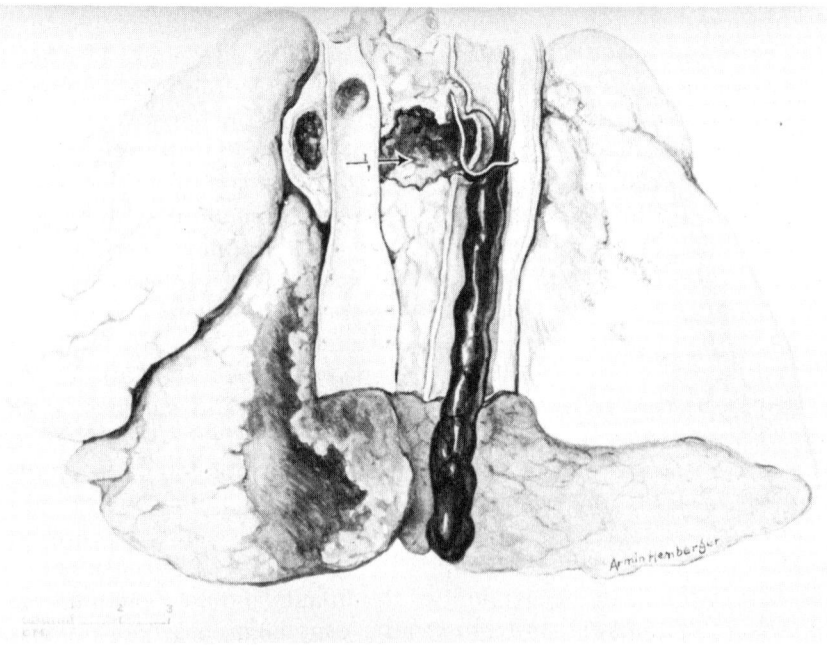

Figure 11–25 Diagrammatic sketch of catastrophic result of wire retained in the esophagus. The wire eroded into the aorta to create a false aneurysm, which ruptured into the esophagus. (Illustration by A. Hemberger, Yale Medical School Art Collection.)

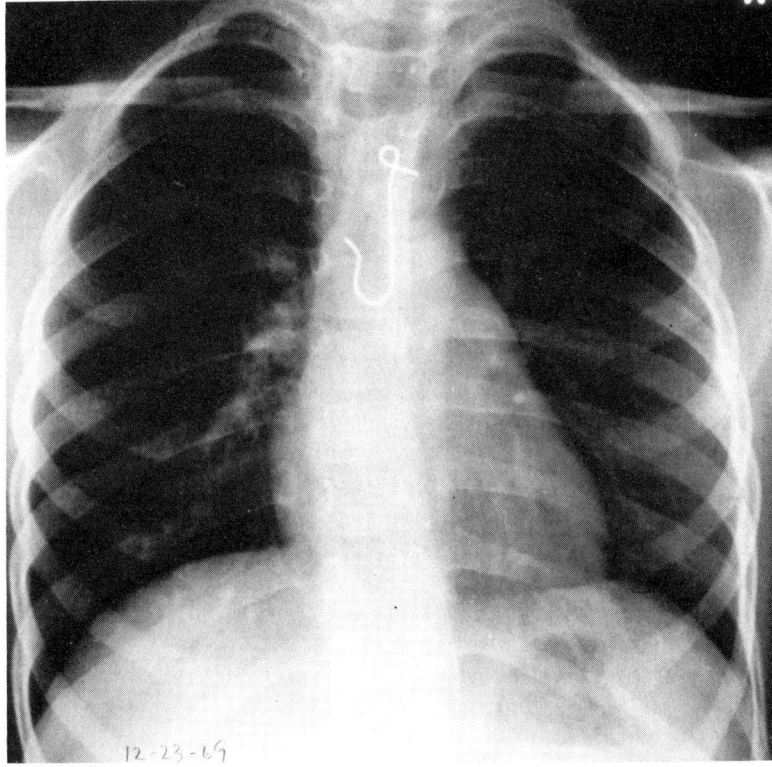

Figure 11–26 Five-year-old boy who accidentally ingested a Christmas tree ornament hanger, which lodged in the mucosa of the upper esophagus.

cervical region, or it may be large and extend to the diaphragm. Radiologic study may be misleading because the mediastinal channels of the diverticula resemble esophageal duplication or true diverticulum (Fig. 11–24). Conservative medical management is usually sufficient, although transcervical drainage may be required.

Foreign Bodies in the Esophagus

Most foreign bodies that are ingested pass uneventfully through the gastrointestinal tract, but some coins, thumbtacks, bones, and other objects become lodged in the esophagus (Figs. 11–25 and 11–26).[28, 98] These snag at the level of the cricopharyngeus, at the aortic arch, or just above the inferior sphincter. Flat objects, such as coins, that lodge in the hypopharynx and cervical esophagus are seen on edge in the lateral film of the neck, whereas those lodged in the upper airway are seen on edge in the frontal film. The infant is given nothing by mouth; if the object is nonopaque, an esophagogram will determine its size and location. Papain and meat tenderizers have been used in attempts to remove a meat bolus by digestion, but they have caused esophageal perforation. Esophagoscopy is the accepted definitive treatment for removal of the foreign body. The patient must be observed in the hospital for 24 hours after treatment for any signs of perforation or continued esophageal obstruction. The chest film or esophagogram should be repeated before the child is discharged.

RUPTURE OF THE ESOPHAGUS OR NEONATAL BOERHAAVE'S SYNDROME

Spontaneous rupture of the esophagus is an extremely rare phenomenon, for when rupture does occur, it is usually secondary to direct traumatic perforation or to necrotizing enterocolitis.[133] Its diagnosis is often overlooked because it presents with the symptoms of a right pneumothorax, which to most examiners connotes a pulmonary origin. True spontaneous rupture is termed Boerhaave's syndrome.[61, 90]

Incidence. Fewer than a dozen cases have been reported.

Etiology and Pathogenesis. In older children and adults, the esophageal tear is preceded by sudden vomiting, coughing, or blunt chest trauma. The left lower lateral wall of the esophagus contains the weakest musculature, and the tear arises in this area. The fact that in the neonate the tear is consistently on the right suggests perhaps a different etiology or an underlying muscular defect. In one of the infants, the tear was above an esophageal web, but in the others no cause could be identified. The lower esophageal sphincter usually remains open during vomiting, but if it is closed during some sudden insult, there is a sharp rise in intraesophageal pressure preceding the tear. Surgical exploration shows a sharp linear tear and no evidence of surrounding esophagitis. There is bacterial contamination of the mediastinum and subcutaneous emphysema. Early pneumothorax is followed by pleural effusion.

Symptoms. The onset in infants is sudden and often follows one or more episodes of vomiting. In two, there was some vomiting, or spitting of blood. In older infants and children, there may be preceding trauma or a paroxysm of coughing, followed by pain on swallowing, vomiting, and respiratory distress. The neonate has only marked respiratory distress with evidence of a pneumothorax: diminished or absent breath sounds, tympanitic percussion of the chest, and retractions and decreased movement of the affected side. There is often subcutaneous emphysema in the neck.

Diagnosis. Chest drainage resembling saliva or containing milk after a feeding is diagnostic, although the early association of subcutaneous emphysema and right pneumothorax should alert the physician to the correct diagnosis. Pneumomediastinum is not common, and early chest films show only tension pneumothorax with or without pleural effusion. Radiologic study of the esophagus with only contrast material shows extravasation along a tract extending into the pleural space. Later there is loculation of the fluid by pleural adhesions. In older children and adults, these findings appear on the left side.

Treatment. Immediate closure of the esophageal tear with chest or mediastinal drainage, antibiotic therapy, and combined gastrostomy and transpyloric feeding will substantially decrease the mortality.

Prognosis. The mortality is about 40 per cent. One of the surviving infants had an esophageal stricture that required dilatations, but the others remained well over several years.

MALLORY-WEISS SYNDROME

Although this syndrome of laceration of the esophagus has been reported in only a few young children, its frequency is probably underestimated, for the diagnosis is confirmed only by endoscopy.[26, 81, 91a]

Etiology. The laceration of the esophagus results from forceful or prolonged vomiting.

Pathology and Physiology. The laceration is located at the esophagogastric junction and cardia of the stomach. The tear is sometimes double, extending only through the mucosa along the longitudinal axis of the organ. There is little inflammatory reaction or fibrosis, but some granulation tissue is apparent with healing. Bleeding is most intense when the gastric as well as the esophageal mucosa is involved.

Symptoms. There is a history of vomiting, either of several acute episodes or of several days' duration. Suddenly the vomitus contains small or large amounts of blood. In one patient, dark blood alternated with bright red blood. In some patients there is a history of achalasia or hiatus hernia.

Diagnosis. Accurate diagnosis is made by visualization of the laceration, which can be actively bleeding or covered with a serofibrinous clot.

Treatment. The medical treatment consists of gastric aspiration to alleviate gastric distention. Gastric hypothermia, vasopressin, and passage of a Sengstaken-Blakemore tube have been used without great success. If hemostasis does not occur, the tear must be sutured. Gelfoam embolization of the left gastric artery has also been effective.[91a]

Prognosis. In adults the mortality is as high as 25 per cent, but in infants it is probably much lower. Recovery usually follows a benign course with rapid cessation of bleeding.

INTRAMURAL DIVERTICULA OF THE ESOPHAGUS

Intramural diverticulosis of the esophagus is an acquired esophageal disease related to primary obstruction and disordered motor function of the esophagus.

Incidence. Approximately 50 instances of this disorder are reported in adults and children who developed intermittent feeding difficulties during the second year of life.[46] It has recently been described in an infant.

Etiology. All the adult patients had a previous history of foreign body in the esophagus, stricture, or disordered motility.[141] The diverticula most likely result from disordered esophageal motility, although *Candida* infection and reflux have also been proposed as etiologic factors. There is a slight male predominance.[157, 158]

Pathology. The diverticula are usually located along the site of a stricture, but in one patient they were located below it. They are of the acquired type, are lined by an intact mucosa, and extend into the submucosa but not into the muscularis. There is some inflammatory reaction in the esophageal submucosa in 90 per cent, submucosal fibrosis in 17 per cent, and columnar-lined mucosa in 6 per cent.

Symptoms. There is a long history of intermittent feeding difficulties before significant dysphagia develops. In some infants there is a history of removal of a foreign body or ingestion of a caustic.

Diagnosis. The radiologic diagnosis is established only after dysphagia is severe, and the x-ray shows an esophageal stricture with walls containing multiple small diverticula. There is some resemblance to the radiologic changes in esophageal moniliasis, but there is no evidence of *Candida* infection.[165] The stricture is either small or large enough to involve half the esophageal length. Esophageal motility studies show noncoordinated waves and hypocontractility in 80 per cent.

Treatment. Relief of the primary cause of esophageal obstruction will improve the dysphagia and lead to a decrease in the number of diverticula.

Prognosis. The prognosis is excellent.

CORROSIVE ESOPHAGITIS

Inquisitive infants cannot discriminate between what is safe and what is unsafe to put in their mouths, and consequently caustic burns are a significant problem in the young child.[19] Corrosive commercial alkalis, such as lye, Dran-O, and Liquid-plumr, are those most frequently ingested. Concentrated sodium hydroxide is a severely damaging agent that produces deep burns through liquefaction necrosis of the esophageal mucosa and its underlying tissue. Weaker alkaline solutions, such as ammonia, cause burns, but they are less likely to lead to stricture formation.[34] Crystals are less often associated with esophageal burns because they cause such pain in the mouth. Esophagitis has been caused by radiation and Adriamycin therapy[101] and by immunodeficiency disorders.[150]

Ingestion of acid is less frequent and rarely causes severe esophagitis, since acids produce coagulation necrosis of only the superficial layers of the esophagus. Strong acid does damage the stomach and duodenum and can even cause perforation of these organs.

Pathology. Because of liquefaction necrosis, alkalis penetrate deeply into the esophageal muscle layers,[78] often destroying the full thickness. Perforation may occur rapidly as a direct result of the burn, or it may be delayed. An intense inflammatory reaction further damages the esophagus and can extend into the mediastinum. Bacterial invasion of the mediastinum occurs even without demonstrable perforation. As healing progresses, granulation tissue replaces the necrotic tissue and fibrous tissue replaces the damaged muscle — all leading to stricture formation.

Pathophysiology. Early dysphagia, within the first 48 hours, is caused by inflammatory edema, which may be so severe as to completely obstruct the esophagus. Late dysphagia is due to stricture.

Symptoms. The infant who has ingested a caustic agent is frightened. He cries, coughs, and spits. A bottle of the ingested material is usually close at hand. Burns are present on the lips and in the oropharynx. Only a third of children with such burns have esophageal burns. The more severe the oral burns, the more likely the possibility of esophageal injury. Conversely, there may on rare occasions be severe esophageal injury with no evidence of burns in the mouth.

Course and Management. The child must be admitted to the hospital and observed for at least 48 hours. A chest film is obtained, and intravenous fluids are administered. He is given nothing by mouth. Some investigators prefer early esophagoscopy (within 12 hours),[144a] but under our present program we delay it until 48 hours after injury lest instrumentation enhance any edema about the arytenoids and cause respiratory obstruction. By 48 hours, burned areas are covered by fibrin patches and are more easily identified. Esophagoscopy is performed under general anesthesia, and the esophagoscope is passed only as far as burn can be visualized. Any further advancement of the instrument increases the risk of perforation. If there is no evidence of an esophageal burn, the patient is discharged and seen in one month for reevaluation. Some investigators do not perform endoscopy but do a celiotomy to determine gastric burn.

If there is an esophageal burn, an oral, broad-spectrum antibiotic is administered for ten days. Steroids[120] (2 mg per kg per day of prednisone) are administered daily, and the dose is tapered over three weeks. Their efficacy is still questioned. Forty-eight hours after the burn the patient can usually swallow; clear liquids are offered first, with subsequent advance to a soft diet. Aspiration pneumonia is a complication most common during the first 48 hours.

Because early cine-esophagography can give false negative results, this study is withheld for several weeks. By the end of the first week, barium swallow shows some deep esophageal ulcerations. Over the next several weeks, the radiologic picture is marked by residual ulceration and an apparent stiffness of the esophageal walls without stricture formation. Peristalsis is deficient, probably because of periesophageal inflammation. The final stage is one of fibrosis and stricture formation, which can involve any portion of the esophagus and may progress over many months.

Steroid therapy must be started within the first few days in order to counteract edema and inhibit fibroplasia. Antibiotics are given to forestall bacterial invasion of the esophageal wall, which is believed to play a role in the pathogenesis of stricture. Some advocate immediate steroid-antibiotic treatment to be continued for ten days without the use of endoscopy. To us, this seems unnecessary if an esophageal burn is not present. If there is no evidence of stricture within the first weeks after the burn, the patient is still evaluated monthly for one year.

Complications. As mentioned, the most frequent complication within the first 48 hours is aspiration pneumonia.

First- and second-degree burns are rarely followed by stricture, but this complication does develop after severe burns in nearly half of untreated patients between three weeks and six months after the burn (Fig. 11–27). Combined steroid-antibiotic treatment has reduced the incidence of stricture to between 4 and 13 per cent. Treatment is discussed in the next section. If there is severe necrosis of the esophagus, esophagectomy and later colon interposition may be necessary.

Disordered esophageal motility persists from nine days to two years after lye ingestion. Peristaltic contractions after a swallow are weak or absent, or else there are many repetitive contractions, causing some dysphagia.

Other Cause of Esophagitis

Esophagitis has been noted in children with immune deficiency and neutropenia and has been associated with Adriamycin and radiation therapy for childhood malignancy.

ACQUIRED ESOPHAGEAL STRICTURE

Esophageal stricture is most often caused by esophagitis due to the reflux of acid gastric contents into the esophagus through an incompetent lower esophageal sphincter, as in chalasia, hiatus hernia, or congenital short esophagus.[94] Acquired strictures follow the ingestion of caustic alkalis, the use of nasogastric tubes, and meningococcemia[19] and are also associated with the skin disease epidermolysis bullosa.

Pathology. All levels of the esophagus are equally vulnerable to acid-peptic digestion, but the area nearest the source of the digestive solution is that most severely injured. Bile combined with acid reflux is more severe than that due to acid alone. Superficially, the mucosal lesions form and tend to heal by regeneration of the mucosa, while the inflammatory process continues within the deeper layers of muscularis and heals by fibrosis. Esophagitis has been shown to decrease the lower esophageal sphincter, and this further perpetuates reflux.

Symptoms. There is by definition an event antecedent to stricture development: either ingestion of a caustic substance or a history of chronic or intermittent regurgitation or vomiting. There is first some difficulty in swallowing solids or semi-solids and later difficulty in swallowing liquids. The infants choke during feeding attempts and eventually cannot swallow even their own oral secretions at rest. As caloric and fluid intake is cut off, weight loss is evident. Urination and defecation decrease in frequency.

Diagnosis. The history is typical for the diagnosis of stricture, but the final diagnosis is made by esophagography. In the typical stricture that develops after reflux esophagitis, one first sees gastroesophageal reflux or a hiatus hernia or both. Esophagitis can develop in the absence of demonstrable reflux, however. Rarely seen in children is an intermediate stage marked by distal esophageal edema and ulceration. The pathognomonic abnormality is progressive esophageal stricture, usually distal, although it can extend the entire length of the esophagus. There may be shortening of the esophagus, with partial thoracic stomach.

Treatment. A short stricture is treated successfully with dilatations. During and after treatment the infants are maintained in the semi-erect position and given small, frequent feedings.[56] If bougienage is unsuccessful, or if the stricture is long, esophageal reconstruction with protection of the interposed colon by vagotomy and pyloroplasty might be necessary.[70] Some have reported success with local injection of steroids, but the consensus does not favor this procedure.[120]

Prognosis. Unless the primary cause for stricture formation is relieved, the stricture will recur and progress in extent.

ESOPHAGEAL VARICES

Esophageal varices are not often encountered in infants, but they are becoming an increasingly frequent cause of upper gastrointestinal bleeding in children.

Etiology and Pathology. Esophageal varices are large, dilated veins in the submucosal layer of the lower esophageal wall that develop as a result of portal hypertension. This is secondary to obstruction of the portal or splenic venous blood flow. The causes of portal hypertension are best examined according to the site of the obstruction. The two major causes are prehepatic block, usually due to portal vein thrombosis, and cirrhosis, due to chronic liver disease. In children the former is twice as common as the latter.[91, 112, 117]

Extrahepatic portal vein obstruction is

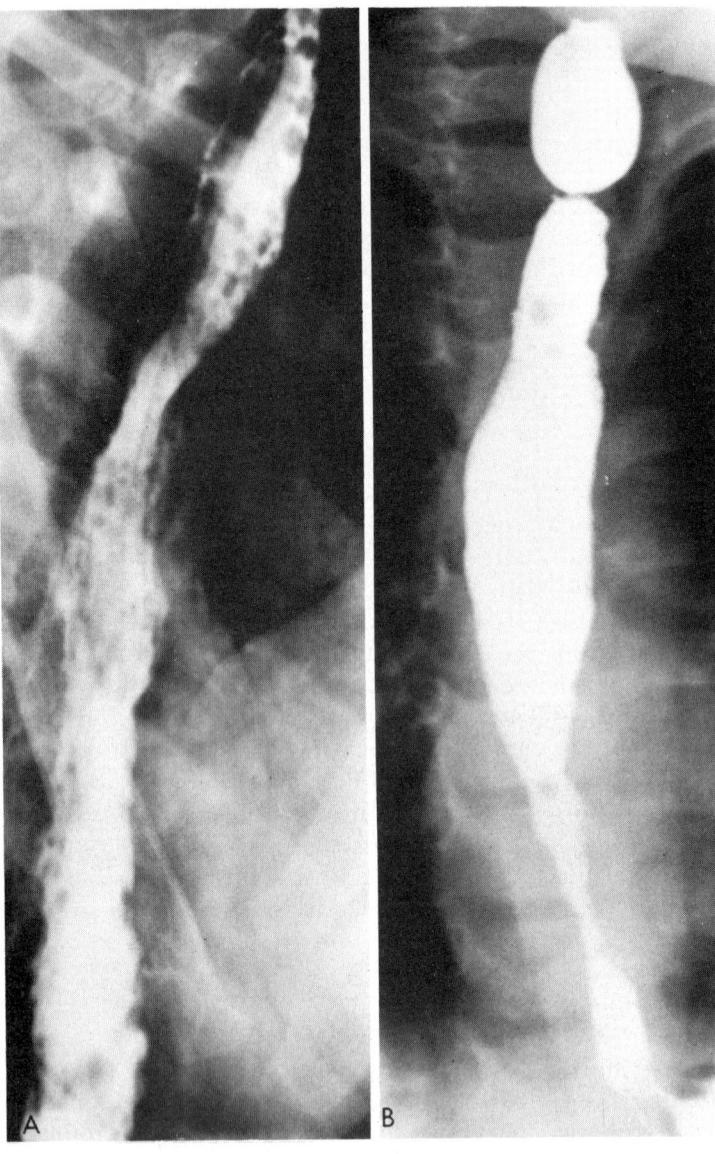

Figure 11–27 Three-year-old girl who developed an esophageal stricture after ingesting Dran-O. *A*, Barium swallow 12 days after ingestion demonstrates edema and ulceration of the esophageal wall without evidence of stricture. *B*, Repeat study nine weeks later shows a tight stricture of the upper esophagus with irregular narrowing of the lower esophagus, representing a stage of active fibrosis.

Illustration continued on opposite page

usually due to thrombosis, fibrosis, or congenital malformation of the portal or splenic vein. Portal vein thrombosis is now recognized as a complication of exchange transfusion and umbilical vein catheterization.[92] When such obstruction follows an illness in which there has been high fever and dehydration, it is termed acquired bland thrombosis; when it follows an infectious process such as omphalitis, peritonitis, or sepsis, it is termed septic thrombosis.[3, 83, 153] Intrahepatic portal vein obstruction follows primary liver disease in which fibrosis and scarring within the liver parenchyma

obstruct the normal blood flow and divert it into anastomotic channels connecting the portal and systemic circulations.

Normally, blood circulates from the portal system through sinusoids of the liver into the hepatic vein and into the inferior vena cava. In portal hypertension, the normal blood flow from the gastric coronary veins into the splenic vein reverses, and collaterals open between the esophageal and gastric veins (Fig. 11–28) through shunts which are probably existent but nonfunctional in health. Veins from the lower esophagus, cardia, and fundus of the stomach drain into the left gastric vein and to the azygos and superior vena cava. A similar situation develops with the collaterals about the umbilicus and in the region of the internal hemorrhoidal veins. As increased portal pressure is transmitted through patent esophageal submucosal collaterals, these usually small veins become dilated and tortuous. Varices in young infants follow intrauterine viral infection with portal hypertension as caused by cytomegalovirus or portal vein thrombosis.

Symptoms. Massive hematemesis is the most frequent presenting symptom. An unusual presentation of esophageal hemorrhage is bleeding per rectum or melena. The onset of hemorrhage in children with portal vein thrombosis is earlier than in those with cirrhosis, but it usually does not occur before the age of five years. Bleeding episodes are often precipitated by a febrile illness, but some suspect that aspirin is responsible, rather than the illness. Less frequent presenting symptoms and findings are sple-

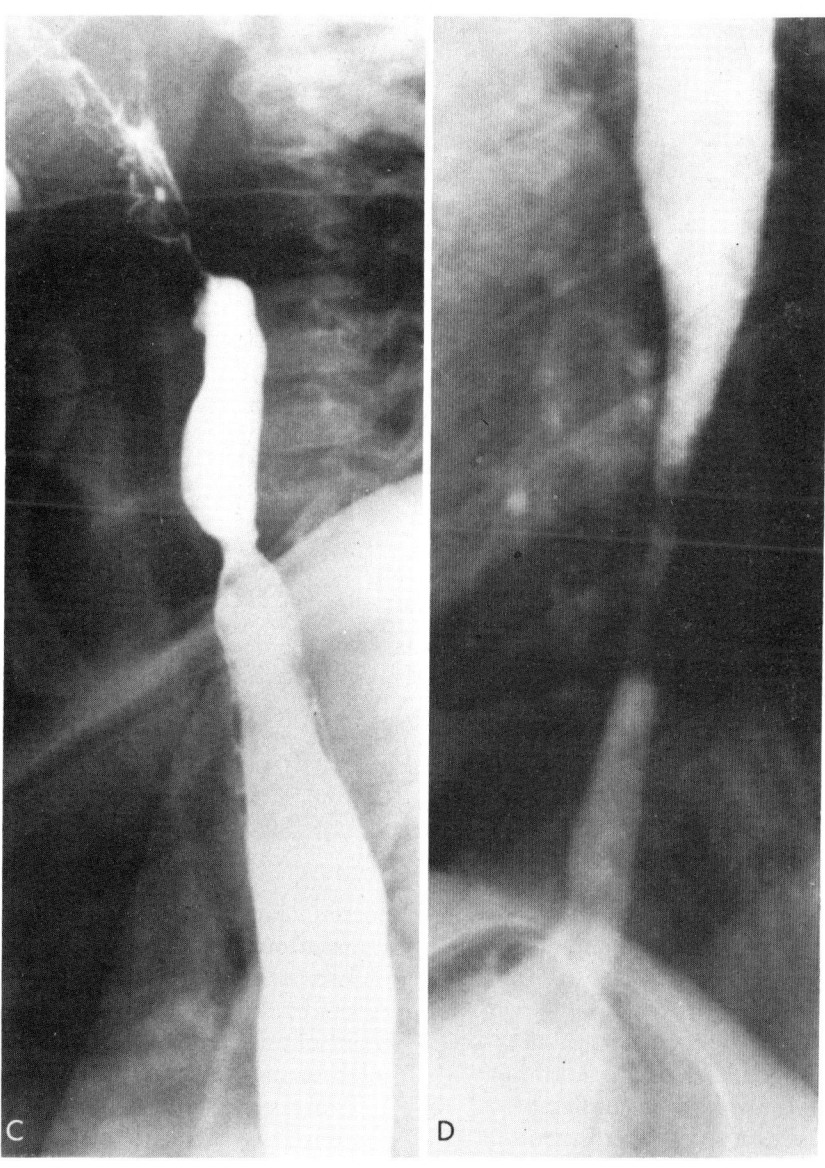

Figure 11–27 Continued C and *D,* Study done one year later and after several dilatations. The child had significant dysphagia, although the localized stricture in the upper esophagus is less tight than in the earlier study. A long segment of distal esophagus remains narrowed.

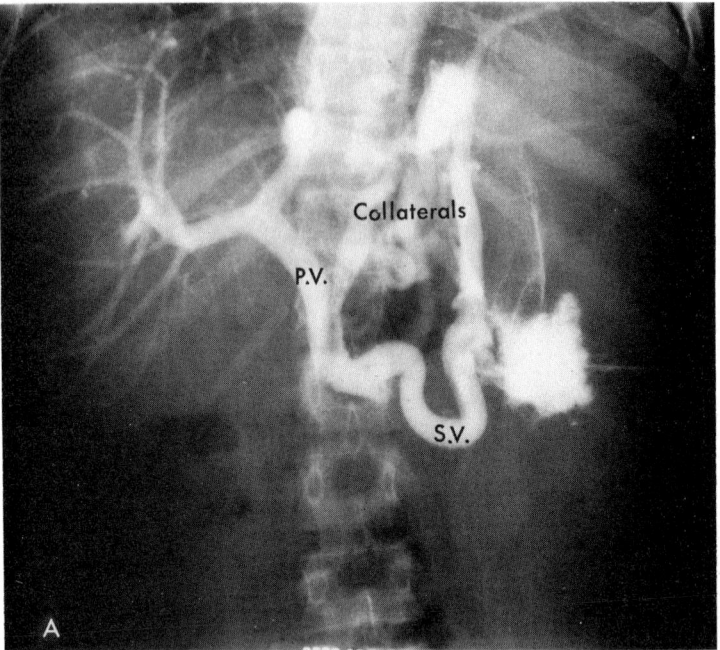

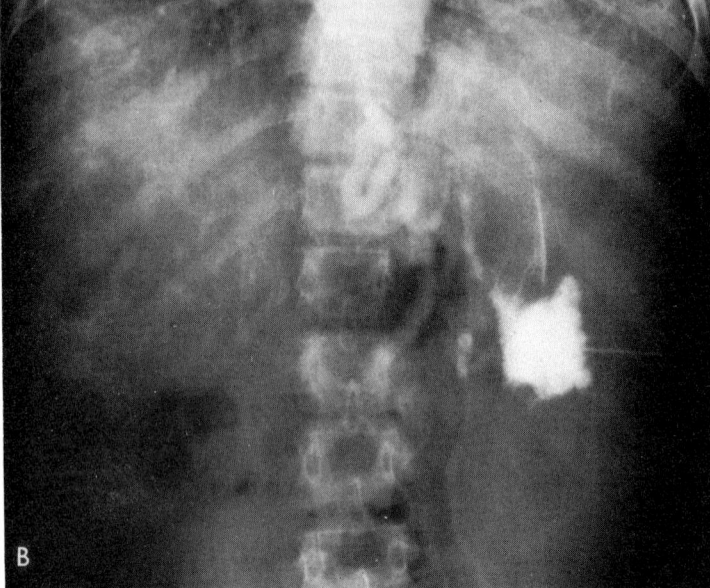

Figure 11–28 This 14-year-old boy had a known history of Wilson's disease and a recent upper gastrointestinal bleed. Barium swallow demonstrated esophageal varices. The splenoportogram defines the dense collection of dye in the left upper quadrant *(A)* representing collection of contrast material within the spleen. There is good opacification of the splenic vein (S.V.) and of the portal vein (P.V.), both of which are patent. Coursing toward the diaphragm are a group of collateral vessels in and around the fundus of the stomach. *B*, A later film from the same study showing several tortuous veins in the midline ascending as esophageal varices.

nomegaly, collateral circulation over the abdomen, fever, ascites or hepatomegaly, and clubbing.

The clinical history in infants with extrahepatic portal vein obstruction is often relatively innocent, and the patient is without symptoms until the onset of a bleed. An early neonatal history of respiratory distress, omphalitis, or exchange transfusion can be elicited. Some children are anemic for months to years before the gross bleed

occurs. The occasional infant has growth retardation and ascites during the first year of life. The ascites subsides as a result of recanalization of the thrombus or development of adequate collateral circulation, but anemia and growth retardation persist.

Those with intrahepatic obstruction have demonstrated prior symptoms of liver disease or cystic fibrosis. Hepatic disorders causing this degree of portal obstruction are hepatic or biliary cirrhosis, the focal biliary cirrhosis of cystic fibrosis, congenital hepatic fibrosis, Wilson's disease, and Gaucher's disease. Hepatomegaly either is present at the time of examination or has been noted before demonstration of varices. If the liver is very cirrhotic, it is no longer palpable.

Examination of the abdomen may reveal the caput medusae, a ring of dilated vessels about the umbilicus. Sigmoidoscopy will demonstrate internal hemorrhoids or a blue to purple coloration of the rectal mucosa. If ascites is present, the abdomen is dull to percussion and a fluid wave can be elicited. Hepatomegaly or splenomegaly or both should arouse immediate suspicion of varices as the cause of bleeding. If the patient is examined immediately after a bleed, the portal system is decompressed and the spleen is no longer palpable. Examination must be repeated after the blood volume has been restored. A disordered sensorium in the child with liver disease signals hyperammonemic encephalopathy precipitated by the bleed.

Diagnosis and Management. Frequently the bleeding has stopped by the time the child arrives at the hospital. One is justified in watching the patient closely at first and managing him conservatively. Vital signs are monitored, and fresh blood is given to maintain the hematocrit between 30 and 35 per cent. Small amounts of oral antacids help to coat the esophagus and alkalinize any refluxed gastric contents. If the infant is vomiting or unresponsive, a nasogastric tube is passed into the stomach and gentle continuous suction is applied to it.

Immediate laboratory studes must include tests of liver function and clotting and ceruloplasmin concentration. Nearly half of those patients with extrahepatic obstruction have hematologic evidence of hypersplenism, such as thrombocytopenia, pancytopenia, or neutropenia. The cirrhosis of cystic fibrosis is focal, so that liver function tests are usually normal. In all of the other liver diseases they are almost always abnormal.

When the vital signs are stable, endoscopy should be performed to determine whether bleeding is actually due to varices. Radiologic examination is helpful not only to demonstrate varices but also to exclude other causes of upper gastrointestinal bleeding, such as peptic ulcer or hiatus hernia. Some report good results from cineradiography examinations with the infant drinking regular barium; others prefer to take multiple films after the infant ingests a barium paste, which coats the esophagus (Fig. 11–29). These techniques are not infallible, for even in the adult there is a poor correlation between radiologic findings and those found at esophagoscopy. The most valuable study is splenoportography and measurement of splenic pulp pressure (which in most is over 200 mm saline). Ideally, this should be done prior to surgery by the percutaneous route when the patient is stable and while there is time to evaluate the films. It can be performed at the time of surgery, however. Water-soluble contrast material is injected into the splenic pulp and rapid filming of the abdomen is performed over 20 to 30 seconds. This technique permits visualization of the portal vein anatomy and any collateral circulation. A pulp pressure of 30 cm saline or H_2O or greater indicates portal hypertension. It has been noted that the risk of bleeding is not consistently related to increased portal pressure; however, most patients with levels under 25 mm H_2O do not bleed, and those with pressures over 40 mm Hg do. Any abnormality of the blood clotting mechanism contraindicates performance of this examination by the percutaneous route. Selective celiac-axis aortography demonstrates portal circulation in the venous phase. Suprahepetic portal vein obstruction cannot be demonstrated by splenoportography but is shown by contrast study of the inferior vena cava or hepatic veins. Such studies are technically difficult in those under two years of age.

If significant bleeding persists or recurs after blood replacement, sedation and rest and intermittent doses of intravenous Pitressin are used.[130] A dose of 2 to 4 milliunits per kg per minute in 5 per cent dextrose is administered over a 20- to 30-minute period every 4 hours for 24 hours. The drug causes constriction of the splanchnic arterioles and decreases portal flow and esophageal ve-

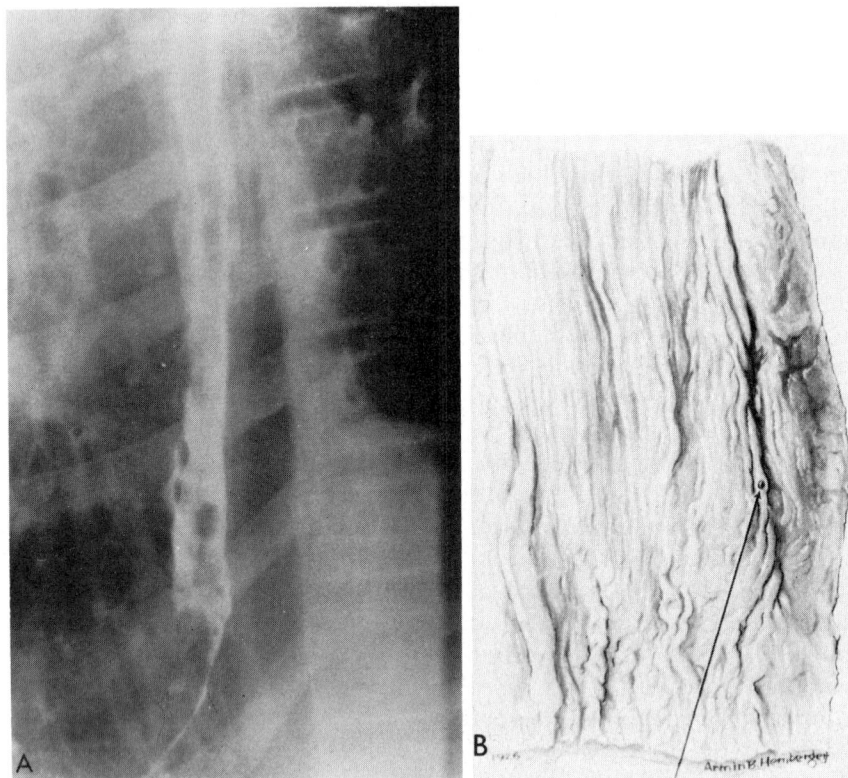

Figure 11–29 Twelve-year-old boy with cystic fibrosis, biliary cirrhosis, and esophageal varices. The varices are clearly seen as nodular filling defects in the barium column. These may be more evident if the patient performs the Valsalva maneuver during the study. *B*, Diagrammatic representation of esophageal varices with punctate bleeding site *(arrow)*. (Illustration by A. Hemberger, Yale Medical School Art Collection.)

nous pressures. A second course of Pitressin can be given if bleeding resumes. Constant infusion of drug in a dose of 0.2 to 0.4 unit per ml per minute over several days into the superior mesenteric artery controls variceal bleeding by decreasing superior mesenteric blood flow and, secondarily, portal pressure. This technique, used in adults, seems rather drastic for the small child, and recent studies show little difference from peripheral therapy. Ischemic necrosis of the bowel may be a complication of Pitressin as well as hypertension, bradycardia, water retention, and arrhythmia.

The Sengstaken-Blakemore tube is placed in the esophagus to control bleeding that persists despite the aforementioned measures. A chest film determines the accurate placement of the balloon in the lower esophagus. It is intermittently deflated at 6-hour intervals over a 24-hour period to avoid pressure necrosis of the esophagus. The balloon is then deflated, and the tube is

left in place for the next 12 to 24 hours while the patient is observed for bleeding. If bleeding persists or recurs, the only recourse is surgery, but the immediate surgical management is aimed at stopping the bleeding; shunting should not be attempted as an emergency procedure. Transesophageal and transgastric ligation of the varices or injection of sclerosing agents is a safe palliative procedure. Ligation is followed by bleed-free periods of three months to two years.[85a] Techniques using direct cautery of the bleeding vessels or spraying of hemostatic agents are being evaluated.

Some advocate resection of the lower esophagus with esophagogastrectomy and interposition of a jejunal or colonic segment and vagotomy and pyloroplasty. Such a procedure removes the acid- and pepsin-producing regions of the stomach and separates the communications between portal and venous systems. It carries both a high mortality and a high incidence of postoperative reflux esophagitis and is not recommended for the small child. The entire goal of management is to maintain the child until he is large enough for a shunting procedure. Ascites developing during this period is managed by salt restriction and administration of intravenous albumin and diuretics. Children with known liver disease should have serum ammonia monitored and dietary protein adjusted accordingly.

Shunting procedures were originally looked upon with favor. Results of long-term follow-up have not proved promising, however, for bleeding recurs within three months to six years in about 70 per cent of patients.[97] With splenorenal shunts there is a tendency to thrombosis, or else the anastomosis is too small to reduce the portal pressure adequately. Shunting has been performed in one-year-old infants, but it is best to wait until the child is five or six years of age or 60 to 70 pounds, when the vessels are larger and there is less technical difficulty and risk of thrombosis.[34] The best operation for those with cirrhosis is the portacaval shunt, which in these children seems to prevent further hemorrhage. If the splenic vein measures 1 cm or more in diameter, a splenorenal shunt is also effective and is more physiologic because the liver continues to receive blood from the intestine. Since the portacaval shunt bypasses the flow of blood from intestine to liver, there is a significant incidence of postshunt hepatic encephalopathy, which may become apparent several years after surgery. Shunting is most difficult in patients with portal vein thrombosis, for the splenic vein is often small or occluded. Either the superior mesenteric vein to inferior vena cava, or mesocaval, anastomosis or the central splenorenal shunt described by Clatworthy is the procedure of choice. Splenectomy is not indicated in the treatment of portal hypertension.

Since there is a high rate of shunt thrombosis and since some varices, such as those related to cavernous transformation of the portal vein or to biliary atresia, may decrease with time, other means of therapy have been investigated. Lilly[45] has recently used staged endoscopic sclerosis of varices with injection of 5 per cent sodium mor-

rhuate as temporizing therapy in seven children, with no rebleed noted at two-year follow-up.

Management of patients with varices that have never bled is controversial.[129] Cirrhotic patients with portal hypertension have no better survival after prophylactic shunt.[118] Our belief is that children should be managed expectantly. The figures of Arcari and Lynn[6] indicate that no children have died during their first bleed, and only 1 of 42 did so after a second one — indicating that early surgical intervention may be delayed.

All patients with known esophageal varices should be cautioned to avoid ingestion of salicylates.

Prognosis. The prognosis varies with the underlying disease but in general is poor.[34] The mortality in those managed medically is about 40 per cent within the first few years of the first major bleed and 20 to 30 per cent in those managed surgically.[6] Rebleeding occurs in 55 to 85 per cent of those whose varices were ligated without shunting. In the series of Meyers and Robinson,[91] 7 of 47 children died, 6 because of underlying liver disease. Alagile and Odievre[3] report thrombosis of the shunt in 5 of 35 children with prehepatic portal hypertension. Of 47 operated on for intrahepatic portal hypertension, thrombosis of the shunt occurred in only three, but eight died of liver failure.

Causes of Disordered Peristalsis

Central nervous system disease
  vascular
  demyelinating
  degenerative
  injury
Myasthenia gravis
Intramural esophageal disease
  ganglia — achalasia
           Chagas' disease
  tumor — diffuse leiomyoma
  irritation — GE reflux
          Candida esophagitis
          caustic burns
  myopathy — collagen disease
          thyrotoxicosis
          muscular dystrophies
          ocular dystrophy

REFERENCES

1. Absolon, K. D., Finney, A., Waddill, G. M., Jr., and Hatchett, C.: Esophageal reconstruction colon transplant in two brothers with epidermolysis bullosa. Surgery 65:832, 1969.
2. Addison, J., and Rice, M. S.: The association of dyskeratosis congenita and Fanconi anemia. Med. J. Aust. 1:797, 1965.
3. Alagile, D., and Odievre, M.: Liver and Biliary Tract Disease in Children. New York, John Wiley & Sons, 1978, p. 262.
4. Allen, M. S., and Thomson, S. A.: Congenital diaphragmatic hernia in children under 1 year of age: a 24 year review. J. Pediatr. Surg. 1:156, 1966.
5. Al-Rashid, R. A., and Harned, R. K.: Dysphagia due to leukemic involvement of the esophagus. Am. J. Dis. Child. 121:75, 1971.
6. Arcari, F. A., and Lynn, H. B.: Bleeding esophageal varices in children. Surg. Gynecol. Obstet. 122:101, 1961.
7. Ardran, G. M., and Kemp, F. H.: Normal and disturbed swallowing. Prog. Pediatr. Radiol. 2:151, 1969.
8. Armstrong, R. G., Lindberg, E., Stanford, W., Takamoto, R. M., Wolf, R. D., and Dietz, J. W.: Traumatic pseudodiverticulum of the esophagus in the newborn infant. Surgery 47:844, 1970.
9. Ashcraft, K. W., and Holder, T. M.: The story of esophageal atresia and tracheoesophageal fistula. Surgery 65:332, 1969.
9a. Axelrod, F., Schneider, K., Ament, M., Kutin, N., and Fonkalsrud, E.: Gastroesophageal fundoplication and gastrostomy in familial dysautonomia. Ann. Surg. 195:253, 1982.
10. Aziskhan, R., Tapper, D., and Eraklis, A.: Achalasia in childhood: a 20 year experience. J. Pediatr. Surg. 15:452, 1980.
11. Bakwin, H., Galenson, E., and LeVine, B. E.: Roentgenographic appearance of esophagus in normal infants. Am. J. Dis. Child. 68:243, 1944.
12. Ballantine, T. V., Fitzgerald, S., and Grosfeld, J.: Trans-thoracic esophagomyotomy for achalasia in childhood. J. Pediatr. Surg. 15:457, 1980.
12a. Bar-Maor, J. A., Shoshany, G., and Monies-Chass, I.: Use of cimetidine in esophageal atresia with lower tracheoesophageal fistula. J. Pediatr. Surg. 16:8, 1981.
13. Barner, H.: Esophageal atresia and tracheoesophageal fistula: preoperative assessment and reduced mortality. Ann. Thorac. Surg. 28:54, 1979.
14. Barousse, A. P., Esposito, M. O., Mandel, S., and Martinez, F. S.: Congenital Chagas' disease in a non-endemic area. Medicina 38:611, 1978.
15. Barrett, N. R.: The lower esophagus lined by columnar epithelium. Surgery 41:881, 1954.
15a. Bastian, J. F., and Kaufman, I. A.: Herpes simplex esophagitis in a healthy 10 year old boy. J. Pediatr. 100:426, 1982.
16. Basu, R., Forshall, I., and Rickham, P. O.: Duplications of the alimentary tract. Br. J. Surg. 47:477, 1960.
17. Bell, M. J., and Ternberg, D.: Antenatal diagnosis

18. of diaphragmatic hernia. Pediatrics 60:738, 1973.
18. Berdon, W. E., and Baker, D. H.: Vascular anomalies and the infant lung: Rings, slings and other things. Semin. Roentgenol. 7:39, 1972.
19. Bernischke, K.: Time bomb of lye ingestion. Am. J. Dis. Child. 135:17, 1980.
20. Berry, B. E., and Ochsner, J. L.: Perforation of the esophagus. J. Thorac. Cardiovasc. Surg. 65:1, 1973.
21. Bismuth, H., and Franco, D.: Portal diversion for portal hypertension in early childhood. Ann. Surg. 183:496, 1976.
22. Blackburn, W. R., and Amoury, R. A.: Congenital esophago-pulmonary fistula without esophageal atresia: an analysis of 260 fistulas in infants, children and adults. Rev. Surg. 23:153, 1966.
22a. Bloss, R. S., Aranda, J. V., and Beardmore, H. E.: Congenital diaphragmatic hernia: pathophysiologic and pharmacologic support. Surgery 89:518, 1981.
23. Blumberg, J. B., Stevenson, J. K., Lemire, R., and Boydon, E. A.: Laryngotracheoesophageal cleft, the embryologic implications: review of the literature. Surgery 57:559, 1965.
23a. Bosher, L. P., and Shaw, A.: Achalasia in siblings. Am. J. Dis. Child. 135:709, 1981.
24. Botha, G. M. S.: The gastro-esophageal region of infants. Arch. Dis. Child. 33:78, 1958.
25. Bouslog, J. S.: The gastrointestinal tract in children. Radiology 28:683, 1937.
26. Bouyala, J. M., Gonggryp, N., Seriat-Gauthier, B., and Pages, M.: Le syndrome de Mallory-Weiss chez l'enfant. Ann. Chir. Infant. 13:313, 1972.
26a. Boyle, J. T., Cohen, S., and Watkins, J. B.: Successful treatment of achalasia in childhood by pneumatic dilatation. J. Pediatr. 99:35, 1981.
27. Breton, R. J., Zachary, R., and Spitz, L.: Preventable death in oesophageal atresia. Arch. Dis. Child. 53:276, 1978.
28. Brooks, J. W.: Foreign bodies in the air and food passages. Ann. Surg. 175:720, 1972.
29. Brown, R. E., Madge, G. E., and Howell, J. R.: Congenital short esophagus in the newborn. Am. J. Dig. Dis. 15:863, 1970.
30. Carre, I. J., and Astley, R.: The fate of partial thoracic stomach. Arch. Dis. Child. 35:484, 1960.
31. Chatrath, R. R., el-Shafie, M., and Jones, R. S.: Fate of hypoplastic lungs after repair of congenital diaphragmatic hernia. Arch. Dis. Child. 46:633, 1971.
32. Christie, D., and Knauss, T. A.: Gastrointestinal manifestations of "acquired dysautonomic" syndrome. J. Pediatr. 94:605, 1979.
33. Clarke, T. A., Coe, U. R., Feldman, B., and Papile, L.: Esophageal perforations in premature infants and comments on the diagnosis. Am. J. Dis. Child. 134:367, 1980.
34. Clatworthy, H. W.: Extrahepatic portal hypertension. In Child, C. G. (ed.): Portal Hypertension. Philadelphia, W. B. Saunders Company, 1974, p. 243.
35. Cohen, S.: Motor disorders of the esophagus. N. Engl. J. Med. 301:184, 1979.
36. Davies, M. R., and Coyes, S.: The flaccid trachea

and tracheoesophageal congenital anomalies. J. Pediatr. Surg. 13:363, 1978.

37. Dent, J.: What's new in the esophagus. Dig. Dis. Sci. 26:161, 1981.

38. Dieter, R. A., Jr., Riker, W. L., and Holinger, J.: Pedunculated esophageal hamartoma in a child. J. Thorac. Cardiovasc. Surg. 59:851, 1970.

39. Dodds, W. J., Dent, J., Hogan, W., Patel, G., Toouli, J., and Arndorfer, R. C.: Paradoxical lower esophageal sphincter contraction induced by cholecystocininoctapeptide in patients with achalasia. Gastroenterology 80:327, 1981.

40. Eckardt, V. F., Adami, B., Hucker, H., and Leeder, H.: The esophagogastric junction in patients with asymptomatic lower esophageal mucosal ring. Gastroenterology 79:426, 1980.

40a. Ein, S., Barker, G., Olley, P., Shandling, B., Simpson, J., Stephens, C., and Filler, R.: Pharmacologic treatment of newborn diaphragmatic hernia: 2 year evaluation. J. Pediatr. Surg. 15:384, 1980.

41. Eklof, O., Ekstrom, G., Eriksson, B. O., Michaelsson, M., Stephenson, O., Soderlund, S., Thoren, C., and Wallgren, G.: Arterial anomalies causing compression of the trachea and/or the esophagus. Acta Paediatr. Scand. 60:81, 1971.

42. Emery, J. L., and Haddadin, A. J.: Gastric-type epithelium in the upper esophageal pouch in children with tracheo-esophageal fistula. J. Pediatr. Surg. 6:449, 1971.

42a. Florent, C., Chagnon, J. P., Vivet, P., Brun, J. G., Cattan, D., and Bernier, J. J.: Esophageal ulceration due to doxycycline. Gastroenterologie Clin. Biol. 4:888, 1980.

43. Fonkalsrud, E., and Ament, M.: Surgical management of esophageal stricture due to recessive dystrophic epidermolysis bullosa. J. Pediatr. Surg. 12:221, 1977.

44. Forshall, I.: Less common herniae through the diaphragm of infants and children. Proc. R. Soc. Med. 59:212, 1966.

45. Frates, R. E.: Roentgen signs in laryngotracheo-esophageal cleft. Radiology 88:484, 1967.

46. Fromkes, J., Thomas, F., Mekhicor, H., Caldwell, J., and Johnson, J.: Esophageal intramural pseudodiverticulosis. Dig. Dis. 22:690, 1977.

47. Goodwin, C., Ashcraft, K., Holder, T., Johnson, R., and Amoure, R.: Esophageal atresia with double tracheoesophageal fistula. J. Pediatr. Surg. 13:269, 1978.

48. Goyal, R., Glancy, J., and Spiro, H. M.: Lower esophageal ring. I. N. Engl. J. Med. 282:1298, 1970.

49. Goyal, R., Glancy, J., and Spiro, H. M.: Lower esophageal ring. II. N. Engl. J. Med. 282:1355, 1970.

50. Goyal, R., Bauer, J., and Spiro, H. M.: The nature and location of lower esophageal ring. N. Engl. J. Med. 284:1175, 1971.

51. Grosfeld, J., O'Neill, J. A., Jr., and Clatworthy, H. W.: Enteric duplications in infancy and childhood: an 18-year review. Ann. Surg. 172:83, 1970.

52. Grossman, H. J., Limosani, M. A., and Shore, M.: Megacolon as a manifestation of familial autonomic dysfunction. J. Pediatr. 49:284, 1956.

53. Gryboski, J. D.: The swallowing mechanism of the neonate. I. Esophageal and gastric motility. Pediatrics 35:445, 1965.

54. Gryboski, J. D., Thayer, W. R., Jr., and Spiro, H. M.: Esophageal motility in infants and children. Pediatrics 31:382, 1963.

55. Haddadin, A., and Emery, J. L.: Pulmonary retention simulating pneumonia as a cause of death in children with tracheoesophageal fistula. Surgery 70:311, 1971.

56. Haller, J. A., Jr., Andrews, H. G., White, J. W., Tamer, M. A., and Cleveland, W.: Pathophysiology and management of corrosive burns of the esophagus: results of treatment in 285 children. J. Pediatr. Surg. 6:578, 1971.

57. Haller, J. A., Jr., Brooker, A. F., Talbert, J. L., Baghdassarian, O., and Vanhoutte, J.: Esophageal function following resection. Studies in newborn puppies. Ann. Thorac. Surg. 2:180, 1966.

58. Hallewell, J. D., and Cole, T. B.: Isolated head and neck symptoms due to hiatus hernia. Arch. Otolaryngol. 92:488, 1970.

59. Handelman, N., and Nelson, T.: Association of milk precipitins with esophageal lesions causing aspiration. Pediatrics 34:699, 1964.

60. Hanson, E. L., Daly, J., and Davis, D.: Ulceration associated with an islet of columnar epithelium in the mid-esophagus: new evidence for an acquired etiology of Barrett's syndrome. J. Pediatr. Surg. 5:370, 1970.

61. Harrell, G. S., Friedland, G. W., Daily, W. J., and Cohn, R. B.: Neonatal Boerhaave's syndrome. Radiology 95:665, 1970.

62. Harrison, M. R., Bjordal, R., Langmark, F., and Knutrud, O.: Congenital diaphragmatic hernia: the mortality. J. Pediatr. Surg. 13:220, 1978.

62a. Harrison, M. R., and de Lorimer, A. A.: Congenital diaphragmatic hernia. Surg. Clin. North Am. 61:1023, 1981.

63. Henderson, S. G.: The gastrointestinal tract in the healthy newborn infant. Am. J. Radiol. 48:302, 1942.

64. Herbst, J., Friedland, G. W., and Zboralske, F. F.: Hiatal hernia and "rumination" in infants and children. J. Pediatr. 78:261, 1971.

65. Hernalatha, V., Batcup, G., Brereron, R. J., and Spitz, L.: Intrathoracic foregut cyst associated with esophageal atresia. J. Pediatr. Surg. 15:178, 1980.

65a. Heyman, M., Bequist, W. E., Fonkalsrud, E. W., Lewin, K., and Ament, M. E.: Esophageal muscular ring and the VACTERYL association: A case report. Pediatrics 67:683, 1981.

65b. Hicks, L., and Mansfield, P. B.: Esophageal atresia and tracheoesophageal fistula; Review of 13 years' experience. J. Thorac. Cardiovasc. Surg. 81:358, 1981.

66. Hillemeier, A. C., Touloukian, R., McCallum, R., and Gryboski, J. D.: Esophageal web — a previously unrecognized complication of epidermolysis bullosa. Pediatrics 67:678, 1981.

67. Holder, T. M., and Ashcraft, K. W.: Esophageal atresia and tracheoesophageal fistula. Ann. Thorac. Surg. 9:445, 1970.

67a. Holder, T. M., and Ashcraft, K. W.: Development in the care of patients with esophageal atresia and tracheoesophageal fistula. Surg. Clin. North Am. 61:1051, 1981.

68. Holder, T. M., Cloud, D. T., Lewis, J. E., Jr., and Pilling, G. P., IV: Esophageal atresia and tracheoesophageal fistula. Pediatrics 34:542, 1964.

69. Hurwitz, A., Duranceau, A., and Haddad, J. K.: Disorders of Esophageal Motility. Philadelphia, W. B. Saunders Company, 1979.

70. Imbrie, J. D., and Doyle, P.: Laryngotracheoesophageal cleft. Laryngoscope 79:1252, 1969.

71. Kabuto, T., Taniguch, K., Iwanga, T., Terasawa, T., Tateish, R., and Tamguchi, H.: Diffuse leiomyomatosis of the esophagus. Dig. Dis. Sci. 25:388, 1980.

71a. Johnston, D., Koehler, R., and Balfe, D. M.: Clinical manifestations of epidermolysis bullosa dystrophica. Dig. Dis. Sci. 26:1144, 1981.

72. Katz, J., Gryboski, J. D., Rosenbaum, H., and Spiro, H.: Dysphagia in children with epidermolysis bullosa. Gastroenterology 52:259, 1967.

73. Kaufmann, H. J.: Candida esophagitis in children with malignant disorders. Ann. Radiol. 13:157, 1970.

74. Kehrer, B., Oesch, A., and Bettex, M.: Manometric studies of esophageal motility in infants with hiatus hernia: J. Pediatr. Surg. 7:499, 1972.

75. Keitel, H. G., and Zeigra, S. R.: Regurgitation in the full-term infant: a controlled clinical study. Am. J. Dis. Child. 102:749, 1961.

76. Kenisberg, K., and Gwinn, J.: The retained sac in repair of posterolateral diaphragmatic hernia in the newborn. Surgery 57:894, 1965.

77. Kiesewetter, W.: Tracheoesophageal fistula in parent and offspring. Am. J. Dis. Child. 134:896, 1980.

78. Kirsh, M., Peterson, A., Brown, J., Orringer, M., Ritter, F., and Sloan, H.: Treatment of caustic injuries of the esophagus. Ann. Surg. 188:675, 1979.

78a. Klein, M. D., Waltner, J., Ball, W., and Kosloske, A.: Schatzki ring in a newborn. Pediatrics 68:1884, 1981.

79. Koberle, F.: Enteromegaly and cardiomegaly in Chagas' disease. Gut 4:399, 1963.

80. Langman, J.: Oesophageal atresia accompanied by a remarkable vessel anomaly. Arch. Chir. Neerl. 4:39, 1952.

81. Larniell, J., and Weyandt, T.: Mallory-Weiss syndrome in two children. J. Pediatr. 92:583, 1978.

82. LaSalle, E., Andrassy, R., VerSteg, K., and Ratner, I.: Congenital tracheoesophageal fistula without esophageal atresia. J. Thorac. Cardiovasc. Surg. 78:583, 1979.

83. Lauridsen, W. B., Enk, B., and Bammeltof, T.: Oesophageal varices as a late complication to neonatal umbilical vein catheterization. Acta Paediatr. Scand. 67:633, 1975.

84. Lell, W. A.: Is congenitally short esophagus truly a rare clinical entity? Ann. Otol. 69:1114, 1960.

85. Leonardi, H., Shea, J., Crozier, R., and Ellis, F. H.: Diffuse spasm of the esophagus. Clinical, manometric and surgical considerations. J. Thorac. Cardiovasc. Surg. 74:736, 1977.

85a. Lilly, J.: Endoscopic sclerosis of esophageal varices in children. Surg. Gynecol. Obstet. 152:513, 1981.

86. Lind, J. F., Blanchard, R. J., and Guyda, H.: Esophageal motility in tracheoesophageal fistula and esophageal atresia. Surg. Gynecol. Obstet. 123:557, 1966.

87. Linde, L. M., and Westover, J. L.: Esophageal and gastric abnormalities in dysautonomia. Pediatrics 29:303, 1962.

87a. Mangla, J.: Barrett's esophagus: An old entity rediscovered. J. Clin. Gastroenterol. 3:347, 1981.

88. Matsumoto, Y., Ogowa, K., Yamamoto, T., Kimura, K., and Kawai, Y.: Extremely rare types of esophageal atresia: two case reports of membranous atresia and multiple atresia of the esophagus. Surgery 71:795, 1972.

89. McDonald, G., Brand, D. L., and Thorning, D. R.: Multiple adenomatous neoplasms arising in columnar lined (Barrett's) esophagus. Gastroenterology 72:1317, 1977.

90. Meyers, N. A.: Neonatal rupture of the esophagus. Ann. Chir. Infant. 13:213, 1972.

91. Meyers, N. A., and Robinson, M. J.: Extrahepatic portal hypertension in children. J. Pediatr. Surg. 8:467, 1973.

91a. Michel, L., Serrano, A., and Malt, R.: Mallory-Weiss syndrome. Ann. Surg. 192:716, 1980.

92. Mitra, K. S., Kumar, V., Datta, D. V., Rao, P. N., and Sand, K.: Extrahepatic portal hypertension: review of 70 cases. J. Pediatr. Surg. 13:51, 1978.

93. Moncreiff, A., and Wilkinson, R. H.: Sucrosuria with mental defect and hiatus hernia. Acta Paediatr. 43:(Suppl. 100) 495, 1954.

94. Monero, J., Cortex, L., and Blesa, E.: Peptic esophageal stenosis in children. J. Pediatr. Surg. 8:475, 1973.

95. Moody, F. G., and Garrett, J. M.: Esophageal achalasia following lye ingestion. Ann. Surg. 170:775, 1969.

96. Murphy, W. J., and Gellis, S. G.: Torticollis with hiatus hernia in infancy. Am. J. Dis. Child. 131:564, 1977.

97. Mutchnick, M. G., Lerner, E., and Conn, H. O.: Portal systemic encephalopathy and portalcaval anastomosis: a prospective, controlled investigation. Gastroenterology 66:1005, 1974.

98. Nagaraj, H. S., Mullen, P., Groff, D. B., et al.: Iatrogenic perforation of the esophagus in premature infants. Surgery 86:583, 1979.

99. Neuhauser, E., Harris, G. B., and Berrett, A.: Roentgenographic features of neurenteric cysts. Am. J. Roentgenol. 79:235, 1958.

100. Newman, A., and Ko, S.: Bilateral neurofibroma of the intrathoracic vagus associated with von Recklinghausen's disease. Am. J. Roentgenol. Radium Ther. Nucl. Med. 112:389, 1971.

101. Newberger, P. E., Cassady, J. R., and Jaffe, N.: Esophagitis due to Adriamycin and radiation therapy for childhood malignancy. Cancer 42:417, 1978.

102. Nix, T. E., Jr., and Christianson, H. B.: Epidermolysis bullosa of the esophagus: report of

two cases and review of the literature. South. Med. J. 58:612, 1965.

103. O'Bannon, R. P.: Congenital partial atresia of the esophagus associated with congenital diverticulum of esophagus: report of a case. Radiology 47:471, 1946.

104. Oeconomopoulos, C. J., and Swenson, O.: Duplications of the gastrointestinal tract. J. Pediatr. 60:361, 1962.

105. Oesch, I., Heliksen, M., Shemata, D., Hutchins, G., and Haller, J. A.: Esophageal reconstruction with free jejunal grafts. J. Pediatr. Surg. 15:433, 1980.

106. Okamato, E., Iwasaki, T., Katukani, I., and Ueda, T.: Selective destruction of myenteric plexus: its relation to Hirschsprung's disease, achalasia of the esophagus and hypertrophic pyloric stenosis. J. Pediatr. Surg. 2:444, 1967.

107. Okamoto, E., and Ueda, T.: Embryogenesis of intramural ganglia of the gut and its relation to Hirschsprung's disease. J. Pediatr. Surg. 2:437, 1967.

108. Okihe, N., Payne, W., Neufeld, D., et al.: Esophagomyotomy versus forceful dilatation for achalasia of the esophagus: results in 899 patients. Ann. Thorac. Surg. 28:119, 1979.

108a. O'Neill, J., Holcomb, G. W., Jr., and Neblett, W.: Recent experience with esophageal atresia. Ann. Surg. 195:739, 1982.

109. Parker, A., Christie, D., and Cahill, J.: Incidence and significance of gastroesophageal reflux following repair of esophageal atresia and tracheoesophageal fistula and the need for anti-reflux procedures. J. Pediatr. Surg. 14:5, 1979.

110. Perlman, M., Banadyl, S., and Saggi, E.: Neonatal diagnosis of familial dysautonomia. Pediatrics 63:238, 1979.

111. Pietsch, J. B., Stokes, K., and Beardmore, H.: Esophageal atresia with tracheoesophageal fistula: end-to-end versus end-to-side repair. J. Pediatr. Surg. 13:677, 1978.

112. Pinkerton, J. A., Holcomb, G. W., Jr., and Foster, J. H.: Portal hypertension in childhood. Ann. Surg. 175:870, 1972.

113. Powers, W.: Further experience with intragastric oxygen measurement to diagnose H-type tracheosophageal fistula. Pediatrics 63:668, 1979.

114. Putnam, T. C.: Esophageal atresia: critical analysis of 39 cases. Arch. Surg. 114:288, 1979.

115. Randolph, J., Altman, R. P., and Anderson, K.: Selective surgical management based upon clinical status in infants with esophageal atresia. J. Thorac. Cardiovasc. Surg. 74:335, 1977.

116. Raffensperger, J.: Gastrointestinal tract defects associated with esophageal atresia and tracheosophageal fistula: surgical management. Arch. Surg. 101:241, 1970.

117. Raffensperger, J. G., Sholnik, A. A., Boggs, J. D., and Swenson, O.: Portal hypertension in children. Arch. Surg. 105:249, 1972.

118. Resnick, R. H., Iber, F., Ishihara, A., Chalmers, T. C., and Zimmerman, H.: A controlled study of the therapeutic portacaval shunt. Gastroenterology 67:843, 1974.

119. Riley, C. M., Day, R. L., Greeley, D. M., and Langford, W. S.: Central autonomic dysfunction with defective lacrimation. Report of five cases. Pediatrics 37:435, 1966.

120. Rosenberg, N., Kunderman, P. J., Vroman, L., and Moolten, S. E.: Prevention of experimental lye strictures of the esophagus by cortisone. Arch. Surg. 63:147, 1951.

121. Roberts, A. H., and Bamforth, J.: The pharynx and esophagus in ocular muscular dystrophy. Neurology 18:645, 1968.

122. Rohatgi, M., Shandling, B., and Stephens, C. A.: Hiatal hernia in infants and children: results of surgical treatment. Surgery 69:456, 1971.

122a. Ruff, S., Campbell, J., Harrison, M., and Campbell, T.: Pediatric diaphragmatic hernia: 11-year experience. Am. J. Surg. 139:641, 1981.

123. Rutgers, L., and Verhaegen, K.: Intravenous miconazole in the treatment of chronic esophageal candidiasis. Gastroenterology 72:316, 1977.

124. Sabiston, D. C., Jr., and Scott, H. W., Jr.: Primary neoplasms and cysts of the mediastinum. Ann. Surg. 136:777, 1952.

124a. Salzman-Mann, C., Harnosh, M., Sivasubramanian, K., Bar-Maor, A., Zinder, O., Avery, G., Watkins, J., and Harnosh, P.: Congenital esophageal atresia; Lipase activity is present in the esophageal pouch and stomach. Dig. Dis. Sci. 27:124, 1982.

125. Saunders, R. L.: Combined anterior and posterior spina bifida in a living neonatal female. Anat. Rec. 87:255, 1943.

126. Sawyer, P.: Partial thoracic stomach and esophageal hiatus hernia in infancy and childhood. Am. J. Dis. Child. 90:421, 1955.

127. Scheer, C. W., and Linville, J. L.: Congenital diaphragmatic hernia through foramen of Bochdalek. Arch. Surg. 91:823, 1965.

128. Schmidt, R., Alkan, W. J., Moses, S., Mundel, G., and Roizen, S.: A clinical entity simulating familial dysautonomia in a North African Jewish family. J. Pediatr. 76:283, 1970.

129. Schuster, R. S., Scwachman, H., Toyama, W., Rubino, A., and Taik-khaw, K.: The management of portal hypertension in cystic fibrosis. J. Pediatr. Surg. 12:201, 1977.

130. Shaldon, C., and Sherlock, S.: The use of vasopressin (Pitressin) in the control of bleeding from oesophageal varices. Lancet 2:222, 1960.

131. Sheft, D. J., and Shrago, G.: Esophageal moniliasis. JAMA 213:1859, 1970.

132. Shepard, R., Fenn, S., and Sieber, W. K.: Evaluation of esophageal function in postoperative esophageal atresia and tracheoesophageal fistula. Surgery 59:608, 1966.

133. Shepard, R., Raffensperger, J., and Goldstein, R.: Pediatric esophageal perforation. J. Thorac. Cardiovasc. Surg. 74:261, 1977.

134. Shultz, E. H., Jr.: Achalasia in children as a cause of recurrent pulmonary disease. J. Pediatr. 59:522, 1961.

135. Similä, S., Kokkonen, J., and Kasai, M.: Achalasia sicca, juvenile Sjögren's syndrome with achalasia and gastric hyposecretion. Eur. J. Pediatr. 129:175, 1978.

135a. Slater, G., and Sicular, A. A.: Esophageal perforations after forceful dilatation in achalasia. Ann. Surg. 195:186, 1982.

136. Smiley, T. B., Caves, P. K., and Porter, D. C.: Relationship between posterior pharyngeal pouch and hiatus hernia. Thorax 25:725, 1970.

137. Smith, A. A., and Dancis, J.: Catecholamine release in familial dysautonomia. N. Engl. J. Med. 277:61, 1957.

138. Smith, A. A., Hirsch, J. I., and Dancis, J.: Response to infused methacholine in familial dysautonomia. Pediatrics 36:225, 1965.

139. Smith, E. I.: The early development of the trachea and esophagus in relation to atresia of the esophagus and tracheoesophageal fistula. Contr. Embryol. Washington, D.C., Carnegie Institute (# 245) 36:41, 1957.

140. Snyder, W. H., and Greaney, E. M.: Congenital diaphragmatic hernia, 77 consecutive cases. Surgery 57:576, 1965.

140a. Spitz, L., Ali, M., and Brereton, R. J.: Combined esophageal and duodenal atresia: experience of 18 patients. J. Pediatr. Surg. 16:4, 1981.

141. Starinsky, R., Manor, A., Pajewsky, M., and Varsano, J.: Intramural esophageal diverticulosis in an infant. Isr. M. Med. Sci. 16:604, 1980.

142. Stillman, A., Larter, W., and Goldman, D.: Longitudinal esophageal bands associated with esophageal aperistalsis. Gastroenterology 74:592, 1978.

143. Strawczinski, H., Beck, I., McKenna, R., and Nickerson, G. H.: The behavior of the lower esophageal sphincter in infants and its relationship to gastroesophageal regurgitation. J. Pediatr. 64:17, 1964.

144. Strobel, C., Byrne, W., Ament, M. E., and Euler, A.: Correlation of esophageal lengths with height. J. Pediatr. 94:81, 1979.

144a. Suwaga, C., Mullins, R. J., Lucas, C. E., and Liebold, W. C.: The value of early endoscopy following caustic ingestion. Surg. Gynecol. Obstet. 153:533, 1981.

145. Tarnay, T. J., Chang, C. H., Nugent, R. G., and Warden, H. E.: Esophageal duplication with spinal malformation. J. Thorac. Cardiovasc. Surg. 59:293, 1970.

146. Teiziera, A., Teiziera, G., Macedo, U., and Prato, A.: Acquired cell-mediated immunodepression in acute Chagas' disease. J. Clin. Invest. 62:1132, 1978.

147. Tornwall, L., Lind, J., Peltonen, T., and Wegelius, C.: The gastrointestinal tract of the newborn. II. Functional disturbances of the motility. Ann. Paediatr. Fenn. 5 (Suppl. 5):15, 1959.

148. Totten, R. S., Strout, A. P., Humphreys, G. H., and Moore, R. L.: Benign tumors and cysts of the esophagus. J. Thorac. Surg. 25:606, 1953.

149. Touloukian, R. J., and Pickett, L.: Operative management of esophageal atresia by end-to-side anastomosis and ligation of the tracheoesophageal fistula. Conn. Med. 34:783, 1970.

149a. Urrutia, J., Antonmarrei, S., and Cordero, L.: Pseudodiverticulum of the esophagus in the newborn infant. Am. J. Dis. Child. 134: 417, 1980.

150. Vanderhoff, J., Rich, K. C., Steihm, R., and Ament, M. E.: Esophageal ulcers in immunodeficiency with elevated levels of IgM and neutropenia. Am. J. Dis. Child. 131:551, 1977.

151. Van Trappen, G., Van Goldsenhoven, G. E., Verbeke, S., Van den Berghe, G., and Van den Broucke, J.: Manometric studies in achalasia of the cardia, before and after pneumatic dilatations. Gastroenterology 45:317, 1963.

152. Visalli, J. A.: Congenital short esophagus. Surgery 56:1137, 1964.

153. Vorhees, A. B., Jr., and Price, J. B., Jr.: Extrahepatic portal hypertension, a retrospective analysis of 127 cases and associated clinical implications. Arch. Surg. 108:338, 1974.

154. Waller, S. L., Misiewicz, J. J., Anthony, P. P., and Gummer, J. W. P.: In vitro pharmacologic and histopathologic studies on human cardiac sphincteric muscle from achalasic and control patients. Am. J. Dig. Dis. 16:566, 1971.

154a. Warren, J., Evans, K., and Carter, C. O.: Offspring of patients with tracheoesophageal fistula. J. Med. Genet. 16:338, 1979.

155. Watkins, E., Jr., and Hering, A. C. L.: Compression of the trachea and esophagus by anomalous great vessels. Diagnosis and treatment 1761–1961. Surg. Clin. North Am. 41:821, 1961.

156. Weenklas, C. G. H.: Pathogenesis of intrathoracic gastrogenic cysts. Am. J. Dis. Child. 83:500, 1952.

157. Weller, M. H.: Intramural diverticulosis of the esophagus: report of a case in a child. J. Pediatr. 80:281, 1972.

158. Weller, M. H., and Lutzker, S. A.: Intramural diverticulosis of the esophagus associated with postoperative hiatal hernia, alkaline esophagitis and esophageal stricture. Radiology 98:373, 1971.

158a. Werlin, S., Dodds, W., Hogan, W., Glicklich, M., and Arndorfer, R.: Esophageal function in esophageal atresia. Dig. Dis. Sci. 26:796, 1981.

159. Westerley, C. R., Herbst, J., Goldman, S., et al.: Inheritance of infantile achalasia. J. Pediatr. 87:243, 1975.

159a. Winckler, K.: Tetracycline ulcers of the oesophagus — endoscopy, histology and roentgenology in 2 cases and review of the literature. Endoscopy 13:225, 1981.

160. Woolf, L. I., and Norman, A. P.: The urinary excretion of amino acids and sugars in early infancy. J. Pediatr. 50:271, 1957.

161. Worman, L. W., Hurley, J. D., Pemberton, A. H., and Narodick, B. G.: Rupture of the esophagus from external blunt trauma. Arch. Surg. 85:333, 1963.

162. Wyndham, N.: The significance of gastric mucosa in the esophagus. Br. J. Surg. 43:409, 1956.

Chapter Twelve

THE STOMACH AND PEPTIC ULCER DISEASE

DEVELOPMENT AND MEASUREMENT OF NEUROMOTOR AND SECRETORY FUNCTION

The stomach arises from the foregut at about four weeks' gestation as a saccular dilatation behind the heart. As the esophagus elongates, the stomach moves downward into the abdomen, and, as the dorsal surface grows more rapidly than the ventral one, the greater and lesser curvatures form as it undergoes rotation and differentiation. Myeloblasts, present at eight to nine weeks, extend caudally until, at 14 to 15 weeks, circular muscle is oriented into bundles in the body of the stomach. By four to five months the pyloric muscle is complete. The longitudinal muscle layer appears over the entire stomach by 11 to 12 weeks. By four and one-half weeks, vagal trunks reach the developing stomach sac and are followed within a few weeks by the sympathetic fibers. These join the vagal trunks, and both extend with the developing stomach to innervate it completely by nine weeks of gestation. Nerve fibers increase through gestation, and by seven months, nerve plexuses within the stomach are of mature type.

Although primitive gastric pits are noted in the developing gastric sac at six weeks, truly differentiated gastric cells do not appear until 11 weeks. By the end of the first trimester, the gastric epithelium has differentiated into gastric pits and glands that contain chief and parietal cells. At three to five months, the fetal stomach produces pepsinogen I, pepsin, acid, cathepsin, gastrin, and renin, and after 32 weeks, pepsinogen II. As the fetus matures, antral gastrin, first noted as G-34 in type, changes to G-17, and when the fetus reaches 21 cm, typical gastrin-producing G cells are present in the antrum.[36] Generally, enzyme activity is maximal in the fundus and increases until the time of delivery. After feeding, enzyme levels rise sharply so that those at two days are four times those of the neonate. Glandular mucoprotein fractions, measuring 15 to 26 mg per dl in the neonate, rise to 48 to 110 mg/per dl in children between two months and eight years of age. Plasma pepsinogen levels are higher during the first week of life than in older infants. Gastric peptic activity is one-fifteenth that of the adult during the first ten days of life and by four months is half that of the adult, paralleling maximal acid output. Intrinsic factor is present by 14 weeks and increases significantly between 14 and 25 weeks.[3] After birth, secretion increases until at two weeks it reaches half that of the adult and at three months, nears adult levels. Lipase activity is provided by lingual lipase and lipoprotein lipase and bile salt–stimulated lipase from human milk.

The major functions of the stomach are to retain, partially digest, and propel food into the small intestine. Of the four divisions, the cardia is that proximal to the esophagus and contains glands with only a few parietal cells, chief cells, and mucous cells. The fundus and the body contain the major digestive glands: parietal cells, producing hydrochloric acid and some blood group substances; chief cells, producing pepsinogen; mucous cells; cells that produce intrinsic factor; and surface epithelial cells. The antrum, extending from the body beyond the angulus to the pylorus, contains glands that secrete blood group substances, gastrin, gastrone, electrolytes, and proteases. Prostaglandins of the E and I types provide cytoprotection for the gastric mucosal cells.

GASTRIC MOTILITY AND EMPTYING

Gastric emptying has been assumed to begin between the fourth and fifth fetal months. It has been demonstrated in one distressed human fetus at 25 weeks and in the normal fetus between 31 and 32 weeks.[36] Emptying has been evaluated in the neonate using dilution techniques, contrast radiology, and, recently, radionuclide scanning.[24, 25, 102, 211] Results differ and must be interpreted according to the technique used. Generally, emptying is prolonged by increased osmolarity, the addition of solids, decreased pH, and increased fat content or elongation of the carbon chain on the fatty acid.[193] Medium-chain triglycerides seem to prolong gastric emptying in the adult but not in the infant. Extremes of emptying have ranged from 1 1/2 to 24 hours, with more than 40 per cent of term infants having an emptying time of greater than eight hours. In 30 per cent it is less than five hours, and in 27 per cent it ranges between five and eight hours.[31, 94, 186] Several investigators have shown the major portion of gastric emptying to fix a monoexponential curve, similar to that of liquid emptying in the adult. During the first 20 minutes, however, gastric emptying is different, being rapid in the majority of infants studied but delayed in some. The delayed early emptying is seen more often in infants taking cow's milk formula than in those taking breast milk or glucose. As determined by nuclide studies, normal infants three to six months old empty 35 to 56 per cent of formula from their stomach by one hour.[102]

Premature infants taking glucose or water have been shown to empty their stomachs in less than five hours, but required seven to eight hours after taking milk. Although these infants have often been considered to have delayed gastric emptying, recent studies have not shown this to be so. Indeed, the half-times of gastric emptying for premature infants and neonates have fallen into the range described for adults. Evidence is controversial as to whether increasing the volume of a feed increases gastric emptying. In most studies, posture has had an effect, with more rapid emptying in the semi-recumbent (two and one-half hours) and right lateral positions than in the prone and supine ones (ten hours).[26]

The most detailed radiologic studies of gastric emptying and motility were performed by Tornwall et al. in 1958.[211] They found that there is no radiologic evidence of peristalsis during the first few days of life and that gastric emptying is accomplished by "tonus" and final contractions of the musculature. Later, ring-shaped peristaltic waves begin in the distal half of the body of the stomach and travel to the pylorus. Contrast material reaches the pylorus in 90 seconds if the infant is in the prone or right-sided position and in 9 to 27 minutes if he is recumbent or in a left-sided position.[100] Good peristaltic waves are apparent by the time the infant is three months old. Our own motility studies in premature infants and neonates less than 12 hours old showed broad, bell-shaped waves measuring 10 to 13 mm in height and lasting 0.8 to 4 seconds. These are neither rhythmic nor progressive. After 24 hours, progressive gastric peristaltic waves are present. In the young infant, small peristaltic waves are seen in the fundus as a progression of esophageal peristalsis. They disappear after several months and their function is not known, although we have speculated that they serve to propel the bolus away from the gastroesophageal sphincter.[92]

The stomach fills by an active rather than a passive process.[211] This "receptive relaxation" is a reflex response in which intraluminal pressure rises gradually as the intragastric volume increases. A gastric wave propagated through the distal half of the stomach is the physiologic determinant of antral peristalsis and ends in "antral systole," a simultaneous contraction of the antrum and pylorus that initiates duodenal contraction.[35, 39, 112] Located primarily in the longitudinal muscle, the wave has two components: The first and most important is a triphasic wave occurring regularly every 20 seconds, and the second is a potential that occurs only with peristalsis.[5, 47] The antral slow wave is slowed by adrenergic drugs, hastened by cholinergic ones, and disrupted by vagotomy or transection of the stomach.[117, 145] Peristaltic waves propagate through the circular muscle and increase in intensity as they near the pylorus. The fundus regulates liquid, and the antrum, solid emptying. Gastric emptying of liquids is abnormal in infants with severe gastroesophageal reflux.[102]

GASTRIC SECRETION

Basal Gastric Secretion and Gastrin

Immediately after birth the gastric contents are alkaline, but within the first hour of life, acid production begins, decreasing the pH from 3.6 to 2.5.[57, 210] This finding, first considered to represent early achlorhydria, is actually due to ingested alkaline amniotic fluid. The rapid fall in pH is correlated with high cord levels of gastrin (mean 135 pg per ml), 13 per cent of which are greater than 200 pg per ml. Cord gastrin levels are significantly higher than maternal ones, indicating that the infant himself manufactures the hormone during the first hours of life. The highest gastrin values are found in infants born to mothers with sickle cell anemia, and there is no correlation between cord gastrin and type of delivery of Apgar score. Unlike the case in older children, serum gastrin levels do not decrease with fasting beyond eight hours. Between three and five hours of age, mean gastrin measures 76 to 155 pg per ml; between one to three days, 151 pg per ml; and between 1.4 and 22 months, 101 pg per ml. All values are higher than the means of 41 to 49 pg per ml reported in the adult.[62, 63]

Basal acid secretion during this period of hypergastrinemia is low when calculated as mEq per kg, measuring 0.010 to 0.22 mEq per kg; by six hours of age, however, basal acid secretion equals that of older controls. By 48 hours, the gastric pH varies between 3 and 1 and eventually stabilizes at 3.2. Achlorhydria or hyperacidity do occur in a few infants. The classic studies of Miller[159] note a gradual decrease in acidity from birth until about the tenth day of life. Acidity then remains stable until the third or fourth week, when it gradually rises. This period of early decreased acidity is corroborated by additional studies with histamine stimulation. By three to four years, gastric acidity approaches normal adult levels.[77]

The situation is somewhat different in premature infants, one third of whom have alkaline gastric contents for the first 12 hours of life and one fifth of whom produce no acid for ten days.[7, 96, 220] In most, however, gastric acidity reaches a maximum by four days. Miller noted the greatest percentage of achlorhydria in the smallest premature infants and correlated this with poorly developed gastric mucosa.[159] Others have not found such a correlation and noted a rapid increase in the gastric acidity of premature infants by six hours of age, with a gradual decrease in acidity over the following two weeks.

Stimulated Gastric Secretion

Hydrochloric acid is secreted at a constant concentration by the parietal cells and then diluted by other gastric secretions to its final concentration. Histamine stimulates the parietal cells, and its use affords a meas-

Table 12–1 Gastric Secretion in Infants*

	1 DAY	3–8 DAYS	10–11 DAYS	14–17 DAYS	25–32 DAYS	67–110 DAYS	OVER 4 YEARS
Gastric Juice ml.	3.3 (0.8–9.3)	3.7 (1.3–4.7)	4.0 (2.0–5.4)	6.4 (1.5–12.0)	3.1 (3.0–3.2)	13.4 (7.1–19.9)	42.5 (35–50)
Titratable Acid							
concentration mEq/L	8.1 (4.2–16.7)	14.4 (9.2–26.0)	34.4 (20.6–55.0)	26.7 (15.4–35.0)	26.4 (10.0–45.3)	34.8 (19.6–50.0)	114.2 (110–117)
output mEq/hr	0.03 (.01–.09)	0.06 (.01–.12)	0.12 (.11–.15)	0.19 (.04–.37)	0.08 (.03–.14)	0.47 (.14–.65)	4.88 (3.89–5.88)
mEq/hr/kg	0.01 (0–.03)	0.02 (0–.03)	0.04 (.04–.05)	0.05 (.01–.09)	0.02 (0–.06)	0.10 (.03–.14)	—
Pepsin							
concentration PE† mg/ml	0.04 (0–.07)	0.05 (0–.09)	0.12 (.09–.14)	0.14 (.12–.16)	0.10 (.07–.12)	0.12 (.06–.18)	0.45 (.41–.50)
output PE mg/hr	0.18 (0–.53)	0.21 (.11–.44)	0.46 (.29–.67)	0.88 (.20–1.46)	0.32 (.21–.38)	1.34 (1.25–1.44)	18.5 (14–29.8)
PE mg/hr/kg	0.04 (0–.19)	0.06 (0–.12)	0.15 (0.11–0.22)	0.24 (.06–.36)	0.08 (.06–.10)	0.28 (.23–.32)	—
Intrinsic Factor							
concentration ng B_{12}/ml	6.8 (3–15)	20.2 (4.7–31)	36.6 (15.2–59.4)	28.7 (23.4–34.2)	38.4 (14.5–53.5)	33.0 (18.7–59.9)	86.3 (74–98)
output ng, B_{12}/ml	22.5 (4.6–79)	78.0 (6.1–127)	156.8 (30.4–243)	172.4 (51–280)	118.0 (46–165)	430.5 (133–659)	3757.0 (1970–7613)
ng B_{12}/hr/kg	7.1 (1.2–26.4)	24.1 (1.7–45.6)	51.7 (11.3–81.2)	48.3 (17–74)	31.2 (10.8–43.6)	90.0 (26.6–146)	—

*From Agunod, M., et al.: Correlative study of hydrochloric acid, pepsin and intrinsic factor secretion in newborns and infants. Am. J. Dig. Dis. 14:400, 1969.

†PE = pepsin equivalent

ure of the total number of cells available to produce the maximal acid output (MAO) of the stomach. Stimulants such as Histalog, which has none of the side effects of histamine, or pentagastrin, a synthetic gastrin-like pentapeptide, are now being used in place of histamine.[129, 150] The largest study of Histalog-stimulated secretion of infants was undertaken by Agunod et al.,[3] and the data are tabulated in Table 12–1. As noted, during the first day of life the outputs of HCl, pepsin, and intrinsic factor are low; they increase until the third week of life, decline briefly between three and four weeks, and rise thereafter. Basal and pentagastrin-stimulated secretion in one- and two-day-old infants shows little variation with mean volumes of 7 and 6.9 ml per hour, basal acid outputs (BAO) measuring 0.1, and maximal acid outputs (MAO) measuring 0.12 and 0.13 ml per kg per hour. The mean basal pH at one day of age was 3.06, as compared with 3.12 at two days of age. The absence of a rise in acid production after stimulation suggests that the gastric mucosa was responding maximally in the resting state. Until three months of age, gastric output is more a function of age than of weight, but thereafter it correlates best with weight. In one study of ten infants whose mean age was 21 months, the maximal acid output for those of low weight was 0.88; for those of medium weight, 1.62; and for those of high weight, 2.02 mEq per kg per hour.[37, 63]

Technique for Gastric Analysis

Acid output is described by pH and total acid, which includes free hydrochloric acid and that combined with protein, phosphates, and organic acids. Basal acid secretion (BAO) is measured in 15-minute aliquots over one hour and represents the unstimulated gastric secretion. Its absence is not of great significance. Maximal acid output (MAO) is the gastric response to stimulation. Histalog, 0.5 to 1 mg per kg, or pentagastrin, 2 to 6 μg per kg, is injected intramuscularly, and the stimulated secretion is measured over four 15-minute periods. The two highest 15-minute figures

are totaled and multiplied by two to measure the peak and output (PAO). The BAO and MAO ratio is normally about 30 per cent, and a figure greater than 60 per cent represents, in older children and adults, the increased basal secretion seen only in the Zollinger-Ellison syndrome or with retained gastric antrum.

Gastric secretion is affected by a number of factors that either stimulate or inhibit it.[113] The vagal stimulus arises in the cortex or subcortical areas and travels through the anterior hypothalamus, the medulla, and the vagal nerves to the stomach. Acetylcholine, released at the nerve synapse, or epinephrine increases secretion. Vagal stimulation of the antrum initiates gastrin release. (Vagotomy, on the other hand, does not inhibit, but rather stimulates, gastrin release.) Hypoglycemia through vagal stimulation causes gastric hypersecretion, and the gastric response to intravenous insulin is used as an index of completeness of vagotomy. Conversely, intravenous glucose or glucagon inhibits gastric secretion. Emotions have been considered to affect gastric secretion, but this is not well documented.

Gastrin is one of the most important stimuli of secretion.[150] In maximal concentration in the antrum, it is present also in the small intestine and pancreas and in small amounts in the fundus of the stomach.[88] The major circulatory gastrin is termed big gastrin and has a molecular weight of 7000. There are probably numerous forms of gastrin both smaller and larger than the original hepadecapeptide gastrin; a larger "big, big gastrin" has been isolated from jejunal mucosa. Gastrin is formed in the pyloric antrum after antral distention or when protein or peptides come in contact with parietal cells and, acting by a direct cholinergic effect,[201] cause them to release gastrin, which then enters the circulation and stimulates acid and water output and, to a lesser extent, pepsin release. Studies indicate that histamine stored in the gastric mucosa in bound form is liberated to stimulate gastric secretion. Histidine decarboxylase is activated by the decreased mucosal histamine stores or by endogenous gastrin to replenish bound histamine. The role of intestinal gastrin is not known, but its concentration in the duodenum is significant and its release is perhaps stimulated by intraluminal protein. Hypersecretion and increased gastrin occur after extensive intestinal resection (the short gut syndrome).

Gastric secretion is inhibited by intravenous glucose or glucagon and by vagotomy. Factors that decrease or inhibit gastrin release decrease secretion; for example, an acid pH of the antrum (below 2.5) or duodenum, or the enzymes secretin or cholecystokinin.

CONGENITAL MALFORMATIONS

CASCADE STOMACH

Although the cascade stomach is considered a normal variant by adult gastroenterologists, it has received essentially no attention by pediatric gastroenterologists. In 15 years, only one instance of this deformity in a child who presented with the chief complaint of chest pain has been seen at Yale.

It has been given a number of eponyms: "cascade stomach," "hourglass stomach" or "cup and spill stomach." Anatomically, the fundus is redundant and hangs posteriorly over the body of the stomach to form a pouch when the patient is erect. During a radiologic examination, this phenomenon becomes apparent after enough barium is given to fill the pouch and then overflow in a cascade fashion into the body of the stomach (Fig. 12–1). Most often described in tall, slender individuals, it is believed to represent a congenital anomaly.

Symptoms are often caused by aerophagia because the pouch is unable to permit eructation and the stomach distends significantly. A left splenic syndrome has also been associated with this anomaly, in which gas is trapped in the splenic flexure. The dilated stomach and diaphragm elevation that it causes may stimulate angina pectoris. In our patient, a rather unexpected finding was the presence of barium refluxed into the esophagus, and it was believed that this was responsible for her pain.

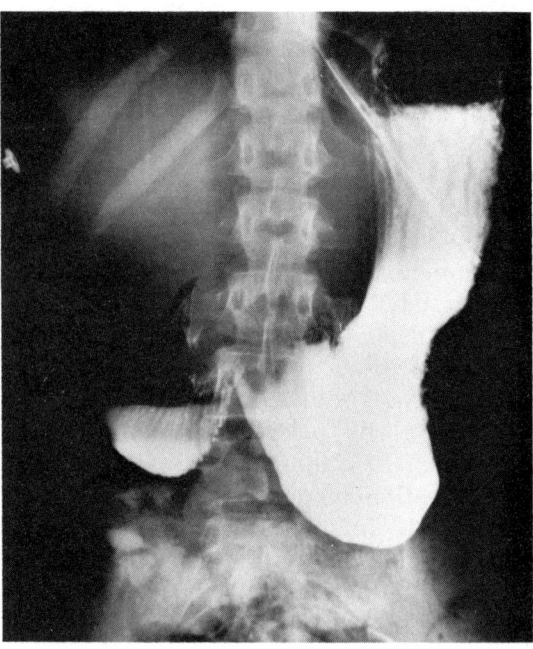

Figure 12–1 Cascade stomach. Also termed the "cup and spill" stomach, it is characterized by anterior displacement of the medial portion of the stomach. Barium drops into the distal part of the cardiac portion and appears to spill over into the remaining medial portion and antrum.

HYPOPLASIA OF THE STOMACH AND CONGENITAL MICROGASTRIA

A hypoplastic stomach, or microgastria, occurs in unusual instances because of faulty separation of the primitive foregut, as in tracheal agenesis or tracheoesophageal fistula.[50] In other circumstances, there are no associated esophageal defects.[23, 184, 189]

Incidence. Fifteen cases of congenital microgastria unassociated with tracheal lesions have been reported in the literature.

Etiology. In such instances, an arrest probably occurs during descent and rotation of the stomach, for the stomach is usually not rotated and remains in a sagittal position.

Pathology. The stomach remains tubular in shape, and its segments are not differentiated. The esophagus above is dilated.

Symptoms. If the abnormality is associated with tracheal lesions, the symptoms are those of the more lethal disorder. Otherwise, there are feeding problems during the first month of life, such as vomiting during or after feedings. Aspiration pneumonia is a recurrent problem. Eventually, the infant limits himself to small feedings and weight gain is retarded.

Asplenia has been an associated finding in all cases in which surgical exploration or autopsy has been done. Other anomalies that occur with congenital microgastria are short duodenum, malrotation, absence of the gallbladder, situs inversus, musculoskeletal anomalies, imperforate anus, Hirschsprung's disease, abnormal lobulation of the lungs, and vaginal atresia.

Diagnosis. Radiologic examination reveals a short, tubular stomach, which in some cases is intrathoracic, and only rarely are gastric segments demonstrable. The gastric aspirate is alkaline. There is usually a hypochromic, microcytic anemia.

Treatment. Small, frequent feedings are readily retained and may have to be continued into adolescence. Gastrostomy has been of little help, but a double-lumen jejunal pouch with distal Roux-en-Y has provided additional reservoir space.

Prognosis. If there are no other severe anomalies, the prognosis is good, although persistent gastroesophageal reflux is a problem.

VOLVULUS OF THE STOMACH

This is a rare occurrence, for the stomach is held securely in place by the gastrophrenic ligaments and the retroperitoneal position of the second portion of the diaphragm. It therefore occurs only when the ligaments are stretched or absent.

Incidence. Over 275 cases have been reported in the literature, with nine being in neonates. Males are affected more often than females.[30, 41, 230]

Etiology. Acute volvulus is sometimes associated with eventration of the diaphragm, elongated gastric attachments, diaphragmatic hernias, congenital bands, or absence of the gastrocolic ligament. Disorders of rotation or conditions causing gas-

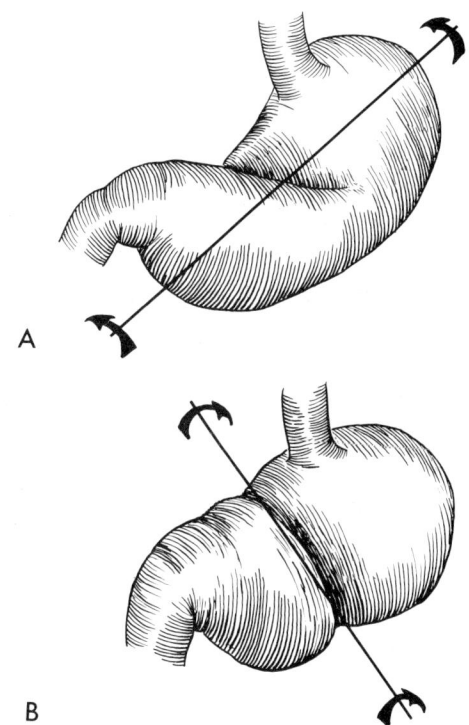

Figure 12–2 Gastric volvulus. A, Organoaxial. The greater curvature passes forward in an anterior direction, as depicted, but may also be displaced posteriorly. B, Mesenterioaxial. The pylorus, or cardia, commonly rotates anteriorly, but the opposite rotation may occur. (From Cole, B. C., and Dickinson, S. J.: Acute volvulus of the stomach in infants and children. Surgery 70:707, 1971. Used by permission.)

tric dilatation are major predisposing factors. Vomiting is believed to precipitate acute gastric volvulus. Several reported patients have had mental retardation and associated asplenia or a mobile spleen.[195]

Pathology. There are two types of volvulus: organoaxial, in which the stomach is rotated upward and about its long axis, and the less common mesenterioaxial type, in which the stomach is rotated from right to left or left to right about the long axis of the gastrohepatic omentum (Fig. 12–2). The torsion is either total, involving the entire stomach except its diaphragmatic attachment, or partial and limited to its pyloric end. The rotating section most often passes anteriorly.

Symptoms. The onset may occur at any time after birth and is usually acute. Nearly half the presentations in childhood are be-

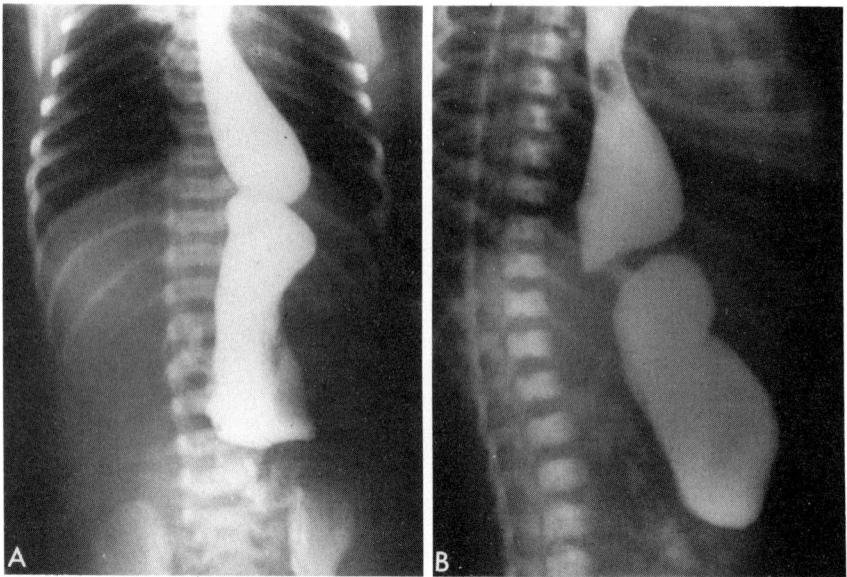

Figure 12–3 A and B (lateral), Contrast examination of an organoaxial volvulus shows a dilated esophagus, medial displacement of the stomach, and deformity of the greater curvature at the site of the twist. (From Cole, B. C., and Dickinson, S. J.: Acute volvulus of the stomach in infants and children. Surgery 70:707, 1971. Used by permission.)

fore one year of age. Vomiting is the major symptom and continues until the gastric contents are emptied. Retching without vomiting indicates extensive volvulus with obstruction near the gastroesophageal junction. The epigastrium is distended and tender, and the infant appears acutely ill and in pain. Hypovolemia and dehydration develop rapidly. If the volvulus is accompanied by a significant diaphragmatic defect in the neonate, respiratory symptoms predominate. In less severe volvulus, the only manifestation may be increasing gastric residuals in the tube-fed infant.

Diagnosis. The first suggestion of this disorder is difficulty encountered in passing a nasogastric tube into the stomach, owing to obstruction. Flat film of the stomach will show gastric distention and two air-filled fluid levels in the upright and lateral films, which represent the portions of the stomach above and below the twist. The position of the gastroesophageal junction is noted to be below its normal location, the stomach lies horizontally, and distention of the antrum, pylorus, and proximal duodenum produces a "beak" in the usual area of the esophagogastric junction. The left diaphragm may be elevated. Contrast studies demonstrate a low-lying gastroesophageal junction, gastric

retention, and obstruction at the pylorus, with twisting of the mucosal folds at the point of rotation and abnormal configuration and position of the greater curvature (Fig. 12–3).

Complications. Gastric perforation occurs in 7 per cent of cases and is either spontaneous or related to gastric ulcer. In a few cases, it is caused by traumatic intubation.

Treatment. Immediate operation is required to correct the volvulus and secure the stomach in a fixed position. Gastrostomy provides postoperative decompression.

GASTRIC DIVERTICULA

Gastric diverticula are unusual in the infant but are occasionally seen in the adult female. They are either congenital, containing all layers of the muscular wall, or acquired, in which case one or more layers are thinned or absent. The acquired form results from increased intragastric pressure, adhesions, or inflammatory or neoplastic disease. Most diverticula lie high in the fundus between the posterior wall and the lesser curvature, where the longitudinal smooth muscle fibers divide into bundles running to the lesser and greater curvatures.

They are less frequently found in the pyloric area and rarely in the fundus or body. Most diverticula are asymptomatic and are discovered in radiologic examinations performed for other reasons. When they do produce symptoms, hemorrhage or signs of acute abdomen due to torsion of the diverticulum or volvulus of the stomach are characteristic.

GASTRIC DUPLICATIONS

Duplication cysts of the stomach are the rarest of the enteric duplications.[115]

Incidence. A review of the literature in 1980 uncovered 84 cases of gastric duplications.[177] These constitute 3.8 per cent of all enteric duplications, with pyloric duplications being most rare. Females are affected twice as often as males.

Etiology. The most familiar theory of the origin of duplication cysts is that there is incomplete resolution of the solid stage of intestinal development at about six weeks' gestation, resulting in a double lumen.[27] Some of the duplications probably result from embryonic dorsal enteric fistulas and faulty separation of the notochord.[16] There is some indication in adults that "double pylorus" may actually represent a fistulous tract from ulcer disease.[87, 118]

Pathology. Most of these cystic or tubular anomalies have a common muscular wall and share a blood supply from the gastroepiploic arteries.[56, 88] The cyst lining contains gastric, intestinal, or pancreatic tissue and is prone to ulceration. Inadequate drainage of gastric-type secretions contributes to local inflammation and perforation.[125] Typically, there is no communication between these duplications, but when they do communicate, the entry is into the stomach, duodenum, or even a Meckel's diverticulum. A few cysts are pedunculated and attached to the stomach by a fibrous strand. Total gastric duplications extend from the cardia to the pylorus.[84] Most of the cysts are located along the greater curvature of the stomach, anywhere from the cardia to the pylorus.

Symptoms. Infants with large cysts or with total gastric duplication vomit during the first few days of life. In more than half, symptoms are present before one year of age. Vomiting occurs soon after feedings and is preceded by irritability and discomfort. If the cyst encroaches upon the pylorus, the vomiting is forceful and resembles that of pyloric stenosis. After vomiting, the infants are comfortable and eager to eat again. A few have no feeding difficulties, and an abdominal mass is palpated during a routine physical examination. Located in the left upper quadrant or near the midline in the epigastrium, the mass becomes progressively larger and firmer as the cyst expands and the inflammatory reaction about it increases. Anemia is present in two thirds of patients, and the stools are positive for occult blood. Weight loss becomes apparent. Melena, rectal bleeding, or hematemesis is evidence of gastric ulceration either within the cyst or at its site of communication with the stomach. Pneumonitis and pleural effusion are unusual complications, occurring only if the cyst perforates and there is a fistulous connection through the diaphragm.

Diagnosis. This anomaly must be differentiated from other causes of pyloric outlet obstruction, such as pyloric stenosis or antral web.[198] The radiologic examination is often negative early, even when there is evidence of active bleeding. Eventually, an intra- or extraluminal mass (Fig. 12–4), an extrinsic pressure defect on the stomach or surrounding viscera, or, rarely, filling of the duplication itself can be demonstrated. Most duplications lie along the greater curvature. Barium enema will reveal deflection of the splenic flexure. Angiography may show increased vascularity in the region of the cyst. There is sometimes a rim of calcification seen in a soft tissue mass that displaces the curvature of the stomach. In distal duplications, a dilated, gas-filled stomach with little air in the intestine below it can be seen. The association of the vertebral anomalies, such as hemivertebrae, or other congenital malformations is suggestive evidence that such a mass or obstructing lesion is a duplication cyst.

Treatment. If the cyst is small, it is excised along with a small margin of adjacent stomach. If it is large, the major part of the

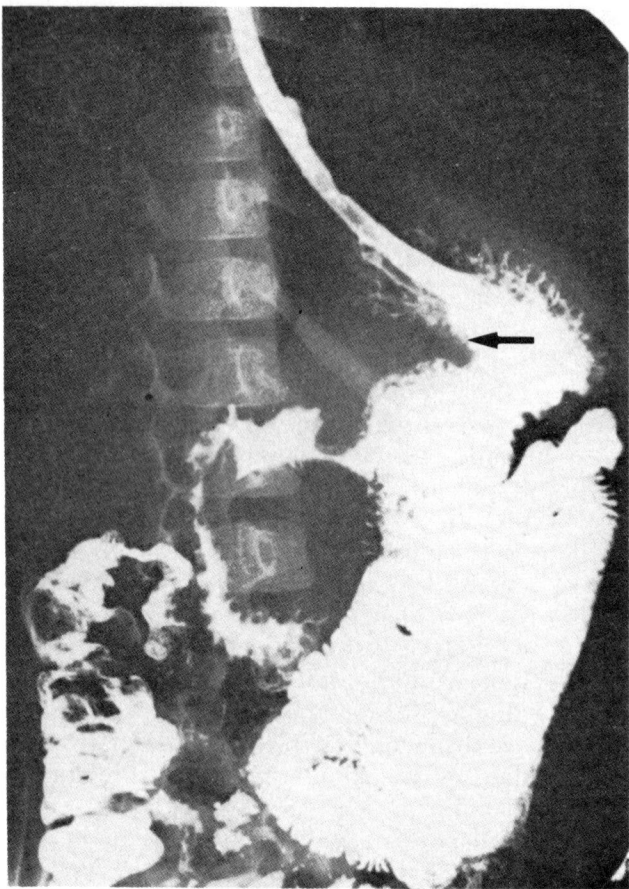

Figure 12–4 This adult male was completely asymptomatic. An upper gastrointestinal series done as part of an executive physical evaluation demonstrated an intramural mass along the upper portion of the lesser curvature of the stomach (*arrow*). Because of this finding he was taken to surgery, at which time an intramural duplication cyst was removed. Histologic examination showed that the lesion was lined with gastric mucosa. (From Gwinn, J. L., and Barnes, G. R.: Radiological case of the month. Am. J. Dis. Child. *113*:581, 1967, Used by permission.)

cyst must be excised and the gastroepiploic vessels preserved. Cyst mucosa that remains against the stomach wall is stripped away to render the residual wall nonfunctioning. Marsupialization of the cyst or extensive gastric resection is to be avoided. The only successful treatment for complete gastric duplication has been creation of a gastrojejunostomy or drainage of the duplication by means of a Roux-en-Y loop of jejunum.[224]

GASTRIC MUCOSAL DIAPHRAGM AND PYLORIC ATRESIA

Gastric mucosal diaphragm and pyloric atresia are variations of the same lesion and have the same embryologic origin.[13, 28] They are therefore discussed as one disease.[52]

Incidence. Atresia in the intestinal tract occurs in about 1 in 10,000 births, and pyloric or prepyloric defects account for less than 1 per cent of the cases.[10, 122, 123] Atresia has been reported in siblings, and both forms affect the sexes equally. It has been described in four infants with epidermolysis bullosa.[174a]

Familial pyloric atresia has been noted in 81 cases and is associated with autosomal recessive inheritance.[209] Alpha-fetoprotein has been elevated in the amniotic fluid. An autosomal recessive type of pyloroduodenal atresia (complex diaphragm) has been described in two siblings in each of three related families.[161] The proximal side of the atresia is lined by gastric mucosa and the distal, by duodenal mucosa. In one instance, a prepyloric diaphragm was covered by squamous epithelium.[136]

Etiology. These congenital membranes are caused by a persistence of the solid-core stage of the embryonic intestine. The reabsorption of ontogenetic occlusion is not constant, and atresia results when this resolution is imperfect. The development of mucosal diaphragm in older persons with peptic ulcer disease suggests an inflammatory origin.

Pathology. The thick membranous septum is located within the pylorus or in the prepyloric antrum.[214] Another membrane is occasionally present in the duodenum. The septum contains a central core of submucosa and thickened muscularis mucosae and is covered by normal gastric mucosa. The epithelial covering may be squamous, or there may be intestinal metaplasia. If the membrane is complete, the condition is pyloric atresia; if the membrane contains an opening — which can vary from minute to sizable — it is known as mucosal diaphragm.[60, 64, 76]

Situs inversus and other intestinal anomalies may be seen with this disorder.

Pathophysiology. Marked gastric distention and signs of pyloric outlet obstruction are caused by pyloric atresia.[198] Partial obstruction caused by a diaphragm produces proximal gastric muscular hypertrophy, gastric dilatation, and edema and hemorrhage of the mucosa.

Symptoms. If the membrane is complete or nearly so, acute gastric obstruction is apparent on the first day of life. Epigastric distention is severe, and the infant vomits clear gastric contents.

Mucosal diaphragm causes symptoms either during the first year or not until childhood or adult life.[143] The delay in onset of symptoms is related to the size of the aperture and to the increased propulsive ability that the stomach develops. Some infants have all the symptoms of pyloric stenosis: gastric distention, visible peristaltic waves traveling over the left upper quadrant, and projectile vomiting after feedings. Others have far milder symptoms and regurgitate small amounts of formula after feeding; only after the baby begins to eat solid food does the situation change, and then it is fairly usual for corn, peas, or other recognizable material to be vomited more than 24 hours after their ingestion. We have seen one patient who vomited corn he had eaten a week before.

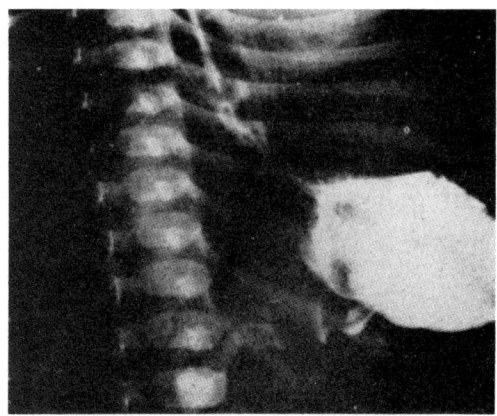

Figure 12–5 This infant girl with a pyloric mucosal diaphragm had passed normal stools but began non-bilious vomiting on the third day of life. X-rays demonstrated a transverse partial obstruction in the distal antrum with apparent elongation of the pyloric canal between the membrane and the faintly opacified duodenum. (From Farman, J., Cywes, S., and Werbeloff, L.: Pyloric mucosal diaphragms. Clin. Radiol. *19*:95, 1968. Used by permission.)

If the lesion is not diagnosed, anorexia, failure to thrive, and emaciation are prominent in older children.

A mass is not palpable unless there is a second diaphragm in the duodenum, in which case a round, firm mass is noted in the epigastrium.

Diagnosis. Upper gastrointestinal examination reveals a delay in passage of barium from the stomach into the duodenum. In cases of complete obstruction, the stomach is greatly dilated and there is no free air below the site of obstruction. A mucosal diaphragm is not always seen in radiologic examinations, especially when it lies in or close to the pylorus, where it can produce a picture resembling that of nonspecific antral spasm. Care must be taken not to obscure the antrum and pylorus with too much barium. When recognized, the diaphragm is a thin, radiolucent line with a stream of barium passing through its central orifice (Fig. 12–5). A "double-bulb" appearance is created as the membrane forms a compartment between itself and the pyloric canal (Fig. 12–6).

Comment must be made about the study of older children with this lesion, in whom weight loss and anorexia are the chief complaints. Small bowel disease is a logical

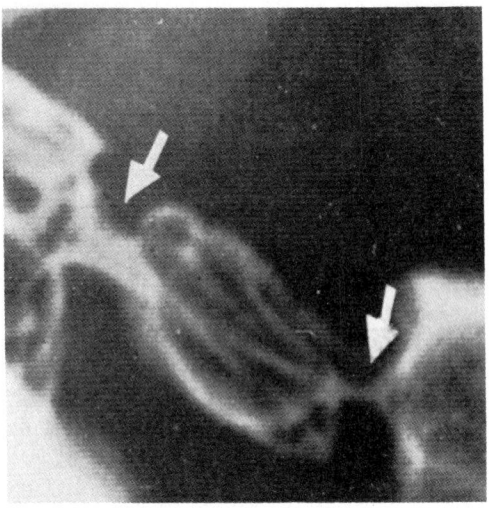

Figure 12–6 The "double-bulb" appearance is produced by the outpouching of distal antrum between the mucosal diaphragm and the pyloric canal (*arrows*). (From Johnson, G. M.: Gastric mucosal diaphragm in a child. Pediatrics 47:916, 1971. Used by permission.)

consideration, and tolerance tests and tests requiring measured urinary excretion rates may well be abnormal because of the prolonged gastric emptying time.

Complications. Peptic ulceration is likely to develop in the chronically dilated stomach and is heralded by anemia and hematemesis or melena.

Treatment. Surgical incision or excision of the diaphragm is curative. If the atresia is complete, gastroenterostomy may be required.

Prognosis. The diaphragm does not recur after surgical treatment. One to six years later, three of four nonoperated infants have had no evidence of web.

CONGENITAL HYPERTROPHIC PYLORIC STENOSIS

Congenital hypertrophic pyloric stenosis is a disease that follows a characteristic pattern and has customarily been said to affect the first-born, male, breast-fed infant. Recent studies indicate that although it is more frequent in males, it does not particularly favor the first-born or the breast-fed.[14, 15, 160]

Incidence. The incidence is generally reported as 4 or 5 per 1000 live births. In a

report from Sweden covering the decade 1950 to 1959, the incidence was only 1.9 per 1000,[219] but no such decrease in incidence has been reported in the United States. The disease tends to be familial[21, 22, 67]; in families in which one parent is affected, the incidence rises to 6.9 per cent.[151] A mother who had pyloric stenosis has a four times greater chance of having an affected infant than does a father who had the disease. An autosomal dominant form of the disease has been described in one large kindred.[72a] The overall incidence in twins is 20 times greater than that in the general population,[155] but the condition is unusual in identical twins and most unusual in identical female twins.[65, 67] Caucasian populations are most often affected. One study has reported a seasonal incidence, with cases clustered in infants born in April and May and in October and November.[104]

Etiology and Pathology. Although possibly congenital, this disorder usually does not become evident until the baby is several weeks old.[5] Its pathogenesis is still not well defined, but the most popular theory is one of hypertrophy of the circular smooth fibers of the pyloric sphincter secondary to spasm of the sphincter or perhaps to peptic ulcer disease.[105, 106] Some factors suggest that environment plays a part in the development of the disease: a greater incidence in the first-born, a later onset in those born in hospitals than outside as well as in those fed every four as contrasted with those fed every three hours in premature infants, and in those in whom oral feeding is delayed. Wallgren[219] examined the upper gastrointestinal tract of 1000 normal male neonates, and although all were normal, five went on to develop pyloric stenosis.

Lynn[142] has proposed that milk curds propelled against a spastic pyloric canal cause edema of the mucosa and submucosa, producing further narrowing of the canal. Secondary work hypertrophy of the pyloric and gastric musculature increases the obstruction. Certainly, a negative radiologic examination in an infant suspected of having pyloric stenosis can become positive days to weeks later. Arguing against theories of environmental contributions is the finding of pyloric stenosis in stillborn infants and in a seven-month fetus.

Bacterial cultures of pyloric tissue taken at surgery have always been sterile, although the perivascular infiltrate of leukocytes in the muscularis of infants in whom symptoms have been present for only a short time suggests an inflammatory etiology.[1]

Some would like to implicate the nervous system, since the pylorus is innervated separately through the hepatic branch of the right vagus and its motor function is independent of that of the rest of the stomach. The ganglion cells have been variously described, from normal to decreased or normal but immature.[11, 75, 95, 169]

Hypergastrinemia has been implicated in pyloric stenosis, but the majority of studies have shown no significantly increased gastrin levels.[85, 95, 111] Interestingly, levels of gastrin were far higher one to two weeks after surgery.

Functionally, the innermost muscular layer of the stomach is weak and incomplete at the pylorus, consisting of a thick inner circular coat and a thinner outer longitudinal layer.[12] The circular muscle is continuous with that of the stomach but is separated from that of the duodenum by a thin fibrous septum. Many of the longitudinal muscle fibers continue into the duodenum, but nearly half dip into the pyloric sphincter to reinforce it. In this disease, the circular layer is greatly hypertrophied and the pylorus is thick, firm, and elongated. The stomach is dilated and, in cases of long duration, contains hypertrophied muscle layers and superficial mucosal ulcerations.

The hyperbilirubinemia sometimes associated with pyloric stenosis is of the indirect type and is attributed to increased intra-abdominal pressure,[167, 206] which causes diminished portal flow and a compensatory increase in hepatic arterial flow. Decreased glucuronyl transferase activity associated with decreased portal flow has been documented. It has been suggested that this may represent mild Gilbert's disease.[4]

Pathophysiology. The classic clinical example of metabolic alkalosis has always been the infant with pyloric stenosis.[8, 119, 120]

The constant vomiting of gastric juice containing hydrochloric acids, sodium, potassium, chloride, and water produces this outcome. The hydrogen ion concentration of gastric juice in this age group is 65 to 80 mEq. The characteristic changes of elevated blood pH, PCO_2 and serum bicarbonate, with decreased chloride and potassium, are reached through a series of events. Early vomiting causes a mild metabolic alkalosis, in which the serum bicarbonate increases to compensate for chloride losses. The kidney excretes an alkaline urine containing sodium and potassium bicarbonate to conserve chloride and maintain blood pH. As gastric losses continue and sodium and potassium are excreted by the kidneys in their compensatory attempts, anion losses are increased. Then, as the kidneys attempt to conserve sodium, the excretion of bicarbonate is decreased. Gastric losses are isotonic, but insensible water loss continues and a relative water deficit develops. At this point, bicarbonate levels vary from 28 to 39 mEq per liter, and ketones and organic and inorganic acids accumulate. If this alkalosis progresses until the bicarbonate level is greater than 40 mEq per liter, urinary potassium loss increases and the kidney can no longer correct the metabolic imbalance.[42] All these changes are not truly reflected in serum electrolyte measurements because there is extracellular volume concentration and serum potassium can seem misleadingly normal or elevated. The blood urea nitrogen is increased with dehydration. Shallow, irregular breathing develops as a mild degree of respiratory compensation takes place.

Since surgery increases the severity of alkalosis because of an aldosterone effect that inhibits the renal excretion of base, time spent in correcting the electrolyte imbalance before operation is time well spent.

Symptoms. The full-term infant typically manifests symptoms between the second and sixth weeks of life.[218] In some, however, the onset of vomiting occurs as early as one week after birth, and in others it appears much later, in one case as late as three and one-half years of age.[123] The vomiting is at first intermittent, increasing in frequency and severity until it follows every feeding and is projectile in character. It reaches such intensity that formula is carried to the far end of the crib or across the room. The vomitus contains sour formula or clear gastric contents. As the lesion is established and less food and water make their way through the pylorus, the number of stools decreases and urination becomes scanty. Weight loss is light or severe, depending upon the duration and severity of symptoms.

Diagnosis. The diagnosis is made easily in most cases on the basis of the history and physical examination. Although malnourished, the infant is active, irritable, and eager to feed. He drinks ravenously, and peristaltic waves are seen to travel across the left upper quadrant to the right and to end just beyond the midline. The waves are best seen during or after feeding and increase in intensity until vomiting occurs. This is the time when the pyloric tumor is best palpated, i.e., when the stomach is emptied of fluid and air. The mass of hypertrophied muscle is firm and small and is more the size of a pit than of the "olive" often used in descriptions. Its positioning is variable; it is generally palpated just to the right of the midline above the umbilicus, but it is sometimes high, under the liver edge, or low, at the level of the umbilicus. One must palpate gently to avoid contraction of the rectus abdominis muscles.

In the premature infant, diagnosis is more difficult, for the onset of symptoms is later, between 32 and 87 days of age.[227] The disease is not rare in premature infants, affecting 3.5 per cent. The course is milder and the onset more insidious. Although it becomes persistent, vomiting is not of the projectile type, and the gastric waves are not diagnostic, for they may be seen in normal premature infants with poorly developed abdominal musculature. The pyloric tumor is easily palpated.

Persistent, projectile vomiting with its associated metabolic changes occurs only with lesions at the pylorus. Hypochloremic metabolic alkalosis has been reported in infants treated for persistent fetal circulation with tolazoline. Although pyloric stenosis is the most common anomaly, antral web, pylorospasm, and pyloric duplication must all be considered. If the mass is easily palpable, further diagnostic studies are not necessary.[128] An infant who does not have a palpable mass or who is not alkalotic warrants further study, for in reviewing our last 40 patients with a diagnosis of pyloric stenosis, we found two with bicarbonate levels of less than 27 mEq per liter in whom operation had revealed no disorder.

Studies of gastric motility show an increased frequency and amplitude of contractions.[92] Rhythmic bell-shaped waves increase in height until vomiting occurs (Fig. 12–7).

Radiologic studies provide the diagno-

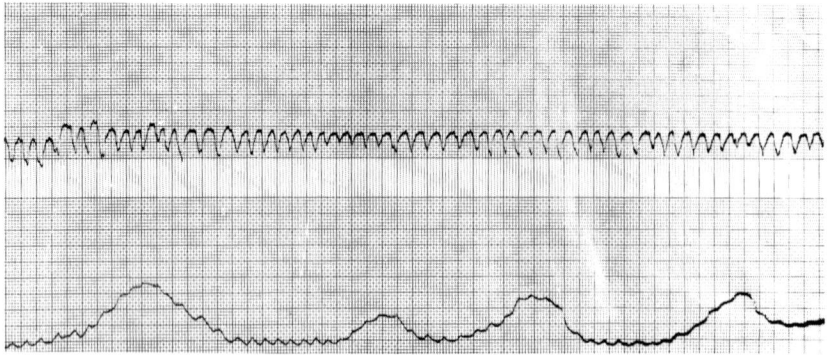

Figure 12–7   Motility tracing from an infant with pyloric stenosis. This four-week-old infant was studied in the resting and fasting states. The upper lead, in the esophagus, records the deflections of respiration. The lower lead, in the stomach, demonstrates rhythmic bell-shaped waves that are not present in recordings from normal infants.

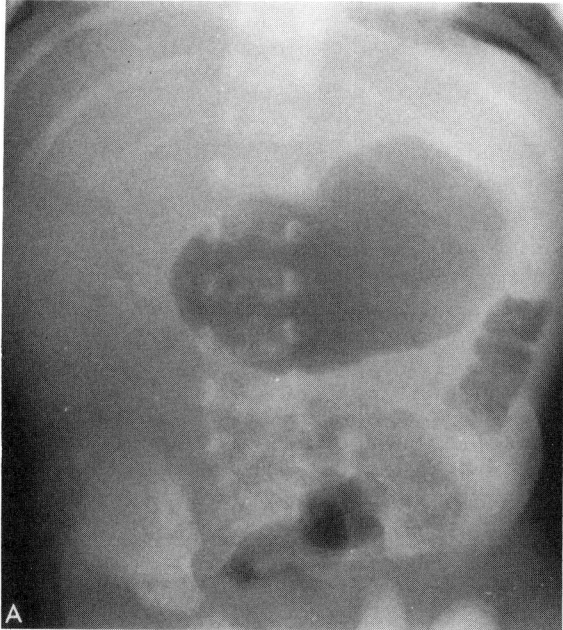
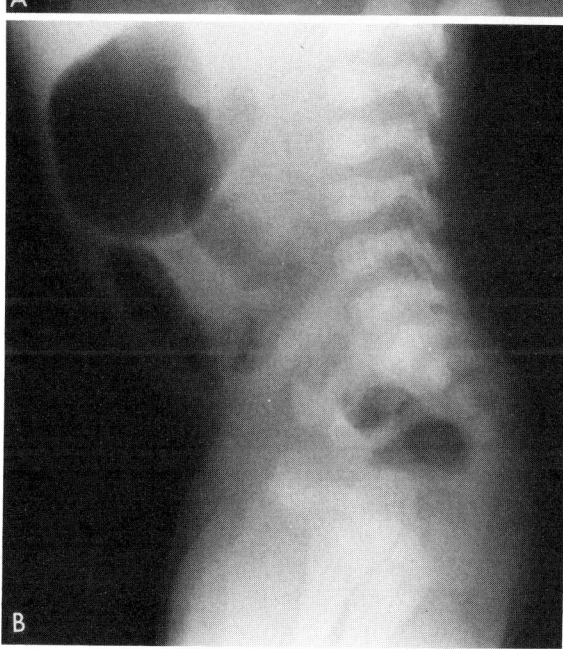

Figure 12–8 One-month-old boy with a two-day history of vomiting and a palpable olive. *A*, Anteroposterior view. There is distention of the stomach with only a small amount of gas seen more distally in the gastrointestinal tract. *B*, On the lateral view, abrupt narrowing of the pylorus can be seen projected just behind the body of the stomach.

sis.[191, 204] Flat film of the abdomen shows a dilated, air-filled stomach and a nondilated pyloric canal. There are only small amounts of gas distal to the stomach (Fig. 12–8). Associated gastric emphysema has been noted in three patients.[134] Contrast studies are reserved for cases in which the clinical diagnosis is in question. The study is best performed after aspiration of the stomach. Barium is injected through a nasogastric tube under fluoroscopic control until moderate gastric filling is attained. Greater distention of the stomach is unnecessary and not only obscures visualization of the pyloric canal but also can induce vomiting. Barium should be removed through the nasogastric tube after the study is completed. A number of radiologic signs are described (Fig. 12–9).[147, 171, 182] (1) The pyloric canal is vertically oriented or swings upward and to

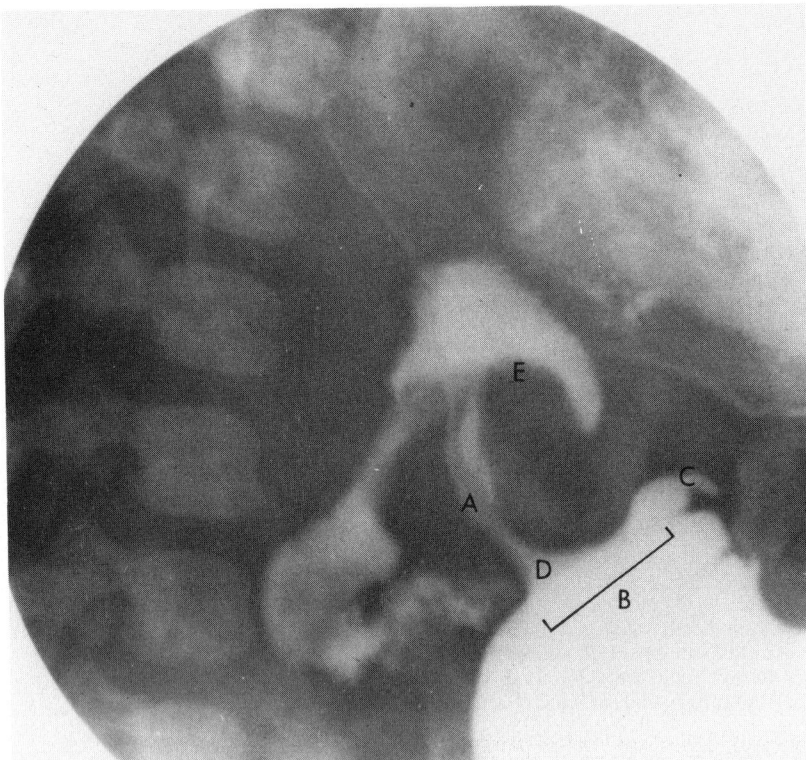

Figure 12–9   Upper gastrointestinal series from a five-week-old boy with a short history of vomiting after feedings. A spot film of the pylorus and duodenum demonstrates several of the roentgenographic findings associated with hypertrophic pyloric stenosis. *A,* The pyloric canal is narrowed (string sign), and there seem to be several tracks of barium in the canal (double-track sign). *B,* The distal part of the pylorus is straightened by pressure from the hypertrophied muscle (shoulder sign). *C,* The distal lesser curvature ends in a superior projection (pyloric tit). *D,* The proximal pyloric canal may appear as a projection from the distal stomach (beak sign). *E,* The hypertrophied muscle produces a curved impression on the base of the duodenal bulb.

the left before entering the duodenal bulb. There is an exaggerated curve of the stomach. (2) The elongated and narrowed canal produces a "string sign." (3) A "double-track" sign is caused by longitudinal ridges of mucosa that are squeezed into the lumen of the pylorus and surrounded on both sides by barium. This is the most reliable diagnostic finding, and its presence allows differentiation from pylorospasm, which can also produce a string sign. (4) The "shoulder sign" is the rather squared-off appearance of the distal antrum where it is impressed upon the "olive." (5) The point at which the lesser curvature of the stomach abuts the "olive" is represented by a sharp angulation or projection, which is termed the pyloric tit. (6) The "beak sign" is a small projection of barium in the proximal end of the pyloric canal caused by the abrupt transition from antrum to pyloric canal. (7) After some contrast material has passed from the stomach into the duodenum, a rounded invagination of the base of the bulb is sometimes evident. This is termed the umbrella sign, and it is caused by impression from the distal end of hypertrophied muscle. Delayed gastric emptying is a constant finding in all studies.

Treatment. It is advisable to take the time needed to correct the alkalosis so that the bicarbonate is less than 30 mEq per liter, since those operated upon before this is done have a higher incidence of postoperative vomiting. Hydration is first accomplished, with 0.45 per cent normal saline in 5 per cent dextrose. After the infant is voiding well and the urine specific gravity approaches 1.010, a maintenance solution containing 2 to 4 mEq per liter of potassium is substituted. Some centers advocate the use of ammonium chloride, but this can be dangerous. Ultimate metabolic recovery depends upon rehydration with adequate electrolyte replacement.

Definitive treatment is pyloromyotomy, which carries an operative mortality of less than 1 per cent. Oral feedings are begun four to six hours after surgery, when the infant is awake, alert, and sucking well. Beginning with clear fluids, the diet is increased to full-strength formula over 24 hours.

There are some proponents of medical treatment of this disease with methylscopolamine, but this agent seems effective only in the milder cases and its use prolongs the hospital stay.[43, 52]

Prognosis. Gastric motility is decreased during the first 24 hours after surgery but returns to normal within 26 to 30 hours.[185] There is no immediate change in the radiologic picture except for an improvement in gastric emptying time. Postoperative vomiting may occur, particularly in infants with preoperative hematemesis, and there is endoscopic evidence of esophagitis. Shortening and widening of the pyloric canal is not always evident until six months after surgery, but despite the persistence of radiologic abnormalities, the infants are asymptomatic. In later life, however, two thirds of patients studied had periodic epigastric burning or symptoms of acid regurgitation. Most had no radiologic abnormality, but there was evidence of increased fasting gastric secretion and the pentapeptide-stimulated volume was 40 per cent above normal, although peak acid output was not increased.[200, 205, 221]

Many of the patients treated medically have had symptoms of dyspepsia, vomiting, or epigastric heaviness, and gastric ulcers have developed in some.[169, 223]

CONGENITAL CYSTIC DISEASE OF THE STOMACH

We have seen congenital cystic dysplasia in the stomach of a one-month-old infant who died of pneumonia. There was cystic cavitation of the walls of the stomach. The cysts, located in the submucosa, were lined by squamous or cuboidal epithelium and filled with thick, homogeneous material. The mucosa was atrophic in some areas, as was the muscularis.

ECTOPIC PANCREATIC TISSUE

Ectopic pancreatic tissue in the stomach has been described by endoscopic examination and biopsy in a child with abdominal pain and upper gastrointestinal bleeding.[44]

FAMILIAL JUVENILE POLYPOSIS OF THE STOMACH

Familial gastric polyposis is a newly described entity, distinct from other polyposis syndromes in that no other gastrointestinal organs are involved.[222]

Incidence. Five cases had been reported by 1979: two siblings in one family and three (two siblings, one mother) in another.

Etiology. Although probably an inherited disorder, the genetic transmission has not yet been defined.

Pathology. Innumerable polyps of varying size carpet the gastric mucosa from cardia to pylorus, being largest and most numerous distally. Histologically, some show cystic dilatation of glands, and others a glandular structure with abundant columnar-lined tubules. The stoma is edematous and infiltrated with polymorphonuclear cells, plasma cells, and lymphocytes, but the muscularis is not involved. There is hypoacidity as well as evidence of enteric protein loss.

Symptoms. Anemia of an iron-deficient type may be the only symptom, but edema is evident later. All patients had suboptimal intelligence and atypical brown hair.

Differential Diagnosis. Gastric polyps are also present in diffuse juvenile polyposis and familial polyposis. In these disorders, however, polyps are present elsewhere in the gastrointestinal tract. Very rarely, polypoid lesions of the antrum represent Menetrier's disease.

MOTOR ABNORMALITIES OF THE STOMACH

PYLOROSPASM AND ANTRAL SPASM

These neuromuscular disorders of infancy are characterized by intermittent vomiting and may simulate pyloric stenosis and gastroesophageal reflux.

Incidence. Their existence as a clinical entity is doubted by many, but some experienced practitioners have no reservations about their reality.

Pathology. No anatomic changes have been noted.

Etiology. These are transient disorders of neuromuscular function to which hyperactive or tense infants are particularly prone. They may, indeed, represent dysfunction of the entire upper gastrointestinal tract, as noted in children with severe gastroesophageal reflux.

Symptoms. Vomiting often begins between the first and fourth weeks and is intermittent or, rarely, continuous. Schaffer and Avery[184] stress that such infants are unable to tolerate more than 1 1/2 to 2 ounces of formula at a feeding. Sometimes a gastric bubble may be seen in the left upper quadrant during feeding, but visible peristaltic waves are minimal or absent. No masses or tumors are palpated, although Craig[45] described a mass discovered after painstaking examination.

Diagnosis. Radiologic examination of the stomach with contrast material produces variable results; there may be a delay in gastric emptying, or the stomach may empty rapidly. Pyloric or antral spasm is noted, and there is a decreased gastric capacity. It is sometimes difficult to distinguish pylorospasm from the early stages of pyloric stenosis, although the pyloric canal is not lengthened. Refractory cases should be examined by endoscopy to rule out pyloric channel ulcer, antral ulcer, or antral erosions.

Treatment. Most infants respond dramatically to atropine. Beginning with 1 drop of a 1:1000 solution 15 minutes before feeding, the dose is increased daily by 1 drop until flushing occurs. The previous day's dosage is established as the permanent one. Antihistamines have not promoted consistent improvement. A two-week treatment period is usually required before the drug can be discontinued. Bentyl (dicyclomine hydrochloride), 1/2 teaspoon three to four times daily, has provided dramatic relief of symptoms in some patients.

Prognosis. There is usually no recurrence of symptoms.

FAMILIAL DYSAUTONOMIA AND OTHER DISORDERS

Familial dysautonomia is discussed in detail under esophageal disease. Gastric as well as esophageal motility disorders are present and consist of moderate to marked pylorospasm with or without decreased gastric peristalsis and prolonged emptying time.[137]

Delayed gastric emptying is also found in infants with central nervous system disease, malnutrition, intestinal pseudo-obstruction, and gastroesophageal reflux. It has also been noted in patients with oral gastroenteritis.[153a]

ACQUIRED LESIONS OF THE STOMACH

GASTROJEJUNOCOLIC FISTULA

This extremely rare disorder has to date been accompanied by a mortality rate of 100 per cent.

Etiology. The lesion is secondary to gastric ulceration, abdominal surgery, or erosion by a gastrotomy tube or umbilical vein catheter.

Symptoms. After one of the causative events, repeated vomiting and intractable diarrhea develop. If there is enough inflammatory reaction about the fistula, there is a palpable epigastric mass.

Diagnosis. Barium enema is the first diagnostic examination to be performed but does not always demonstrate the fistula. Examination of the upper gastrointestinal tract shows gastrojejunal or gastrocolic passage of contrast material.

Treatment. Surgery is poorly tolerated in these critically ill babies. Ileostomy or transverse colostomy should be performed as a first-stage procedure, and hyperalimentation should be provided until the infant's condition improves. Traumatic fistulas have been shown to heal during periods of hyperalimentation. Later, continuity of the gastrointestinal tract can be established.

ACUTE GASTRIC DILATATION

Acute gastric dilatation can occur in any critically ill child and has been described in the terminal stages of leukemia, in diabetes, in anorexia nervosa, and with hypokalemia. Of special interest to the pediatrician is gastric dilatation in infants who are in a body cast.[29]

Etiology. Although the cause is not known, most investigators believe that paralytic ileus of the stomach with functional outlet obstruction is present. Forced immobilization is a recognized cause of gastric dilatation and is termed the cast syndrome. This is presumably due to compression of the duodenum by the superior mesenteric artery. Abdominal trauma and severe pain also precede this event.[165]

Pathology and Pathogenesis. Acute gastric dilatation causes increased portal venous pressure and increased fluid losses into the stomach, small bowel, and mesentery.[174] Mechanical pressure by the stomach on the abdominal vena cava and angulation of the cava at the diaphragmatic hiatus decrease venous return to the heart and lead to reduced cardiac output and stroke volume.[54] These factors in combination with the fluid losses contribute to the development of shock.[61] Elevation of the diaphragms causes respiratory embarrassment. Air-swallowing secondary to pain or apprehension further increases distention. Cast immobilization impairs belching and exacerbates the condition. As distention increases, so does angulation of the gastroduodenal junction, which causes partial or complete outlet obstruction.

Symptoms. Massive abdominal distention develops in a very sick infant in a cast. Respiratory distress is evidenced as tachypnea and grunting respirations, but the lung fields are clear to auscultation. Percussion reveals elevated diaphragms. Small quantities of liquid flow effortlessly from the mouth. The abdomen is tightly distended and tympanitic in its upper half. Unless the gastric distention is relieved, cardiovascular collapse follows.

Diagnosis. Plain film of the abdomen shows a huge, dilated, air-filled stomach. The diaphragms are elevated (Fig. 12–10).

Treatment. Passage of a nasogastric tube decompresses the stomach immediately. If a cast surrounds the abdomen, a window must be cut in it. Any electrolyte imbalances must be corrected, and the status of hydration and electrolytes must be monitored for several days after decompression because of the possibility of additional losses into the gastric wall and lumen. Nasogastric suction is continued for several days to a week, until gastric motility is functional.

INTERSTITIAL GASTRIC EMPHYSEMA

Interstitial gastric emphysema, reported as an autopsy finding in a premature infant,[208] was considered of traumatic origin and the result of continuous gavage feedings. The disorder was asymptomatic during life. The stomach was distended and contained bloody mucoid material. There were clusters of emphysematous cysts in an area where the submucosa was destroyed.

PEPTIC ULCER DISEASE AND GASTRIC EROSIONS

Peptic ulcer disease in the infant is unlike that in older children, being most often acute and far more serious.[170] The onset is sudden, and the ulcerations tend to erode through the muscularis into blood vessels, causing massive hemorrhage or perforation or both. Because of the early superficial nature of the ulcer, it is often not demonstrated radiologically. Similar symptoms are produced by hemorrhage erosions.[23, 24]

Incidence. The incidence in infants is difficult to determine. A review of nine major series of peptic ulcer disease or upper gastrointestinal bleeding in childhood pub-

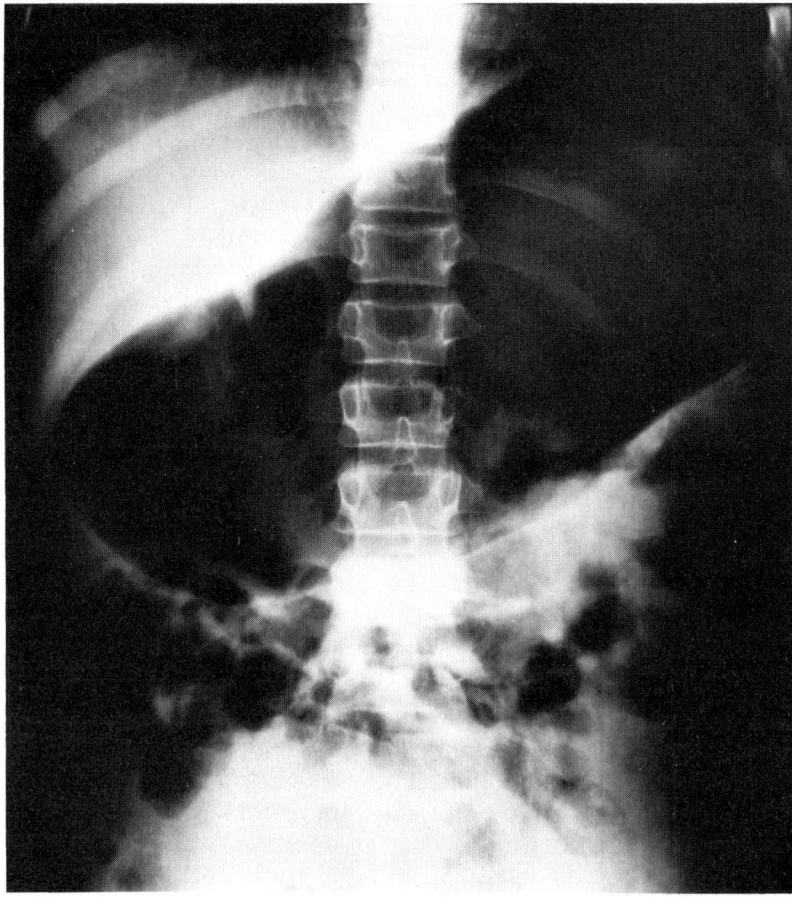

Figure 12–10   This 14-year-old boy with known diabetes mellitus was admitted to the hospital for treatment of ketoacidosis and complained of abdominal pain. The plain film of the abdomen demonstrates a dilated stomach. Although older diabetics may have chronic gastric dilatation on a neurotrophic basis, the specific cause of it in association with acute ketoacidosis is not known.

lished before 1971 accumulated 969 patients.[18, 19, 46, 116, 170, 188] Ninety-seven, or 10 per cent, were under two weeks of age; 47 had gastric ulcers, 21 had duodenal ulcers, and 29 had duodenal and pyloric lesions. In 164 infants two weeks to one year of age, there were 25 gastric and 92 duodenal ulcers; 46 had both duodenal and pyloric ulcers, and 1 had gastric and duodenal ulcers. In 1976, Curci et al.[46] reviewed 116 children with ulcers. In infants under six months of age, six ulcers were due to stress and one to body casting; one patient had a chronic ulcer. Only one child 7 to 12 months of age had an ulcer, and that was considered to be chronic. Three ulcers occurred in infants one to two years old; one was related to stress, one to steroid therapy, and one was chronic. Similarly, Puri et al.[178] in 1978 described duodenal ulcers in four children one and one-half to five years old and stressed persistence of symptoms in those treated medically.

The incidence in neonates may well be on the increase, since critically ill infants are now surviving situations that would have precluded life a decade ago. The frequency of diagnosis, particularly of acute ulcers, has increased significantly with the use of endoscopy.[44]

There is usually no predilection for sex in infancy. In older children, however, ulcer is more common in males than in females, in whites than in blacks, and in urban populations than in rural ones.

Etiology and Pathogenesis

ACUTE ULCERS AND EROSIONS.   Most ulcers in infants are acute and are related to neonatal anoxia, marasmus, drugs, dehydration, sepsis, meningitis, hypoglycemia, cold, trauma, impairment of the vascular supply, or chronic overdistention of the stomach.[68] These are usually stress-type ulcers. A few whose etiology is unknown are termed acute primary ulcers.[9]

STRESS ULCERS. Most stress ulcers are *not* associated with increased gastric acidity, and it has been thought that endogenous ACTH or cortisol production contributes to ulceration by altering gastric mucus and decreasing its resistance to proteolysis.[58] Increases in blood histamine and in gastric histidine decarboxylase in animals that acquire stress ulcers suggest that histamine plays a role in this type of ulcer development. Pretreatment of such animals with histamine inhibitors prevents ulcer formation. Stress promotes ischemic changes in the mucosa, which are at first generalized and then focal. The arteriovenous anastomoses in the submucosal vessels contract to cause localized ischemia, microvascular breakage, and necrosis of the surface epithelial cells.[97] Only small quantities of acid are needed to damage the ischemic mucosa. Once disruption of the gastric mucosal barrier has occurred, there is back-diffusion of H^+ into the gastric mucosa, which in turn leads to tissue histamine release.

CUSHING'S ULCERS. These follow head trauma or central nervous system disease and are associated with gastric hyperacidity.

CURLING'S ULCER. Curling's ulcer, estimated to occur in 25 per cent of burn patients, may be a sequela of hemorrhagic gastritis present in the early burn period. Gastric secretion is normal.[176]

DRUG-INDUCED EROSIONS AND ULCERATION. These are caused by a variety of drugs, which either stimulate gastric secretion or damage the mucosal barrier. Erosions or ulcers have been noted in patients taking aspirin, nonsteroidal anti-inflammatory agents, tetracycline, erythromycin, aminophylline, and alcohol.

ANTIPYRETIC AND ANTI-INFLAMMATORY DRUGS. The relationship between salicylate ingestion and gastrointestinal bleeding was established 20 years ago, when it was shown that the oral ingestion of as little as 5 grains caused approximately 3 ml of blood loss in the adult.[194, 199] The major effect of salicylates is upon the gastric mucosa, with aqueous preparations most rapidly absorbed. Aspirin seems to damage gastric mucosa only in an acid environment, where salicylate in an un-ionized form is lipid-soluble and penetrates the luminal cellular lipid membrane. Within the cell, where the pH is less acid, the drug changes to an ionized form that interferes with cellular metabolism: decreasing ATP, increasing cation and decreasing anion permeability of the fundus, and decreasing prostaglandin synthesis. Increased mucosal permeability and back-diffusion of acid lead to liberation of histamine and increased mucosal blood flow. Aspirin does not increase gastric secretion and, indeed, may even lower it, interfering with stimulated secretion.

Hematologically, salicylates increase the prothrombin time by decreasing hepatic synthesis of factor VII and prolong the bleeding time by causing abnormalities of platelet aggregation.

The aspirin-induced erosions are diffuse with serpiginous edges. Powdered residue may be seen adhering to the erosions. Lesions have not been seen with acetaminophen usage.

Nonsteroidal anti-inflammatory agents may case gastritis through their effect upon prostaglandin synthetase, but their effects are less marked than those of salicylates.

Exogenous ACTH and cortisone increase the incidence of peptic ulcer two to three fold[49] through several mechanisms: inhibition of mucus secretion, alteration of mucus composition,[79] and increased gastrin secretion. If there is an urgent need for steroids, they may be given in the lowest dose possible.

Bile salts cause peptic erosions and ulceration by damaging the gastric mucosal barrier and decreasing mucosal blood flow.[171]

Reserpine in small doses does not affect gastric secretion but in large doses increases it within a period of hours.[98]

Tolazine, used in the neonate for therapy of persistent fetal circulation, causes gastric hypersecretion by enhancing the effect of histamine and stimulating pepsin, acid, and volume. Increased secretions may lead to hypochloremic metabolic alkalosis through gastric losses of chloride. Other complications are hyperperistalsis, diarrhea, and gastrointestinal bleeding.

Pathology. The ulcers are single or multiple and situated in the stomach, duodenum, or both.[44] Duodenal ulcers are located in the posterior duodenum above the ampulla of Vater. The lesions associated with trauma and stress are classified as diffuse erosions of the gastric mucosa with little surrounding reaction, multiple punctate erosions throughout the stomach, and a single punched-out ulcer having little surrounding reaction.[83] These ulcers are typically destructive and erode rapidly. There is no inflammatory reaction or thickening of the gastric or duodenal wall. Erosion into a mural blood vessel results in hemorrhage, and erosion through the organ wall, in perforation.

Symptoms. The onset of symptoms in infants under one month of age is dramatic and marked by hemorrhage, perforation, or both. (Perforation of a gastric ulcer has occurred even *in utero*.)[131] There is often a history of preceding illness or anoxia at birth. Although the infant appears stable for several hours or days, massive abdominal distention and shock develop without warning, or he vomits or passes bright red blood per rectum. The distended abdomen becomes tympanitic, and the normal area of liver fullness is lost. If there is an inguinal hernia, air distends the scrotal sac. In cases of hemorrhage, hematemesis is as frequent as rectal bleeding. If the bleeding is slow, blood is acted upon by gastric contents, the vomitus resembles coffee grounds and the stools are black and tarry. The bowel sounds are hyperactive with bleeding but disappear in the presence of perforation and peritonitis. Fever, leukocytosis, anemia, and tachycardia precede circulatory collapse. In extremely ill infants, however, symptoms may be minimal and overshadowed by those of the primary disease.

Rarely, duodenal ulcer in the neonate presents as high intestinal obstruction.

Case History. T.B., a three-week-old white male infant, was admitted because of poor weight gain and regurgitation. He was born after a full-term pregnancy, and the delivery was uncomplicated. Weight at birth was 3200 gm, and at the time of admission it was 2700 gm. During the second week of life, the baby began to regurgitate every feeding of breast milk. Weight loss was apparent upon admission, for he had wasting of the extremities and gluteal muscles. Vital signs, serum electrolytes, and cultures from the nose, throat, blood, and stool were normal. He tolerated clear liquids and increasing strengths of Nutramigen. On the fourth hospital day he suddenly exhibited tachycardia, passed a dark red stool, and vomited blood. The hemoglobin fell from 12 to 8 gm per dl and the hematocrit from 38 to 24 mm. Despite continuous nasogastric suction and blood transfusions the bleeding continued briskly and the hemoglobin dropped to 6 gm per dl over the next 24 hours. Radiologic study of the stomach and duodenum showed no lesion, and emergency laparotomy was performed. A large posterior duodenal ulcer was bleeding from an eroded vessel at its base and had penetrated to the pancreas. The bleeding point was ligated, and the perforation was closed. The infant recovered without complications and at one year had no evidence of hypersecretion.

Diagnosis. A history of birth trauma, anoxia, infection, or central nervous system disease will point to peptic ulcer as the underlying cause of gastrointestinal bleeding or perforation. In severely burned children, Curling's ulcer is likely to develop between 8 and 15 days after injury. Return of blood through the nasogastric tube indicates bleeding from the esophagus, stomach, or duodenum. Gastric secretion studies are not valid during active bleeding, and stimulation is contraindicated. In any case, because of wide variation in normal values these studies are of little diagnostic help.[213]

Because the radiologic diagnosis of ulcer disease requires demonstration of an ulcer crater or associated duodenal deformity, it is of little value in detecting the acute superficial ulcer.[132] Radiographic study is, however, of value in ruling out esophageal varices or peptic esophagitis, chalasia, or gastric bezoar. Deep ulcerations are not visualized if the lesion is acute and unassociated with inflammation or fibrosis. Apparent spasm or hypertonicity of the antrum, pylorus, or duodenum is sometimes seen in studies of normal infants and does not constitute evidence of ulcer disease in the absence of a demonstrable crater.

Endoscopy is of value in identifying the site of upper gastrointestinal bleeding (see Chapter One). Selective celiac and mesenteric arteriography is being used increasingly to localize actively bleeding sites in the gastrointestinal tract. Serial x-ray filming after injection of contrast material into the selected vessel demonstrates the point of extravasation and is followed by persistence of an opaque blush in the lumen of the viscus after the contrast material has disappeared from the vascular structures. Isotope studies do not localize a site of bleeding, since the blood-bound isotope extravasated into the gastrointestinal lumen is measured either in the gastric aspirate or in the stool.

Perforation of the ulcer with resulting pneumoperitoneum produces a characteristic radiographic appearance, but similar findings also occur in spontaneous gastric rupture, intestinal perforations, and necrotizing enterocolitis.

Treatment. Perforations, either free into the peritoneum or posterior into the pancreas, are accompanied by a rapid decline of the baby's condition and should be treated by immediate plication of the ulcer and ligation of bleeding points. Because the infantile ulcer is usually acute, surgical management should not involve wide resection. Medical therapy and use of cimetidine[32] are discussed under upper gastrointestinal bleeding in Chapter Seven.[108] In patients operated, the mortality is about 20 per cent.[162]

Chronic Peptic Ulcer

This type of ulcer is usually seen in infants a year old or more and is far less common than the acute ulcer.[157]

Etiology. There is undoubtedly a familial tendency, for chronic ulcer has a higher than expected frequency in persons of blood group O and is two and a half times more frequent in siblings of ulcer patients. The parietal cell mass and the maximal acid output are increased in patients with duodenal ulcer. Basal gastrin levels are not elevated, but the postprandial gastrin output is greater in the ulcer patient than in the normal person. In children, postprandial values may be elevated for age but may not approach normal values for adults. Ischemia resulting from stress is probably an important factor in the genesis of this type of ulcer as well as of the acute type.

Pathology. The chronic infantile ulcers have well-defined zones of fibrosis, inflammatory reaction, and endarteritis obliterans. There is some erosion of muscularis at the ulcer base. In infancy the ratio of duodenal to gastric ulcer is 2:1, but in older children it is 7:1. Five per cent of patients have both gastric and duodenal ulcers.

Symptoms. The history is long and vague, with feeding difficulties, regurgitation, pain, or vomiting persisting for several weeks or months. Pyloric channel ulcer may cause cyclic vomiting. The correct diagnosis is usually not considered until perforation or hemorrhage complicates the picture. Posterior penetrating ulcers produce a secondary pancreatitis that causes severe epigastric pain and abdominal rigidity.[78]

The typical ulcer symptoms of the adult — pain relieved by eating and recurring one to two hours after meals, or pain that awakens the patient late at night — are not apparent in children until they reach six or more years of age.[166]

Diagnosis. The signs of chronic infantile ulcer are identical to those of the adult in radiologic examinations (Fig. 12–11): the ulcer crater, thickening of the surrounding gastric or duodenal wall, and folds radiating about the crater like a corona. Local spasm may produce a persistent notch deformity of the opposite wall of the stomach in cases of gastric ulcer, or a bizarre deformity of the duodenal bulb in cases of duodenal ulcer — causing difficulty in distinguishing spasm from scarring. Gastric and duodenal motility is increased or decreased, and there is often transient or persistent pylorospasm as well as gastric retention of secretions or barium. In infants, most studies of stimulated gastric secretion and fasting or stimulated gastrin levels fall within the normal range.

Treatment. Medical management consists of offering small, frequent feedings; formula, milk, gelatins, and creamed soups are ideal and palatable. Initially, antacids

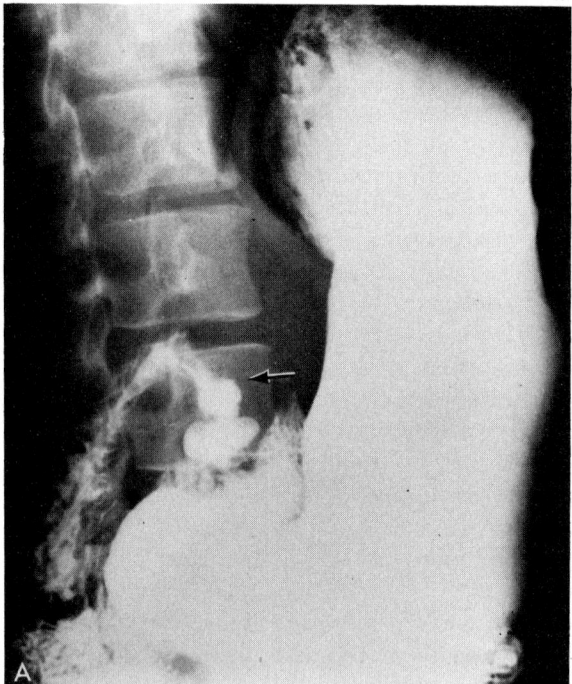

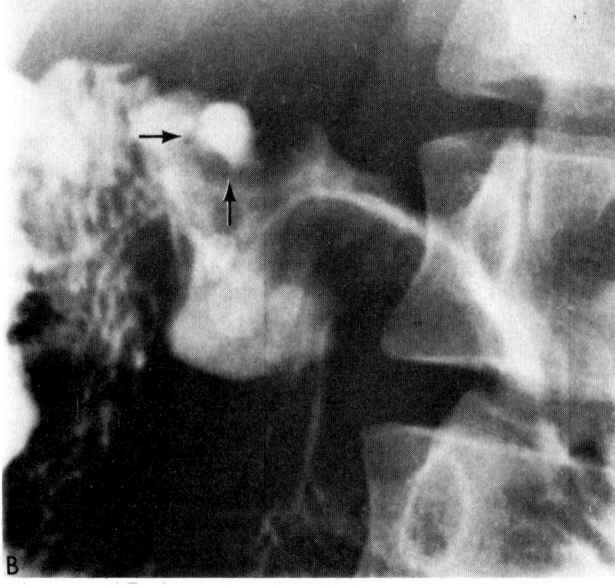

Figure 12–11 Upper gastrointestinal series from a 15-year-old girl with a one-day history of nausea and vomiting followed by hematemesis. Both parents had gastrointestinal bleeding secondary to duodenal ulcer when they were in their thirties. A repeat contrast study on this girl after seven weeks of medical therapy was normal. *A*, The overhead film demonstrates a spastic, contracted duodenal bulb (*arrow*). *B*, A compression spot film shows the ulcer crater filled with barium (*arrows*). The lucent halo surrounding the ulcer represents thickening and edema of the adjacent duodenum. The apparent difference in size between the upper and the lower half of the duodenal bulb is a manifestation of spasm in the superior recess.[162, 163]

may be required in hourly or two-hourly dosage (2 to 3 ml). Those containing magnesium hydroxide may cause diarrhea, and those containing aluminum hydroxide may cause constipation. Cimetidine, a histamine receptor antagonist, in dosage of 10 to 20 mg per kg will decrease gastric secretion but should be used only in refractory cases. Anticholinergics are avoided because they lower LES pressure, and salicylates are contraindicated. In cases of hemorrhage or per-foration, plication of the ulcer with vagotomy and pyloroplasty is recommended. Subtotal gastrectomy has been performed in some infants and has been followed by relatively normal growth and development.[162, 163]

Prognosis. Chronicity is the rule for this ulcer; one quarter to one half of the patients eventually require surgery for hemorrhage, perforation, or duodenal obstruction secondary to scarring.[42]

Peptic Ulcer and Associated Diseases

Up to 18 per cent of patients with chronic pancreatitis or cystic fibrosis incur peptic ulcer.[20] We have performed gastric analyses on 20 children with cystic fibrosis and peptic ulcer disease or epigastric complaints and have found no evidence of hyperacidity; others have noted hypersecretion. Ulcer most likely results from the presence of unbuffered acid in the duodenum. An increased incidence in uremic patients (9 per cent) has been noted and associated with hypergastrinemia from decreased renal clearance of the hormone.[123, 164]

The effect of carbon dioxide on gastric secretion is not clear, but there is an increased incidence of ulcer in patients with chronic pulmonary disease or cyanotic heart disease.

Hyperparathyroidism[53] and duodenal ulcer are related beyond normal coincidence, and most of the patients do not have gastric hyperacidity. Experimentally, a serum calcium level of greater than 12 mg per dl stimulates gastric secretion, and a level less than 7 mg per dl results in no free acid in basal secretions.

The multiple endocrine adenoma syndrome consists of multiple tumors or hyperplasia of endocrine glands. It is familial and is transmitted as an autosomal dominant with variable penetrance. The patients generally present in adolescence or young adult life with tumors or hyperplasia of the thyroid, parathyroid, pancreas, pituitary, or adrenal glands. In those with peptic ulcer disease, bleeding or perforation frequently develops.

The *Zollinger-Ellison syndrome,* consisting of single or multiple peptic ulcerations and watery or steatorrheal stools in association with a non–insulin-secreting tumor of the pancreas,[2, 5, 11] probably represents one variant of the multiple adenoma syndrome. It has not yet been described in infancy. Blood gastrin levels are elevated, and there is hypertrophy and thickening of the gastric rugal folds. The mucosal folds of the duodenum and jejunum are similarly thickened. Characteristically, the peptic ulcerations are atypical in location, occurring in the prepyloric, lower duodenal, or jejunal region. Gastric analysis reveals an increased basal secretion with little or no rise after histamine stimulation, resulting in a MAO to BAO ratio of 0.6 or less. There is increased pancreatic basal secretion and a greatly increased secretion after secretin stimulation. This is due to either increased pancreatic secretory mass or increased endogenous secretin. The diagnosis is usually considered only after a course of unsuccessful medical therapy for peptic ulcer. Calcium or secretin infusion increases gastric secretion and blood gastrin levels in these patients but not in those with hypersecretion of other origins.[51] An accurate diagnosis is essential because total gastrectomy is the only successful treatment.[73] In most cases the pancreatic tumor is not resectable. Gastrectomy not only eliminates hypersecretion but also is followed by visible regression of metastases.[73, 74] Normal growth and development have followed surgery in older children, with atropine helpful in controlling diarrhea. Cimetidine may also be of value in controlling hypersecretion.

Diffuse cutaneous mastocytosis, a variant of urticaria pigmentosa, is a skin disease of mast cell proliferation and infiltration.[198a] The skin manifestations are primary, but other organs, including the gastrointestinal tract, are involved. Because of increased histamine release, peptic ulcer is the major gastrointestinal complication. Increased transit time and thickened mucosal folds are radiologic findings. Cromolyn, a mast cell membrane–stabilizing agent, will decrease systemic symptoms.

Eosinophilic gastritis — see eosinophilic gastroenteritis.

GASTRIC PERFORATION

Neonatal Gastric Perforation

This emergency is the most common hollow viscus perforation in the neonate.[6, 107]

Incidence. The exact incidence of gastric perforation is unknown, but approximately 200 cases have been reported in newborns. Since isolated cases are often not reported, the condition is undoubtedly more common than is suggested by the literature.

Etiology. In a few cases, obvious causes for the perforation are found: nasal catheter oxygen administration or feeding tubes.[17, 40, 69, 99, 103, 152, 203, 217] peptic ulcer, necrotizing enterocolitis, or gastric distention secondary to pyloric atresia.[138, 139, 175, 190] More unusual cases of perforation have been associated with hemorrhage into the gastric wall, foreign body,[147] abscess, or gastromalacia.[148]

One favored theory is that perforation occurs through a congenital defect in the gastric musculature.[121, 156, 158] Normally, the stomach wall of infants is thinner near the cardia, and circular muscle in this area contains several gaps, most of which are in the region of the greater curvature.[59, 81] Some speculate that muscle gaps result from gastric dilatation, but these are not found in all infants with dilated stomachs.[101] Further evidence against a congenital defect in gastric musculature is provided by experimental work that shows muscle retraction as a phenomenon secondary to perforation.[109]

Silbergleit and Berkas[192] postulate that traumatic delivery causes a gastric tear, which fills with swallowed amniotic fluid. During the first few days, gastric distention increases with feedings until ultimately the stomach perforates. Experimentally determined pressures required to cause rupture of the infant stomach range between 55 and 320 mm Hg. It is unlikely that such pressures are attained in any clinical situation, except perhaps in infants receiving nasal oxygen or those who are inappropriately ventilated.

Recent evidence indicates that necrotizing or, more aptly, ischemic enterocolitis is one of the major factors contributing to gastric perforation.

Pathology. The perforation is usually a sharp linear tear along the anterior margin of the greater curvature. There is submucosal hemorrhage and often necrosis of the gastric wall, which is either localized at the area of perforation or generalized, involving nearly the entire stomach. The capillaries are dilated and there are recently thrombosed blood vessels, but inflammatory infiltrate is minimal. The edges of the perforation contain mucosa and submucosa but the muscularis is retracted 2 to 10 cm from the edge. Gastric ulceration, if present, is multiple.

Symptoms. More than half the infants are premature or have had one or more anoxic episodes shortly after delivery. After this event, all seems well for the first few days until the infant begins to vomit and refuses feedings. Symptoms usually appear between the third and fifth days but may occur as early as the second and as late as the eighth day. There is distention of the abdomen, which increases until it is firm and tense and the infant is critically ill and anxious. Respiration is compromised by elevation of the diaphragms, and respiratory distress and even cyanosis result. The lungs are either clear on auscultation or contain rales and coarse rhonchi. On percussion, the upper half of the abdomen is tympanitic and the lower half is dull. The usual area of liver dullness becomes obliterated. Bowel sounds are either hyperactive or, as peritonitis develops, absent. Dissection of intraperitoneal air sometimes causes scrotal swelling and flank crepitus. In a few cases, there is pitting edema of the abominal skin.

Diagnosis. If there is a significant amount of bleeding from the perforation, anemia occurs. Once bacterial contamination of the peritoneum has taken place, there is elevation of the white blood cell count. For any infant with acute abdomen, plain radiologic films must be taken in the erect and lateral decubitus views as well as in the supine positions. The diagnosis of perforated viscus is established in the erect film by demonstration of free air under the diaphragm and above the dome of the liver, and in the lateral decubitus film by the demonstration of free air in the anterior abdomen under the peritoneal fat. Intraperitoneal fluid is evident and there are dilated loops of small bowel, but an air-fluid level usually is not present. Under no circumstances should barium be instilled into the stomach (Fig. 12–12).

Treatment. A nasogastric tube is passed immediately to decompress the stomach and aspirate gastric contents. This aids in preventing further contamination of the peritoneal cavity as the anterior perforations are not confined by omental sacs. A tension

Figure 12–12 Abdominal distention developed in this newborn male on the third day of life, at which time the plain films of the abdomen were obtained. At subsequent surgery, a perforation along the greater curvature of the stomach was found and repeated. Postoperatively the infant did poorly, and he died several days later. At autopsy the major findings were the intact repaired perforation and multiple areas of liver infarction. There was no evidence of necrotizing enterocolitis or other bowel abnormalities. *A,* A supine film of the abdomen shows generalized areas of lucency representing free gas within the peritoneum. This is most evident where the intraperitoneal lucency contrasts with the water density of the lateral abdominal wall, and gas can be seen outlining the outside of a loop of bowel in the left lower quadrant. The arrow indicates the falciform ligament surrounded by gas along the anterior abdominal wall. *B,* The erect film demonstrates a large amount of gas under both hemidiaphragms with a long air-fluid level across the entire mid-abdomen. This is sometimes referred to as the saddlebag sign because of apparent draping of the lucent gas shadow over upper abdominal viscera. The arrows indicate portal vein gas in the periphery of the liver. This probably results from dissection of gas into small vessels in the wall of the stomach.

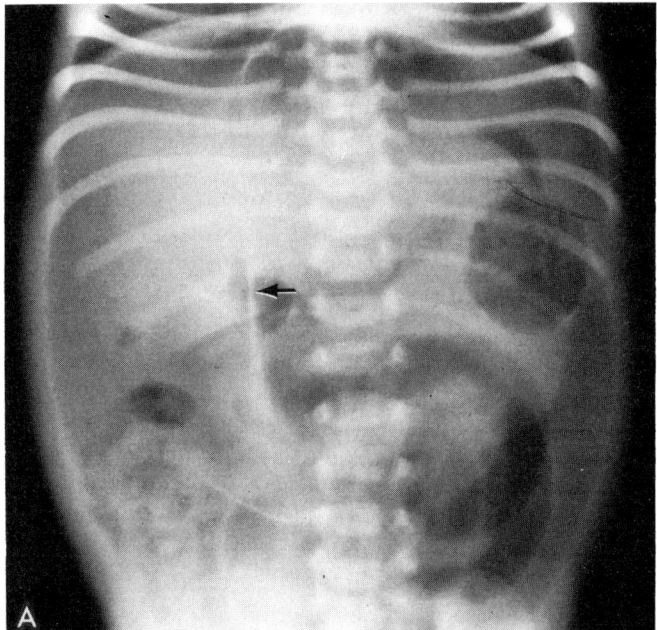

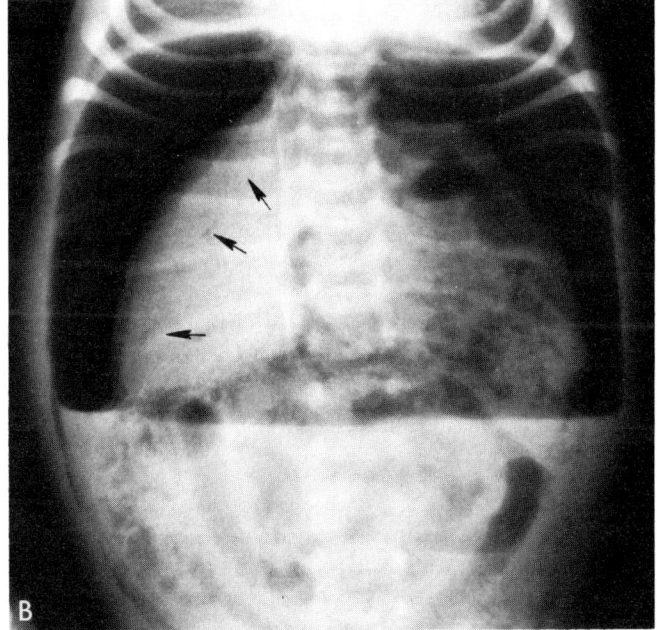

pneumoperitoneum causing severe respiratory distress can be relieved by paracentesis. Vitamin K, fluid and electrolytes, and antibiotics are administered, but the immediate and definitive treatment is operative intervention with closure of the perforation. Other sites of perforation must be sought before the stomach is closed. If there is a significant degree of hemorrhagic necrosis, distal, proximal, or even total gastrectomy may be required. Because duodenal atresia can cause gastric dilatation and perforation, the surgeon should establish patency of the duodenum before closing the stomach.

Complications. Perforation may develop at another site during the first few postoperative days.

Prognosis. The prognosis is directly related to the time of diagnosis and operation. More than half the infants who are operated upon within 12 hours of the onset of symptoms survive, compared with only one quarter of those operated upon later. Most survivors who have had the perforation closed without other procedures have had no problems. Most infants who have undergone partial gastrectomy, and particularly those with distal partial gastrectomy, have had excellent growth and development. Proximal gastrectomy and esophagogastrostomy, however, are often associated with poor growth and with peptic esophagitis.[162, 163]

Spontaneous Gastric Perforation in Older Infants

As in the neonate, gastric perforation may be associated with peptic ulceration or with Cushing's or Curling's ulcers. However, gastric perforation in the mobile infant must always arouse suspicion of ingestion of a strong acid or alkali. Less common causes are excessive eating or drinking or ingestion of bicarbonate after a large meal.[133] In such instances, ischemic necrosis from extreme gastric dilatation precedes the tear.[180] Often, however, no antecedent event or factor can be identified. The diagnostic procedures and treatment are as for gastric perforation in the neonate.

ACUTE TRANSIENT GASTROENTEROPATHY OF CHILDHOOD OR MENETRIER-LIKE DISEASE

This disorder is erroneously referred to in the literature as Menetrier's disease, but it is a totally different entity and must stand alone. Menetrier's disease is a chronic, unremitting lesion of the adult that may ultimately be associated with gastric carcinoma, whereas this disorder in children is self-limited.[206a]

Incidence. Sixteen cases have been reported in the literature to 1981, and our institution sees one approximately every three to four years. All cases have occurred in children ten years of age or younger.[34]

Etiology. The etiology is as yet unknown, although infectious and viral mechanisms may well be involved. Viral infec-

tion has been suspected in a number of the patients whose illnesses were preceded by a viral upper respiratory or gastrointestinal infection. In two, cytomegalic inclusion bodies were identified in the gastric mucosa and in two others, CMV titers in the serum were elevated. Allergy has been suggested by a fairly constant peripheral and intestinal eosinophilia and by increased numbers of IgE immunocytes in the gastric mucosa.[34]

Pathophysiology. Gastrointestinal protein loss is evidenced by measurement of intravenous radioisotope losses through the stool and shortened albumin half-life. Endoscopically and radiologically, the gastric folds are large and thickened and the duodenal folds are edematous. Rarely, there are polypoid lesions of the antrum. Biopsy of the fundus shows hyperplasia of the gastric mucosa with elongation and tortuosity of the foveolar pits, and cystic dilatation of the basilar portions of the mucous glands. Serum gastrins are usually normal, and gastric hyposecretion is present.

Symptoms. The child has usually been entirely well until after a viral syndrome, when he has failed to return to previous health, complaining of anorexia and fatigue. Within a week to ten days, some epigastric pain, anorexia, and edema are noted. Vomiting is frequent; hematemesis, although noted, is rare. Respiratory distress due to pleural effusion may occur in those with anasarca. The physical examination is positive for peripheral edema or anasarca.

One third of patients have a mild, normocytic, normochromic anemia, and two thirds have peripheral eosinophilia. The serum albumin and globulins are decreased, and transport proteins, such as ceruloplasmin or transferrin, are also diminished. Liver and renal function is normal.

Differential Diagnosis. The absence of proteinuria will rapidly differentiate this from the nephrotic syndrome, but the disease must still be distinguished from Zollinger-Ellison syndrome, intestinal lymphangiectasia, lymphoma, and allergic gastroenteritis.[127]

Diagnosis. Measurement of radioisotope losses from the intestine are now extremely difficult to perform because of un-

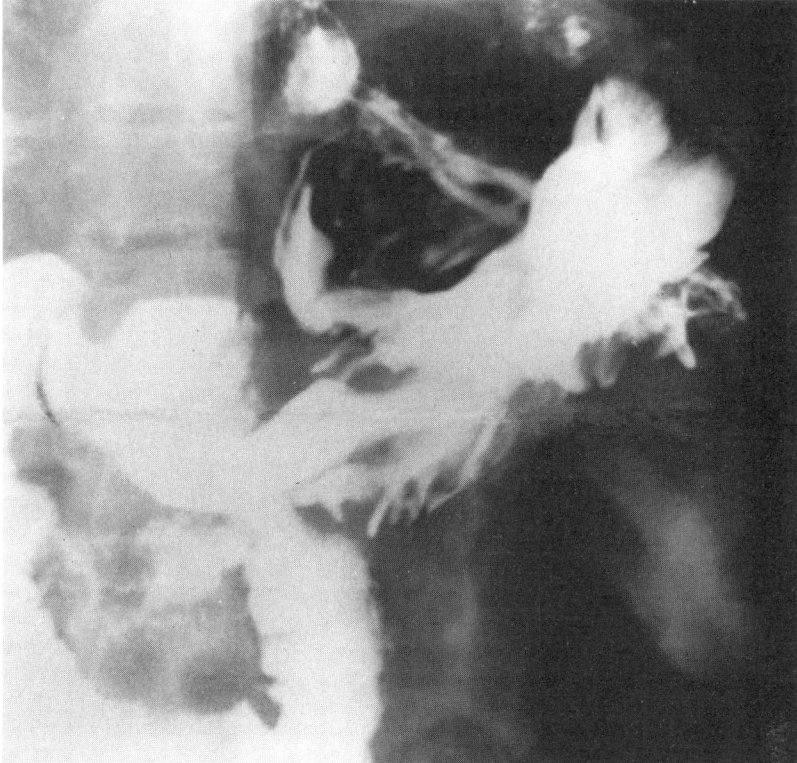

Figure 12–13 This four-year-old boy presented with vomiting, weight loss, and unexplained ankle edema. After gastric biopsy, the microscopic examination showed mucosal thickening and eosinophilic infiltration. Upper gastrointestinal series demonstrates bizarre thickening of the gastric mucosal folds with sparing of the antral portion of the stomach and a normal small bowel.

availability of commercial isotope. The fecal excretion of alpha-1-antitrypsin is a current simple means of quantitating enteric protein loss. Radiologic examination of the upper gastrointestinal tract will demonstrate large edematous mucosal folds of the stomach and duodenum, and biopsy will provide evidence of the characteristic histologic change (Figs. 12–13 and 12–14).

Treatment. Time and minimal supportive therapeutic measures lead to complete recovery. If respiratory compromise due to pleural effusion is present, intravenous albumin is indicated. Otherwise, a high-protein, salt-poor diet, supplemented by medium-chain triglycerides, will provide nutritional support during the acute phase of the illness.

Prognosis. The acute disease persists for ten days to six weeks and is followed by complete recovery. Radiologic examination and biopsy performed several months after recovery are normal.

NONDISTENSIBLE ANTRUM

A thickened, nondistensible antrum may result from ulcer disease, even in the child under two years of age (Fig. 12–15). It is also a complication of chronic granulomatous disease of childhood, the thickening being due to local inflammation and granulomas.[86] Intravenous or oral methicillin or oxacillin has been successful in some cases (Fig. 12–16). Other lesions that may cause antral narrowing are eosinophilic granuloma and eosinophilic gastritis.

GASTRIC BEZOARS

Bezoars are large ball-like collections of material within the stomach. They are of varied composition and etiology.

Incidence. Although the actual incidence is unknown, gastric bezoars are being described with increasing frequency in the

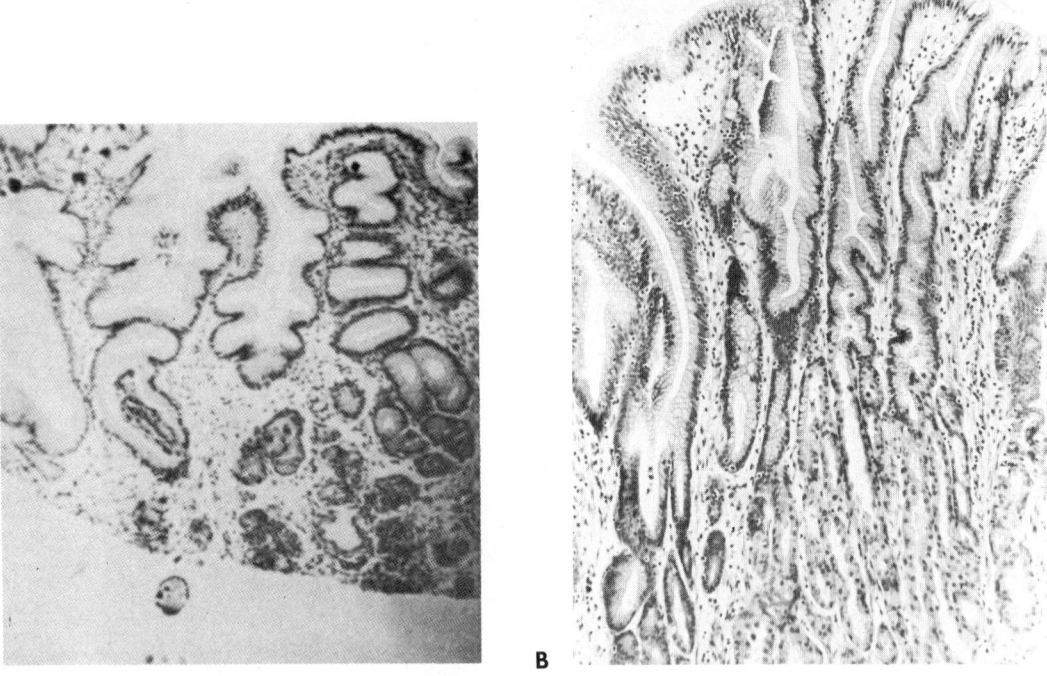

Figure 12–14 A, Gastric biopsy from patient with acute transient gastroenteropathy. The biopsy taken from the fundus of the stomach shows tortuous glands that are compressed in their basal regions. There is a moderate infiltrate of eosinophils and mononuclear cells in the lamina propria. B, Gastric biopsy from an adult with Menetrier's disease. Note the long, tortuous glands and similarities to the acute transient type. (A from Herskovic, T., Spiro, H. M., and Gryboski, J. D.: Acute transient gastrointestinal protein loss. Pediatrics 4:818, 1968. Used by permission.)

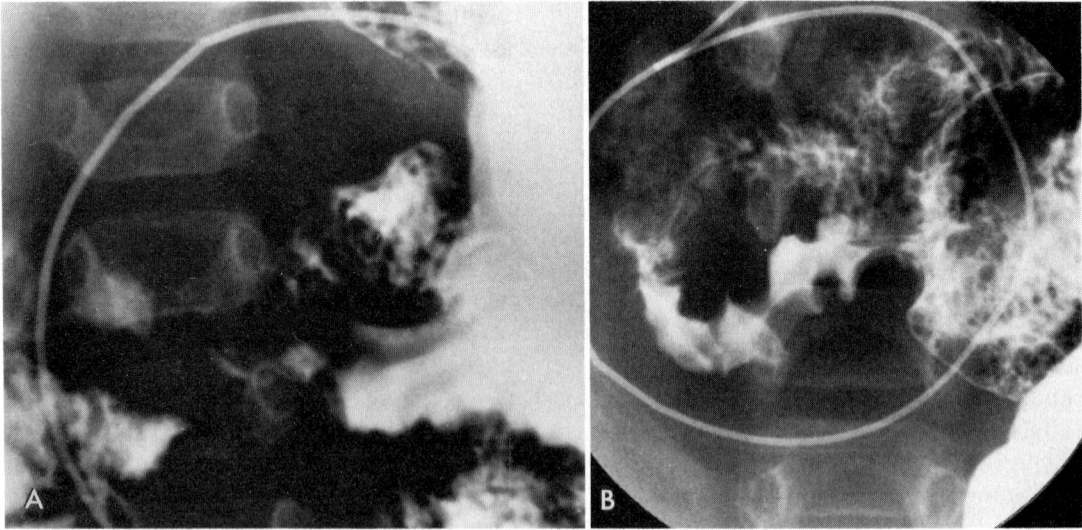

Figure 12–15 A, A 14-month-old child who was admitted with fever and hematemesis. The patient had *E. coli* sepsis, and radiologic examination showed an ulcer in the distal antrum. B, Study three months after treatment for 12 weeks with cimetidine when symptoms of gastric distress persisted after feeding. Note lack of distensibility of antrum. Antral biopsy revealed considerable fibrosis.

infant. In a seven-year period, Grosfeld et al.[89] accumulated a series of 40 bezoars, 31 of which were in premature infants.

Etiology and Pathology. Milk bezoars, or lactobezoars, may develop in full-term infants given improperly diluted formula. In two of our patients, the mothers had retained the 1:1 dilution when switching from liquid to powdered formula. The increase in lactobezoars is, however, largely in premature infants taking high-density, 24 calorie per ounce formula containing lactose, casein, and medium-chain triglycerides. Rarely do those taking formula containing 80 per cent casein and 20 per cent whey develop bezoars. Delayed gastric emptying is related to prematurity, respiratory distress, myotonic dystrophy,[126] supine position, and ingestion of medium-chain triglycerides. This lesion is related to "milk curd" obstruction in the ileum.

Symptoms. Typically, infants are less than 33 weeks' gestation, have a mean birth weight of 1500 gm, and three quarters have been anoxic at birth. They exhibit no gastrointestinal symptoms until 5 to 32 days of age. They have been tube-fed a hypercaloric formula. Mild abdominal distention and increasing gastric residuals after feeding become progressively marked. Eventually, vomiting develops and physical examination reveals a mass in the epigastrium or left upper quadrant. In the presence of mucosal irritation the gastric aspirate may contain blood.

Differential Diagnosis. The symptoms may resemble those of gastric outlet obstruction.

Diagnosis. Plain and erect films of the abdomen show gastric distention and an intraluminal, dense, homogeneous mass or cast, that is occasionally outlined by a halo of air. As noted in Figure 12–17, mucoid secretions accumulated from outlet obstruction may mimic bezoar. In very ill children, pneumatosis has been noted in the fundus.

Treatment. Although some bezoars may resolve spontaneously, those presenting in infancy require treatment. Uncomplicated cases are managed by discontinuation of feedings and gentle gastric lavage with saline for 24 hours. Hydration is maintained by intravenous fluids. Subsequent feedings should contain 20 calories per ounce in predigested formula or one with a 60:40 whey to casein ratio. Radiologically, bezoars have resolved in 5 to 15 days.

Complications. Gastric perforation is a complication in 11 to 14 per cent of infants. Extension of the bezoar into the small bowel may be a cause of persisting symptoms.

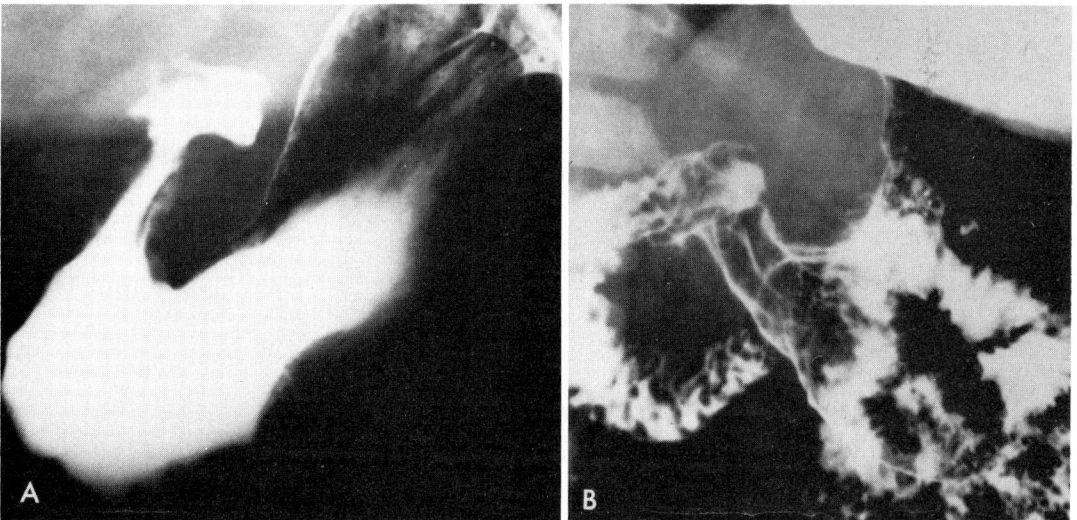

Figure 12–16 A two-year-old male with chronic granulomatous disease of childhood. Upper gastrointestinal study was performed because of recurrent vomiting. *A,* Narrowed, nondistensible antrum is evident in barium examination as well as persistent narrowing of antrum and thickened proximal duodenal folds. *B,* Clinical improvement followed three weeks of oral oxacillin therapy.

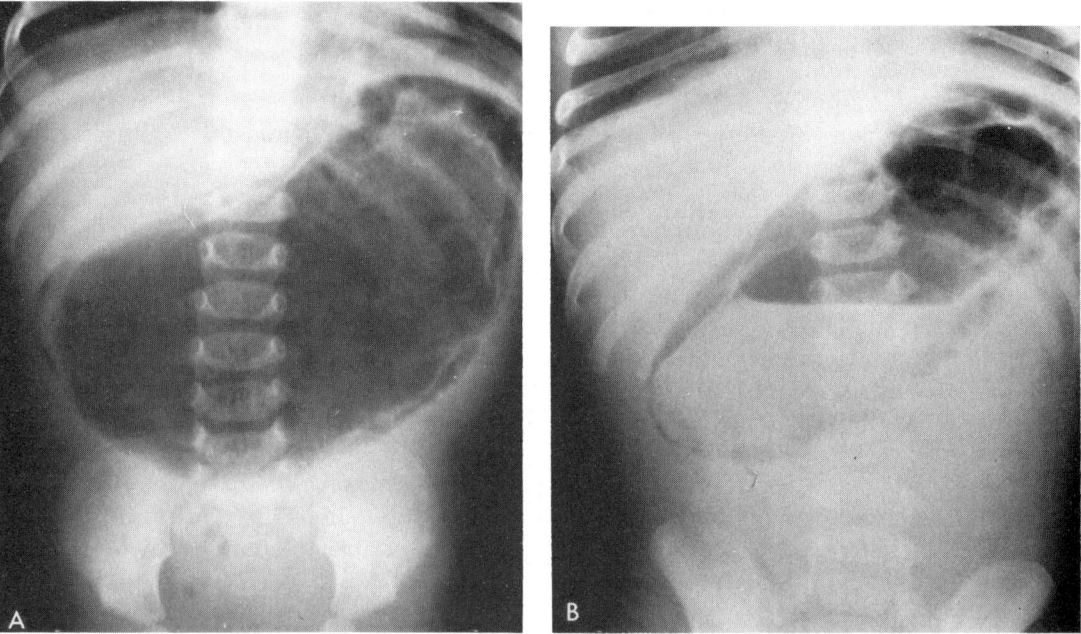

Figure 12–17 A young infant with vomiting of recent onset. *A,* The supine film demonstrates a distended stomach filled with an ill-defined, mottled density. This appearance could be mistaken for a gastric bezoar. *B,* The erect film shows that the density within the stomach represents liquid gastric content. Because of persistent vomiting, the infant was taken to surgery and was found to have hypertrophic pyloric stenosis with a large mucous cast in the stomach.

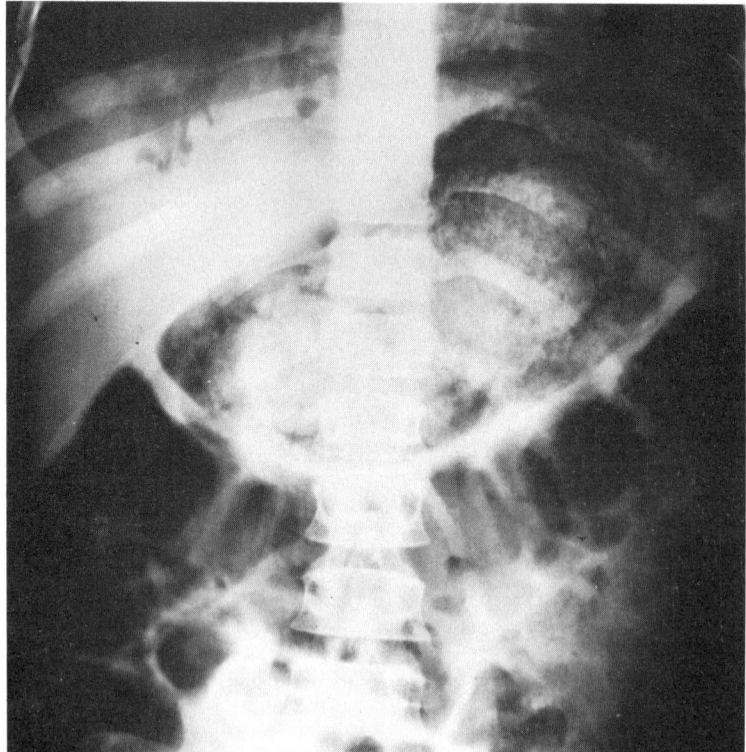

Figure 12–18 Trichobezoar in a mentally retarded child who ingested her own hair and that from other children. A large, shaggy mass is outlined by gas within the slightly distended stomach.

Trichobezoar and Phytobezoar

Trichobezoar of matted hair is more common in older children and particularly those with psychiatric problems. They have been seen in children as young as 15 months. The majority occur in females, although now that boys are wearing longer hair the ratios may equalize. Phytobezoars are composed of vegetable matter, skins, and seeds and, lately, bubble gum. These are the least frequently encountered bezoars and develop in patients with neurologic disease, those taking anticholinergic medications that delay gastric emptying, and those without teeth.

Symptoms. The onset of symptoms is vague, consisting of ill-defined upper abdominal pain, weight loss, and anorexia. Hematemesis is rare but, when present, indicates gastric ulceration.

Diagnosis. The margins of these bezoars are shaggy, and the center is mottled. They tend to mat against the gastric mucosa, and contrast studies may be required for their definition (Figs. 12–18 and 12–19).

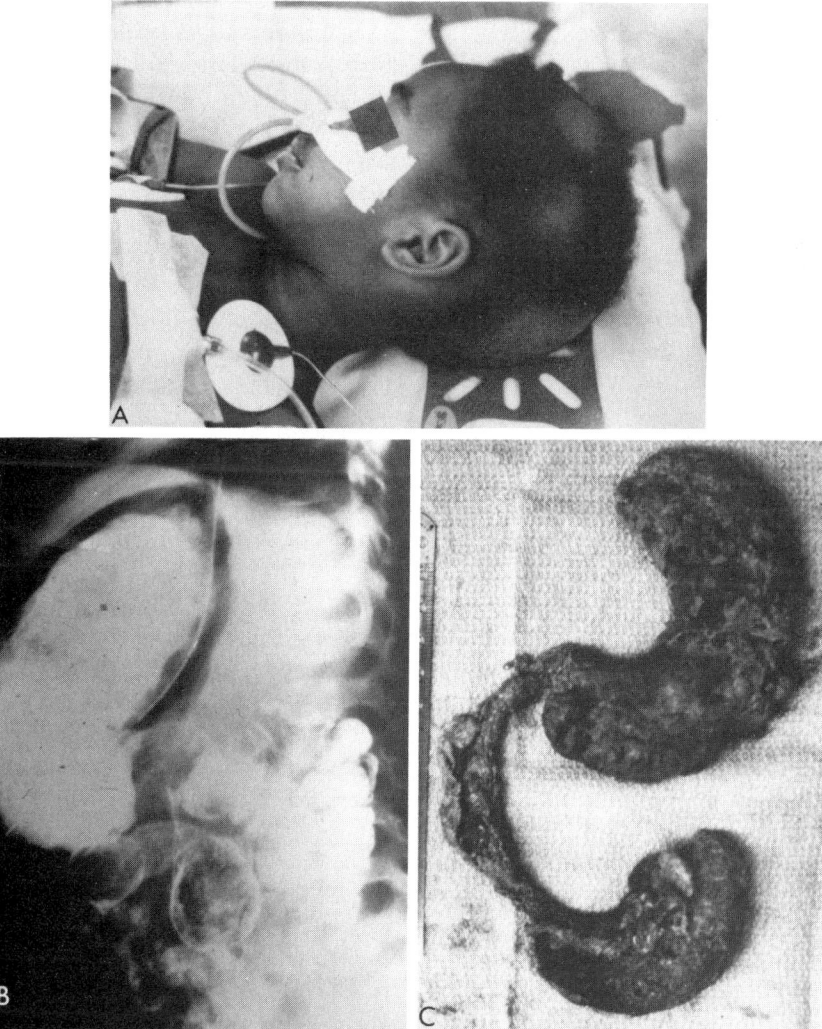

Figure 12–19   This two-year-old female with a one-year history of pica was admitted to the hospital with anorexia and intermittent vomiting of three months' duration and constant vomiting for three days. *A,* Although there was no history of hair ingestion, the area of the scalp from which the hair had been pulled was readily apparent. *B,* Radiologic examination of the upper gastrointestinal tract shows a large bezoar filling the stomach and extending into the duodenum. *C,* The surgical specimen consisted of a large bezoar composed of matted hair. (Courtesy of John Seashore, M.D.)

Treatment. Some may resolve spontaneously over weeks to months. Small feedings containing digestive or mucolytic enzymes (Cotazym, Viokase, or Mucomyst) sometimes dissolve the bezoar and may be used if there is no outlet obstruction. If the bezoar is symptomatic or does not dissolve, extraction by gastrotomy is recommended.

Medication Bezoars

Antacid bezoars may develop in infants treated for upper gastrointestinal bleeding or esophagitis with intragastric or frequent oral administration of aluminum hydroxide products. Those who for some reason, such as renal disease, are fluid-restricted, are most susceptible. Gastric lavage with saline is usually effective in dissolving the bezoar within ten days.

INGESTION OF TOXIC SUBSTANCES

CORROSIVE GASTRITIS FROM ALKALIS OR ACIDS

Burns of the stomach follow the ingestion of acid and strong alkalis. The amount of burn is related more to the concentration of the swallowed solution than to the quantity, although both are important. Some of the common household corrosives are toilet bowl and jewelry cleaners, antirust products, disinfectants, furniture and floor polishes, waxes, electric dishwasher preparations, and detergents. Total gastric necrosis has followed the ingestion of muriatic acid, tinning paint, and lye.[66]

Pathology. Gastric acidity usually protects the stomach against alkali burns, but if a strong alkali is ingested, gastric burns develop in 10 to 20 per cent of cases. Alkalis cause a liquefying necrosis and saponification of tissue fat, which begin at the moment of contact and continue for one to four days. The inflammatory reaction is intense, with small vessel thrombosis and bacterial infiltration of the muscular layers. During the next five to seven days, there is edema and sloughing of the necrotic tissue and the beginning of a granulation and fibrotic healing response. During the third and fourth weeks, as the inflammatory reaction subsides and fibrous tissue contracts, scarring, stricture, and adhesion formation can be extensive enough to cause pyloric stenosis.

Concentrated acids spare the esophagus in 80 to 94 per cent of cases. They produce a coagulation necrosis with a protective eschar, so the damage is far more superficial than that caused by alkali. Damage is greatest when the stomach is empty. Because pylorospasm causes retention of the acid, damage is maximal in the prepyloric region. Damage beyond the pylorus, although unusual, may extend as far as the ileum.

Symptoms. As in the case of esophageal burns, the infant chokes, gags, and attempts to spit out the corrosive. Burning pain extending from the mouth to the stomach makes him cry, and he vomits blood-tinged material or has frank hematemesis.[207] The temperature rises quickly, and tachypnea, tachycardia, and hypotension signal cardiovascular collapse. In cases of total gastric necrosis, the bowel sounds become hypoactive and the abdomen is distended and tense.

Diagnosis. A chest film and three-way examination of the abdomen will reveal mediastinitis or gastric perforation. It is not advisable to use contrast material during the acute stage of the burn. The residual effects of a gastric burn are evident after the third or fourth week; contrast study then shows a narrowed gastric antrum that does not distend, loss of the normal mucosal pattern, and, perhaps, pyloric stenosis.[72]

Treatment. Emergency treatment depends upon the type of agent that has been ingested. Dilute vinegar or orange juice is given to those who have swallowed alkali; milk or egg white is given in the case of ingestion of acid. If the treatment is instituted within two hours of ingestion, cautious lavage will dilate any residual caustic material. The patient is observed carefully for signs of esophageal or gastric perforation.[93, 146] In cases of total gastric necrosis, gastrectomy is indicated.[181, 187]

Complications. Weeks to years after acid ingestion, symptoms of gastric outlet obstruction may appear.[38] Most patients are achlorhydric. Treatment in such instances requires a limited gastric resection.

ACUTE IRON POISONING

Iron ingestion is one of the more common causes of poisoning in late infancy and childhood, for ferrous sulfate tablets are often part of the medicinal supplies of young mothers. At least ten 300 mg tablets of ferrous sulfate are required to produce a serum iron level of 400 to 500 μg per dl, with the most severe symptoms developing when the ingested dose is greater than 20 tablets (6 gm). Enteric-coated preparations are particularly dangerous because of the prolonged release of iron.[225, 226]

Pathology. The oral lethal dose is 200 to 250 mg per kg of elemental iron, but as little as 130 mg has been fatal. Iron affects the gastric mucosa directly, causing edema, ulceration, hemorrhage, and necrosis of the gastric wall. Congestion and ulceration of the small bowel are noted in fatal cases. Because of the damage to intestinal mucosa, iron absorption increases and the problem is compounded.[216]

Pathophysiology. Absorbed iron, perhaps as ferritin, causes postarteriolar dilatation and venous pooling.[110] There are increased peripheral resistance, increased hematocrit, and decreased blood volume and central venous pressure. Eventually, diminished cardiac output and shock lead to hypoperfusion and acidosis.

After plasma transferrin is saturated, iron is taken up by the liver, first by the Kupffer cells and then by the mitochondria of the hepatic parenchymal cells to cause lipid peroxidation and abnormalities of the Krebs cycle and electron transport system.

Symptoms. Acute iron poisoning has been divided into four stages. The first stage is noted within six hours and consists of vomiting, abdominal pain, diarrhea, seizures, lethargy, and coma. Symptoms are moderate when the serum iron is less than 300 μg per dl and severe when 500 μg per dl or more. All who died were at some time in shock, semicomatose, or comatose. The second stage of 24 to 48 hours is quiet. The third stage (in major ingestions) occurs at 12 to 48 hours, with shock, convulsions, and hypoglycemia. Liver damage may be evident. Stage 4 is one of late sequelae: pyloric or antral stenosis, cirrhosis, and neurologic damage.

Diagnosis. The diagnosis, suspected from a history of iron ingestion, is confirmed by the serum iron level, which is increased far above the normal range of 52 to 112 μg per dl. The level does not always correlate with symptoms, for coma has been known to develop with levels of less than 450 μg per dl. The highest levels occur two to four hours after ingestion, but later when they result from enteric-coated preparations.

Treatment. The stomach should be emptied immediately, either by gastric lavage or by emesis induced by ipecac and 2 gm of deferoxamine mesylate given intramuscularly.[149] Lavage does not always remove the enteric-coated tablets. Sodium bicarbonate, phosphate-containing substances, or milk should be added to the gavage solution because each of these reacts with iron to form insoluble iron complexes. Two gm of deferoxamine mesylate per liter of water plus $NaHCO_3$ to alkalinize is used to lavage the stomach. Following this, 10 gm deferoxamine in 50 ml of water with bicarbonate is left in the stomach. A flat film of the abdomen will detect any residual tablets.

This treatment is all that is required for the mild case. More aggressive treatment with chelators or even exchange transfusion is required for toxic infants. The chelating agent desoxyferramine has a high specificity for iron with a stronger affinity for ferric than ferrous ions, with which it complexes at pH 6 or above. This agent is itself toxic, and its dosage must be monitored. It is excreted by the kidneys as ferrioxamine. Serial urine specimens are examined; brown urine represents large quantities of ferrioxamine. The child with symptoms of acute poisoning with a positive urine or an elevated serum iron level should be treated intravenously with 10 to 15 mg per kg per hour of deferoxamine in saline or lactated Ringer's solution. Plasma or blood is used to combat shock, and treatment is continued until the urine is negative and there are no symptoms. The same dose of chelator is given intravenously over the next 12 hours. When serum levels of iron fall below 500 μg per dl, there is no discoloration of the urine. Serum iron concentration can fall precipitously at this point, and fatalities can occur if the level falls below 45 μg per dl.

Complications. An early complication is hypoglycemia, which becomes apparent about four hours after ingestion. Later complications, occurring after three or more weeks, are pyloric stenosis and stricture.

Prognosis. The mortality in severely affected infants used to be 50 per cent, but use of chelators has reduced the mortality by half.

Secondary iron poisoning, or hemachromatosis, is due to iron overload from increased hemoglobin destruction or often-repeated transfusions. Desoxyferramine therapy has always been successful in treating this type of iron toxicity. During treatment, a rise in serum iron is to be expected as the iron is mobilized from the tissues.

Congenital iron overload has been reported in two siblings who had increased tissue stores of iron, peculiar facies, hypotonia, and polycystic kidneys and who died of respiratory disease within the first few months of life.[193]

CALCIUM CHLORIDE GASTRITIS

This type of gastritis is rare in the infants, but care must be taken to administer calcium in 1 to 2 per cent solutions, for concentrations of 15 per cent cause necrosis and calcification of the gastric mucosa. Chelating agents may be of some value in treating this condition.

TUMORS OF THE STOMACH

Gastric tumors are extremely rare in infancy, and most of those reported have been benign. Malignant tumors have included lymphoma, adenocarcinoma, leiomyosarcoma, and rhabdomyosarcoma.[71, 80, 144, 197, 202, 229]

Adenomas and hamartomas most often present with only anemia and occult blood loss.[29a]

TERATOMA

Incidence. In 1969, DeAngelis[48] compiled 17 cases of this gastric tumor, all of which occurred in boys and 13 of which occurred in infants less than one year of age. By 1981, 46 gastric teratomas had been reported in infants, with the first cases occurring in females. In contrast, extragastric teratomas are more usual in females.[33, 45, 48, 179]

Pathology. These tumors are extremely large, measuring 10 to 20 cm in diameter. They contain both cystic and solid areas and are often hemorrhagic. All three germ layers may be represented, and one tumor contained nervous, respiratory, gonadal, urologic, and intestinal tissue as well as bone and cartilage. These masses occur anywhere in the stomach and may involve the entire organ or simply part of the wall. The largest tumor, removed from a 45-day-old infant, weighed 990 gm. In one instance, the tumor extended into the mediastinum.

Symptoms. The tumor may be suspected immediately after birth if it is large enough to cause difficulties in delivery. Many infants have no associated symptoms other than an enlarging left upper quadrant mass associated with abdominal distention. Less often, hematemesis, melena, constipation, anorexia, or fever is a complication of the tumor.

Diagnosis. Plain film of the abdomen is helpful when dense areas of calcification, bone, or teeth are seen in the region of the stomach. Flecks of calcification without other densities may be seen in neuroblastoma and Wilms' tumor. Examination with barium shows a bulky defect within the stomach. Unfortunately, the tumor has not always been detected in radiologic studies of very young infants.

Treatment. In most instances, excision of the tumor and adjacent stomach wall has been possible. Very large tumors require partial or total gastrectomy.

Prognosis. Since all of these tumors are benign, the outlook is excellent. Forty-two of the 46 patients have fully recovered following resection.

SMOOTH MUSCLE TUMORS

Fewer than 50 smooth muscle tumors of the stomach have been reported, the youngest patient being a two and one-half-year-old female with a leiomyosarcoma. Of 34 cases reported in 1973, 14 were benign and 20 were malignant. The *leiomyoma,* consisting of smooth muscle bundles and whorls, is estimated to account for 2.5 per cent of gastric tumors in all age groups. The malignant tumors cannot always be differentiated histologically or by history. The tumors are asymptomatic until they cause hematemesis, epigastric pain, or anemia, at which time a mass can usually be palpated.

Because leiomyosarcoma occurs anywhere within the stomach, there is some question as to whether it arises from the leiomyoma, which originates in the proximal stomach. The tumors grow outward into the serosa as well as inward into the lumen, so that radiologic studies show a polypoid defect or one with a dumbbell contour. Central ulcerations of the lesion are noted in both tumors as they outgrow their vascular supply. Treatment for the benign form is wedge resection, and for the malignant one, limited excision or subtotal gastrectomy. Metastasis to liver and regional nodes occurs in two thirds of patients with leiomyosarcoma. Only one quarter of patients achieve a five-year survival.

LIPOMA

Lipoma, a benign fatty tumor, causes symptoms because of ulceration of the overlying gastric mucosa; therefore, gastric hemorrhage is the presenting symptom. Radiologic examination shows the tumor to be smooth and rounded. It is cured by simple local excision.

LYMPHOMA

This tumor exists in two types, both of which are highly malignant. *Lymphosarcoma* has been reported in a two-year-old child who had vomiting, abdominal pain, and anorexia for several weeks. The tumor consisted of densely packed cells resembling lymphocytes. *Reticulum cell sarcoma* was described in an infant whose only symptoms were abdominal distention and increased venous pattern over the abdomen. These tumor cells are larger and contain more cytoplasm than lymphosarcomas and tend to be pleomorphic. They have several different radiologic appearances: a deep solitary ulcer, a polypoid lesion, or a diffuse infiltration of the stomach wall causing hypertrophic gastric folds. The folds are typically not rigid, and peristalsis extends through them. Both forms are treated by total or partial excision, followed by chemotherapy or radiation. The prognosis for cure is minimal.

GASTRIC DISPLACEMENT

This is solely a radiologic finding but deserves mention because it is helpful in the diagnosis of other abdominal lesions.[90] Liver enlargement produces medial and either anterior or posterior displacement of the stomach. Splenic enlargement displaces the stomach medially or inferiorly and anteriorly.[70] Pancreatic masses cause anterior and superior displacement with widening of the duodenal loop. Multicystic kidney, hydronephrosis, neuroblastoma, and Wilms' tumor also displace the stomach in an anterior and upward direction. Pressure defects from omental or mesenteric cysts depend upon their site of origin.

Less common causes of gastric displacement or impression are abscess, teratoma, duplication cyst, and colonic distention.[183] Filling defects in the region of the antrum are caused by solitary cysts of the liver, choledochal cysts, or a left-sided gallbladder. Ectopic spleen in the pancreas can cause an indentation of the fundus and resemble an intrinsic mass, whereas normal

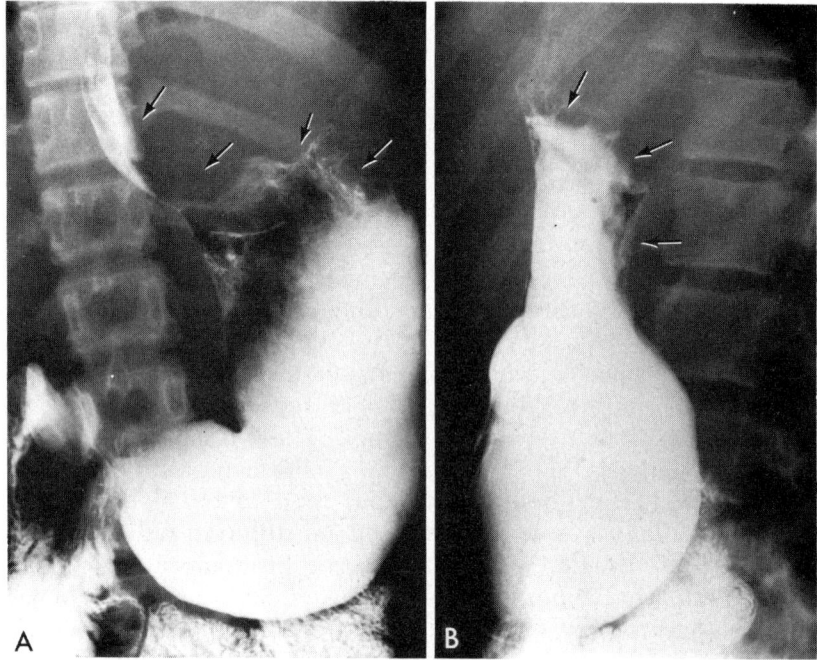

Figure 12–20 This young girl had been struck in the abdomen several weeks before she was admitted to the hospital with left upper quadrant pain and tenderness and fever. At the time of surgery, an infected splenic hematoma was found and the spleen was removed. *A,* Anteroposterior view of the stomach during upper gastrointestinal series demonstrates inferior displacement of the gastric fundus (arrows). The distortion of the wall of the stomach is the result of edema secondary to the adjacent inflammation, but a similar change may be seen with dissection of blood through the gastrosplenic ligament. *B,* The lateral view of the abdomen shows inferior and anterior displacement of the gastric fundus (arrows).

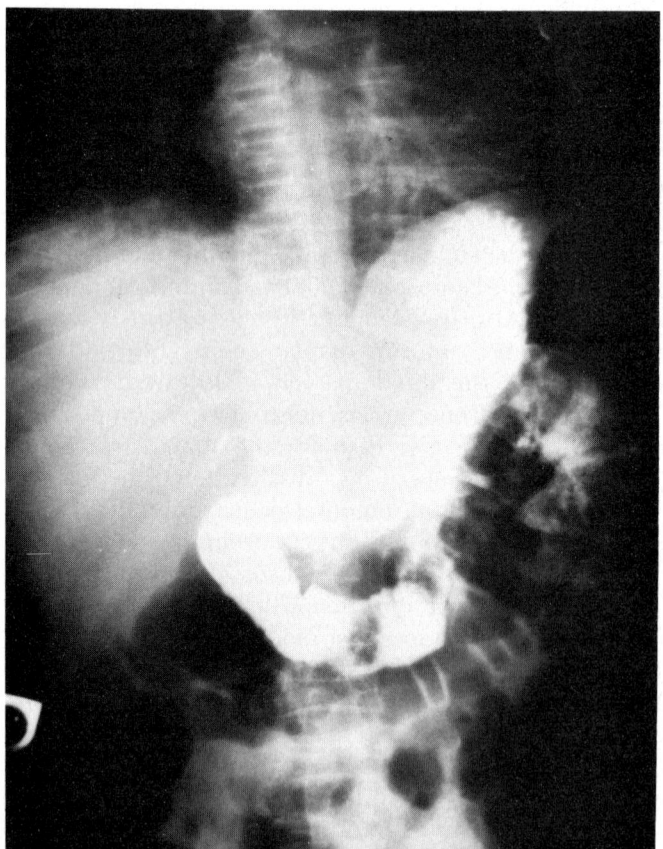

Figure 12–21 An upper gastrointestinal series from a child with hepatomegaly shows displacement of the stomach to the left and an impression along the lesser curvature from the enlarged liver.

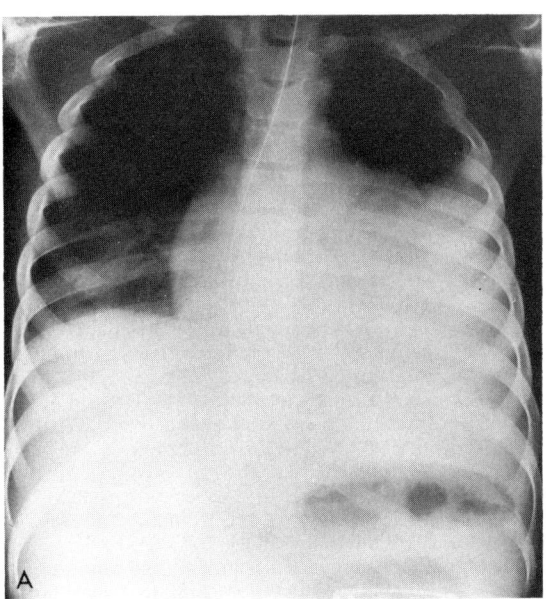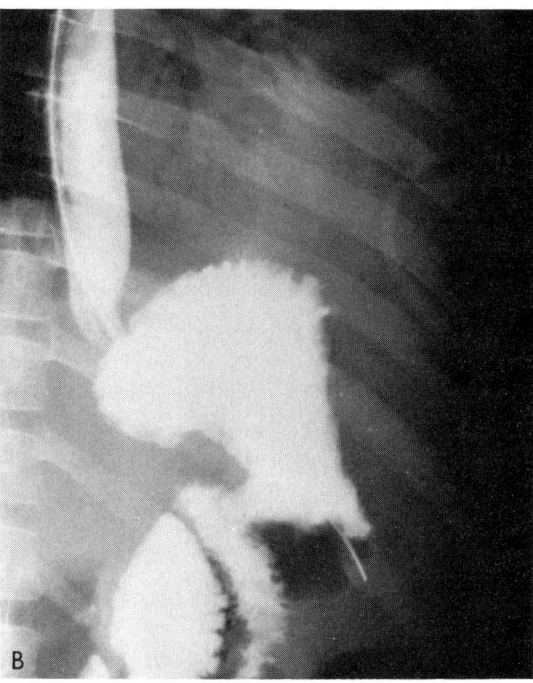

Figure 12-22   Gastric displacement caused by a left subdiaphragmatic abscess in a boy who had undergone partial resection of the small bowel because of regional enteritis one week earlier. *A*, Chest film shows a large left pleural effusion and a small amount of pleural fluid on the right side. The shadow of the left hemidiaphragm cannot be identified because of the fluid. *B*, A contrast study demonstrates medial displacement of the stomach by an extrinsic mass. The sharply outlined bronchial air shadows indicate that there is an associated inflammatory process in the left lower lobe of the lung.

spleen may indent the cardia (Figs. 12-20 to 12-22).[22]

INTRAMURAL GASTRIC HEMATOMA

Intramural hemorrhage due to primary bleeding disorders or to anticoagulant therapy may occur anywhere within the gastrointestinal tract but is seen most often in the colon.[82] Rarely, intramural hemorrhage develops within the gastric wall, where it presents as a left upper quadrant mass. The differential diagnosis includes gastric tumors and splenic hematoma. The diagnosis may be resolved by radiologic examination, which will show a filling defect in the stomach, and by transverse and longitudinal ultrasonography, which will define the size and characteristics of adjacent organs.

Treatment consists of correction of the underlying disease, replacement of blood and clotting factors, and gastrointestinal rest. Resolution of the mass is apparent within several days to weeks.

FOREIGN BODY IN THE STOMACH

Most foreign bodies that reach the stomach will pass through the pylorus without difficulty, provided they are of reasonable size and shape. Fortunately, most are radiopaque and weekly fluoroscopy or flat plate will monitor their position. Generally, small coins, marbles, and screws require several weeks to pass, whereas larger objects and coins require up to several months.

If the object has not passed through the pylorus after four weeks, radiologic examination of the upper gastrointestinal tract should be performed to rule out obstruction from an antral web or persistent narrowing of old pyloric stenosis.

REFERENCES

1. Adams, J., Hyde, W., Procianoy, R., and Rudolph, A.: Hypochloremic metabolic alkalosis following tolazoline-induced gastric hypersecretion. Pediatrics 65:298, 1980.

2. Adeyeml, S., Ein, S., and Simpson, J.: Perforated stress ulcer in infants. A silent threat. Ann. Surg. 190:707, 1979.

3. Agunod, M., Yamaguchi, N., Lopez, R., Luhby, A. L., and Glass, G. B.: Correlative study of hydrochloric acid, pepsin and intrinsic factor secretion in newborns and infants. Am. J. Dig. Dis. 14:400, 1969.

4. Alagile, D., and Odievre, M.: Liver and biliary tract disease in children. New York, John Wiley & Sons, 1978, p. 36.

5. Alarotu, H.: Preclinical stage of infantile hypertrophic pyloric stenosis. Am. J. Dis. Child. 72:371, 1946.

6. Amadeo, H. H., Ashmore, H. W., and Aponte, G. E.: Neonatal gastric perforation caused by congenital defects of the gastric musculature. Surgery 47:1010, 1960.

7. Ames, M. D.: Gastric acidity in the first ten days of life of the prematurely born baby. Am. J. Dis. Child. 100:122, 1960.

8. Atkins, E. L., and Schwartz, W. B.: Factors governing correction of the alkalosis associated with potassium deficiency: the critical role of chloride in the recovery process. J. Clin. Invest. 41:218, 1962.

9. Avery, G., Randolph, J. G., and Weaver, T.: Gastric response to specific disease in infants. Pediatrics 38:874, 1966.

10. Becker, J. M., Schneider, K. M., and Fischer, A. E.: Pyloric atresia. Arch. Surg. 87:413, 1963.

11. Belding, H. H., III, and Kernonhan, J. W.: A morphologic study of the myenteric plexus and musculature of the pylorus with special reference to the changes in hypertrophic pyloric stenosis. Surg. Gynecol. Obstet. 97:322, 1953.

12. Benson, C. D. (ed.): Pediatric Surgery. Chicago, Year Book Medical Publishers, 1962.

13. Benson, C. D., and Coury, J. J.: Congenital intrinsic obstruction of the stomach and duodenum in the newborn. Arch. Surg. 62:856, 1951.

14. Benson, C. D., and Lloyd, J. R.: Infantile pyloric stenosis. A review of 1120 cases. Am. J. Surg. 107:429, 1964.

15. Benson, C. D., and Warden, M. J.: 707 cases of congenital hypertrophic pyloric stenosis. Surg. Gynecol. Obstet. 195:348, 1957.

16. Bentley, J. F. R., and Smith, J. R.: Developmental posterior enteric remnants and spinal malformations. Arch. Dis. Child. 35:76, 1960.

17. Berg, R. B., Schuster, S. R., and Colodny, A. H.: The use of gastrostomy in feeding premature infants. Pediatrics 33:287, 1964.

18. Berg, R. M.: Peptic ulcers in children. South. Med. J. 54:325, 1961.

19. Berg, R. M., Berg, H. M., Eriksen, J. A., and Levi, W. F.: Peptic ulcers in children. Lancet 80:423, 1960.

20. Bernard, E., Israel, L., and Debris, M.: Le role de la mucoviscidose dans la pathogenie de l'association emphyseme-ulcere digestif. Presse Med. 70:861, 1962.

21. Bilodeau, R. G.: Inheritance of hypertrophic pyloric stenosis. Am. J. Roentgenol. Radium Ther. Nucl. Med. 113:241, 1971.

22. Bishop, H. C., and Hope, J. W.: Pyloric stenosis. Post-operative roentgen studies and their clinical significance. J. Pediatr. 60:62, 1962.

23. Blank, E., and Chisolm, A. J.: Congenital microgastria, a case report with a 26 year follow-up. Pediatrics 51:1037, 1973.

24. Blumenthal, I., Ebel, A., and Pildes, R.: Effect of posture on the pattern of stomach emptying in the newborn. Pediatrics 63:532, 1979.

25. Blumenthal, I., Ebel, A., and Pildes, R.: Stomach emptying in the newborn. Pediatrics 66:487, 1980.

26. Bouslog, J. S., Cunningham, T. D., et al.: Roentgenologic studies in the infant's gastrointestinal tract. J. Pediatr. 6:234, 1935.

27. Bremer, J. L.: Diverticula and duplication of the intestinal tract. Arch. Pathol. 38:132, 1944.

28. Bronsther, B., Nadeau, M., and Abrams, M.: Congenital pyloric atresia. Surgery 69:130, 1971.

29. Byrne, J. J., and Cahill, J. M.: Acute gastric dilatation. Am. J. Surg. 101:301, 1961.

29a. Buts, J., Gosseye, S., Claus, D., de Montpelier, C., and Nyakabasa. M.: Solitary hyperplastic polyp of the stomach. Am. J. Dis. Child. 135:848, 1981.

30. Campbell, J.: Neonatal gastric volvulus. Am. J. Radiol. 132:723, 1979.

31. Cavell, B.: Gastric emptying in preterm infants. Acta Paediatr. Scand. 68:725, 1979.

32. Chhatriwalla, Y., Colon, A., and Scanlon, J.: The use of cimetidine in the newborn. Pediatrics 65:301, 1980.

33. Chiba, T., Suzuki, A., Hebiguchi, T., Kato, T., and Kasar, M.: Gastric teratoma extending into the mediastinum. J. Pediatr. Surg. 15:191, 1980.

34. Chouraqui, J. P., Roy, C. C., Brochu, P., Gregoire, H., Morin, C., and Weber, A.: Menetrier's disease in children: report of a patient and review of sixteen other cases. Gastroenterology 80:1042, 1981.

35. Christensen, J.: The controls of gastrointestinal movements: some old and new views. N. Engl. J. Med. 285:85, 1971.

36. Christie, D. L.: Development of gastric function during the first month of life. In Lebenthal, E. (ed.): Textbook of Gastroenterology and Nutrition in Infancy. Vol. I. New York, Raven Press, 1981, p. 109.

37. Christie, D. L., and Ament, E. E.: Gastric acid hypersecretion in children with duodenal ulcer. Gastroenterology 71:242, 1976.

38. Cochran, S. T., Fonkalsrud, E. W., and Gyepes, M. T.: Complete obstruction of gastric antrum in children following acid ingestion. Arch. Surg. 113:308, 1978.

39. Code, C. F., Szurszewski, J. H., and Kelly, K.: A concept of motor control by the pacesetter potential in the stomach and small bowel. Am. J. Dig. Dis. 16:601, 1971.

40. Cohn, R., and Sunshine, P.: Gastrostomy in the premature and newborn infant. Arch. Surg. 96:933, 1968.

41. Cole, B. C., and Dickinson, S. J.: Acute volvulus of the stomach in infants and children. Surgery 70:707, 1971.

42. Commons, R. R.: Study of alkalosis. I. Renal function during and following alkalosis resulting from pyloric obstruction. J. Clin. Invest. *29*:169, 1950.

43. Corner, D. B.: Hypertrophic pyloric stenosis in infancy treated with scopolamine nitrate. Arch. Dis. Child. *30*:377, 1955.

43a. Cowton, J. A. L., Beattie, T. J., Gibson, A. A. M., Mackie, R., Skerrow, C. J., and Cockburn, F.: Epidermolysis bullosa in association with aplasia cutis congenita and pyloric atresia. Acta Paediatr. Scand. *71*:155, 1982.

44. Cox, K., and Ament, M. E.: Upper gastrointestinal bleeding in children and adolescents. Pediatrics *63*:408, 1979.

45. Craig, W. S.: Palpable contractile tumors in the newly born. Arch. Dis. Child. *30*:484, 1955.

46. Curci, M., Little, K., Sieber, W. K., and Kieswetter, W.: Peptic ulcer disease in childhood re-examined. J. Pediatr. Surg. *11*:329, 1976.

47. Daniel, E. E., and Irwin, J.: Electrical activity of the stomach and upper intestine. Am. J. Dig. Dis. *16*:602, 1971.

48. DeAngelis, V.: Gastric teratoma in a newborn infant. Surgery *66*:794, 1969.

49. Desbaillets, L., and Menguy, R.: Influence of corticotrophic hormone on the secretion of gastric mucus. Surg. Forum *17*:291, 1966.

50. Devi, B., and More, J. R.: Total tracheopulmonary agenesis. Acta Paediatr. Scand. *55*:107, 1966.

51. Deveney, C., Deveney, K., Jaffe, B., Jones, R., and Way, L.: Use of calcium and secretin in the diagnosis of gastrinoma. Ann. Intern. Med. *87*:680, 1977.

52. Dineen, J., and Redo, S.: Pyloric obstruction due to mucosal diaphragm. Surgery *53*:674, 1963.

53. Donegan, W. L., and Spiro, H. M.: Parathyroids and gastric secretion. Gastroenterology *38*:759, 1960.

54. Doppman, J., Rubinson, R. M., Rockoff, S., Vasco, J., Shapiro, R., and Morrow, A.: Mechanism of obstruction of the infradiaphragmatic portion of the inferior vena cava in the presence of increased intra-abdominal pressure. Invest. Radiol. *1*:37, 1966.

55. Dreiling, D. A., and Greenstein, A.: Pancreatic function in patients with Zollinger-Ellison syndrome. Am. J. Gastroenterol. *58*:66, 1972.

56. Duhamel, B.: Concerning the embryology of intestinal duplications. Ann. Chir. Infant. *8*:55, 1967.

57. Ebers, D. W., Smith, D. I., and Gibbs, G. E.: Gastric acidity on the first day of life. Pediatrics *18*:800, 1956.

58. Eiseman, B., and Heyman, R. L.: Stress ulcers — a continuing challenge. N. Engl. J. Med. *282*:372, 1970.

59. Elders, M., and Hughes, E.: Rupture of the stomach. Clinical and experimental study. Lancet *86*:104, 1966.

60. Elshafie, M., Stidham, G., Klippel, C. H., Katzman, G. H., and Weinfield, I.: Pyloric atresia and epidermolysis bullosa letalis: a lethal combination in 2 premature newborn siblings. J. Pediatr. Surg. *14*:446, 1980.

61. Englers, H. S., Kennedy, T., Ellison, L., Purvis, J., and Mortex, W.: Hemodynamics of experimental acute gastric dilatation. Am. J. Surg. *113*:194, 1967.

62. Euler, A., Ament, M. E., and Walsh, J.: Human newborn hypergastrinemia: an investigation of prenatal and perinatal factors and their effects on gastrin. Pediatr. Res. *12*:652, 1978.

63. Euler, A., Byrne, W., Meis, P., Leake, R., and Ament, M. E.: Basal and pentagastrin stimulated acid secretion in newborn human infants. Pediatr. Res. *13*:36, 1979.

64. Farman, J., Cywes, S., and Werbeloff, L.: Pyloric mucosal diaphragms. Clin. Radiol. *19*:95, 1968.

65. Fenwick, T.: Familial hypertrophic pyloric stenosis. Br. Med. J. *2*:13, 1953.

66. Finney, D., Schnaufer, C., and Stafford, E. S.: Total gastrectomy in an infant made necessary by ingestion of tinning paint. Ann. Surg. *151*:891, 1960.

67. Finsen, U. R.: Infantile hypertrophic pyloric stenosis: unusual familial incidence. Arch. Dis. Child. *54*:720, 1979.

68. Floyd, C. H.: Duodenal ulcer with intestinal obstruction in a newborn. J. Pediatr. *54*:369, 1959.

69. Fonkalsrud, E.: Intestinal obstruction from gastrostomy tube in infants. J. Pediatr. *69*:908, 1966.

70. Font, R. G., Sparks, R., and Herbert, G. A.: Ectopic spleen mimicking an intrinsic fundal lesion of the stomach. Am. J. Dig. Dis. *15*:49, 1970.

71. Franchini, M.: A rare case of gastric sarcoma in a child. Minerva Chir. *21*:165, 1966.

72. Franken, E. A.: Caustic damage of the gastrointestinal tract: roentgen features. Am. J. Roentgenol. Radium Ther. Nucl. Med. *118*:77, 1973.

72a. Fried, K., Avir, S., and Nisenbaum, C.: Probable autosomal dominant infantile pyloric stenosis in a large kindred. Clin. Genet. *20*:328, 1981.

73. Friesen, S. R.: Effect of total gastrectomy on the Zollinger-Ellison tumor: Observations by second-look procedures. Surgery *62*:609, 1967.

74. Friesen, S. R.: A gastric factor in the pathogenesis of the Zollinger-Ellison syndrome. Ann. Surg. *168*:483, 1968.

75. Friesen, S. R., Boley, J. O., and Miller, D. R.: The myenteric plexus of the pylorus: its early normal development and its changes in hypertrophic pyloric stenosis. Surgery *39*:21, 1956.

76. Gerber, B. C.: Prepyloric diaphragm: an unusual abnormality. Arch. Surg. *90*:472, 1965.

77. Ghai, O., Singh, M., Walia, B., and Gadeker, N. G.: An assessment of gastric acid secretory response with maximal augmented histamine stimulation in children with peptic ulcer. Arch. Dis. Child. *40*:77, 1965.

78. Glynn, P. J.: Chronic gastric ulcer in an infant treated by gastrectomy. Aust. N.Z. J. Surg. *40*:256, 1971.

79. Goksen, Y., and Hardy, J. D.: Effects of cortisone on parietal cells and acid secretion. Gut *7*:406, 1967.

80. Golden, T., and Stout, A. P.: Smooth muscle

tumors of the gastrointestinal tract and retroperitoneal tract tissues. Surg. Gynecol. Obstet. 73:784, 1941.

81. Gonzalez-Crussi, F., Staphithanoda, P., and Ramchand, S.: Spontaneous gastric rupture in infants and children. Am. J. Dig. Dis. 15:463, 1970.

82. Gordon, R., d'Avignon, M., Storch, A., and Eyster, E.: Intramural gastric hematoma in a hemophiliac with an inhibitor. Pediatrics 67:417, 1981.

83. Gottlieb, G., Chu, F., and Sharlin, H. S.: Perforation of a gastric ulcer associated with intracranial hemorrhage in a newborn infant. Radiology 54:595, 1950.

84. Gray, D. H.: Total reduplication of the stomach: a rare anomaly. Aust. N.Z. J. Surg. 41:130, 1971.

85. Grochowski, J., Szafran, H., Sztefko, K., Janik, A., and Szafran, Z.: Blood-serum immunoreactive gastrin level in infants with hypertrophic pyloric stenosis. J. Pediatr. Surg. 15:279, 1980.

86. Griscom, N., Kirkpatrick, J., Jr., Girdany, B., Berdon, W., Grand, R., and Mackie, G.: Gastric antral narrowing in chronic granulomatous disease of childhood. Pediatrics 54:456, 1974.

87. Grosfeld, J. L., Boles, E. T., Jr., and Reiner, C.: Duplication of pylorus in the newborn: a rare cause of gastric outlet obstruction. J. Pediatr. Surg. 5:365, 1970.

88. Grosfeld, J. L., O'Neill, J. A., and Clatworthy, H. W., Jr.: Enteric duplications in infancy and childhood: an 18 year review. Ann. Surg. 172:83, 1970.

89. Grosfeld, J. L., Schreiner, R., Franken, E., Lemons, J., Ballantine, T. V., Weber, T. R., and Gresham, E. M. L.: The changing pattern of gastrointestinal bezoars in infants and children. Surgery 88:425, 1980.

90. Grossman, H., and Redo, F.: Unusual causes of gastric displacement. Radiology 87:725, 1966.

91. Grossman, M. I.: Physiological role of gastrin. Fed. Proc. 27:1312, 1968.

92. Gryboski, J. D., Thayer, W. R., and Spiro, H. M.: Esophageal motility in infants and children. Pediatrics 31:382, 1963.

93. Gryboski, W. A., Page, R., and Rush, B.: Management of total gastric necrosis following lye ingestion. Ann. Surg. 161:469, 1965.

94. Gupta, M., and Brans, Y. W.: Gastric retention in neonates. Pediatrics 62:26, 1978.

95. Hamburg, M., Mignon, M., and Ricour, C.: Serum gastrin levels in hypertrophic pyloric stenosis of infancy. Arch. Dis. Child. 54:208, 1979.

96. Harries, J. J., and Fraser, A. J.: The acidity of gastric contents of premature babies during the first fourteen days of life. Biol. Neonate 12:186, 1968.

97. Hase, T., and Moss, B. J.: Microvascular changes of gastric mucosa in development of stress ulcers in rats. Gastroenterology 65:224, 1973.

98. Haverback, B. J., Stevenson, T. B., Sjoerdsma, A., and Terry, L. L.: The effect of reserpine and chlorpromazine on gastric secretion. Am. J. Med. Sci. 230:601, 1955.

99. Haws, E. B., Sieber, W. K., and Kieswetter, W. B.: Complications of tube gastrostomy in infants and children. Ann. Surg. 164:284, 1966.

100. Henderson, S. G.: The gastrointestinal tract in the healthy newborn infant. Am. J. Roentgenol. 48:302, 1942.

101. Herbut, P. A.: Congenital defect in the musculature of the stomach with rupture in the newborn infant. Arch. Pathol. 36:91, 1943.

102. Hillemeier, A. C., Lange, R., McCallum, R., Seashore, J., and Gryboski, J. D.: Delayed gastric emptying in infants with gastroesophageal reflux. J. Pediatr. 98:190, 1981.

103. Holder, I., Leape, L., and Ashcraft, K.: Gastrostomy: its use and dangers in pediatric patients. N. Engl. J. Med. 286:1345, 1972.

104. Ho-Man Kwok, R., and Avery, G.: Seasonal variation of congenital hypertrophic pyloric stenosis. J. Pediatr. 70:963, 1967.

105. Horton, B. T.: Pyloric musculature with special reference to pyloric block. Am. J. Anat. 41:197, 1928.

106. Horton, B. T.: Pyloric musculature with special reference to the musculature, myenteric plexus and lymphatic vessels. Arch. Surg. 22:438, 1931.

107. Inouye, W., and Evans, G.: Neonatal gastric perforation. Arch. Surg. 88:471, 1964.

108. Jackson, C. R.: Gastroduodenal perforations in the newborn: report of four cases treated surgically with three survivors. Am. J. Surg. 28:244, 1962.

109. James, D. H.: Spontaneous rupture of the stomach. J. Pediatr. 58:849, 1961.

110. James, J.: Acute iron poisoning: assessment of severity and prognosis. J. Pediatr. 77:117, 1970.

111. Janik, J. S., Akbar, A. M., and Burrington, G.: The role of gastrin in congenital hypertrophic pyloric stenosis. J. Pediatr. Surg. 13:151, 1978.

112. Jansson, G.: Extrinsic nervous control of gastric motility: an experimental study in the cat. Acta Physiol. Scand. (Suppl.) 326:1, 1969.

113. Johnson, L. R.: Control of gastric secretion: no room for histamine. Gastroenterology 61:106, 1971.

114. Judd, D. R., Heimberger, I., Vellios, F., and Waldhausen, J. A.: Zollinger-Ellison syndrome in adolescents. Surgery 54:673, 1963.

115. Kammerer, G. T.: Duplications of the stomach resembling hypertrophic pyloric stenosis. J.A.M.A. 207:2101, 1964.

116. Karlstrom, F.: Peptic ulcer in children in Sweden during the years 1953 to 1962. Ann. Paediatr. 202:218, 1964.

117. Kelly, K. A., and Code, C. F.: Effect of transthoracic vagotomy on canine gastric electrical activity. Gastroenterology 57:61, 1969.

118. Kelley, M. E., Mohtashemi, H., Patel, S., and Gupta, R.; report of a double pylorus. Dig. Dis. Sci. 25:807, 1980.

119. Kildeberg, P.: Metabolic alkalosis in hypertrophic pyloric stenosis. Dan. Med. Bull. 10:245, 1963.

120. Kildeberg, P.: Metabolic alkalosis in hypertrophic pyloric stenosis. Clinical significance and treatment. Acta Paediatr. 53:132, 1964.

121. Kneiszl, F.: Some data on the etiology of gastric rupture in the newborn. Biol. Neonate 4:201, 1962.

122. Konvolinka, C. W., and Steward, R.: Pyloric atresia. Am. J. Dis. Child. 132:903, 1978.

123. Konvolinka, C. W., and Wermuth, C. R.: Hypertrophic pyloric stenosis in older infants. Am. J. Dis. Child. 122:76, 1971.

124. Kornfield, H. J.: Pyloric atresia and its repair. Surgery 51:569, 1962.

125. Kremer, R. M., Lepoff, R. B., and Izant, R. J.: Duplication of the stomach. J. Pediatr. Surg. 5:360, 1970.

126. Kuiper, D. H.: Gastric bezoar in a patient with myotonic dystrophy: a review of the gastrointestinal complications of myotonic dystrophy. Am. J. Dig. Dis. 16:529, 1971.

127. Lachman, R. S., Martin, D. J., and Vawter, G. F.: Thick gastric folds in childhood. Am. J. Roentgenol. Radium Ther. Nucl. Med. 112:83, 1971.

128. Ladd, P., Ware, W. E., and Pickett, L.: Congenital hypertrophic pyloric stenosis. JAMA 131:647, 1946.

129. Lari, J., List, J., and Deuthrie, H. L.: Response to pentagastrin in children. J. Pediatr. Surg. 3:682, 1968.

130. Lari, J., Lister, J., and Duthie, R.: Response to gastric pentapeptide in children. J. Pediatr. Surg. 3:682, 1968.

131. Lee, W. E., and Wells, J. R.: Perforation in utero of a gastric ulcer. Ann. Surg. 78:36, 1923.

132. Lemak, L. R.: Roentgenological manifestations of gastroduodenal ulceration in the newborn. Am. J. Roentgenol. 66:191, 1951.

133. Lemmon, W. T., and Paschal, G. W., Jr.: Rupture of the stomach following ingestion of sodium bicarbonate. Ann. Surg. 114:997, 1941.

134. Lester, P., Budge, A., Barnes, J., and Kirks, D.: Gastric emphysema in infants with hypertrophic pyloric stenosis. Am. J. Roentgenol. 131:421, 1978.

135. Liebman, W. M., and Samloff, M.: Fetal pepsinogens in human amniotic fluid. Biol. Neonate 33:174, 1978.

136. Liechte, R. E., Mikkelsen, W. P., and Snyder, W. H.: Prepyloric stenosis caused by congenital squamous epithelial diaphragm — resultant infantilism. Surgery 53:670, 1963.

137. Linde, L. M., and Westover, J.: Esophageal and gastric abnormality in dysautonomia. Pediatrics 29:303, 1962.

138. Linkner, L. M., and Benson, C. D.: Spontaneous perforation of the stomach in the newborn. Ann. Surg. 149:525, 1959.

139. Livaditis, A., and Omkian, L.: Gastric perforation in the neonate. Acta Paediatr. 52:595, 1963.

140. Lucaya, J., Perez-Candela, V., Aso, C., and Calvo, J.: Mastocytosis with skeletal and gastrointestinal involvement in infancy. Radiology 131:363, 1979.

141. Lynch, A., Shaw, H., and Milton, G. W.: Effect of aspirin upon gastric secretion. Gut 5:230, 1964.

142. Lynn, H. B.: The mechanism of pyloric stenosis and its relationship to preoperative preparation. Arch. Surg. 81:453, 1960.

143. Lynn, H. B., and Espinas, E. E.: Intestinal atresia. Arch. Surg. 79:357, 1959.

144. Mahour, G., Isaacs, H., and Chang, L.: Primary malignant tumors of the stomach in children. J. Pediatr. Surg. 15:603, 1980.

145. Martinson, J.: Studies on the efferent vagal control of the stomach. Acta Physiol. Scand. (Suppl.) 255:1, 1968.

146. Maull, K., Scher, L., and Greenfield, L.: Surgical implications of acid ingestion. Surg. Gynecol. Obstet. 148:895, 1980.

147. McCollough, W. E.: Foreign body in the stomach of a premature infant. J. Pediatr. 60:277, 1962.

148. McCormick, W. F.: Rupture of the stomach in children. Review of the literature and report of seven cases. Arch. Pathol. 67:416, 1959.

149. McEnergy, J. T., and Greengaard, J.: Treatment of acute iron ingestion with desferrioxamine in 20 children. J. Pediatr. 68:773, 1966.

150. McGuigan, J. E.: On the distribution and release of gastrin. Gastroenterology 64:497, 1973.

151. McKeown, T., and MacMahon, B.: Infantile hypertrophic pyloric stenosis in parent and child. Arch. Dis. Child. 30:497, 1955.

152. Meekar, I. A., and Snyder, W. H.: Gastrostomy for the newborn surgical patient. Arch. Dis. Child. 37:159, 1962.

153. Meelin, G. W., Santulli, T. V., and Altman, H. S.: Congenital pyloric stenosis: a controlled evaluation of medical treatment utilizing methyl-scopolamine-nitrate. J. Pediatr. 66:649, 1965.

153a. Meeroff, J. C., Schreiber, D. S., Trier, J. S., and Blacklow, N. R.: Abnormal gastric motor function in viral gastroenteritis. Ann. Intern. Med. 92:370, 1980.

154. Menguy, R., and Masters, Y. F.: Effects of aspirin on gastric mucous secretions. Surg. Gynecol. Obstet. 120:92, 1965.

155. Metrakos, J. D.: Congenital hypertrophic pyloric stenosis in twins. Arch. Dis. Child. 27:351, 1953.

156. Meyer, J. L., III: Congenital defect in musculature of the stomach resulting in spontaneous gastric perforation in the neonatal period. J. Pediatr. 51:416, 1957.

157. Michener, W. M., Kennedy, R. L., and DuShane, J. W.: Duodenal ulcer in childhood: ninety-two cases with follow-up. Am. J. Dis. Child. 100:814, 1960.

158. Millar, T. M., Bruce, J., and Patterson, J. R.: Spontaneous rupture of the stomach. Br. J. Surg. 44:513, 1957.

159. Miller, R. A.: Observations on the gastric acidity during the first month of life. Arch. Dis. Child. 16:22, 1941.

160. Miller, R. F., and Ostrum, H. W.: Hypertrophic pyloric stenosis in infants. Am. J. Roentgenol. 54:17, 1945.

161. Mishlany, H., Idriss, A., and derKaloustian, V.: Pyloroduodenal atresia: an autosomal recessive disease. Pediatrics 62:419, 1968.

162. Morden, R., Schullinges, J., Mollitt, D., and Santulli, T.: Operative management of stress ulcers in children. Ann. Surg. 196:18, 1982.

163. Moore, T. C.: Gastrectomy in infancy and childhood. II. Results of an international survey. Ann. Surg. 162:91, 1965.

164. Moorthy, A. V., and Chesney, R.: Peptic ulcer in uremic children. J. Pediatr. 92:419, 1978.

165. Morris, C. R., Ivy, A. C., and Maddock, W. G.: Mechanism of acute abdominal distention. Arch. Surg. 55:101, 1947.

166. Muggia, A., and Spiro, H. M.: Childhood peptic ulcer. Gastroenterology 37:715, 1959.

167. Nakai, H., and Margaretten, W.: Protracted jaundice associated with hypertrophic pyloric stenosis. Pediatrics 29:198, 1962.

168. Nielsen, O. S.: Congenital pyloric stenosis as a factor predisposing to the ulcer syndrome. Acta Paediatr. 43:432, 1954.

169. Nielsen, O. S.: Histologic changes of the pyloric mesenteric plexus in infantile pyloric stenosis. Acta Paediatr. 45:636, 1956.

170. Nuss, D., and Lynn, H.: Peptic ulceration in children. Surg. Clin. North Am. 51:945, 1971.

171. O'Brien, P., and Silen, W.: Effects of bile salts and aspirin on the gastric mucosal blood flow. Gastroenterology 64:246, 1973.

172. O'Neill, J. A., Jr., Pruitt, B. A., Jr., Moncreif, J. A., and Switzer, W. E.: Studies related to the pathogenesis of Curling's ulcer. J. Trauma 7:275, 1967.

173. Papasova, M. P., Nagai, T., and Prosser, C. L.: Two-component slow waves in smooth muscle of cat stomach. Am. J. Physiol. 214:695, 1968.

174. Passi, R. B., Kraft, A. R., and Vasko, J. S.: Pathophysiologic mechanisms of shock in acute gastric dilatation. Surgery 65:298, 1969.

174a. Peltier, F. A., Tschen, E. H., Raimer, S. S., and Kuo, T. T.: Epidermolysis bullosa fetalis associated with congenital pyloric atresia. Arch. Dermatol. 117:728, 1981.

175. Pertsemilidis, D.: Neonatal gastric perforation. J. Mt. Sinai Hosp. 31:97, 1964.

176. Pruitt, B. A., Jr., Foley, F. D., and Moncreif, J. A.: Curling's ulcer: a clinical pathology study of 323 cases. Ann. Surg. 172:523, 1970.

177. Pruksapong, C., Donovan, R., Pinit, A., and Heldrich, F.: Gastric duplication. J. Pediatr. Surg. 14:83, 1980.

178. Puri, P., Boyd, E., and Guinney, E.: Duodenal ulcer in childhood: a continuing disease in adult life. J. Pediatr. Surg. 13:525, 1978.

179. Purvis, J., Miller, R., and Blumenthal, B.: Gastric teratoma: first reported case in a female. J. Pediatr. Surg. 14:86, 1979.

180. Rees, J. R., and Redo, S. F.: Neonatal gastric necrosis and perforation treated by gastrectomy and esophagogastric anastomosis. Surgery 64:472, 1968.

181. Robothan, J. L., and Lietman, P. S.: Acute iron poisoning. Am. J. Dis. Child. 134:875, 1980.

182. Rodbro, P., Krasilnikoff, P. A., and Bitsch, V.: Gastric secretions of pepsin in early childhood. Scand. J. Gastroenterol. 2:257, 1967.

183. Roviralta, E., Martinez-Mora, J., and Casasa, J.: Syndrome of "gastrocolic interference." Rev. Esp. Pediatr. 22:309, 1966.

184. Schaffer, A. J., and Avery, M. E.: Diseases of the Newborn. Ed. 3. Philadelphia, W. B. Saunders Company, 1971.

185. Scharli, A. F., and Leditschke, J. F.: Gastric motility after pyloromyotomy in infants: a reappraisal of postoperative feeding. Surgery 64:1133, 1968.

186. Schell, W. B., Karelitz, S., and Epstein, B. S.: Radiographic study of gastric emptying in premature infants. J. Pediatr. 62:342, 1963.

187. Scher, L., and Greenfield, L. J.: Surgical implications of acid ingestion. Surg. Gynecol. Obstet. 148:895, 1979.

188. Seagram, C. G. F., Stephens, C. A., and Cummings, W. A.: Peptic ulceration at the Hospital for Sick Children, Toronto, during the 20 year period 1949–1969. J. Pediatr. Surg. 8:407, 1973.

189. Shackelford, G., McAlister, W., Brodeur, A., and Ragsdale, E.: Congenital microgastria. Am. J. Roentgenol. Radium Ther. Nucl. Med. 118:72, 1973.

190. Shaw, A., Blanc, W. A., Santulli, T. V., and Kaiser, G.: Spontaneous rupture of the stomach in the newborn: a clinical and experimental study. Surgery 58:561, 1965.

191. Shuman, F. I., Darling, D. B., and Fisher, J. H.: The radiographic diagnosis of congenital hypertrophic pyloric stenosis. J. Pediatr. 71:70, 1967.

192. Silbergleit, A., and Berkas, E. M.: Neonatal gastric rupture. Minn. Med. 49:65, 1966.

193. Silverio, J.: Gastric emptying time in the newborn and nursing. Am. J. Med. Sci. 247:732, 1964.

194. Silvoso, G. R., Ivey, K. G., Butt, J. H., et al.: Incidence of gastric lesions in patients with rheumatic disease on chronic aspirin therapy. Ann. Intern. Med. 91:517, 1979.

195. Singleton, A. C.: Chronic gastric volvulus. Radiology 34:53, 1940.

196. Singleton, E. B., and Faykus, M. H.: Incidence of peptic ulcer as determined by radiologic examination in the pediatric age group. J. Pediatr. 65:858, 1964.

197. Skandalakis, J. E., Gray, S. W., and Shepard, D.: Smooth muscle tumors of the stomach. Surg. Gynecol. Obstet. 110:209, 1960.

198. Sloop, R. D., and Montague, A. C.: Gastric outlet obstruction due to congenital pyloric mucosal membrane. Ann. Surg. 165:598, 1967.

198a. Soter, A. F., and Wasserman, S.: Oral sodium cromoglycate in the treatment of systemic mastocytosis. N. Engl. J. Med. 301:465, 1979.

199. Spiro, H. M., and Milles, S.: Clinical and physiologic implications of the steroid induced peptic ulcer. N. Engl. J. Med. 263:286, 1960.

200. Spitz, L: Vomiting after pyloromyotomy for infantile hypertrophic pyloric stenosis. Arch. Dis. Child. 54:886, 1979.

201. Stadil, F., and Rehfeld, J. G.: Release of gastrin by epinephrine in man. Gastroenterology 65:210, 1973.

202. Stefan, H., and Rejlek, J.: Large lipoma of the stomach with ulceration and massive hemorrhage. Cesk. Pediatr. 21:246, 1966.

203. Steigman, A. J., Cruise, M. O., and Falkner, F. J.: Results with a trial of increased caloric feeding in premature infants. Am. J. Dis. Child. 100:794, 1960.

204. Steinicke, O., and Roselgaard, M.: Radiography of stomach in hypertrophic pyloric stenosis. Acta Paediatr. 48:245, 1959.

205. Steinicke, O., and Roselgaard, M.: Radiographic follow-up in hypertrophic pyloric stenosis. Acta Paediatr. 49:4, 1960.

206. Stevens-Rocmans, C., and Moyson, F.: Association d'ictere et de stenose hypertrophique du pylore. Arch. Fr. Pediatr. 20:723, 1963.

206a. Stillman, A. E., Sieber, O., Manthei, U., and Pinnas, J.: Transient protein-losing enteropathy and enlarged gastric rugae in childhood. Am. J. Dis. Child. *135*:21, 1981.

207. Strode, E. C., and Dean, M. L.: Acid burns of the stomach — report of two cases. Ann. Surg. *131*:801, 1950.

208. Sznejder, M. A.: Interstitial gastric emphysema in newborn infants due to polyvinyl feeding tube. J. Pediatr. *66*:126, 1965.

209. Tan, K. L., and Murgusau, J. J.: Congenital pyloric atresia in siblings. Arch. Surg. *105*:100, 1973.

210. Thomson, J.: The volume and acidity of the gastric contents in the unfed newborn infant. Arch. Dis. Child. 26:558, 1951.

211. Tornwall, L., Lind, J., Peltonen, T., and Wegelius, C.: The gastrointestinal tract of the newborn. Ann. Paediatr. Fenn. *4*:219, 1958.

212. Touloukian, R., Berdon, W., and Amoury, R.: Surgical experience with necrotizing enterocolitis in the infant. J. Pediatr. Surg. *4*:77, 1969.

213. Tudor, R.: Peptic ulcerations in childhood. Pediatr. Clin. North Am. *14*:109, 1967.

214. Tunell, W., and Smith, E. I.: Antral web in infancy. J. Pediatr. Surg. *15*:152, 1980.

215. Vengusamy, S., Pildes, R., Raffensperger, J., Levine, H., and Cornblath, M.: A controlled study of feeding gastrostomy in low birth weight infants. Pediatrics *43*:815, 1969.

216. Vitale, L., Opitz, J. M., and Shahidi, N. T.: Congenital and familial iron overload, N. Engl. J. Med. *280*:642, 1969.

217. Wagner, E. A., Jones, D. V., Koch, C. A., and Smith, C. D.: Polyethylene tube feeding in premature infants. J. Pediatr. *41*:79, 1952.

218. Wallgren, A.: Preclinical stage of infantile hypertrophic pyloric stenosis. Am. J. Dis. Child. *72*:371, 1946.

219. Wallgren, A.: Is the rate of hypertrophic pyloric stenosis declining? Acta Paediatr. *49*:530, 1960.

220. Wangel, A. G., and Callender, S. T.: Gastric secretion in the premature infant. Gut 9:249, 1968.

221. Wanschner, B., and Jensen, H. E.: Late follow-up studies after operation for congenital hypertrophic pyloric stenosis. Scand. J. Gastroenterol. 6:597, 1971.

222. Watanabe, A., Nagashima, H., Motoi, M., and Ogowa, K.: Familial juvenile polyps of the stomach. Gastroenterology 77:148, 1979.

223. Wellmann, K. F., Kagan, A., and Fang, H.: Hypertrophic pyloric stenosis in adults. Gastroenterology *46*:601, 1964.

224. White, J. J., and Morgan, W. W.: Improved operative technique for gastric duplication. Surgery 67:522, 1970.

225. Whitten, C. F., Cheny, Y., and Gibson, G. W.: Studies in acute iron poisoning. II. Further observations in desferrioxamine in the treatment of acute experimental iron poisoning. Pediatrics 38:102, 1966.

226. Whitten, C. F., Gibson, G. W., Good, M. H., Goodwin, J., and Brough, A. J.: Studies in acute iron poisoning. I. Desferrioxamine in the treatment of acute iron poisoning: clinical observations, experimental studies and theoretical considerations. Pediatrics *36*:322, 1965.

227. Wilson, M.: Pyloric stenosis in premature infants. J. Pediatr. 56:490, 1960.

228. Wolf, S., Telander, R. L., Dozois, R., and Go, L. W.: Increased meal-stimulated gastric acid secretion and serum gastrin after extensive small bowel resection in puppies. J. Pediatr. Surg. *12*:921, 1977.

229. Wurlitzer, F. P., Mares, A., Isaacs, H., Jr., Landing, B., and Woolley, M.: Smooth muscle tumors of the stomach in childhood and adolescence. J. Pediatr. Surg. 8:421, 1973.

230. Ziprowski, M., and Teek, R.: Gastric volvulus in childhood. Am. J. Radiol. *132*:921, 1979.

231. Zollinger, R. M., Tompkins, R., Amerson, J. R., Endahl, G., Kraft, A., and Moore, F.: Identification of the diarrheogenic hormone associated with non-beta islet cell tumors of the pancreas. Ann. Surg. *168*:502, 1968.

Chapter Thirteen

THE PERITONEUM, ABDOMINAL WALL, AND OMPHALOMESENTERIC DUCT

NEONATAL ASCITES AND PERITONITIS

ASCITES AND PRENATAL ABDOMINAL ENLARGEMENT

Prenatal abdominal enlargement in the fetus is an immediate problem for the obstetrician for it causes dystocia, which, if extreme, requires fetal abdominal paracentesis to facilitate delivery.[92] Rh incompatibility was formerly a cause of fetal ascites, but this now is relatively uncommon.[126] Abdominal dystocia is most often caused by obstructive uropathy, particularly posterior urethral valves, ureterocele, ureteral stenosis, or atresia. The mortality has approached 50 per cent. This type of ascites generally results from transudation of urine into the peritoneum, but a few cases have been caused by ruptured perinephric cysts.[16, 83] Urinary ascites has been described in the absence of obstruction in five cases and was associated with a mortality of 20 per cent. Meconium peritonitis ranks second as the cause of this type of abdominal distention and is discussed separately. Perhaps third in frequency is hydrometrocolpos, a disease in which cervical and vaginal secretions accumulate because their outflow is obstructed. This is most often caused by imperforate hymen and, rarely, by vaginal atresia; it is relieved by incision of the hymen or, in the latter case, by plastic repair. Rare causes of abdominal enlargement are cytomegalic inclusion disease, chylous ascites,[89, 108] polycystic kidneys or liver, Wilms' tumor, neuroblastoma, anterior meningocele,[75] subcapsular hematoma of the liver,[77] mesenteric constriction from malrotation,[51] and eosinophilic ascites. Ascites may be diagnosed prenatally by ultrasonography.[27, 38, 46, 116] Now, with the advent of fetal surgery, the prognosis may be improved.

CHEMICAL PERITONITIS

Meconium Peritonitis

Meconium peritonitis develops from intestinal perforation during the last trimester of fetal life or in the immediate neonatal period. During this time the meconium is sterile and produces only a foreign body reaction in the peritoneum.[8, 9, 31, 72] It may present as a giant cyst.[66]

Incidence. Several hundred cases have been reported, and neonatal centers see one or more per year.

Etiology. This type of peritonitis is associated with intestinal atresias or with the

260

meconium ileus of cystic fibrosis. It results from perforation or tear of the bowel proximal to a site of obstruction. Other disorders with which it is found are volvulus, congenital bands, mesenteric hernia, intussusception, Meckel's diverticulum, imperforate anus, meconium plug, enteric duplications, enteritis, and ischemic enterocolitis. In some cases in which there is no evidence of obstruction, an intrauterine vascular accident followed by perforation is postulated.[94]

Pathology. Meconium forms by the end of the third intrauterine month, after the fetus has begun to swallow, and is present in the rectum by the fifth month. If intrauterine intestinal obstruction is a factor, there is maternal polyhydramnios and sometimes abdominal dystocia.

Meconium peritonitis has been divided into three types. The *fibroadhesive type,* the most common, is due to a chemical peritonitis caused by digestive enzymes. There is extensive fibroblastic reaction forming a dense, adherent membrane in which calcium is deposited. The membrane may seal off the site of perforation. In this type, adhesions can cause extrinsic obstruction. The *cystic type* results when there is no seal over the perforation and the bowel loops are fixed to form a cystic cavity, which seals off the rest of the intestine from the perforation. Meconium continues to enter the cyst, which becomes filled with exudate and lined by a calcified peel. The *generalized type* occurs with perinatal perforation. There is bacterial peritonitis because the meconium contains enteric flora. Calcium plaques float freely in the peritoneal cavity and have not had time to become embedded in the intestinal wall. There are multiple fibrinous adhesions.

Symptoms. The baby is born with abdominal distention or develops it rapidly after birth. He is obstipated and vomits bilious material. He may pass one or two small meconium stools but no more after that. There is ascites and, in the male, scrotal swelling (Figs. 13–1 and 13–2). The veins over the abdomen are distended, and there is paraumbilical ecchymosis. Hypothermia, cyanosis, and shock appear within

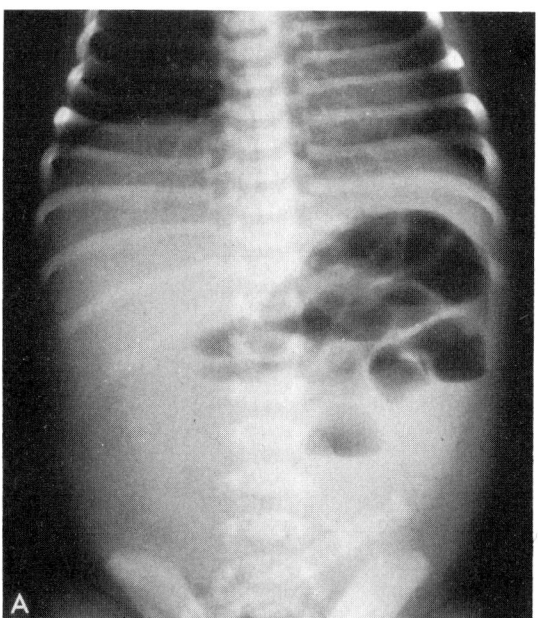

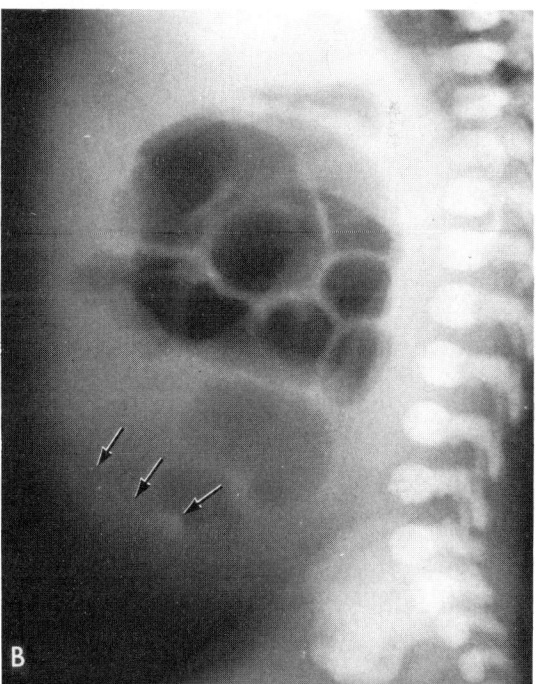

Figure 13–1 Meconium peritonitis and obstructing adhesions. The patient is a three-month-old infant, previously well, who presented with vomiting and abdominal distention. Plain films showed a pattern of mechanical obstruction and some intra-abdominal calcifications. At surgery, matted adhesions were found to produce small bowel obstruction and were presumed to represent an intrauterine perforation and peritonitis with postnatal complications. The infant did not have cystic fibrosis. A, Erect film shows dilated loops with air-fluid levels. Faint calcifications in the right lower quadrant are present. B, Irregular calcifications are better seen in the lateral view *(arrows).*

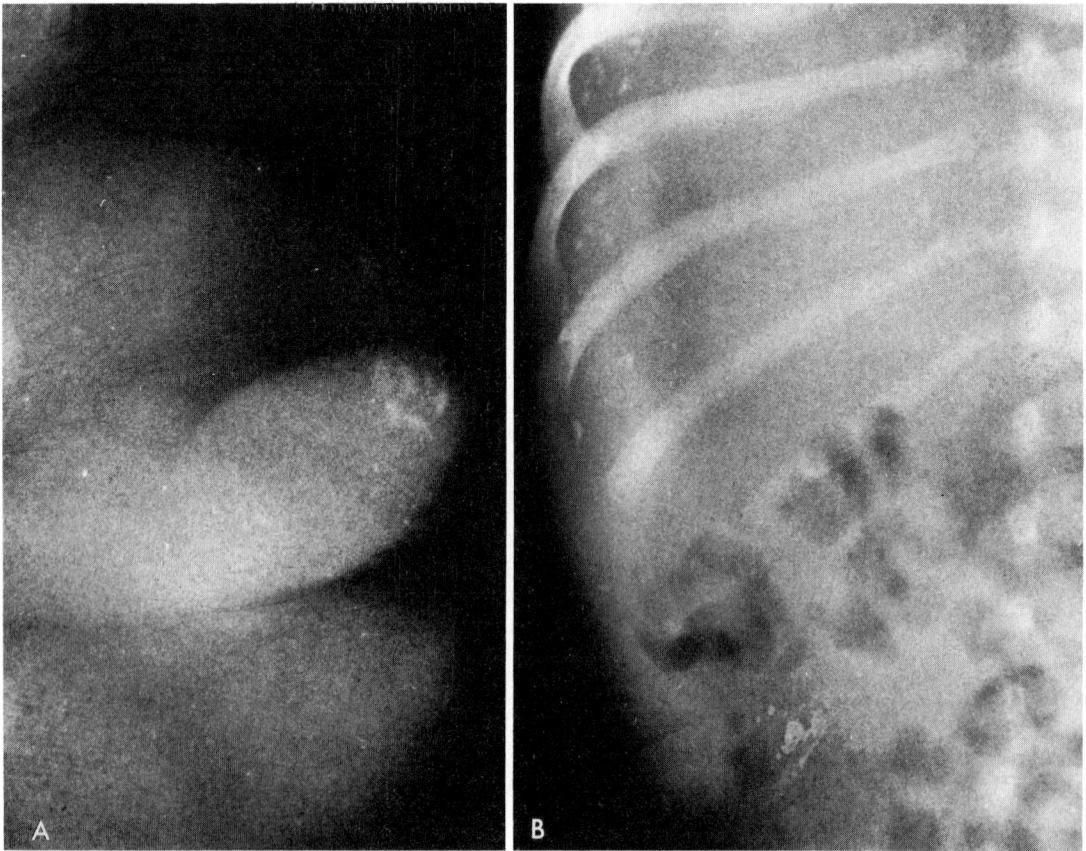

Figure 13–2   *A,* Scrotal calcification in infant with meconium peritonitis. *B,* Intra-abdominal calcification in same infant.

minutes to hours after the abdominal distention, and pneumoperitoneum is present if the perforation occurs at or after birth. As the abdominal distention increases, the respirations are labored and edema in the flanks is noted. A rare baby will have only abdominal distention and hydroceles and will appear quite well otherwise. After several weeks, firm, calcified scrotal masses replace the hydrocele fluid.

Diagnosis.   Unless there is a family history of cystic fibrosis, this entity cannot be distinguished from other forms of peritonitis or ascites. The radiologic findings are characteristic, however. The plain abdominal film has an opaque ground-glass appearance with a scattering of flecks or sizable masses of calcium. Intraluminal concretions are present in some. If there are calcifications in the scrotum, they are pathognomonic. Pneumoperitoneum is present if the perforation is recent. The localized cystic type is illustrated in Figure 13–3.

Treatment.   Emergency medical treatment consists of nasogastric suction, administration of oxygen and intravenous antibiotics, and restoration of body temperature. Surgical treatment depends upon the type of peritonitis — lysis of adhesions for the fibroadhesive type, decortication for the cystic type. In all, areas of abnormal bowel must be removed whenever possible.

Prognosis.   The mortality is high, for up to 90 per cent of infants weighing less than 5 pounds die. Mortality is increased further in those with neonatal rupture. Unresected or matted bowel functions poorly if it is not removed at surgery. During the last decade, the survival of infants treated definitively by surgery has risen in one series to 55 per cent.[109]

Bile Peritonitis

The disease in the infant is unlike the fulminating peritonitis in the adult, which

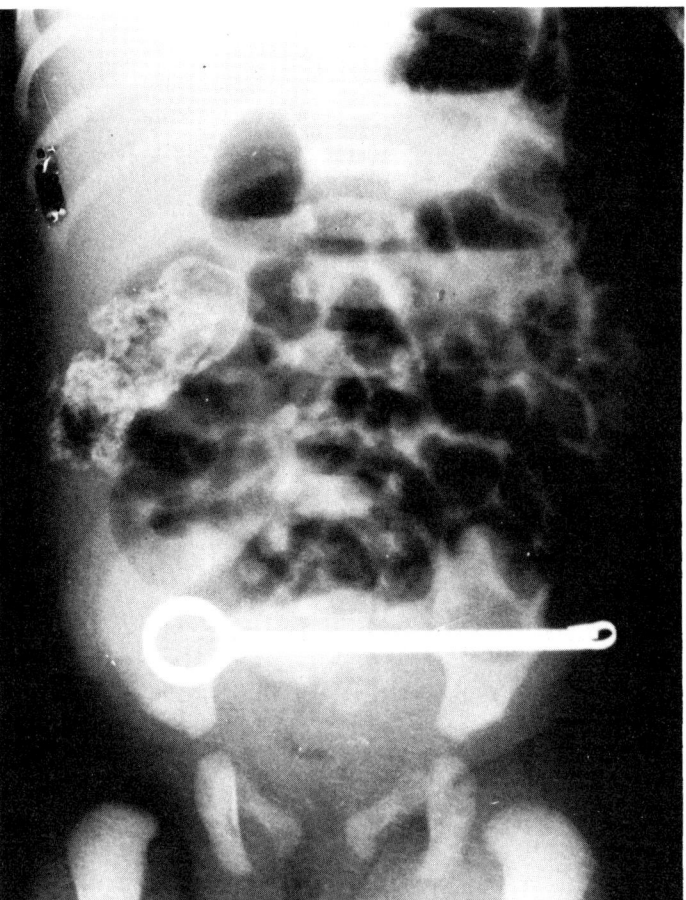

Figure 13–3 Meconium abscess in a neonate. This male infant was found at neonatal examination to have a hard abdominal mass to the right of the umbilicus. Plain film of the abdomen demonstrates dense calcification, mostly localized to the right abdomen. At surgery, an abscess was found adherent to loops of bowel, liver, and anterior abdominal wall. After bowel loops were freed and the abscess collection removed, an old perforation of the terminal ileum was identified and repaired. The infant did not have cystic fibrosis.

carries a 50 per cent mortality. Bile ascites might be a more appropriate term, for infants have little in the way of acute symptoms.[14, 19, 22, 23, 41]

Incidence. Several dozen cases have been reported.

Etiology and Pathology. This type of ascites results from perforation of the biliary tree, usually on the anterior aspect of the common duct or at the junction of the gallbladder and the cystic duct. Perforated choledochal cyst and gallstones have been other findings. There is usually little tissue reaction, although there is some walling-off of bile by a false sac resembling a choledochal cyst. In one infant, there was so much necrotic reaction above the perforation that the biliary tree could not be identified.

Symptoms. The onset occurs during the first few weeks of life. Some infants, however, are thought to have physiologic jaundice, and the correct diagnosis is considered only after three to six weeks, when abdominal distention and inguinal hernias develop and pale-colored stools are passed. Indeed, hernia is often the only reason parents bring the infant to the pediatrician. Most affected infants feed vigorously and grow well. A few babies have more acute symptoms — anorexia, vomiting, abdominal distention, and the habit of drawing up their legs as if in pain. In only one of the reported cases was there abdominal tenderness, fever, and shock. There is evidence of fluid in the abdomen, but the liver and spleen are not enlarged. The bowel sounds may be hypoactive or absent.

Diagnosis. All the causes of ascites and jaundice must be considered, but the combination of prolonged neonatal jaundice, acholic stools, and ascites in a fairly well baby should suggest bile peritonitis. Ascites is not one of the early signs of biliary atresia. It is found, although rarely, in some cases of neonatal hepatitis of great severity and in the extremely infrequent congenital cirrhosis or syphilitic hepatitis. Differentiation of bile peritonitis from these diseases on clinical grounds alone is not possible, although the jaundice is less severe than one would suspect with acholic stools. Diagnosis depends upon the discovery of bile-stained fluid on abdominal paracentesis or, if the scrotum is distended with fluid, on scrotal tap. HIDA liver scan may show extravasation of the compound into the peritoneum.

Treatment. Exploration of the biliary tree is indicated. The perforation is closed, and an anastomosis establishing free drainage from the gallbladder or common duct to the duodenum is constricted.

Fibrinous Chronic Peritonitis from Vaginal Secretions

Hydrometrocolpos is a cause of abdominal dystocia resulting from dilatation of the fetal female genital tract by retained cervical and vaginal secretions. In rare instances it leads to aseptic peritonitis.[16]

Incidence. The incidence is 1 in 16,000 female births.

Etiology. The usual cause is imperforate hymen or, less often, atresia of the vagina due to incomplete resolution of the central, solid-core stage in the entire or lower vagina.

Pathology. The abdomen is filled by a large cystic vagina and a dilated cervix and uterus. Mechanical obstruction of the urethra results in bladder distention. The genital secretions overflow through the fallopian tubes and the peritoneal cavity fills with clear or milky fluid. Fibrinous inflammation covers the parietal and visceral peritoneum, and the intestines are crowded into the flanks.

Symptoms. After a delivery complicated by dystocia or prolonged labor, cyanosis, respiratory distress, and abdominal distention are present in the infant at birth. The hymen or the perineum or both bulge, or no vagina at all can be identified. A fluid wave is present in the abdomen, and sometimes the large abdominal mass produces an inferior vena cava syndrome with edema of the lower extremities.

Diagnosis. Radiologic plain films of the abdomen show bulging of the flanks, separation of loops of bowel by free fluid, and compression of loops in the right and left lower quadrants. Cystourethrography shows anterior displacement of the bladder, lateral deviation of the ureters, and hydronephrosis. Posterior displacement of the rectum is revealed by barium enema.

Treatment. Laparotomy, drainage, relief of the vaginal obstruction, and lysis of adhesions are performed.

Prognosis. Most of these infants have died.

Chylous Ascites

Chylous ascites is a rare disorder that is less frequent in the infant than in the older child, in whom it is related to trauma or neoplasm.[29, 42, 43, 63]

Incidence. Only 55 cases had been gathered by 1962, and sporadic cases have been reported in the literature since then. The disease is twice as common in males as in females, and other members of the family often have disturbances in lymphatic drainage.[79]

Etiology and Pathology. In many neonates the pathogenesis is never discovered, but one factor that has been identified is congenital malformation of the lymphatics, which obstructs the proximal flow of lymph. Among those autopsied or subjected to laparotomy have been found failure of peripheral channels to communicate with central ones, congenital occlusion of the thoracic duct with cyst formation and perforation, lymphatic obstruction in the ileal mesentery, defect in the lymphatic channels at the root of the mesentery, and obstruction of the mesentery by a band of congenital venous remnants. Adhesions following surgery have caused obstruction of the mesentery of the ileum in neonates.

Only 10 per cent of patients with chylous ascites have lymphedema of the extremities. The severe hypoproteinemia that accompanies the disease is due to loss of plasma proteins through the gastrointestinal tract, for with lymphatic obstruction there is increased pressure in the lymphatics and exudation of lymph into the intestinal lumen. The ascitic fluid is rich in protein (up to 19 gm per dl) and fat (up to 18 gm per dl) and contains electrolytes in the same proportion as serum.[96]

Symptoms. The infant's abdomen is swollen at birth or becomes so over the first few days or weeks. Lymphedema, if present, sometimes precedes abdominal swelling. The infant eats well, but as ascites increases a venous pattern develops over the abdominal wall and there is scrotal, pedal, sacral, and periorbital edema. The nutritional status deteriorates, and malnutrition is evident in muscular wasting. Respiratory distress is related either to an associated chylothorax or to pneumonitis. As globulins as well as albumin are lost through the bowel wall, there is a secondary hypogammaglobulinemia. Intercurrent bacterial infections are frequent.

Diagnosis. Differentiation from other causes of ascites is made by paracentesis, which yields the typical milky chylous fluid. Radiologic examination may show thickening of the bowel wall and separation of small bowel loops by intraperitoneal fluid. Examination of the small bowel with barium shows edema of the bowel wall and some segmentation and flocculation of barium. Small bowel biopsy demonstrates dilated lymphatic channels in the intestinal lamina propria, but this does not determine the site of lymphatic block. Lymphangiography is the most definitive technique to demonstrate abnormalities or absence of lymphatic channels. The procedure is not without hazard, however, for we have seen complete obstruction develop after such a study in two patients with partial lymphatic obstruction. Balance studies determine quantitative fecal fat and nitrogen losses, and radioactive protein studies quantitate enteric losses and albumin turnover.

Treatment. If no etiologic factor is demonstrated, the treatment is conservative, using paracentesis for relief of abdominal discomfort or respiratory distress, but only when necessary because it further depletes the protein pool.[125] A low-fat diet reduces the rate of formation of ascitic fluid; the formula Pregestimil, composed of medium-chain triglycerides, is ideal. Intravenous re-

turn of the chylous ascitic fluid has lessened alimentary demands in some patients.[123]

Laparotomy is indicated when the ascites continues to accumulate after 10 to 12 months.

Prognosis. Most patients undergo a sustained or permanent remission.

BACTERIAL PERITONITIS

Bacterial peritonitis results from gastrointestinal spillage through perforated or necrotic bowel or through hematogenous or lymphatic seeding of the peritoneum with bacteria.

Primary Peritonitis

Primary peritonitis is that which occurs without a primary intra-abdominal source of infection.[40, 49]

Incidence. In the neonatal period, males are affected twice as often as females, but in older children, girls are affected four times as often as boys. Before antibiotics were developed, this disease accounted for 10 per cent of cases of acute abdomen in children, but now this figure is less than 1 per cent. In the last ten years only two cases have been seen in New Haven, and 33 cases have been reported from Boston Children's Hospital since 1950.

Etiology. The accepted cause of primary peritonitis is hematogenous or lymphatic spread of bacteria to the peritoneum. In one third of the cases the bacteria cultured from the peritoneum are found in the nose, throat, blood, or urine; in 60 per cent the bacteria originated in sites other than these or there was a history of preceding upper respiratory infection.[7] In females, retrograde spread of bacteria through the fallopian tubes may take place. The serum gamma globulin was less than normal in 75 per cent of the Boston children who were tested at the time of infection. Fowler[34] reviewed 97 cases seen between 1925 and 1955 and found, as have others, that the causative organisms were pneumococcus and hemolytic streptococcus, whereas those isolated from patients during the last 15 years were gram-negative organisms. Staphylococcal peritonitis occurred in 6 patients of 33 studied since 1950 in Boston.

Predisposing factors are genitourinary infection, upper respiratory infection, and hypogammaglobulinemia. Typically, this was a disease complicating nephrosis in the presteroid era.

Symptoms. There is usually a preceding history of otitis, pharyngitis, or urinary tract infection. The baby may not seem terribly ill until he suddenly becomes listless or extremely irritable. Vomiting accompanies abdominal distention, the temperature rises rapidly to 103 to 104° F, and tachycardia and tachypnea occur. In some there is diarrhea, and the bowel sounds, though present, are decreased. Normal stools and audible bowel sounds do not preclude the diagnosis, however. The abdomen is tender to palpation, and a fluid wave can be elicited. In a few cases the onset is insidious, with abdominal pain localized to the lower quadrants and only mild abdominal distention. Leukocytosis is present, with counts sometimes rising over 20,000 cells per cubic millimeter.

Diagnosis. Because of its rarity the diagnosis is not often considered, the disease being most often confused with appendicitis or perforated viscus with secondary bacterial contamination. Aspiration of the peritoneal fluid with recovery and identification of pneumococci or other organisms in pure culture is diagnostic. The recovery of mixed organisms suggests perforation and warrants surgical exploration. Radiologic examination of the abdomen shows intraperitoneal fluid and dilated loops of bowel and is of most help in ruling out the presence of free intraperitoneal air.

Treatment. Penicillin is effective in treating pneumococcal or streptococcal peritonitis and must be continued for ten days. Ampicillin (Polycillin) or cephalothin (Keflin) is used to treat gram-negative infection until the results of sensitivity studies are known. Methicillin or one of the oxacillins is used for staphylococcal peritonitis. Continuous nasogastric suction is applied until clinical improvement is apparent and bowel sounds are again active.

Prognosis. With vigorous care and antibiotic therapy the mortality has fallen from 45 per cent to less than 8 per cent.

Tuberculous Peritonitis

This becomes increasingly rare as the incidence of tuberculosis decreases.

Etiology. Some decades ago the bovine strain of *Mycobacterium tuberculosis* was responsible for the great majority of cases of tuberculous peritonitis. Bacteria contained in infected cow's milk penetrated the intestinal wall and caused caseating mesenteric lymphadenitis and peritonitis. With the elimination of bovine tuberculosis in the United States this form has virtually disappeared. The few cases that do appear stem from either swallowing of bronchial secretions or hematogenous spread from a primary focus, usually in the lung and mediastinal lymph nodes.[84]

Pathology. Tuberculous gastrointestinal disease takes a variety of forms: esophageal stricture, pyloroduodenal obstruction, intra-abdominal mass, malabsorption and protein-losing enteropathy, small bowel strictures, colonic lesions resembling Crohn's disease, ischiorectal fistula, or peritonitis.

A dry form of tuberculous peritonitis consists of dense inflammatory exudate and adhesions between loops of bowel. Fecal fistulas may develop and may even communicate with the umbilicus. In the moist form there is ascites, the fluid being yellowish and serous with a high protein content. Miliary tubercles are present in both types.

Symptoms. The onset of the disease is usually insidious, with fever, anorexia, weight loss, vomiting, and abdominal pain. There can be diarrhea, constipation, or dysuria, and when ascites develops the abdomen is tense and distended.

Diagnosis. The chest film is positive in only about half the patients. A Mantoux or tine test is usually positive, but it can be negative. The differential diagnosis includes bacterial peritonitis and all of the causes of ascites. Abdominal paracentesis is not often helpful because acid-fast bacteria are seldom isolated. Peritoneoscopy will demonstrate caseating tubercle follicles

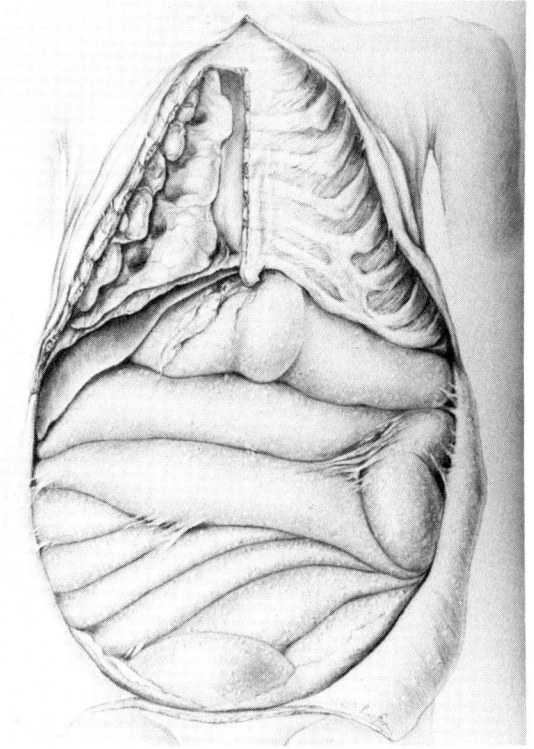

Figure 13–4 Tuberculous peritonitis with tubercles scattered through the peritoneum. Fibrous adhesions are noted between loops of bowel. (Illustration by A. Hemberger. Yale University School of Medicine Collection.)

studding the peritoneal surface, and biopsy will confirm the diagnosis (Fig. 13–4).

Treatment. The treatment is as for miliary tuberculosis with isoniazid and streptomycin or para-aminosalicylic acid. Evacuation of the ascites fluid makes the child more comfortable. The addition of steroids to the antituberculous regimen has given better results in treatment.

Secondary Bacterial Peritonitis

This is actually the most common form of peritonitis in infants beyond the neonatal period and is secondary to direct contamination of the peritoneum by gram-positive organisms from the skin or gram-negative organisms from the intestinal tract after a penetrating injury or perforation.[86, 88]

Etiology. Bacterial peritonitis results from transmural spread from enterocolitis or gastroenteritis, from perforation of a viscus or gangrenous bowel, from gastroschisis or

ruptured omphalocele, or from sepsis. It is the usual form of presentation in neonatal appendicitis.[106a] One source unique to the newborn is spread from the infected umbilicus to the peritoneum via thrombosed umbilical vessels or perivascular connective tissue.[35]

Pathology and Pathophysiology. Depending upon the organisms present, the peritoneal fluid is either purulent or serosanguineous, and a fibrinous exudate covers the intestinal serosa. Pooling of fluid in the bowel loops and, in cases of perforation, in the peritoneal cavity, creates a large third space and hypovolemia. Fever, by increasing work expenditure, leads to increased cardiac output, which on occasion results in cardiac failure.[13, 18, 20a] Late renal failure is another complication. The pathogens are usually gram-negative organisms, e.g., *Escherichia coli*, *Klebsiella* or *Pseudomonas*, and *Streptococcus faecalis*. Rarely, fungi are isolated.

The process is generalized because, unfortunately, walling-off of the infection into an abscess does not occur in the young infant.

Symptoms. The diagnosis is sometimes obscured by symptoms of underlying obstructive disease. In less complicated cases there is anorexia, vomiting, constipation or, at times, diarrhea, and increasing abdominal distention. The infant appears acutely ill, in pain, and apprehensive. His respiration is labored, and he lies quietly with his knees flexed. The abdomen is dull to percussion, and a fluid wave is elicited. The abdomen is tender to palpation and often, but not always, rigid. In the early stages peristalsis is present and hyperactive, but as peritonitis develops the abdomen becomes silent. The temperature is usually in the range of 102° F, but the affected premature infant or the neonate may be hypothermic. Leukocytosis is usually evidenced by a count of above 15,000 cells per cubic millimeter, but development of leukopenia with a marked shift to the left is a poor prognostic sign.

Diagnosis. Diagnosis requires differentiation between primary and secondary peritonitis. In both, radiologic examination shows a generalized distention of bowel loops and separation of the loops by homogeneous material. Edema of the bowel wall, obliteration of the psoas shadow, and the peritoneal fat line all signify peritonitis, but the only certain distinguishing sign is pneumoperitoneum, which represents a perforated viscus.[80] Contrast studies are contraindicated. If the question remains unresolved after radiologic examination, paracentesis is helpful if it yields fluid which by stain and culture contains one organism.

Treatment. Immediate medical treatment consists of nasogastric suction, correction of hypovolemia and electrolyte imbalance, and antibiotic therapy with penicillin or ampicillin and broad-spectrum drugs such as kanamycin or gentamycin. Metronidazole has proved extremely effective in the treatment of anaerobic infections. The patient should be maintained in Fowler's position in an attempt to localize the infected peritoneal fluid in the lower quadrants, away from the liver and diaphragms. Laparotomy is performed as soon as dehydration and electrolyte and acid-base problems have been corrected. Hypothermia lowers the metabolic demands during the first few days of treatment.

HYPERSENSITIVITY PERITONITIS

An eosinophilic peritonitis has been reported in young children in whom gradual abdominal distention, nausea, abdominal pain, vomiting, diarrhea, weight loss, and ascites developed.[1, 87] There is a peripheral eosinophilia, reaching levels as high as 34 per cent; the bone marrow is normal except for increased numbers of eosinophils. Surgical exploration reveals chronic lymphadenitis and eosinophilic infiltration of the muscle and connective tissue of the appendix, with obliteration of its lumen; on peritoneal biopsy a hypersensitivity necrotizing angiitis, probably representing an allergic reaction and excessive bowel histamine release, is found. The disease is self-limited and subsides within two to four weeks.

This disorder has been associated with eosinophilic gastroenteritis of three types:

(1) mucosal disease with iron deficiency, intestinal blood loss, and hypoproteinemia; (2) muscle layer disease leading to obstructive symptoms; and (3) subserosal disease. Eosinophilic ascites has also been described with vasculitis, lymphoma, and allergy.

A more serious and often lethal form, termed the hypereosinophilic syndrome, is associated with eosinophilia, fibroplastic endocarditis, hepatomegaly, and splenomegaly as well as small bowel disease.

CANDIDA PERITONITIS

Candida peritonitis has been reported in two infants, both of whom were receiving broad-spectrum antibiotics: One had congenital heart disease and had undergone cardiac catheterization, and the other had ileal perforation.[60]

This form of peritonitis usually develops after perforation, intestinal surgery, or chronic dialysis and usually occurs in older children and adults. The diagnosis is made by culture of the organism from peritoneal fluid. Although adults are treated by surgical drainage or lavage with antifungal agents, these infants were treated systemically with amphotericin B. One also received intravenous 5-fluorocytosine as well as intraperitoneal lavage. Both infants died.

DISEASES OF THE PERITONEUM

PNEUMOPERITONEUM AND GASTROINTESTINAL PERFORATION

Neonatal gastrointestinal perforation is a catastrophic event with a multitude of causes.[11] Gastric perforation, discussed in Chapter 12, has ranked in some series as the most common form. In other series, intestinal obstruction is rated the major cause, with rupture of the ileum more common than that of jejunum or colon.[71] Perforated appendix and Meckel's diverticulum are next in order.[12] In the large bowel, cecal perforation has been noted as a spontaneous occurrence. Colonic perforations are idiopathic,[115] are secondary to localized muscular defects or ulcerative or necrotizing colitis,[121] or may occur through a pseudo-diverticulum. Stercoral ulcers developing over a bolus of hard feces cause some perforations of the sigmoid. Recently, perforation of the colon has been reported to follow exchange transfusion, and the pathologic findings were those of necrotizing enterocolitis. Finally, rectal perforation can result from the vigorous introduction of a thermometer.

Symptoms. Gastrointestinal perforation is more common in infants who have had an episode of anoxia or whose mothers have had significant bleeding or a prolonged, difficult labor.[53] The onset of symptoms is sudden, with extreme abdominal distention, dyspnea, cyanosis, and vomiting. Less frequent manifestations are anorexia, hematemesis, and rectal bleeding. There are edema and erythema of the anterior abdominal wall, hypothermia, and collapse. The abdomen is tense and tympanitic to percussion, and the bowel sounds are decreased and, later, absent. The normal area of liver dullness is obliterated.

Diagnosis. The diagnosis is established by three radiographic views of the abdomen. In the erect film, air is present under the diaphragm (5 ml of air is all that is required for a positive film in the older child, and probably half that amount is adequate in the neonate). If air is present in large amounts, it separates the liver from the diaphragm and increases the distance between the fundus and the right diaphragm. In the lateral supine film, a collection of air lies anterior to the viscera and below the peritoneal fat fold. In the supine film the "football sign" is helpful.[105] The falciform ligament is outlined against the radiolucent abdominal air, which is in the shape of a large bubble, sometimes termed the air-dome sign. The association of intraperitoneal fluid indicates perforation.

Pneumoperitoneum is not always associated with perforation, and other diseases must be considered.[3] *Clostridium welchii* in an intraperitoneal abscess can produce free peritoneal air. Pneumatosis cystoides intestinalis can occur without perforation. Pneumoperitoneum has on rare occasions complicated pneumothorax and pneumomediastinum secondary to the obstruction of massive aspiration, hyaline membrane disease, or too vigorous resuscitation at birth. It is likely that in tension pneumothorax air dissects through the aortic and inferior vena caval openings in the diaphragm, flows down around the smaller vessels, and forms subserosal air cysts that rupture to cause pneumoperitoneum. This form of pneumoperitoneum resolves spontaneously but does so more rapidly if the tension pneumothorax is relieved.

Treatment. If fluid as well as air is present, early laparotomy is indicated. If there is only pneumoperitoneum and evidence of tension pneumothorax, pneumomediastinum, or both, the pneumothorax should be treated and the infant thoroughly evaluated for perforation before exploration is undertaken. Bell et al. have found that more than half of their infants with neonatal peritonitis and perforation had multiple organisms and one third had positive blood cultures.[7] The most frequently isolated organisms were *Escherichia coli* and *Bacteroides*, sensitive generally to gentamicin and clindamycin.

Prognosis. The prognosis of neonatal perforation improves with earlier diagnosis; at present a survival rate of 50 per cent is possible.[68]

GAS IN THE PORTAL VEIN

Gas in the portal vein usually carries a grave prognosis. In most cases it is a manifestation of gastrointestinal mucosal damage or dead bowel.

Incidence. Forty-three cases were reported between 1955 and 1971[4] and sporadic cases have been noted since.

Etiology. This finding has been associated with Clostridial enteritis, gastroenteritis, necrotizing enterocolitis, and sepsis and has been documented after umbilical vein catheterization and peroxide enema. It is postulated that after catheterization or enema, luminal gas under tension passes

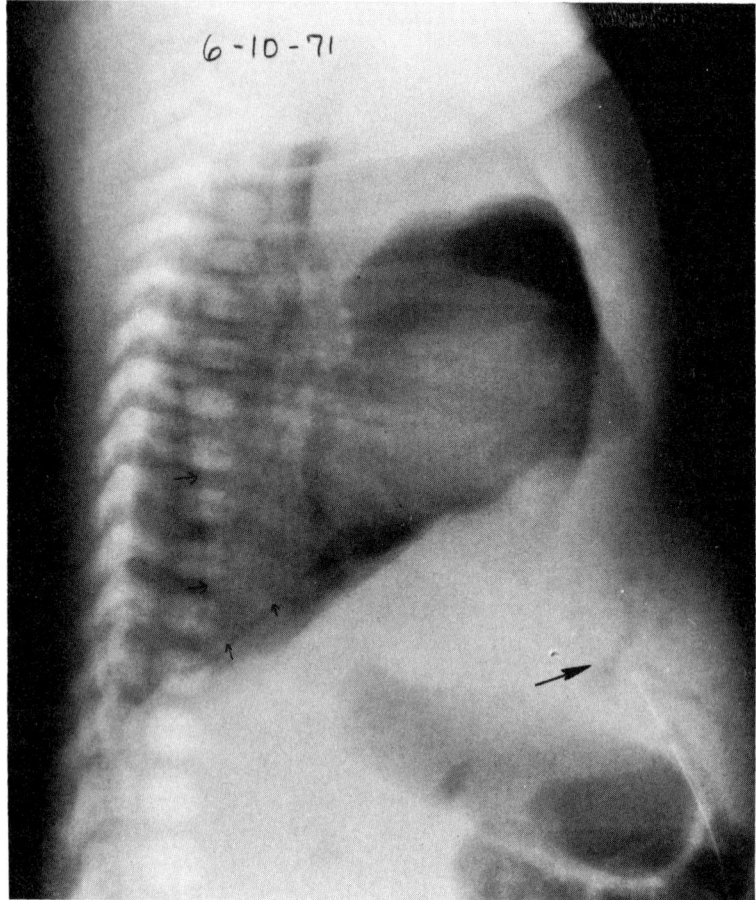

Figure 13–5   Gas in the portal vein seen as a pattern of branching linear, lucent areas extending toward the periphery of the liver *(large arrow)*. Gas in the biliary tree tends to remain in a more central distribution. In this patient, gas was inadvertently introduced during umbilical vein catheterization and was of benign consequence. Also present are a large anterior pneumomediastinum and pneumothorax. The edge of partially collapsed lung is noted by small arrows.

through the bowel and into the mesenteric veins and portal system. Many patients with this finding have positive blood cultures for gas-forming organisms. In some, however, no pathologic findings in the gastrointestinal tract can be demonstrated.

Pathology. The gas accumulates in branches from the porta hepatis to the edge of the liver, where it outlines the peripheral portal radicals. Gas can also be found in the bowel wall, mesenteric, and portal veins in some patients.

Symptoms. Except in cases in which umbilical catheterization or peroxide enema has been performed, the clinical findings are rather nonspecific. The infant often has a sudden onset of gastroenteritis and bloody stools as well as abdominal distention. One fifth of those reviewed by Arnon and Fishbein had underlying congenital anomalies, ranging from esophageal atresia to imperforate anus, for which they had had prior surgery.[4]

Diagnosis. Radiologic examination of the right upper quadrant is the only way of establishing the diagnosis, and the examiner must specifically look for portal gas. Radiolucent branchings extend from the porta hepatis throughout the liver (Fig. 13–5).

Treatment. As soon as the diagnosis is established and blood has been withdrawn for culture, broad-spectrum antibiotic therapy is instituted. The organisms most frequently isolated have been *Escherichia coli, Aerobacter, Proteus, Candida,* and *Salmonella.* Early surgical intervention is recommended.

Prognosis. The survival rate is reported to be 14 per cent, except in those with portal gas from umbilical catheterization, in whom it is 50 per cent.

INTERNAL ABDOMINAL HERNIAS

True internal hernias occur when small intestine resides in an anomalous fossa and is contained in a true sac. Other hernias in which the intestine is not covered by a sac are considered "false hernias."

Incidence. An exact incidence is not known, but these hernias are extremely rare.

Etiology. True internal hernias form during abnormal rotation of the colon, when the small intestine becomes encased in an anomalous fold of peritoneum. In the false hernias, there are mesenteric defects that are caused by atrophy and resorption of a poorly vascularized region of mesentery.

Pathology. True hernias are classified as paraduodenal, pericecal, intersigmoid, or internal supravesical. Those due to a defect in the mesentery are either transmesenteric or perimesenteric, usually involve the region of the terminal ileum (Treves's fold), and are the most common of the internal hernias of childhood.

Symptoms. Unfortunately, these hernias are asymptomatic until the infant has signs of intestinal obstruction. Constipation, vomiting, and increased distention occur. Colicky abdominal pain is reflected by periods of crying and drawing up of the legs alternating with short periods of comfort. The bowel sounds are at first hyperactive but become hypoactive and eventually absent if strangulation of bowel follows its incarceration.

Diagnosis. Intussusception, malrotation, and volvulus are among the first diagnoses considered. Usually the radiologic plain films show only partial or complete intestinal obstruction with dilated, fluid-filled loops of small bowel.

Treatment. Nasogastric suction decompresses the gastrointestinal tract, but the definitive treatment is surgical reduction of the hernia and repair of the mesentery.

Prognosis. The mortality is as high as 50 per cent, since strangulation of these hernias is common.

DISEASES OF THE OMENTUM AND MESENTERY

The omentum is a fatty apron covering a large part of the intestine in the adult. In the infant and young child, it is shorter and may reach only over the transverse colon.

OMENTAL INFARCTION

Primary segmental infarction of the omentum is usually a disease of men in late adult life, but since it may occur in children it deserves mention.

Incidence. In a large review of the literature in 1959, 46 cases had been reported, 14 per cent of them in children. No large series has been reported since. There is no predilection for either sex.[54]

Pathogenesis. This type of infarction usually follows trauma or sludging of the venous omental circulation. Anomalies in venous drainage may explain the localization of the infarct to the right lower quadrant. Recently, omental infarction due to omental herniation has been reported as a complication of intrauterine transfusion.[73]

Pathology. There is hemorrhage into and polymorphonuclear infiltration of the omentum, with engorgement of the blood vessels. The peritoneal cavity contains serosanguineous fluid.[90]

Symptoms. There is increasing nausea and abdominal pain for one to six days before the diagnosis is made. One third of the patients vomit. Abdominal tenderness is diffuse but maximal in the right lower or even the right upper quadrant. There is mild leukocytosis and temperature elevation.

Diagnosis. This disease is usually mistaken for appendicitis, and the diagnosis is made at the time of operation.

Treatment. The infarcted omentum is removed to prevent fibrosis and the development of adhesions.

OMENTAL CYSTS

Omental cysts sometimes present as an acute surgical event but most often cause progressive abdominal enlargement as their only symptom. Similar in origin to mesenteric cysts, they are one quarter to one fifth as common.[25, 74, 80a]

Incidence. Several hundred cases have been reported, and one quarter have been in children.[80a, 122]

Etiology. Many cysts are undoubtedly congenital and result from embryonic mesodermal and lymphatic abnormalities, but others are acquired, resulting from trauma, neoplasms, or infection of mycotic, parasitic, or tuberculous origin.

Pathology. The cysts vary in size from small to extremely large and are usually filled with clear amber fluid. Less often the contents are milky. They are usually single and multilocular, but some have been multiple. The wall is fibrous, with inner mesothelial cells ranging from endothelial to high columnar in form. The covering is mesothelial. Acquired cysts have no lining. New or old bleeding into the cyst cavity may be evident, and, rarely, cysts contain calcification. Most are contained within the omentum, but others arise from a pedicle. Malignant change is unusual and, if present, is usually a low-grade sarcoma.

Symptoms. The asymptomatic cysts are usually diagnosed later in life. Acute symptoms are fewer than in infants with mesenteric cysts and result from complications such as torsion, infection, rupture, hemorrhage, or obstruction of other organs.[85] The youngest patient was a one-day-old infant who had lethargy and abdominal distention. There is progressive abdominal enlargement, and a flank mass (right) is palpable. If extremely large, the cyst mimics ascites and may cause enteric protein loss. Hemorrhage into the cyst causes diffuse abdominal pain, vomiting, and, perhaps, rectal bleeding. The abdomen is tense, and the bowel sounds hypoactive. Fever is moderate, and there is usually leukocytosis. Young infants may, however, be leukopenic.

Diagnosis. The signs of acute surgical abdomen occur only in children with omental cysts and resemble those of acute appendicitis or perforated appendix. If abdominal guarding and rigidity are marked, the mass may not be palpable. Radiologic examination may or may not show a soft tissue mass and displacement of bowel, and lateral films will show the mass anterior to the intestines. Calcification is rare. Contrast studies of large and small bowel show displacement of loops in 75 per cent of patients. Intravenous pyelography will show pressure effects upon bladder or ureter. The echogram will localize a fluid-filled cyst.

Treatment. Excision of the cyst with preservation of as much omentum as possible is curative.

Prognosis. Treatment is definitive, for these cysts do not occur.

MESENTERIC CYSTS

Mesenteric cysts are extremely unusual and vary in the symptoms they produce. Most common in children under ten years of age, they may be recognized at any age and have been reported in the neonate. Such lymphangiomatous cysts usually occur in the neck or axilla.[6, 80, 80a]

Incidence. In 1978, Grosfeld's group[6] reported 11 cases in a 40-year review, and six cases were reported in an 11-year survey in Spain. Approximately 700 cases have been reported in the literature. The incidence is greater in males than in females.

Etiology. Mesenteric cysts are believed to represent lymphangiomatous malformations of proliferating lymphatic tissue with no available drainage route. Rarely, they develop as a result of inflammation, hemorrhage, or stasis and may best be considered lymphatic hamartomas.[122]

Pathology. These cysts may arise from the mesocolon or mesentery. In half of the patients, they occur in the mesentery of the small intestine and mostly in the ileum. Next in frequency are those in the lesser sac; more unusual are those in jejunal mesentery or mesocolon. The cysts are usually solitary and multilocular, measure from several millimeters to a size that fills the abdomen, and contain from 50 ml to 3 liters of fluid. The fluid may be serous (chemically resembling plasma) or chylous and, occasionally, hemorrhagic. Chylous-type cysts are most often located in the small bowel mesentery.[74]

Histologic examination shows a fibrous wall lined by endothelial cells; at times, smooth muscle is present. Some cysts have caused gastrointestinal protein loss, hypoproteinemia, and edema. In one patient the cyst communicated freely with the thoracic duct.

Symptoms. Sixty-three per cent of Gros-

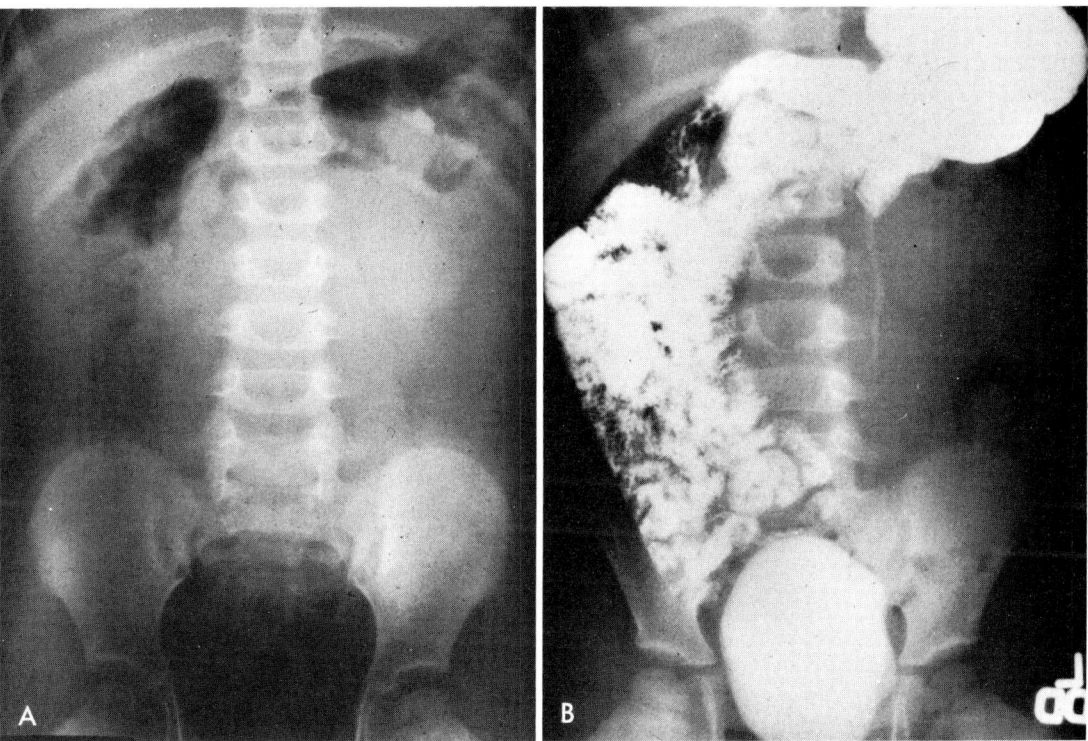

Figure 13–6 *A*, Mesenteric cyst in a neonate born with abdominal distention. *B*, Displacement of bowel loops by cyst.

feld's patients presented before 30 months of age. The symptoms may be acute or chronic. An acute presentation as the result of volvulus or perforation is signaled by the sudden onset of abdominal pain, distention, and vomiting or shock (Fig. 13–6). Complete or partial obstruction is caused by mechanical compression of the intestine. A smooth, movable, nontender abdominal mass is present in more than half of the patients. It is usually palpated in the right abdomen.

Occasionally, gradual abdominal enlargement in an otherwise well child may be the only complaint.

Diagnosis. Plain films of the abdomen will show partial or complete small bowel obstruction or splaying of bowel loops by a dense mass or will suggest ascites. Barium enema will show displacement of the colon and ileocecal region by a mass, and studies of the small bowel will show displacement and compression of small bowel loops. Ultrasonography will define the cystic structure of the mass. Arteriography will demonstrate angulation and splaying of mesenteric vessels about the lesion.

Treatment. Surgical excision or enucleation of the cyst is ideal therapy, but if bowel wall or its vasculature adheres to the cyst, segmental resection of mesentery and bowel is necessary.

Complications. Hemorrhage into or rupture of the cyst may occur spontaneously or follow trauma. Torsion of the cyst, intestinal volvulus, obstruction of the intestine or urinary tract, and malignant degeneration of the cysts are recognized complications.

DISEASES OF THE UMBILICUS

The umbilical cord, which provides sustenance and oxygen to the developing fetus and removes waste products, undergoes involution after birth. The gelatinous cord material dries, the umbilical arteries contract, and their inner layers undergo aseptic necrosis. The stump separates after a week or so, and granulation tissue followed by epithelium covers the umbilicus.

SINGLE UMBILICAL ARTERY

This phenomenon has an overall incidence of 0.9 per cent, with 1.2 per cent of the cases occurring in whites and 0.5 per cent in blacks.[36] The overall incidence of associated congenital anomalies was first reported at 28.6 per cent, with renal anomalies the most frequent type. However, in a later study of nearly 40,000 infants, the mortality was 14 per cent. Half of the dead infants had associated anomalies, but the incidence of cardiovascular and urinary anomalies was not higher than that in other dead malformed infants without single umbilical artery. Of the survivors, four years later only 4 per cent had associated anomalies, the most common of which was inguinal hernia. Since many urinary tract anomalies are relatively silent, it is wise to examine the urine of affected infants periodically and to order intravenous pyelography if there is any evidence of urinary tract disease.

OMPHALITIS

Infection of the umbilicus causes persistent serous, serosanguineous, or purulent drainage from the umbilical stump. Erythema and induration surround the umbilicus. In nursery populations the causative organisms are most often gram-negative, although occasionally the cultures are positive for staphylococcus or streptococcus. In the latter case, bright red erysipeloid skin changes spread from the umbilicus. Infants born in underdeveloped countries may acquire the tetanus bacillus through the umbilicus.

Mild omphalitis with little induration and persistent discharge as the only manifestation responds rapidly to topical application of bacitracin or neomycin ointments. If there is any periumbilical inflammation or systemic infection, broad-spectrum antibiotics appropriate to the organism cultured must be given. Thrombophlebitis, sepsis, or metastatic infection to bone or lung may complicate even the slightest umbilical infection. If septic umbilical arteritis develops, the umbilicus drains purulent material as long as the artery is patent externally.[33] If the internal end of the artery is patent, septicemia results. If the infection spreads through the mantle, it causes peritonitis, and if along the artery, scrotal or thigh abscesses.

UMBILICAL GRANULOMA

Umbilical granuloma forms after separation of the cord and resembles a small, red, velvety nubbin that is solid and has no central orifice. Serous or serosanguineous material drains from the umbilical stump. This lesion responds well to desiccation with alcohol sponges or silver nitrate cauterization. Schaffer prefers sprinkling borax powder into the umbilicus daily for five and ten days after the morning bath.[103]

ABERRANT TISSUE IN THE UMBILICUS

This usually represents aberrant gastric mucosa and is sometimes termed aberrant umbilical stomach,[120] although ectopic pancreas and intestinal tissue have also been reported in the umbilicus.[50] There is either a chronically indurated draining umbilicus or a laterally placed indurated area surrounded by a cystic or solid mass. The diagnosis of ectopic gastric tissue is neatly made by testing the pH of the drainage; it is acid if gastric tissue is present. Treatment is excision of the mass or indurated area and, if necessary, of the umbilicus.

UMBILICAL POLYP

Umbilical polyp represents the mucosal remnants of the omphalomesenteric duct and appears as a small cherry-red mass on the umbilicus after the cord has separated. The remnants secrete mucus, and although there is granulation tissue, the polyp is more moist than a granuloma. A biopsy specimen is composed of intestinal mucosa. Cautery or excision of the polyp is followed by complete healing in several weeks. If the area does not heal, a search for a patent omphalomesenteric duct must be made.

ANOMALIES OF THE OMPHALOMESENTERIC DUCT

These anomalies are estimated to occur in up to 1 per cent of newborns and represent failure of complete obliteration of the omphalomesenteric duct.

PATENT OMPHALOMESENTERIC DUCT

In this type of enteroumbilical fistula there is a complete patency between the small bowel and the umbilicus.

Incidence. Approximately 200 cases have been reported in the literature.[37]

Etiology. Very early in the development, the yolk sac is large and connects directly to the coelom on the ventral surface of the embryo. It is formed from entoderm, and the overlying vitelline vessels are derived from mesoderm.[63, 64] In the three-week embryo the isthmus of the yolk sac draws out to form the omphalomesenteric duct, which is incorporated into the umbilical cord. The yolk sac becomes smaller, and between the fourth and tenth weeks the intestine moves out of the abdominal cavity and returns. After this, the duct obliterates, and by five months all that remains is a fibrous strand that detaches, atrophies, and is absorbed. It is during these last stages of dissolution that the duct anomalies are formed. Patency of the entire duct causes this anomaly.[102]

Symptoms. A small bulge is sometimes noted in the area of the umbilicus at birth, but symptoms usually are not apparent until the cord has dried and separated. The patent duct resembles a granuloma but is actually protruding intestinal mucosa. It exudes a mucoid or bloody discharge, some gas, and, rarely, fecal material. Probing will reveal an orifice in the center of the lesion.

Diagnosis. Injection of radiopaque material into the duct will permit visualization of a connection with the small bowel (Fig.

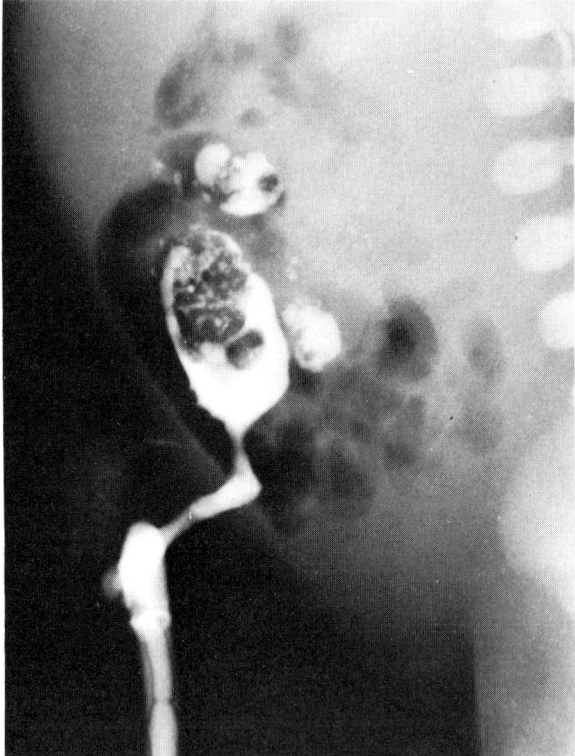

Figure 13–7 Patent omphalomesenteric duct in an infant with purulent discharge from the umbilical stump. A lateral film of the abdomen was obtained after contrast material had been injected into the draining orifice and demonstrates communication between the umbilicus and small bowel.

13–7). Diagnostic pneumoperitoneography will demonstrate urachal or omphalomesenteric duct remnants (Fig. 13–8).

Complications. Omphalitis and periomphalitis are likely to develop in the excoriated skin surrounding the duct. There is usually not a great deal of enteric fluid loss, but if the duct is widely patent it can function as a high ileostomy, and fluid and electrolyte losses can be severe.

One quarter to one fifth of the cases are complicated by prolapse of the small bowel through the fistula, causing obstruction and strangulation.[10] Internal volvulus sometimes develops about the fixed connections of the duct.

Treatment. The defect must be repaired surgically before complications develop.[65] The duct is clamped at its base and resected, and the enterotomy is closed.

Prognosis. In uncomplicated cases the mortality is about 17 per cent, but if prolapse has occurred, it rises to about 87 per cent.

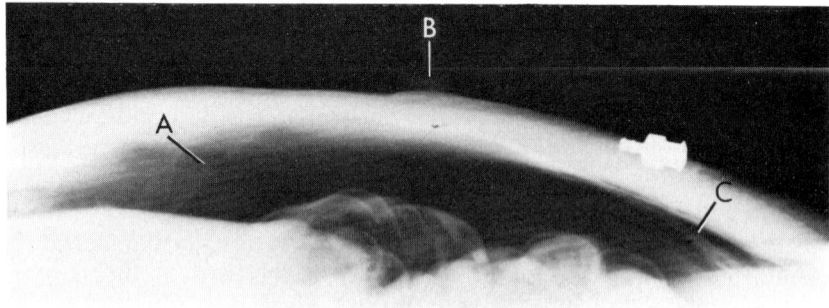

Figure 13–8 Normal diagnostic pneumoperitoneum in an infant with similar symptoms of purulent drainage from the umbilicus. This technique employs the instillation of nitrous oxide into the peritoneal cavity. The inside of the abdominal wall is outlined by gas. A represents the remnant of the umbilical artery and B, the umbilicus. C is the shadow of umbilical vein remnants. No mass or band is present in the umbilical region.

the population, Meckel's diverticulum is three to four times more common in males.

Etiology. The diverticulum results from failure of the intestinal end of the omphalomesenteric duct to obliterate.[64]

Pathology. Located most often in the terminal ileum, Meckel's diverticulum can be encountered anywhere in the small bowel up to 100 cm from the ileocecal valve. It is rarely seen in the jejunum and hardly ever in the duodenum. The diverticulum is on the antimesenteric border of the bowel and lies free or is connected by its tip to the umbilicus by a fibrous band. The lumen of the diverticulum is usually narrow, but in a few cases it is wide. Its length may vary from 1 to 10 cm (Fig. 13–10).

It is a true diverticulum with a complete wall. In 20 to 50 per cent of those operated on, the diverticulum contains ectopic mucosa, which is most commonly gastric mucosa that replaces or overlies the intestinal mucosal lining. Less often, the lining is pancreatic or a combination of pancreatic and gastric tissue. Very rarely, the lining is of duodenal mucosa.

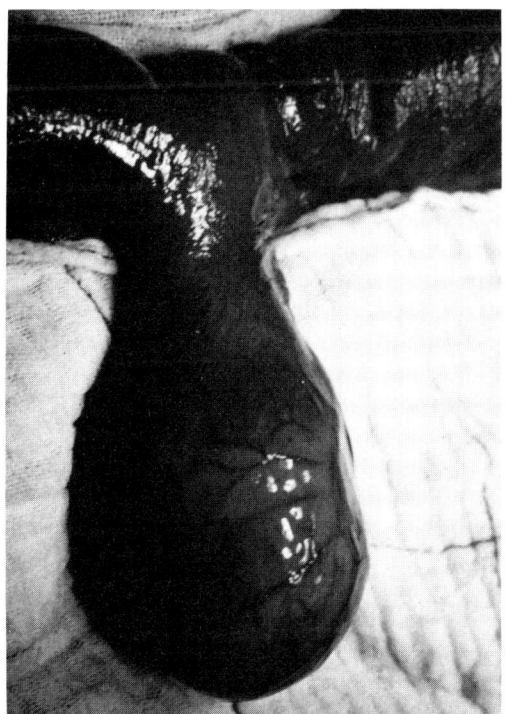

Figure 13–10 Surgical specimen of Meckel's diverticulum arising from the distal ileum.

The gastric mucosa, through acid and pepsin production, causes ulceration of the adjacent ileal mucosa, with resultant hemorrhage or perforation. Nodules of pancreatic tissue in the diverticulum or inversion of the diverticulum serve as a lead point for intussusception.

Symptoms. Hemorrhage or intestinal obstruction is the usual mode of presentation in children under two years of age. The classic description of bleeding from Meckel's diverticulum is the alternate passage of dark and bright blood. This does not hold true in the infant, however, in whom massive lower gastrointestinal bleeding and shock develop. A few pass tarry stools and have anemia from chronic blood loss. Rarely, a mother reports that her baby has passed currant-jelly stools. Usually the bleeding is painless. We have seen one patient and heard of another in whom hematemesis was associated with Meckel's diverticulum. Although this finding seems illogical, there was no recurrence of bleeding after removal of the diverticulum.

Low intestinal obstruction is caused by intussusception or by volvulus of the small bowel or diverticulum about the fibrous remnant of the vitelline duct. The diverticulum tends to invert and cause intussusception more often in infancy than in later life.

If diverticulitis develops, there is fever, leukocytosis, and tenderness and guarding in the right lower quadrant, all of which arouse suspicion of appendicitis. With perforation of the diverticulum, there is an increase in temperature and white blood cell count. The abdomen becomes rigid, and bowel sounds decrease or disappear.

Diagnosis. If there is no preceding history of intermittent bleeding, the differential diagnosis includes polyp, duplication cyst, peptic ulcer, colitis, and bleeding disorders. A negative gastric aspirate rules against a high bleeding site. Barium enema, even when it extends into the terminal ileum, does not always demonstrate Meckel's diverticulum. When the lesion is evident, it fills as a saccular collection of barium arising from the antimesenteric border of bowel. (Duplication cysts arise from the mesenteric border — Fig. 13–11.) Ulcer-

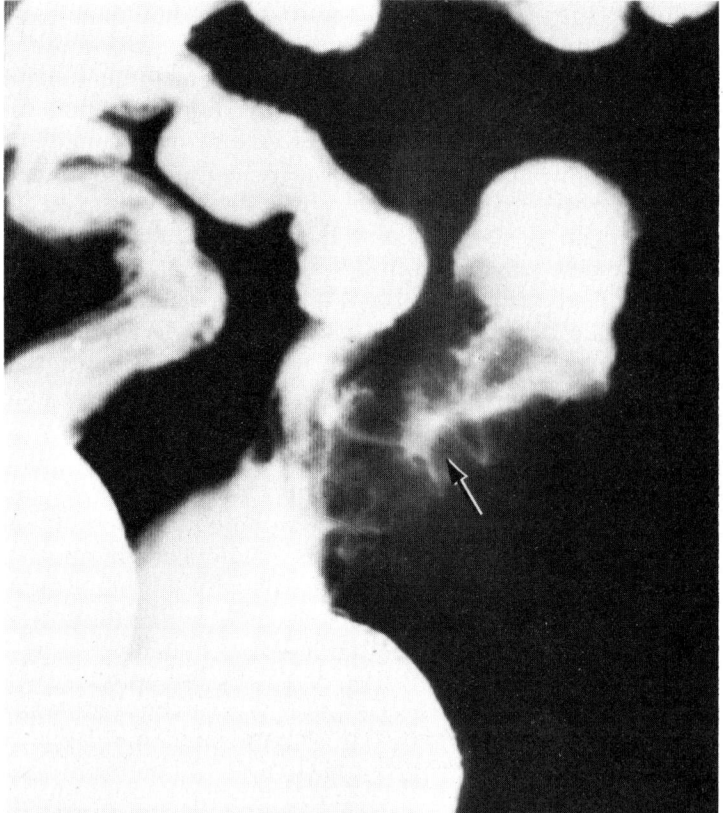

Figure 13–11 Meckel's diverticulum in a five-year-old who presented with rectal bleeding and falling hematocrit. Barium study of the small bowel demonstrates Meckel's diverticulum in the distal ileum, seen as a side branch from the segment of bowel in the center of the photograph. The collection of barium indicated by the arrow represents an ulcer. The diverticulum was surgically removed and found to contain ectopic gastric mucosa and an adjacent ulcer crater.

ation is often evident within the diverticulum.

If a lesion cannot be identified, scanning of the abdomen with the radionucleide technetium-99m sodium pertechnetate, which has a particular affinity for parietal cells of the gastric, thyroid, and salivary glands, demonstrates increased uptake of the isotope if the diverticulum is lined by gastric mucosa.[26] Oral potassium perchlorate or intravenous sodium iodide is used as premedication, and 100 μc per kg of isotope is injected intravenously. The abdomen is scanned twice, 30 minutes and 3 hours later. The majority of the isotope is excreted in the urine within 24 hours. False positive test results do occur, but a refinement in the technique using scinti-imaging decreases their incidence.[58, 59, 114] False negatives may occur in instances of extremely brisk bleeding.

It is so difficult to identify the cause of rectal bleeding in infants that there is a good deal of controversy about how extensive a work-up for rectal bleeding should be. It is our preference that radiologic examination and scan should be performed in any infant who has a significant bleed.

Treatment. Surgical treatment consists of excision of the diverticulum, removal of the fibrous cord, and closure of the ileum.

Sarcoma has been reported in a Meckel's diverticulum in a four-day-old infant operated on for intestinal perforation.[17] The intestine was perforated at the base of the diverticulum, and pathologic study showed the wall of the diverticulum to be infiltrated with spindle cell tumor.

ABDOMINAL WALL DEFECTS AND HERNIAS

UMBILICAL HERNIA

This common defect is still one in which opinions differ with respect to management.

Incidence. The incidence of umbilical hernia has been reported at 84 per cent in premature infants weighing less than 1500 gm and at 20.5 per cent in those weighing

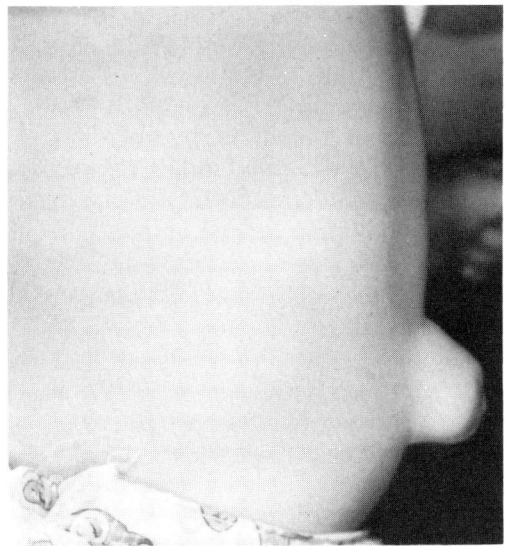

Figure 13–12 Lateral view of the abdomen of a two-year-old male with umbilical hernia. (Courtesy of L. Pickett, M.D.)

41.6 per cent in infants under one year and of 15.9 per cent at four years. A familial incidence is common. It is a frequent concomitant defect in Down's syndrome, hypothyroidism, and Hurler's syndrome.

Etiology and Pathology. There is incomplete fascial closure of the umbilical ring, although the defect is entirely covered by skin and subcutaneous tissue. As the contents of the cord involute, the hernia becomes apparent.

Symptoms. The hernia is visible at birth or just after the cord has separated. It appears as a fullness in the umbilical region, which increases with crying or straining. The hernia varies from the size of a fingertip to that of an orange (Fig. 13–12) and frequently increases significantly during the first few months of life. The width of the ring defect varies from 0.5 to 5 cm, and a small diastasis recti is often palpable. The sac may contain only omentum, but when herniated bowel occupies it, the sac feels soft and silky and the hernia is reduced with a gurgling sound (Fig. 13–13).

between 2000 and 2500 gm. An increased incidence is noted also in term infants of large birth weight. Umbilical hernia is more prevalent in blacks, with an incidence of

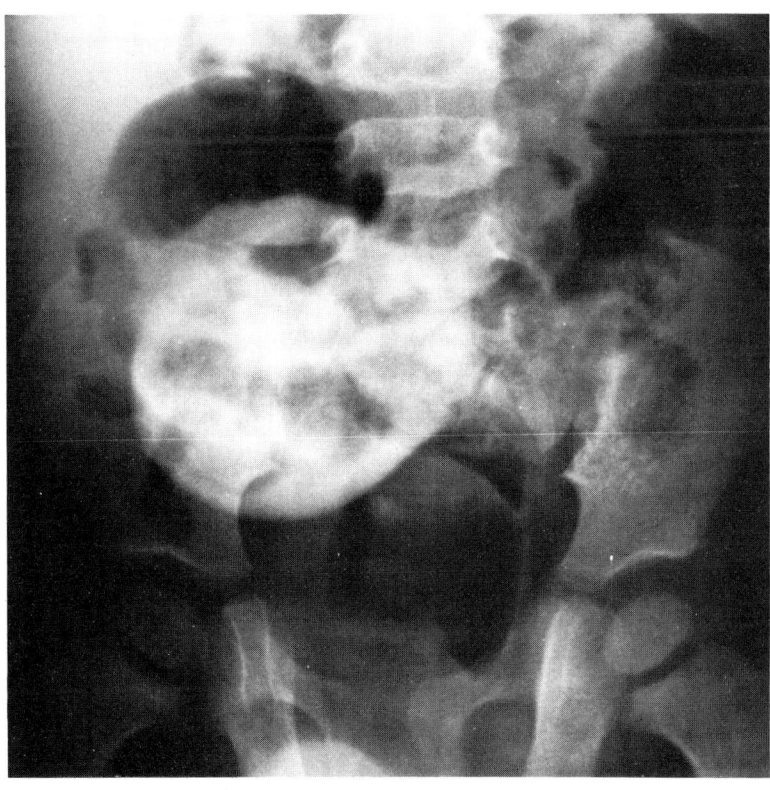

Figure 13–13 Plain film of the abdomen of an infant with a large umbilical hernia. The round density projected over the right sacroiliac area is the protruding hernia sac. The margins are clearly defined, since it is surrounded by air.

Very rarely, omentum becomes incarcerated, causing exquisite localized tenderness and pain. Intestinal obstruction from incarceration and strangulation of small bowel is unusual but can occur.

Treatment. Most umbilical hernias close spontaneously within the first year of life and should not be treated.[46a] Taping of a hernia has its advocates, but there is no conclusive evidence that it hastens closure of the defect.

Small bowel obstruction at any age mandates hernia repair without delay. Defects 5 cm or larger should be repaired within the first few years of life. If the hernia is still present when the child is two to three years of age, and the defect measures 1.5 cm or greater, repair is indicated. Haller et al.[48] feel that all umbilical hernias persisting after two years of age should be repaired, since the mortality in incarcerated umbilical hernias in adult women is significant. Small defects may become large umbilical hernias in the pregnant woman.

Little has been said about the psychologic aspects of hernias that persist beyond two years of age, but protrusion of a hernia can subject the little boy wearing only shorts in warm weather to ridicule by his peers.

Hamartoma within an umbilical hernia of a neonate has been reported.[106] The herniation, originally diagnosed as omphalocele, had skin covering the mass. The sac contained tissue composed of subcutaneous tissue and cartilage.

CONGENITAL ABSENCE OF THE ABDOMINAL MUSCULATURE

Deficiency of the abdominal musculature is recognized at birth because the infant has the typical "prune belly," in which the skin of the abdominal wall is flaccid and wrinkled.[91] Although it is not very significant in itself, the defect is associated with long and tortuous ureters, hydronephrosis, and a distended, thickened bladder (Fig. 13–14).

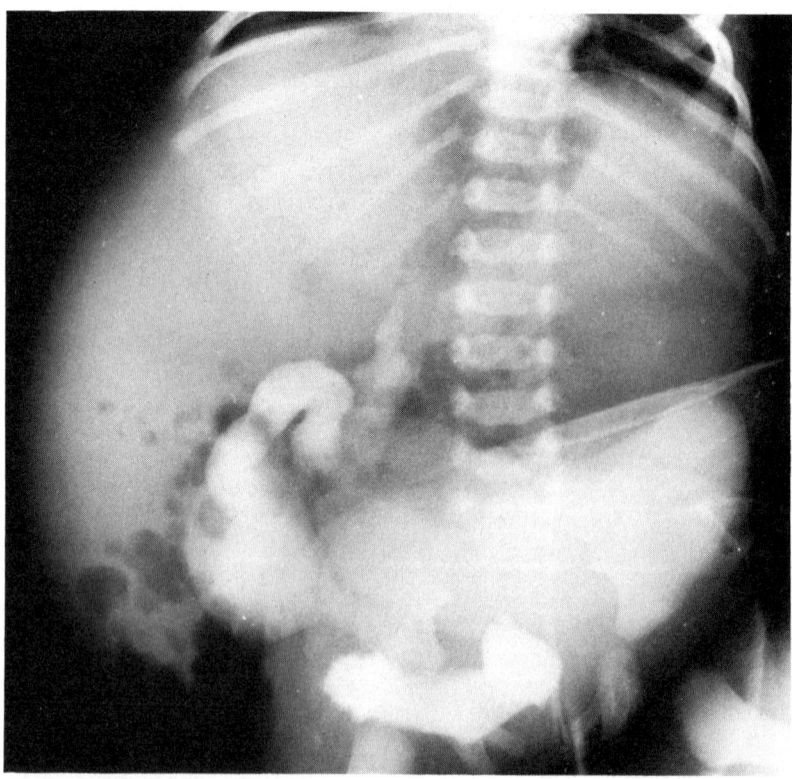

Figure 13–14 Infant with "prune belly" due to deficiency of the abdominal musculature. Intravenous pyelogram shows a thickened bladder, massive, twisted hydroureters, and hydronephrosis.

Other associated anomalies are undescended testes, lower extremity malformations, patent urachus, and congenital heart disease. This defect is usually an isolated happening in a family, but its occurrence in twin males has been reported; one of them also had an omphalocele. It is debatable whether absence of the musculature is due to a primary developmental defect in the abdominal musculature or is secondary to bladder outlet obstruction,[86a] but it is likely that faulty embryogenesis dates to the tenth fetal week, when the abdominal wall and genitourinary tract are forming. Treatment entails urinary tract decompression by cystostomy and nephrostomy or ureterostomies and later revision of the bladder neck and ureters. The prognosis is poor; half these infants die before the end of the first year. The disease has been associated with Turner's syndrome, and, in such infants, urinary tract anomalies are less severe.[73a]

SMALL OMPHALOCELE OR UMBILICAL CORD HERNIA

The small omphalocele is located at the umbilicus and is caused by the same embryologic defect as its larger counterpart. It develops late, near the tenth week, when most of the bowel has returned to the abdominal cavity.

Symptoms. This mass, also evident at birth, is in some cases covered by a membrane of peritoneum and amnion, which may rupture antenatally or during delivery. In less obvious cases, the mass projects into the base of the cord and appears as a small swelling in this location.

Diagnosis. If the diagnosis needs further confirmation, radiologic examination of the lateral position may show some loops of small bowel within the mass. Similar swellings may be Wharton's cysts or hematomas.

Complications. Complications result from clamping the cord too close to the abdomen.[67] In two infants, this was discovered to be the case after they vomited bilious material. At laparotomy, cecum and appendix were found to have been clamped in the omphalocele. Another infant studied at four months had a draining granulomatous nodule on the umbilicus. Injected radiopaque material entered a fistulous tract and opacified the cecum.[100]

BECKWITH-WIEDEMANN SYNDROME (EMG SYNDROME)

This syndrome has been recognized only in the last 15 years and is mentioned because omphalocele is so often associated with it.[20, 95]

Incidence. Nearly 100 cases have been described. Although usually not familial, it has affected three siblings in one family.

Pathogenesis. Diencephalic dysfunction is postulated as the cause of the giantism, but it does not account for all the features of the syndrome.

Pathology and Symptoms. These babies have giantism, macroglossia, microcephaly, omphalocele, and visceromegaly of the pancreas and liver and sometimes of the kidneys and spleen. Recently, adrenal hyperplasia and fibroadenoma of the breast have been reported. Less frequent anomalies are malrotation, diaphragmatic and ear malformations, and hemihypertrophy. Eight types of cardiac anomalies have been described in patients. Renal lesions have been defined as medullary sponge kidney. Histologic examination shows hyperplasia and immaturity of the kidneys and pancreas, islet cell hyperplasia, and cytomegaly of the adrenal cortex.[118]

Hypoglycemia is symptomatic in the neonatal period and persists for up to six months. It can usually be treated medically with steroids or diazoxide, but hemipancreatectomy may be necessary.

Prognosis. Long-term follow-up is not available in most cases. Even though the hypoglycemia is controlled, there is some evidence of mental retardation. Malignancy seems to be associated, for 17 patients have been reported with 14 malignant and 5 benign tumors.[110] Most frequently associated tumors are nephroblastoma and adrenal and hepatic neoplasms.

VESICOINTESTINAL FISSURE AND OMPHALOCELE

This extremely rare defect occurs in 1 in 200,000 live births.[32] It consists of exstrophy of the bladder and ileocecal portion of the gut, imperforate anus, and absence of a major portion of the colon. There may be phallic, genital, and vertebral anomalies. The lesion results from an arrest in development of the urogenital and gastrointestinal systems in the third and fourth weeks of fetal life. Most infants are born prematurely and have a large area of exposed bladder mucosa on the lower abdominal wall and an omphalocele superior to it. A blind, short colon enters through an inferior orifice. Treatment consists of complicated plastic procedures that will not be discussed here.

GASTROSCHISIS

Although most consider gastroschisis to be of a different congenital origin than omphalocele, its presentation and problems are similar (Table 13–1).

Incidence. Gastroschisis has been estimated to occur in 1:6300 to 1:50,000 live births, often in first-born infants.[93] It has occurred in siblings in less than 17 per cent of cases. It is thought to be inherited as an autosomal dominant trait in such cases.[99] A few series report a predominance of males, but in most, males and females are affected equally. Association with genetic abnormalities is unusual. The incidence of this disorder is increasing as is the association with prematurity and young maternal age.[39]

Etiology. The generally accepted etiology is failure of development of the somatopleure of the lateral fold of the abdomen after the bowel has returned to the peritoneal cavity and the umbilical ring has formed.[47, 107] This theory has been questioned, however, and it has been suggested that gastroschisis results from rupture of the amniotic membrane at the base of the umbilical cord during or after the physiologic period of herniation. A third proposal is intrauterine rupture of an incarcerated hernia into the cord. Moore recently noted that 78 per cent of associated defects in 278 infants represented jejunoileal disruption and were largely ileal atresia in type. Other abnormalities, such as renal aplasia or hypoplasia of the gallbladder, suggest a vascular interruption of the omphalomesenteric artery.[55, 82] Whatever the etiology, if the muscular defect occurs late, the peritoneal cavity is of normal size and there is little serosal reaction in the intestine. Such is usually not the case, for the defect occurs most often in early fetal life and perhaps even before innervation and differentiation of the abdominal wall. The abdominal cavity is small, and there is extensive serosal reaction in the exposed bowel.

Pathology. The defect in gastroschisis is paraumbilical, and there is normal insertion of the umbilical cord into the anterior abdominal wall. Most defects are on the right and measure 1.5 to 2.5 cm. The margins are rounded and smooth. Eviscerated organs are nonrotated, nonfixed intestine and include small bowel or even the entire gastrointestinal tract. No sac covers the organs, and the edematous bowel loops are covered by a green, fibrinous peel (Fig. 13–15), which is composed of fibrogelatinous mem-

Table 13–1   Characteristics of Gastroschisis and Omphalocele

	GASTROSCHISIS	OMPHALOCELE
Site of defect	lateral	midline
Prematurity	40–67%	10 to 30%
Other malformations	23%	66%
Cardiac	8.5%	52%
Chromosomal	0%	sporadic to 4%
Intestinal atresia	15%	0%
Mortality	12%	34%

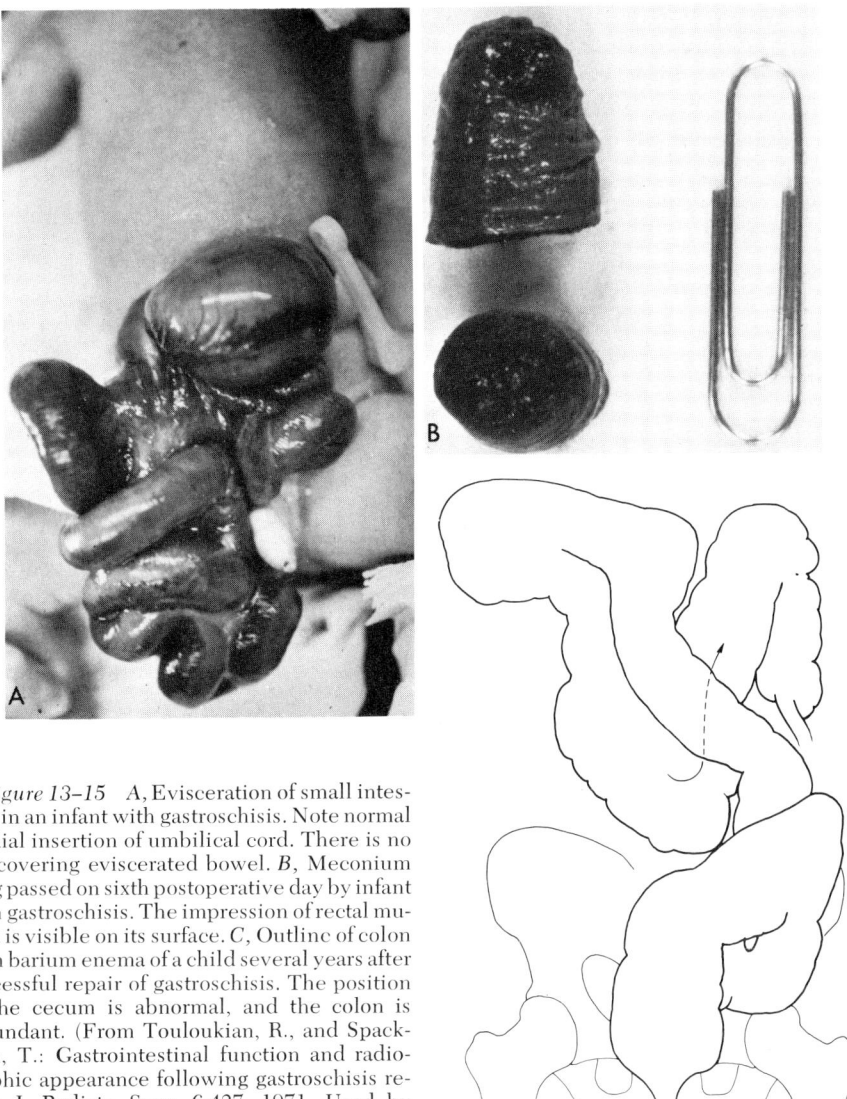

Figure 13–15 *A,* Evisceration of small intestine in an infant with gastroschisis. Note normal medial insertion of umbilical cord. There is no sac covering eviscerated bowel. *B,* Meconium plug passed on sixth postoperative day by infant with gastroschisis. The impression of rectal mucosa is visible on its surface. *C,* Outline of colon from barium enema of a child several years after successful repair of gastroschisis. The position of the cecum is abnormal, and the colon is redundant. (From Touloukian, R., and Spackman, T.: Gastrointestinal function and radiographic appearance following gastroschisis repair. J. Pediatr. Surg. 6:427, 1971. Used by permission.)

brane containing squamous cells and vernix. Peritonitis is present, and the midgut is shortened. The mesentery appears pulseless, and no peristalsis is visible. Malrotation, intestinal atresia, or stenosis is present in 25 per cent of patients. Seventy-five per cent of the babies are premature.

Symptoms. At first glance, the defect can be confused with ruptured omphalocele, but on closer inspection it is seen to be paraumbilical and associated with normal insertion of the cord.

Treatment. The treatment and problems are similar to those of ruptured omphalo-

cele.[56, 76a] Fluid losses are increased owing to antenatal peritonitis. Intravenous hyperalimentation will sustain the infant through a prolonged postoperative ileus. As in omphalocele, the placement and multistage sequential removal of synthetic material are used to promote enlargement of the abdominal cavity and avoid later repair of ventral hernia.[30, 42a] Use of Silastic has aided rapid reduction of bowel into the abdominal cavity. Enlargement of the defect is critical to prevent compression of the vascular supply. Complete removal of the prosthesis and fascial closure can usually be accomplished within two weeks. On the other hand, Savage and Davey recommended creation of a planned transverse ventral hernia with later repair of the hernia.[101] Primary repair with short-term ventilation is associated with fewer complications.[9a]

Prognosis. The mortality, previously about 40 per cent in the best infant care centers, has now been reduced to 6.2 per cent.[113] There is a great deal of concern preoperatively about bowel viability in the pulseless mass of exposed intestine, but an amazing return of function can be expected, although prolonged ileus may require continuous nasogastric suction. Postoperative evacuation of meconium occurs between 4 and 17 days after surgery and is heralded by the passage of a meconium plug bearing

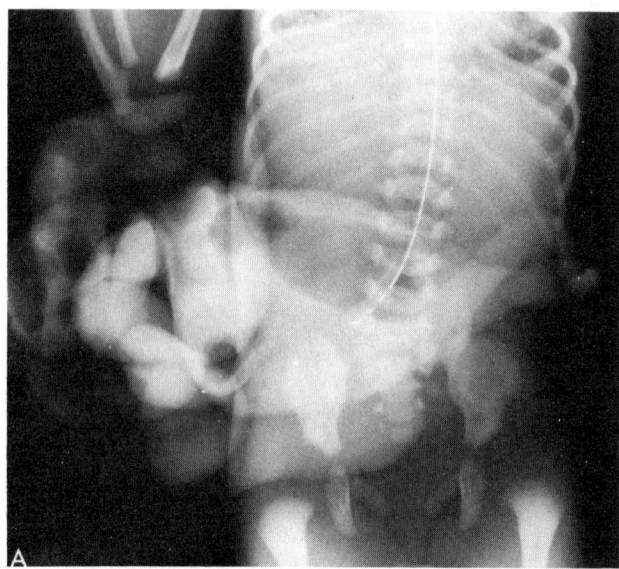

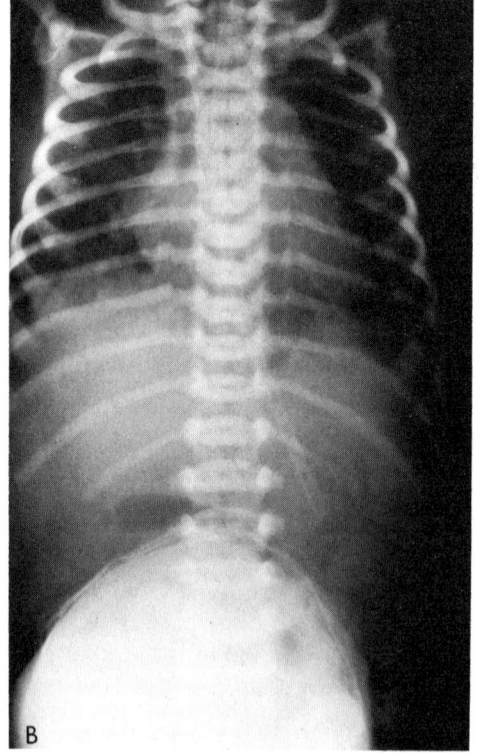

Figure 13–16 Newborn infant with paraumbilical evisceration without peritoneal cover. This represents a case of gastroschisis. *A*, Plain film shows a portion of air-filled stomach and multiple loops of small bowel outside the abdominal cavity. *B*, The initial surgical procedure consisted of construction of a Silastic bag to protect the viscera and repair the abdominal wall defect. The prosthesis is represented as a radiodense area projected over the lower abdomen. Portions of the Silastic were sequentially removed over several weeks to allow the abdominal cavity to accommodate the replaced viscera.

Illustration continued on opposite page

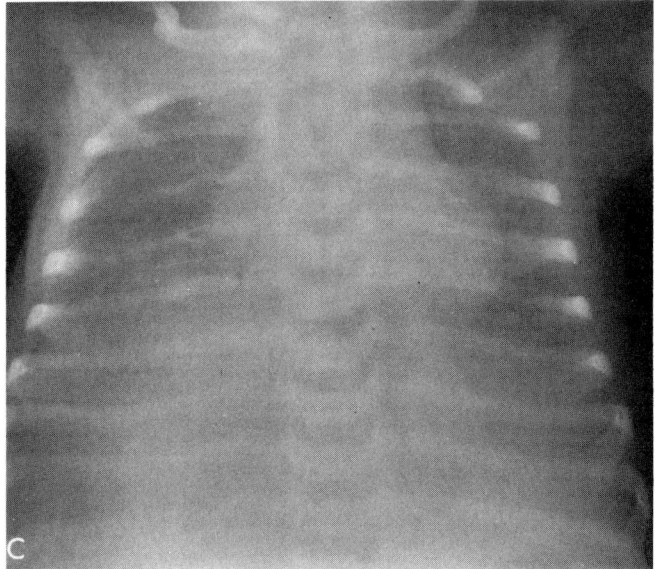

Figure 13–16 Continued C, Chest film after complete removal of the prosthesis demonstrates elevation of the diaphragms resulting from replacement of the viscera within the small abdominal cavity.

impressions of rectal mucosa (Fig. 13– 15*B*). Gentle saline enemas sometimes induce passage of this inspissated plug. Feedings are then begun and increased rapidly to provide adequate caloric requirements.

Touloukian and Spackman[117] studied six infants one and one-half to six years after treatment and found that all grew normally and attained at least the twenty-fifth percentiles for height and weight; some surpassed them. Radiologic examination demonstrated nonrotation of the gut without evidence of intestinal obstruction. The authors postulate that adhesions create a fortuitous plication of the intestine (Fig. 13–16).

Numerous studies have noted shortness of the bowel to a third or a half of its normal length. This is apparently reversible, for in the same group of children, the small and large intestine later appeared of normal length. In these patients the colon was redundant and seemed longer than normal.[116]

Complications. Major complications are sepsis due to exposure of the eviscerated bowel to bacterial contamination, ileus, necrosis, perforation, and malabsorption.

OMPHALOCELE

Omphalocele is a grostesque anomaly of the abdominal wall that is noted at birth and requires prompt treatment. There is a large central defect with bowel protruding through it into a clear sac of peritoneum[61, 76a] (Table 13–1).

Incidence. This anomaly occurs in 1 in 3000 to 1 in 9000 live births. An autosomal sex-linked inheritance is suggested, as omphalocele has been reported in four males in two family generations. It is associated with genetic disorders such as the Beckwith-Wiedemann syndrome and trisomies of chromosomes 13, 18, and 21.[52]

Pathogenesis. The defect occurs between 8 and 11 weeks of fetal life and results from failure of the intestines to return to the abdominal cavity from the umbilical cord. A failure in development in the upper abdominal wall is postulated.

Pathology. In this central defect, which may measure from several centimeters to several inches, there is no umbilical ring. In some infants it extends from the umbilical area to the xiphoid. The cord inserts at the apex of the sac, which contains intestine and, often, liver. The peritoneal cavity is underdeveloped since it has never contained growing intestine. The rectus muscles approximate each other behind the herniated mass and lie close to the vertebral bodies. Malrotation or atresia complicates one third of cases and extragastrointestinal anomalies, chiefly cardiovascular or genitourinary, are common. The peritoneal and

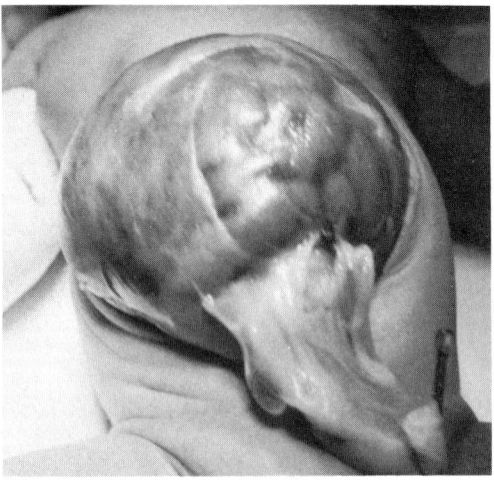

Figure 13–17   Large omphalocele. Note central insertion of cord. (Courtesy of L. Pickett, M.D.)

amniotic membranes covering the viscera may rupture.

Symptoms and Diagnosis. Many of the infants are born prematurely, and the defect is easily recognized at birth (Figs. 13–17 and 13–18). Hypothermia resulting from heat loss through the exposed viscera is significant. Associated anomalies produce their usual symptoms and signs. Total serum proteins and particularly albumin and immunoglobulin G are decreased.[44]

Treatment. Until relatively recently, all cases were operated upon immediately. The eviscerated organs were covered with moist compresses and the gastrointestinal tract was decompressed by continuous nasogastric suction. The baby was given vitamin K and, if the sac was ruptured, antibiotics for peritonitis.

Treatment and prognosis are directly related to the size of the omphalocele.[104] If the base measures less than 8 cm and contains no liver, primary skin closure without suturing of the underlying fascia is performed; the fascia is closed a month later.[124] There is some controversy about whether an intact sac should be opened and the bowel explored for malrotation or atresia, but this decision is one to be made by the surgeon.

If the defect is large and the abdominal cavity is small, a tight abdominal skin closure presents dangers of elevation of the

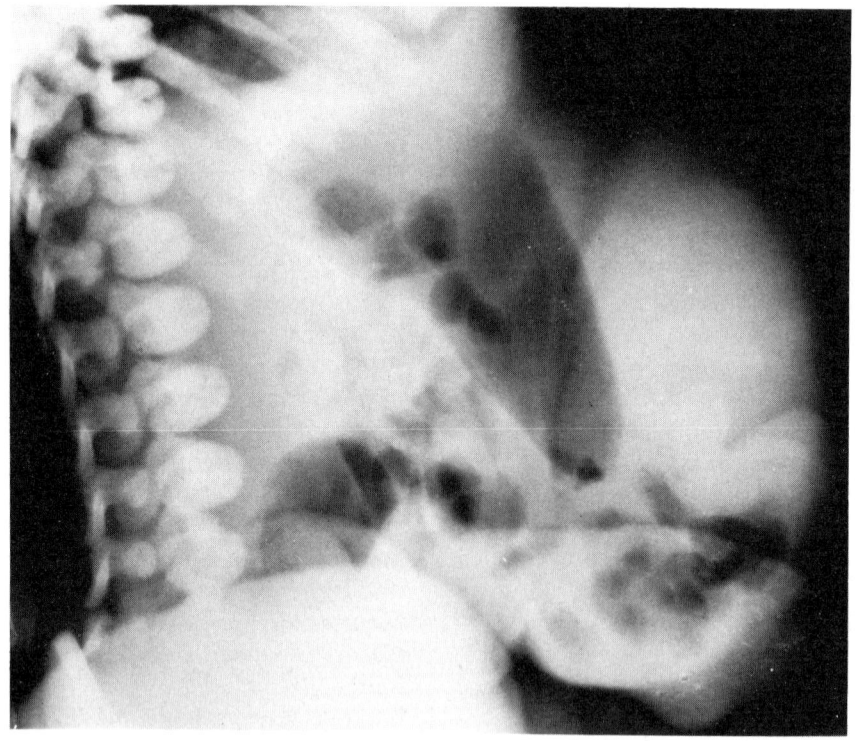

Figure 13–18   Neonate with large omphalocele. A portion of stomach and multiple air-filled bowel loops are seen within the extra-abdominal peritoneal sac.

diaphragms and respiratory embarrassment, interference with venous return, and intestinal ileus or necrosis. Suprahepatic obstruction of the vena cava, due to posterior displacement of the inferior vena cava with increase in its angulation through the diaphragm, has been described. The result was occlusion and Budd-Chiari syndrome.[15] In addition, the procedure leaves a large ventral hernia that must be repaired, and the problems of an underdeveloped abdominal cavity remain.

For these reasons, medical management has come into vogue. For the uncomplicated large omphalocele, some advocate daily painting of the sac with 2 per cent Mercurochrome to allow epithelialization from the periphery until the sac is covered with granulomatous tissue in six to eight weeks.[28] Because mercury intoxication has been reported with this method, other topical medications are being tried.

Good results have also followed staged repairs and silver nitrate dressings. The abdominal opening is enlarged to extend from xiphoid to symphysis pubis, and the mass is delivered into the abdomen. A nonelastic synthetic material, Teflon mesh, Silastic, or polymer membrane, is used to cover the omphalocele and supplies controlled intra-abdominal pressure. After five or six days the abdominal cavity increases considerably in size, and the prosthesis is gradually made smaller to reduce the mass back into the enlarging abdomen. With this method, pulmonary ventilation, venous return, and intestinal integrity are not compromised. The membrane is usually removed in three weeks.

If the sac has ruptured before birth, the intestines are matted, purple, and covered by fibrin, but in many instances the bowel is viable, and all attempts should be made to preserve it.[111]

Prognosis. The mortality in infants with small omphaloceles is in the range of 30 per cent; it rises to 73 per cent if the base of the defect is greater than 8 cm and the liver as well as bowel is eviscerated. As conservative and staged repairs for large defects have gained popularity, the overall survival has increased to 70 per cent.[113]

INGUINAL HERNIA

Inguinal hernia results from failure of closure of the processus vaginalis. This is patent in 80 to 90 per cent of newborns but closes in over half during the first year of life. A true hernia exists only when part of the abdominal contents enter the sac.[1a, 5, 98]

Incidence. The reported incidence of inguinal hernia varies from 0.6 to 4 per cent. Many infants have a family history of hernia, with at least 20 per cent of other family members affected. The incidence in twins under three years old is 4 per cent; the concordance for hernia is 18 per cent in monoxygotic twins and 25 per cent in dizygotic twins.

Symptoms. Most hernias are noted within the first three months of life and are located on the right side. The majority are indirect in type. Very rarely does a direct inguinal hernia occur.[119] Mothers note the hernia as a soft lump that appears in the infant's groin when he cries or strains and disappears when he relaxes. A communicating hydrocele that is small in the morning and enlarges during the day strongly suggests the association of hernia. When the lump is present, the infant is irritable.

Diagnosis. The diagnosis is a clinical one, and hydrocele is the primary condition to be differentiated from hernia. A good history is of value, for the mass is not always visualized by the pediatrician. The cord seems thickened to palpation and has a silky feel as the examining finger rolls over it. The testis is sometimes not fully descended and is not palpable in the scrotum. In the female, herniated ovary is palpated as a small nubbin. Both inguinal areas must be examined, for hernia is often bilateral.[70] Preoperative herniography has proved useful in demonstrating a contralateral hernia if it is present,[45] but hematoma of the bowel and cellulitis of the abdominal wall have been subsequent complications.[21]

Treatment. Unless there is marked prematurity or severe illness, a hernia should be repaired when it is discovered. In many reported series, contralateral hernia is found in 20 to 48 per cent of cases when the opposite side is explored.[78] Probing of the opposide side with a Baker dilator reduces the need for surgical exploration in all but positive cases and has been accurate in detecting contralateral hernia in all the cases in which it has been used,[63a] but the technique is difficult.

Complications. Incarceration of the hernia occurs at any age but is most common at about 11 months. Hernias incarcerate more on the right side than on the left and more often in female and in black patients than in white males.[97] Surgical reduction should be performed, for the incidence of complications in those reduced by nonoperative means is 19 per cent as compared with 1.5 per cent in those operated upon.[21, 98a] Retroperitoneal lymphangioma herniated through the inguinal canal has been found in three children.[62]

FEMORAL HERNIA

Femoral hernias are extremely rare in infancy and throughout childhood, having an incidence of less than 0.5 per cent.[12, 57]

Symptoms and Pathology. Femoral hernias are often diagnosed after repair of what was thought to be a simple inguinal hernia. The symptoms are similar to those of inguinal hernia: a bulge in the groin that fluctuates in size. Careful examination, however, reveals the bulge to be inferior to the inguinal canal and to Poupart's ligament. A patent processus vaginalis is common in both types of hernia. A femoral hernia may be overlooked during a typical inguinal repair in which the transversalis fascia is not routinely incised, for the femoral hernia appears under the inguinal canal. If the transversalis fascia is sutured to Poupart's ligament, as in inguinal hernia repair, the femoral canal may enlarge. It is conceivable that some femoral hernias are actually created in this fashion.

Treatment. Repair consists of reduction of the hernia and suturing of the transversalis fascia to Cooper's ligament.

PELVIC HERNIA

The pelvic hernia is most often seen in the postpartum female and is extremely rare in infancy, although several cases have been reported.[24] The hernias may be sciatic, perineal, lumbar, obturator, or internal in type. Characteristically, one buttock is larger than the other and contains a soft mass. There is often a history of loose stools. During rectal examination, the finger passes toward or into the buttock. Barium enema will show a barium-filled rectum displaced into the buttock. Treatment is repair through an oblique buttock incision.

REFERENCES

1. Adams, H. W., and Mainz, D. L.: Eosinophilic ascites. Dig. Dis. Sci. 22:40, 1977.
1a. Altman, R. P., Randolph, J. G., and Anderson, K.: Pediatric surgery. In Schwartz, S., Shires, G. T., Spencer, F., and Storer, E. H. (eds.): Principles of Surgery. McGraw-Hill Book Company, New York, 1979, p. 1631.
2. Androulakis, J. A., Gray, S., Lionakis, B., and Skandelakis, G.: The sex ratio of Meckel's diverticulum. Am. Surg. 35:455, 1969.
3. Aranda, J. V., Stern, L., and Dunbar, J. S.: Pneumothorax with pneumoperitoneum in a newborn infant. Am. J. Dis. Child. 123:163, 1972.
4. Arnon, R. G., and Fishbein, J. F.: Portal venous gas in the pediatric age group. J. Pediatr. 79:255, 1971.
5. Bakwin, H.: Indirect inguinal hernias. J. Pediatr. Surg. 6:165, 1971.
6. Ballantine, T., and Grosfeld, J. L.: Mesenteric cysts in infancy and childhood. Surg. Gynecol. Obstet. 147:182, 1978.
7. Bell, M., Ternberg, J., and Bower, R.: The microbial flora and antimicrobial therapy of neonatal peritonitis. J. Pediatr. Surg. 15:569, 1980.
8. Bendel, W. J., Jr., and Michel, M. L., Jr.: Meconium peritonitis: review of the literature and report of a case with survival after surgery. Surgery 34:321, 1953.
9. Birtch, A. G., Coran, A. G., and Gross, R. E.: Neonatal peritonitis. Surgery 61:305, 1967.
9a. Bower, R., Bell, M., Ternberg, J., and Cobb, M.: Ventilatory support and primary closure of gastroschisis. Surgery 91:52, 1982.
10. Brown, A. G., and Cain, F. G.: Evagination of ileum through patent omphalomesenteric duct. Am. J. Surg. 79:339, 1950.
11. Brown, D. R., and Keenan, W. J.: Pneumoperitoneum without gastrointestinal perforation in a neonate. J. Pediatr. 85:377, 1974.
12. Burke, J.: Femoral hernia in childhood. Ann. Surg. 166:287, 1966.
13. Burke, J. F., Pantoppidan, H., and Welch, C. E.: High output respiratory failure: an important cause of death ascribed to peritonitis or ileus. Ann. Surg. 158:581, 1963.
14. Byrne, J. J., and Bottomley, G. T.: Bile peritonitis in infancy. Am. J. Dis. Child. 85:694, 1953.
15. Carlton, G., Towne, B., Bryan, R., and Chang, J.: Obstruction of the suprahepatic inferior

vena cava as a complication of giant omphalocele repair. J. Pediatr. Surg. *14*:733, 1979.

16. Ceballos, R., and Hicks, G.: Plastic peritonitis due to neonatal hydrometrocolpos. J. Pediatr. Surg. *5*:63, 1970.

17. Chatterjee, C. R.: Sarcomas of Meckel's diverticulum. Can. J. Surg. *13*:163, 1970.

18. Clowes, G. H., Vucinic, M., and Weidner, M. G.: Circulatory and metabolic alterations associated with survival or death in peritonitis. Ann. Surg. *163*:866, 1966.

19. Clover, H. D.: Perforation of the biliary tract due to gallstones in infancy. Ann. Surg. *160*:226, 1964.

20. Combs, J. T., Grunt, J. A., and Brandt, I. K.: New syndrome of neonatal hypoglycemia: association with visceromegaly, macroglossia, microcephaly and abnormal umbilicus. N. Engl. J. Med. *275*:236, 1966.

20a. Condon, R. E.: Peritonitis and intraabdominal abscesses. *In* Schwartz, S., Shires, G. T., Spencer, F., and Storer, E. H. (eds.): Principles of Surgery. McGraw-Hill Book Company, New York, 1979, p. 1397.

21. Ducharine, J., Guttman, F., and Molijak, M.: Hematoma of bowel and cellulitis of the abdominal wall complicating herniography. J. Pediatr. Surg. *15*:318, 1980.

22. Danelatos-Athanassiadis, C., Tsakagiannis, E., Karpouzas, I., Mousatos, G., and Katerelos, C.: Bile peritonitis in infancy. Helv. Paediatr. Acta *25*:655, 1970.

23. Davies, P. A., and Elliot-Smith, A.: Bile peritonitis in infancy. Arch. Dis. Child. *30*:174, 1955.

24. Doig, C. M., and Nixon, H. H.: Pelvic hernias in children. J. Pediatr. Surg. *7*:44, 1972.

25. Dugas, J. E., Jr., Burke, E. L., and Oms, L.: Primary idiopathic segmental infarction of the greater omentum. Am. J. Gastroenterol. *31*:382, 1959.

26. Duszynski, D. P., Jewett, T. C., and Allen, J. E.: Tc 99m Na pertechnetate scanning of the abdomen with particular reference to small bowel pathology. Am. J. Roentgenol. Radium Ther. Nucl. Med. *113*:258, 1971.

27. Effman, E., and Griscom, N. T.: Neonatal gastrointestinal masses arising late in gestation. Am. J. Roentgenol. *135*:681, 1980.

28. Ein, S., and Shandling, B.: A new nonoperative treatment of large omphaloceles with a polymer membrane. J. Pediatr. Surg. *13*:255, 1978.

29. Fawcitt, J., and Goldberg, H. M.: Chylous ascites in infancy. Br. J. Surg. *46*:175, 1958.

30. Fonkalsrud, E. W.: Selective repair of neonatal gastroschisis based on degree of visceroabdominal disproportion. Ann. Surg. *191*:139, 1980.

31. Fonkalsrud, E. W., Ellis, D. G., and Clatworthy, H. W., Jr.: Neonatal peritonitis. J. Pediatr. Surg. *1*:227, 1966.

32. Fonkalsrud, E. W., and Linde, L.: Successful management of vesicointestinal fistula. J. Pediatr. Surg. *5*:30, 1970.

33. Forshall, I.: Septic umbilical arteritis. Arch. Dis. Child. *32*:25, 1957.

34. Fowler, R.: Primary peritonitis: changing aspects. Aust. Paediatr. J. *7*:73, 1971.

35. Friedman, A. B., Abellara, R. M., Lidsky, I., and

36. Lubert, M.: Perforation of the colon after exchange transfusion in the newborn. N. Engl. J. Med. *282*:769, 1970.

36. Froelich, L., and Fujikura, T.: Follow-up of infants with single umbilical artery. Pediatrics *52*:6, 1973.

37. Fox, P. F.: Uncommon umbilical anomalies in children. Surg. Gynecol. Obstet. *92*:95, 1951.

38. Garb, M., and Riseborough, J.: Meconium peritonitis presenting as fetal ascites on ultrasound. Br. J. Radiol. *53*:602, 1980.

39. Gierup, J., and Lundquist, Z.: Gastroschisis: a pilot study of its incidence and the possible influence of teratogenic factors. Z. Kinderchir. *28*:39, 1979.

40. Golden, G. T., and Shaw, A.: Primary peritonitis. Surg. Gynecol. Obstet. *135*:513, 1972.

41. Goswitz, J. T., and Kimmerling, R.: Perforated choledochal cyst with bile peritonitis in an infant: case report and surgical management. Surgery *59*:878, 1966.

42. Gribetz, D., and Kanaf, F.: Chylous ascites in infancy. Pediatrics *7*:632, 1951.

42a. Grosfeld, J., Dawes, L., and Weber, T. R.: Congenital abdominal wall defects — current management and survival. Surg. Clin. North Am. *61*:1037, 1981.

43. Gross, J. I., Goldenberg, V. E., and Humphreys, E. M.: Venous remnants producing neonatal chylous ascites. Pediatrics *27*:408, 1961.

44. Gutenberger, J., Miller, D., Dibbins, A., and Gitlin, D.: Hypogammaglobulinemia and hypoalbuminemia in neonates with ruptured omphaloceles and gastroschisis. J. Pediatr. Surg. *8*:353, 1973.

45. Guttman, F. M., Bertrand, R., and Ducharme, J. C.: Herniography and the pediatric contralateral inguinal hernia. Surg. Gynecol. Obstet. *135*:551, 1972.

46. Hadlock, F. B., Deter, R. L., Garciapratt, J., Athey, P., Carpenter, R., Hinkley, C. M., and Park, S. K.: Fetal ascites not associated with Rh incompatibility. Am. J. Roentgenol. *134*:1275, 1980.

46a. Hall, D., Roberts, K., and Charney, E.: Umbilical hernia: what happens after five years? J. Pediatr. *98*:415, 1981.

47. Haller, A., Kehrer, B., Shaker, I., Shermeta, D., and Wyllie, R. G.: Studies of the pathophysiology of gastroschisis in fetal sheep. J. Pediatr. Surg. *5*:627, 1974.

48. Haller, A., Morgan, W., Stumbaugh, S., and White, J.: Repair of umbilical hernia in childhood to prevent adult incarceration. Am. Surg. *37*:245, 1971.

49. Harken, A., and Shochat, S.: Gram-positive peritonitis in children. Am. J. Surg. *125*:769, 1973.

50. Harris, L. E., and Wenzl, J. E.: Heterotopic pancreatic tissue and intestinal mucosa in the umbilical cord. N. Engl. J. Med. *268*:721, 1963.

51. Hertzel, J., and Volsted-Pedersen, P.: Congenital ascites due to mesenteric vessel constriction caused by malrotation of the intestines. Acta Paediatr. Scand. *68*:281, 1979.

52. Havalad, S., Noblett, H., and Speidel, B. D.: Familial occurrence of omphalocele suggesting sex-linked inheritance. Arch. Dis. Child. *54*:142, 1979.

52a. Hillemeier, A. C., Hen, J. J., Riely, C., Dolan, T., and Gryboski, J. D.: Meconium peritonitis and increasing sweat chloride determinations in a case of familial progressive intrahepatic cholestasis. Pediatrics 69:325, 1982.

53. Hoffman, S., and Petrausch, P.: Perforation of the gastrointestinal tract in infancy and early childhood. Dtsch. Med. Wochenschr. 93:1503, 1968.

54. Holden, M. P.,: Primary idiopathic segmental infarction of the greater omentum. J. Pediatr. Surg. 7:77, 1972.

55. Hoyme, H., Higginbottom, M., and Jones, K.: The vascular pathogenesis of gastroschisis: intrauterine interruption of the omphalomesenteric artery. J. Pediatr. 90:288, 1981.

56. Hrabovsky, E., Boyd, B., Savrin, R., and Boles, E. T., Jr.: Advances in management of gastroschisis. Ann. Surg. 169:244, 1980.

57. Immordino, P. A.: Femoral hernia in infancy and childhood. J. Pediatr. Surg. 7:40, 1972.

58. Jaros, R., Schussheim, A., and Levy, L.: Preoperative diagnosis of bleeding Meckel's diverticulum utilizing 99m technetium pertechnetate scinti-imaging. J. Pediatr. 82:45, 1973.

59. Jewett, T. C., Jr., Duszynski, D. O., and Allen, J. E.: The visualization of Meckel's diverticulum with 99m Tc-pertechnetate. Surgery 68:567, 1970.

60. Johnson, D. E., Conroy, M. M., Foker, J. E., Ferrieri, P., and Thompson, T. R.: Candida peritonitis in the newborn infant. J. Pediatr. 87:298, 1980.

61. Jones, P.: Exomphalos: review of 45 cases. Arch. Dis. Child. 38:180, 1963.

62. Kafka, V., and Novak, K.: Multicystic retroperitoneal lymphangioma in an infant appearing as inguinal hernia. J. Pediatr. Surg. 5:573, 1970.

63. Kessel, I.: Chylous ascites in infancy. Arch. Dis. Child. 27:79, 1952.

63a. Kiesewetter, W. B., and Oh, K. S.: Unilateral inguinal hernias in children. Arch. Surg. 115:1443, 1980.

64. Kittle, C. F., Jenkins, H. P., and Dragstedt, L. B.: Patent omphalomesenteric duct and its relation to the diverticulum of Meckel. Arch. Surg. 54:10, 1947.

64a. Klein, M. D., Kosloske, A., and Hertzler, J.: Congenital defects of the abdominal wall: A review of the experience in New Mexico. JAMA 245:1643, 1981.

65. Kling, S.: Patent omphalomesenteric duct: surgical emergency. Arch. Surg. 96:545, 1968.

66. Kodawole, T. M., Bankhole, M. A., Glurin, E. O., and Familusi, J. B.: Meconium peritonitis presenting as giant cysts in neonates. Br. J. Radiol. 46:964, 1973.

67. Landor, J. H., Armstrong, J., Dickerson, O., and Westerfeld, R.: Neonatal obstruction of bowel caused by accidental clamping of small omphalocele. South. Med. J. 56:1236, 1963.

68. Lasserre, J., Saintsupery, G., Letac, R., and Besset, J. C.: The prognosis in neonatal peritonitis based on 32 cases. Ann. Chir. Infant. 9:77, 1968.

69. Leonidas, J. C., Kopel, F. B., and Danese, C. A.: Mesenteric cyst associated with protein loss in the gastrointestinal tract. Am. J. Roent-

genol. Radium Ther. Nucl. Med. 112:150, 1971.

70. Levy, J. L., Jr.: Evaluation of transperitoneal probing for detection of contralateral inguinal hernias in infants. Surgery 71:412, 1972.

71. Lloyd, J. R.: The etiology of gastrointestinal perforation in the newborn. J. Pediatr. Surg. 4:77, 1969.

72. Lorimer, W. S., Jr., and Ellis, D. G.: Meconium peritonitis. Surgery 60:470, 1966.

73. Low, R. A., and Grant, J. C.: Intrauterine transfusion complicated by omental herniation of the newborn. J. Pediatr. Surg. 7:62, 1972.

73a. Lubinsky, M., Doyle, K., and Trunca, C.: The association of prune belly with Turner's syndrome. Am. J. Dis. Child. 134:1171, 1980.

74. Lucaya, J., Herrera, M., and Espax, R. M.: Mesenteric and omental cysts in children: report of 8 cases and review of the literature. Ann. Radiol. 21:161, 1978.

75. Maciejewski, A.: Anterior meningocele presenting as abdominal swelling. J. Pediatr. Surg. 7:48, 1972.

76. MacMillan, R., Schullinger, J., and Santulli, T. V.: Pyourachus: an unusual surgical problem. J. Pediatr. Surg. 8:387, 1973.

76a. Mayer, T., Black, R., Matlak, M., and Johnson, D.: Gastroschisis and omphalocele. An eight-year review. Ann. Surg. 192:783, 1980.

77. Maze, A., Lieber, M. A., and Aballi, A.: Neonatal subcapsular hematoma of the liver presenting as an abdominal mass. Clin. Pediatr. 18:307, 1979.

78. McGregor, D. B., Halverson, K., and McVay, C. B.: The unilateral pediatric inguinal hernia: should the contralateral side be explored. J. Pediatr. Surg. 15:313, 1980.

79. McKenry, J. B. J., Lindsay, W. K., and Gerstein, M.: Congenital defects of the lymphatics in infancy. Pediatrics 19:21, 1957.

80. Miller, R. E.: Perforated viscus in infants. A new roentgen sign. Radiology 74:65, 1960.

80a. Molander, M. L., Mortensson, W., and Uden, R.: Omental and mesenteric cysts in children. Acta Paediatr. Scand. 71:227, 1982.

81. Mollitt, D., Ballantine, T. V., and Grosfeld, J.: Mesenteric cysts in infancy and childhood. Surg. Gynecol. Obstet. 147:182, 1978.

82. Moore, T. C.: Gastroschisis and omphalocele.: clinical differences. Surgery 82:561, 1977.

83. Murphy, D., Simmons, M., and Guiney, E. J.: Neonatal urinary ascites in absence of urinary tract obstruction. J. Pediatr. Surg. 13:629, 1978.

84. Novis, B. H., Bank, S., and Marks, I. N.: Gastrointestinal and peritoneal tuberculosis. S. Afr. Med. J. 47:365, 1973.

85. Oliver, G. A.: The omental cyst: a rare cause of the acute abdominal crisis. Surgery 56:588, 1964.

86. Orme, R. L., and Eades, S. M.: Perforation of the bowel in the newborn as a complication of exchange transfusion. Br. Med. J. 4:349, 1968.

86a. Pagon, R., Smith, D., and Shepard, T.: Urethral obstruction malformation complex. A cause of abdominal muscle deficiency and the "prune belly." J. Pediatr. 94:900, 1979.

87. Papermaster, T. C., Nelson, E., and Krivit, W.:

Eosinophilic peritonitis: report of 2 cases. Lancet 87:473, 1967.

88. Parrish, R. A., Sherman, R. T., and Wilson, H.: Gastroenteric perforation in newborns. Ann. Surg. 159:244, 1964.

89. Perriello, V. A., and Flemma, R. J.: Lymphangiomatous omental cyst in infancy masquerading as ascites. J. Pediatr. Surg. 4:227, 1969.

90. Perry, J., Jr.: Primary segmental infarction of the omentum in children. Surgery 56:584, 1964.

91. Peterson, D. S., Fish, L. S., and Cass, A.: Twins with congenital deficiency of the abdominal musculature. J. Urol. 107:670, 1972.

92. Radman, M.: Dystocia due to fetal abdominal enlargement. Obstet. Gynecol. 19:481, 1962.

93. Rangarathnam, C. S., Lal, R. B., and Swenson, O.: Gastroschisis. Arch. Surg. 98:742, 1969.

94. Rickham, P. P.: Peritonitis in the neonatal period. Arch. Dis. Child. 30:23, 1955.

95. Roe, T., Kershnar, A., Weitzman, J., and Madrigal, L. S.: Beckwith's syndrome with extreme organ hyperplasia. Pediatrics 52:372, 1973.

96. Rosen, F., Smith, D., Earle, R., Jr., Janeway, C. A., and Gitlin, D.: The etiology of hypoproteinemia in a patient with congenital chylous ascites. Pediatrics 30:696, 1962.

97. Rowe, M. I., and Clatworthy, H. W.: Incarcerated and strangulated hernias in children: a statistical study of high risk factors. Arch. Surg. 101:136, 1970.

98. Rowe, M. I., Copelson, L. W., and Clatworthy, H. W.: The patent processus vaginalis and the inguinal hernia. J. Pediatr. Surg. 4:102, 1969.

98a. Rowe, M. I., and Marchildon, M. B.: Inguinal hernia and hydrocele in infants and children. Surg. Clin. North Am. 61:1137, 1981.

99. Salinas, C., Bartoshesky, L., Otherson, B., Leape, L., Feingold, M., and Jorgenson, R.: Familial occurrence of gastroschisis. Am. J. Dis. Child. 133:515, 1979.

100. Sandborn, W. D., and Shafer, A. D.: Appendiceal umbilical fistula. J. Pediatr. Surg. 4:461, 1967.

101. Savage, J. P., and Davey, R. B.: The treatment of gastroschisis. J. Pediatr. Surg. 6:148, 1971.

102. Scaletter, H. E., and Mazursky, M. M.: Congenital entero-umbilical fistula due to a patent vitelline duct. J. Pediatr. 40:310, 1952.

103. Schaffer, A. J., and Avery, M. E.: Diseases of the Newborn. Ed. 3. Philadelphia, W. B. Saunders Company, 1971.

104. Schuster, S. A.: A new method for the staged repair of large omphaloceles. Surg. Gyncol. Obstet. 124:837, 1967.

105. Schwarz, E.: Roentgen signs of pneumoperitoneum in the newborn. Am. J. Roentgenol. 85:714, 1961.

106. Scobie, W. G., and Eckstein, H. B.: Umbilical hernia with associated hamartoma in a neonate. J. Pediatr. Surg. 6:73, 1971.

106a. Shaul, W.: Clues to the early diagnosis of neonatal appendicitis. J. Pediatr. 98:473, 1981.

107. Shaw, A.: The myth of gastroschisis. J. Pediatr. Surg. 10:235, 1975.

108. Singh, S., Baboo, M. L., and Pathak, I. C.: Cystic lymphangioma in children. Surgery 69:947, 1971.

109. Smith, B., and Clatworthy, H. W., Jr.: Meconium peritonitis: prognostic significance. Pediatrics 27:967, 1961.

110. Sotelo-Avila, C., and Gooch, W. M.: Neoplasms associated with Beckwith-Wiedemann syndrome. In Rosenberg, H. S., and Bolande, R. P. (eds.): Perspectives in Pediatric Pathology. Vol. 3. Chicago, Year Book Medical Publishers, Inc., 1976.

111. Stone, H. H., and Hester, R., Jr.: Management of complicated omphaloceles. Am. Surg. 37:224, 1971.

112. Stone, H. H., Sanders, S. L., and Martin, J. D., Jr.: Perforated appendicitis in children. Surgery 69:673, 1971.

113. Stringel, G., and Filler, R.: Prognostic factors in omphalocele and gastroschisis. J. Pediatr. Surg. 14:515, 1978.

114. Taucher, J., Bryant, D., and Gruenther, R.: False positive scan for Meckel diverticulum. J. Pediatr. 92:1022, 1978.

115. Thomas, C. S., and Brockman, S. K.: Idiopathic perforation of the colon in infancy. Ann. Surg. 164:853, 1966.

116. Touloukian, R. J., and Hobbins, J. C.: Maternal ultrasonography in the antenatal diagnosis of surgically correctible fetal anomalies. J. Pediatr. Surg. 15:373, 1980.

117. Touloukian, R. J., and Spackman, T.: Gastrointestinal function and radiographic appearance following gastroschisis repair. J. Pediatr. Surg. 6:427, 1971.

118. Verdis, R., Drayer, J. I., Montolia, J., Levine, L. S., and Laragh, J. W.: Hypertension and medullary sponge kidneys in an adolescent with Beckwith-Wiedmann syndrome. J. Pediatr. 91:761, 1977.

119. Vidik, T., and Marshall, D.: Direct inguinal hernias in infancy and early childhood. J. Pediatr. Surg. 15:846, 1980.

120. Wachter, H. E., and Elman, R.: Aberrant umbilical stomach. Am. J. Dig. Dis. Child. 87:204, 1954.

121. Waldenhausen, J. S., Herendeen, T., and King, H.: Necrotizing colitis of the newborn: common cause of perforation of the colon. Surgery 54:365, 1963.

122. Walker, A. R., and Putnam, T. C.: Omental mesenteric and retroperitoneal cysts: a clinical study of 33 cases. Ann. Surg. 178:13, 1973.

123. Warwick, W., and Good, R. A.: Intravenous alimentation with chylous ascitic fluid. J. Pediatr. 56:387, 1960.

124. Wesselhoeft, C. W., and Randolph, J. G.: Treatment of omphalocele based on individual characteristics of the defect. Pediatrics 44:101, 1969.

125. Whittlesey, R. H., Ingram, P. R., and Riker, W.: Chylous ascites in childhood. Ann. Surg. 142:1013, 1955.

126. Wynne, J. M., Cywes, S., Reteif, P. J., and Louw, J. H.: Ascites in the newborn. S. Afr. Med. J. 42:919, 1968.

Chapter Fourteen

THE LIVER AND BILIARY TREE

INTRODUCTION

Jaundice is more common in infancy than at any other time in life, and elevated serum levels of unconjugated bilirubin in the neonate are of special concern because of the danger of kernicterus. Maturational and physiologic aspects of bilirubin metabolism were presented in Chapter Six. Intrinsic liver disease and clinical conditions that influence production, transport, uptake, conjugation, and enterohepatic circulation of bilirubin will be discussed in this section. Table 14–1 is a classification for the differential diagnosis of noncholestatic and cholestatic jaundice in infancy.

PHYSIOLOGIC JAUNDICE

Physiologic jaundice, a transient benign condition, is the most common cause of neonatal jaundice. Serum bilirubin usually increases to 6 mg per dl by the second to third day of life and rarely exceeds 12 mg per dl except in the premature infant. For most infants, the jaundice clears within seven days. Physiologic jaundice should be carefully differentiated from pathologic jaundice by the following criteria:[2] (1) elevated indirect bilirubin prior to 36 hours of age, (2) total bilirubin of greater than 12 mg per dl, and (3) persistent jaundice beyond the eighth day of life, especially with a direct bilirubin value of greater than 1.5 mg per dl.[39]

Incidence. The incidence is variable because the neonate may not be obviously

jaundiced until the serum bilirubin concentration exceeds 6 mg per dl. Clinical jaundice is noted in approximately 15 per cent of normal newborn infants.[1]

Etiology. There is probably no single cause of physiologic jaundice.[1, 1a, 3] Delayed conjugation of bilirubin occurs regularly because of immaturity of glucuronyl transferase enzyme and poor phosphorylation of glucuronic acid. Other neonatal factors include bilirubin overproduction secondary to increased catabolism of fetal hemoglobin; delayed cellular transport of bilirubin because of decreased cytoplasmic transport proteins; and increased intestinal reabsorption of unconjugated bilirubin because of high levels of neonatal stool β-glucuronidase and diminished gut flora, responsible for deconjugation and reduction of bilirubin, respectively.

Treatment. No treatment is necessary for most neonates, but hypoalbuminemic, premature infants are at greater risk for deposition of bilirubin in neuronal tissues and may require therapy, including exchange transfusion.

NONCHOLESTATIC JAUNDICE (UNCONJUGATED HYPERBILIRUBINEMIA)

OVERPRODUCTION OF BILIRUBIN

Etiology. Rh and ABO incompatibilities can produce severe hemolysis in the neonate and should be suspected when jaundice occurs during the first 36 hours of

Table 14–1 Differential Diagnosis of Jaundice in Infancy

NONCHOLESTATIC JAUNDICE	CHOLESTATIC JAUNDICE

Bilirubin Overproduction
 Sepsis
 Rh/ABO incompatibility
 Hematoma (birth trauma)
    Cephalhematoma
    Subdural hematoma
 Drugs (e.g., vitamin K)
 Polycythemia
    Maternal-fetal or fetofetal transfusion
    Delayed clamping of umbilical cord
 Erythrocyte defects
    Congenital spherocytosis
    Congenital nonspherocytic anemias
    (e.g., G-6-PD deficiency)
 Hemoglobinopathies
 Physiologic jaundice
	Idiopathic Cholestatic Jaundice
	 Hepatocellular cholestatic jaundice
	    (or hepatocellular cholestasis)
	 Ductal cholestatic jaundice
	    (or ductal cholestasis)
	    Biliary atresia
	    Biliary hypoplasia
	    Paucity of the intrahepatic bile ducts
	    Choledochal cyst

Impaired Transport of Bilirubin
 Hypoxia
 Acidosis
 Drugs (e.g., sulfa, ASA)
 Serum free fatty acids
    Fat emulsions
 Hypoalbuminemia of prematurity
	Inherited Cholestatic Jaundice
	 Familial cholestasis syndromes
	    Benign recurrent cholestasis
	    Recurrent cholestasis with lymphedema
	    Progressive intrahepatic cholestasis
	    (e.g., Byler's disease)
	    Inborn errors in bile acid metabolism
	 Metabolic hepatocellular cholestasis
	    Galactosemia
	    Hereditary fructose intolerance
	    Hereditary tyrosinemia
	    Cystic fibrosis

Impaired Hepatic Uptake
 Decreased sinusoidal perfusion
    Diminished venous flow after birth
    Post-term patent ductus venosus
 Gilbert's syndrome
 Physiologic jaundice
	Alpha$_1$-antitrypsin deficiency
	    Glycogen storage disease
	 Other storage diseases
	    Niemann-Pick disease
	    Gaucher's disease
	    Cholesterol ester storage disease
	    Wolman's disease

Impaired Conjugation
 Breast milk jaundice
 Lucey-Driscoll syndrome
 Drugs (e.g., chloramphenicol)
 Hypoglycemia
 Hypothyroidism
 High intestinal obstruction
 Glucuronyl transferase deficiency
    (types I and II)
 Physiologic jaundice
	Inherited "Noncholestatic" Jaundice
	 Dubin-Johnson syndrome
	 Rotor syndrome
	
	 Acquired Cholestatic Jaundice
	 Sepsis
	 Other infections
	    Bacterial
	    Congenital (TORCH)
	    Viral (e.g., hepatitis A, B)
	    Parasitic (e.g., toxoplasmosis)
	 Chemical liver injury (e.g., drugs)

Enterohepatic Circulation
 Delayed passage of meconium
    Low intestinal obstruction
     Ileal atresia
     Hirschsprung's disease
    Cystic fibrosis
 Decreased intestinal motility
 Physiologic jaundice
    Negligible intestinal bacterial flora
    Presence of intestinal β-glucuronidase	

life.[1-3] Early, rapid elevation of indirect bilirubin may also occur in the infant with bacterial or viral *sepsis*. The presence of a *hematoma* or *polycythemia*, for example, following delayed clamping of the umbilical cord, can potentially lead to hemolysis because of the increased red blood cell mass, and this more chronic process may be overlooked as the cause of hyperbilirubinemia. *Vitamin K* produces hemolysis by acting as an oxidizing agent, especially in infants with glucose-6-phosphate dehydrogenase (G-6-PD) deficiency, which is usually not a clinical problem until after the neonatal period. *Hereditary spherocytosis* and *hemoglobinopathies* are other congenital hemolytic syndromes that cause chronic unconjugated hyperbilirubinemia in infancy.[4]

Clinical Evaluation. Jaundice may be associated with hepatomegaly. Early pallor and splenomegaly suggest significant hemolytic disease, and neurologic signs and symptoms indicate kernicterus, a severe central nervous system disorder resulting from deposition of unconjugated bilirubin in the brain.

Diagnosis. Blood group typing of infant and mother and direct Coombs test will establish the diagnosis of fetomaternal incompatibility. For ABO incompatibility, the direct Coombs test may be negative; hence, the presence of spherocytes in blood smears is an important diagnostic observation. A family history of splenomegaly or hemolysis suggests congenital spherocytosis when maternal agglutination antibodies are not demonstrated. The reticulocyte count and hemoglobin concentration are usually abnormal. Most importantly, the serum bilirubin concentration requires careful monitoring during the early hours of life.

Treatment. The risk of kernicterus and milder forms of neurologic and developmental damage may be related to the duration of unconjugated hyperbilirubinemia greater than 15 mg per dl.[23] However, a variation in susceptibility to neurologic damage is now recognized, and premature infants with serum bilirubin levels of less than 10 mg per dl may develop kernicterus. This is probably related to clinical factors that potentiate the central nervous system toxicity of bilirubin, such as acidosis, hypoalbuminemia, hypoglycemia, septicemia, and administration of drugs that interfere with bilirubin binding and transport. Rigid therapeutic guidelines have consequently not been established, but excellent general treatment reviews are available for unconjugated hyperbilirubinemia.[4, 46] In general,

the bilirubin-binding capacity of albumin in hyperbilirubinemia is not helpful in determining the risk of kernicterus, although intravenous infusion of albumin, especially prior to exchange transfusion, increases the number of sites available for potential binding of the unconjugated molecule.[35]

Exchange transfusion is indicated for acute or chronic hemolysis when the serum indirect bilirubin concentration exceeds 20 mg per dl in full-term neonates or 10 mg per dl in premature infants. This is the most effective method of controlling hyperbilirubinemia, and it requires double blood volume replacement with whole blood. Postpartum Rh immunoprophylaxis has reduced the incidence of hemolytic disease and subsequent requirement for transfusion therapy, but this is not a consideration for the sick premature infant without Rh immunization who may develop kernicterus at comparatively low bilirubin levels.

Phototherapy is more efficacious than exchange transfusion for nonhemolytic jaundice[45] and may help prevent a rapid increase in serum bilirubin to exchange levels, but effectiveness in prevention of kernicterus has not been established. There is controversy regarding the indications for commencement of phototherapy; nomograms are now available[16] but are not generally accepted over existing phototherapy protocols. It has been emphasized that this form of therapy is never routine and should be reserved for premature infants and term infants with high serum bilirubin concentrations, i.e., 20 mg per dl.[29, 31] The mechanism of action is probably photo-oxidation of bilirubin in exposed skin at appropriate light wavelengths (400 to 500 μ) and increased excretion of bilirubin in bile.[40] Photodegradation products occurring in patients are not well defined but are considered less toxic than unconjugated bilirubin.[38] Unnecessary treatment should be avoided, however, because of well-recognized or potential side effects: abdominal distention, increase in insensible water loss, diarrhea with increased intestinal motility or lactose intolerance,[37] retinal damage, hemolysis, unusual bronzing of the skin ("bronze baby" syndrome),[26, 40] and alteration of intracellular DNA.[41] *Phenobarbital* should not be used routinely for prevention or treatment of hyperbilirubinemia. If given to the mother a few days prior to parturition, this drug may lower peak bilirubin concentrations in the neonate, but it does not enhance the effect of phototherapy.[17]

IMPAIRED TRANSPORT OF BILIRUBIN

Etiology. Certain drugs contribute to indirect hyperbilirubinemia, and central nervous system dysfunction may occur at lower than usual serum bilirubin concentrations. For example, aspirin and sulfonamides cause bilirubin displacement from secondary albumin-binding sites. The primary albumin-binding sites can also be blocked by high serum concentrations of free fatty acids,[1] the main metabolic product of soybean fat emulsion (e.g., Intralipid or Liposyn). The latter mechanism may be responsible, in part, for the hyperbilirubinemia secondary to breast milk, which has a high concentration of fatty acids. High molar ratios (i.e., greater than six) of free fatty acids to albumin have been shown to cause significant displacement of bilirubin from albumin. In addition, hypoproteinemic premature infants have decreased levels of albumin for bilirubin binding, and they are often hypoxemic and acidotic, clinical conditions that further enhance bilirubin displacement from albumin.

Diagnosis. Attention to factors that contribute to elevated indirect bilirubin levels, such as drugs, acidosis, hypoxemia, and prematurity, is necessary to decrease the risk of neonatal encephalopathy.

IMPAIRED HEPATIC UPTAKE OF BILIRUBIN

Etiology. Diminished hepatic sinusoidal perfusion or persistent patency of the ductus venosus occurs in sick neonates, especially those with respiratory distress syndrome; both these conditions result in decreased hepatic uptake of bilirubin, as in Gilbert's disease.

IMPAIRED CONJUGATION OF BILIRUBIN

A number of physiologic processes affect the hepatic conjugation mechanism. Like physiologic jaundice and Gilbert's syndrome, they are not all pathologic conditions that lead to significant elevation of bilirubin.

Breast Milk Jaundice[33]

Incidence. Unconjugated hyperbilirubinemia occurs in approximately 1 per cent of breast-fed children and usually does not exceed 20 mg per dl.

Etiology. Oral administration of pregnane-3,20-diol has been shown to cause hyperbilirubinemia in neonates but not in older infants. This unusual steroid is found in the breast milk of some mothers with hyperbilirubinemic infants; it is thought to compete with bilirubin for glucuronyl transferase enzyme conjugation,[25] but *in vitro* studies do not always demonstrate the abnormality of bilirubin conjugation. More recent evidence suggests that excess fatty acids in breast milk and, perhaps, lipoprotein lipase[36a] cause displacement of bilirubin from albumin-binding sites.[1]

Clinical Evaluation. Jaundice usually appears between the sixth and eighth days of life in a thriving infant and recedes following discontinuance of breast feeding, or several weeks after birth with continued ingestion of breast milk.

Treatment. Hyperbilirubinemia usually does not recur if breast feeding is reinstituted after five or six days. Breast feedings may be continued despite moderate jaundice because kernicterus has not been reported with this form of hyperbilirubinemia. However, prudence would dictate consideration of a short discontinuance of breast milk because of the more subtle neurologic or developmental insults secondary to hyperbilirubinemia.

Prognosis. Breast milk jaundice is a benign condition.

Lucey-Driscoll Syndrome[6]

This is a rare familial cause of hyperbilirubinemia associated with early onset of marked hyperbilirubinemia[6] and affecting all babies of certain mothers.

Etiology. The serum of these infants and mothers contains an undefined inhibitor of glucuronyl transferase, which is not present in breast milk and which appears early in the second trimester. Although the inhibitor is found in the sera of all pregnant women, it is three to five times higher in these mothers.

Symptoms. Jaundice develops in the first week of life, and serum bilirubin concentrations may reach as high as 65 mg per dl to cause central nervous system damage. The condition may be confused with breast milk jaundice.

Treatment. Depending upon severity, the treatment consists of phototherapy or exchange transfusion.

Congenital Hypothyroidism[30]

The mechanism of jaundice in hypothyroidism is unknown, although there may be a delay in the maturation of hepatic glucuronyl transferase. Thyroid studies are necessary in all infants with unconjugated hyperbilirubinemia, for hypothyroidism is a treatable disease and jaundice clears after appropriate therapy with thyroid hormone.

Jaundice with High Intestinal Obstruction

Etiology. Some infants with pyloric stenosis and other less common forms of intestinal obstruction (e.g., duodenal atresia) develop unconjugated hyperbilirubinemia.[14] The incidence may be as high as 8 to 10 per cent. The precise mechanism for the hyperbilirubinemia is not known, but it may be related to vomiting, fasting, and hypoglycemia.[9] Diminished glucuronyl transferase activity has recently been demonstrated in these jaundiced infants compared with non-

jaundiced infants having similar surgical problems.[27]

Treatment. The jaundice rapidly clears after surgical correction of the anatomic problem.

Miscellaneous

Etiology. HYPOGLYCEMIA. Glucose is a substrate for glucuronic acid, which participates in the synthesis of bilirubin glucuronide with glucuronyl transferase enzyme. Hence, hypoglycemia secondary to decreased caloric intake (e.g., vomiting, fasting) or specific diseases (e.g., early galactosemia, infant of diabetic mother) may cause a reciprocal increase in serum unconjugated bilirubin levels.[31] Infants with low blood glucose also have elevated levels of epinephrine and glucagon, both of which stimulate hepatic heme oxygenase with subsequent conversion of heme to biliverdin and an increased bilirubin load.[8]

DRUGS. Chloramphenicol and novobiocin compete for glucuronyl transferase and therefore can potentially decrease bilirubin conjugation in the young infant.

Enterohepatic Circulation

Etiology. Clinical conditions leading to lower intestinal obstruction (e.g., ileal atresia or Hirschsprung's disease) and decreased intestinal motility promote the increased enterohepatic circulation of unconjugated bilirubin.[20] High levels of intestinal β-glucuronidase and diminished gut flora in the first days of life further increase the intestinal absorption of the unconjugated molecule.

INHERITED INDIRECT HYPERBILIRUBINEMIAS

Glucuronyl Transferase Deficiency (Crigler-Najjar Syndrome)

In 1952, Crigler and Najjar described a syndrome characterized by familial, nonhemolytic, indirect hyperbilirubinemia occurring in the newborn and often associated with kernicterus. This syndrome is more aptly termed chronic nonhemolytic hyperbilirubinemia due to glucuronyl transferase deficiency.[7, 17]

Incidence. More than 60 cases are now documented in the literature.

Etiology and Pathogenesis. This syndrome is due to a deficiency of glucuronyl transferase activity and is divided into two types. In type I, the bile is colorless and contains no bilirubin. There is no evidence of enzyme activity. It is inherited as an autosomal recessive trait, and there is extensive consanguinity and inbreeding in the families. The serum bilirubin rise is severe, and death often results in infancy from neurologic damage. In type II, inherited as an autosomal dominant trait with incomplete penetrance, small amounts of glucuronide appear in yellow bile. The serum bilirubin does not rise as significantly as in the type I form, for the bilirubin is eliminated by transfer of the unconjugated form across the intestinal mucosa and is excreted in the bile as the glucuronide or in the form of polar, azonegative derivatives of bilirubin. In both forms, bilirubin turnover studies are normal and the bilirubin curve shows a rapid decline in plasma content for the first day, followed by a slower exponential disappearance. The role played by the Y and Z proteins in this condition is not yet known. Histologically, the liver remains normal save for the development of pigment-filled bile canaliculi. It is suggested that type I represents total absence of enzyme, and type II, a defect in addition of the second molecule of glucuronic acid.

Symptoms. The disease arises in a well infant and is noted only when severe jaundice unassociated with hemolysis appears during the first few days of life. If untreated, it leads to neurologic manifestations of kernicterus. Many infants die of neurologic damage within the first few weeks or months, but others survive into adulthood. Signs of neurologic deterioration may appear as late as the sixteenth to the eighteenth year.[12, 13]

Diagnosis. The diagnosis is made after other causes of hemolytic disease have been ruled out. In type I, the bilirubin ranges between 20 and 45 mg per dl, whereas in type II it varies between 8 and 22 mg per dl. Liver biopsy reveals essentially normal tissue.

Treatment. In the neonate, exchange transfusion is the only effective treatment for maintaining the bilirubin level below that at which kernicterus occurs. Type I disease does not respond to phenobarbital therapy, and phototherapy has not been followed by dramatic reduction in bilirubin, perhaps because of the large tissue deposits of bilirubin. Phenobarbital is often used for patients with type II disease but is perhaps not necessary, because once the hazard of kernicterus is past, there is usually little danger from hyperbilirubinemia. If desired, phenobarbital may be given, 10 mg per kg per day in three divided doses, and bilirubin levels will fall to between 1 and 2 mg per dl. Experimental data suggest that extracorporeal phototherapy or perfusion over albumin-conjugated agarose columns may ultimately be of benefit in maintaining low bilirubin levels.[36] It is even suggested that auxiliary liver transplantation may in the future be used in treatment of this disorder.

Chronic Nonhemolytic Unconjugated Hyperbilirubinemia (Gilbert's Disease, Idiopathic Unconjugated Hyperbilirubinemia, or Constitutional Hepatic Dysfunction)

All cases of chronic unconjugated hyperbilirubinemia have at one time or another been classified under the term "Gilbert's syndrome," but, strictly speaking, this disease should not be considered a major cause of neonatal jaundice since bilirubin elevation associated with it seldom exceeds 4 or 5 mg per dl.[18]

Incidence. The disease must be fairly common, for Levine and Klatskin[28] collected from their own experience 366 patients who displayed a wide variety of infectious and metabolic disorders. The true disease is probably inherited as an autosomal dominant trait, with males affected more often than females.

Etiology. The etiology remains unknown, although some postulate it to be a defect in the handling of conjugated bilirubin or a defect in bilirubin uptake.[25] Indocyanine green is handled normally in some, but in others, abnormally. UDPG glucuronyl transferase is 10 to 30 per cent of normal.

Pathology. Histologically, the liver is normal or reflects an underlying disease.[15] The level of bilirubin fluctuates considerably and shows a reciprocal relationship with the caloric intake.[18, 32]

Symptoms. Mild, persistent hyperbilirubinemia may be noted during early infancy, and the level fluctuates during childhood. The disease is more common in boys and lessens in intensity with age. Associated symptoms are vague abdominal pain, nausea, and, rarely, constipation or diarrhea. These and the jaundice are aggravated by fatigue or intermittent illness.[21, 24]

Diagnosis. The diagnosis rests largely upon elimination of other causes of jaundice, the most important of which is hemolysis. This is not as simple as it may seem, for, unfortunately, red cell survival studies in patients with Gilbert's disease show that 42 per cent have evidence of mild hemolysis, although it is not of great enough significance to increase the bilirubin if liver function is otherwise normal. A mild conjugated hyperbilirubinemia occurs occasionally in patients with congestive heart failure, thyrotoxicosis, and polycythemia and as a frequent residual of viral hepatitis. It may occur after portacaval but not after splenorenal shunts. Jaundice is often increased by fasting.

Liver function tests are normal except for a mild elevation of bilirubin and an impaired bilirubin tolerance. The accepted criteria for diagnosis are a direct bilirubin of less than 0.3 mg per dl and an indirect bilirubin of greater than 1.5 mg per dl. BSP clearance is impaired.[10]

Treatment. Adequate caloric intake and frequent feedings will cause a fall in bilirubin, but it is not known whether the abdominal pain is alleviated. Phenobarbital also will lower the serum bilirubin level.

INHERITED CONJUGATED HYPERBILIRUBINEMIA

Dubin-Johnson Syndrome (Sprinz-Nelson Syndrome, Chronic Idiopathic Jaundice with Unidentified Pigment in Liver Cells, Familial Conjugated Hyperbilirubinemia)

Patients with this syndrome have hyperbilirubinemia, mainly of the direct-reacting

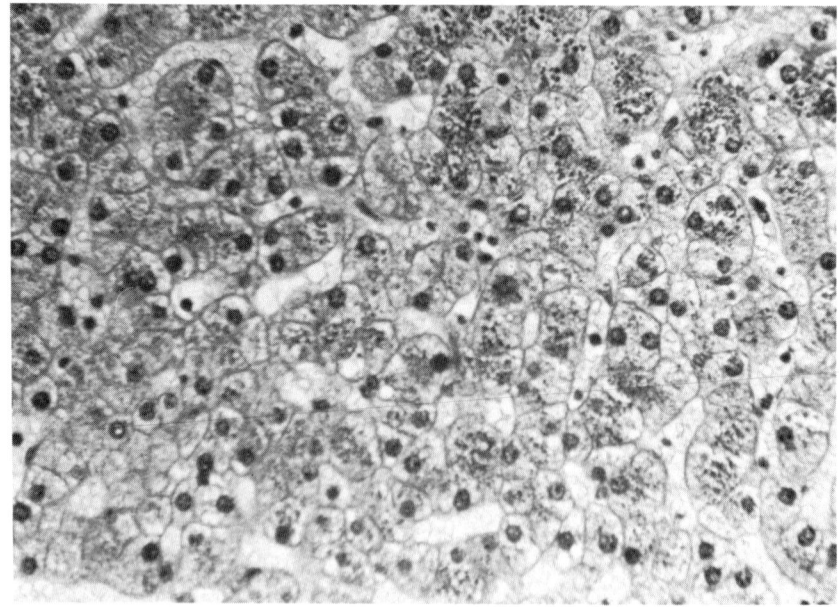

Figure 14–1   Dubin-Johnson pigment. Coarse brown-black pigment is found in the hepatocytes.

type, increased urine bile (conjugated bilirubin) and urobilinogen, nonvisualizing gallbladder at cholecystography, and a granular brown pigment in hepatocytes that gives the liver a black color on gross inspection.[19, 41]

Incidence. This syndrome may be the most common familial form of jaundice.

Etiology and Pathology. There is some controversy about whether this disease is inherited as an autosomal recessive or an autosomal dominant trait with variable expressivity. Not all patients with abnormal pigment in their liver cells have hyperbilirubinemia, and so accurate family studies must include liver biopsy. Consanguinity is reported in up to 45 per cent of parents of afflicted individuals. Males are affected more often than females and have more severe disease with an earlier onset.

The defect is one in which the hepatocyte is unable to transport certain organic anions into the bile. Supporting this hypothesis is the fact that the transport maximum (Tm) for BSP is virtually zero in the Dubin-Johnson syndrome (normal, 9 mg per minute), whereas the storage capacity for BSP is normal (67 mg per dl). No abnormality of production, hepatic uptake, or conjugation of bilirubin can be demonstrated, and the extrahepatic biliary tract is entirely normal. Other dyes such as rose bengal, methylene blue, and indocyanine green as well as cholecystographic dye are also retained by the liver. Bile salt excretion is normal, therefore rendering the jaundice noncholestatic. The only abnormality in liver histology is the presence of a coarsely granular amorphous brown pigment in the cytoplasm of the centrilobar hepatocytes, as shown in Figure 14–1. The Kupffer cells are normal, and there is no inflammation or necrosis. Histochemical staining does not differentiate this pigment from lipofuscin. Recent evidence suggests it to be melanin-like, composed of polymerized,[44] oxidized catecholamine metabolites. If acute viral hepatitis develops, the pigment disappears.

Symptoms. Jaundice may be noted at birth, but the diagnosis frequently is delayed until much later in life. Indeed, the onset may be acute, often occurring at the time of an intercurrent illness. There is often a family history of jaundice, and as many as three patients with this condition have been reported from one family. Generalized constitutional symptoms, such as weakness, fatigue, anorexia, nausea, and vomiting as well as right upper quadrant pain, may be present. The liver may be slightly enlarged and occasionally tender. A bleeding tendency due to decreased factor VII has been described in some patients.

Diagnosis. The only liver function tests that are abnormal are those concerned with hepatic excretory function. There is hyperbilirubinemia up to 6 mg per dl (conjugated bilirubin constitutes 36 to 86 per cent), prolonged BSP retention, and nonfilling of the gallbladder even with a double dose of iodinated dye. After administration of BSP, the normal fall is followed by a rise 30 to 45 minutes later owing to the appearance of BSP-conjugated glutathione. The stools are pale, and the urine is dark because of bile and urobilinogen. Serum uroporphyrinogen is normal, but urinary coproporphyrin is abnormal, with increased coproporphyrin I and decreased III.[41]

Treatment. No treatment is necessary. Estrogens and anabolic steroids should be avoided, as they inhibit conjugated bilirubin excretion.

Rotor Syndrome

Rotor and associates have described a syndrome that appears to be identical with the Dubin-Johnson syndrome except that there is no abnormal pigment in the liver cells and the gallbladder usually is visualized normally on cholecystography. Urinary coproporphyrin I is only minimally elevated. Despite these differences, the two may be related entities, since each syndrome has been reported in the same family.

Lethal Familial Cholestatic and Pigmentary Liver Disease

A new disease affecting four males from a family of North African descent has been described, which includes arthrogryposis, renal dysfunction, and cholestatic jaundice.

Earlier, a nonfamilial type of arthrogryposis associated with hepatic calcifications was reported.[34]

Occurring as a sex-linked disorder, this condition includes arthrogryposis and low insertion of the thumbs, which are noted at birth. The infants fail to gain weight and become jaundiced after several weeks. Urinary tract disease is evidenced by polyuria, glycosuria, proteinuria, calcinuria, ketonuria, and hyperchloreuric acidosis. Death occurs within several weeks to months.

Post-mortem examination revealed atrophy of peripheral muscles, alterations of anterior horn motor neurons, capsulosynovial fibrosis of the joints, renal tubular cell degeneration with nephrocalcinosis, and black pigment within the liver cells. The pigment had chemical characteristics similar to that of the Dubin-Johnson syndrome.

CHOLESTATIC JAUNDICE (CONJUGATED HYPERBILIRUBINEMIA)

Conjugated bilirubin, a nontoxic product of heme catabolism, represents only a small fraction of bile, but elevated serum concentrations suggest bile secretory failure, referred to as cholestasis. More importantly, hepatic excretion of organic anions, such as bilirubin, is dependent primarily on movement of bile acid and H_2O across the canaliculus, a bile secretory membrane. Physiologic and morphologic cholestasis are defined as a reduction in bile flow and the histologic presence of bile pigment in canaliculi and hepatocytes, respectively. They are regularly associated with hyperbilirubinemia — hence, the term "cholestatic jaundice." This problem may be secondary to anatomic abnormalities of large bile ducts (extrahepatic) or smaller intralobular ducts (intrahepatic). Also, functional diminution of intrahepatic bile flow occurs after damage to the canalicular membrane, especially in the young infant with immature bile acid synthesis. Various idiopathic, inherited, and acquired conditions responsible for cholestatic jaundice will be discussed in this section (Table 14–1). Long-term follow-up is necessary, for Ghisan et al.[74] reported four infants, two of whom had biopsy-proven paucity of bile ducts; one was well at three years, and the other developed biliary atresia. Two others had bile duct proliferation and later had a paucity of bile ducts.

IDIOPATHIC CHOLESTATIC JAUNDICE

Hepatocellular Cholestatic Jaundice

Neonatal hepatitis is a misleading term because it implies an infectious disease process, e.g., viral hepatitis, when it is well known that a number of noninfectious liver diseases of infancy, such as alpha$_1$-antitrypsin deficiency and galactosemia, may have similar clinical and morphologic features suggestive of hepatitis.[109] Therefore, neonatal hepatitis should be considered only as an exclusion diagnosis for undefined (idiopathic) hepatocellular cholestatic disorders or as an infectious disease of the liver in the neonatal period.

Incidence. The precise incidence is not known, but idiopathic hepatocellular cholestasis represents the diagnosis for the majority of children with persistent liver dysfunction in the early months of life.

Pathology. The histopathologic features of hepatocellular cholestasis include liver cell necrosis, bile stasis, fibroblast proliferation, variable inflammatory cell infiltration, extramedullary hematopoiesis, and giant cell transformation.[58] Multinucleated giant cells (Fig. 14–1) appear regularly in hepatocellular disease occurring in the first three months of life. These cells were once considered to be the hallmark of hepatocellular cholestasis, but they have been demonstrated in as many as 15 to 50 per cent of patients with ductal cholestasis.[70, 88] It has been suggested that giant cell transformation may be a response of the infant liver to viral injury; however, it is generally believed to be a nonspecific response to various types of hepatic injury. Portal signs of biliary obstruction are usually absent, especially bile duct proliferation, and hypoplastic bile ducts can be noted in some patients.

Table 14–2 Idiopathic Cholestatic Jaundice: Diagnostic Studies

IMMEDIATE	LESS URGENT
Bilirubin (total and direct)	Aminotransferases (SGPT, SGOT)
Prothrombin time	Serum bile acids
Total protein, albumin	Serologic studies
Blood glucose	Hepatitis A, B
Serologic studies	Rubella
Syphilis	Cytomegalovirus
Toxoplasmosis	Herpes simplex
Sepsis evaluation	Serum protein electrophoresis
Urine	Sweat electrolytes
Reducing substances (nonglucose)	
Organic acids	
Serum amino acids	

Clinical Evaluation. Clinical symptoms may appear at any time after birth, but poor feeding and failure to thrive are usually noted in the first two weeks of life. These symptoms may be present before the occurrence of jaundice. The typical presentation, however, is that of an unwell, jaundiced infant with hepatomegaly. Splenomegaly is not always present in the early weeks of illness.

Diagnosis. Certain immediate studies are necessary to determine the type and significance of hyperbilirubinemia and to establish an early diagnosis of treatable disease (Table 14–2). These studies include total and direct bilirubin, Coombs' test, hemoglobin, prothrombin time, serum total protein and albumin, blood glucose, evaluation for sepsis, urine for non–glucose-reducing substances and organic acids, serologic studies for toxoplasmosis and syphilis, and serum amino acids. Less urgent studies include serum alanine aminotransferase (glutamic-pyruvic transaminase, or SGPT); serology for hepatitis A and B virus; serology for rubella, cytomegalovirus, and herpes simplex (TORCH); cord serum for IgM; sweat electrolytes; serum bile acids; and a serum protein electrophoretic pattern. Serum protein electrophoresis may reveal an absence of the alpha-$_1$-globulin band suggestive of alpha-antitrypsin deficiency. A low serum antitrypsin level and appropriate protease inhibitor (Pi) phenotype confirm this diagnosis. After coagulation studies are determined to be normal, a percutaneous liver biopsy is safely performed,

and the histologic findings may suggest an etiology for the infant's liver problem. Failure to make a specific diagnosis of hepatocellular cholestasis usually necessitates an evaluation of the patency of the biliary tree (ductal cholestasis); the most accurate nonsurgical laboratory test for determining this is a carefully performed ^{131}I-rose bengal test. Fecal *excretion* of greater than 10 per cent of the injected dose rules out biliary atresia.[110]

Treatment. Hepatocellular cholestasis may lead to fat malabsorption because of inadequate intestinal bile acids for critical micellar concentration. Medium-chain triglycerides supplement caloric intake because they are easily absorbed without micellar solubilization, and intake of fat-soluble vitamins (A, D, E, K) should be increased to twice the recommended daily allowance. Cholestyramine (2 to 4 gm TID) and phenobarbital (3 to 5 mg/kg/day) may improve bile flow by a bile acid–dependent and bile acid–independent mechanism, respectively.[59, 73, 106] Serum calcium and phosphorus must be monitored carefully because of the potential for vitamin D and calcium malabsorption and abnormal hepatic 25-hydroxylation of this vitamin. This is especially important if the infant is treated with phenobarbital, which increases the metabolism of vitamin D.[82, 85] For infants with significant liver disease, oral 1,25-(OH)$_2$ cholecalciferol may be ineffective at a dose of 0.10 mcg per kg per day, but the parenteral dose of 0.20 mcg per kg per day is usually effective treatment of the metabolic bone disease. In general, daily require-ments of vitamin D increase to at least 2000 IU for the infant with liver disease. Daily vitamin K (2.5 to 5.0 mg) therapy is some-times necessary to treat a prolonged prothrombin time and subsequent bleeding complications.

Prognosis. More significant complica-tions arise when the hepatocellular chole-stasis is severe and prolonged. Other factors related to an unfavorable prognosis are the early appearance of portal fibrosis, coexis-tence of systemic disease, and the presence of a similar cholestatic syndrome in a sib-ling.[67] Furthermore, surgery has an adverse effect on infants with hepatocellular chole-stasis. Death may occur after exploratory laparotomy, and a greater number of pa-tients develop chronic liver disease follow-ing surgery compared with those who are not operated upon. Progressive liver failure, in addition to cirrhosis and portal hyperten-sion, occurs in approximately 30 per cent of infants with idiopathic cholestasis. These patients may well have had unrecognized alpha$_1$-antitrypsin deficiency.

DUCTAL CHOLESTATIC JAUNDICE

Biliary Atresia

Incidence. Extrahepatic biliary atresia is the most common form of ductal cholesta-sis.[57] It is not rare, and the estimated in-cidence varies from 1 in 8000 to 1 in 20,000 live births.

Etiology. Until recently, biliary atresia was considered a developmental malforma-tion, separate and distinct from other types of cholestasis such as acquired "neonatal hepatitis."[102] It was suggested that during organogenesis of bile ducts around the fifth to eighth week of embryonic development, there was a failure of recanalization of the solid epithelial cord resulting in atresia of the extrahepatic biliary tree. This was sup-ported by reports of the extrahepatic bile ducts appearing as fibrous cords, the finding of associated anomalies in as many as 25 per cent of patients with biliary atresia, and the association of biliary atresia with trisomy chromosomal disorders. This maldevelop-

ment hypothesis, however, does not corre-late with the rare occurrence of biliary atre-sia in aborted fetuses or autopsied premature infants, in addition to the lack of associated abnormalities of the pancreas, an organ that also develops from the foregut endoderm.

Since Rolleston's report of biliary atresia resulting from "descending cholangitis," numerous investigators have suggested that this bile duct problem may be an acquired defect of early or late gestation. How-ever, it was not until the concept of "infantile obstructive cholangiopathy" was introduced that biliary atresia was seriously considered as an acquired problem with a possible relationship to hepatocellular cho-lestasis.[50,91] Developmentally, the fetus seems to be affected at between 150 and 155 days' gestation. A study from Texas has identified time-clusters for babies born with this lesion to have had their susceptible gestation period in times of intense agricul-tural activity in the state; the role of toxins has been suggested.[108a] It has been reported in association with rubella virus. This un-proved hypothesis implies that ductular in-flammation and cholestasis lead to fibrosis of the biliary epithelium.[74] There is little evidence that biliary atresia is both a devel-opmental malformation and an acquired cholestatic lesion, but overlap of diagnos-tic features (histologic and chemical) along with the presence of hepatitis and biliary atresia in certain chromosomal abnormal-ities lends support to this possibility.[87] Recently, it has been reported in a child with the fetal alcohol syndrome[70c] and in another with the polysplenia syndrome and abnormal cilia.[108c]

Pathology. The majority of patients with biliary atresia have lesions of the hepatic ducts adjacent to the liver hilus ("noncor-rectable"), the remainder being complete or incomplete lesions more distal to the hilus ("correctable").[63] This form of ductal chole-stasis may involve the intrahepatic ducts as well, and the gallbladder is often hypoplas-tic or absent.[71a,90a] The histologic lesion is similar to that of hepatocellular cholestasis, with prominent vesiculation of hepatocytes and the presence of multinucleated giant cells (Fig. 14–2). There may be decreased

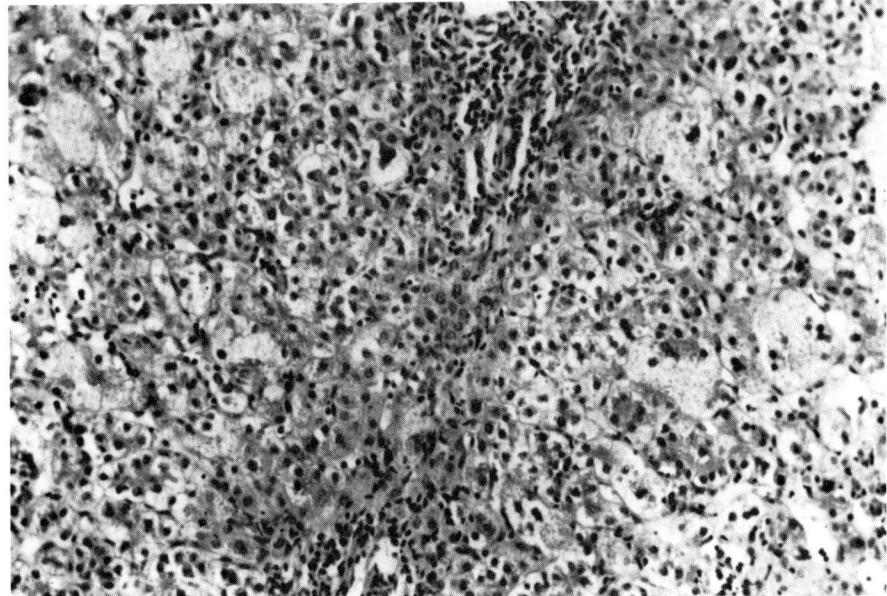

Figure 14–2   Liver biopsy specimen from a neonate with giant cell hepatitis. H & E, × 10, portal areas.

or absent portal bile ducts, but tortuous, interconnecting, proliferated bile ducts (Fig. 14–3) are noted in extrahepatic atresia, which would be unusual in the liver of an infant with hepatocellular cholestasis.[66]

Clinical Evaluation. There seems to be no familial incidence or association with prematurity. Unlike patients with hepatocellular cholestasis, most infants with biliary atresia are apparently well until jaundice persists beyond the first week of life.

Meconium and the early stools are frequently of a normal color, but they gradually become clay-colored and the urine darkens. Jaundice increases with time and assumes a greenish tint, particularly apparent in the sclerae, and usually does not fluctuate as the liver enlarges and becomes hard and firm. Fluctuations in jaundice and in bilirubin levels do not preclude the diagnosis. The stools may intermittently have color. Splenomegaly, ascites, and portal hypertension

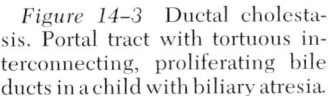

Figure 14–3 Ductal cholestasis. Portal tract with tortuous interconnecting, proliferating bile ducts in a child with biliary atresia.

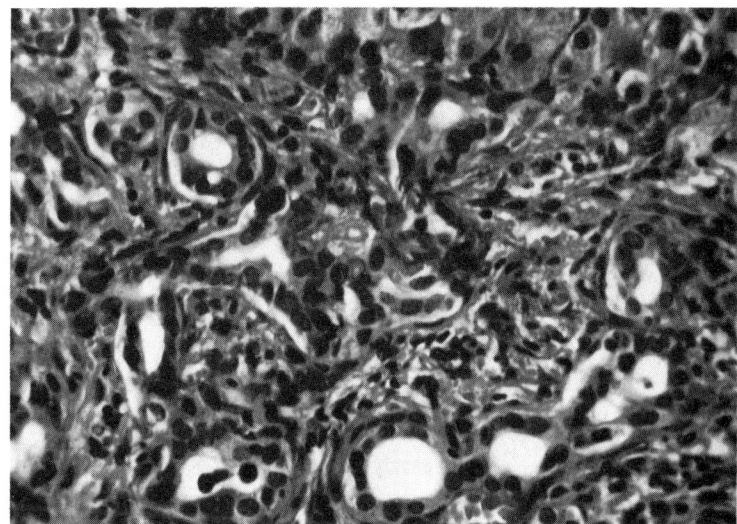

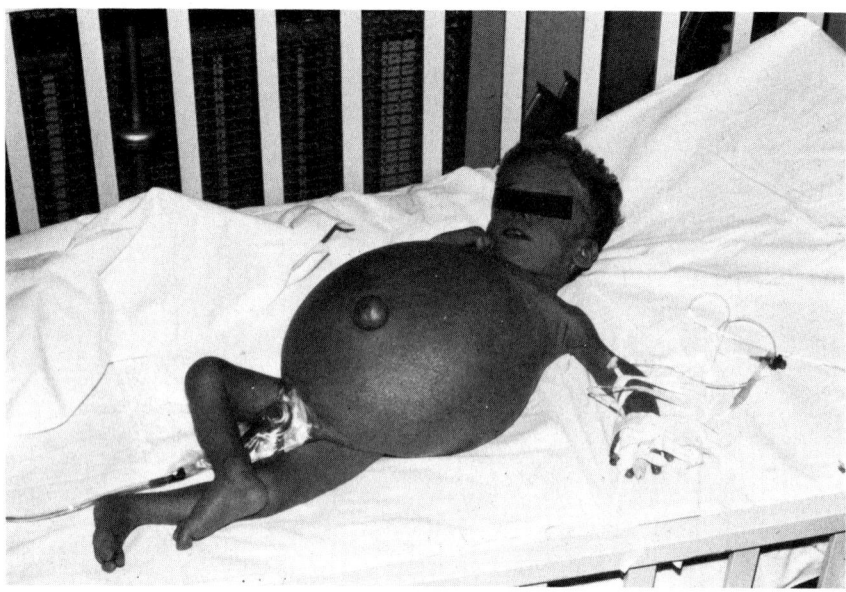

Figure 14–4 A 15-month-old white male in the terminal stages of biliary atresia. Deep jaundice is apparent even in a black-and-white-photograph. The abdomen is markedly distended, and there is a secondary umbilical hernia. Edema and malnutrition are evident.

occur as cirrhosis progresses over the first months of life (Figs. 14–4 and 14–5). Malabsorptions lead to malnutrition and vitamin deficiencies. Pruritus is exhibited by children over three months of age. Progressive neuromuscular disease is a result of vitamin E deficiency and responds to treatment with alpha-tocopherol.[77a] Severe zinc and magnesium deficiencies exist and may persist even after surgery in those with progressive disease.[156a]

Diagnosis. Routine liver function tests are usually not helpful in differentiating biliary atresia from other cholestatic syndromes of infancy. A SGOT value under 500 units suggests atresia rather than hepatitis. Hence, after appropriate studies designed to rule out treatable causes of hepatocellular cholestasis have been performed, it is important to determine the degree of biliary obstruction by *[131]I-rose bengal excretion in stool*. Intravenous injection of radiolabeled rose bengal is followed by separately collecting stool and urine for 72 hours; this is best accomplished in females and males by placement of a Foley bladder catheter. The

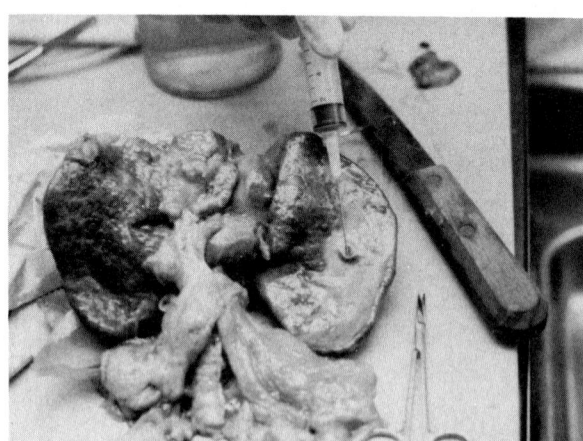

Figure 14–5 Post-mortem liver of an infant with biliary atresia showing cirrhosis with nodularity and large bile lakes (syringe is aspirating bile from a lake).

diagnostic value of this test can be enhanced by pretreatment of the infant with cholestyramine, since this resin binds to the rose bengal dye and increases its fecal excretion in the presence of a patent biliary tract. Complete obstruction of extrahepatic bile ducts is suggested if the rose bengal excretion in stool is less than 10 per cent. The rose bengal scan does not provide a quantitative analysis of biliary excretion; therefore, it is a less reliable test, especially because of the potential failure to observe radionuclide in the gut after small quantities of radiolabeled rose bengal traverse hypoplastic bile ducts. Similarly, the PIPIDA scan can also be misinterpreted because biliary secretion of conjugated imidodiacetic acid may be markedly decreased in the presence of hypoplastic ducts or damage to the hepatocyte canalicular membrane.[92, 99] Visual inspection of duodenal fluid has recently been recommended as an effective method to differentiate ductal and hepatocellular cholestasis and may prove to be a reliable indicator of bile duct patency.[77] An *ultrasound* examination can display the gallbladder, but the sensitivity of sonography must be improved before the narrow or normal bile ducts of infants can be reliably visualized by this technique.

The following *special laboratory tests* may help suggest the diagnosis of ductal cholestasis: Serum 5′-nucleotidase, more specific and sensitive for hepatobiliary disease than alkaline phosphatase, is reported to be significantly increased with active bile duct proliferation and associated bile salt retention; normal values average 4.0 units/L; those in hepatitis 14 IU/L, and those in biliary atresia, 58.5 IU/L. Serum lipoprotein-X, an abnormal low-density lipoprotein of cholestasis, decreases in the serum after the patient with hepatocellular cholestasis is primed with cholestyramine because bile acids are preferentially synthesized by the liver (after loss in the gut lumen) rather than lipoproteins; increased serum lipoprotein-X[101] presumably occurs in the infant with a nonpatent biliary tree because of progression of disease and inability of bile acids to pass to the intestines for binding with cholestyramine.[96] Serum

alpha-fetoprotein, a developmental protein similar to albumin, is usually greater than 35 μg per ml in infants with hepatocellular cholestasis.[52] In contrast, serum concentrations of less than 10 μ per ml suggest the diagnosis of biliary atresia or other types of ductal cholestasis. Finally, the usefulness of serum bile acid concentrations for infants with cholestasis will increase with greater availability of techniques for their measurement, especially the sulfated secondary bile acid, lithocholic acid.[54, 84] Secretory IgA is increased in the serum.[76] Gamma glutamyl transpeptidase may separate patients with atresia from those with other forms of liver disease. Mean levels in hepatitis are 183 ± 54 IU/L; in biliary atresia, 760 ± 492 IU/L; and in alpha$_1$-antitrypsin deficiency, 1725 ± 921 IU/L. Levels over 300 IU/L identified 6 of 7 infants with atresia.[112b]

The *liver biopsy* is an important part of the work-up for biliary atresia, although the rate of diagnostic error with percutaneous or operative liver biopsy is significant.[80] If the accumulated data suggest complete biliary obstruction, then operative cholangiogram should be performed immediately. An equivocal diagnostic work-up demands prompt medical therapy for two weeks with cholestyramine and phenobarbital in an effort to enhance bile flow and obviate the need for surgery. In this situation, careful follow-up is essential, including serial laboratory tests and repeat liver biopsy, with reconsideration of laparotomy because of persistently abnormal tests and undefined cholestasis.

Treatment. The Kasai portoenterostomy is used for the surgical treatment of biliary atresia.[51, 51a, 55, 60, 70a, 88] This procedure for "noncorrectable" biliary atresia usually requires the presence of patent intrahepatic bile ducts ($> 150 \mu$) if successful resumption of bile flow is to be expected.[63] However, bile flow has been demonstrated in a few infants with no histologic evidence for bile ducts at the porta hepatis (Fig. 14–6).[72] Surgery should be performed before the infant reaches three months of age to maximize the opportunity for bile drainage and to allow surgery in an infant with ongoing liver damage and lower portal venous pressures.[69, 97]

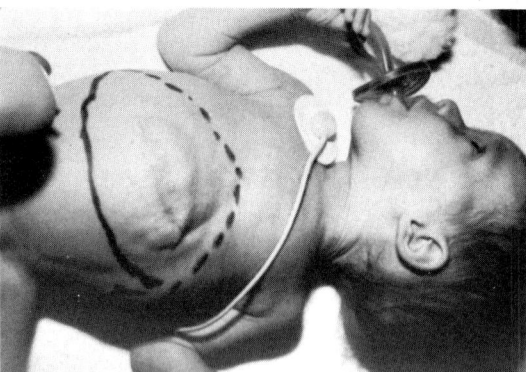

Figure 14–6 A three-month-old infant after porto-enterostomy for biliary atresia.

In spite of adequate postoperative bile drainage, it is now recognized that many patients with noncorrectable biliary atresia develop recurrent cholangitis and progressive cirrhosis with portal hypertension, ascites, and esophageal varices. Obviously, persistent hepatocellular dysfunction may be as important as postoperative bile drainage in these patients, and infants with advanced cirrhosis and portal hypertension are not helped by the portoenterostomy surgery. The "correctable" type of biliary atresia is more amenable to surgical correction because the most common lesion is cystic dilatation of the ducts adjacent to the liver hilus, but long-term survivors after porto-enterostomy are infrequently reported.[56] Those who have established drainage and subsequently decreased their bile flow often benefit from reoperation with curettage.[108b]

Prognosis. The prognosis for infants with biliary atresia correlates with expert surgical treatment performed by surgery teams interested in biliary microsurgery. The operative management of biliary atresia has recently been reviewed, and the results suggest a better outlook for the future. In the best Japanese units, bile drainage is reported in almost 90 per cent of patients and the five-year survival rate is 36 per cent.[49, 50, 105] In North America, the overall results are less satisfactory but are beginning to approach the success rate reported by Kasai. Hepatic copper, which is elevated, decreases after surgery. Postoperative cholangitis leads to deteriorating liver function; this continues to be a major problem despite surgical advances and occurs in over 50 per cent of successful portoenterostomies.[85, 86] Aminoglycosides and Bactrim are the most suitable antibiotics for treatment because of high biliary levels that are achieved. All conduits are colonized by colonic flora by one month. Liver transplantation is the only opportunity for survival for many patients with end-stage liver disease.[98] In one large series of children with liver replacement, biliary atresia was the most common indication for operation and the one-year survival has been 62 per cent since 1976.[108] The average life expectancy for infants with untreated biliary atresia is between 16 and 19 months. Cholestyramine in dosage of 1 gm administered four times daily is effective in relieving pruritus. Intramuscular vitamin K, water-soluble vitamins, and medium-chain triglycerides serve as nutritional supplements.

Biliary Hypoplasia

Etiology. Cessation of bile flow can occur in infants with hepatocellular cholestasis. This is poorly understood, but it has been shown that inflamed bile ductules, which make a network around larger bile ducts, gradually become obliterated, with subsequent decrease in flow of bile. If diminution of bile flow persists, progressive intrahepatic biliary hypoplasia (small, patent ducts) may develop. This dynamic pathologic process can potentially lead to an absolute decrease in number (paucity) or complete disappearance of bile ducts (atresia). Intrahepatic biliary hypoplasia, paucity of the intrahepatic bile ducts, and intrahepatic biliary atresia are clinical terms that are used interchangeably. Obviously, they are different anatomic entities and may be associated with extrahepatic biliary atresia.

Hypoplastic intrahepatic ducts are found in children with the arteriohepatic dysplasia syndrome; these infants with familial cholestasis have associated cardiovascular disorders (peripheral pulmonic stenosis), osseous abnormalities (vertebral arch defects), mental retardation, and characteristic facies (prominent forehead, hypertelorism). Antitrypsin deficiency is another inherited disease with a high incidence of biliary hypoplasia, in addition to a recently described familial cholestatic syndrome in two siblings with an apparent inborn error of cholic acid synthesis. Most important are the acquired infectious insults of the liver, which may lead to hypoplasia of bile ducts and subsequent cholestasis.

Clinical Evaluation and Diagnosis. The clinical course is characterized by early pruritus and later appearance of xanthoma, which are secondary to high serum levels of bile acids and cholesterol, respectively. Otherwise, the course is variable because of different degrees of hypoplasia and hepatocyte damage. Along with identification of specific clinical features, the histologic evaluation of an adequate sample of liver tissue usually confirms the diagnosis. ^{131}I-rose bengal excretion in stool is greater than 10 per cent.

Treatment. Treatment with choleretic agents such as cholestyramine and phenobarbital can dramatically improve the patient's symptoms.

Prognosis. The prognosis is poor if the cholestasis is severe, prolonged, and secondary to an acquired infectious disease, such as that caused by rubella virus. Cirrhosis and portal hypertension appear early in some patients, but in others there may be a lack of development of portal fibrosis until the second decade of life. Overall survival of patients with intrahepatic biliary hypoplasia is longer than for those with extrahepatic biliary atresia; some children will survive beyond the second decade to adulthood.

Choledochal Cyst

Incidence. This is the uncommon form of ductal cholestasis. The estimated incidence is 1 in 13,000 to 1 in 15,000 live births. It is four times more frequent in Japan than elsewhere, and one third of reported cases are in Orientals. Females are affected three to four times more often than males.[104]

Etiology. The etiology is uncertain. It may be a congenital defect secondary to unequal recanalization of bile ducts during late embryogenesis; this perhaps leads to a weakness of the bile duct muscle wall. It has also been suggested that biliary tree damage occurs because of regurgitation of pancreatic enzymes into the common bile duct due to an anomalous junction of the pancreaticobiliary system.[53, 93] The cysts measure 8 to 14 cm in diameter, although they can attain massive proportions with capacities to 8 liters.

Pathology. The cyst walls are composed of dense fibrous connective tissue with little muscle or epithelial lining. When lining is present, it is columnar in type and resembles that of normal bile ducts. Cysts can occur throughout the biliary tract and are single or multiple dilatations involving both extrahepatic and intrahepatic ducts. The gallbladder is always present and usually of normal size, although it may become fibrotic. Depending upon the degree of obstruction, biliary cirrhosis may be found.

Various classifications have been devised to categorize the different cysts according to certain anatomic characteristics. The older classification of anomalies of the extrahepatic tree contains types I, II, and III, which correspond to types A1, A2, and A3 of a more recent classification. The first type, A1, represents a congenital cystic dilatation of the common bile or hepatic duct, which is associated with a normal intrahepatic biliary tree, a dilated tract above the dilatation, a sharp beginning and end of the dilatation, and a narrowing of the common bile duct. The cystic dilatation begins proximally at the level of the cystic duct and rarely extends into the wall of the duodenum. The second type, A_2, a congenital diverticulum of the common bile duct, is rare and arises laterally from the wall of the common duct. The biliary tree is otherwise normal and only slightly dilated. A third type, A_3, is also rare and involves the intraduodenal part of the common bile duct and is termed a choledochocele. The common and pancreatic ducts empty from it, and it is lined by duodenal mucosa. Type B includes extrahepatic and intrahepatic dilatation and type C, intrahepatic communicating cysts. Todani et al.[111] in 1977 offered a new system of classification for anomalies of the biliary tree.

I. Common
   A. Choledochal cyst
   B. Segmental dilatation
   C. Diffuse dilatation
II. Diverticulum type in the entire extrahepatic duct
III. Choledochocele
IV. Multiple cysts
   A. In intra- and extrahepatic ducts
   B. In extrahepatic ducts
V. Intrahepatic cysts

Symptoms. Clinical recognition depends upon cyst size and the presence of biliary obstruction. The onset of symptoms may occur at any age. In young infants the symptoms resemble those of neonatal hepatitis or biliary atresia, with prolonged jaundice, acholic stools, and dark urine. Often, a large, firm mass is palpable under the liver edge. If untreated, jaundice may subside gradually, only to recur intermittently. One of our patients had, by 18 months of age, seen three dermatologists for treatment of pruritus for four months before mild icterus developed.

In older children, colicky epigastric pain, nausea, and vomiting are major complaints, and jaundice is not always present. In most, careful palpation will reveal a mass under the right costal margin. The mass may even fill the epigastrium and reach to the umbilicus.

Although the classic diagnostic triad is considered to be jaundice, pain, and a right

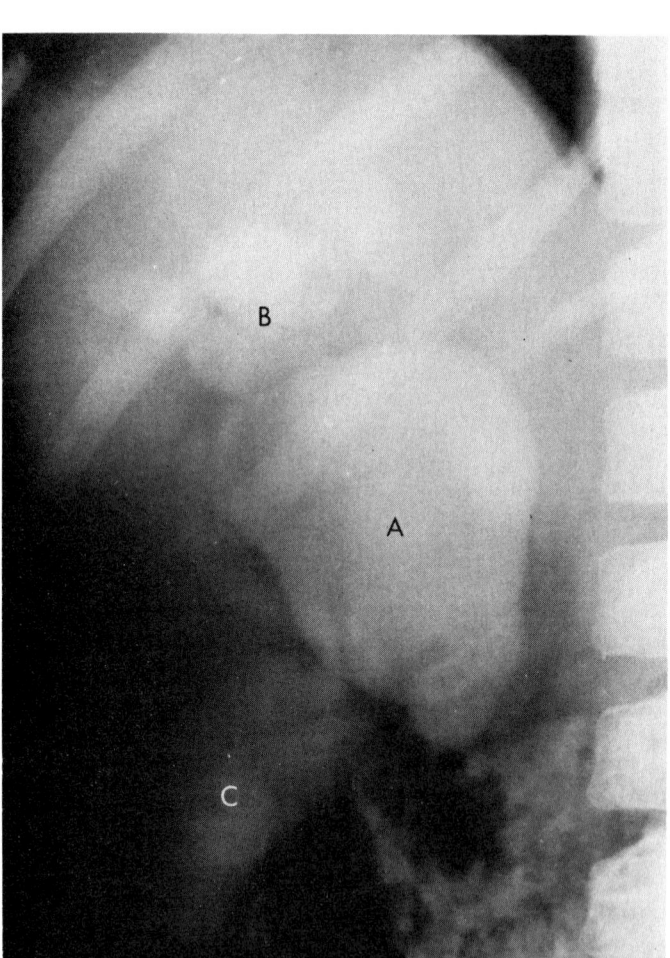

Figure 14–7 Choledochal cyst demonstrated by intravenous cholangiogram in a child with increasing jaundice. The cystic dilatation of the hepatic duct is marked *A*. Dilated hepatic ducts within the liver are marked *B*. *C* indicates a normal gallbladder.

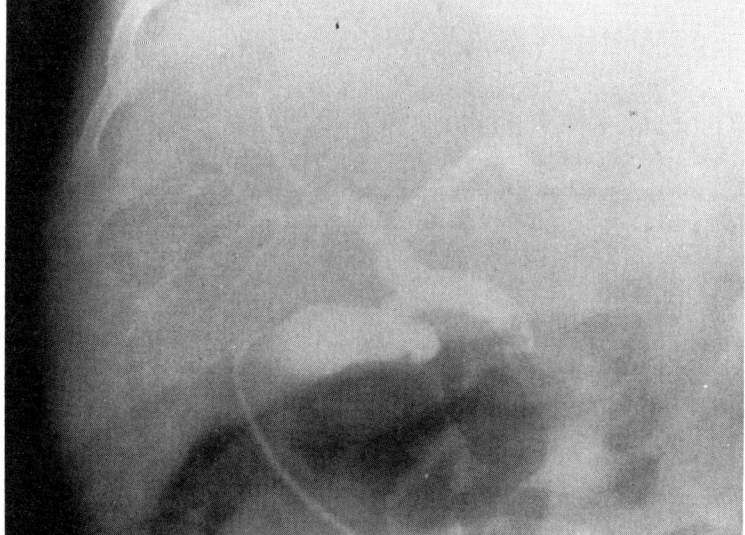

Figure 14–8 Cholangiogram showing distal common bile duct obstruction due to choledochocele adjacent to duodenum. Results of liver biopsy were compatible with a diagnosis of biliary atresia.

upper quadrant mass, all of these signs are present in only 26 per cent of patients. Jaundice alone occurs in 67 per cent, pain in 60 per cent, and mass in 50 per cent. Because the symptoms are intermittent and the cyst periodically decreases in size, the clinical diagnosis may be extremely difficult.

Very rarely, the cyst presents as hematemesis due to esophageal varices that have developed as a result of portal hypertension. An extremely unusual presenting symptom is pancreatitis, which may or may not be due to obstruction of the pancreatic duct.

Diagnosis. Liver function tests are compatible with the diagnosis of biliary obstruction, but there may be mild to moderate elevations of the transaminases. The upper gastrointestinal radiologic examination may show displacement of the proximal duodenum downward and to the left.[103] Cholangiogram may be worthless in the jaundiced patient, but in the nonjaundiced one, dye may visualize a small cyst (Figs. 14–7 and 14–8). In a large cyst, the dye may be so diluted that visualization is blunted. Ultrasonography has proved highly successful in revealing a cystic mass in the biliary tree. A HIDA scan may show a rounded area of absent uptake, which fills later after the agent has been excreted by the liver (Fig. 14–9). Arteriography is of little help, for

these cysts contain few large vessels. Operative cholangiogram at the time of surgery will define the cystic structure and its relation to the biliary tree.

Complications. Biliary cirrhosis and portal hypertension develop from prolonged extrahepatic obstruction in untreated cases, but are relieved after surgery. Hematemesis from varices may appear as early as two and one-half years of age. Occasionally, calculi develop within the cyst. An extremely rare complication is cyst rupture after trauma, infection, or necrosis

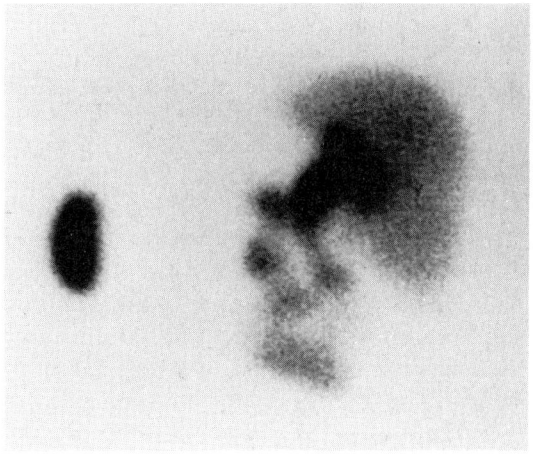

Figure 14–9 HIDA scan of the liver showing (*left*) filling defect in the liver and (*right*) residual agent remaining in the choledochal cyst after the bulk of material had been excreted by the liver.

of the wall. A late and serious complication is the development of adenocarcinoma within the cyst.

Treatment. Complete excision of the cyst followed by choledochojejunostomy is the treatment of choice.[89,90] Choledocho-cyst-jejunostomy should not be performed because of a high risk of cholangitis. Simple aspiration of the cyst is unacceptable.

Prognosis. Untreated choledochal cyst leads to progressive biliary obstruction and cirrhosis.

SEGMENTAL DILATATION OF THE EXTRAHEPATIC DUCTS

Segmental dilatations of the extrahepatic ducts other than choledochal cysts are infrequently mentioned in textbooks of surgery or gastroenterology, although they are recognized causes of biliary tract disease in infancy and adulthood.

Incidence. Glenn and McSherry[75] reported 15 cases of their own and speculated that well over 500 cases of all types of biliary tract cysts have been reported in the literature. The disease is more common in females than in males.

Etiology. Segmental dilatations probably result from pressure changes in bile ducts in regions where there is maldevelopment of the fibromuscular and subserous layers of the duct wall. Short, intermittent pressure rises, related to periods of increased bile flow, may produce dilatation without obstructive jaundice.

Pathology. All of the 15 patients that Glenn and McSherry studied in detail had segmental dilatation that involved all or part of the extrahepatic tree, and two thirds had involvement of the intrahepatic tree as well. Most had calculi within the gallbladder, common duct, or intrahepatic dilatations. Suppurative cholangitis or hepatic abscess often complicated the disease. Microscopic examination of the cyst walls revealed absence of subserous or fibromuscular layers.

Symptoms. The onset of symptoms occurred at any time from the early months of life to late adulthood. Signs of biliary tract disease, such as right upper quadrant pain,

fever, and vomiting, were common in all age groups, although jaundice was more common in infants than in older patients. A mass was often palpated in the right upper quadrant.

Diagnosis. Oral or intravenous cholangiography will usually define a cystic dilatation in the larger extrahepatic ducts, but operative cholangiography must be performed to determine abnormalities within the intrahepatic ductal system.

Treatment. If cholangitis or hepatic abscess is present, the first line of treatment is surgical drainage of the biliary tree, and correction of the underlying lesion is deferred. Excision of the cysts is the ideal therapeutic procedure. If this is not possible, cystoduodenostomy will accomplish drainage in many cases and cystojejunostomy with Roux-en-Y anastomosis will accomplish decompression of the biliary tract when there is extensive intrahepatic and extrahepatic disease.

Prognosis. Long-term follow-up is not available in most of these patients; second operations for recurrent cholangitis and cholelithiasis will be required in many cases.

CONGENITAL SEGMENTAL DILATATIONS OF THE INTRAHEPATIC BILIARY TREE

Congenital segmental dilatations of the intrahepatic tree occur as two types: simple dilatation, otherwise known as Caroli's disease, and another type associated with periportal fibrosis.[61]

Caroli's Disease

This form of simple dilatation of the intrahepatic tree is characterized by segmental, usually saccular, dilatation of the intrahepatic bile ducts.

Incidence. Between 15 and 20 cases had been reported in the literature to 1973, mainly in adults, and since that time the disease has been recognized in young children and even infants.

Etiology. The disease is considered due

to a congenital hypoplasia of the fibromuscular, subserosal, and submucosal components of the duct wall. Inheritance is probably of an autosomal recessive type affecting mostly males. It may be associated with hepatic fibrosis.

Pathology. The liver is only moderately enlarged, and the surface, which has a spongy, pitting feel to the finger, contains no visible cystic lesions. Large rather than small ducts are most involved in the segmental ectasia, with dilated and rounded superficial ducts measuring between 10 and 45 mm in diameter. The deeper dilatations are separated by stretches of normal ducts, and some appear ovoid. Unlike the cysts of polycystic disease, all cysts contain bile. Liver biopsy shows a normal lobular parenchyma with small portal tracts that contain only a single biliary tract, one or two small veins, and one or two arteries. Sclerosis is minimal, and there is no inflammatory change. The larger portal tracts, which are not reached by the biopsy needle, show ectasia of the biliary canals, which are lined by a hyperplastic and folded cylindric epithelium. The tunica externa contains masses of adenomatous biliary glands.

Two associated diseases are cystic spongiosis of the renal medulla, in which the renal cysts are usually not clinically significant, and cystic disease of the pancreas.

Pathophysiology. The bile contains low concentrations of pigment and bile salts but normal or increased levels of electrolytes; the bile from one patient contained urobilinoids and biliverdin but no bilirubin. One study has shown the bile volume to be greatly increased to 2400 to 2900 ml per day, as compared with normal excretions of 700 to 1200 ml per day.

Symptoms. The time of onset can vary from birth to middle age. The symptoms resemble those of ascending cholangitis with a history of spiking fevers, mild or no jaundice, cramping abdominal pain, and tenderness in the right upper quadrant. Patients may be symptom-free for years between attacks. Sepsis is one of the more common causes of death. Young children with extensive cyst formation may have failure to thrive secondary to malabsorption. Rarely, the young child may have fevers of unknown origin for one to two years before

the cause is localized to the liver. A few may have hepatomegaly, steatorrhea, and failure to thrive.

Diagnosis. The disease is usually confused with cholecystitis or liver abscess, and the diagnosis is rarely made preoperatively. The laboratory findings are not diagnostic and show an elevated alkaline phosphatase value and usually normal liver function. Cholangiography usually shows stones within the intrahepatic ducts as well as dilated hepatic and common ducts and low-density shadows over the liver parenchyma, which are most frequent near the liver surface. Arteriography demonstrates a chessboard pattern of rounded, air-filled cavities. Scanning with technetium-99m shows loss of interlobular uptake, and ultrasonography may detect dilated ducts.[70b] The technique of "skinny needle" transhepatic cholangiography has proved a particularly effective diagnostic tool for demonstrating saccular dilatations of the intrahepatic ducts (Fig. 14-10).

Complications. Intracavitary lithiasis is the most important complication and predisposes these patients to obstruction, cholangitis, and other infections, such as liver abscess, subphrenic abscess, pericarditis, and sepsis. If hepatic fibrosis is also present, hypersplenism and esophageal varices develop within several years.

Treatment. Therapy is unsatisfactory and includes removal of stones when they occur and long-term prophylactic administration of broad-spectrum antibiotics to prevent cholangitis. Analgesics and antispasmodics may provide some relief of pain during the acute attacks. Operation is of little help because the lesions are too high for surgical correction. A new technique of transhepatic decompression of the biliary tree has provided drainage.[112a] Rarely, if the disease is limited to one lobe, partial hepatectomy is attempted. Choledochal-jejunal anastomosis, if possible, decreases stasis and facilitates the evacuation of calculi. Urinary tract infections must be treated promptly.

Prognosis. If infection can be controlled, these patients without evidence of hepatic fibrosis survive well into adult life because they do not have cirrhosis and portal hypertension.

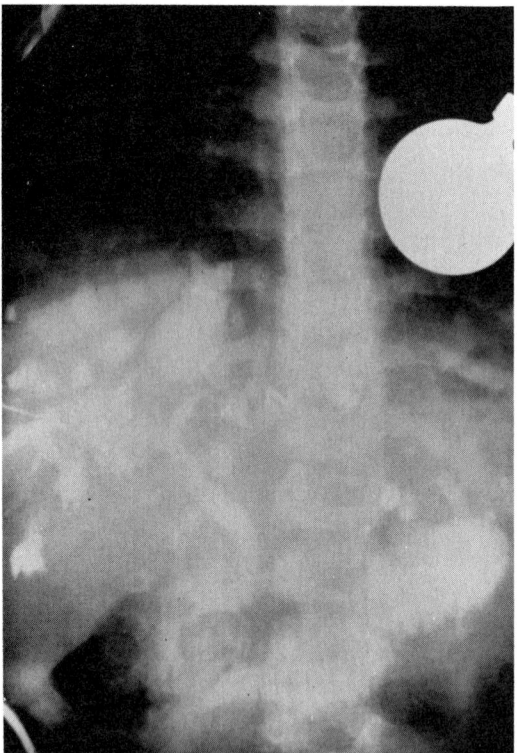

Figure 14–10 Transhepatic cholangiogram in a three-year-old male with Caroli's disease. Massive saccular dilatations within the liver represent dilated intrahepatic ducts.

SEGMENTAL DILATATION OF THE INTRAHEPATIC BILIARY TREE AND PORTAL HYPERTENSION

This form of the disease, associated with periportal fibrosis, is more common than the simple form and is usually seen in children. Much of the information is derived from necropsy reports because it is usually fatal.

Incidence. Although this form is more common than the simple one, its exact incidence is unknown. That both forms may occur within the same family indicates a recessive autosomal inheritance, with some predilection for males.

Etiology. The etiology is similar to that for the simple form.

Pathology. The liver is enlarged and hard, and there is no evidence of regenerating nodules with this form of cirrhosis. There is a great deal of fibrosis with particular involvement of the portal areas, where there is hyperplasia of the small dilated biliary branches. It is the ectasia and hyperplasia of these smaller branches that cause portal hypertension, splenomegaly, and esophageal varices. Changes in the larger ducts resemble those seen in the simple form. Infantile renal medullary spongiosis is an associated finding in most cases.

Symptoms. Signs of portal hypertension are the major manifestations of this disease. Hepatosplenomegaly, hypersplenism and anemia, esophageal varices, and upper gastrointestinal hemorrhage appear at any time from infancy through childhood. Cholangitis is encountered less often.

Prognosis. These patients usually die in late childhood from hematemesis or liver failure.

CONGENITAL HEPATIC FIBROSIS

Congenital hepatic fibrosis is a relatively silent form of liver disease that is recognized only after portal hypertension and esophageal varices become symptomatic.

Incidence. Fewer than 200 patients have been reported.

Etiology. Nearly half of the cases are familial, and the others, sporadic. Half involve only the liver, and the others are associated with polycystic disease of the kidneys. The etiology is unknown, but it may represent one end of the spectrum of Caroli's disease.

Pathology. The liver grossly resembles that of cirrhosis, being firm and nodular. Interlobular bile ducts are abnormal, and connective tissue is strikingly increased. Hepatic architecture in areas unaffected by fibrosis is relatively normal. The fibrous bands in the liver vary from 100 to 1000 μ and occasionally form a continuous network enclosing liver cell masses. Hyperplastic bile ducts are often present, and the portal veins in triads are decreased, hypoplastic, or compressed. Indeed, the portal hypertension is thought to result from a congenital paucity of the small intrahepatic portal venous branches.

The most common renal lesion is a fusiform or cystic dilatation of tubules, especially in the collecting systems. The tubules are apparently part of the functioning nephrons, since they fill during intravenous pyelography. The appearance is described as renal tubular ectasia or medullary sponge kidney.

Symptoms. There is no preceding history of liver disease until hepatomegaly or splenomegaly or both are noted on routine physical examination. The first symptoms may be upper gastrointestinal bleeding or signs of hypersplenism or urinary tract infection.

Diagnosis. The disease must be differentiated from polycystic disease of the liver. Liver function tests are normal or only minimally deranged. Mild anemia, leukopenia, and thrombocytopenia reflect hypersplenism. The hepatic wedge pressures are normal or only slightly elevated, and hepatic scan shows a homogeneous uptake of isotope. Intravenous pyelography is indicated because the combination of portal hypertension and medullary sponge kidney virtually establishes the diagnosis. This is confirmed by liver biopsy.

Complications. The complications are those of portal hypertension and recurrent renal infection and sepsis. Renal function remains normal.

Treatment. Treatment is symptomatic for urinary infection and for portal hypertension. If splenectomy must be performed for hypersplenism, a splenorenal shunt should be constructed at the time.

Prognosis. Shunt surgery is quite successful because of normal hepatocellular function.

POLYCYSTIC LIVER

Polycystic disease of the liver is usually not diagnosed until later in life, if at all. It is of practical importance as an incidental liver biopsy finding in children.

Incidence. The incidence varies from 0.07 to 0.6 per cent of autopsies.

Etiology. The cysts represent an embryologic maldevelopment due to a failure of involution of excess embryonic intrahepatic bile ducts. They are associated in half the cases with other cystic lesions in the kidneys, spleen, lungs, and pancreas and with cerebral aneurysms.

Pathology. The cysts vary in number from a few to many and in size from microscopic to those containing up to a quart of fluid. Hepatic tissue between the lesions is

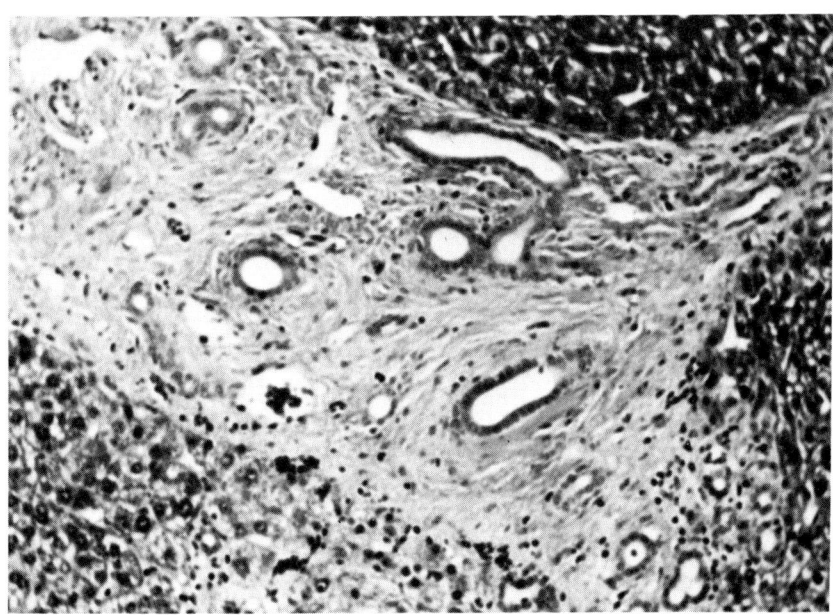

Figure 14–11 Meyenburg complex. Fibrous connective tissue encases large lymphatics and bile ducts. There is a very sharp dividing line between the complex and the liver parenchyma.

normal. Clusters of small bile ducts, known as Meyenburg complexes, are present in the liver lobules separate from the portal triads. These are considered to represent persisting intrahepatic bile ducts that embryologically connect the bile canaliculi and the interlobular bile ducts in the portal septa (Fig. 14–11). Gradual cystic dilatation of these residual ducts ultimately results in the formation of a polycystic liver.

Symptoms. The disease is usually asymptomatic and is diagnosed as an incidental finding in a surgical procedure. Occasionally a large cyst may cause pain or jaundice. In a few cases a large cyst may be palpable; when it is, the liver is not tender.

Diagnosis. Liver function tests are normal, but radiologic examination of the upper gastrointestinal tract or the biliary tree may show evidence of extrinsic compression by a large cyst. Liver scan may show many filling defects within the hepatic parenchyma.

Complications. Infection within a cyst may cause tenderness and fever, and hemorrhage into or rupture of the cyst can cause signs of peritonitis.

Treatment. No treatment is necessary for the disease itself, although its complications require specific surgical therapy.

Prognosis. The prognosis is excellent, for hepatic function usually remains normal.

AGENESIS OF THE GALLBLADDER

Agenesis of the gallbladder has been reported in association with agenesis of the pancreas.

DUPLICATIONS OF THE BILIARY TRACT AND GALLBLADDER

The term "double (or accessory) gallbladder" is applied to the situation in which two or more gallbladders are present.[48] Duplication refers to abortive embryonic rests, representing incomplete structures that are attached to an otherwise normal, hollow organ. Such structures are usually nonfunctional.

Incidence. Only three cases of true duplication of the biliary tract or gallbladder had been reported to 1972.

Etiology. The etiology is the same as for other enteric duplications.

Pathology. The duplications are usually lined with the same mucosa as that of the area of the duplication, although some are lined with gastric or duodenal mucosa. These duplications may involve the hepatic ducts, the biliary tree in the region of the common bile duct, and the gallbladder.

Symptoms. The symptoms reported have been recurrent abdominal pain, intestinal obstruction, and melena. One infant had feeding difficulties and pain from the time of birth. Jaundice is occasionally observed; gastrointestinal bleeding due to hematobilia from peptic ulceration of the biliary mucosa is an unusual complication. The abdomen is tender in the right upper quadrant, and the liver may be enlarged. A soft mass of variable size is palpable in the right upper quadrant.

Diagnosis. The diagosis is usually not made preoperatively, for the lesion is usually confused with cholangitis or choledochal cyst. The serum bilirubin and transaminase values may be elevated, and the gallbladder does not fill in oral or intravenous cholangiography.

Treatment. The reported patients have been successfully treated by removal of the duplication and closure of the duct.

INHERITED CHOLESTATIC JAUNDICE SYNDROMES

BENIGN RECURRENT CHOLESTASIS[71, 112]

This is the least severe of the cholestatic syndromes and is unassociated with any true parenchymal liver disease. It was originally described in 1959 as a new syndrome characterized by intermittent jaundice often appearing during the first year or two of life. Several variations of the disease have been subsequently reported.

Incidence. Approximately 50 cases have been described. Initially all those affected were males from the Faroe Islands who claimed to be related to each other. Although males predominate, the disease does occur in females and is reported in siblings.[47] An autosomal form of transmission has been suggested for the familial form of the disease.

Etiology. The cause is unknown, although a defect in the uptake of organic anions, such as bile acids, has been discovered in those with nonfamilial benign disease. In the familial form, hepatic uptake of some organic anions (e.g., indocyanine green) may be normal or increased.[71, 112]

Pathology. During periods of remission, the liver biopsy is usually normal, although some intercanalicular bile pigment may remain. Tissue obtained during exacerbations shows centrilobar bile stasis and now specific round cell infiltration in the portal areas. Intracellular vesicles have been noted.

Symptoms. Episodes of cholestasis begin as early as one year of age or as late as adult life. Attacks occur every three to four months or every several years and consist of jaundice, pruritus, and passage of light stools and dark urine. Abdominal pain, when it occurs, is usually epigastric and, rarely, pancreatitis complicates the picture. Between attacks, the patients are well and liver function returns to normal.

Physical examination during a symptomatic period reveals only jaundice and cutaneous excoriations. The liver is not enlarged or only moderately so.

Diagnosis. During an attack, the serum bilirubin may rise to 10 to 20 mg per dl, with the major contribution from the conjugated fraction. BSP storage and transport maximum are decreased, and alkaline phosphatase, alpha-2 and beta globulins, and serum bile acids are increased. The SGOT is normal or mildly elevated. Studies of unconjugated bilirubin clearance from plasma are conflicting, with normal rates reported in some patients and extremely rapid rates in others.

Treatment. Cholestyramine may relieve the pruritus, although phenobarbital improves bile acid excretion more effectively.

Prognosis. The clinical course of the disease is benign, and biliary cirrhosis has never been reported.

FAMILIAL INTRAHEPATIC CHOLESTATIC SYNDROMES

This terminology represents several syndromes that are quite disparate and require separate discussion for an understanding not only of the underlying pathophysiology but also of the course and eventual outcome of disease (Table 14–3).[60, 62, 71, 81]

LYMPHEDEMA AND RECURRENT INTRAHEPATIC CHOLESTASIS (NORWEGIAN CHOLESTASIS)[107]

This syndrome, extremely rare, is considered a variant of benign recurrent cholestasis.

Incidence. This disease has been reported in 16 patients in seven families, most of Norwegian extraction.

Etiology. It is postulated that the cholestasis is a result of congenital anomalies of the lymphatic system and of the intrahepatic lymphatics.

Pathology. The liver tissue shows intrahepatic cholestasis and, often, giant cell transformation. At times, there is periportal fibrosis and progression to cirrhosis.

Symptoms. Cholestasis is apparent shortly after birth, and jaundice persists for up to seven years. Hepatomegaly is prominent in the infant. The stools become light and foul-smelling, and growth retardation results from malabsorption. Pedal edema is usually not noted until five or six years of age and becomes progressively worse, occasionally associated with lymphangitis. After a number of years, cholestasis subsides and growth resumes.

The condition may reappear periodically in adult life, precipitated by pregnancy, anesthesia, or infection.

Diagnosis. The laboratory findings are those of obstructive jaundice. The liver biopsy is in no way diagnostic for the dis-

Table 14–3 Differential Characteristics of Cholestatic Disorders

	BENIGN RECURRENT CHOLESTASIS	ARTERIOHEPATIC DYSPLASIA	BYLER SYNDROME	THCA SYNDROME	NORWEGIAN CHOLESTASIS	INTRAHEPATIC BILIARY ATRESIA
Familial	±	+	+	+	+	−
Early death	−	−	+		+	+
Benign liver disease	+	+	−	−	±	−
Cirrhosis	−	−	+late	+	−	+
Jaundice	episodic	clears	persistent	may clear	episodic	persistent
Onset	1 yr.	neonate	1–12 mo.	neonate	neonate	neonate
Other organs	−	heart extremities eyes ± retardation	clubbing areflexia retardation	clubbing eyes	lymphatics areflexia	−
Inheritance	autosomal recessive in some	autosomal dominant	autosomal recessive	autosomal recessive	autosomal recessive	−
Laboratory findings						
Alkaline phosphatase	↑ in attacks	↑ 150–250	↑ 95–150	sl↑	sl↑	↑
SGOT	nl	sl↑	nl	nl	↑	sl↑ (<500)
Cholesterol	nl	↑	↑↓	↑ THCA	↑	↑
Bile acids	nl	↑↓	↑↓	↓ cholate	−	↑
BSP Tm	↓ in attacks					

order, but the lymphangiogram is abnormal, showing numerous collaterals, back flow, and delayed clearance of dye. Rarely, the lymphatics are normal.

Treatment. Therapy is limited to diuretics for edema, cholestyramine or phenobarbital for pruritus, and medium-chain triglycerides for improvement of fat malabsorption.

Prognosis. Many patients live on as adults, although those with cirrhosis die relatively early.

ARTERIOHEPATIC DYSPLASIA

This disorder was first recognized three decades ago but was given its name in 1973 by Watson and Muller. It has been described in further detail by Alagille[49] and by Riely.[100]

Incidence. Although considered quite rare, six patients with this syndrome have been seen at the Yale–New Haven Medical Center in the last decade, one of whom, an adult, had been considered to have inoperable biliary atresia as an infant. Better recog-

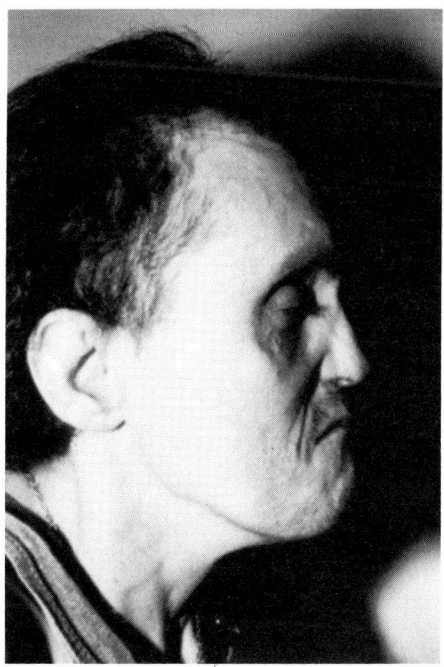

Figure 14–12 Father of a baby with arteriohepatic dysplasia who was diagnosed in infancy as having intrahepatic biliary atresia. (Courtesy of C. Riely, M.D.)

nition of the characteristic facies will undoubtedly lead to increases in diagnosis (Fig. 14–12).

Etiology. In two patients, autosomal dominant transmission has been demonstrated; in one, transmission was from father to son.

Pathology and Pathophysiology. The liver biopsy shows cholestasis and a paucity of intrahepatic bile ducts. The disease does not progress to cirrhosis. Anomalies are present in other organs. The face is atypical, with broad forehead, small maxilla, and pointed chin; cardiac anomalies are associated with peripheral pulmonary stenosis. Osseous anomalies include butterfly vertebrae, shortened ulna, and decreased interpedicular distances in the lumbar spine; the hands are small and the fingers short. In the eyes are anterior chamber anomalies (posterior embryotoxon), choroidal degeneration, and retinal lesions. Delayed motor development and disordered personality may be evident. Renal function studies often show decreased creatine clearance and hyperuricemia.

Symptoms. The neonate demonstrates jaundice of a cholestatic type. By four months, signs of pruritus are noted as excoriations over cheeks and trunk. After about four years the jaundice clears, although xanthomas may develop. The children are essentially asymptomatic from their liver disease, but cardiac problems dominate.

Diagnosis. Laboratory studies show hyperbilirubinemia, predominantly of the conjugated form, hypercholesterolemia, and increased levels of alkaline phosphatase, SGOT, and 5′-nucleotidase. Bile acids are elevated but normal in type.[68] Type II hyperlipoproteinemia is present. In later life, although bilirubin values are normal, the $BSPT_m$ is decreased and liver biopsy shows cholestasis and few intrahepatic bile ducts.

Treatment. Phenobarbital has not proved very effective in ameliorating jaundice and pruritus.

Prognosis. Those patients without severe cardiac disease may live into adult life.

PROGRESSIVE INTRAHEPATIC CHOLESTASIS (BYLER SYNDROME)

This more serious form of intrahepatic cholestasis was described in 1965 in an Amish kindred.[64, 70]

Incidence. The disease is extremely rare but has been reported in patients from the Orient and Europe as well as the United States.

Inheritance. Inheritance is of an autosomal recessive type.

Etiology. It is suggested that the disease is due to a primary secretory failure at the biliary canaliculus; this therapy is supported by the finding of canalicular membrane defects identified by electron microscopy.

Pathology. The liver biopsy may show a paucity of intrahepatic bile ducts, with bile stasis most marked in the centrilobular regions. There is a mild, mononuclear infiltrate in the portal triads, normal hepatic architecture, and a normal extrahepatic biliary tree. Unlike the syndromes discussed previously, the changes progress to cirrhosis. In a few patients, increased serum litholiolic acid has been reported. Multiple system involvement is represented by mental and physical retardation, areflexia, and digital clubbing.

Symptoms. Malabsorption may be the first symptom of disease, with jaundice and pruritus appearing between several months and one year of age. Although the pruritus is intense, the jaundice does not progress in intensity and, indeed, may fluctuate. The abdomen becomes progressively enlarged, and the liver and spleen are palpable. Rickets is a frequent sequela of fat malabsorption and is often accompanied by vitamin K deficiency. Kayser-Fleischer rings have been noted in those with long-standing disease.

Meconium peritonitis was a unique presentation in one patient who had increasingly elevated sweat chloride with age, and no evidence of cystic fibrosis. Another group of patients had thick skin, prominent eyes, short fingers and toes, and convex nails.

Diagnosis. The serum conjugated bilirubin and bile acids are always elevated, and the prothrombin time is often prolonged. Transaminases and alpha and beta globulins are only modestly elevated. Alkaline phosphatase and 5'-nucleotidase values are increased. Cholesterol and gamma globulin levels are characteristically normal.

The $BSPT_m$ is markedly decreased (less than 1 mg/min), and abnormal transport has been reported in the fathers of two patients and in two pregnant mothers. The cholangiogram may show a normal or dilated extrahepatic tree but an attenuated intrahepatic one; ^{131}I-rose bengal excretion in the stool is usually greater than 20 per cent. The quantitative fecal fat is increased and serum dihydroxy and trihydroxy bile salts are increased.

Treatment. Malabsorption is treated with a medium-chain triglyceride supplemented diet and double-dose water-soluble vitamins. Phenobarbital in dosage of 6 mg per kg per day lowers serum bilirubin and decreases pruritus but does not affect serum bile acids.

THE THCA SYNDROME

This cholestatic syndrome is characterized by high levels of [3, 7, 12 trihydroxy-5 β-cholestan-26-orc acid] (THCA) in the bile and serum. It was reported in two siblings who developed progressive intrahepatic cholestasis in the neonatal period and died by two years of age. Growth retardation, retinal degeneration, and rickets were associated findings. An autosomal recessive inheritance is presumed, and defective metabolism of trihydroxycoprostamic acid to cholic acid has been shown. The liver biopsy shows a paucity of bile ducts and, eventually, cirrhosis. Phenobarbital has proven ineffective in treating the jaundice.

OTHER SYNDROMES

A cholestatic syndrome has been described in two siblings with an apparent inborn error of cholic acid synthesis.[76] Alpha-1-antitrypsin and acquired infectious insults may result in hypoplasia of the bile ducts and cholestasis. Cholestasis associated with peripheral or central hyperalimentation is discussed elsewhere.[55a, 275a]

INFECTIOUS LIVER DISEASE

NEONATAL HEPATITIS

Since neonatal hepatitis represents an infection of the liver during the first three months of life, a variety of causes and manifestations are present. Infectious agents may be introduced to the fetus through the placenta, to the neonate at delivery, or by postnatal exposure.[114, 115] The causes of neonatal hepatitis are listed in Table 14–4.

VIRAL HEPATITIS

At least three and perhaps four forms of traditional viral hepatitis exist: A, B, and one or two types of non-A, non-B.

Hepatitis A (Ha)

This virus has not been associated with disease in the neonate but is the major cause of epidemic hepatitis in young children.[114]

Etiology and Epidemiology. The virus is a 27 nm particle excreted in the stool and present in the blood during viremia. The incubation period is 15 to 40 days: Virus is excreted two to three weeks before jaundice develops and for seven to eight days after.

Table 14–4 Causes of Neonatal Hepatitis

Hepatitis B
Rubella
Coxsackie
Echo II
Adenovirus
Varicella
Epstein-Barr
Herpes
Toxoplasmosis
Cytomegalovirus
Psittacosis
Syphilis
Tuberculosis

Viremia persists from the onset of fecal excretion of virus to two to three days after the onset of jaundice. Epidemics have been attributed to poor sanitation, i.e., fecal material contaminating hands, food, or water provides a source of infection, with shellfish providing a viral reservoir. Transmission may also rarely occur through blood transfusion or contaminated needles.

The virus may be identified by immuno-electron microscopy in stool. Infected serum or stool has produced disease in chimpanzees and monkeys, but the organism has not yet been grown in culture. Antigen (HA Ag) is detected transiently in the serum. Antibody (HA Ab) is detected one to four weeks after the onset of disease using complement-fixation and immune adherence techniques. Peak titers occur weeks later and remain for years. Immunity is permanent.

Pathology. The changes are similar to those described in detail for hepatitis B. Although rare, fulminant hepatitis may be due to the A virus, and severe clotting abnormalities and transient hepatic fibrosis have been reported in anicteric infection.

Hepatitis B (Hb)

This form of hepatitis, long termed serum, or long-incubation, hepatitis, has had over the last decade a variety of antigen classifications. Called the serum hepatitis, or MS_2, antigen, it was for some time termed Australia antigen, after its initial identification in 1963 in an aborigine. Today, a number of antigen-antibody systems are defined for this virus.[115]

Hb_sAg is the surface antigen of the virus, which has five antigenic determinants, a, y, d, w, and z. The antigen is manufactured in the cytoplasm of liver cells and is detectable in 75 to 85 per cent of infected patients for approximately eight weeks during the course of clinical illness. The diagnosis is best made by seroconversion. Within a month after remission of disease, the antigen is barely measurable. However, it persists in chronic carriers, in serum, semen, and breast milk.[118]

Hb_sAb, the antibody to surface antigen, appears at the end of clinical illness and may persist for several years.

Hb_cAg, or core antigen (27 nm in diameter), is the antigen of the core of the Dane particle (42 mn in diameter), the circulating virus; viral replication takes place in the nuclei of hepatocytes. Antigen has been identified in the liver, but not in the serum, during acute infection or in the chronic carrier state.

Hb_cAb, the antibody to core antigen, however, is present in the serum of patients with acute hepatitis before antibody to surface antigen. It persists for seven to eight months. In chronic carriers, titers remain elevated.

Epidemiology. The Hb antigen is present in the blood during acute infection along with the spheroid Dane bodies. Transmission of disease to the infant may be parenteral, through blood products (except albumin and gamma globulin) or infected needles; through the placenta or during delivery by ingestion of contaminated blood or amniotic fluid; or, later, through the oral route. The incubation period is about 8 weeks after parenteral exposure and 12 weeks after exposure by the oral route.

Mothers with active hepatitis during the early months of pregnancy do not deliver infants who develop antigenemia,[136] probably because of transplacental transmission of antibody (Hb_s Ab), which binds antigen and prevents proliferation of the virus *in utero*. The highest risk is to infants whose mothers have active, antigen-positive hepatitis during the last trimester of pregnancy.[150, 158] Fifty to 70 per cent of these receive surface antigen (Hb_s) and may become chronic carriers. The transmission of hepatitis virus from asymptomatic chronic carrier (Hb_s Ag)[114] mothers is not constant and is dependent upon the presence of other antigens or antibodies. Maternal Hb_e Ag is associated with a higher incidence of infant Hb_s Ag and development of chronic liver disease.[142, 152, 162] In contrast, the presence of Hb_e Ab is not usually associated with transmission of disease.[142] Hepatitis has been described in some infants, however, after several months.[120]

Some infants have extremely mild disease but become Hb_s Ag-positive at about two months and remain so for several years.

Administration of hepatitis B immune globulin (0.5 ml/kg initially followed by 0.16 ml/kg monthly for six months) to infants

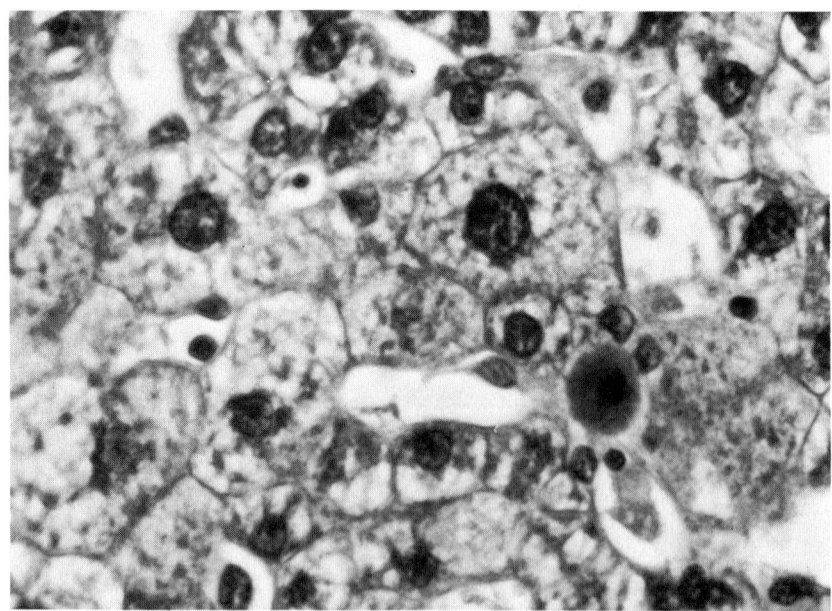

Figure 14–13. Acidophilic body. Cytoplasm is relatively homogeneous and stains bright red with hematoxylin and eosin or with Masson trichrome. The nucleus is pyknotic.

born of Hb$_s$ Ag-positive mothers resulted in no cases of hepatitis and no carriers as compared with a 25 per cent carrier rate in control infants.

Non-A, Non-B Hepatitis

This is one or possibly two forms of hepatitis resembling serum hepatitis (Hb) but in which no antigen or antibody has been identified. Viral particles may be seen, however, in liver cells, and virus-like particles have been found in fibrinogen and in the circulation of apparently healthy blood donors.[135a, 163] These are capable of inducing non-A, non-B hepatitis in humans and chimpanzees after a shorter incubation period than hepatitis B (one to five weeks). Infected serum may transmit the agent four to five weeks after inoculation. These agents are now responsible for more than 80 per cent of transfusion-related infections and liver disease in renal transplant patients,[153, 160] and are also transmitted by Factor VIII concentrates used for patients with congenital coagulation disorders.[116a]

Pathology. Both infectious and serum hepatitis are capable of producing two different and distinct histologic lesions. In the more common "classic" form, necrosis and inflammation are distributed in random fashion through the liver lobule. The necrotic areas consist of acidophilic bodies (Fig. 14–13) and cell dropout (Fig. 14–14), whereas the inflammatory reaction is usually represented by a mixture of lymphocytes, monocytes, and polymorphonuclear leukocytes (Fig. 14–15). Perhaps the best way to understand the distribution of the disease in classic hepatitis is to say that this page is the liver and the distribution of necrosis is what would happen if this book were hit by buckshot from a shotgun. Some areas of necrosis are central, some midzonal, and some portal, but the distribution is throughout and random. When this histologic lesion is seen (Fig. 14–16), one can be assured that the patient will not die of the acute disease and that cirrhosis will never develop.

In about 5 per cent of patients with icteric hepatitis a different histologic pattern develops, in which not only are necrosis and inflammation distributed in a random fashion through the liver lobule but in addition there are intralobular and interlobular bridges of necrosis. These bridges extend

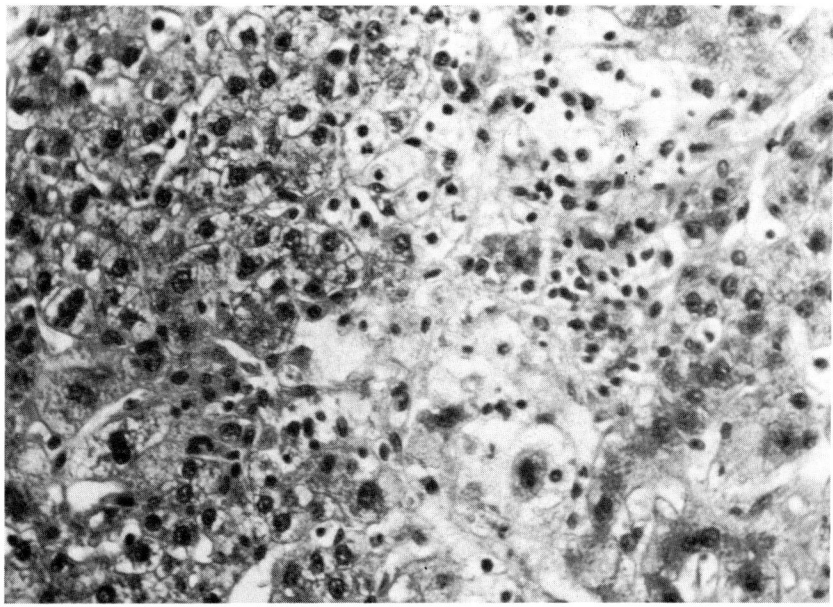

Figure 14–14 Cell dropout in a patient with viral hepatitis. In this area liver cells are seen on the left, but on the right only shells remain. There is a modest inflammatory exudate as well.

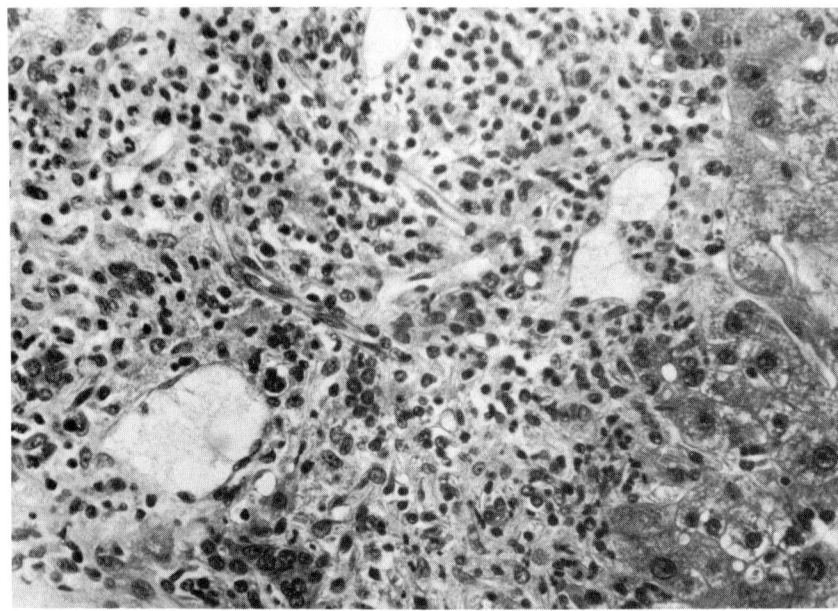

Figure 14–15 Inflammatory reaction. This patient with viral hepatitis has an intense infiltrate in the portal triad, consisting of round cells and polymorphonuclear leukocytes.

between two central veins, between two portal triads, or between a central vein and a portal triad. In other words, the shotgun has gone off again, but so has a machine gun. When this bridging necrosis is seen, the prognosis is entirely different: About 20 per cent of these patients will die of hepatic failure within several months, 30 per cent will have postnecrotic cirrhosis, and only 50 per cent will recover normal liver function. This bridging necrosis is often called sub-

acute hepatic necrosis (SHN), subacute hepatitis, or acute yellow atrophy. There is evidence that when this lesion is secondary to infectious and not serum hepatitis, it tends not to progress to cirrhosis or to cause fetal liver failure. Clinical parameters assist one in differentiating classic hepatitis.

Electron microscopy has demonstrated virus-like particles in liver biopsy tissue of patients with unresolved disease, and hepatitis B antigen-antibody immune complexes

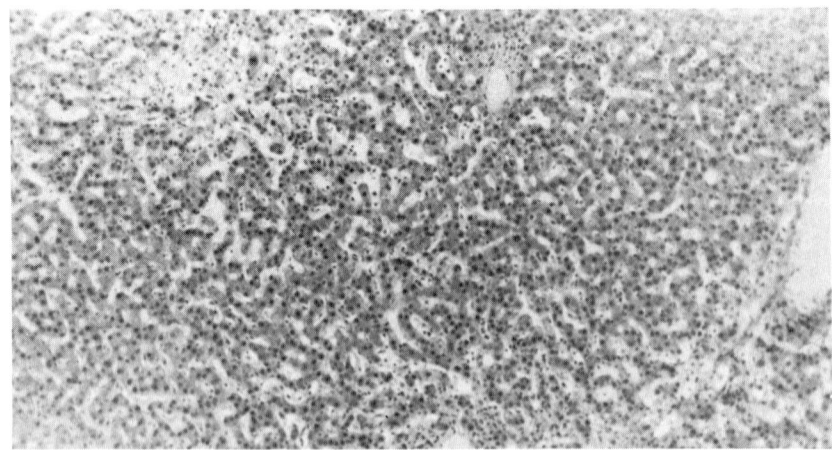

Figure 14–16 Classic hepatitis. Note the random distribution of inflammation and necrosis.

are found in some of the Kuppfer cells during the acute stages of hepatitis.

Symptoms. In both conditions, the onset of the illness can be dated with precision only from the development of jaundice or dark urine. Before these clinical signs develop, however, there are marked changes in hepatic function, and constitutional symptoms may be present. Prospective studies indicate that for every case of icteric viral hepatitis, three to five cases of anicteric disease go undetected clinically.

In the icteric cases, nonspecific constitutional symptoms of generalized fatigue, malaise, and anorexia may occur one to three weeks before jaundice is seen. Muscle pain, morbilliform rash, urticaria, fever, arthralgia, and frank arthritis may also precede the development of jaundice in some cases and are usually associated with hepatitis B. Nausea, vomiting, diarrhea, and abdominal pain, especially in the right upper quadrant and epigastrium, are more common symptoms and herald the onset of jaundice by one to three days. The liver may be tender but is not palpably enlarged. During this period of anicteric disease, the serum transaminase levels may be greatly elevated, indicating severe hepatocellular damage. Indeed, the transaminase level has often reached its peak and is falling at a time when the bilirubin levels are still rising. In patients with serum hepatitis, hepatitis B surface antigen may appear in the serum as early as two months before the onset of jaundice and disappear when the jaundice becomes obvious. The antigen is detectable earlier after parenteral transmission of serum hepatitis than after oral transmission. In the typical case of *icteric viral hepatitis,* serum bilirubin levels rise for up to two weeks after either dark urine or jaundice is clinically evident (jaundice does not become clinically evident until the bilirubin level is above 2 mg per dl). Once the bilirubin level has reached its peak, it may be four weeks before it falls below 2 mg per dl. Indirect hyperbilirubinemia may persist for many months, however, even when the patient is asymptomatic, when liver function tests are normal, and when the histologic picture in the liver has returned to normal.

Most patients with viral hepatitis are reasonably asymptomatic except for mild fatigue within a week after the onset of jaundice. The liver is enlarged and somewhat tender to percussion. Rarely, patients may suffer considerable gastrointestinal distress consisting of persistent nausea and vomiting that results in severe dehydration.

Although the typical course of viral hepatitis as outlined consists of an eight-week illness, there are perhaps more exceptions to this than to the rule of two weeks of anicteric dysfunction, two weeks of increasing jaundice, and two weeks of resolving jaundice. During the period of increasing jaundice, the stools are light, the urine is dark, and the bilirubin and serum transaminase values are elevated. The indirect and direct bilirubin levels are initially increased, but as jaundice clears, the chemical abnormalities return toward normal, the stools regain their color, and the urine lightens. One common variant in the course is the development of cholestatic hepatitis; when this occurs, alkaline phosphatase levels may rise considerably and jaundice may persist for inordinately long periods. In addition, pruritus may become a prominent feature, presumably owing to the retention of bile salts. The degree of cholestasis is correlated with the level of serum bilirubin and the length of time it has been elevated. Coma, ascites, and edema are associated with subacute hepatic necrosis.

Thus far, no distinction can be made between hepatitis A, B, or non-A, non-B in regard to clinical course except for the incubation period. There does appear to be a difference in the severity of the diseases, with long-incubation hepatitis being the most serious condition.[117a] Some patients, especially those with serum hepatitis, may incur a serum sickness–like syndrome, characterized by a macular, measles-like rash, angioneurotic edema, urticaria, arthralgia, and even frank arthritis simulating rheumatoid arthritis. In some of these patients there is a markedly depressed level of serum complement and high titers of hepatitis B surface antigen. This illness is thought to be due to circulating immune complexes containing the hepatitis B surface antigen.

Since viral hepatitis is a systemic disease, pancreatitis, myocarditis, mild nephritis, headache, myalgia, a Guillain-Barré syndrome,[159a] and irritability may all be part of the clinical picture. In fact, diarrhea, abdominal pain, and sore throat are often predominant symptoms of the anicteric phase. One peculiar complication is aplastic anemia, which usually appears after the liver function has returned to normal, and is usually fatal.

A fulminant form of the disease may occur in 0.1 to 0.2 per cent of all cases. Typically, encephalopathy occurs shortly after jaundice appears and within one to three weeks, signs of acute liver failure develop.

Differential Diagnosis. Half of the infants with nonhemolytic jaundice will have some viral hepatitis, and a quarter will have malformations of the bile ducts. The rest will have jaundice due to a variety of causes including sepsis, syphilis, cytomegalic inclusion disease, congenital rubella, toxoplasmosis, cystic fibrosis, galactosemia or alpha-$_1$-antitrypsin deficiency. Both neonatal hepatitis and biliary atresia are common in patients with the D-trisomy and Down's syndrome. If the jaundice is prolonged and there is a picture of obstruction, the distribution changes: More than half the cases are due to biliary atresia, 15 per cent to erythroblastosis, and the rest to a miscellaneous group of disorders including viral hepatitis, which affects half of these remaining patients.

LABORATORY TESTS. The hemoglobin and hematocrit are usually normal, although in a few patients, red blood cell survival is shortened. The total white blood cell count is normal, although there may be leukopenia early in the course of the illness and many of the lymphocytes appear atypical. The erythrocyte sedimentation rate is normal in hepatitis B and increased in other forms.[153] Urinary urobilinogen is increased before and early in the icteric period but disappears as the stools become acholic. There is occasional proteinuria. Bilirubinuria is present early in the disease and disappears as jaundice becomes more apparent. The serum bilirubin shows an early increase in direct bilirubin in the preicteric stage and an increase to usually less than 10 mg per dl total bilirubin during the icteric phase, with elevation of indirect bilirubin as well as of direct.

Measurement of serum transaminase is one of the most popular tests used to follow the progression of viral hepatitis; the level may rise to several thousand units during the acute illness, usually returning to normal as the illness subsides, although some patients may show a secondary rise or a persistence of elevated values for several months. The serum alkaline phosphatase value may be normal or slightly elevated; marked elevations reflect cholestasis or biliary obstruction.

Measurements of alpha-fetoprotein are of assistance in differentiating between neonatal hepatitis and biliary atresia.[160a, 164] Concentrations of 40 mg per dl are found in the serum of infants with hepatitis, but this protein is usually absent from the serum of infants with biliary atresia. Conversely, the 5′-nucleotidase is elevated in infants with biliary atresia and is usually normal in those with hepatitis. The radioactive rose bengal test is used to detect biliary obstruction. In a study of 24 children with chronic hepatitis B infection, IgG bound to liver cells paralleled activity of virus replication, but not the severity of the lesions. Virus persisted in those on immunosuppressive medication.[158a]

LIVER BIOPSY. In neonatal hepatitis the liver biopsy characteristically shows giant cell transformation of hepatocytes (Fig. 14–17), in which several liver cells fuse so that one giant cell contains many nuclei. There are feathery degeneration of the cytoplasm of the liver cells, scattered foci of necrosis and inflammation, cholestasis, and, occasionally, deposition of iron in hepatocytes. Giant cell transformation, previously thought to be specific for hepatitis, may also be seen in biliary atresia as well as in many other forms of liver disease affecting infants. This seems to be, in the neonate, a nonspecific way in which the liver reacts to injury. The hepatic lesions of viral hepatitis that is acquired later in infancy are those described earlier under pathology.

Unfortunately, the liver biopsy is not

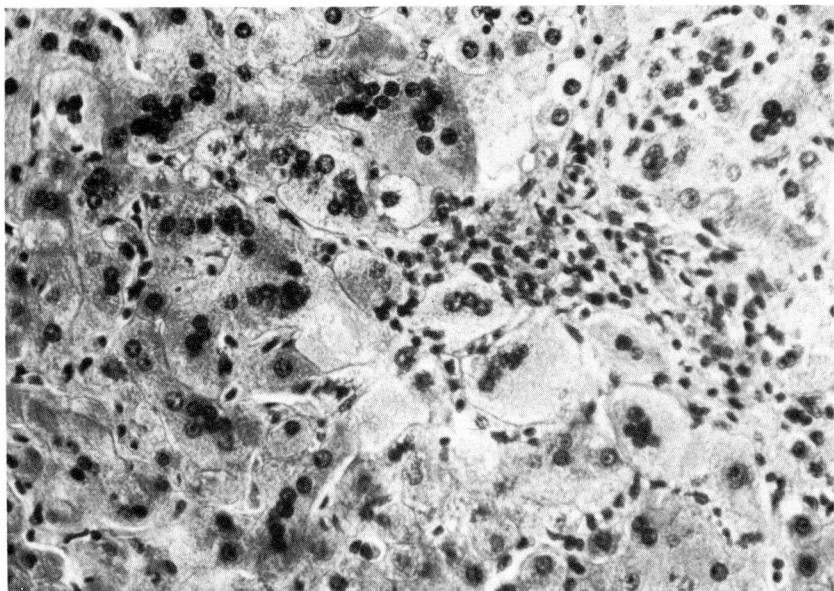

Figure 14–17 Giant cell hepatitis. This infant with viral hepatitis has large, multinucleated hepatocytes. In this section there is also a rather intense inflammatory reaction.

always successful in differentiating atresia from hepatitis, and, under selected circumstances, surgical exploration is necessary. In older infants with hepatitis the indications for biopsy are coma, ascites, an insidious onset, rising bilirubin level for more than two weeks, failure of bilirubin to return to less than 2 mg per dl after ten weeks, prolongation of the prothrombin time more than two or three seconds over normal, low serum albumin, or elevated serum globulin. Bilirubin levels greater than 30 mg per dl or hyperbilirubinemia of longer than two weeks' duration, prolongation of the prothrombin time, and a history of symptoms for more than two weeks before the development of jaundice are suggestive, but not conclusively diagnostic, of bridging necrosis. Subacute hepatic necrosis is also seen in anicteric infections and can progress to cirrhosis without the patient's ever becoming jaundiced. Such patients are detected only incidentally or through prospective epidemiology studies.

Exploratory laparotomy as a diagnostic technique has been employed with caution in infancy, for cirrhosis developed in one third of infants with hepatitis in whom exploration was carried out. A recent retro-spective analysis has shown that nonfamilial sporadic neonatal hepatitis is not adversely affected by surgical exploration. Those infants with the familiar type of idiopathic obstructive neonatal jaundice, however, do have a significant morbidity and mortality that is most likely related to their underlying disease.

Treatment. Rest during the acute stage of the disease is not difficult to enforce, because at this time the children feel sick enough to remain quiet. As they improve, we permit ambulation as long as the tests reflect improvement in liver function, for there is no definite evidence that bed rest prevents cirrhosis. Dietary restrictions are usually not necessary, although carbohydrate-containing substances such as hard candy, soda, and juices provide a good source of glucose during the early anorectic phase of the disease. Some children are intolerant of fatty foods, and if this is the case, these foods should be restricted. Adequate protein is certainly necessary during the recovery period. Depression of the prothrombin time is an indication for intramuscular vitamin K. If nausea and vomiting are of such severity as to cause dehydration, intravenous fluid replacement for one or two days will usually alleviate these symptoms. If they persist, a two- or three-day course of steroid therapy is often of great benefit. Cholestatic hepatitis is a benign complication and does not require steroids. Itching, the major complaint, can be brought under excellent control by cholestyramine, an anion-exchange resin that binds bile salts in the intestine to ultimately deplete the bile salt pool and leach the bile salts from the skin. The medication has a sand-like consistency and is made palatable by mixing with a small amount of orange or grape juice, applesauce, or grape jelly. It is given in three or four divided doses to a total of 3 to 4 gm per day for the infant or 9 to 12 gm for the adult.

Steroids are not used in the treatment of classic viral hepatitis,[129] but our practice is to use them for patients whose biopsy findings show bridging necrosis. Their long-term effect in promoting survival or preventing cirrhosis is not yet known, although it is clear that one immediate effect is to restore ill patients to relatively normal function. Two mg or more per kg of prednisone daily (in four divided doses) is begun as soon as the biopsy is interpreted, and this dose is tapered rapidly to about one third of the original amount as soon as transaminase levels have returned to normal or have stabilized at the lowest level possible. Then further tapering is attempted at two-week intervals. If rebound occurs, the steroids are increased until the transaminase value again returns to normal and are tapered to the last level that was capable of maintaining the liver function near normal. At this point, an every-other-day program is adopted, with doubling of the maintenance dose on the second day and discontinuation on alternate days. At this point some physicians add azathioprine (Imuran) at a dose of 0.75 to 1 mg per kg per day, but there is no clear evidence that the average patient benefits from its use.

HEPATIC COMA. The overall fatality rate for those with acute viral hepatitis in whom hepatic coma develops is about 90 per cent. The positive prognostic factor seems to be age, for some young patients survive. Numerous procedures have been used to treat coma: exchange transfusion, cross circulation, and *ex vivo* liver perfusion.[145] The only therapy that has met with any real success is administration of massive doses of steroids, given twice daily as 50 to 100 mg intravenous prednisone and intramuscular ACTH (10 U). The usual hepatic coma regimen of neomycin by mouth or gastric tube four times a day and as retention enema twice a day is also employed. With this vigorous approach the mortality falls to about 70 per cent. Steroid dosage, if used, is decreased as soon as the patient wakens. Antacid therapy must be given to prevent the development of gastritis; magaldrate (Riopan), low in sodium, is ideal for this purpose. Lactulose, a disaccharide not split within the intestine, produces an osmotic diarrhea and is of some help in preventing ammonia accumulation.

Prophylaxis. In patients exposed to viral hepatitis, 0.01 to 0.02 ml of gamma globulin per pound is effective in preventing or modifying the disease.[135, 137] In endemic areas, the chances of acquiring hepatitis are decreased if the individuals receive gamma globulin every six months. Its efficacy is dependent upon the titer of hepatitis B surface antigen antibody. A vaccine for hepatitis B is now available and may prove effective in preventing disease in infants born to mothers who are chronic carriers.

RUBELLA

Intrauterine infection with rubella virus has become a less important cause of neonatal hepatitis because of maternal immunization practices. It still occurs, however, and has recently been described in an outbreak in Chicago.[138a] Even some immunized mothers, exposed to rubella virus, may deliver a child with the congenital rubella syndrome. Characteristically, hyperbilirubinemia is of the conjugated type.[125]

Incidence. The incidence of hepatitis in congenital rubella is estimated at 20 per cent.

Etiology. The rubella virus passes through the placenta as early as the first trimester.

Pathology. Examination of the liver demonstrates a giant cell hepatitis and focal areas of necrosis or severe cholestasis or both. Although areas of necrosis can be large, there is usually no bridging. Periportal inflammation and bile duct proliferation are common when there is cholestasis. These changes may be present in the absence of apparent liver disease. Other changes seen in this disease are portal or periportal fibrosis, reduction in the bile ductules, and giant cell transformation. Biliary atresia also seems to be prevalent in these infants. As in viral hepatitis, the atresia may be a separate lesion or the end result of involvement of the bile ducts by the hepatitis process.

Symptoms. Clinically, the birth weight falls below the norm for date, and there is a high incidence of neonatal purpura, thrombocytopenia, cataracts, deafness, palatal and cardiovascular anomalies, mental retardation, and splenomegaly. There are some abnormalities in thymic cell–mediated immune mechanisms.

Diagnosis. As stated, there is an indirect hyperbilirubinemia in addition to laboratory evidence of hepatitis. The rubella virus can be cultured from the nasopharynx and liver as well as from other body tissues and fluids. An elevated rubella antigen titer in the blood is presumptive early evidence of congenital rubella infection. Maternal titers should also be examined.

Prognosis. Recovery from the hepatitis is relatively common, and death due to liver disease is rare. Deaths in this syndrome are related to cardiovascular disease or to hemorrhage.

CYTOMEGALIC INCLUSION DISEASE

While cytomegalic inclusion disease virus can produce a congenital disease with central nervous system, pulmonary, hematopoietic, and hepatic involvement resembling any other form of neonatal hepatitis, cytomegalovirus hepatitis can also occur in debilitated patients and in those who are immunologically deficient as a result of immunosuppressive therapy.[143a] In older children and adults, it produces a disease that resembles infectious mononucleosis.[131]

Incidence. Maternal infection with cytomegalovirus is estimated at 5 per cent. Inapparent infection in neonates approximates 1 per cent.

Etiology. The virus may cross the placenta early or late in pregnancy or may be transmitted during delivery.

Pathology. The liver shows giant cell transformation, scattered foci of necrosis and inflammation, periportal inflammation,

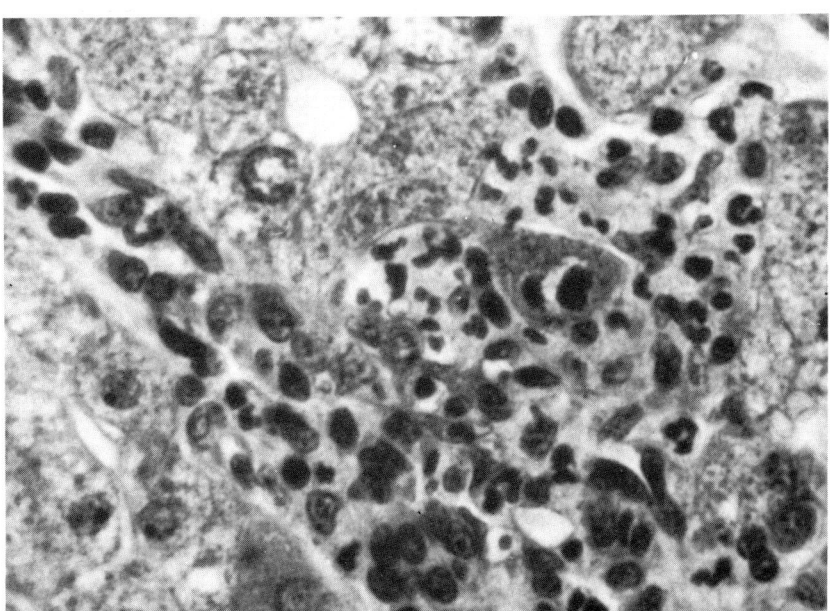

Figure 14–18　Cytomegalic inclusion disease. Typical cell with halo around inclusion is surrounded by polymorphonuclear leukocytes.

and bile stasis. Large intranuclear inclusions surrounded by a clear halo (Fig. 14–18) are pathognomonic of the disease and are seen sparsely scattered in hepatocytes, bile duct epithelium, and Kupffer cells.

Symptoms. These babies are often premature, and jaundice, edema, ascites, hemolytic anemia, thrombocytopenia, and hepatosplenomegaly develop soon after birth. Central nervous system involvement is reflected in mental retardation, motor disorders, and chorioretinitis.

Diagnosis. Cells containing large intranuclear inclusions can be found in the urinary sediment. The virus can be isolated from urine or diagnosed by a rising titer of complement-fixing antibodies. Cord serum–specific IgM antibodies seem to correlate well with infection, being positive in 89 per cent of babies with congenital infection and in highest titer in those with clinical disease.[129a] It is usually recoverable from the mothers of affected infants. Calcifications within the brain are noted in films of the skull.

Treatment. There is no known treatment for this disease. Development of a vaccine may significantly alter the incidence of the disease in the future.[125a, 130a]

Prognosis. If the disease is severe, the prognosis is poor, but if it is mild, survival is often accompanied by mental retardation and microcephaly.

VARICELLA

In most cases of neonatal varicella, the mother has contracted chickenpox near term and the baby is born with a varicella-like rash. A congenital varicella syndrome results when the mother contracts the disease early in pregnancy. Liver disease has not been a major component of either syndrome, but since it may occur, it will be described briefly.

Etiology and Pathology. Liver disease associated with varicella infection is caused by a direct viral action on the hepatic parenchyma, causing focal liver cell necrosis with giant cells and free hyaline bodies. Epithelioid granulomas with or without necrosis may occur.[124]

Symptoms. In the usual neonatal infection, the infant is born with the typical varicella-like rash or it develops during the first few days of life. A few days later, as the lesions progress, hepatomegaly and icterus appear and the stools become light and the urine dark. Infants with the congenital varicella syndrome have a low birth weight, microphthalmia, cataracts, hypotrophic limb or limbs, chorioretinitis, and encephalomyelitis.

Diagnosis. The virus is not usually isolated from these infants, but elevated varicella-zoster antibody titers are present in mother and infant. The liver function tests are compatible with those of acute hepatitis. Cord immunoglobulin M is increased.

Treatment. There is no treatment for the hepatitis or for the varicella infection. Nonimmunized mothers exposed before delivery or infants born to such mothers should be immunized with hyperimmune varicella plasma.[127]

Prognosis. Complete recovery from the liver disease is the usual outcome. Ara-A (adenine arabinoside) may prove to be of value.

HERPES SIMPLEX

Disseminated herpes simplex infection occurs in neonates whose mothers have genital type 2 herpesvirus infection and who have no circulating antibody to the virus. It is less often acquired after exposure to the oral type 1 virus, and recent studies suggest that it can be acquired transplacentally. It is usually associated with generalized herpetic disease.

Pathology. The liver shows extensive hepatocellular necrosis as well as giant cell transformation of hepatocytes and acidophilic intranuclear inclusions. Typical changes of encephalitis are present in the brain.

Symptoms. Intrauterine infection is suggested at birth in a microcephalic infant with vesicles over his body. In babies who are infected at birth, typical vesiculopustular eruptions over the face, neck, trunk, and arms develop during the first week of life. Twitching and frank seizures herald encephalitis in those most severely affected. A few babies have fever, respiratory distress, and frank gastrointestinal hemorrhage. Those with hepatitis become jaundiced within several days of the initial eruption and have hepatomegaly.

Diagnosis. The virus can be cultured directly from the skin or throat.

Treatment. Treatment with ara A (adenine arabinoside) is new but has provided dramatic results in some cases in a dosage of 10 to 20 mg per kg per day. Prevention is achieved by cesarean delivery.[120]

Prognosis. Intrauterine infection is associated with mental retardation, microcephaly, and cerebral anomalies. In the acquired form, a mild infection is followed by good recovery with only mild neurologic sequelae; most infants with severe infection usually die within two weeks, however.

COXSACKIE B VIRUS

Coxsackie B virus causes a wide spectrum of disease and is occasionally associated with hepatitis.

Etiology and Pathology. The liver shows scattered foci of inflammation, necrosis, giant cell transformation, and cholestasis. This infection may be acquired transplacentally as well as directly.

Symptoms. Infection in the young infant is typically characterized by severe myocarditis. The baby suddenly becomes extremely ill with tachycardia, fever, dyspnea, and perhaps signs of encephalitis. Hepatomegaly associated with jaundice signifies viral hepatitis rather than the enlarged liver of cardiac failure. Symptoms in older children are usually milder and vary from aseptic meningitis to pleurodynia to myocarditis. There is usually a pharyngitis or conjunctivitis and occasionally a morbilliform rash. The liver may be somewhat tender, but jaundice is absent or mild.

Diagnosis. Isolation of the virus confirms the diagnosis. Liver function tests may show the severe derangements of hepatitis in infants, but in older children they are usually normal.

Prognosis. Hepatic necrosis, meningoencephalitis, or cardiac failure may result in the infantile infection, but in most older children the liver disease clears spontaneously.

INFECTIOUS MONONUCLEOSIS

Infectious mononucleosis is now believed to be due to infection by the Epstein-Barr virus, which is also associated with the development of lymphomas in older children and of pharyngitis in infants.

Pathology. Although jaundice is not always present in this disease, the liver is usually involved to some degree. The major lesions are in the portal triads, where there is a marked inflammatory reaction consisting of mononuclear cells and lymphocytes. In some cases, plasma cells, polymorphonuclear leukocytes, and eosinophils are seen, and reticuloendothelial proliferation is common. Acidophilic bodies are usually sparse. As a generality, the inflammatory reaction vastly predominates over the amount of necrosis. Some patients also have a marked endophlebitis involving the central veins. Bile stasis is observed in most of the jaundiced patients. Although the histologic lesion of infectious mononucleosis is often indistinguishable from that of viral hepatitis, the extent of the inflammatory reaction when juxtaposed to the paucity of necrosis serves as a major differential feature between the two disorders. A considerable amount of regenerative activity usually is noted.

Symptoms. The only symptoms in young children may be a severe exudative pharyngitis or signs of a mild encephalitis, with a low-grade fever. Jaundice occurs in only 5 to 10 per cent of patients. There is generalized lymphadenopathy, mild hepatomegaly and liver tenderness, and splenomegaly.

Diagnosis. The mononucleosis spot test is the most specific test and should be employed in all cases of hepatitis. It may not become positive until the third or fourth week of illness, and so repeated determinations may be necessary to establish the diagnosis. Bilirubin levels are increased in nearly one quarter of the patients, but the elevation is mild. The serum transaminase levels are increased in a much larger percentage and on occasion may exceed 2000 units. BSP retention is abnormally prolonged, and alkaline phosphatase levels are elevated.

Treatment. Rest until jaundice and hepatic tenderness subside will help to shorten the recovery period.

Complications. There are no clearly documented reports of mononucleosis going on to chronic liver disease such as cirrhosis. Liver function tests usually return to normal within two months, but abnormalities may persist for as long as two years in a few patients. The major potential fatal complication of this disease is splenic rupture, which may occur after trivial trauma such as abdominal palpation. Severe left upper quadrant pain and the development of peritoneal signs in a patient with lymphadenopathy, fever, and lymphocytosis should alert the clinician to this entity. Occasionally, abdominal pain is seen as a consequence of the rare development of pancreatitis.

MISCELLANEOUS INFECTIONS

Psittacosis, reovirus, echovirus II, and adenovirus are rare causes of hepatitis in children.[141] Campylobacter hepatitis has been noted in an agammaglobulinemic patient.[161]

CONGENITAL TOXOPLASMOSIS

As in infants infected by cytomegalovirus, this disease is a systemic one, associated with findings of intrauterine infection and septicemia.[157, 159b]

Etiology. Infection by *Toxoplasma* organisms occurs transplacentally, and it is estimated that there are 2500 subclinical cases per year.[159b]

Pathology. There are microcephaly, chorioretinitis, intracranial calcifications, extramedullary hematopoiesis, and hepatitis in severely affected infants. The liver tissue shows bile stasis, periportal mononuclear infiltration, and, occasionally, anular cirrhosis.

Symptoms. Many infants have mild illness with only hepatitis, but those with severe disease show predominantly central nervous system and liver symptomatology. Microcephaly, hypotonia, and poor suck are noted often at birth, and 40 per cent of the infants have conjugated hyperbilirubinemia.

Diagnosis. The organism may be identified in the placenta or in the spinal fluid using Wright's stain. A positive Sabin-Feldman dye test is confirmatory. Hemagglutination titers are unreliable, for they may not rise until six months of age.

Treatment. Prophylactic treatment with sulfonamides is given to mothers who are infected. Infected infants are treated with pyrimethamine, sulfadiazine, and folic acid or pyrimethamine and trisulfapyrimidines for at least three weeks.

Prognosis. Infants with mild disease, treated early, have a good prognosis, but those with severe central nervous system damage show little improvement.

BACTERIAL INFECTIONS

Bacterial infection is occasionally associated with abnormalities of liver function, especially increased transaminase levels and hyperbilirubinemia.[130] It has been previously stated that gram-negative sepsis and pyelonephritis are common causes of jaundice in the newborn and reflect chemically a regurgitative type of jaundice with an increase in direct and indirect bilirubin. The liver lesion is one of cholestasis with hepatocellular damage that varies from slight to severe. Jaundice may be an early manifestation of scarlet fever or may accompany other hemolytic streptococcal infections. Liver lesions associated with streptococcal disease are of two types: (1) centrilobular lesions probably due to circulating toxin, and (2) scattered focal areas of hepatocellular necrosis due to direct bacterial invasion. Gonorrhea, which is being seen increasingly in adolescents and even in young children, may be associated with perihepatitis due to invasion of the peritoneal cavity by the gonococcus. Culture of liver biopsy material will yield the organism, and the fluorescent test for gonococcal antibody is positive. This type of perihepatitis, known as the Fitz-Hugh–Curtis syndrome, is characterized by the development of adhesions between Glisson's capsule and the anterior peritoneal surface. These thin adhesions cause a characteristic pain in the region of the liver that resembles pleuritic pain, for it is worsened by deep inspiration, coughing, sneezing, or bending over. In addition, they produce a friction rub.

Hepatic function is often impaired during pneumococcal infections, but only nonspecific changes are seen in the liver. Liver involvement also occurs in *Salmonella*,[144a] *Brucella, Listeria,* and *Clostridium* infections. Tubercular infection will be discussed in the section on infiltrative liver disease.

SYPHILIS

Congenital syphilis producing advanced cirrhosis has been well described in the past, but it is almost never seen in the United States today, presumably because of the frequent use of serologic testing during pregnancy.[116]

Etiology. The disease is caused by transplacental transmission of the spirochete.

Symptoms. Severely affected infants are usually born prematurely and are extremely ill, often apneic. Maculopapular diffuse skin lesions may be present at birth or may develop after several weeks. Rhinitis, with ulceration of the skin and nasal cartilage, is usually present between the second and sixth weeks. Jaundice and hepatomegaly appear within days to weeks. In less severely affected infants, the disease goes unrecognized for months, during which time a foul, purulent nasal discharge persists and the baby fails to gain weight.

Diagnosis. All infants with unexplained neonatal jaundice should be subjected to serologic testing. Since the antibody may be passively acquired, the STS may remain positive for months; however, it is not positive in normal infants beyond the third month. A positive TPI may persist for six months. A change in titers is most helpful when one cannot differentiate active infection from acquired antibody. The *Treponema* organisms can be recovered from moist skin lesions. Bone lesions, such as osteochondritis, dactylitis, and periostitis, although not clinically apparent, are readily recognized in radiologic examinations. Diffuse pneumonitis is caused by the spirochete, as is massive liver invasion. The liver biopsy shows miliary gummas with foci of necrosis and inflammation, intralobar fibrosis, mononuclear infiltrate, cirrhosis, and spirochetes.

Treatment. Benzathine penicillin G, 50,000 units per kilogram in a single injection, or aqueous procaine penicillin, 10,000 units per kilogram in daily intramuscular injections for ten days, will eradicate the spirochete. Erythromycin and tetracycline are alternative antibiotics that can be used if for some reason penicillin is contraindicated.

PYOGENIC LIVER ABSCESS

Pyogenic liver abscess is an uncommon disorder that is most often seen in children receiving steroids or immunosuppressive agents, or in those with chronic granulomatous disease due to defective leukocyte function, dysgammaglobulinemia, sepsis with hepatic seeding of bacteria, or pyelophlebitis following omphalitis, umbilical vein catheterization, or perforations of the bowel, especially acute appendicitis.

Incidence. Thirteen cases of solitary liver abscess had been reported in the American and British literature to 1973; the overall incidence of hepatic abscesses in children is 0.38 per cent.[119, 122] By 1981, 37 cases had been reported in neonates.[141a]

Etiology. The etiology has changed since the antibiotic era began. Cases reported before 1940 developed in children with distant foci of infection, such as pneumonia, otitis, and cutaneous burns, and were most often caused by *Staphylococcus aureus*. Since the introduction of antibiotics, liver abscess has been more often related to umbilical catheterizations or immunologic abnormalities, and the predominant organisms have been enteric bacilli, with *Candida* second in frequency. Rarely, abscess follows bowel perforation.

Pathology. Most patients have multiple abscesses, and nearly half have abscess formation in other organs. Microscopically, these are areas of necrosis surrounded by polymorphonuclear cells, mononuclear cells, and occasional lymphocytes. Fibrous tissue is present among surrounding hepatocytes.

Symptoms. The usual systemic signs and symptoms of infection are present (tachypnea, cyanosis, intermittent apnea), and the liver is often quite tender to palpation and extends below the costal margin. Jaundice occurs in 10 to 25 per cent of patients. Abdominal pain and vomiting are present. Compression of the liver with the hands placed anteriorly and posteriorly causes severe pain; this contrasts with the tenderness of hepatitis, which is most severe when the liver is compressed laterally.

Diagnosis. There is a marked leukocytosis with an increase in band forms. Liver function tests are quite nonspecific and mimic any infiltrative disease with mild hyperbilirubinemia, increased alkaline phosphatase values, and modestly increased transaminase levels. Hepatic angiography and radioisotope liver scanning employing such agents as ^{99m}Tc sulfur colloid are most helpful in suggesting the diagnosis.

Treatment. Pyogenic liver abscesses are fatal unless treated, and, unfortunately, the diagnosis is often missed simply because it is not considered. Therapy entails a combination of surgical drainage and antibiotic administration. Since the most common organisms are staphylococci and enteric bacteria, ampicillin and methicillin, given intravenously in a dosage of 200 to 300 mg per kg per day in four divided doses, are probably the best agents to employ unless the causative bacterium has been identified by culture. Drainage tubes inserted at the time of surgery usually must be left in the abscess cavity until drainage has ceased.

PARASITIC INFECTION

The Visceral Larva Migrans Syndrome (Eosinophilia-Hepatomegaly Syndrome Due to Parasites)

Parasitic infection causing the visceral larva migrans syndrome results in hepatomegaly, jaundice, eosinophilia, and hyperglobulinemia.[149]

Etiology and Pathology. The syndrome is most often caused by larval migration of *Ascaris lumbricoides* or *Toxocara canis*, but occasionally it has followed infestation by *Capillaria hepatica*, *Ascaris suis*, and *Strongyloides*. After migration through the lung the swallowed larvae reach the small intestine, from which they may migrate up the biliary tree. Invasion of the liver radicles is relatively rare, but once worms are entrapped in the distal radicle they cannot return; they survive for a month or more to cause a massive eosinophilic inflammation and granuloma formation with typical epithelioid and giant cells. Abscesses may result.

Symptoms. The disease is most common during the first three years of life in children who have an affinity for eating dirt. Often there is some contact with young puppies. The first symptoms are chronic paroxysmal cough, wheezing, and fever. These are shortly followed by anorexia and bouts of colicky abdominal pain. A few patients become jaundiced and a quarter of them have seizures. Some are malnourished, but others grow and develop normally. Most of these children have some degree of hepatomegaly and the liver is tender. The abdomen is enlarged. Pulmonary rales and wheezes are diffuse. The retinal lesions, which resemble retinoblastoma, may appear years later.

Diagnosis. Plain films of the abdomen often show the linear configuration of the worms within the intestine, and films taken after a barium swallow may outline the digestive tracts of the worms. Chest films show a patchy or peribronchial pneumonitis, which may change from day to day. The white blood count is elevated and sometimes reaches 100,000, with at least 30 per cent and perhaps 90 per cent eosinophils. The serum albumin is low, and the total gamma globulin and immunoglobulin M levels are increased. Liver function tests are normal or only slightly impaired. Precipitating, hemagglutinating, or flocculating antibodies against worm extract are identified in the patient's serum.

Complications. Liver abscess is a major complication of hepatic infestation and is characterized by deterioration of the clinical condition, elevation of temperature, and increase in hepatic tenderness.

Treatment. In past years the disease was considered self-limited and was not treated, but now that they are available, diethylcarbamazine citrate and thiabendazole should be used. Surgical drainage is required for the management of liver abscess.

Amebiasis

Amebiasis is discussed in detail elsewhere, but it must be noted that infection of the liver may occur with active or inactive colonic disease. The parasites reach the liver through the portal vein and initially cause symptoms of hepatitis as they produce focal infarction. Later, the smaller abscesses fuse into the larger, more typical liver abscesses. In the Far East, hepatic involvement is estimated to occur in 25 per cent of patients who are infected.

The clinical presentation is one of fever, hepatomegaly, and liver tenderness, with or without jaundice. Right pleuritic involvement occurs with or without pulmonic disease. Leukocytosis is present, but liver function tests may be normal. Liver scan and ultrasonography will reveal the abscesses; the diagnosis may be confirmed by high hemagglutination and immunofluorescent titers. Rapid treatment is imperative, using metronidazole, 30 to 50 mg per kg per day for at least ten days. Although the organisms are eliminated, defects may persist for months on scan or ultrasonograph.

Other Parasitic Diseases

Hepatic involvement from schistosomes, liver flukes, and hydatid disease is unusual in the infant. *Ascaris lumbricoides* may invade the common bile duct to cause biliary obstruction or cholangitis, and, very rarely, *Giardia lamblia* may cause cholecystitis or hepatic granulomas.

REYE'S SYNDROME

In 1963 a new syndrome was described that is characterized by encephalopathy and hepatomegaly.[146] Pathologically, there is fatty degeneration of the viscera without any specific anatomic change in the brain. This disease, now known as Reye's syndrome, is a well-defined disorder occurring exclusively in children, usually following a prodromal illness characterized by cough, coryza, and fever; the family history discloses that other family members have recently recovered from chickenpox or adenovirus or coxsackievirus infection. Vomiting in the anicteric child that follows varicella or an upper respiratory infection may be associated with abnormal liver function and may represent a mild form of Reye syndrome.[153a]

Incidence. The early sporadic case reports are now being supplanted by series of several dozen cases. The disease has been reported in siblings and in such instances has been associated with the BW-38 antigen.[154]

Etiology. The etiology remains unknown, although one must speculate whether it is a result of direct viral infection or a later autoimmune-type phenomenon. Influenza B virus, reovirus, varicella, parainfluenza virus, coxsackieviruses A and B, and adenovirus 3 have all been implicated.[139] With certainty, its incidence is increased in children who have taken aspirin for treatment of nonspecific symptoms.[143b, 155] In older children the disorder predominates in Caucasians from nonurban environments, but infants may be nonwhite or from lower socioeconomic or urban communities. The majority of cases are reported from the United States and Thailand. Aflatoxin B has been found in the tissue of 22 of 23 Thailand patients,[148] and pyrrolizidine intoxication has mimicked Reye's syndrome.[126]

Pathology and Pathophysiology. On liver biopsy, diffuse, severe fatty infiltration of hepatic parenchymal cells and little hepatocellular necrosis are found. Kupffer cells may be increased in size and number. Frozen sections stained with Sudan demonstrate numerous fat droplets, many of which are microvesicular. Mitochondrial ultrastructure is significantly altered. Only minor nonspecific changes are seen on neuropathologic examination, including cerebral edema and neuronal lesions.

Coma is due to hepatic encephalopathy, and blood ammonia levels are frequently elevated. Hypoglycemia is relatively common. There seems to be a typical pattern of hyperaminoaciduria which can differentiate Reye's syndrome from severe hepatitis, with elevation of glutamine, alanine, α-amino-N-butyrate, and lysine.[147] Ornithine transcarbamylase and carbamyl phosphate synthetase deficiencies have caused Reye-like syndromes and certainly any patient with recurrent symptomatology should be evaluated for one of these inherited metabolic disorders. A patient with a Reye-like picture presented with cold agglutinin, autoimmune hemolytic anemia. Hypertyraminemia has also been described.[143]

Symptoms. This syndrome must be suspected in any child recovering from a viral illness in whom vomiting, stupor, and lethargy develop. Breathing abnormalities, i.e., tachypnea and apnea, and early seizures are common in infants. After hours or days of these prodromal symptoms, muscle rigidity, spasticity, hyperactivity, delirium, hallucinations (stage I), and seizures appear. Hyperventilation seems to be of central origin and leads to respiratory acidosis. On examination, fever, hepatomegaly, and occasionally the remains of a macular rash are seen. Jaundice is not always apparent and indeed may be absent. Stage II coma, although representing stupor and failure to arouse to painful stimuli, still maintains avoidance reactions. In the more severe cases, the initial stage of hyperactive reflexes progresses to marked depression of cerebral and brainstem functions with decerebrate rigidity, paralysis of extraocular movements, fixed dilated pupils, failure to respond to pain (stage III), respiratory failure, and complete flaccidity of musculature (stage IV). A bleeding disorder can manifest itself as gastrointestinal hemorrhage. The development of papilledema is a poor prognostic sign and signifies increasing intracranial pressure. Coma may persist, even with treatment, for days or longer than a week. Spontaneous decline in the blood ammonia level usually precedes the return of consciousness, which is often sudden. Survivors usually have no recollection of their ordeal except to express gratitude that they are free of headache.

Diagnosis. Liver function tests must be obtained and a specimen for blood ammonia drawn as soon as the disease is suspected. Ammonia levels rise well above 100 μg per dl. The transaminase value is usually markedly elevated and the bilirubin only mildly so (4.0 mg/dl). The blood ammonia is elevated in most patients as is the CPK; the prothrombin activity is decreased, and the blood sugar often is low. Cerebrospinal fluid is normal.

Treatment. Treatment is essentially supportive. Ten per cent glucose in electrolyte solution is given intravenously to combat hypoglycemia. Immediate treatment of hyperammonemia consists of intragastric neomycin and lactulose. Exchange transfusion, still employed at some centers, has decreased mortality.[117] However, at the Yale–New Haven Hospital, the combination of intracranial pressure monitoring, intravenous mannitol, barbiturate coma, and controlled ventilation has further decreased mortality.[140] Because of the similarity of the hyperaminoacidemia to that seen in ornithine transcarbamylase deficiency, some centers administer citrulline early and report prompt decreases in ammonia levels.

Prognosis. When the syndrome was first described, 50 to 75 per cent of the patients died. With the advent of exchange transfusion, mortality was decreased to 30 to 70 per cent.[134] Using the supportive therapy described at Yale, only 3 of the last 41 patients have expired — a rate of only 7 per cent.

The development of pancreatitis indicates a poor prognosis, for all of our patients who did so, died.[128] Recurrence of Reye's syndrome has been reported.[144]

LIVER DISEASE IN UREA CYCLE ENZYME DEFICIENCIES

LaBrecque et al.[138] reviewed the liver pathology of patients with ornithine transcarbamylase (OTC) and carbamyl phosphate synthetase I (CPS) deficiencies. They noted that, although five of six homozygous males with OTC deficiency died within the first few days of hyperammonemia,[151] the liver histology was normal. Nearly all heterozygous females and adults had abnormalities despite normal liver function, however: nine with steatosis and eight with focal cell necrosis and inflammation. Patients with CPS deficiency had normal histology. In neither disorder did the histologic picture resemble that of Reye's syndrome.

DRUG AND TOXIC HEPATITIS

DRUG-INDUCED HEPATIC DISEASE

A full discussion of drug and toxic hepatitis is beyond the scope of this book, and reference should be made to standard treatises on the subject.[188] However, general principles should be stated for the guidance of the clinician, and some specific examples, particularly common in children, will be cited. Some drugs cause severe hepatocellular damage, and others, cholestasis.

An hepatotoxic substance is a chemical that produces liver injury in all subjects after an incubation period measured in minutes or hours. In general terms, the greater the amount of toxin, the greater will be the hepatic injury. The type of lesion that develops is characteristic for the specific toxin and can be reproduced in experimental animals. For example, carbon tetrachloride affects man, rat, mouse, and many other animals and characteristically causes massive central necrosis and fatty infiltration of the liver that usually can be distinguished

from lesions caused by other toxic agents. The effect of carbon tetrachloride on the hepatocyte reaches its maximum within four hours. Thus, the transaminase level rises rapidly because of massive hepatocyte injury. However, there is no continuation of the injury once the initial insult is over, and the transaminase level decreases at a rate consistent with the half-life of transaminase in the circulating blood. In the case of serum glutamic oxaloacetic transaminase, the half-life in the circulation is about 21 hours.

In contrast to toxic hepatitis, drug-induced hepatitis is due to chemicals that cause hepatic injury in only a small fraction of exposed persons, usually 1 in 100 to 100,000. The latent period is quite variable, often measured in days or even weeks. There is no correlation between the amount of chemical ingested and either the incidence or the severity of the hepatic lesion. The histologic lesion cannot be reproduced in experimental animals. This has important implications when new drugs are introduced for human use, since animal testing reveals only hepatotoxicity and does not determine whether or not the drug will result in drug-induced hepatitis. The histologic lesion seen in drug-induced hepatitis is quite variable and may mimic extrahepatic obstruction when cholestatic hepatitis is its primary feature, or viral hepatitis when hepatocellular necrosis predominates. A predominance of lymphocytic and monocytic infiltration and reticuloendothelial proliferation with a paucity of necrosis favors the diagnosis of drug hepatitis. In those with severe cholestatic hepatitis, bile lakes (Fig. 14–19), which are seen in only a minority of patients, provide the only clue to the diagnosis of extrahepatic obstruction. In some, extrahepatic signs and symptoms of hypersensitivity, including pruritus, morbilliform rash, hives, angioneurotic edema, arthralgia, arthritis, fever, and eosinophilia, may provide the clues to the diagnosis of drug-induced hepatitis which is clearly idiosyncratic.

The causes of drug-induced hepatitis are legion. As a generality, any chemical that produces any sort of allergic reaction in man

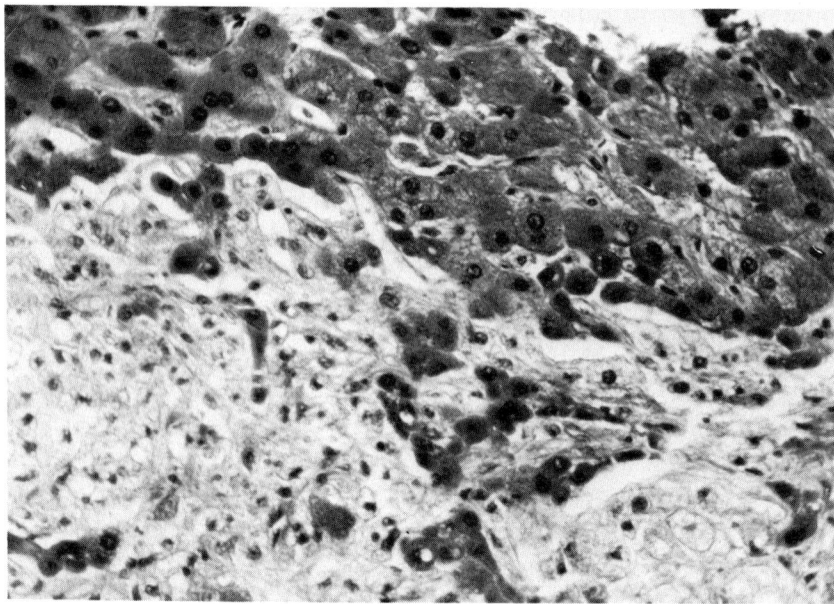

Figure 14–19   Bile infarct. Patient has extrahepatic biliary obstruction. Note foamy degeneration of liver cells.

will ultimately be reported to cause a drug-induced hepatitis in man.

A few toxic chemicals need to be singled out in this presentation because of their frequent occurrence in children.

Pyrrolizidine Alkaloids

Pyrrolizidine alklaloids are found in a number of plants belonging to the *Senecio*, *Crotalaria*, and *Heliotropium* families.[165, 168] These plants are worldwide in distribution, and the alkaloids contained therein are known to produce severe liver damage leading to cirrhosis in grazing animals. Cirrhosis following ingestion of these plants has also been described in man. Malnutrition appears to enhance the likelihood of liver injury from these agents. In children, ingestion of the pyrrolizidine or *Senecio* alkaloids results in endophlebitis of the hepatic vein with the consequent development of veno-occlusive disease that mimics the Budd-Chiari syndrome. This has been especially common in Jamaican children following the ingestion of "bush teas" used for folk medicinal purposes, which contain the alkaloids. Pathologically, endophlebitis is seen involving both large and small hepatic veins. The veins may be thrombosed. There usually is intense congestion of the central portion of the liver lobule, with atrophy and destruction of liver cells followed by the development of pericentral hepatic fibrosis. Clinically, patients experience severe epigastric pain followed within a few days by rapidly accumulating ascites. Patients may outgrow their clothing or their belts within two or three days. Although about one half of the patients die within the first few months of the illness, the remainder progress to clinical recovery over a period of one or two years. Presumably, recovery occurs because hepatic vessels recanalize. The onset of *Senecio* poisoning may also be insidious, with hepatosplenomegaly being the most common sign and hepatocellular failure and hematemesis being the most common cause of death.

Antibiotics

The antibiotic novobiocin causes an increase in the level of unconjugated bilirubin in the serum owing to interference with glucuronyl transferase activity. This toxic effect of novobiocin seems especially common in neonates. Novobiocin probably also interferes with bilirubin uptake and excretion by the hepatocyte, since BSP retention is abnormally prolonged. It can also produce hypersensitivity reactions leading to a mild drug-induced hepatitis. However, massive hepatic necrosis also has been described. *Penicillin* and its synthetic derivatives, such as ampicillin, oxacillin, and carbenicillin, may cause a parenchymal-type hepatitis of an allergic nature. *Isoniazid* (and, similarly, iproniazid) is associated with hepatic disease in approximately 7 per cent of children.[166a, 167, 180] It is uncommon in infancy, and there may be an increased frequency with age. The toxic effects are due to acetylated metabolites, acetylisoniazid and acetylhydrazine. Jaundice may not develop for months after the onset of therapy, and the severity of liver disease correlates with continued use of the drug. *Sulfonamides* may rarely cause parenchymal necrosis, and cholestatic hepatitis has been reported after methoprim-sulfamethoxazole administration.[181] Erythromycin estolate may cause cholestasis.

Chlortetracycline, oxytetracycline, and tetracycline given orally produce fatty infiltration of the liver. Characteristically, the fat is in the form of fine vacuoles that are distributed diffusely throughout the liver parenchyma. Liver function usually remains normal. Large doses of tetracycline given intravenously may give rise to a much more severe form of liver injury. In addition to the fat, Kupffer cells contain large amounts of pigment and debris, indicating preceding necrosis of liver cells. Although most commonly seen in pregnant women with pyelonephritis treated with intravenous tetracycline, this condition is also seen in children and has a mortality rate of around 80 per cent. Clinically, abdominal pain, nausea, vomiting, and jaundice are the predominant symptoms. Liver function studies show an increase in serum bilirubin, alkaline phosphatase, and transaminase levels. Pancreatitis and renal failure may be serious complications. Amylase and lipase levels in serum may be increased in those patients in whom pancreatitis develops. Uremia and metabolic acidosis may occur in patients with renal failure.

Immunosuppressive Agents

Azathioprine and 6-Mercaptopurine. Antimetabolites, such as azathioprine (Imuran) and its parent compound 6-mercaptopurine, are frequently used in the therapy of leukemia and other neoplastic conditions and may cause hepatic injury characterized by jaundice, hepatomegaly, dark urine, light stools, and increased serum levels of bilirubin, alkaline phosphatase, and transaminase. Usually, toxicity to 6-mercaptopurine does not occur unless the dose level is above 2.5 mg per kg of body weight daily, and it is reversible upon cessation of therapy. Occasionally, however, the toxic hepatitis is progressive and fatal. Bile duct proliferation, periportal inflammation, bile stasis, and periportal acidophilic bodies are the most common histologic abnormalities caused by these purine antagonists.

Methotrexate. Methotrexate (amethopterin) is a folic acid antagonist used in the treatment of leukemia, lymphoma, psoriasis, and a variety of neoplastic disorders. Mild hyperbilirubinemia, modest increases in transaminase levels, decreases in serum albumin levels, and the development of ascites, edema, and hepatomegaly may follow its administration. Pathologically, there is marked periportal fibrosis. Initially, the liver injury was thought to be due to the destruction of the leukemic process in the liver, with fibrosis replacing the formerly infiltrated area. However, periportal fibrosis also occurs when methotrexate is used to treat psoriasis and other conditions not known to affect the liver. Thus, the current view is that methotrexate is a hepatotoxin. Continuation of treatment may result in progressive liver injury leading ultimately to cirrhosis. Upon cessation of methotrexate therapy, the liver lesion occasionally resolves.

Aflatoxin

Aspergillus flavus is a fungus that grows on peanuts (ground nuts) and produces a toxin known as aflatoxin. In experimental animals fed aflatoxin, focal areas of hepatic necrosis, fatty infiltration, bile duct proliferation, central vein endophlebitis, and, ultimately, cirrhosis and hepatoma are known to develop. Protein deficiency increases the hepatotoxic effect of the aflatoxin. Aflatoxin has been implicated in human disease only recently. In India, cirrhosis in children with a peak incidence at three years occurs quite frequently and is characterized by hepatomegaly, jaundice, edema, and ascites. Ultimately, hepatocellular failure with hepatic coma develops. Aflatoxin has been identified in the urine of some patients with Indian childhood cirrhosis and may be important in its etiology. Recently, a group of children with kwashiorkor treated with a high-protein flour made from peanut meal and contaminated with aflatoxin were found to have a cirrhosis histologically identical with Indian childhood cirrhosis. The role of aflatoxin in Reye's syndrome in Thailand is under current investigation.

Corticosteroids

Corticosteroids consistently produce fatty infiltration of the liver but do not cause changes in hepatic function. However, one case of massive fatty infiltration of the liver following prednisone administration in a child who died of fat embolism has been described.

Cimetidine may cause cholestasis in infants and may also interfere with the hepatic metabolism of such drugs as Valium.[173]

Halothane and Methoxyflurane

Halothane (Fluothane) and methoxyflurane (Penthrane) are halogenated hydrocarbons that are not hepatotoxic to man or experimental animals. There is, however, convincing evidence that they cause drug hepatitis, usually subacute hepatic necrosis. Histologically, the lesion mimics viral hepatitis. These agents produce other manifestations of hypersensitivity in some persons and an associated decrease in intrahepatic arterial circulation. Most patients develop serum antimitochondrial antibodies. Halothane-induced hepatitis occurs in 1 in 10,000 patients in whom it is used and is

fatal in 50 per cent. In those exposed to halothane for the first time, the onset of symptoms averages seven days. After multiple exposures the latent period becomes shorter, even to within one hour of inhaling the agent. The onset is acute, with shaking chills and fever over 102° F, and is followed in two to four days by dark urine, light stools, and deepening jaundice. Anorexia, nausea, vomiting, abdominal pain, rash, leukocytosis, and eosinophilia accompany the acute illness. Edema, ascites, and hepatic coma can quickly supervene and usually indicate a fatal outcome. The overall mortality is 50 per cent. Steroids are of benefit if given before the development of coma. Methoxyflurane appears to act in a similar fashion.

Despite the fact that it causes bridging necrosis in a few patients, halothane is perhaps the most desirable of all anesthetics currently in use because of the low postoperative mortality attendant to its use. The low anesthetic morbidity and mortality appear to outweigh its potential harm as a cause of hepatic necrosis. Nevertheless, certain precautions should be employed. Halothane should not be used in low-risk surgical procedures, and it should not be used when multiple exposures to the anesthetic agent are necessary. The reason for this is that the risk of halothane-induced hepatitis is at least twice as great after multiple exposures as it is after a single exposure. Finally, halothane should not be employed in patients who have previously received the agent and had either postoperative hepatitis or unexplained postoperative fever. Unfortunately, the practice of using halothane for multiple minor surgical procedures in children continues, and no data are yet available to show whether this results in sensitization that will be troublesome later in life.

Antipyretics

Aspirin-induced hepatitis has been associated with the long-term use of this agent for arthritic disorders, but the liver may also be affected by juvenile rheumatoid arthritis.[166, 188a] Elevations of transaminase values have been reported in 50 per cent of patients taking salicylates for rheumatic fever. Most children with elevated transaminases have had serum salicylate levels greater than 25 mg per dl.[169, 184] Hepatic necrosis, however, has been caused only by massive overdose.

Similarly, hepatocellular injury follows only massive doses of *acetaminophen*. Peak plasma levels are reached after 30 minutes from the syrup and in 60 to 120 minutes from the tablets. The sulfate conjugate is the primary metabolite in the infant, whereas glucuronide conjugates predominate in the adult. Neither acetaminophen nor its major conjugates are hepatotoxic, so that damage is postulated from a minor metabolite that leads to glutathione depletion. Acetylcysteine (Mucomyst) is administered within 24 hours after ingestion (20 per cent solution diluted 1:3 in soda or fruit juice) in a dosage of 140 mg per kg orally for loading followed by 70 mg per kg orally every four hours for 17 doses (72 hours). (Toxic levels of acetaminophen are above 100 μg per ml.)[174, 176, 178] Gold therapy for rheumatoid arthritis has caused cholestasis.[177]

Anticonvulsant Drugs

Anticonvulsant therapy is frequently employed in pediatric practice because of the high incidence of seizure disorders. Dilantin has produced drug hepatitis; in all cases, other manifestations of hypersensitivity have accompanied the liver disorder.[175] Hepatosplenomegaly occurs, with or without jaundice. Although hepatocellular dysfunction is usually observed on liver function testing, the hepatitis may be primarily cholestatic. Very rarely, fulminant hepatocellular necrosis develops and is usually fatal.[179a]

Phenobarbital only rarely causes drug hepatitis, and in all cases skin rash has been associated with the condition. *Trimethadione* (Tridione) therapy has also been reported to cause hepatitis. *Phenacemide* (Phenurone) produces perhaps the highest incidence of hepatitis, and up to 10 per cent of the cases described have been fatal. Since abnormalities of liver function may precede clinical signs of hepatitis, patients given Phenurone should have frequent serum transaminase determinations to detect the early onset of liver abnormalities. *Valproic acid* causes cholestatic hepatitis and diffuse hepatocellular injury, and when it is used concurrently with other anticonvulsants, hepatic function should be carefully monitored.[182, 186]

Ritalin, used for control of hyperactivity, is often associated with elevation of transaminase.

Estrogens

Therapy with estrogen and C-17 alkyl-substituted steroids causes jaundice in some females but is rarely used in infancy.

HYPERALIMENTATION

Hepatocellular and canalicular cholestasis has been noted in infants receiving intravenous alimentation.[170, 183, 185] Periportal inflammatory infiltrates with a predominance of eosinophils are occasionally noted, suggesting an idiosyncratic reaction. Although the precise mechanism is unknown, a toxic insult is possible in these sick infants, who may be premature, malnourished, and on multiple drugs. The possible causes of cholestasis include decreased bile acid synthesis because of relative amino acid deficiency, inadequate stimulation of post-canalicular bile flow via duodenal secretion in the child with minimal oral alimentation, and metabolically induced cholestasis secondary to hyperammonemia.[171] The discovery of hepatocellular dysfunction should not lead one to assume that the alimentation fluid is necessarily the source of the hepatic insult before appropriate investigations are completed, e.g., sepsis work-up. If at all possible, the rate of administration is not increased because of the potential for further metabolic impairment, but cessation of central or peripheral parenteral alimentation is not generally indicated. Infusion of soybean oil emulsion (Intralipid) does not cause definite liver damage but must be carefully monitored in the neonatal period because fatty acids cause displacement of bilirubin from albumin-binding sites.[172] Also, deposition of pigment is reported in reticuloendothelial and hepatic cells, the significance of which is not known. Reduction of the protein load is often followed by improvement.

Thirty per cent of patients treated for two or more weeks will develop some type of liver disease.[55a, 64a] Fatty changes are noted in 74 per cent. After three weeks of treatment, there is bile duct proliferation; between 11 and 90 days, portal fibrosis; and after 90 days, severe changes and cirrhosis. Many livers contain PAS-positive material. Cholelithiasis is an additional complication.[169a]

Cirrhosis may develop in small, premature infants as early as 60 days. Hepatocellular carcinoma has been reported in one 900-gram (birth weight) infant who received hyperalimentation for 395 days. He developed cirrhosis at 5 months and carcinoma at 25 months.[225a]

Drug Injury. In addition to cholestasis and hepatonecrosis, the patterns of drug injury include chronic active liver disease, which is occasionally noted with methyldopa, sulfonamide, or nitrofurantoin therapy. Resolution of the acute liver injury occurs a few days after withdrawal of the drug; corticosteroid therapy is not indicated.

Vitamin Injury. *Vitamin A* in high, chronic dosage may cause hepatitis and periostitis. Cirrhosis and perisinusoidal steatosis have been long-term sequelae.

HYPERTHERMIA

Hyperthermia is commonly associated with hyperbilirubinemia and clinical jaundice. The artificial induction of fever (106.7° F for seven hours) results in clinical jaundice in at least 20 per cent of patients. Similar findings are seen in association with the hyperpyrexia of heat stroke. Jaundice is occasionally seen during acute febrile illnesses in children. In fatal cases, central liver necrosis with little inflammatory reaction is found histopathologically. The cause of the liver injury is probably related to anoxia.

RADIATION HEPATITIS

Virtually all patients who receive more than 3500 rads of x-ray therapy over the liver incur radiation hepatitis, and in some it occurs with a smaller exposure. The usual clinical picture is development of pain over the liver, hepatomegaly, ascites, and intense jaundice two to six weeks after the radiation treatment. Central lobular hemorrhage, congestion, and necrosis are the usual pathologic findings. Children may be more sensitive to radiation injury than adults, since as little as 2000 rads have been associated with its development. Radiation hepatitis may progress to fibrosis and death.

CONGENITAL HEART DISEASE

Infants dying in the first month of life of congenital heart disease display a high incidence of central and midzonal necrosis of the liver at autopsy.[187] Coarctation of the aorta and hypoplastic left heart syndrome are the most common congenital anomalies associated with the liver necrosis. As a result of the severe hepatic dysfunction, bleeding disorders are common and may be the cause of death. Histologically, central passive congestion of the liver is not seen and the hepatic lesion appears to be mainly due to anoxia.

JUVENILE RHEUMATOID ARTHRITIS

Still's disease is a term that has been applied to the varied clinical picture seen in rheumatoid arthritis of childhood.[179] Still's triad refers to arthritis, splenomegaly, and lymphadenopathy. These terms emphasize the frequency of extra-articular manifestations of the disease, especially the splenomegaly. Less well appreciated is the fact that juvenile rheumatoid arthritis can present as an acute illness that mimics viral hepatitis. Fever, rash, malaise, anorexia, massive hepatomegaly, and arthralgia are the acute clinical features. Laboratory workup usually discloses leukocytosis, increased bilirubin and transaminase levels, and impaired BSP excretion. Pleuritis and pericarditis may complicate the clinical course. Histologically, the liver shows only periportal inflammation and reticuloendothelial proliferation.

SICKLE CELL ANEMIA

Tests of liver function are usually abnormal in patients with sickle cell anemia and tend to worsen as the patient gets older. Hepatomegaly develops and liver function worsens during periods of crisis; malaise, anorexia, and fatigue are common. SGOT levels may be over 1000 and bilirubin over 30, and the prothrombin time becomes prolonged. Bilirubin elevations are of both direct and indirect reacting components; this indicates that hepatic dysfunction rather than hemolysis is the cause. Histologically, red blood cell aggregates are seen in the hepatic sinusoids, especially pericentrally. On the portal side of the agglutinates, sinusoidal dilatation is seen. Electron microscopic examination of hepatocytes suggests anoxic liver injury. Phagocytosed red cells are often seen in Kupffer cells, and bile stasis may be a prominent feature. Cirrhosis is rare, but when it is seen, it resembles hemochromatosis because of the marked increase in stainable iron.

CHRONIC HEPATITIS AND CIRRHOSIS

Liver disease, in some instances, pursues a chronic course of varying severity from the mildest chronic persistent hepatitis to cirrhosis, the major causes of which are listed in Table 14–5.

CHRONIC PERSISTENT HEPATITIS

This disorder implies hepatitis persisting longer than the usual ten-week course of viral hepatitis; it is characterized by periodic episodes of fatigue, anorexia, epigastric distress, and liver tenderness.

Pathology. Histologically, one sees the classic hepatitis lesion with spotty necrosis and inflammation scattered through the liver lobule. The portal zones are normal or only slightly thickened, and there is no bridging.

Diagnosis. The liver function tests show moderate increases in transaminases, bilirubin, and gamma globulin, but serum albumin is normal.

Treatment. Treatment is not required for this lesion.

Prognosis. Although liver function abnormalities may persist for years, the outlook is optimistic, for spontaneous remission will occur eventually.

CHRONIC ACTIVE HEPATITIS

One of the most confusing areas of liver disease today is in the nomenclature of chronic active hepatitis, with classifications based on pathology, clinical course, serologic abnormalities, and other imprecise measurements. Synonyms have included subacute hepatitis, subacute hepatic necrosis, chronic aggressive hepatitis, lupoid or plasma cell hepatitis, Kunkel hepatitis, and hypergammaglobulinemic hepatitis.[195] It seems best to term the disease "chronic active hepatitis," with attention to the presence of hepatitis B antigen, lupus erythematosus (LE) cells, smooth muscle antibody, and antinuclear factor as well as to the actual histology of the liver.

Incidence. The true incidence is unknown, although it is accepted that 10 per cent to 30 per cent of patients with acute hepatitis B will progress to chronic active hepatitis.

Etiology. As noted, one tenth to one third of these patients have hepatitis B antigenemia. Morphologic and biochemical changes may resemble those of Wilson's disease, primary biliary cirrhosis, or drug hepatitis. This form of hepatitis may be associated with autoimmune disorders such as thyroiditis or colitis, suggesting an autoimmune origin.

Pathology. A variety of morphologic changes may occur in the liver. During

Table 14–5   Diseases That Cause Cirrhosis

POSTNECROTIC CIRRHOSIS	BILIARY CIRRHOSIS
Infectious hepatitis	Intrahepatic and extrahepatic
Serum hepatitis	atresias
Congenital or neonatal diseases	Choledochal cyst
Rubella	Familial intrahepatic cholestasis
Cytomegalic inclusion disease	Cholangitis
Syphilis	Cystic fibrosis
Herpes simplex	Ulcerative colitis
Toxoplasmosis	
Coxsackievirus B infection	
Chronic active hepatitis	
Hepatic fibrosis	
Genetic diseases and metabolic disorders	
Alpha$_1$-antitrypsin deficiency	
Wilson's disease	
Galactosemia	
Tyrosinemia	
Cystinosis	
Porphyria hepatica	
Fructose intolerance	
Hemochromatosis — primary	
or secondary	
Sickle cell disease	
Histiocytosis X	
Rendu-Osler-Weber disease	
Lipid storage diseases	
Glycogen storage diseases	
Gangliosidosis	
Hurler's disease	
Hyperpipecolatemia	
Jamaican veno-occlusive disease	
Indian cirrhosis	
Kwashiorkor — protein malnutrition	
Hemangioendothelioma	
Drugs and toxins	

inactive periods, the biopsy shows relatively normal architecture with some round cell infiltration in the portal areas, small amounts of piecemeal necrosis of liver cells, and blurring of the limiting plate. In active disease, the biopsy specimen resembles that of subacute necrosis, with more marked piecemeal necrosis and cellular infiltrate and the additional presence of bridging between portal triads and hepatic veins and lobules and cellular collapse (Fig. 14–20). B cells are increased in the liver in chronic hepatitis of unknown cause.[194]

Symptoms. In infants, as in adults, females are affected more often than males, in a ratio of four to one, and the disease may occur as early as six months of age. The onset is associated or not with jaundice and is usually insidious. Hepatosplenomegaly, spider angiomas, and palmar erythema are noted, and occasionally there is tenderness over the liver. Systemic manifestations in-clude diarrhea, pleurisy, pericarditis, glomerulonephritis, myocarditis, and diabetes mellitus. Unremitting nosebleeds secondary to hypoprothrombinemia may be the only presenting symptom in young children. If the LE factor becomes positive or an antinuclear factor develops, the disorder is termed lupoid hepatitis and carries a slightly worse prognosis. Hypergammaglobulinemia is the rule and a false positive VDRL may be noted. The liver decreases in size as cirrhosis progresses.

Diagnosis. The disease must be differentiated from chronic persistent hepatitis. Usually, the bilirubin is increased owing to the conjugated fraction, and transaminase levels increase significantly. Even a mild elevation of transaminase implies progression of disease and should be considered highly abnormal. The albumin is normal or low as are the clotting factors. Anti–smooth muscle and antiendoplasmic

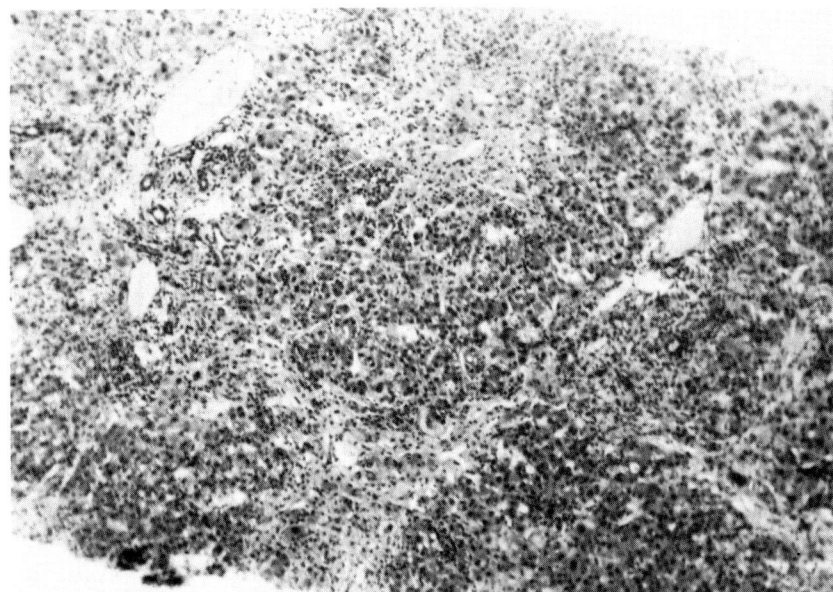

Figure 14-20 Subacute hepatic necrosis. A bridge of necrosis extends between the portal triads on the left to the triad on the right.

reticulum antibodies are present in the serum.

Treatment. There is no question that steroid therapy is of value in the treatment of this disease, and therapy is initiated if bridging necrosis is present on biopsy or if liver function abnormalities have persisted for longer than three months.[189, 199] Prednisone is given in a dosage of 2 mg per kg per day in four divided doses and continued until liver function tests are at or near normal levels. Steroids are gradually tapered over the following weeks to an alternate-day schedule and maintained for 18 to 24 months. If there is no response to steroids within six weeks, azathioprine, in a dosage of 1.5 mg per kg per day, is added to the schedule. Such treatment will promote remission or conversion to chronic persistent hepatitis. In some series, treatment has been required for four to ten years before the disease becomes quiescent. Remissions are frequent, and the mortality approaches 20 per cent.

POSTNECROTIC CIRRHOSIS

Cirrhosis is irreversible end-stage liver disease characterized by widespread fibrosis and a nodular parenchyma that interferes with hepatocellular nutrition and alters hepatic hemodynamics.[190] The precise etiology of infantile cirrhosis is often not known, although it may be associated with idiopathic hepatocellular and ductal cholestasis (e.g., biliary atresia); with inherited cholestasis or genetically transmitted metabolic disease, such as galactosemia, hereditary fructose intolerance, tyrosinemia, or antitrypsin deficiency; and with acquired cholestasis, such as viral hepatitis or chronic active hepatitis. Cirrhosis may be "active" with hepatocellular necrosis (poorly compensated) or "inactive" (compensation),[190] therefore, treatment of the underlying disease may influence the severity of the cirrhosis (e.g., dietary elimination of lactose for the infant with galactosemia). Prevention of cirrhosis is the optimal goal; otherwise, treatment is supportive or directed against the complications of this slowly progressive process.

Pathology. The liver is enlarged or shrunken but is usually firm and nodular, having a reddish-yellow color. Histologically, broad, narrow bands of connective tissue traverse the liver and represent both collapsed stroma and enhanced fibroblastic activity. Portal triads may coalesce, but some central veins remain (Fig. 14-21).

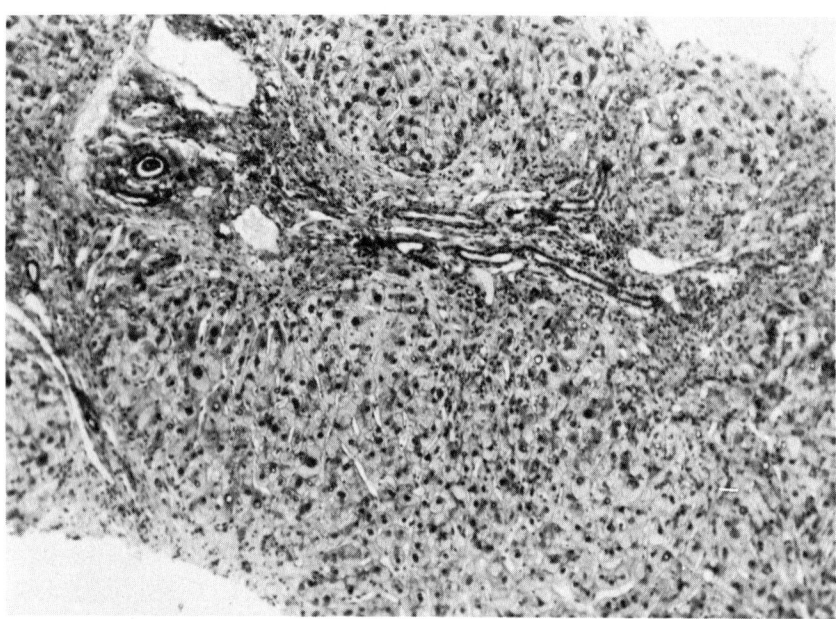

Figure 14–21   Postnecrotic cirrhosis. A thin band of connective tissue traverses this section and totally distorts the architecture.

Symptoms.   The history may fail to disclose previous liver disease, although one may elicit symptoms such as failure to thrive, anorexia, dark urine, or bleeding diatheses. Signs of chronic liver disease, such as palmar erythema, spider angiomas, parotid swelling, and splenomegaly, may be observed. The abdominal veins are dilated and ascites is present in advanced disease.

Diagnosis.   Persistent elevations of the transaminase, hypoalbuminemia, and hypergammaglobulinemia as well as hypoprothrombinemia all indicate cirrhosis, and the development of hypersplenism and esophageal varices document it. The definitive diagnosis is by liver biopsy.

Treatment.   If the biopsy indicates active parenchymal disease, the administration of prednisone as described earlier may be indicated. Otherwise, the treatment is that for liver failure, as indicated by hyperammonemia or bleeding abnormalities. In addition to an adequate intake of fat-soluble vitamins, a diet high in protein (2 gm/kg/day) and carbohydrate should be encouraged for the patient without liver failure. Hypochromic anemia secondary to blood loss or splenic hemolysis may be severe enough to require blood transfusions. Thrombocytopenia is usually the first indicator of hypersplenism, and leukopenia can lead to serious infection, but impaired coagulation is the major hematologic complication of cirrhosis. Decreased activity of vitamin K–dependent coagulation factors and thrombocytopenia are serious problems for the poorly compensated infant with cirrhosis; parenteral vitamin K (5 to 10 mg/dose), fresh frozen plasma (10 ml/kg/dose), and platelet concentrates may need to be administered to decrease the potential of blood loss.

Bleeding from *esophageal varices* requires prompt diagnosis and aggressive management (see Chapter Eleven).

Ascites[199] is another serious complication of cirrhosis and subsequent portal hypertension that will often diminish when the infant is placed on a low-sodium diet (1 to 2 gm/day). Pharmacologic diuresis can be dangerous because of rapid reaccumulation of ascitic fluid and precarious effective blood volume. Spironolactone (3 mg/kg/day) is one of the safest drugs for mobilization of ascites because of its potassium-sparing effect and its ability to inhibit aldosterone. However, urine electrolytes must be carefully evaluated during therapy with this diuretic; if urine sodium continues to be less than 15 mEq/L after 72 hours, the dose may be doubled and subsequently increased to 10 mg per kg per day. Chlorothiazide (20 to 30 mg/kg/day) is added to the therapeutic regimen if spironolactone is not effective. Furosemide and ethacrynic acid are used only if the ascites continues to be refractory. Complications of diuretic therapy include excessive reduction in plasma volume, hyponatremia, hypokalemia, and encephalopathy. Paracentesis may be necessary to provide symptomatic relief from dyspnea and abdominal distress; salt-poor albumin (1 gm/kg/dose) is usually infused during this procedure. Decompressive portal shunts and the continuous peritoneovenous shunt (of LeVeen)[193] are rarely considered for infants with intractable ascites.

Hepatic coma (portal-systemic encephalopathy) may be precipitated by gastrointestinal bleeding, electrolyte abnormalities, excessive dietary protein, infection, and certain drugs (especially sedatives, analgesics, and diuretics). Protein catabolism is minimized by cleansing the bowel of blood, providing less dietary protein, and sterilizing the colon with antibiotics such as neomycin (100 mg/kg/day), which suppress growth of bacteria that produce proteolytic enzymes. Lactulose, 10 gm TID or titrated to a point of loose stools, will also decrease blood ammonia because its bacterial degradation causes an increase in intestinal acidity and the pH gradient favors movement of ammonia into the gut lumen. Theoretically, lactulose and neomycin are mutually exclusive. Exchange transfusions, hemoperfusion with activated charcoal, and parenteral steroids have not been therapeutically effective.[191] Because of their small size, most infants with end-stage chronic liver disease are not candidates for liver transplantation.

INDIAN CHILDHOOD CIRRHOSIS

In tropical areas, especially India, infantile cirrhosis is extraordinarily common.[193a, 196, 197] It is now reported in one sibship in the U.S.A.[139a]

Incidence. The incidence is unknown, although in one 8-year period, 166 cases were seen in Madras, India. A similar disease is seen in the West Indies, where Jamaicans have termed it veno-occlusive disease, but this has been related to aflatoxin ingestion. It may occur sporadically in other parts of the world and has recently been described in Great Britain.

Etiology. Genetic factors may be involved, for there is a familial incidence. Affected children are usually from the Brahman caste and are well nourished.

Pathology. In early cases and in asymptomatic patients, the changes may resemble those of viral hepatitis with mild to severe swelling of liver cells, periportal and intralobular cellular infiltrate of mononuclear cells, "balloon" cells, and rare acidophilic bodies. After several weeks there are rarefaction of cytoplasm and pyknotic nuclear changes. Periportal infiltrates are present, but intralobular ones have decreased and the reticular framework is intact. With persistent disease, parenchymal destruction, heavy intralobular infiltrates, and fibroblasts appear. Later, cirrhosis is the major feature with increased numbers of fibroblasts, proliferation of reticulin and collagen fibers, and areas of regeneration. Inflammatory changes and fatty infiltration are absent. Increased copper concentrations in the liver and orcein-positive deposits in both liver and kidney have been described. The onset is between one and three years of age.

Symptoms. The disease may be entirely asymptomatic until cirrhosis develops. Otherwise it occurs in two forms. *"Posthepatitis"* is initiated as a disease resembling viral hepatitis that fails to clear, and after several months to years, jaundice and hepatomegaly recur along with fever, anorexia, irritability, vomiting, or diarrhea. In *malignant hepatitis* the disease progresses relentlessly to cirrhosis with anasarca and portal hypertension.

Differential Diagnosis. In tropical areas, the disease must be differentiated from kala-azar, malaria, and schistosomiasis.

Diagnosis. The laboratory data are those of hepatitis and, later, cirrhosis.

Treatment. Supportive therapy is given as for other forms of cirrhosis.

Prognosis. The mortality rate approximates 60 per cent, with death occurring weeks to years after the onset of illness.

TURKISH FAMILIAL CIRRHOSIS

Three pairs of siblings with familial cirrhosis have been reported from Turkey: Five were male and one female.[192] Abdominal swelling was noted as early as one year of age. There was usually no history of jaundice prior to the onset of hepatosplenomegaly. Transaminases were modestly or moderately elevated, bilirubin ranged from 0.6 to 2.8 mg per dl, and serum proteins were normal. There was no evidence of infectious, inherited, or metabolic liver disease. Disease did not seem to be progressive.

INHERITED AND METABOLIC HEPATOCELLULAR DISEASES

GALACTOSEMIA

Galactosemia is of major concern in the neonate as a cause of jaundice, for if untreated, it may lead to cirrhosis, severe brain damage, and cataracts.

Incidence. In different areas of the world, the incidence of galactosemia is estimated from 1 in 10,000 to greater than 1 in 100,000. In a Massachusetts study in which more than 177,000 patients were screened, only two cases were found.[245] Double heterozygosity for the Duarte variant and galactosemia is less rare (1:3750), and it is suggested that the Duarte and galactosemic genes are allelic with the normal one. These patients are asymptomatic as neonates, and red blood cell transferase is approximately 17 per cent of normal.[243a]

Etiology. The disease is inherited as an autosomal recessive form and affects males more often than females. Usually, infants lack the enzyme galactose-1-phosphate uridyl transferase which is necessary for the conversion of galactose to glucose. New variants are galactose-1-phosphate uridyl transferase sensitive to product inhibition by glucose-1-phosphate[222] and uridine diphosphate galactose-4-epimerase deficiency.[213, 219a, 236] Galactokinase deficiency can also cause hyperbilirubinemia and cataracts, owing to failure of conversion of galactose to galactose-1-phosphate, but symptoms are later in developing.

Pathology and Pathophysiology. The cerebral and renal lesions are well described elsewhere; they are due to the accumulation of galactose-1-phosphate in erythrocytes, lens, kidney, and liver. In the liver there are fatty infiltration of hepatic cells, focal necrosis, and cirrhosis. Hypoglycemia develops after administration of galactose.[230]

Symptoms. The clinical hallmarks of the disease include hepatosplenomegaly, cataracts, and mental retardation. Affected infants may be normal at birth or may already have an enlarged liver or spleen or both. After a few days of milk ingestion, vomiting and diarrhea occur, and this is often followed by severe dehydration. Jaundice and hepatosplenomegaly usually are pronounced by the end of the first week. Cataracts may appear as early as a few days after birth, and mental retardation is often evident within a few weeks. Because of inadequate caloric intake, growth retardation is common. Ascites is a poor prognostic sign and indicates severe liver disease and hypoproteinemia. Purpura is another manifestation, and hemolysis contributes to the jaundice. Untreated, these infants die of hepatic failure or bacteremia.

Diagnosis. The urine is positive by Clinitest for reducing substances but is negative to Clinistix, which measures glucose. The diagnosis is made by assay of red blood cell transferase. Liver function tests are generally abnormal.[224] A prenatal diagnosis is possible by enzyme assay of fetal erythrocytes.

Treatment. Since the major source of galactose in the diet is lactose, milk and milk products must be eliminated. Milk ingestion should also be restricted in pregnant women who have previously had infants with the disease. Liver failure has been successfully treated by exchange blood transfusion.

Prognosis. Patients remain asymptomatic when they follow the diet but experience diarrhea or vomiting with dietary indiscretions. If the condition is diagnosed and treated early in life, abnormal liver function tests return to normal and cataract formation is reversed or stopped. Growth retardation seems to persist, however. If the disease is diagnosed late, the chances are good that portal hypertension has developed and mental retardation persists.

HEREDITARY FRUCTOSE INTOLERANCE

This rare inborn error of metabolism was first described in 1956 as a familial disorder characterized by symptoms of hypoglycemia following the ingestion of foods containing fructose.[208]

Incidence. The incidence is estimated to be 1 in 40,000, and transmission is of an autosomal recessive form.

Etiology and Pathophysiology. There is a deficiency of fructose-1-phosphate aldolase (and, rarely, fructose 1,6-diphosphate aldolase) with subsequent accumulation of fructose and fructose-1-phosphate in body tissues. In the liver are prominent steatosis, pseudoacinal (glandular) distribution of liver cells, and hepatic cell necrosis. Portal or lobular fibrosis may not be obvious early in the disease, but deposition of fibrous tissue progresses if the infant is not treated.

Symptoms. The onset of symptoms is usually in the first few months of life, when juices or fruits are added to the diet. Drowsiness, convulsions, pain, sweating, or even coma are immediate sequelae to ingestion of fruits or sugar. In a few patients, bloating, nausea, and vomiting are the major manifestations. Some children evidence mental retardation. Older children demonstrate a distinct aversion to sweets.

Diagnosis. Hypoglycemia following fructose ingestion is diagnostic. After fructose administration, glucagon will not produce hyperglycemia.[246a]

Treatment. Therapy consists of elimination of fructose from the diet.

TYROSINEMIA

This disorder of protein metabolism is associated with cirrhosis.[204, 215]

Incidence. The incidence is probably greater than 1 in 100,000 in most countries.

Etiology. Tyrosinemia is inherited as an autosomal recessive disease whose enzymatic defect is poorly understood. A deficiency in parahydroxy phenyl pyruvic acid oxidase activity, which causes an increase in plasma tyrosine, has been demonstrated.

Pathophysiology. The disorder has been associated with ocular abnormalities, mental retardation, or skin keratoses in some families, and with cirrhosis in others.

Symptoms. Elevated tyrosine levels may cause apathy and, eventually, mental retardation. Symptoms develop earlier in infants taking high-protein feeds. Some children may show no symptoms until six months of age, when cirrhosis, rickets, and renal disease are obvious.

Diagnosis. Elevated serum alpha-fetoprotein levels are common as well as elevated serum tyrosine and, perhaps, methionine. Renal disease is represented by aminoaciduria, glycosuria, and phosphaturia (Fanconi syndrome). Amino acids are elevated in the urine.

Treatment. A low tyrosine, phenylalanine, and methionine diet may improve the renal lesions but not the hepatic disease.

Prognosis. There is an increased incidence of hepatoma in later childhood, and therefore these patients should be followed closely with periodic liver scans.[252]

WILSON'S DISEASE

This inborn error of copper metabolism results in copper excess that leads to severe hepatic and neurologic disease. This accounts for its synonym, hepatolenticular degeneration, described by Wilson in 1912.[242, 247]

Incidence. The gene frequency is estimated at 1 in 500 births, giving the disease an incidence of about 1 in 1 million live births.

Inheritance. Family studies indicate that Wilson's disease is inherited as an autosomal recessive trait. Although primarily seen in Caucasians, it may occur in all nationalities; we have seen two affected brothers from one family in Trinidad.

Etiology. The exact genetic abnormality is not yet clearly defined, but the end result is excessive deposition of copper in most body tissues, particularly the brain, liver, and kidneys. Copper seems to be the most likely cause of the nephrotoxicity and of brain degeneration and necrosis, but it is not absolutely clear that copper is the cause of hepatic necrosis.

A decrease in serum ceruloplasmin has been documented in most patients with Wilson's disease; normal levels of this protein have been reported in some patients, however, especially in adolescents presenting with chronic active hepatitis who are subsequently found to have Wilson's disease. The ceruloplasmin molecule in affected patients does not seem to be structurally different from that of normal subjects. That the liver is definitely involved in the etiology of Wilson's disease is shown by the fact that after liver transplantation, patients no longer require copper chelation therapy. Significantly in the homozygote and partially in the heterozygote, the incorporation of copper into ceruloplasmin is impaired. Biliary excretion of copper is decreased in patients with the disease. One current hypothesis suggests that there is a defect in lysosomal function, resulting in defective excretion of copper into bile. However, against this theory is the fact that early in the disease lysosomal copper is not increased. A second theory suggests that metallothionein, a low molecular weight binding protein in the liver, has an abnormally high affinity for copper and causes its retention within the liver, thereby rendering the metal unavailable for incorporation into ceruloplasmin or for excretion into bile.

Pathology and Pathophysiology. To understand the events of Wilson's disease we must first consider the normal mechanisms of copper metabolism. Copper is essential to homeostasis, being incorporated into a variety of oxidative enzymes: cytochrome c oxidase, superoxide dismutase, and ceruloplasmin. Excessive copper, however, is toxic to the body, presumably through its inhibitory action upon ATPase. The daily diet contains 2 to 5 mg of copper, probably half of which is absorbed through the stomach and proximal small bowel. Thirty to 70 per cent of that which is absorbed passes through the portal vein to the liver, where it is incorporated into proteins. Some copper passes through the liver and appears in the serum complexed with albumin, and with a lesser quantity complexed with amino acids.

Amounts of copper exceeding those required by the body are excreted primarily through the bile, although small quantities are excreted through the urine. In the bile, copper complexes with taurocholate and with low and large molecular weight proteins. There is some evidence that, as with bile salts, an enterohepatic circulation for copper exists. Bound copper is not absorbed in the proximal small bowel, but later, in the distal ileum, after the bile salt complex is split, copper is absorbed from the distal ileum.

The liver is the chief organ for storage as well as for excretion of copper, and, although it and the central nervous system contain the greatest copper concentrations, muscle and bone contain over half of total body copper because of their relative mass. Small amounts of copper are bound by metallothionein, which is present in the cytosol and lysosomes of hepatocytes. Ceruloplasmin is the major binding protein of copper. This blue plasma protein is an alpha$_2$ globulin containing 6 to 8 atoms of copper. It functions as an oxidase enzyme, oxidizing ferrous to ferric ions. By the incorporation of copper into its molecule during synthesis, it serves to remove the metal from the liver. Because the copper is irreversibly bound to the enzyme it is not available for exchange within the body, and ceruloplasmin cannot therefore be considered a transport protein. In the normal subject, the oral administration of radiolabeled copper (^{64}Cu) is followed in one to two hours by a peak in serum radioactivity of the label, reflecting absorption from the gut.

The counts decrease, but as the label is incorporated into ceruloplasmin, a second peak appears at 48 hours after ingestion.

In the normal subject, serum copper representing copper bound to ceruloplasmin and that small percentage (5 per cent) bound to albumin measure 70 to 160 μg per dl. Serum ceruloplasmin measures 25 mg per dl, and urinary copper excretion is less than 50 μg in 24 hours. Hepatic copper is normally less than 250 μg per gm dry weight.

In Wilson's disease the serum copper is low, often below 20 μg per dl, probably owing to increased copper excretion in the urine. Copper absorption, however, seems to be normal, and after a loading dose the serum copper rises to greater than normal values and urinary copper excretion increases. The serum ceruloplasmin is low, because of its decreased synthesis by the liver. Normal values, however, have been reported in some affected individuals. Isotope studies show a failure of the second serum rise in copper to indicate its appearance in ceruloplasmin. Whole-body isotope studies using cupric chloride show a prolonged whole-body turnover of copper in both homozygotes and heterozygotes, and this is correlated with hepatic retention, diversion to muscle, impaired incorporation into ceruloplasmin, and abnormal partitioning of radioactive copper into red blood cells. Furthermore, biliary excretion of copper is significantly decreased. An abnormal copper-binding protein has been isolated from liver samples of patients with the disease. This high-avidity, copper-binding protein may perhaps be a primary gene product.

The pathophysiologic consequences of the disease are multiple. Hepatic copper content rises, and liver histology extends through a spectrum ranging from normal to cirrhotic. The liver biopsy contains some fat, glycogen nuclei, and Mallory bodies in addition to fine fibrous septa. Some patients, particularly adolescents, will have biopsy findings indistinguishable from those of chronic active hepatitis. Central nervous system involvement is reflected by deposition of copper in the caudate and lenticular nuclei, which may progress to softening and cavity formation. Copper is deposited along the posterior margin of the cornea near the limbus, resulting in the classic Kayser-Fleischer rings.

In the kidney, copper deposition causes a variety of lesions affecting primarily the renal tubules. An early degenerative arthritis has been reported, although the cause is unknown.

Symptoms. The clinical onset of Wilson's disease is rare before six years of age and may occur as late as the fifth decade of life. We have seen one patient in whom liver disease and jaundice were evident at two years of age. Most patients under the age of ten present classically with liver disease, and the neurologic manifestations appear later. Occasionally a child will demonstrate only central nervous system symptoms, and very rarely the disease presents solely as an acute hemolytic anemia.

The liver dysfunction can present as acute viral hepatitis, chronic active hepatitis, cirrhosis, or chronic cholestasis of childhood. In a fulminant form it may present as ascites and advance rapidly to hepatic coma. Some asymptomatic children simply present with upper gastrointestinal hemorrhage secondary to esophageal varices and portal hypertension. Often Wilson's disease is discovered in the evaluation of a child with few hepatic symptoms who has been discovered to have abnormal liver function tests.

Neurologic involvement fulfills the original description of hepatolenticular degeneration. The first signs are insidious, with deviations from normal behavior resulting in personality changes that may require psychiatric referral. Eventually a parkinsonian picture may appear, with drooling, mask-like facies, and loss of fine motor control reflected first in handwriting. Athetoid movements suggesting chorea may be the first sign, and such may eventually progress to a state of decerebrate rigidity. Others demonstrate a "wing-beating" tremor.

Some patients may present with unexplained acute hemolytic anemia, although this manifestation often accompanies a presentation of acute hepatitis. The hemolysis appears related to an acute loss of copper from tissues, after which the increased serum and red blood cell copper damages the erythrocytes and causes autohemolysis, decreased erythrocyte glutathionine levels, and inhibition of glucose-6-phosphate dehydrogenase and glutathione reductase. In addition, increased Heinz body formation occurs after exposure of red blood cells to acetylphenylhydrazine. Episodes of anemia of this type are seen early in the disease before hepatic and neurologic manifestations are obvious, or after cessation of penicillamine therapy. In short, they occur during periods of rapid body accumulation of copper.

Renal involvement is a late manifestation, with both glomerular and tubular function affected. Most characteristic is a Fanconilike syndrome, with renal tubular acidosis, aminoaciduria, glycosuria, hyperuricosuria, and calciuria. Hematuria has also been described.

Arthralgia, described by some patients, is related to osteoarthritis or osteoporosis with rickets and even pseudofractures. In the rare patient, azure lunulae, or blue moons, of the nails as well as sunflower cataracts develop. Most patients, if untreated after the first decade, will eventually develop Kayser-Fleischer rings of the cornea.

Diagnosis. Many of the findings once considered pathognomonic for the diagnosis of Wilson's disease are now recognized to occur in other disorders, primarily those associated with cholestasis, such as familial intrahepatic cholestasis, biliary atresia, and primary biliary cirrhosis. The disease, however, must be suspected in any patient with atypical neurologic disease or with hepatitis that has become chronic.

Slit-lamp examination of the eyes provides a rapid confirmation of Kayser-Fleischer rings if they are present. A low serum ceruloplasmin value is strongly suggestive of the disease, but this protein may be low in other forms of liver disease, in acute liver failure, or in protein-losing diseases such as the nephrotic syndrome. Furthermore, some patients may have normal levels of ceruloplasmin or protein-losing enteropathy. The serum copper is low and urinary copper high, but, again, these findings may be present in other forms of liver disease. Meticulous care must be taken in collections of samples to prevent copper contamination. The 24-hour urine copper excretion is extremely helpful and a penicillamine-loading test is often used for screening patients.[247] One gm of penicillamine is given orally, and the urine is collected in a copper-free container over the next 24 hours. Normal controls excrete less than 30 to 50 μg of copper in 24 hours; homozygotes, more than 100 μg in 24 hours. Hepatic copper levels are the most important diagnostic criteria, and hepatic copper is well above the normal of 50 μg per gm dry weight. Increased hepatic copper is also present in cholestatic diseases but rarely reaches the levels attained in patients with Wilson's disease. This is not an absolute diagnostic tool, for rarely one encounters a patient with Wilson's disease who has a normal hepatic copper level.

Radiolabeled copper studies, although limited to investigative use because of their cost, provide helpful data in the diagnosis of atypical patients. The second peak of isotope in the serum affecting incorporation of copper into ceruloplasmin is present in patients with cholestatic disease but not in those with Wilson's disease. Patients who are heterozygote carriers for Wilson's disease show a subnormal second peak.

As noted previously, liver histology may show a variety of pathologic change, although specific stains may show increased copper. Recently, however, electron microscopy has demonstrated mitochondrial changes considered specific for Wilson's disease.

Detection of the heterozygote is essential to prevent progression of the disease, which can be totally aborted by the institution of early therapy. Obviously, liver function, ceruloplasmin, and copper studies are the first line of investigation after slit-lamp examination of the eyes. However, it must be remembered that ceruloplasmin levels may be normal in this disease and may be increased by stress or by estrogens, such as in birth control pills. Therefore, liver biopsy for histology and copper quantitation remain the major diagnostic tests for the carrier as well as for the patient with overt disease.

Treatment. Screening of infants should probably be performed in high-risk areas where there is considerable intermarriage. Therapy is extraordinarily effective, for penicillamine chelates copper and the copper chelate is excreted in the urine. If treatment is instituted at an early stage, symptoms can be totally reversed. The drug is administered orally in four divided doses, starting at a level of 0.25 to 0.50 gm per day. It is increased over several weeks to a final dosage of 1.5 to 2 gm per day. It must be continued indefinitely and administered as in the dextroisomer Cuprimine. Pyridoxine hydrochloride, 50 mg daily, is also given to prevent pyridoxine deficiency. Some physicians also give potassium sulfide three times daily for the first year to bind any dietary copper within the intestine. Since the penicillamine also binds iron, supplemental iron may be indicated. Because of the widespread use of copper piping, all patients should have their drinking water analyzed for copper; if the water contains more than 0.1 mg per liter, distilled or bottled water should be substituted. A low-copper diet restricts chocolate, nuts, shellfish, dried fruits, mushrooms, and liver. Since table salt contains 0.7 mg of copper per 100 gm, it is advisable to use analytic-grade sodium chloride.

The quantitative excretion of urinary copper is monitored, and when this has decreased to near-normal levels, the drug is decreased to a maintenance level of 1 gm per day.

Occasionally, sensitivity reactions to penicillamine occur and include the nephrotic syndrome, fever, rash, and neutrophilic agranulocytosis. These reactions usually develop within the first six weeks of treatment and resolve when the drug is discontinued and the patient treated with prednisone in a dosage of 1 to 2 mg per kg. After one to two weeks, the drug is reinstituted and steroids continued for another week or two. Symptoms usually do not recur. A late complication of fatal Goodpasture's syndrome has been reported after two to three years of drug intake.

Prognosis. Treatment early in life can prevent liver and brain disease. Even when treatment is initiated after the disease is well developed, neurologic and hepatic function may return to normal and the patient may survive in a reasonable state of good health. If there is severe brain cavitation, therapy will arrest the progress of the disease but will not reverse it. Screening must be performed on all family members; if asymptomatic patients are detected, treatment must be initiated.

PIPECOLIC ACIDEMIA AND HEPATOMEGALY

In 1968, increased serum pipecolic acid was identified in a child with neuropathy and hepatomegaly. Since then, several more patients have been identified. During the first few months of life, diarrhea and vomiting develop and, later, hepatomegaly and motor retardation with nystagmus and hypotonia. The liver shows cells in the portal area with vacuolated nuclei, foci of necrosis, and increase in connective tissue around central veins. There is atrophy of striated muscle and neuronal degeneration.

CYSTIC FIBROSIS

Although this is the most common genetic disease in Caucasians (1:1500), the incidence of associated liver disease is low and primarily represents steatosis or biliary cirrhosis.[210, 234, 249, 251]

Incidence. Liver disease occurs in 10 to 30 per cent of patients with cystic fibrosis.

Pathology. Focal biliary cirrhosis has been found as early as the third day of life. The usual change in infancy is mild periportal fibrosis, mild bile duct proliferation, and moderate inflammation. In long-standing disease, the bile ducts are plugged with inspissated eosinophilic material and are surrounded by fibrosis, inflammatory reaction, and biliary proliferation. Twenty to 30 per cent of patients have abnormalities of the gallbladder, varying from microgallbladder, a nonfunctioning organ, or one with cholelithiasis. The organ is lined with tall columnar epithelial cells and does not show inflammatory change. There is increased staining of mucicarmine-positive cells. The bile is white and viscous. Infant jaundice is attributed to bile duct compression.[251]

Symptoms. Persistent jaundice is unusual but may be associated with increased enterohepatic circulation of bilirubin (meconium ileus), drug hypersensitivity, or common duct inflammation secondary to inspissation of biliary secretions.

Diagnosis. Because of the focal nature of the lesion, liver function tests are usually normal until the disease progresses to cirrhosis. A liver biopsy may be needed to establish the diagnosis. Serum glutamyl transpeptidase (SGGT) is considered to be the most sensitive indicator of liver disease associated with cystic fibrosis, but normal levels are reported even with significant abnormalities.

Treatment. Cholestasis due to inspissated secretions may respond to choleretic agents, especially phenobarbital, which stimulates bile acid–independent flow.

Prognosis. This is always related to the infant's pulmonary dysfunction, although esophageal varices may cause serious bleeding.

ALPHA₁-ANTITRYPSIN DEFICIENCY

Alpha$_1$-antitrypsin is the major protease inhibitor of the extracellular fluids, accounting for 90 per cent of the alpha$_1$-globulin fraction of normal plasma proteins.[229, 244, 248] Alpha$_1$-antitrypsin deficiency, a genetic defect of glycoprotein metabolism, is the most common metabolic disorder associated with liver disease in infants. The alleles of the principal gene are collectively known as the protease inhibitor (Pi) system. The allele products (Pi phenotypes) are designated by letters according to the electrophoretic mobility of the protein, e.g., Pi M (medium-fast), Pi S (slow), and Pi Z (ultraslow) and number at least 26. For the infant with the most common phenotype, Pi M, there is a normal concentration of antitrypsin in the serum; in contrast, the patient with Pi Z has a deficient quantity of the antitrypsin protein.[233]

Incidence and Etiology. The incidence of the Pi Z phenotype varies in different parts of the world and ranges from 1 in 1500 to 1 in 3400.[232] The incidence of disease in individuals with a Pi Z phenotype is not precisely known; however, the association of the Z allele with liver disease in infants and with early-onset emphysema in adults has been clearly established. Deficiency of the antitrypsin protein may be inherited as an autosomal recessive trait or by a codominant allele pattern. It is estimated that up to 18 per cent of infants with neonatal hepatitis may have this disorder.

Pathophysiology. The general histologic findings are similar to those of other forms of hepatocellular cholestasis, including intracellular or canalicular bile retention and giant cell formation. Damage is due to presumed release of proteolytic enzymes from white blood cells. These accumulate in the liver and result in proteolysis. But the distinctive pathologic feature is intracellular periodic acid–Schiff (PAS)–positive, diastase-resistant globules in periportal hepatocytes (Fig. 14–22); these globules contain alpha$_1$-antitrypsin and are located in the endoplasmic reticulum. This suggests that the antitrypsin protein cannot be secreted out of the hepatocyte, perhaps because of an aberrant molecular configuration, thus leading to a decrease in serum antitrypsin. The relationship between liver cell antitrypsin accumulation and manifestations of liver disease is unknown. One could speculate, however, that exogenous or endogenous protease (e.g., intestinal bacterial or Kupffer cell protease) may gain access to the portal circulation and cause hepatocyte damage in the absence of antitrypsin (protease inhibitor) or cause the liver to become more vulnerable to hepatotoxic agents.[207a] This could ultimately lead to biliary hypoplasia (proliferation of bile ductules and bile duct

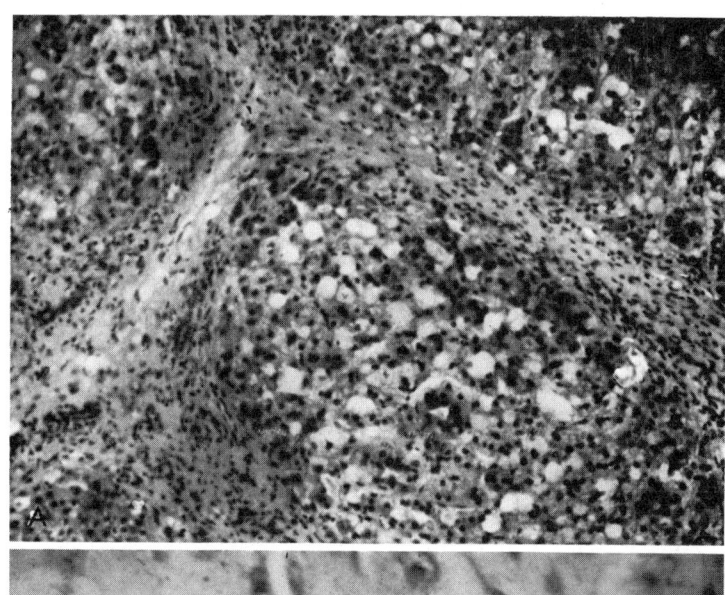

Figure 14–22 A, Alpha-1-antitrypsin deficiency. Periportal hepatocytes with distinctive intracellular periodic acid–Schiff (PAS) positive material. *B*, Early areas of fibrosis. *C*, Immunofluoresent staining with anti–alpha-1-antitrypsin.

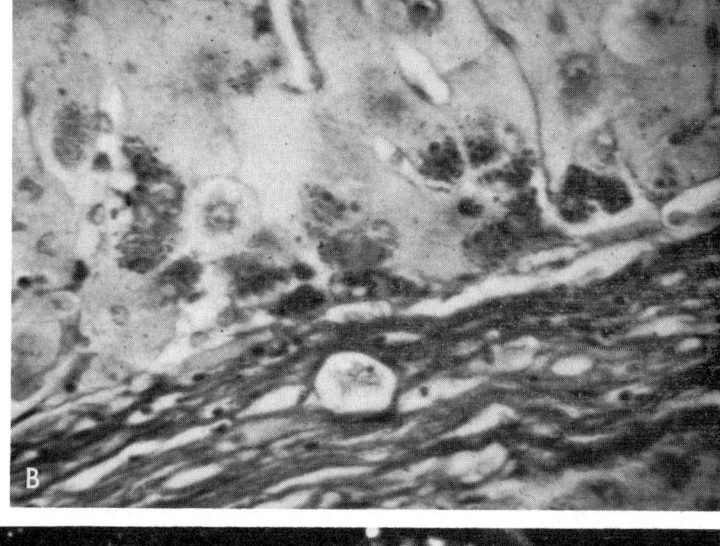

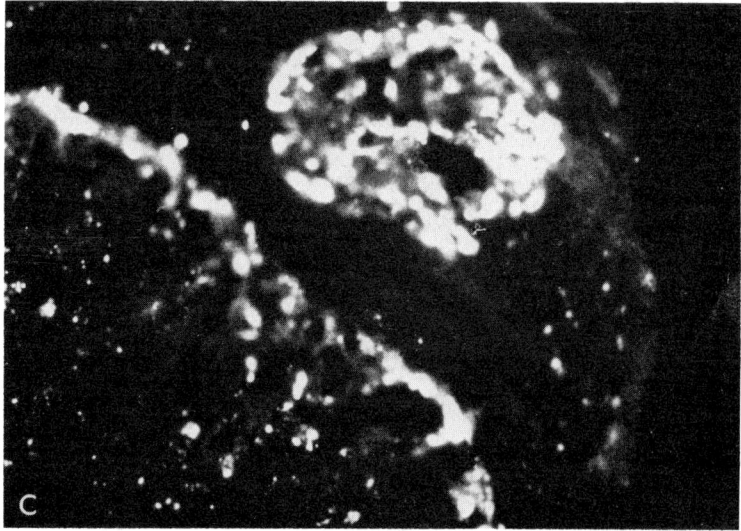

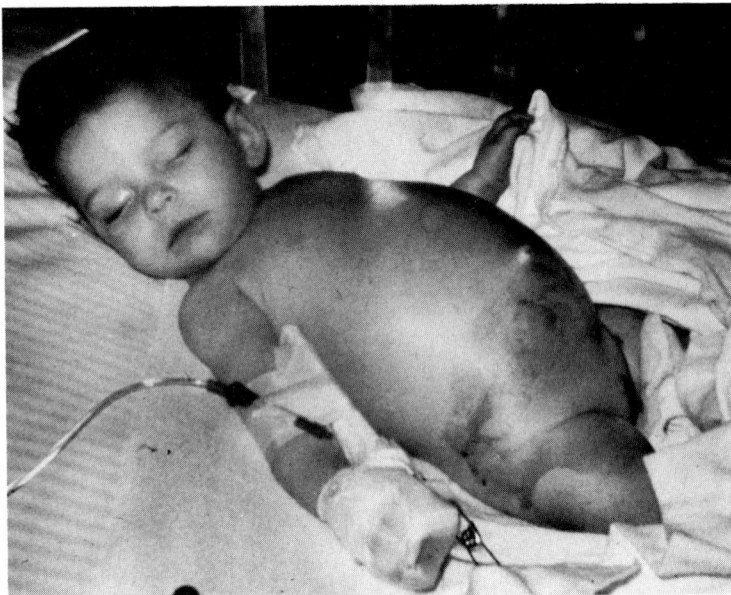

Figure 14–23 End-stage of alpha-1-antitrypsin deficiency in an infant admitted for ascites with no history of jaundice.

hypoplasia have both been noted), portal fibrosis, and cirrhosis. Cholestasis has occurred in the Pi SZ type.[239]

The PAS-positive material may be absent in the neonate with disease, but usually appears within several months. It is not totally specific for the disease since it has been observed in alcoholic cirrhosis and liver disease from hyperalimentation.[234a]

Clinical Evaluation. The usual presentation in infancy is hepatocellular cholestasis or neonatal hepatitis with jaundice and hepatomegaly, although the occasional infant may present with hallmarks of cirrhosis with no prior history of jaundice (Fig. 14–23).

Diagnosis. Simple observation of a diminished or absent alpha$_1$ globulin peak in the serum protein electrophoresis pattern suggests the diagnosis.[211] Diagnosis is then confirmed by a decreased serum alpha$_1$-antitrypsin concentration and protease inhibitor (Pi) typing. Normal values are 250 μg per ml or more, whereas those of affected infants are well below 100. Values in carriers lie between the two. Recently, mild liver disease has been observed in carriers.

Treatment. No specific treatment is available, but it is essential to identify infants at risk and provide proper genetic counseling to the family, for parents have a 0.25 probability of producing a homozygote infant with each pregnancy. Liver transplantation has been used for older children with end-stage liver disease due to antitrypsin deficiency, and studies are in progress using alpha$_1$-antitrypsin infusion.[220] Studies using replacement therapy with alpha$_1$-antitrypsin have been promising in adults with pulmonary disease.[215a]

Prognosis. The prognosis is extremely variable. Despite persistence of mild hepatocellular dysfunction, clinical improvement may occur in some infants a few months after birth. Others may die of cirrhosis rapidly. Biliary cirrhosis and portal hypertension eventually develop in some older children. Not all infants with Pi ZZ have liver disease; 50 per cent without neonatal hepatitis had intermittently abnormal liver function, and 15 per cent had a permanent abnormality.[223]

ZELLWEGER SYNDROME[209, 216]

Infants with this very rare autosomal recessive problem, also known as the cerebrohepato-renal syndrome, may present in early infancy with hepatocellular cholestasis. The major clinical manifestations are signs of central nervous system dysfunction, especially hypotonia; renal insufficiency; and liver dysfunction. This progressively lethal disease is associated with abnormal mitochondria and deficiency of peroxisomes. Cardiac lesions are patent ductus arteriosus and patent foramen ovale. Increased iron stores have been demonstrated in some infants with iron concentrated in hepatocytes or reticuloendothelial cells. A few infants have agenesis of the thoracic lobes of the thymus and pancreatic islet cell hyperplasia with hypoglycemia.

GLYCOGEN STORAGE DISEASES

The rare glycogen storage diseases are characterized by the accumulation of glycogen in the liver, muscles, and kidneys.[226, 237] Types I, II, III, IV, and VI are the major glycogenoses with liver involvement; the specific enzyme deficiencies and clinical characteristics are noted in Table 14–6.

Type I

Type I glycogen storage disease (hepatorenal glycogen storage disease, von Gierke's disease) is characterized by a deficiency of glucose-6-phosphatase activity and is inherited as an autosomal recessive trait.[240] It is a severe disease because of significant hypoglycemia and abnormal platelet function leading to seizures and bleeding.

Pathology and Pathophysiology. This enzyme deficiency causes an accumulation of glycogen in the liver because glucose-6-phosphate cannot be hydrolyzed to free glucose. Other organs affected are the kidney and intestine. Excessive lactate accumulates, urate secretion is inhibited, and hyperuricemia develops. Blood glucose may fall precipitously and cause ketosis and acidosis. The liver biopsy specimen shows marked infiltration of the hepatic cells with glycogen and fat and enlarged and vacuolated nuclei. The accumulated glycogen is normal in structure.

Symptoms. Hepatomegaly is discovered in the newborn period and persists through-

out life. As glycogen accumulates, enlargement of the buccal fat pads gives the infant's face a Kewpie-doll appearance (Fig. 14–24). Bruises over the body are common, and growth retardation becomes obvious as the baby grows older, becoming a short, rather adipose child with poor muscle development. Xanthomas and lipemia retinalis develop later in life. Sweating is relatively common during periods of hypoglycemia. As uric acid accumulates, gouty arthritis becomes an additional problem. Diarrhea is a complication of later childhood.

Diagnosis. There is fasting hypoglycemia that is unresponsive to epinephrine and glucagon, and there are marked elevations in serum lactate, pyruvate, uric acid, triglycerides, phospholipids, and cholesterol. Results of liver function tests are usually normal although the transaminases at times may rise into the hundreds. The definitive diagnosis is made by demonstration of absence or greatly reduced enzyme activity in liver tissue.

Treatment. Therapy has been unsatisfactory, although frequent feedings containing glucose are used to control the hypoglycemia. Continuous nocturnal intragastric feedings is the treatment of choice, but long-term therapy may be difficult to maintain.[217, 227a] Recently, portacaval shunt has been advocated, since it has been shown to reduce liver glycogen and result in the delivery of glucose-rich blood to peripheral

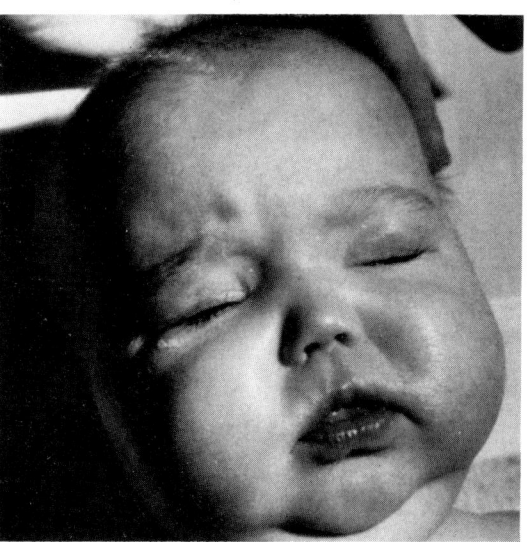

Figure 14–24 Typical facies of infant with glycogen storage disease. (Courtesy of Caroline Riely, M.D.)

Table 14–6   Differentiation of Glycogen Storage Diseases*

TYPE	CIR-RHOSIS	MUSCLE	BRAIN	HEART	BLOOD SUGAR RESPONSE	HYPO-GLYCEMIA	LIVER BIOPSY
I. Hepatic glucose-6-phosphatase deficiency	–	–	–	–	Minimal	+	Glycogen in nuclei. Large vacuoles in cytoplasm. Mosaic pattern.
II. Lysosomal α-glucosidase deficiency	–	+	–	+	Normal	–	Cells mildly enlarged. Glycogen in lysosomes. No mosaicism.
III. Amylo-1, 6-glucosidase deficiency	–	±	–	±	Increases immediately after eating—low fasting	–	Increased nuclear glycogen droplets in cytoplasm. Fibrous septa. Little fat.
IV. Amylo-1, 4 → 1, 6-transglucosidase or brancher enzyme deficiency	+	+	+	+	Variable	+	Large cytoplasmic vacuoles. Fibrous septa. Amylopectin deposits mainly at periphery of lobules.
V. Absence of muscle phosphorylase	–	+	–	–	Normal	–	Normal
VII. Absence of phosphorofructokinase	–	+	–	–	Normal	–	Normal
VI. Decreased phosphorylase	–	–	–	–	Basically non-responsive	–	Lipid droplets in cell cytoplasm. Most changes at periphery of lobule. Mosaic pattern.
VIII. Low phosphorylase activity but normal levels	–	–	+	–	Normal	–	Irregular size of glycogen-filled cells. Localized mosaic pattern in periphery.
IX. Deficient phosphorylase kinase	–	–	–	–	Normal	–	Irregular size of glycogen-filled hepatocytes. Largest hepatocytes are periportal. Some fibrous septa.
IXc. Deficient phosphokinase	–	+	–	–	Normal		
X. Deficient AMP-dependent kinase	–	+	–	–	No rise	–	Largest glycogen-distended cells near portal areas.

*From McAdams, A. J., Hug, G., and Bove, K.: Glycogen storage diseases, Types I to X. Hum. Pathol. 5:463, 1974. Used by permission.

tissue before it can reach the liver. This drastic procedure needs further evaluation.

Prognosis. Liver adenomas may develop in childhood.

Type II

Type II glycogen storage disease (generalized glycogenosis, Pompe's disease) is due to a deficiency of lysosomal alpha-1,-4-glucosidase and is also inherited as an autosomal recessive trait.

Pathology. Glycogen accumulates in most tissues, particularly in cardiac muscle and liver. Accumulation occurs within the lysosomes. These patients have hepatomegaly, but not cholestasis, in addition to cardiomegaly and myopathic hypotonia.

Symptoms. Generalized hypotonia is the presenting complaint. The muscular weakness resembles that of amyotonia congenita. The tongue is often enlarged, and the infant resembles a cretin. Progressive cardiac enlargement eventually results in cardiac failure, and death occurs by six months of age.

Diagnosis. Chest films and electrocardiograms indicate bilateral ventricular enlargement. The results of carbohydrate metabolism studies are normal, and the diagnosis is established by the finding of increased glycogen content in skeletal muscle. Specific enzyme deficiency is identified in muscle and fibroblasts.

Treatment. There is no treatment for this disease, and cardiac failure is treated as it develops.

Type III

Type III glycogen storage disease (limit dextrinosis, Cori's disease) is due to a deficiency of amylo-1,6-glucosidase, or the debrancher enzyme, and is a milder disease than type I. Inheritance is of an autosomal recessive type, and there is a higher incidence of muscle and liver involvement.

Pathology. Structurally abnormal glycogen resembling limit dextrin accumulates in the liver and other organs as in the type I disease, but it causes only moderate hepatomegaly.

Symptoms. Hepatomegaly is present early on, and, unlike type I disease, there is also splenomegaly. Cardiomegaly, myopathy, and hypoglycemia may also develop, but acidosis due to lactic acid accumulation and ketosis is rare. The liver sometimes returns to normal size at puberty.

Diagnosis. Serum transaminase levels are frequently elevated, and mild cirrhosis has been described. Although the serum lipids are somewhat increased, the uric acid usually remains normal. The definitive diagnosis is made by analysis of the erythrocytes for excessively branched glycogen and of the leukocytes, muscle, or fibroblasts for debrancher enzyme activity. Blood sugar is increased by epinephrine and glucagon after short periods of fasting but not after fasts of 12 hours or more.

Treatment. Therapy is limited to frequent feedings, with a high-protein meal before bedtime to prevent hypoglycemia. Continuous nocturnal intragastric feeds improve hypoglycemic syndromes. Portacaval shunting has been performed successfully in several patients.

Prognosis. The disease can be well controlled medically to provide for normal growth and development. However, less fortunate infants develop cirrhosis, myopathy, and nocturnal hypoglycemia, and a few, liver adenoma.

Type IV

Type IV glycogen storage disease (amylopectinosis or Andersen's disease) is a defect of glycogen synthesis rather than of degradation. Its mode of genetic transmission is unknown, but it results in hepatocellular dysfunction.

Pathology. The deficiency of brancher enzyme or phosphorylase causes an accumulation in the liver, kidneys, intestine, muscle, and other tissues of straight-chain insoluble polysaccharides, which resemble amylopectin.

Symptoms. Hepatomegaly is present in the first few months of life and is noted about the same time as a failure to gain weight. Muscle tone is poor. Progressive cirrhosis develops. Splenomegaly becomes apparent as portal hypertension manifests itself as anemia or bleeding esophageal varices.

Diagnosis. There is mild hypoglycemia, and liver function test results are compatible with those in cirrhosis. The glycogen of red blood cells and tissue stains as starch rather than as glycogen.

Treatment. Treatment is aimed toward the hepatic failure and the fluid accumulation that usually occurs but is ineffective in its long-term results.

Prognosis. The disease is uniformly fatal within the first five years of life.

Types V and VII

Types V and VII are limited to muscle and will not be discussed in this text.

Type VI

In Type VI glycogen storage disease (Hers' disease), increased hepatic glycogen accumulates as a result of reduced, but not absent, phosphorylase activity. The disease tends to occur in families and involves both sexes. Unfortunately, some patients have been placed in this category despite having normal phosphorylase activity and no other defined enzyme defect. Thus, the category has become a wastebasket, although it is probably the most common form of abnormal glycogen metabolism.

Pathology. After glucagon accumulates in the liver cells, hepatomegaly develops but regresses in later childhood.

Symptoms. As in the other forms, hepatomegaly, growth retardation, and increased concentrations of liver glycogen are the major manifestations of the disease.

Diagnosis. Blood sugar is often low, and blood lactate is normal or increased. The serum lipid levels are elevated. The blood sugar response to glucagon or epinephrine is variable and not diagnostic of the disease; definitive diagnosis is made only by phosphorylase assay of the leukocytes or liver tissue.

Treatment. No therapy is usually required. Five asymptomatic children have been reported who have hepatomegaly and increased liver glycogen concentrations but slow activation of phosphorylase owing to phosphorylase-d-kinase deficiency. These patients have responded to glucagon administration, with shrinkage of liver size.

Prognosis. The prognosis is excellent for hypoglycemia, and seizures are not a problem.

Type VIII

This form of glucogenosis is associated with severe central nervous system degeneration. The basic biochemical defect remains obscure, although there is low liver phosphorylase activity in the presence of normal levels of total liver phosphorylase.

Pathology. Zones of irregularly enlarged cells form localized mosaic plaques in the periphery of the lobules. Glycogen is concentrated in the cytoplasm and is not stored in the nuclei. There is no evidence of hepatic fibrosis. Excessive accumulations of the alpha form of glycogen are present in the axon cylinders and the synaptic vessels of the nervous system.

Symptoms. The infants appear normal at birth but within a few weeks develop hepatomegaly and signs of central nervous system degeneration, such as truncal ataxia, hypotonia, and nystagmus. Eventually, spasticity and decerebrate rigidity herald death.

Diagnosis. There are mild abnormalities of liver function, but the blood sugar responses to glucagon and to epinephrine are normal. There is no evidence of hypoglycemia. Urinary catecholamines are usually increased. The diagnosis is confirmed by the demonstration of low liver phosphorylase activity in the presence of normal enzyme levels.

Prognosis. The disease is uniformly fatal in infancy or in early childhood.

Type IX

This type of glycogenosis is associated with two distinct forms: one that is inherited as a sex-linked recessive and the other as an autosomal recessive trait. The biochemical defect of low phosphorylase activity is due to a deficiency of phosphorylase kinase. Other organ systems are not involved.

Pathology. The hepatocytes are irregularly distended by intracytoplasmic glycogen, and the largest cells are found in the periportal areas. Low-grade inflammatory changes and septa formation are seen throughout the tissue.

Symptoms. The only manifestation of the disease is hepatomegaly, which may be noted at birth. Development may be entirely normal, although a few children are growth retarded.

Diagnosis. The serum bilirubin, transaminase, and alkaline phosphatase may be mildly increased, and the cholesterol is elevated. The blood sugar response to glucagon is normal, but that to epinephrine is abnormal. Liver biopsy shows increased cytoplasmic glycogen, and enzyme assay shows low phosphorylase and phosphorylase kinase activities.

Prognosis. The ultimate prognosis is unknown, but the majority of these children have survived at least into early adult life.

Type IXc[223a]

This variant of type IX has been reported in a four year old boy and his two female siblings and differs in that muscle and erythrocytes are involved, as well as liver.

Pathology. Liver glycogen is greatly increased, and phosphorylase activity is decreased to 20 per cent of normal levels. Liver biopsy shows essentially normal liver architecture but increased glycogen in the hepatocytes. Occasional fat droplets are noted, but there is no evidence of cirrhosis. Gastrocnemius biopsy specimen shows increased glycogen and decreased PK activity, and, similarly, the PK activity of erythrocytes and granulocytes is reduced.

Symptoms. The index patient in this family presented with hepatomegaly, growth retardation, and jaundice at age four years. Physical examination revealed generalized muscular hypotonia but normal psychomotor development. The facies was doll-like. The two sisters had protuberant abdomens in infancy, but these became less prominent with age. They, likewise, had doll-like facies, but their growth was normal.

Diagnosis. Serum bilirubin is either normal or mildly increased. The transaminases may be elevated, and cholesterol, triglycerides, and total lipids are increased. Definitive diagnosis rests upon liver and muscle biopsy with enzyme analyses.

Type X

This rarest of the glycogen storage diseases presents with asymptomatic hepatomegaly and is due to deficient cyclic AMP–dependent kinase.

Pathology. The glycogen-distended hepatocytes are irregular in size, with the largest cells lying adjacent to the portal areas. The nuclei are not involved, and occasional cytoplasmic vacuoles are present within the cells. Septa formation is prominent, but inflammatory reaction is not a factor. Increased glycogen is also present in muscle and lies between the sarcolemma and the muscle fibers.

Symptoms. Hepatomegaly from early childhood is the only symptom.

Diagnosis. The diagnosis rests upon scrutiny of the liver and muscle biopsy specimens, with the demonstration of low phosphorylase activity and normal total phosphorylase content.

GRANULOMATOUS DISEASE OF CHILDHOOD

This inherited disease is characterized by suppurative lymphadenitis, hepatomegaly, splenomegaly, recurrent pneumonitis, chronic lung disease, liver abscess, and eczematoid dermatitis in areas near the abscesses or about the orifices. The organisms usually involved in these infections are *Staphylococcus*, *Serratia marcescens*, gram-negative enterococci, *Aerobacter aerogenes*, and the *Klebsiella* species.

Incidence. More than 100 cases have been reported since the illness was first described in 1952.

Inheritance. All of the patients originally reported were males, and an x-linked mode of inheritance was reported. More recent reports, however, described the disease in females as well, and so in some cases an autosomal recessive inheritance is probable. Although most of the patients have been of Caucasian origin, there have been a few black children among the group.

Pathology and Pathogenesis. Granulomatous disease of childhood is caused by a defect in the phagocytes that leaves them unable to kill certain bacteria.[207b] Abnormalities in the vacuolization of the cells and in the kinetics of their ingestion of bacteria have been noted. The neutrophils cannot form peroxide and have a decreased NADH oxidase activity. A number of steps are involved in the oxidative reactions of phagocytosis and can be condensed into three processes: increased oxygen uptake, increased hydrogen peroxide production, and increased hexose monophosphate shunt activity. The hydrogen peroxide forms a bactericidal system by reacting with a halide, iodine, and myeloperoxidase to produce iodination and bacterial death. In granulomatous disease, myeloperoxidase is released but the C_1 of glucose is not oxidized to carbon dioxide and there is no formation of peroxide. Therefore, those bacteria that produce peroxide and have no catalase to destroy it, i.e., *Streptococcus*, pneumococcus, and *Lactobacillus*, are phagocytized and die within these abnormal cells. Organisms that produce peroxide and also catalase to destroy it, i.e., *Candida, Staphylococcus, Serratia marcescens*, and gram-negative enteric organisms, survive in the abnormal cells and invade the reticuloendothelial system, whose cells have the same metabolic defect.

Typical granulomas and abscesses develop in infected sites. The granulomas contain yellow or tan pigmented, lipid-filled histiocytes. Liver biopsy shows granulomas with necrotic centers that contain cellular debris, polymorphonuclear leukocytes, giant cells, and pigment-laden macrophages. The small bowel structure is not affected, but the villi contain the same pigmented cells as well as PAS-positive histiocytes. Rectal biopsy tissue contains pigmented cells, giant cells, and granulomas, but there is no evidence of necrosis, although perianal fistulas are sometimes present. Pulmonary involvement is either segmental or diffuse.

Symptoms. In most patients, symptoms develop before the second year, with suppurative lymphadenopathy the most common finding. Hepatosplenomegaly, dermatitis, and pneumonitis are present in the majority of patients. Nearly half have hepatic or perihepatic abscesses, and one third have osteomyelitis. Rhinitis, stomatitis, and diarrhea are lesser complaints. Four out of one group of nine patients had overt gastrointestinal symptoms; two had steatorrhea and six had vitamin B_{12} malabsorption. The course of disease is one of chronic infection leading to severe debilitation.

Diagnosis. This disease must be differentiated from the hypogammaglobulinemias and agammaglobulinemias. Neutrophilic leukocytosis, hypergammaglobulinemia, and anemia of the normochromic-normocytic type are characteristic. Serum immunoglobulins are usually normal, but immunoglobulin A deficiency has been described. Some patients have a failure of lymphocyte transformation after phytohemagglutinin stimulation, and a serum inhibitor of chemotaxis and an abnormal inflammatory response as tested by a skin window have been demonstrated in one patient. Radiologic examination of the chest reveals pulmonary infiltrates, and of the abdomen, calcifications within the liver (Fig. 14–25). The diagnosis is made by demonstration of the defect in hydrogen peroxide formation by phagocytes and abnormal vacuolization of the cells during phagocytosis. Nitroblue tetrazolium, a yellow dye that is normally reduced to purple color inside the phagocytic vacuoles, is not affected by leukocytes from patients with granulomatous disease. Intermediate values in dye reduction have been obtained from cells of some mothers of patients, but others have had normal values. Diagnosis using fetal fibroblasts has been made *in utero*.[212]

Treatment. Intensive treatment of infections is the only available therapy. Some children have fared extremely well taking continuous gantrisin or sulfamethoxazole/trimethoprim.[243b] Granulocyte infusion has been used effectively for the treatment of aspergillosis in one patient.

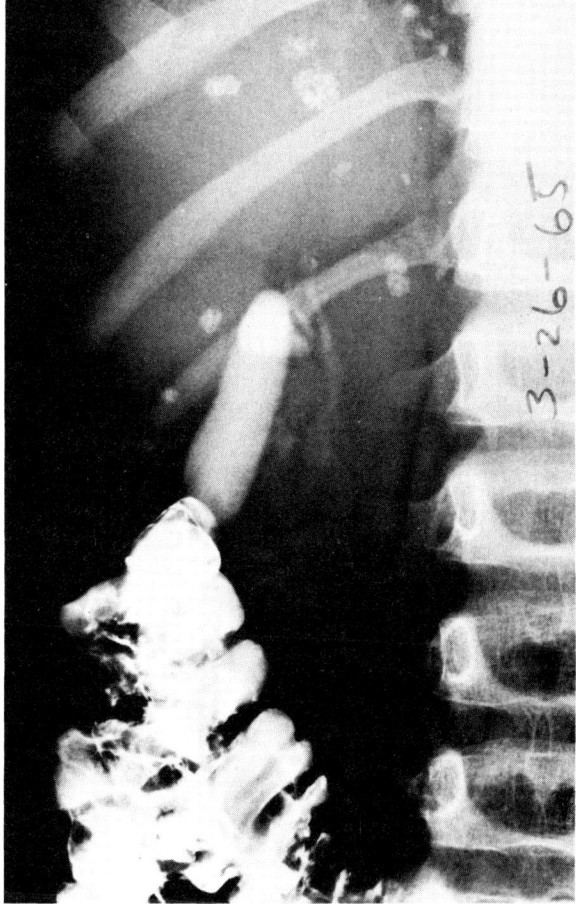

Figure 14–25 Calcified hepatic granulomas in a child with chronic granulomatous disease of childhood. The relationship of these densities to the opacified gallbladder and hepatic flexure of the colon can be seen.

Prognosis. The ultimate prognosis is poor; of one series of 92 patients, half were dead before their twelfth birthday.

Caution. Immunization against tuberculosis is contraindicated in these patients, for disseminated BCG infection can develop after vaccination. *In utero* diagnosis may be established by measurement of NBT reduction by cultured amniotic cells.

Job's Syndrome[201, 219]

This variant of chronic granulomatous disease affects red-haired and fair-skinned females. Its inheritance is presumed to be autosomal recessive or x-linked[228] in type, and in some patients it is due to a deficiency of glutathione peroxidase. The pathology and course are similar to those of granulomatous disease, but recent evidence indicates that sulfonamide administration increases the phagocytosis of white blood cells and leads to a decrease in the incidence of infection.

LIPID STORAGE DISEASES

Niemann-Pick Disease

This lipid storage disease is due to lysosomal sphingomyelinase deficiency.[205]

Incidence and Inheritance. Several hundred cases have been reported, with children of Jewish origin affected in an autosomal recessive form of inheritance.

Etiology and Pathology. Five variants of the disease have been described, with type

A, the most common infantile form, causing hepatosplenomegaly during the first year of life. These infants may have hepatocellular dysfunction, but this is more common in types B and D. Sphingomyelinase is responsible for the cleavage of phosphorylcholine from sphingomyelin. In its absence, sphingomyelin and comparable amounts of cholesterol accumulate in the reticuloendothelial system to produce an abundance of "foam" cells, large histiocytes with cytoplasm full of lipid droplets. They are most prominent in liver, spleen, and marrow. Histologic examination of the liver shows these cells in the sinusoids along with inflammation, fibrosis, and bile retention. Destruction of ganglion cells and demyelinization occur in the central nervous system of type A patients.

Symptoms. Affected infants are normal at birth but fail to gain weight. Hepatosplenomegaly and lymphadenopathy develop within the first few months of life. Some infants become markedly jaundiced. Feeding difficulties represent the onset of neurologic disease, which eventually progresses to a generalized deterioration of motor and mental function, rigidity of the body and extremities, and seizures. Many infants

seem to be deaf. Those with severe liver disease have marked abdominal distention, ascites, and edema. A cherry-red spot may be seen in the macula of the eye. In other infants, the onset of the disease is delayed and the course more prolonged and milder.

Diagnosis. Central nervous system deterioration in the presence of hepatosplenomegaly, particularly in a Jewish child, strongly suggests the disorder. Though not entirely specific for this disease, foam cells are present in bone marrow and in rectal and liver biopsy tissue. Chemical analysis and enzyme assay in white blood cells are required for certain diagnosis. Radiologic examination of the chest shows a "honeycomb" pattern in the lung fields. Liver function may be mildly or severely impaired.

Treatment. There is no known effective therapy.[205]

Prognosis. Some patients die in infancy, but others with mild disease may survive to adulthood.

Gaucher's Disease

This lipid storage is due to a deficiency of the enzyme β-glucosidase with resultant

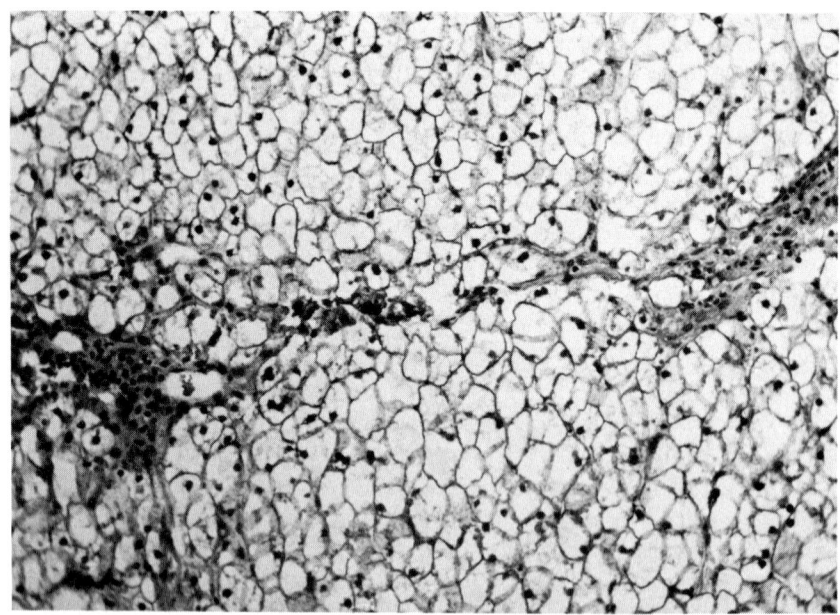

Figure 14–26 Gaucher's disease. The nucleus remains in the center of the vacuolated liver cells. There is some fibrosis and inflammation apparent in this section.

accumulation of glucosyl ceramide in reticuloendothelial tissue. Liver, spleen, lymph node, lung, and bone involvement is common, and the major manifestations of the disease are hypersplenism, bone pain, and pathologic fractures.

Inheritance. The pattern of inheritance is varied, with all autosomal or dominant expression.

Pathology. Three forms occur, including the acute neuropathic type (type 2), which usually leads to death by two years of age. Lipid-filled Gaucher cells are large, with eccentric nuclei and whorls of fibrils or filaments in the cytoplasm (Fig. 14-26). They involve all reticuloendothelial cell areas, which also accumulate glucosyl ceramide. Liver histology is abnormal, showing Gaucher cells with "wrinkled" cytoplasm about central hepatic veins and in sinusoids. Hepatic fibrosis may be evident, and eventually cirrhosis, portal hypertension, and ascites develop in all forms of the disease. Extramedullary erythropoiesis in the liver and spleen contribute to the increasing size of these organs.

Symptoms. Manifest after six months of age, in the usual chronic form of the disease, there are relatively few early symptoms other than an enlarged liver and spleen and seizures. In long-standing cases, hypersplenism, joint pain and deformities, and pulmonary hypertension develop in addition to cirrhosis. In patients in whom the onset of hepatosplenomegaly occurs before one year of age and in those with the acute form, there is significant neurologic disease with ocular palsies, brainstem involvement, spasticity, and anemia. Feeding difficulties are of neurologic origin, and eventually decerebrate rigidity renders the infant incapable of feeding.

Diagnosis. The diagnosis is made by finding the typical Gaucher cells in the bone marrow aspirate. Characteristically, the serum acid phosphatase value is elevated, and liver function abnormalities are common.

Treatment. There is no specific treatment for this disorder. Enzyme replacement therapy has been ineffective. Gavage feeding is necessary in infants with severe neurologic impairment, and steroid therapy may provide some improvement in joint pain and in hypersplenism. Enzyme replacement has been attempted through renal transplantation.[218]

Prognosis. Death before two years of age is the rule for those with the acute, early-onset form, but those with the chronic form survive well into adult life.

Hepatic Cholesterol Ester Storage Disease

A familial disorder has been described in which cholesterol esters accumulate in the liver and produce an orange-yellow discoloration of that organ owing to deficiency of acid lipase.[203, 207, 243] Hepatosplenomegaly is found on physical examination, but there is no other clinical evidence of chronic liver disease. A separate cirrhosis is seen pathologically, and enlarged liver cells are filled with fat droplets. Long-term follow-up is not available, and the cause of this abnormality in lipid metabolism is not known. However, bile salt metabolism is deranged, as evidenced by a decrease in deoxycholic acid and a decreased ratio of cholic to chenodeoxycholic acid in the bile.

Wolman's Disease

Wolman's disease occurs in early infancy and has been uniformly fatal.

Inheritance. Inheritance is of the autosomal recessive type, and several siblings may be affected.

Etiology. This disorder also represents a deficiency of lysosomal acid lipase, with accumulation of cholesterol esters and triglycerides in many organs of the body.[235]

Pathology. The liver and spleen are enlarged and contain deposits of cholesterol and its esters and of triglycerides. Similar deposits are present in lymph nodes, adrenal glands, and intestinal mucosa. Histologic study of the liver shows fat-laden hepatocytes and Kupffer cells, particularly near the portal areas, as well as portal fibrosis. The small bowel mucosa appears yellow, greasy, and granular. There are loss of villous structure, mucosal atrophy, and infiltrate of lipid-filled histiocytes in the lamina propria. Calcification and bilateral enlargement of the adrenals are characteristic of the disease. Histiocytes are found in thymus and bone marrow and in vacuolated lymphocytes in the peripheral blood.

Chemically, the liver contains 3 to 20 times the normal amount of cholesterol but normal phospholipids and glycolipids. The normal liver contains 1 to 1.5 per cent wet weight as triglyceride or neutral fat, but in this condition it constitutes 10 per cent. The spleen contains four- to fivefold increases of cholesterol, and lesser increases are noted in thymus, lung, and kidney. The gray matter of the brain contains one and one-half to two times normal cholesterol but that in white matter is normal. Myelination is abnormal.

Symptoms. In contrast to cholesterol ester storage disease, these infants are acutely ill during the first weeks of life with vomiting, chronic diarrhea, jaundice, failure to thrive, and progressive hepatosplenomegaly. One infant was normal until the age of five months, when symptoms appeared: She also had alpha- and beta-hypolipoproteinemia. The disease progresses rapidly, and death usually occurs within the first year of life.

Familial Neonatal Hepatosteatosis[241]

This is a similar disorder of undetermined etiology. In this condition, however, significant fatty infiltration and necrosis of hepatocytes are present at birth and lead to early hepatocellular dysfunction and death.

The Liver in Abetalipoproteinemia

Although the major manifestations of abetalipoproteinemia are chronic diarrhea, mental retardation, and abnormalities in the retina, the clinical picture may also include hepatomegaly and abnormal liver function. The disorder is discussed in detail in Chapter Sixteen; liver manifestations will be noted here.[242]

Pathology. Using both light and electron microscopy, Partin et al. have described liver biopsy changes produced in one infant by different dietary regimens.[234b] Pale, white-yellow tissue was obtained when the patient was taking a skim milk diet. The hepatocytes were distended by large fat droplets that displaced the nuclei. Focal accumulations of inflammatory cells were scattered throughout the lobules surrounding hepatocytes or fatty lakes. Early changes of fibrosis were evident in the ramifications of the portal tracts. The fat was neutral lipid. Biopsy taken several months after supplementation of medium-chain triglycerides (MCT) showed a slight reduction in the fat droplet population. Connective tissue plates were present but did not bridge the entire liver lobule. After one year of the MCT-substituted diet, liver biopsy showed micronodular cirrhosis and alcohol hyalin within the hepatocytes.

Symptoms. Liver disease is asymptomatic in patients with abetalipoproteinemia.

Diagnosis. Hepatomegaly or signs of liver dysfunction in such patients should suggest fatty liver infiltration or cirrhosis. Liver biopsy will demonstrate fatty infiltration.

Treatment. The disease is treated by a low-fat diet, although the value of MCT substitution is questionable if the liver is incapable of secreting endogenous triglyceride.

Prognosis. Liver biopsy changes have been described in only one patient, and the ultimate course of the liver disease is not yet known.

Sea-Blue Histiocyte Disease[221]

This hereditary disorder of lipid metabolism is transmitted as an autosomal recessive trait and has been reported in one family.

Etiology and Pathogenesis. The biochemical nature of this lipid disorder is not yet known. The reticuloendothelial system contains histiocytes with granules in the cytoplasm that stain bright blue with Wright's or Giemsa's stain. Foam cells may or may not be present in liver biopsy tissue.

Symptoms. The disease resembles other lipid storage disorders, with splenomegaly, hepatomegaly, pulmonary infiltrates, and thrombocytopenia as the main symptoms. The natural history is not yet known, and there is no effective therapy.

Fatal Familial Histiocytosis with Eosinophilia[202]

This extremely rare disease has been described in infants and established by history in others who were related and died in infancy.

Etiology. The disease is familial, with an autosomal recessive type of inheritance. The etiology is unknown, although there is a primary immune deficiency and thymic dysplasia. Because the disease resembles the graft-versus-host reaction, it is postulated that perhaps maternal-fetal transfer of immunologically competent cells triggers the reaction in these babies. Another consideration is that the disease represents a variant of the Letterer-Siwe syndrome.

Pathology. There is depletion of lymphocytes in the thymus, lymph nodes, spleen, and lamina propria of the intestine. Hassall's corpuscles are absent from the thymus, and there is an abnormal myeloid-erythroid ratio in the bone marrow, with a preponderance of eosinophils. Bizarre histiocytes proliferate in bone marrow, lymph nodes, and skin. Immunoglobulins are present in only small amounts or not at all. The liver and myocardium are infiltrated by histiocytes.

Symptoms. These infants are well until the third or fourth week of life, when a diffuse maculopapular rash, lymphadenopathy, and hepatosplenomegaly develop. Respiratory infections and septicemia lead to death within the first six months.

Diagnosis. The combination of low levels or absence of immunoglobulins, myeloid hyperplasia of the bone marrow with eosinophilia, and a hypoplastic thymus suggests this diagnosis.

Treatment. Antibiotics and steroids have been given but have not influenced the course of the illness. Antimetabolite therapy has proven temporizing but not curative.

Other Reticuloendothelioses

Histiocytic proliferation in the reticuloendothelial system, as in Letterer-Siwe disease, Hand-Schüller-Christian disease, and histiocytosis X, causes hepatomegaly and hepatocellular damage and, in some cases, cirrhosis.

GANGLIOSIDOSIS

Generalized Gangliosidosis[231]

Generalized gangliosidosis (GM$_1$, gangliosidosis type I) is a disorder resulting in the accumulation of ganglioside GM$_1$ in histiocytes and neurons along with accumulations of keratin sulfate and sialomucopolysaccharides.

Incidence. In 1969, 18 patients with this disorder were reviewed by O'Brien; since that time a number of additional cases have accumulated, enabling two types of disease to be defined.

Inheritance. The disease is inherited as in an autosomal recessive with no predilection for sex or ethnic group.

Etiology and Pathology. The disease is due to a deficiency of beta-galactosidase, an enzyme that aids in the catalysis of ganglioside GM$_1$ and the catabolism of mucopolysaccharide. This deficiency results in the accumulation of the ganglioside and of mucopolysaccharide similar to keratin sulfate. The mucopolysaccharide is stored primarily in the visceral histiocytes, and the ganglioside, in the neurons, renal glomeruli, spleen, and liver. Mucopolysaccharide accumulates in connective tissue and interferes with the normal process of bone maturation.

Symptoms. Psychomotor abnormalities are present at birth, for the infant is hypoactive and hypotonic and feeds poorly. There is facial and peripheral edema and a peculiar facies with frontal bossing, low-set ears, depressed nasal bridge, wide upper lip, and maxillary hyperplasia. The wrists and ankles are prominent. In type I disease, hepatosplenomegaly is apparent after six months, and after that time there is a rapid physical and neurologic deterioration. Macular cherry-red spots are present in 50 per cent. Death is usually caused by pneumonia.

Diagnosis. Radiologic changes in the spine and the upper extremities are evident with type I disease and resemble those of Hurler's syndrome. The long bones are wider in the midshaft and taper at the ends. The humerus is cloaked by subperiosteal new bone. The lymphocytes in the peripheral blood contain three or four vacuoles, and foamy mononuclear cells are present in the marrow, spleen, liver nodes, and urinary sediment. Urinary mucopolysaccharides are normal or only slightly increased. Decreased beta-galactosidase activity is noted in urine and in skin tissue.

Treatment. There is no effective treatment.

Prognosis. Death within two years is the ultimate outcome.

DISORDERS OF MUCOPOLYSACCHARIDE METABOLISM

A variety of mucopolysaccharide disorders are associated with hepatomegaly. Hurler's syndrome, Hunter's syndrome, deficiencies of aryl sulfatase A and B, and I-cell disease are all characterized by similar coarse features, some degree of mental retardation, skeletal abnormalities, and hepatomegaly.

INFILTRATIVE DISEASE

In general terms, infiltrative diseases are great mimics of other hepatic disorders, especially biliary obstruction. Although the liver may grow to gigantic size in infiltrative disease owing to fat, tumors, or leukemic infiltrate, ordinarily its size is normal or only slightly increased. Signs of chronic liver disease are rare. When they occur, liver function abnormalities usually include rises in serum bilirubin levels (which may be quite high), increased BSP retention, and increased alkaline phosphatase and

5'-nucleotidase levels. Serum transaminase levels seldom rise above 300 units. Unless the cause of the infiltrative disease is obvious, diagnosis usually rests upon liver biopsy.

FATTY INFILTRATION OF THE LIVER (STEATOSIS)

Accumulation of hepatic fat (steatosis) occurs in infants with protein and other forms of malnutrition.[225, 227, 228] This may result from deficient lipoprotein synthesis and decrease in transport of triglyceride from the liver cell. Normally, 4 to 5 per cent of the net weight of the liver is fat, including phospholipids, cholesterol, cholesterol esters, fatty acids, and triglycerides. In steatosis, triglyceride content may reach 40 to 50 per cent of liver weight. In abnormal metabolic states or after administration of hormones (glucagon, steroids, growth hormone, epinephrine) or antibiotics, steatosis also occurs. Fatty acids are mobilized from adipose tissue when there is decreased availability of glucose or insulin. It also occurs in obesity or when there is decreased lipoprotein formation. A modest degree of fatty infiltration of the liver is common in a wide variety of hepatic disorders and has been seen at one time or another in virtually every liver disease. An unusual roentgenographic finding in infants is a "radiolucent liver." The condition does not progress to cirrhosis, although periportal fibrosis is occasionally seen. Intracellular lipid droplets are seen on light microscopy; the vacuoles vary in size but are usually large (macrovesicular) and nuclear displacement is not uncommon.

The diagnosis may be suggested by historical factors noted above. Alkaline phosphatase and 5'-nucleotidase measures may be quite elevated, and the SGOT normal or mildly increased. Radionuclide studies using xenon uptake by the liver may demonstrate fatty infiltration, as may the CAT scan. A histologic diagnosis may be necessary.

Treatment is the restoration of adequate nutrition.

TRAUMATIC INJURIES OF THE LIVER

LACERATION

Liver laceration may occur at birth from the trauma of a difficult delivery or at any time of life from sharp or blunt abdominal injury.[257a] Male premature infants with antepartum complications are particularly prone to injury.[262b]

Symptoms. Acute laceration is accompanied by the rapid development of anemia, shock, and hemoperitoneum. Delayed rupture follows liver trauma and is manifest as much as five days later, when intrahepatic hemorrhage leads to rupture of the liver capsule. In such cases there is pain in the right upper quadrant and tenderness preceding the catastrophe. Some infants present simply with hypovolemic shock.

Diagnosis. Abdominal distention and signs of peritoneal irritation in association with profound anemia and shock must suggest intra-abdominal hemorrhage. A four-quadrant tap of the abdomen will indicate intraperitoneal hemorrhage, but laparotomy is the most direct diagnostic measure.

Treatment. In most cases the laceration can be sutured and bleeding controlled.

POST-TRAUMATIC BUDD-CHIARI SYNDROME[266]

Automobile injury in a 15-month-old infant resulted in hepatic laceration. Three weeks later, ascites with increased alkaline phosphatase and mildly elevated transaminase values developed. Treatment was peritoneovenous shunt.

NEOPLASMS

PRIMARY TUMORS OF THE LIVER

Primary tumors of the liver are the third most frequent solid abdominal tumor seen in children, and approximately half of them are malignant. Unlike the situation in adults, malignant tumors in children are not usually associated with underlying cirrho-

sis.[265] Evidence now suggests that incorporation of hepatitis B virus into the hepatocyte plays a role in the development of liver tumors.[257a]

Hepatoma or Hepatoblastoma

Primary carcinoma of the liver, or hepatoma, although rare, is seen in children under two and over ten years of age.[261, 262a]

Incidence. Its incidence in all ages ranges between 0.2 and 1.0 per cent. It is more frequent in African blacks and in Orientals and is twice as common in males as in females. The majority of tumors present before one year of age. A familial occurrence has been reported.[255]

Etiology. Although there is no known cause for tumors originating in young children, many adults have a preceding history of cirrhosis. Hepatoma has recently been reported two decades after irradiation of the liver for the treatment of hepatic hemangiomas. In a few instances the tumors are associated with neonatal hepatitis, cholestasis, cirrhosis, or biliary atresia.[258, 269, 275a] A developmental aberration during gestation is likely, for this lesion has been recognized in premature infants.

Pathology. Hepatomas are either large, solitary, massive lesions with perhaps smaller nodules about them or multiple nodules scattered through the liver.[264] It is not known whether the latter form represents one tumor of multiple origin or metastases from the original site. If the tumor is localized, it most often involves the right lobe and metastases are less frequent than in tumors of multiple origin, in which metastases to the right atrium and lungs are found in a third of the cases.

The tumors are soft, fatty, and yellow or yellow-green in color. Microscopically, the tumor cells resemble those of the adult form but are smaller and more tightly packed (Fig. 14–27). Parenchymal cells are arranged in cords or sheets separated by endothelial or tumor-lined vascular channels. Mitotic figures are not conspicuous, and necrosis is common. The stroma, which varies from scant to moderate in amount, is mature. Some tumors are mixed, embryonal or teratoid, and may contain primitive vas-

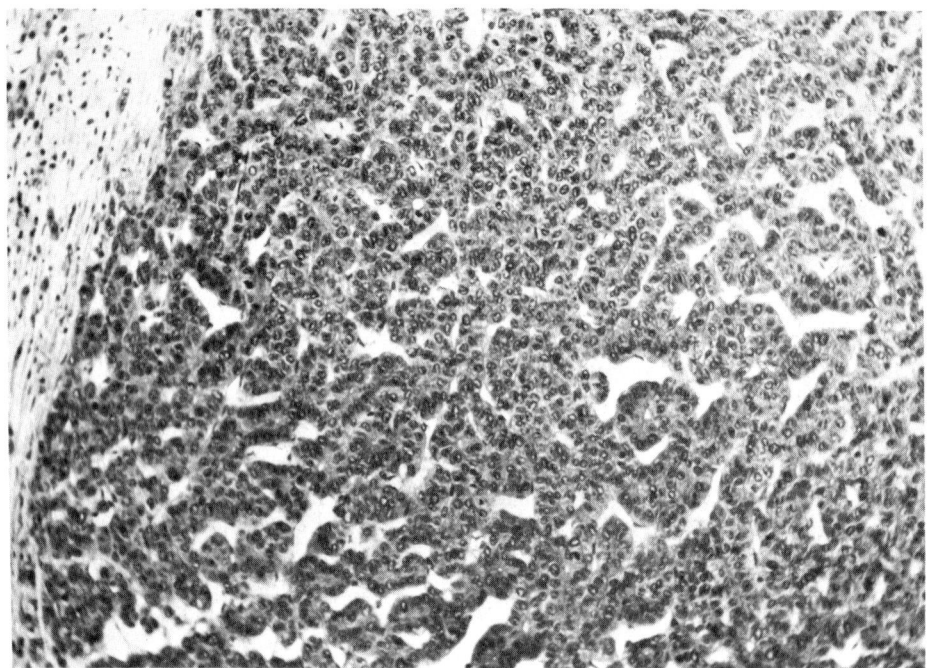

Figure 14–27   Hepatoma. Arrangement of these small malignant cells simulates the usual liver cord structure.

cular structures, osteoid or bone. If bile duct cells predominate, the tumor is termed cholangiocarcinoma, and if a sarcomatous stroma or bone is present, it is termed embryonal cell carcinoma or hepatoblastoma (Fig. 14–28). Tumors of mesodermal origin, such as hemangiosarcoma, rhabdomyosarcoma, lymphangiosarcoma, or fibroangiosarcoma, are extremely rare. All of these tend to invade either the portal or the hepatic veins.

Symptoms.   In most children, symptoms appear before the age of two years, and the initial complaint is of a protuberant abdomen or a visible abdominal mass. Pain in the right upper quadrant is occasionally noted before the mass is detected. Anorexia, weight loss, vomiting, and diarrhea all are associated but nonspecific complaints. In a few cases, periodic vomiting or diarrhea may be the only symptom. Some older children note a pleuritic type of pain or dull ache in the upper abdomen or under the right shoulder. Even precocious puberty in male infants with elevated serum gonadotropins has been caused by hepatoma.[268] A large, nontender mass is visualized and pal-

pated in the right upper quadrant, or asymmetric hepatomegaly is noted. Ascites, edema, and splenomegaly occur late in the disease. Spontaneous rupture of the tumor produces hemoperitoneum and all the physical findings of acute peritonitis. Symptoms produced by metastases to lungs, peritoneum, diaphragm, kidney, spleen, pleura, or pericardium depend on the site of implantation.

Diagnosis.   Laboratory examination reveals anemia of the normocytic type, an increased erythrocyte sedimentation rate, and hypercholesterolemia, with values between 400 and 600 mg per dl. Flat film of the abdomen shows a large soft tissue mass in the right upper quadrant, which may or may not contain scattered calcifications, and demineralization of the bones. The presence of alpha$_1$-fetoprotein (which is normally present in fetal serum and disappears before birth) in the serum is a rather specific diagnostic test for hepatoma. It is present in 80 per cent of patients with the hepatocellular type of tumor, but it does rarely occur in patients with embryonal cell tumors of the gonads, primitive gastrointes-

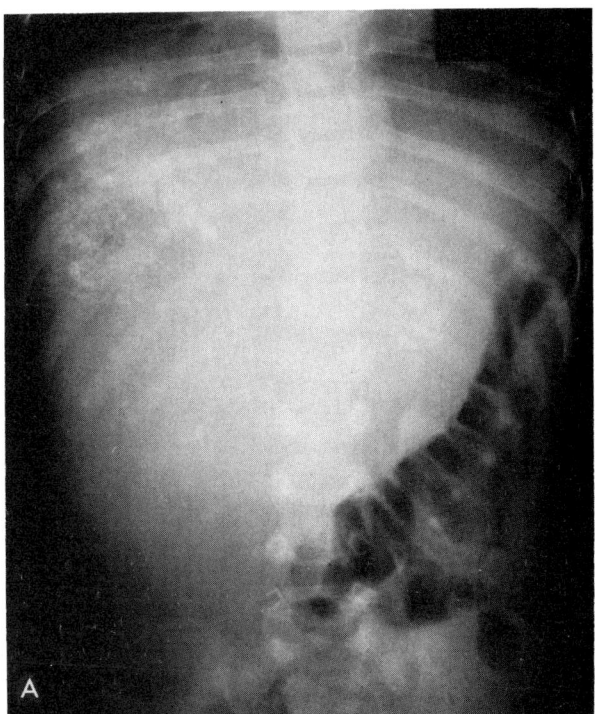

Figure 14-28 A one-year-old girl who presented with increasing abdominal girth was shown by biopsy to have cholangiocarcinoma of the liver. *A*, Frontal view of the abdomen shows displacement of loops of bowel by a huge mass filling more than half the abdominal cavity. Scattered calcifications are seen throughout the mass. *B*, Lateral view shows calcifications more clearly.

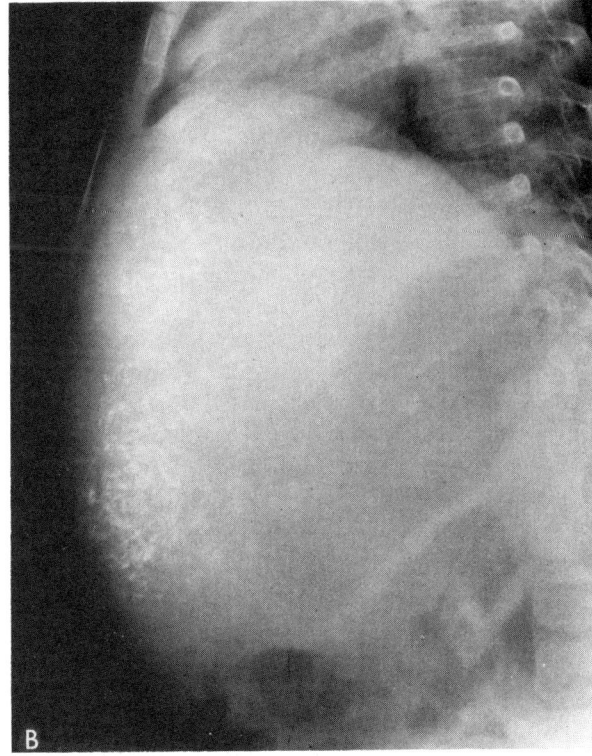

tinal tumors, or tyrosinemia with cirrhosis. Liver function tests are normal. Intravenous pyelogram will rule out the more common neuroblastoma or nephroblastoma that may invade or displace the liver.[273] Ultrasonography will confirm hepatomegaly, and a technetium liver scan will reveal a filling defect. Hepatic arteriography and venocavography are necessary procedures to carefully define the mass prior to surgery. Operative biopsy will distinguish the tumor.[263]

Treatment. Radiation and chemotherapy have not proved very successful in treating this tumor, and aggressive surgical procedures — lobectomy or even liver transplantation — are the only truly encouraging therapeutic approaches. Recently, preoperative Adriamycin has been shown to be effective in prolonging survival.[254]

Prognosis. Some two-year survivals have followed radiation therapy, but survivals of six to seven years are reported after hepatic lobectomy.[262, 270] In most patients, long-term results are not encouraging; even in those with transplanted livers, tumor recurrences develop, and most patients are dead within one to two years after treatment. The alpha-fetoprotein is an index of tumor activity because it disappears from the serum after complete tumor removal or after liver transplantation. Its persistence or reappearance signifies remaining or recurring tumor.

Hamartomas

These benign tumors account for a quarter of primary liver tumors and represent a congenital malformation, since the tumors are composed of tissue normally present in the liver.[260, 272, 274] They are therefore termed cystic lymphangioma, mesenchymal hamartoma, or cystic or solitary hepatobiliary hamartoma. Some classifications also include focal nodular hyperplasia, liver cell adenoma, and solitary cyst of the liver.

Pathology. The tumor tissue contains collagenous connective tissue, cellular bile ducts, lymph channels and liver cells, pseudocysts, or true cysts with mesothelial cells (Fig. 14–27). There is no evidence of malignant change.

Symptoms. Symptoms are usually obvious by the second year and consist of rapid abdominal enlargement, abdominal pain, vomiting, constipation or diarrhea, and eventual emaciation. A large cystic mass is palpable in the right upper quadrant.

Diagnosis. Plain films of the abdomen reveal a large homogeneous mass in the right upper quadrant and do not permit differentiation of the lesion (Fig. 14–28). Isotope scanning of the liver will reveal a filling defect. The results of liver function tests are normal.

Treatment. Surgical exploration with excision of the tumor is curative.

Prognosis. The outlook is one of complete recovery, because there is no associated cirrhosis.

VASCULAR TUMORS

Infantile hemangioendothelioma and cavernous hemangioma occur in childhood, hemangioma being the most common.[257, 267, 275]

Hemangiomas

These vascular tumors represent congenital malformations of the cavernous or generalized hemangioendothelioma type. Although they are pathologically benign, they are potentially lethal to the young infant for they can produce high-output heart failure as a result of arteriovenous shunting, hemoperitoneum from rupture, or exsanguination from thrombocytopenia and clotting factor deficiencies.

Incidence. These are the most common benign hepatic tumors of childhood, but they are extraordinarily rare in adults. The infantile hemangioendotheliomas are more common than the cavernous type.

Pathology. The generalized hemangioma appears as multiple gray-white tumor masses that contain red centers, while the cavernous hemangioma is single and large (Fig. 14–29). Both are lined by blood-filled endothelial channels; in one third of cases there are extrahepatic hemorrhagic nodules that are not metastatic but represent independent, multicentric growths. If large, they receive a significant portion of the cardiac output.

Symptoms. The onset of symptoms is in the immediate neonatal period or during the first few weeks of life. Many babies (58 to 78 per cent) have associated hemangiomas of the skin. Jaundice has been reported in association with hepatic hemangioma (Fig. 14–30) in the young infant, but it is usually not a prominent feature of this le-

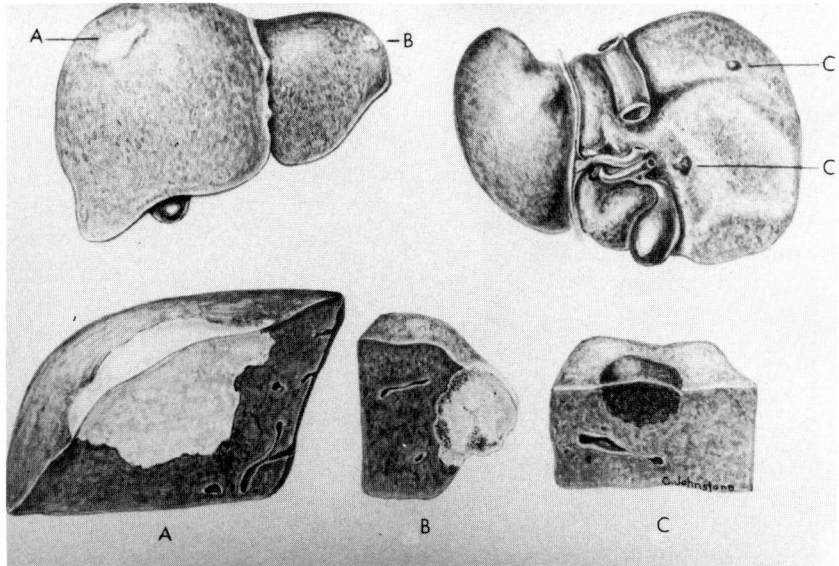

Figure 14–29 Artist's representation of organizational stages of hepatic hemangiomas. The lesions progress from C on the right — active, patent, vascular tumors — to B in the center — partially organized tumors — to A on the left, completely scarred and organized hemangiomas. (Courtesy of C. Johnstone).

sion. Some infants have vomiting and abdominal distention and appear pale, while in others (55 to 59 per cent) cardiac failure or massive gastrointestinal bleeding suddenly develops. The major physical finding is a mass in the right upper quadrant (78 to 81 per cent). If coagulation disorders are severe, there are petechiae and ecchymoses.

Complications. Death may result from progressive growth of the tumor with rupture and intraperitoneal hemorrhage.

Diagnosis. The development of bleeding or cardiac failure in an infant with cutaneous hemangiomas should immediately suggest the diagnosis. Some infants have elevated bilirubin and many have alpha-

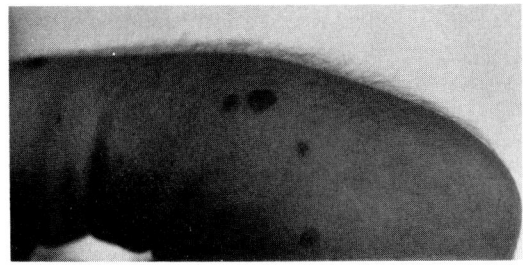

Figure 14–30 Hemangioma of arm of infant with hepatic hemangiomatosis.

fetoprotein levels that reach into the thousands. Flat film of the abdomen shows a mass in the right upper quadrant, and examination of the upper gastrointestinal tract with barium may show displacement of the stomach by an extrinsic mass. Anemia and thrombocytopenia are present owing to trapping of platelets in the arteriovenous shunts. A consumption coagulopathy with decreased factors V and VII and fibrinogen can often be demonstrated. An arteriogram will outline the vascular malformation (Fig. 14–31). Ultrasonography may determine the extent of the lesion without invasion.

Treatment. As with the cutaneous lesions, there is spontaneous regression of hepatic hemangioma with time (Fig. 14–29), but if the infant has symptoms, immediate treatment must be initiated. Radiation, in a dose of 400 to 600 rads over ten days, has been used, but the danger of irradiation hepatitis and hepatoma must be kept in mind.[271] Good results have followed therapy with prednisone in a dose of 20 to 40 mg every other day for one month, followed by a rest period and resumption of the same course over the next four to five months. Hepatic lobe or wedge resection has been performed with good success in localized lesions, and, in unresectable cases, hepatic

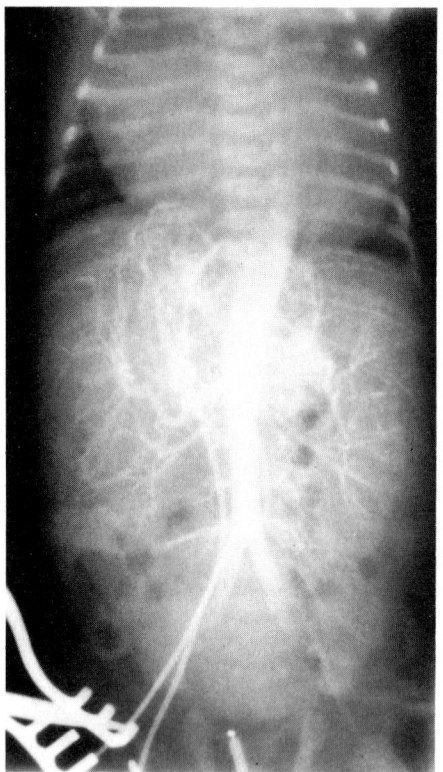

Figure 14–31 Arteriogram of an infant with severe congestive heart failure secondary to a large hepatic hemangioma. Severe hepatomegaly is noted in the film, and the hemangioma is demonstrated by opacification of the vessels within the lesion in the right lobe of the liver.

multifocal hepatocellular necrosis. It has been associated with tuberculosis, tumor, uremia, pemphigus, septic shock, and androgenic steroid administration. The etiology is not certain: Some consider it a congenital malformation, and others feel that the primary event is hepatocellular necrosis or dilatation of sinusoids leading to central atrophy. There is a spectrum of chemical abnormalities, with results of liver function tests ranging from normal to markedly elevated.

METASTATIC TUMORS

Virtually any tumor that metastasizes can metastasize to the liver. In these situations, the presenting complaints may be attributable more to the primary lesion, but they may relate to the hepatic metastases. In infants and children, Wilms' tumor and neuroblastoma are perhaps the most common metastatic tumors seen in the liver. It is important to make the diagnosis of neuroblastoma, since this lesion, even when metastatic, responds quite well to radiation therapy.

In the young infant, hepatomegaly may rarely be due to lymphatic leukemia infiltration.

artery ligation or embolization has proved lifesaving.[257] Alpha-fetoprotein values may be helpful in following regression of the lesion.

Prognosis. Once the initial danger is past, the lesions cause no difficulty in later life.

Focal Nodular Hyperplasia

This benign tumor of the liver is associated with slowly progressive deposition of fibrous tissue and sometimes requires surgical intervention because of the potential for portal hypertension.

Peliosis Hepatitis

Peliosis hepatitis is a condition characterized by blood-filled spaces in the liver and

AMYLOIDOSIS

Hepatic involvement is seen in 60 to 80 per cent of cases of amyloidosis. Primary amyloidosis, with widespread deposits of amyloid involving muscle, blood vessels, and heart is occasionally seen in children, especially in those with the familial form of the disease. Rarely, hepatic signs and symptoms such as jaundice, hepatomegaly, ascites, and edema are seen, but usually the liver function remains normal or is only minimally deranged. An abnormal peak in the alpha$_2$-globulin area on protein electrophoresis is common in the familial form of the disease.

Secondary amyloidosis occurs in patients with chronic diseases, but as these are becoming more amenable to treatment, fewer cases of this type are being seen. The liver is frequently involved in conjunction with the spleen, kidney, and adrenal glands. Although hepatomegaly is common, hepatic failure and abnormal liver function are rare. Secondary amyloidosis occasionally resolves after treatment of the underlying disease. The only certain way of establishing the diagnosis is by the demonstration of amyloid in tissue from biopsy of the liver, kidney, or rectal mucosa. There is no known therapy for amyloidosis other than the treatment of any underlying disease.

GRANULOMAS

Granulomatous involvement of the liver in children is in no way different from that seen in the adult and is more commonly due to sarcoidosis, tuberculosis, histoplasmosis, or toxoplasmosis. Rare infectious causes of granuloma are brucellosis, syphilis, tularemia, influenza B, Q fever, and *Mycoplasma* infection. Fungal diseases are caused by *Candida*, *Actinomyces*, *Nocardia*, *Cryptococcus*, and *Aspergillus*.

ACQUIRED LESIONS OF THE BILIARY TREE

DISEASES OF THE GALLBLADDER

Cholelithiasis

Cholelithiasis is rare during childhood and, when it occurs, affects most often the postpubertal child. In contrast to the situation in the adult, in the child it is usually associated with some underlying disease such as hemolysis or infection.

Incidence. The disease is extremely rare in infancy, only sporadic cases having been reported.[285] Even at this young age, females are affected more often than males.

Etiology. Genetic factors are of some importance, because in older children there is often a family history of gallstones. Abnormalities in the quantity and quality of bile salts, particularly lithogenic acid, are reported in some ethnic groups that have a high incidence of gallstones. Certainly, cho-

lelithiasis seems to develop in patients who have had previous abdominal surgery for infection and in those with hyperbilirubinemia or hypercholesterolemia. Gallstones have been reported in fetuses and infants with hemolytic disease of the newborn, and the hemolysis of sickle cell and Wilson's diseases is associated with an increased incidence of cholelithiasis. Stasis by itself is probably not a factor in the production of stones, although congenital anomalies of the biliary tree, as noted in previous sections, are associated with cholelithiasis. In small premature infants who have received long-term hyperalimentation, however, stasis may play a role in the genesis of cholelithiasis.

Pathology. The stones are usually located in the gallbladder and usually do not obstruct the cystic or the common duct, although Lilly has reported four infants with common duct stones and biliary tract atresia or stasis.[282]

Symptoms. Abdominal symptoms are most common, with recurrent abdominal pain being the major complaint. During acute attacks, nearly half the children vomit and two thirds become jaundiced. The pain becomes colicky and localizes in the right upper quadrant. In a few instances the pain may radiate to the right lower quadrant or into the back to simulate appendicitis or even pancreatitis. Small children usually have no history of fatty food intolerance.

Physical examination shows an acutely ill, febrile infant who is jaundiced. There is tenderness and guarding in the right upper quadrant, but the remainder of the abdomen is essentially soft and nontender.

Diagnosis. Leukocytosis varies from moderate to marked, and urinalysis is normal. The alkaline phosphatase value may be elevated, but the results of liver function tests are usually normal. If the patient is studied between attacks, all of the laboratory studies may be normal. Plain film of the abdomen may show opaque calculi in the right upper quadrant, but nonopaque stones are not visualized. Oral cholecystography, with use of a double dose of contrast medium if necessary, is the preferred means of diagnosis and will demonstrate the calculi within the gallbladder. Ultrasonography is of value in the jaundiced patient.[276]

Treatment. Cholecystectomy is the treatment of choice and is usually curative. If spherocytosis is an associated disease, splenectomy should be performed during surgery or at a later date.

Prognosis. Approximately 5 per cent of patients suffer from a recurrence of symptoms owing to new stones or stenosis of the common duct.

Acute Hydrops of the Gallbladder

Noncalculous distention of the gallbladder occurs in the absence of biliary tract infection or stones.

Incidence. The disease is extremely rare but is being recognized with increased frequency, particularly as part of Kawasaki's disease (mucocutaneous lymph node syndrome). Males are affected twice as often as females.[284, 286, 289] Recently, we have seen significant hydrops in several small premature infants receiving hyperalimentation.

Etiology. The etiology is unknown, although hyperplastic lymph nodes are often noted in the region of the cystic and common bile ducts. In a few cases there have been abnormalities of the cystic duct, such as atresia, torsion, or stenosis. The disorder has been associated with upper respiratory infection, salmonella infection, cervical adenitis, and streptococcal and pseudomonas sepsis.[286a, 288a] It may develop after cardiac surgery. In the premature infant this disorder may be due to a combination of poor motility, lack of enteral stimulation, and hyperalimentation. Although it can never be considered normal and must be watched carefully, the hydropic gallbladder in the premature infant may resolve spontaneously after the introduction of oral feeds.[281a]

Pathology. The gallbladder wall is edematous and contains some evidence of fibrosis and mild inflammation.

Symptoms. The disease presents as an acute illness. All patients have abdominal pain, which in 93 per cent is localized to the right upper quadrant; 75 per cent of patients vomit, and 55 per cent have a palpable mass in the right upper quadrant.

There may be a history of an upper respiratory infection for a few days before the acute attack, but in most cases the disease resembles intussusception or acute appendicitis with abscess. There is little or no fever or jaundice.

Diagnosis. The diagnosis is usually made by ultrasonography. At the time of surgery there is no evidence of intestinal disease and only a large edematous gallbladder, which is filled with white, yellow, or green bile. Cultures of the bile and mesenteric lymph nodes are usually sterile.

Treatment. The treatment of choice is cholecystectomy.

Prognosis. Surgical excision of the gallbladder is curative, although in those in whom only drainage has been performed, gallbladder function has returned to normal.

Acute Gangrenous Cholecystitis or Acute Acalculous Cholecystitis

Acute cholecystitis unassociated with cholelithiasis is far more unusual than that associated with gallstones and is often encountered with systemic disease.

Incidence. By 1968 only nine cases had been reported in children under three years of age, but by 1979, Glenn had collected 139 patients.[279] The condition is more common in males than in females.[288, 290]

Etiology. Primary cholecystitis has been associated with such infectious diseases as typhoid fever, typhus, diphtheria, scarlet fever, shigellosis, viral gastroenteritis, pneumonia, and respiratory infections. Anaerobic diphtheroids have been cultured from one infant. In a few cases, parasitic infestation with *Giardia lamblia* or *Ascaris lumbricoides* has involved the gallbladder. It has been reported after trauma and burns. Malformations of the biliary tree that cause stasis and increased mucus production are often considered in the etiology of cholangitis, but their role is not well documented. It has been suggested that spasm of the sphincter of Oddi causes regurgitation of pancreatic juice.

Pathology. The gallbladder is acutely inflamed and distended and often contains punctate necrotic areas. It is filled with dark bile and contains no calculi. Microscopically, there is polymorphonuclear leukocytic infiltrate of the mucosa and muscularis. Fibrosis is minimal. Adjacent lymph nodes show an inflammatory reticular hyperplasia.

Symptoms. The clinical findings resemble those of gastroenteritis or appendicitis, with a history of nausea, vomiting, and anorexia over several days accompanied at first by diarrhea and later by obstipation. Abdominal pain is at first periumbilical and may be colicky or constant. The physical examination shows guarding and tenderness in the right upper quadrant. Jaundice may or may not be present, and the infant is usually febrile.

Diagnosis. Laboratory studies show leukocytosis, and if jaundice is present the chemical abnormalities are of the obstructive type, with elevations of the alkaline phosphatase and direct-reacting bilirubin. During the acute attack, the gallbladder is not visualized during oral cholecystography but may be noted as abnormal on ultrasonography.

Treatment. The treatment is cholecystectomy after operative cholangiography.

Prognosis. The outlook is excellent because the surgical procedure is curative, but if the disorder is recognized and treated, mortality may reach 65 per cent.

SPONTANEOUS PERFORATION OF THE EXTRAHEPATIC BILE DUCTS

This event is considered by some to be the second most common cause of surgical jaundice in the infant, after biliary atresia.[283]

Incidence. Fifty-five cases of spontaneous perforation of the extrahepatic bile ducts have been reported over the past 20 years.[283]

Etiology and Pathogenesis. The etiology is unknown, although stenosis of the distal common duct, stones, and sludging of bile have been implicated in the pathogenesis of rupture. These are not entirely likely, however, for dilatation of the ducts or gallbladder has not been found at the time of surgery. Another theory, of localized embryonic malformation of the wall of the common duct, is attractive because the site of rupture is usually the juncture of the cystic and common ducts.

Pathology. The perforation is usually localized, as already stated, near the junction of the common and cystic ducts. An inflammatory sac surrounds the perforation in half the cases and is filled with dark green fluid. Bile peritonitis is an additional finding in most infants, and stones are reported in one fifth of them.

Symptoms. The disease is found exclusively in infancy and has not been reported during the first few days of life and only rarely after 20 weeks. Symptoms occur most often in those between one and three months of age, when a normal infant becomes irritable and somewhat anorectic. After several days, jaundice, low-grade fever, vomiting, pale and perhaps watery stools, and ascites focus attention on the liver and biliary tree.

Diagnosis. There is moderate leukocytosis, and liver function test results are usually normal except for elevation of both direct and indirect bilirubin. Preoperative diagnosis can be made by intravenous cholangiography and by rose bengal scan. Cholangiography shows extravasation of contrast material from the bile ducts into a sac-like structure. Scanning of the liver one hour after injection of iodine-131 rose bengal shows normal hepatic uptake of the isotope, but the repeated scan, taken 24 hours later, shows isotope concentrated under the diaphragm and free in the peritoneal cavity.

Treatment. Medical therapy is uniformly unsuccessful, and immediate surgical treatment is indicated to prevent secondary infection. Operative cholecystography is followed by drainage of the area of perforation with several soft rubber drains. Exploration of the ducts is not attempted, and the gallbladder is left in place. Spontaneous closure of the leak after 25 days has been demonstrated by tube cholecystography. Fat-free formulae or parenteral hyperalimentation eliminate the oral stimulus to bile flow during the healing period.

Volvulus of the Gallbladder

An abnormal mesenteric attachment may predispose to volvulus of the organ. The onset is often acute, with vomiting and epigastric or right upper quadrant pain mimicking cholecystitis. Therapy consists of immediate surgical intervention to avoid necrosis.

TRAUMATIC INJURIES

Traumatic Hemobilia

This emergency situation arises after trauma or battering.

Etiology. Rarely, this lesion is due to an aneurysm of the hepatic artery, but it most often results from blunt injury that leads to the formation of intrahepatic pseudocysts that suddenly empty into the biliary tree.

Symptoms. As in the case of pancreatic pseudocysts, these lesions are difficult to relate to trauma for they develop days to weeks after the initial injury. The symptoms are sudden colicky pain in the right upper quadrant, melena, or hematemesis. Jaundice is uncommon.

Diagnosis. If a bleeding site is not evident, retrograde cholangiography should be done if the patient's size is adequate. Ultrasonography may define abnormalities of the ducts or a hematoma. Scintiscanning or angiography is sometimes of help in delineating the site of bleeding.

Treatment. The only treatment is surgical, with removal of the edges of the cystic cavity and drainage of the lesion.

Avulsion of the Bile Ducts

This is another lesion that immediately follows application of heavy force to the abdomen, causing a tear in the distal bile ducts.[277]

Symptoms. After abdominal trauma there is diffuse epigastric pain that is local-

ized to the right upper quadrant. Peritonitis develops as blood and bile flow into the abdomen.

Treatment. Surgical treatment consists of drainage and repair of the tear.

Acquired Bile Duct Stricture

Biliary stricture has been reported as a sequela of blunt trauma.[280]

Pseudocholedochal Cyst

This type of cyst results from injury to the common duct during abdominal surgery and has been reported in only one infant. The symptoms, diagnosis, and treatment are similar to those described for choledochal cyst.[277]

TUMORS OF THE BILIARY TREE

Tumors of the biliary tree are extremely rare in childhood.

Incidence. Benign tumors are more common than malignant ones. Papillomas are the most common of the benign tumors, with adenomas and fibromas next in frequency. Malignant tumors have been reported in patients with choledochal cysts and biliary atresia, the most common being sarcoma botryoides,[284a, 287] 25 cases of which have been reported. Other tumors are rhabdomyosarcoma and cholangiocarcinoma.[281]

Symptoms. The onset of symptoms may occur at any time of life, although malignant tumors usually are symptomatic within the first six years. Pruritus and jaundice are the major findings, and a mass in the right upper quadrant may or may not be palpable.

Diagnosis. Laboratory tests are compatible with those of obstructive jaundice. Cholangiography will demonstrate an obstructive lesion in the biliary tree, often in the ampullary region.

Treatment. The treatment for benign tumors is excision, and that for malignant ones, excision followed by radiotherapy.

Prognosis. The prognosis is excellent for benign tumors, but malignant ones are generally fatal. Of the 25 patients with sarcoma botryoides, 24 died between 5 and 16 months after surgical excision and only one patient has survived for four years after surgery.[287]

REFERENCES

Physiologic Jaundice

1. Hardy, J. B., and Peeples, M. D.: Serum bilirubin levels in newborn infants. Distributions and associations with neurological abnormalities during the first year of life. Johns Hopkins Med. J. 128:265, 1971.

1a. Maisels, M. J.: Jaundice in the newborn. Pediatr. Rev. 3:305, 1982.

2. Odell, G. B.: Neonatal jaundice. In Popper, H., and Schaffner, F. (eds.): Progress in Liver Disease. New York, Grune & Stratton, 1976, pp. 457–475.

3. Odell, G. B.: Physiologic hyperbilirubinemia in the neonatal period. N. Engl. J. Med. 277:193, 1967.

Noncholestatic Jaundice or Indirect Hyperbilirubinemia

4. Alagille, D., and Odièvre, M.: Hyperbilirubinemia in the newborn. In Liver and Biliary Tract Disease in Children. New York, John Wiley & Sons, 1979, pp. 18–42.

5. Andrew, G., Chan, G., and Schiff, D.: Lipid metabolism in the neonate. II. Effect of intralipid on bilirubin binding in vitro and in vivo. J. Pediatr. 88:279, 1976.

6. Arias, I. M., Wolfson, S., Lucey, J. M., and McKay, R. J.: Transient familial neonatal hyperbilirubinemia. J. Clin. Invest. 44:1442, 1965.

7. Arias, I. M., Gartner, L. M., Cohen, M., Ezzer, J. B., and Levi, A. J.: Chronic nonhemolytic unconjugated hyperbilirubinemia with glucuronyl transferase deficiency: clinical biochemical, pharmacologic, and genetic evidence for heterogeneity. Am. J. Med. 47:395, 1969.

8. Bakken, A. F., Thaler, M. M., and Schmid, R.: Metabolic regulation of heme catabolism and bilirubin production. I. Hormonal control of hepatic heme oxygenase activity. J. Clin. Invest. 51:530, 1972.

9. Barret, P. V.: Bilirubinemia and fasting. N. Engl. J. Med. 283:823, 1970.

10. Berk, P. D., Blaschke, T. F., and Waggoner, J. G.: Defective bromosulfophthalein clearance in patients with constitutional hepatic dysfunction (Gilbert's syndrome). Gastroenterology 63:472, 1972.

11. Blackburn, M. G., Orzalesi, M. M., and Pigram, P.: The combined effect of phototherapy and phenobarbital on serum bilirubin levels in premature infants. Pediatrics 49:110, 1972.

12. Blaschke, T., Berk, P., Scharschmidt, B., Guyther, J. R., Vergalla, J., and Waggoner, J.: Crigler-Najjar syndrome: an unusual course with development of neurological damage at age eighteen. Pediatr. Res. 8:573, 1974.

13. Blumenschein, S. D., Kallen, R. J., Storey, B., Natzchka, J. G., Odell, G. B., and Childs, B.: Familial nonhemolytic jaundice with late onset of neurological damage. Pediatrics 42:786, 1968.

14. Boggs, J. R., Jr., and Bishop, H.: Neonatal hyperbilirubinemia associated with high obstruction of the small bowel. J. Pediatr. 66:349, 1965.

15. Christina, M., L., Ribeiro, J. C., Pinho, C., and Baptista, A. S.: The fine structure of liver cells of Gilbert's disease. In Proceedings of the 5th Meeting of European Association for Study of the Liver. Berne, 1970, p. 48.

16. Cockington, R. A.: A guide to the use of phototherapy in the management of neonatal hyperbilirubinemia. J. Pediatr. 95:281, 1979.

17. Crigler, J. F., and Najjar, A. V.: Congenital familial nonhemolytic jaundice with kernicterus. Pediatrics 10:169, 1952.

18. Dawson, J., Carrlocke, D. L., Talbot, I. C., and Rosenthal, F. D.: Gilbert's syndrome evidence of morphologic heterogeneity. Gut 20:848, 1979.

19. Dublin, I. N.: Chronic idiopathic jaundice. A review of fifty cases. Am. J. Med. 24:268, 1958.

20. Felsher, B. F., Corpio, N. M., Wooley, M. M., and Asch, M. J.: Hepatic bilirubin glucuronidation in neonates with unconjugated hyperbilirubinemia and congenital gastrointestinal obstruction. J. Lab. Clin. Med. 83:90, 1974.

21. Felsher, B. F., Rickard, D., and Redecker, A. G.: The reciprocal relation between caloric intake and degree of hyperbilirubinemia in Gilbert's syndrome. N. Engl. J. Med. 283:170, 1970.

22. Gartner, L. M., and Arias, I. M.: Studies of prolonged neonatal jaundice in the breast fed infant. J. Pediatr. 68:54, 1966.

23. Gartner, L. M., Snyder, R. N., Chabon, R. S., and Bernstein, J.: Kernicterus: high incidence in premature infants with low serum bilirubin concentrations. Pediatrics 45:906, 1970.

24. Gollan, J. L., Bateman, C., and Billing, B. H.: Effect of dietary composition on the conjugated hyperbilirubinemia of Gilbert's syndrome. Gut 17:335, 1976.

25. Goresky, C. A., Gordon, E. R., Schafler, E. A., et al.: Definition of a conjugation dysfunction in Gilbert's syndrome: studies of the handling of bilirubin loads and of the pattern of bilirubin conjugates secreted in bile. Clin. Sci. Mol. Med. 55:63, 1978.

26. Kopelman, A. E., Brown, R. S., and Odell, G. B.: The "bronze-baby" syndrome: a complication of phototherapy. J. Pediatr. 81:466, 1972.

27. Levine, G., Favara, B., Mierau, G., and Bailey,

W.: Jaundice, liver ultrastructure and congenital pyloric stenosis. Arch. Pathol. 95:267, 1973.

28. Levine, R., and Klatskin, G.: Unconjugated hyperbilirubinemia in the absence of overt hemolysis. Importance of acquired disease as an etiologic factor in 366 adolescent and adult cases. Am. J. Med. 36:541, 1964.

29. Lucey, J.: Neonatal jaundice and phototherapy. Pediatr. Clin. North Am. 19:827, 1972.

30. McGillivray, M. H., Crawford, J. D., and Robey, J. S.: Congenital hypothyroidism and prolonged neonatal hyperbilirubinemia. Pediatrics 40:283, 1967.

31. Maisels, M. J.: Bilirubin: On understanding and influencing its metabolism in the newborn. Pediatr. Clin. North Am. 19:447, 1972.

32. Metreau, J. M., Yvarts, J., Dumeaux, D., and Berthelot, P.: Role of bilirubin overproduction in revealing Gilbert's syndrome: is dyserythropoiesis an important factor? Gut, 19:844, 1978.

33. Newman, A. J., and Gross, S.: Hyperbilirubinemia in breast fed infants. Pediatrics 32:995, 1963.

34. Nezelof, C., Dupart, H. C., Jauber, T. F., and Eliachar, E.: A lethal familial syndrome associating arthrogryposis multiplex congenita, renal dysfunction and a cholestatic and pigmentary liver disease. J. Pediatr. 94:258, 1979.

35. Odell, G. B., Stavey, G. N., and Rosenberg, L.: Studies in kernicterus 3. The saturation of serum protein with bilirubin during neonatal life and its relationship to brain damage at 5 years. J. Pediatr. 76:12, 1970.

36. Odièvre, M., Trivin, F., Eliot, N., and Alagille, D.: Case of congenital nonobstructive, nonhemolytic jaundice: successful long term phototherapy at home. Arch. Dis. Child. 53:81, 1978.

36a. Odièvre, M., and Luzeau, R.: More on breastmilk jaundice. J. Pediatr. 100:671, 1982.

37. Oh, W., and Korecki, H.: Phototherapy and insensible water loss in the newborn infant. Am. J. Dis. Child. 124:230, 1972.

38. Ostrow, J. D., and Branham, R. V.: Photodecomposition of bilirubin and biliverden in vitro. Gastroenterology 58:15, 1970.

39. Powell, L. W.: Clinical aspects of unconjugated hyperbilirubinemia. Semin. Hematol. 9:91, 1972.

40. Rubaltelli, F. F.: Phototherapy, Pediatrics 61:838, 1978.

41. Schimizu, Y., Kondo, T., Kuchiba, K., and Urata, G.: Uroporphyrinogen III cosynthetase in liver and blood in the Dubin-Johnson syndrome. J. Lab. Clin. Med. 89:517, 1977.

42. Schmid, R.: Bilirubin metabolism: State of the art. Gastroenterology 74:1307, 1978.

43. Speck, W. T., Chen, C. C., and Rosenkranz, H. S.: In vitro studies of effects of light and riboflavin on DNA and HeLa cells. Pediatr. Res. 9:150, 1975.

44. Swartz, H. M., Sarna, T., and Varmair, R.: On the nature and excretion of the hepatic pigment in the Dubin-Johnson syndrome. Gastroenterology 76:958, 1979.

45. Tan, K. L.: Comparison of the effectiveness of

phototherapy and exchange transfusion in the management of nonhemolytic neonatal hyperbilirubinemia. J. Pediatr. 87:609, 1975.

46. Vaisman, S. L., and Gartner, L. M.: Pharmacologic treatment of neonatal hyperbilirubinemia. Clin. Perinatol. 2:37, 1975.

Cholestatic Jaundice and Ductal Disease

47. Aagenaes, O., VanderMagen, C. B., and Refsum, J.: Hereditary recurrent intrahepatic cholestasis from birth. Arch. Dis. Child. 43:644, 1969.

48. Akers, D., Favara, B., Franciosi, R., and Nelson, J. M.: Duplications of the alimentary tract: report of three unusual cases associated with bile and pancreatic ducts. Surgery 71:817, 1972.

49. Alagille, D., Odièvre, M., and Gautier, M.: Hepatic ductular hypoplasia associated with characteristic facies, vertebral manifestations, retarded physical, mental and sexual development and cardiac murmur. J. Pediatr. 86:63, 1975.

50. Alpert, L. I., Strauss, L., and Hirschhorn, K.: Neonatal hepatitis and biliary atresia associated with trisomy 17–18. N. Engl. J. Med. 280:16, 1969.

51. Altman, R. P.: The portoenterostomy procedure for biliary atresia: a five year experience. Ann. Surg. 188:351, 1978.

51a. Altman, P. R.: Biliary atresia. Pediatrics 68:896, 1981.

52. Andres, J. M., Lilly, J. R., Altman, R. P., Walker, W. A., and Alpert, E.: Alpha$_1$ fetoprotein in neonatal hepatobiliary disease. J. Pediatr. 91:217, 1977.

53. Arima, E., and Akita, H.: Congenital biliary tract dilatation and anomalous junction of the pancreatico-biliary system. J. Pediatr. Surg. 14:9, 1979.

54. Balistreri, W. F., Suchy, F. J., Farrell, M. K., and Heubi, J. E.: Pathologic versus physiologic cholestasis: Elevated serum concentration of a secondary bile acid in the presence of hepatobiliary disease. J. Pediatr. 98:399, 1981.

55. Barkin, R. M., and Lilly, J. R.: Biliary atresia and Kasai operation: Continuing care. J. Pediatr. 96:1915, 1980.

55a. Benjamin, D.: Hepatobiliary dysfunction in infants and children associated with long-term total parenteral nutrition. Am. J. Clin. Pathol. 76:276, 1981.

56. Bill, A., Haas, J., and Foster, G.: Biliary atresia. J. Pediatr. Surg. 12:977, 1978.

56a. Book, L., Eggert, L., and Matlak, M.: Trace minerals in children with biliary atresia. Pediatr. Res. 16:157A, 1982.

57. Brent, R. L.: Persistent jaundice in infancy. Pediatrics 61:111, 1968.

58. Brough, A. J., and Bernstein, J.: Conjugated hyperbilirubinemia in early infancy. A reassessment of liver biopsy. Hum. Pathol. 5:507, 1974.

59. Campbell, D., and Williams, G. R.: Identification

of the jaundiced infant who is likely to recover without surgical intervention. Ann. Surg. *184*:89, 1976.

60. Caplinsky, C.: Familial cholestatic cirrhosis. Pediatrics *65*:782, 1980.

61. Caroli, J.: Diseases of the intrahepatic biliary tree. Clin. Gastroenterol. *2*:147, 1973.

62. Catlon, D. A.: Intrahepatic biliary atresia. Lancet, *2*:294, 1960.

63. Chandra, R., and Altman, P.: Ductal remnants in extrahepatic biliary atresia: A histopathologic study with clinical correlation. J. Pediatr. *93*:196, 1978.

64. Clayton, R. J., Iber, F. L., Ruebner, B. H., and McCusick, V. A.: Byler disease. Fatal familial intrahepatic cholestasis in an Amish kindred. Am. J. Dis. Child. *117*:112, 1969.

64a. Cohen, C., and Olsen, M.: Pediatric total parenteral nutrition: Liver histopathology. Arch. Pathol. Lab. Med. *105*:152, 1981.

65. Danks, D. M.: Biliary atresia: Lessons from Japan. Lancet *1*:219, 1981.

66. Danks, D. M., Campbell, P., Clarke, A., Jones, P. G., et al.: Extrahepatic biliary atresia. Am. J. Dis. Child. *128*:684, 1974.

67. Danks, D. M., Campbell, P. E., Smith, A. L., and Rogers, J.: Prognosis of babies with neonatal hepatitis. Arch. Dis. Child. *52*:368, 1977.

68. Deleze, G., and Paumgartner G.: Bile acids in serum and bile of infants with cholestatic syndromes. Helv. Paediatr. Acta *32*:29, 1977.

69. DeLorimier, A. A.: Surgical management of neonatal jaundice. N. Engl. J. Med. *288*:1285, 1973.

70. DeVas, R., DeWolf-Peeters, C., Desmel, Y., Eggermont, E., et al.: Progressive intrahepatic cholestasis (Byler's disease). Gut *16*:943, 1975.

70a. Devries, P., and Cox, K.: Surgical treatment of congenital and neonatal biliary obstruction. Surg. Clin. North Am. *61*:987, 1981.

70b. Douilett, P., Brunelle, F., Chaumont, P., Valayer, J., Sassoon, C., and Odièvre, M.: Ultrasonography and percutaneous cholangiography in children with dilated bile ducts. Am. J. Dis. Child. *135*:131, 1981.

70c. Dunigan, T. H., and Werlin, S. L.: Extrahepatic biliary atresia and renal anomalies in fetal alcohol syndrome. Am. J. Dis. Child. *135*:1067, 1981.

71. Gates, G. F., Sinatra, F., Thomas, D., Muhletaler, C., and Gerlock, A. J.: Cholestatic syndromes of infancy and childhood. Am. J. Roentgenol. *134*:1141, 1980.

71a. Gautier, M., and Eliot, N.: Extrahepatic biliary atresia—morphologic study of 98 biliary remnants. Arch. Pathol. Lab. Med. *105*:397, 1981.

72. Gautier, M., Jehan, P., and Odievre, M.: Histological study of biliary fibrous remnants in 48 cases of extra hepatic biliary atresia. Correlation with postoperative bile flow restoration. J. Pediatr. *89*:740, 1976.

73. Ghent, C., Bloomer, J., and Hsia, Y. E.: Efficacy and safety of long term phenobarbital therapy of familial cholestasis. J. Pediatr. *93*:127, 1978.

74. Ghisan, E., LaBrecque, D., and Mitros, E.: Evolving nature of infantile obstructive cholangiopathy. J. Pediatr. *97*:27, 1980.

75. Glenn, F., and McSherry, C. K.: Congenital segmental cystic dilatation of the biliary ductal system. Ann. Surg. *177*:705, 1973.

76. Goldblum, R., Powell, G., and van Sickle, W.: Secretory IgA in serum with obstructive jaundice. J. Pediatr. *97*:33, 1980.

77. Greene, H. L., Helisek, G. L., Roberto, M., and O'Neill, J.: A diagnostic approach to prolonged obstructive jaundice by 24 hour collection of duodenal fluid. J. Pediatr. *95*:412, 1979.

77a. Guggenheim, M., Ringel, S. P., Silverman, A., and Grabert, B. E.: Progressive neuromuscular disease in children with chronic cholestasis and vitamin E deficiency; Diagnosis and treatment with alpha-tocopherol. J. Pediatr. *100*:51, 1982.

78. Hanson, R. F., Isenberg, J. N., Williams, G. C., et al.: The metabolism of 3,7,12 trihydroxy-5B-Cholestan-26-oic acid in two siblings with cholestasis due to intrahepatic bile duct anomalies. J. Clin. Invest. *56*:577, 1975.

79. Hays, D. M., and Kimura, S.: Biliary Atresia: The Japanese Experience. Cambridge, Harvard University Press, 1980, pp. 1–218.

80. Hays, M., Woolley, M. M., Snyder, W. H., Reed, G. B., et al.: Diagnosis of biliary atresia: Relative accuracy of percutaneous liver biopsy, open liver biopsy and operative cholangiography. J. Pediatr. *71*:598, 1967.

81. Heathcote, J., Deodhar, K. P., Scheuer, P. J., and Sherlock, S.: Intrahepatic cholestasis in childhood. N. Engl. J. Med. *25*:801, 1976.

82. Heubi, J. E., Tsang, R. C., Steichen, J. J., and Chan, G. M.: 1,25-Dihydroxy D_3 in childhood hepatic osteodystrophy. J. Pediatr. *94*:977, 1979.

83. Hitch, D. C., and Lilly, J. R.: Identification, quantification and significance of bacterial growth within the biliary tract after Kasai's operation. J. Pediatr. Surg. *23*:563, 1978.

84. Javitt, N., Keating, J., and Grand, R.: Serum bile acid patterns in neonatal hepatitis and extrahepatic biliary atresia. J. Pediatr. *90*:736, 1977.

85. Jung, R. T., Davie, M., Siklos, P., and Chalmers, T.: Vitamin D metabolism in acute and chronic cholestasis. Gut *20*:840, 1979.

86. Kasai, M., Watanabi, I., and Ryaji, O.: Follow up studies of long term survivors after hepatic portoenterostomy for "noncorrectable" biliary atresia. J. Pediatr. Surg. *10*:173, 1975.

87. Landing, B. H.: Considerations of the pathogenesis of neonatal hepatitis, biliary atresia, and choledochal cyst: the concept of infantile obstructive cholangiopathy. Prog. Pediatr. Surg. *6*:113, 1974.

88. Lilly, J. R.: Surgical jaundice in infancy. Ann. Surg. *186*:549, 1977.

89. Lilly, J. R.: The surgical treatment of choledochal cyst. Surg. Gynecol. Obstet. *149*:36, 1979.

90. Longmire, W. P., Mandiolo, S. A., and Gordon, H. E.: Congenital cystic disease of the liver and biliary system. Ann. Surg. *174*:711, 1971.

90a. Lygidakis, N. J.: Histologic changes and intrahepatic biliary abnormalities in extrahepatic biliary tract destruction. Surg. Gynecol. Obstet. 153:532, 1981.

91. McDonald, P. J., Stehman, F., and Stewart, D.: Infantile obstructive cholangiopathy. Am. J. Dis. Child. 133:518, 1979.

92. Miller, J. H., Sinatra, F. R., and Thomas, D. W.: Biliary excretion disorders in infant evaluation using Tc 99 m Pipida. Am. J. Roentgenol. 135:47, 1980.

93. Miyano, T., Suruga, K., and Suda, K.: Abnormal choledocho-pancreatico-ductal junction related to the etiology of infantile obstructive jaundice. J. Pediatr. Surg. 14:16, 1980.

94. Oh, R., Kasai, M., and Takahashi, T.: Intrahepatic biliary obstruction in congenital bile duct atresia. Tohoku J. Exp. Med. 99:129, 1969.

95. Ohi, R., and Lilly, J.: Copper kinetics in infantile hepatobiliary disease. J. Pediatr. Surg. 15:509, 1980.

95a. Pereira, G. R., Sherman, M. S., DiGiacomo, J., Ziegler, M., Roth, K., and Jacobowski, D.: Hyperalimentation-induced cholestasis. Am. J. Dis. Child. 135:842, 1981.

96. Poley, J. R., Smith, E. I., Boon, D. J., Bhatia, M., et al.: Lipoprotein-A and the double ^{131}I-rose bengal test in the diagnosis of prolonged infantile jaundice. J. Pediatr. Surg. 7:660, 1972.

97. Psacharapoulos, H. T., Howard, E. R., Portmann, B., and Mowat, A. P.: Extrahepatic biliary atresia: Preoperative assessment and surgical results in 47 consecutive cases. Arch. Dis. Child. 55:351, 1980.

98. Putnam, C. W., Halgrimson, C. G., Koep, L., and Starzl, T.: Prognosis in liver transplantation. World J. Surg. 1:165, 1977.

99. Riely, C. A., Caride, V. J., Lange, R. C., Gottschalk, A., and Klatskin, G.: The use of ^{99m}Tc HIDA in evaluating pediatric liver disease. Gastroenterology 75:983, 1978.

100. Riely, C.: Familial intrahepatic cholestasis: an update. Yale J. Biol. Med. 52:89, 1979.

101. Ritland, S.: Quantitative determination of the abnormal lipoprotein of cholestasis, LP-X in liver disease. Scand. J. Gastroenterol. 10:5, 1975.

102. Rolleston, H. D., and Hayne, L. B.: A case of congenital hepatic cirrhosis with obliterative cholangitis. Br. Med. J. 1:758, 1981.

103. Rosenfeld, N., and Griscom, N. T.: Choledochal cyst: Roentgenographic techniques. Radiology 114:113, 1975.

104. Saito, A., and Ishida, M.: Congenital choledochal cyst. Prog. Pediatr. Surg. 6:63, 1974.

105. Sawaguchi, S., Akiyama, H., and Nakajam, T.: Long term follow up after radical operation for biliary atresia. In Japan Medical Research Foundation (ed.): Cholestasis in Infancy. Tokyo, University of Tokyo Press, 1980, pp. 371–380.

106. Sharp, H. L., Carey, J. B., White, J. G., and Krivit, W.: Cholestyramine therapy in patients with a paucity of intrahepatic bile ducts. J. Pediatr. 71:723, 1967.

107. Sigstad, H., Aagenaes, O., Bjorn-Hansen, R. W., and Rootwelt, K.: Primary lymphedema combined with hereditary recurrent intrahepatic cholestasis. Acta Med. Scand. 188:213, 1970.

108. Starzl, T. E., Koep, L. J., Schroter, P. J., Halgrimson, C. G., et al.: Liver replacement for pediatric patients. Pediatrics 63:825, 1979.

108a. Strickland, A., and Shannon, K.: Studies in the etiology of extrahepatic biliary atresia timespace clustering. J. Pediatr. 100:749, 1982.

108b. Suruga, K., Miyano, T., Kimura, K., Arai, T., and Kojima, Y.: Reoperation in the treatment of biliary atresia. J. Pediatr. Surg. 17:1, 1982.

108c. Teichberg, S., Markowitz, J., Silverberg, M., Aiges, H., Schneider, K., Kahn, E., and Daum, F.: Abnormal cilia in a child with the polysplenia syndrome and extrahepatic biliary atresia. J. Pediatr. 100:399, 1982.

109. Thaler, M. M.: Cryptogenic liver disease in young infants. In Popper, H., and Schaffner, F. (eds.): Progress in Liver Diseases. New York, Grune & Stratton, 1976, pp. 476–493.

110. Thaler, M. M., and Gellis, S. S.: Studies on neonatal hepatitis and biliary atresia. II. The effect of diagnostic laparotomy on long term prognosis of neonatal hepatitis. Am. J. Dis. Child. 116:262, 1968.

111. Todani, T., Wanatabe, Y., Narusue, M., et al.: Congenital bile duct cysts: classification, operative procedures and review of 37 cases. Am. J. Surg. 134:263, 1977.

112. Van Berge-Hanegauwen, G. P., Ferguson, D. R., Hoffmann, A. F., and DePagter, G. F.: Familial and nonfamilial benign recurrent cholestasis distinguished by plasma disappearance of indocyanine green but not cholyglycine. Gut 19:345, 1978.

112a. Witlin, L., Gadacz, T., Zuidema, G., and Kriedelbaugh, W.: Transhepatic decompression of the biliary tree in Caroli's disease. Surgery 91:205, 1982.

112b. Wright, K., and Christie, D. L.: Use of gammaglutamyl transpeptidase in the diagnosis of biliary atresia. Am. J. Dis. Child. 135:134, 1981.

Infectious Liver Disease

113. Adler, R.: Acute pericarditis and hepatitis B infection. Pediatrics 61:716, 1978.

114. Alagille, D., and Odièvre, M.: Liver and Biliary Tract Disease in Children. New York, John Wiley & Sons, 1979.

115. Alagille, D.: Clinical aspects of neonatal hepatitis. Am. J. Dis. Child. 123:287, 1972.

116. Baker, A. L., Kaplan, M., Wolfe, H., and McGowan, J.: Liver disease associated with early syphilis. N. Engl. J. Med. 284:1422, 1971.

116a. Bamber, M., Murray, A., Arborgh, B., Scheuer, P. J., Kernoff, P. B., Thomas, H. C., and Sherlock, S.: Short incubation non-A, non-B hepatitis transmitted by Factor VIII concentrates in patients with congenital coagulation disorders. Gut 22:854, 1981.

117. Berman, W., Pizzi, F., Schut, L., et al.: The effects of exchange transfusion on intracranial pressure in patients with Reye syndrome. Pediatrics 87:887, 1975.

117a. Borlotti, F., Cadrobbi, P., Crivellaro, C., Bertagglia, A., Alberti, A., and Realdi, G.: Chronic hepatitis type B in childhood—longitudinal study of 35 cases. Gut 22:499, 1981.

118. Boxall, E. H., Flewett, T. H., and Dane, D. S.:

Hepatitis B surface antigen in breast milk. Lancet 2:1007, 1974.

119. Chesid, M. J.: Pyogenic hepatic abscess in infancy and childhood. Pediatrics 62:554, 1978.

120. Committee on the Fetus and Newborn: Perinatal herpes simplex virus infections. Pediatrics 66:147, 1980.

121. Dahlquist, E., and Nordenfelt, E.: Neonatal hepatitis type B. A three year follow-up. Scand. J. Infect. Dis. 6:305, 1974.

122. Dehner, L. P., and Kissane, J. M.: Pyogenic hepatic abscesses in infancy and childhood. J. Pediatr. 74:763, 1969.

123. Dupuy, J. M., Kostewicz, E., and Alagille, D.: Hepatitis B in children. J. Pediatr. 92:17, 1978.

124. Eschar, J., Reif, L., Waron, M., and Alkan, W.: Hepatic lesion in chickenpox. Gastroenterology 64:462, 1973.

125. Esterly, J. R., Slusser, R. J., and Ruebner, A. H.: Hepatic lesions in congenital rubella syndrome. J. Pediatr. 71:676, 1967.

125a. Fleisher, G. R., Starr, S. E., Freidman, H. M., and Plotkin, S. A.: Vaccination of pediatric nurses with live, attenuated cytomegalovirus. Am. J. Dis. Child. 136:294, 1982.

126. Fox, D., Hart, M., Bergeson, P. S., et al.: Pyrrolizidine intoxication mimicking Reye syndrome. J. Pediatr. 93:980, 1978.

127. Gellis, S.: Commentary. In Year Book of Pediatrics. Chicago, Year Book Medical Publishing, Inc., 1978, p. 220.

128. Glassman, M., Tahan, S., Hillemeier, C., Rothstein, P., Shaywitz, B., and Gryboski, J.: Pancreatitis in patients with Reye's syndrome. J. Clin. Gastroenterol. 3:169, 1981.

129. Gregory, P. B., Knauer, C. M., Kempson, R. L., and Miller, R.: Steroid therapy in severe viral hepatitis. A randomized trial. N. Engl. J. Med. 294:681, 1976.

129a. Griffeths, P. D., Stagno, S., Pass, R., Smith, R., and Alford, C. A.: Congenital cytomegalovirus infection: Diagnostic and prognostic significance of the detection of specific IgM antibodies in cord serum. Pediatrics 69:544, 1982.

130. Hamilton, J. R., and Sass-Kortsak, A.: Jaundice associated with severe bacterial infection in young infants. J. Pediatr. 63:121, 1963.

130a. Hanshaw, J.: The launching of a cytomegalovirus vaccine. Am. J. Dis. Child. 136:291, 1982.

131. Henson, D., Grimley, P., and Strano, A.: Postnatal cytomegalovirus hepatitis. Hum. Pathol. 5:93, 1974.

132. Hilty, M. D., McClung, H. J., Haynes, R. E., Romste, C. A., et al.: Reye syndrome in siblings. J. Pediatr. 94:576, 1979.

133. Humphrey, M., Hansen, R., Bradley, D., Nagle, R., and Stillman, A. E.: Severe clotting abnormalities and transient hepatic fibrosis in acute anicteric hepatitis A. J. Pediatr. 95:987, 1979.

134. Huttenlocker, P. R., and Trauner, D. A.: Reye's syndrome in infancy. Pediatrics 62:84, 1978.

134a. Jabor, E., April, M., Selff, L. B., and Gerety, R. J.: Acute non A non B hepatis: prolonged presence of the infectious agent in blood. Gastroenterology 76:680, 1979.

135. Jhaveri, R., Rosenfeld, W., Salazar, J. D., Dosik, H., et al.: High titer multiple dose therapy with HB1G in newborn infants of HBsAg positive mothers. J. Pediatr. 97:305, 1980.

136. Kaitamus, C. A., Demetrois, D., and Matsanoits, N. S.: Australia antigen and neonatal hepatitis syndrome. Pediatrics 54:156, 1974.

137. Kohler, P. F., Dubois, R. S., Merrill, D. A., and Bowes, W. A.: Prevention of chronic neonatal hepatitis B virus infection with antibody to the hepatitis B surface antigen. N. Engl. J. Med. 291:1378, 1974.

138. LaBrecque, D., Latham, P., Riely, C., Hsia, E., and Klatskin, G.: Heritable urea cycle enzyme deficiency liver disease in 16 patients. J. Pediatr. 94:580, 1979.

138a. Lamprecht, C., Schaut, V., Warren, D., Nelson, K., Northrop, R., and Christiansen, M.: An outbreak of congenital rubella in Chicago. JAMA 247:1129, 1982.

139. Landay, S. E.: Varicella hepatitis and Reye's syndrome. Pediatrics 60:746, 1978.

139a. Lefkowich, J., Honig, C., King, M., and Hagstrom, J. W.: Hepatic copper overload and features of Indian childhood cirrhosis in an American sibship. N. Engl. J. Med. 307:271, 1982.

140. Marshall, L. F., Shapiro, H. M., Rausher, A., and Kaufman, N. M.: Pentobarbital therapy for intracranial hypertension in metabolic coma: Reye's syndrome. Crit. Care. Med. 6:1, 1978.

141. Modlin, J. F.: Fatal echovirus disease in premature neonates. Pediatrics 66:775, 1980.

141a. Moss, T., and Pysher, J.: Hepatic abscess in neonates. Am. J. Dis. Child. 135:726, 1981.

142. Okada, K., Kamiyama, I., Inomata, M., Imia, M., et al.: "e" Antigen and anti-e in the serum of asymptomatic carrier mothers as indicators of positive and negative transmission of hepatitis B virus to their infants. N. Engl. J. Med. 294:746, 1976.

143. Orlowski, J. P., Johannsson, J., and Ellis, N.: Encephalopathy and fatty metamorphosis of the liver associated with cold agglutin autoimmune hemolytic anemia. J. Pediatr. 94:569, 1979.

143a. Panjvani, Z. F. K., and Hanshaw, J. B.: Cytomegalovirus in the perinatal period. Am. J. Dis. Child. 135:56, 1981.

143b. Partin, J., Schubert, W. K., and Hammond, J.: Serum salicylate concentration in Reye's disease. Lancet 1:191, 1982.

144. Pichichero, M. E., and McCabe, E. R.: Recurrent Reye's syndrome. Am. J. Dis. Child. 132:1097, 1978.

144a. Prokopowicz, D., and Anaka, J.: Injury of liver in experimental salmonellosis of rabbits infected by Salmonella agona. Acta Hepato-Gastroenterol. 26:17, 1979.

145. Redeker, A. G., and Yamahiro, H. S.: Controlled trial of exchange transfusion therapy in fulminant hepatitis. Lancet 1:3, 1973.

146. Reye, R. D., Morgan, G., and Baral, J.: Encephalopathy and fatty degeneration of the viscera. Lancet 2:749, 1963.

147. Romsche, C., Hilty, M., McClung, J., Kerzner, B., and Reiner, C. B.: Amino acid pattern in Reye syndrome: comparison with clinically similar entities. J. Pediatr. 98:788, 1981.

148. Ryan, N. J., Hogan, G., Hayes, A. W., Unger, P.,

and Siraj, M.: Aflatoxin B: its role in the etiology of Reye's syndrome. Pediatrics 64:71, 1979.

149. Saw, H. S., Somasundaram, K., Kamath, R., and Lumpur, K.: Hepatic ascariasis. Arch. Surg. 108:733, 1974.

150. Schweitzer, I. L.: Vertical transmission of the hepatitis B surface antigen. Am. J. Med. Sci. 270:287, 1975.

151. Shapiro, J. M., Schaffner, F., Tallan, H., and Gaull, G. E.: Mitochondrial abnormalities of liver in primary ornithine transcarbamylase deficiency. Pediatr. Res. 14:725, 1980.

152. Shiraki, K., Yoshihara, N., Sakurai, M., Eto, T., et al.: Acute hepatitis B in infants born to carrier mothers with the antibody to hepatitis B e antigen. J. Pediatr. 97:768, 1980.

153. Silenzi, M.: The ESR in viral hepatitis. Pediatrics 61:4884, 1978.

153a. Sokol, R. J., Heubi, J., Farrell, M., Daugherty, C., Lichtenstein, P., Hug, G., Suchy, F., Balistreri, W.: Reye's syndrome: Primary cause of hepatic dysfunction following varicella or URI. Pediatr. Res. 16:178a, 1982.

154. Squires, J., Keating, J., Schwartz, K., Haymond, M. W., DeVivo, D. C., and Rodney, G.: HLA phenotypes in Reye syndrome patients. Pediatr. Res. 16:178, 1982.

155. Starko, K., Ray, G., Dominguez, L., Stromberg, W., and Woodall, D. F.: Reye's syndrome and salicylate use. Pediatrics 66:859, 1980.

156. Stray-Pedersen, B.: Infants potentially at risk to congenital toxoplasmosis. Am. J. Dis. Child. 134:639, 1980.

157. Tan, K. L.: The reemergence of early congenital syphilis. Acta Paediatr. Scand. 62:601, 1973.

158. Tiku, M. L., and Beutner, K. R.: Hepatitis B e antigen and antibody activity. J. Pediatr. 91:540, 1977.

158a. Trevisan, A., Cadrobbi, P., Crivellaro, C., Bortolotti, F., Rugge, M., and Realdi, G.: Virologic features of chronic hepatitis B virus infection in children. J. Pediatr. 100:366, 1982.

159. Tsuchida, Y., Endo, Y., Saito, S., Kaneko, M., et al.: Evaluation of alpha fetoprotein in early infancy. J. Pediatr. Surg. 13:155, 1978.

159a. Walle, A., and Lehmann, H.: Guillain-Barré syndrome and HBs-Ag–positive acute viral hepatitis. Acta Hepato-Gastroenterol. 28:305, 1981.

160. Ware, A. J., Luby, J. P., Hollinger, B., et al.: Etiology of liver disease in renal transplant patients. Ann. Intern. Med. 91:364, 1979.

160a. Wilson, C., Remington, J., Stagno, S., and Reynolds, D.: Development of adverse sequelae in children with subclinical congenital toxoplasma infection. Pediatrics 66:767, 1980.

161. Wyatt, R., Younoszai, K., and Anuras, S.: Campylobacter fetus septicemia and hepatitis in agammaglobulinemia. J. Pediatr. 91:441, 1977.

162. Yanagida, M., Horiguchi, S., Fugii, T., Okada, K., Nakao, C., Ishikawa, S., Miyakawa, Y., Baba, K., and Mayumi, M.: Failure of maternofetal transmission for small as well as large molecular hepatitis B e antigen. J. Pediatr. 95:76, 1979.

163. Yoshizawa, H., Akahane, Y., Itoh, Y., Iwakiris, S., Kitajima, K., Morita, M., Tanaka, A., Nojiri, T., Shimizu, M., Miyakawa, Y., and Mayumi, S.: Virus-like particles in a plasma fraction (fibrinogen) and in the circulation of apparently healthy blood donors capable of inducing non A/non B hepatitis in humans and chimpanzees. Gastroenterology 79:512, 1980.

164. Zeltzer, P. M.: Alpha fetoprotein in the differentiation of neonatal hepatitis and biliary atresia: current status and implications for the pathogenesis of these disorders. J. Pediatr. Surg. 13:361, 1978.

Drug and Toxic Hepatitis

165. Amla, I., Kamala, C. S., Gopalakrishna, G. S., Jayaraj, P., Sreenivasamurthy, V., and Parpia, H.: Cirrhosis in children from peanut meal contaminated by aflatoxin. Am. J. Clin. Nutr. 24:609, 1971.

166. Bernstein, B. H., Singsen, B. H., King, K. K., et al.: Aspirin induced hepatotoxicity and its effect on juvenile rheumatoid arthritis. Am. J. Dis. Child. 131:659, 1977.

166a. Bistritzer, R., Barilay, Z., and Jonas, A.: Isoniazid-rifampin–induced fulminant liver disease in an infant. J. Pediatr. 97:480, 1980.

167. Black, M., Mitchell, J. R., Zimmerman, H. J., Ishak, K. G., et al.: Isoniazid-associated hepatitis in 114 patients. Gastroenterology 69:289, 1975.

168. Bras, G., Jelliffe, D. B., and Stuart, K. L.: Venoocclusive disease of liver with nonportal type of cirrhosis, occurring in Jamaica. Arch. Pathol. 57:285, 1954.

169. Bulugahapitiya, D. T. D., Hebron, B., and Beck, P. R.: Salicylate hepatitis with acidosis in an infant. Lancet 1:1295, 1979.

169a. Callahan, J., Haller, J., Cacciarelli, A., Slovis, T., and Freidman, A.: Cholelithiasis in infants: Association with total parenteral nutrition and furosemide. Radiology 143:437, 1982.

170. Heird, W. C., Driscoll, J. M., Schullinger, J. N., Greben, B., et al.: Intravenous alimentation in pediatric patients. J. Pediatr. 80:351, 1972.

171. Johnson, J. D., Albritton, W. L., and Sunshine, P.: Hyperammonemia accompanying parenteral nutrition in newborn infants. J. Pediatr. 81:154, 1972.

172. Koga, Y., Swanson, V. L., and Hays, D. M.: Hepatic intravenous fat pigment in infants and children receiving lipid emulsion. J. Pediatr. Surg. 10:641, 1975.

173. Lilly, J. P., Hitch, D. C., and Javitt, N. B.: Cimetidine cholestatic jaundice in children. J. Surg. Res. 24:384, 1978.

174. Mitchell, J. R., Jollow, D. V., Potter, W. Z., Gillette, J. R., et al.: Acetaminophen induced hepatic necrosis. I. Role of drug metabolism. J. Pharm. Exp. Ther. 187:185, 1973.

175. Mullick, F. G., and Ishak, K. G.: Hepatic injury

associated with diphenylhydantoin therapy: A clinicopathologic study of 20 cases. Am. J. Pathol. *74*:442, 1980.

176. Prescott, L. F., Newton, R., Swainson, C. S., Wright, N., et al.: Successful treatment of severe paracetamol overdosage with cysteamine. Lancet *1*:588, 1974.

177. Rhishan, F., Labredque, D., et al.: Intrahepatic cholestasis after gold therapy in juvenile rheumatoid arthritis. J. Pediatr. *93*:1042, 1978.

178. Rumack, B., and Peterson, R.: Acetaminophen overdosage: incidence, diagnosis and management in 416 patients. Pediatrics *62*:898, 1978.

179. Schaller, J. G.: Chronic salicylate administration in rheumatoid arthritis: aspirin "hepatitis" and its clinical significance. Pediatrics *62*:916, 1978.

179a. Spechler, S. J., Sperber, H., Doos, W. G., and Koff, R. S.: Cholestasis and toxic epidermal necrolysis associated with phenytoin sodium ingestion. The role of bile duct injury. Ann. Intern. Med. *95*:455, 1981.

180. Stein, M. T., and Liang, D.: Clinical hepatotoxicity of isoniazid in children. Pediatrics *64*:499, 1979.

181. Stevenson, D. K.: Hepatic injury caused by trimethoprim sulfamethoxazole. Pediatrics *61*:864, 1978.

182. Suchy, F. J., Balistreri, W. F., Buchino, J. J., Sondheimer, J. M., et al.: Acute hepatic failure associated with the use of sodium valproate. N. Engl. J. Med. *300*:962, 1979.

183. Touloukian, R. J., and Seashore, J. H.: Hepatic secretory obstruction with total parenteral nutrition in the infant. J. Pediatr. Surg. *10*:353, 1975.

184. Ulshen, M., Grand, R., Crain, J., and Gelfand, S.: Hepatotoxicity and encephalopathy with aspirin. J. Pediatr. *93*:1034, 1978.

185. Vileisis, R. A., Inwood, R. J., and Hunt, C. E.: Parenteral nutrition associated cholestatic jaundice. J. Pediatr. *96*:893, 1980.

186. Ware, S., and Millward-Sadler, G. I.: Acute liver disease associated with sodium valproate. Lancet *2*:1110, 1980.

187. Weinberg, A. G., and Bolande, R. P.: The liver in congenital heart disease. Effects of infantile coarctation of the aorta and the hypoplastic left heart syndrome in infancy. Am. J. Dis. Child. *119*:390, 1970.

188. Zimmerman, H. G.: Hepatic injury caused by therapeutic agents. *In* Becker, F. J. (ed.): The Liver: Normal and Abnormal Functions. New York, Marcel Dekker, 1974, pp. 225–302.

188a. Zimmerman, H. G.: Effects of aspirin and acetaminophen on the liver. Arch. Intern. Med. *141*:333, 1981.

Chronic Hepatitis and Cirrhosis

189. Arasu, T., Wyllie, R., Hatch, J., and Fitzgerald, J.: Management of chronic aggressive hepatitis in children and adolescents. J. Pediatr. *95*:514, 1979.

190. Conn, H. O.: Cirrhosis. *In* Schiff, L. (ed.): Diseases of the Liver. Philadelphia, J. B. Lippincott Company, 1975, pp. 833–939.

191. Gazzard, B. G., Portmann, B., Weston, M. J., Longley, P. G., et al.: Charcoal hemoperfusion in the treatment of fulminant hepatic failure. Lancet *1*:1301, 1974.

192. Kocak, N., and Ozsoxlu, S.: Familial cirrhosis. Am. J. Dis. Child. *133*:1160, 1979.

193. LeVeen, H. H., Wapnick, S., Grosberg, S., and Kinney, M. J.: Further experience with peritoneo-venous shunt for ascites. Ann. Surg. *184*:574, 1976.

193a. Marinaha, N., Nayuk, N., Roy, S., Kalra, V., and Ghai, O. P.: The role of excess hepatic copper in the evolution of Indian childhood cirrhosis. Indian J. Med. Res. *73*:395, 1981.

194. Miller, D., Dwyer, J., and Klatskin, G.: Identification of lymphocytes in percutaneous liver biopsy cores. Gastroenterology *72*:1199, 1977.

195. Soloway, R. D., Summerskill, W. H. J., Baggenstoss, A. H., and Schoenfield, L.: Lupoid hepatitis, a nonentity in the spectrum of chronic active liver disease. Gastroenterology *63*:458, 1972.

196. Tanner, M. S., Portmann, B., Mowat, A. P., et al.: Indian childhood cirrhosis presenting in Britain with orcein-positive deposits in liver and kidney. Br. Med. J. *2*:928, 1978.

197. Tanner, M. S., Portmann, B., Mowat, A. P., Williams, R., Pandit, A. M., and Brenner, I.: Increased hepatic copper concentration in Indian childhood cirrhosis. Lancet *1*:1203, 1979.

198. Wright, E., Seeff, L., Berk, P., Jones, A., and Plotz, P.: Treatment of chronic active hepatitis. Gastroenterology *73*:1422, 1977.

199. Wyllie, R., Arasu, T. S., and Fitzgerald, J. F.: Ascites: Pathophysiology and management. J. Pediatr. *97*:167, 1980.

Inherited and Metabolic Hepatocellular Diseases

200. Ament, M., and Ochs, H.: Gastrointestinal manifestations of chronic granulomatous disease. N. Engl. J. Med. *288*:382, 1973.

201. Bannatyne, R. M., Kowrin, P. N., and Weber, J. L.: Job's syndrome — a variant of chronic granulomatous disease. J. Pediatr. *75*:236, 1979.

202. Barth, R., Vergara, G., Khutana, S., and Lowman, J.: Rapidly fatal familial histiocytosis associated with eosinophilia and primary immunologic deficiency. Lancet *2*:503, 1972.

203. Beaudet, A., Ferry, G., and Nichols, B.: Cholesterol ester storage disease. J. Pediatr. *90*:910, 1976.

204. Belanger, L., Belanger, M., Price, L., Larochelle, J., et al.: Hereditary tyrosinemia and alpha-1-fetoprotein. I. Clinical tyrosinemia. Pathol. Biol. (Paris) *21*:449, 1973.

205. Brady, R. O., and King, F. M.: Niemann Pick disease. *In* Hers, H. G., and van Hoff, F. (eds.): Lysosomes and Storage Diseases. New York, Academic Press, 1973, pp. 439–451.

206. Brady, R. O., Pentchev, P. G., Gal, A. E., Hillert, S. R., et al.: Replacement enzyme therapy for inherited enzyme deficiency. N. Engl. J. Med. 291:989, 1974.

207. Burke, J. A., and Schubert, W. K.: Deficient activity of hepatic acid lipase in cholesterol storage disease. Science 176:309, 1972.

207a. Carlson, J., Eriksson, S., and Hagerstrand, I.: Intra- and extracellular alpha₁-antitrypsin in liver disease, with special reference to Pi phenotype. J. Clin. Pathol. 34:620, 1981.

207b. Chusid, M. J., and Tomasulo, P. A.: Granulocyte survival in chronic granulomatous disease. Pediatrics 61:556, 1978.

208. Cornblath, M., Rosenthal, I. M., Peisner, S. H., Wybregt, S. H., et al.: Hereditary fructose intolerance. N. Engl. J. Med. 269:1271, 1963.

209. Dank, D. M., Tippett, D., Adams, C., and Campbell, P.: Cerebro-hepatorenal syndrome of Zellweger: report of eight cases with comments on incidence, the liver lesion and a fault in pipecolic acid metabolism. J. Pediatr. 86:382, 1975.

210. DiSant'Agnese, P., and Blanc, W.: A distinctive type of biliary cirrhosis of the liver associated with cystic fibrosis of the pancreas. Recognition through signs of portal hypertension. Pediatrics 18:387, 1956.

211. Fagerhol, M., and Braend, M.: Serum prealbumin polymorphism in man. Science 149:986, 1965.

212. Fikrig, S., Suntharalingam, S., Smithwick, E., and Good, R. A.: Fibroblast nitroblue tetrazolium test and the in-utero diagnosis of chronic granulomatous disease. Lancet 1:18, 1980.

213. Gardner, L.: Uridine diphosphate galactosemia 4-epimerase deficiency. Am. J. Dis. Child. 134:995, 1980.

214. Gatfield, P., Taller, E., Hinton, G., Wallace, A., Abdelnour, G., and Haust, M.: Hyperpipecolatemia: a new metabolic disorder associated with neuropathy and hepatomegaly. Can. Med. Assoc. J. 99:1215, 1968.

215. Gentz, J., Jagenburg, O. R., and Zetterstrom, R.: Tyrosinemia: An inborn error of tyrosine metabolism with cirrhosis of the liver and multiple renal tubule defects. J. Pediatr. 66:670, 1965.

215a. Godek, J. E., Klein, H. G., Holland, P. V., and Crystal, R. G.: Replacement therapy of alpha-1-antitrypsin deficiency — Reversal of protease-antiprotease imbalance within the alveolar structures of PiZ subjects. J. Clin. Invest. 68:1158, 1981.

216. Goldfischer, S., and Moore, C. L.: Peroxisorenal and mitochondrial defects in the cerebro-hepato-renal syndrome. Science 182:62, 1973.

217. Greene, H., Slonim, A., Burr, I., et al.: Type 1 glucogen storage disease: five years of management with nocturnal intragastric feeding. J. Pediatr. 96:590, 1980.

218. Groth, C. G., Collste, H., Dreborg, S., Håkansson, G., Lundgren, G., and Svennerholm, L.: Attempt at enzyme replacement in Gaucher disease by renal transplantation. Acta Paediatr. Scand. 68:475, 1979.

219. Holmes, B., Park, B. H., Malawista, S., Quie, P., Nelson, D., and Good, R. A.: Chronic granulomatous disease in females: a deficiency of leukocyte glutathione peroxidase. N. Engl. J. Med. 283:217, 1970.

219a. Holton, J. B., Gillett, M. G., MacFaul, R., and Young, R.: Galactosemia: A new severe variant due to uridine diphosphate galactose-4-epimerase deficiency. Arch. Dis. Child. 56:885, 1981.

220. Hood, J. M., Koep, L. J., Peters, R. L., Schroter, G. P., et al.: Liver transplantation for advanced liver disease with alpha-1-antitrypsin deficiency. N. Engl. J. Med. 302:272, 1980.

221. Jones, B., Gilbert, E., Zugibe, F., and Thomson, H.: Sea-blue histiocyte disease in siblings. Lancet 2:73, 1970.

222. Lang, A., Groebe, H., Hellkuhl, B., and von Figura, K.: A new variant of galactosemia: galactose-1-phosphate uridylytransferase sensitive to product inhibition by glucose 1-phosphate. Pediatr. Res. 14:729, 1980.

223. Larsson, C.: Natural history and life expectancy in severe alpha1-antitrypsin deficiency, Pi Z. Acta Med. Scand. 204:345, 1978.

223a. Lerner, A., Iancu, T., Bashan, N., Potashnik, R., and Moses, S.: A new variant of glycogen storage disease. Am. J. Dis. Child. 136:406, 1982.

224. Levy, H. L., and Hammersen, G.: Newborn screening for galactosemia and other galactose metabolic defects. J. Pediatr. 92:871, 1978.

225. Lewis, B., Hansen, J. D., Wittman, W., Krut, L., et al.: Plasma free fatty acids in kwashiorkor and the pathogenesis of fatty liver. Am. J. Clin. Nutr. 15:161, 1964.

226. McAdams, A. J., Hug, G., and Bove, B. E.: Glycogen storage disease, types I to X. Criteria for morphologic diagnosis. Hum. Pathol. 5:463, 1974.

227. McLaren, D. S., Bitar, J. G., and Nassar, V. H.: Protein calorie malnutrition and the liver. In Popper, H., and Schaffner, F. (eds.): Progress in Liver Disease. New York, Grune & Stratton, 1973, pp. 527–534.

227a. Michels, V. V., Beaudet, A. L., Potts, V. E., and Montandon, C. M.: Glycogen storage disease: Long-term follow-up of nocturnal intragastric feeding. Clin. Genet. 21:136, 1982.

228. Mills, E. L., Rholl, K. S., and Quie, P. G.: X linked inheritance in females with chronic granulomatous disease. J. Clin. Invest. 66:332, 1980.

229. Morse, J.: Alpha-1-antitrypsin deficiency. N. Engl. J. Med. 299:1045, 1978.

230. Nadler, H. L., Inouye, T., and Hsia, D. Y.: Classical galactosemia: a study of 55 cases. In Hsia, D. Y. (ed.) Galactosemia. Springfield, Ill., Charles C Thomas Publishers, 1969, p. 127.

231. O'Brien, J.: Generalized gangliosidosis. J. Pediatr. 75:167, 1969.

232. O'Brien, M., Burst, N., and Murphy, W.: Neonatal screening for alpha-1-antitrypsin deficiency. J. Pediatr. 92:1006, 1978.

233. Odièvre, M., Martin, J., Hadchouel, M., and Ala-

gille, M.: Alpha-1-antitrypsin deficiency and liver disease in children: phenotypes, manifestations, and prognosis. Pediatrics *57*:226, 1976.

234. Oppenheimer, E. H., and Esterly, J. R.: Hepatic changes in young infants with cystic fibrosis: possible relation to focal biliary cirrhosis. J. Pediatr. *86*:683, 1975.

234a. Pariente, E., Degott, C., Martin, J., Feldmann, G., Potet, F., and Benhamou, J.: Hepatocytic PAS-positive diastase-resistant inclusions in the absence of alpha-1-antitrypsin deficiency—high prevalence in alcoholic cirrhosis. Am. J. Clin. Pathol. *76*:299, 1981.

234b. Partin, J. S., Partin, J. C., Schubert, W., and McAdams, J.: Liver ultrastructure in abetalipoproteinemia. Gastroenterology *67*:107, 1974.

235. Patrick, A. D., and Lake, B. D.: Deficiency of acid lipase in Wolman's disease. Nature *222*:1067, 1969.

236. Pesce, M., and Bodourian, S.: Problems in the diagnosis of transferase and galactokinase deficient galactosemia. Ann. Clin. Lab. Sci. *10*:26, 1980.

237. Pizzo, C. J.: Glycogen storage disease. Pediatrics *65*:341, 1980.

238. Rozenthal, P., Biava, C., Spender, H., and Zimmerman, H. J.: Liver morphology and function tests in obesity and during total starvation. Am. J. Dig. Dis. *12*:198, 1967.

239. Rosenthal, P.: Infantile cholestasis and PiSZ. Am. J. Dis. Child. *133*:1195, 1979.

240. Sann, L., Matthieu, M., Bourgeois, J., et al.: Defective activity of glucose-6-phosphatase in type IB glycogenotypes. J. Pediatr. *96*:691, 1980.

241. Satran, L., Sharp, H. L., Schenken, J. R., and Krivit, W.: Fatal neonatal hepatic steatosis. A new familial disorder. J. Pediatr. *75*:39, 1969.

242. Scheig, R., and Gryboski, J. D.: The liver. *In* Gryboski, J.: Gastrointestinal Problems in the Infant. Philadelphia, W. B. Saunders Company, 1975, pp. 311–449.

243. Schiff, L., Schubert, W., McAdams, A., Spiegal, E., and O'Donnell, J. F.: Hepatic cholesterol storage disease — a familial disorder. Am. J. Med. *44*:538, 1968.

243a. Schwarz, H., Zuppinger, K. A., Zimmerman, A., Dauwalder, H., Scherz, R., and Bier, D. M.: Galactose intolerance in individuals with double heterozygosity for Duarte variant and galactosemia. J. Pediatr. *100*:704, 1982.

243b. Seger, R. A., Baumgartner, S., Tietnauer, L. X., and Gmunder, F. K.: Chronic granulomatous disease — effect of sulfamethoxazole/-trimethoprim on neutrophil microbicidal function. Helv. Paediatr. Acta *36*:579, 1982.

244. Sharp, H. L.: The current status of alpha-1-antitrypsin, a protease inhibitor in gastrointestinal disease. Gastroenterology *70*:621, 1976.

245. Shih, V., Levy, H., Karolewicz, V., Houghton, S., Efron, M., Isselbacher, K., Beutler, E., and MacCready, R.: Galactosemia screening of newborns in Massachusetts. N. Engl. J. Med. *284*:753, 1971.

246. Starzl, T. E., and Putnam, C. W.: Portal diversion for the treatment of glycogen storage disease in humans. Ann. Surg. *178*:525, 1973.

246a. Steinmann, B., and Gitzelmann, R.: The diagnosis of hereditary fructose intolerance. Helv. Paediatr. Acta *36*:297, 1981.

247. Sternlieb, I.: Diagnosis of Wilson's disease. Gastroenterology *74*:787, 1978.

248. Sveger, T.: Antitrypsin deficiency in early childhood. Pediatrics *62*:22, 1978.

249. Valman, H. B., France, N. E., and Wallis, P. G.: Prolonged neonatal jaundice in cystic fibrosis. Arch. Dis. Child. *46*:805, 1971.

250. Van Berge Henegouwen, G. P., Tangedahl, T. N., Hoffman, A., et al.: Biliary secretion of copper in healthy man. Gastroenterology *72*:1228, 1977.

251. Vitullo, B., Rochon, L., Seemayer, T., Beardmore, H., et al.: Compression of the bile ducts in cystic fibrosis. J. Pediatr. *93*:1060, 1978.

252. Weinberg, A. G., Mize, C. E., and Worthan, H. G.: The occurrence of hepatoma in the chronic form of hereditary tyrosinemia. J. Pediatr. *88*:434, 1976.

Trauma and Liver Tumors

253. Alpert, E., Starzl, T. E., Schur, P. H., and Isselbacher, E.: Serum alpha-fetoprotein in hepatoma patients after liver transplantation. Gastroenterology *61*:144, 1971.

254. Andressy, R., Brennau, L. P., Siegel, M., Weitzman, J., Siegel, S., Stanley, P., and Mahour, G.: Preoperative chemotherapy for hepatoblastoma in children. J. Pediatr. Surg. *15*:617, 1980.

255. Aoyama, K., Takada, Y., Mou, S., et al.: Familial occurrence of hepatoblastoma. J. Jpn. Soc. Pediatr. Surg. *15*:1213, 1979.

256. Bord, J. V.: Neuroblastoma metastatic to the liver in infants. Arch. Dis. Child. *57*:879, 1976.

257. Braun, P., Ducharme, J. C., Riopelle, J. L., and Davignon, A.: Hemangiomatosis of the liver in infants. J. Pediatr. Surg. *10*:121, 1975.

257b. Brechot, C., Nalpas, B., Courouce, M., Duhamel, G., et al.: Evidence that hepatitis B virus has a role in liver cell carcinoma in alcoholic liver disease. N. Engl. J. Med. *306*:1384, 1982.

257a. Cooney, D. R.: Splenic and hepatic trauma in children. Surg. Clin. North Am. *61*:1165, 1981.

258. Dahms, B. B.: Hepatoma in familial cholestatic cirrhosis of childhood—its occurrence in twin brothers. Arch. Pathol. Lab. Med. *103*:30, 1979.

259. deLorimier, A. A., Simpson, E. B., Braun, R. S., et al.: Hepatic artery ligation for hepatic hemangiomatosis. N. Engl. J. Med. *277*:333, 1967.

260. Erdon, Z., Hittner, I., and Makoi, Z.: Hamartoma of the liver in a newborn infant. Gastroenterology *30*:272, 1979.

261. Exelby, P. R., Filler, R. M., and Grosfeld, J. L.: Liver tumor in children in the particular reference to hepatoblastoma and hepatocellular carcinoma. J. Pediatr. Surg. *10*:329, 1975.

262. Fegiz, G., Rosati, D., Tonelli, F., et al.: Hepatoblastoma treated by chemotherapy and hepatic lobectomy. World J. Surg. *1*:407, 1977.

262a. Filler, R. M., and Hagen, J.: Liver tumors. Surg. Clin. North Am. *61*:1209, 1981.

262b. French, C., and Waldstein, G.: Subcapsular hemorrhage of the liver of the newborn. Pediatrics *69*:204, 1982.

263. Ishak, K. G., and Glunz, P.: Hepatoblastoma and hepatocarcinoma in infancy and childhood: report of 47 cases. Cancer *20*:396, 1967.

264. Kasai, M., and Wanatabe, I.: Histologic classification of liver cell carcinoma in infancy and childhood and its clinical evaluation. Cancer *25*:551, 1970.

265. Keeling, J. W.: Liver tumors in childhood. J. Pathol. *103*:69, 1971.

266. Klein, M., and Philippart, A.: Post traumatic Budd-Chiari syndrome with late reversibility of hepatic venous obstruction. J. Pediatr. Surg. *14*:661, 1979.

266a. Larcher, V. F., Howard, E. R., and Mowat, A.: Hepatic haemangiomata: Diagnosis and management. Arch. Dis. Child. *56*:7, 1981.

267. Leonidas, J. C., Strauss, L., and Beck, A. R.: Vascular tumors of the liver in newborns. Am. J. Dis. Child. *125*:507, 1973.

268. McArthur, J. W., Toll, G. D., Russfield, A. B., Russ, A. M., et al.: Sexual precocity attributable to ectopic gonadotropin secretion by hepatoblastoma. Am. J. Med. *54*:390, 1973.

269. Okuyama, K.: Primary liver cell carcinoma associated with biliary cirrhosis due to congenital bile duct atresia. J. Pediatr. *67*:89, 1965.

270. Randolph, J., Altman, P., Arensman, R., Mathak, M., and Leikin, S.: Liver resection in children with hepatic neoplasm. Ann. Surg. *187*:599, 1978.

271. Rothman, M., John, M., Inamdar, S., et al.: Radiation treatment of pediatric hepatic hemangiomatosis and coexisting cardiac failure. N. Engl. J. Med. *302*:852, 1980.

272. Shah, J., Goldsmith, H., and Huvos, A.: Hamartomas of the liver. Surgery *68*:778, 1970.

273. Sordahl, O., and Gay, B. B.: Roentgenologic features of a primary carcinoma of the liver in infants and children. Am. J. Roentgenol. *100*:117, 1967.

274. Sutton, C. A., and Eller, J. L.: Mesenchymal hamartoma of the liver. Cancer *22*:29, 1968.

275. Touloukian, R.: Hepatic hemangioendothelioma during infancy: pathology, diagnosis and treatment with prednisone. Pediatrics *45*:71, 1970.

275a. Vileisis, R. A., Sorensen, K., Gonzalez-Crussi, F., and Hunt, C.: Liver malignancy after parenteral nutrition. J. Pediatr. *100*:88, 1982.

Acquired Lesions of the Biliary Tree

276. Buschi, A. J., and Brenbridge, A.: Sonographic diagnosis of cholelithiasis in childhood. Am. J. Dis. Child. *134*:575, 1980.

277. Defans, G., and Pisoni, F.: Rupture of the common hepatic duct after blunt abdominal trauma in childhood. Ital. Chir. Ped. *18*:56, 1976.

278. Fitzgerald, R., Parbhoo, K., and Guiney, E.: Spontaneous perforation of bile ducts in neonates. Surgery *83*:303, 1978.

279. Glenn, F.: Acute acalculous cholecystitis. Ann. Surg. *189*:458, 1979.

280. Kendall, R. S., Chapoy, P. R., Busutil, R. W., Kolodny, M., and Ament, M. E.: Acquired bile duct stricture in childhood related to blunt trauma. Am. J. Dis. Child. *134*:551, 1980.

281. Kulkarni, P., and Beatty, E.: Cholangiocarcinoma associated with biliary cirrhosis due to congenital biliary atresia. Am. J. Dis. Child. *131*:442, 1977.

281a. Leichty, E., Cohen, M., Lemons, J., Jansen, R., and Schreiner, R.: Normal gallbladder appearing as abdominal mass in neonates. Am. J. Dis. Child. *136*:462, 1982.

282. Lilly, J.: Common bile duct calculi in infants and children. J. Pediatr. Surg. *15*:577, 1980.

283. Lilly, J., Weintraub, W., and Altman, P.: Spontaneous perforation of the extrahepatic bile ducts and bile peritonitis in infancy. Surgery *75*:664, 1974.

284. Magilavy, D. B., Speert, D. P., Silver, T. M., and Sullivan, D. B.: Mucocutaneous lymph node syndrome: report of two cases complicated by gallbladder hydrops and diagnosed by ultrasound. Pediatrics *61*:699, 1978.

284a. Mihara, S., Matsumoto, H., Tokunaga, F., Yano, H., Ota, M., and Yamashita, S.: Botryoid rhabdomyosarcoma of the gallbladder in a child. Cancer *49*:812, 1982.

285. Mock, D. M., Perman, J., Rosenthal, P., Harrison, M., and Thaler, M.: Cholelithiasis in a 2 year old child with reflux esophagitis and hiatus hernia. J. Pediatr. *96*:898, 1980.

286. Ney, J., Arvin, A., and Ariagno, R.: Hydrops of the gallbladder. Am. J. Dis. Child. *134*:892, 1980.

286a. Peevy, K. J., and Loiseman, H. J.: Gallbladder distension in septic neonates. Arch. Dis. Child. *57*:75, 1982.

287. Perrelli, L., Calisti, A., Lauriola, L., and Ramno, O.: Sarcoma botryoides of the bile ducts in childhood: diagnosis and therapy. J. Pediatr. Surg. *13*:563, 1978.

288. Pieretti, R., Auldist, A. W., and Stephens, C. A.: Acute cholecystitis in children. Surg. Gynecol. Obstet. *140*:16, 1975.

288a. Schrumpf, J., and Handmaker, H.: Hydrops of gallbladder in a premature neonate. Am. J. Dis. Child. *136*:173, 1982.

289. Slovis, T. L., Hight, D., Philippart, A., and duBois, R.: Hydrops of the gallbladder. Pediatrics *65*:789, 1980.

290. Ternbery, J. L., and Keating, J. R.: Acute acalculous cholecystitis. Arch. Surg. *110*:543, 1975.

291. Wiscombe, J. B.: Biliary rhabdomyosarcoma of childhood. Br. J. Radiol. *52*:1006, 1979.

Chapter Fifteen

THE PANCREAS

INTRODUCTION

Pancreatic disease in infancy is quite rare. Little is known about normal pancreatic development *in utero* and in early infancy, making it difficult to assess the disease state. Much of the existing literature extrapolates the adult or childhood condition to that of infancy. Yet, pancreatic exocrine function in term infants, under physiologic conditions, is thought to be insufficient. The following is a review of the knowledge at present. With increasing investigation, infantile pancreatic disease may be found to be more common than was initially suspected.

PANCREATIC DEVELOPMENT

Pancreatic development begins *in utero* during the fifth week of gestation.[87, 90] The structure destined to become the pancreas arises from two diverticula of the foregut region that is later to become the duodenum. Development of these diverticula is completed by the seventh week of gestation. The diverticula are known as the dorsal and ventral pancreatic buds. The larger dorsal bud is the first to appear and grows rapidly, extending into the dorsal mesentery. The ventral bud is small and develops distal to the dorsal bud. It arises near the insertion of the common bile duct into the duodenum. Owing to the rapid growth of the duodenum, the ventral bud and common bile duct rotate behind the duodenum, which then fuses with the dorsal bud. Most of the pancreas is formed from the dorsal bud. The uncinate process and inferior part of the head of the pancreas are derived from the ventral bud. When the two buds fuse, the pancreatic ducts of each bud anastomose. The main pancreatic duct, also known as the duct of Wirsung, is formed from the ducts of the ventral bud and the distal part of the dorsal bud. The upper portion of the head is drained by the remaining part of the dorsal duct, known as the accessory pancreatic duct, or the duct of Santorini (Fig. 15–1).

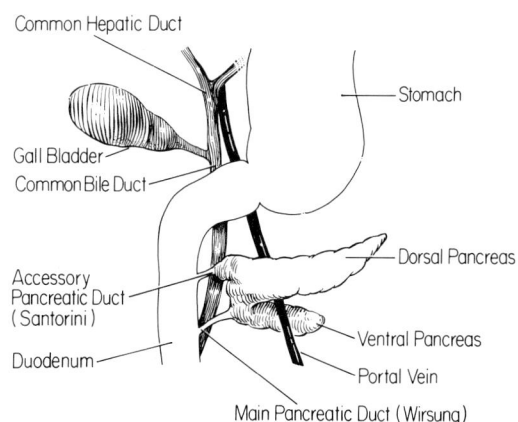

Figure 15–1 Anatomic relationships of the normal pancreas.

In its early origins, the pancreas consists of tubules with blind ends. Pancreatic acini arise from these blind ends during the twelfth week of gestation. The acini are initially solid, but each eventually develops a lumen.

In the fully developed newborn infant, the pancreas lies in the posterior upper abdomen. It is a "hidden" organ, impossible to palpate. It is in immediate proximity to the duodenum, stomach, spleen, ampulla of Vater, common bile duct, portal vein, and superior mesenteric artery. Because of its location, there are often few clinical signs of pancreatic disease. Clinical symptoms and signs are most often referable to the above-mentioned adjacent structures.

PANCREATIC FUNCTION

The pancreas functions to produce the necessary enzymes for the digestion and absorption of food.[151] In addition, it secretes buffer and electrolytes into the duodenum to provide the optimal milieu for enzymatic activity. During the cephalic phase of digestion, which is mediated by the vagus nerve, pancreatic enzymes are mobilized from the acinar cells into the ducts. The intestinal phase of digestion is mediated by secretin and pancreozymin. When an acid substance enters the duodenum, secretin is released from the duodenal mucosa. This, in turn, stimulates the pancreatic secretion of bicarbonate and electrolytes, which neutralizes the duodenal fluid to an optimal pH of 8. The electrolyte concentrations are isotonic to plasma. When protein and fat enter the duodenum, cholecystokinin-pancreozymin is released, stimulating pancreatic enzyme secretion — mostly amylase, lipase, and the proteolytic enzymes. The proteolytic enzymes are secreted in their inactive form to protect the pancreas. The pancreas also secretes a trypsin inhibitor that inactivates any activated trypsin present before it reaches the intestinal lumen, thus preventing autodigestion of the pancreas. In the duodenum, enterokinase activates trypsinogen (inactive trypsin) to trypsin. In turn, activated trypsin activates chymotrypsinogen to chymotrypsin, and procarboxypeptidase to carboxypeptidase. Digestion and absorption of food then proceed.

DEVELOPMENT OF PANCREATIC FUNCTION

As stated earlier, information on the development of normal pancreatic function is incomplete at present. Much of this knowledge is anatomic, but there is little on the normal pancreatic physiology at birth.[31, 70]

The acinar cells of the pancreas contain zymogen granules that secrete digestive enzymes. These granules are present by the twelfth week of gestation, and trypsin activity can be detected by the sixteenth week. Eventually, one can detect trypsin, chymotrypsin, carboxypeptidase, elastase, lipase, and collagenase activity. There is a steep rise in the activity of all enzymes at 28 weeks' gestation. Enterokinase development is most important at this stage. Enterokinase activity cannot be detected until 26 weeks of gestation. This is the same time at which trypsin activity is first detected in the meconium. At birth, enterokinase activity is only 25 per cent of that in babies one year old, and 17 per cent of that in children one to four years of age.

At birth, premature infants (32 to 34 weeks' gestation) have relatively good pancreatic function, although less than that of full-term infants. This is understandable, as it is known that pancreatic enzyme activity is greatly increased from 36 to 40 weeks' gestation. Zoppi et al. documented that one week after birth, premature infants have higher pancreatic enzyme activity than do term infants.[168] It is thought that the pancreatic zymogen granules in the premature infant develop more rapidly in response to increased growth demands. Zoppi et al. also demonstrated pancreatic enzyme induction using different substrates.[168] Small amounts of starch stimulate amylase production, known to be low in newborn infants. High-protein formulae stimulate trypsin and lipase production, whereas a high-fat diet has little or no effect on lipase activity.

Amylase activity is quite low in newborns

and remains so until six months of age. Repeated studies of duodenal fluid with and without secretin-pancreozymin stimulation reveal almost no amylase activity at birth. Yet, babies are able to tolerate starch right from birth. There is much controversy in the literature about the actual digestion of starches by neonates and the possibility of amylase induction by an increased carbohydrate load.

TESTS OF PANCREATIC FUNCTION

The full battery of pancreatic function tests is listed in Table 15–1. Tests are selected based on the clinical indications provided by the patient's presentation.[8]

Stool Examination

A patient presenting with a history of failure to thrive and large, bulky, foul-smelling stools alerts the physician to the possibility of steatorrhea. One can look at the stool stained with Sudan III to assess the number and size of fat globules. The stool can also be examined for the presence

Table 15–1   Pancreatic Function Tests

STOOL
Stool examination for meat fibers and fat
Sudan III staining
72-hour fecal fat collection
Trypsin and chymotrypsin activity

PANCREATIC ENZYMES
Serum amylase
Urine amylase
Amylase-creatinine clearance
Amylase isoenzymes
Serum lipase
Methemalbumin

DIRECT TEST
Secretin-pancreozymin stimulation tests

INDIRECT TEST
Bz-Ty-PABA test

MISCELLANEOUS
Gastrointestinal x-rays
Selenomethionine uptake
Ultrasound
Angiography
CAT scan
ERCP

of meat fibers as evidence of impaired digestion.

In children, stool testing for trypsin and chymotrypsin is more valuable.[15] Absence or low values of these two enzymes is indicative of pancreatic insufficiency, usually cystic fibrosis. Stool cultures should be taken at the same time, as certain bacteria can alter the test results.

The 72-hour fecal fat test is a very reliable one, for children who are fed 40 to 70 gm of fat per day should not excrete greater than 10 per cent of the ingested load. Those under two years of age average less than 3.5 gm of fat per 24 hours.

Stool Trypsin.   Use of the digestion of x-ray film as a rough measurement of trypsin activity provides, if fresh stool is obtained, an idea of the concentration of pancreatic enzyme in the stool. Because of fairly rapid transit in the infant, trypsin is not significantly affected by colonic bacteria. It is normally present in dilutions of 1:100, and its absence from the stool is suggestive of pancreatic insufficiency. Stool cultures must be obtained at the same time, for *Proteus* can also digest gelatin and give a misleading positive result. Titrimetric determinations yield 80 to 742 (average, 219) μg per gm of stool in normal infants and 1.3 to 30 μg in patients with cystic fibrosis.

Stool Chymotrypsin.   Chymotrypsin is also influenced by intestinal transit and by bacterial flora. This test is more sensitive than that for trypsin and is performed with stools obtained for 72-hour quantitative fat determination. Administration of pancreatic extract is discontinued for five days before the test. Normal stools contain 75 to 839 μg per gm of stool, or 3 to 16 mg per kg; those from patients with cystic fibrosis contain 0 to 58 μg per gm of stool, or 2 mg per kg or less. Normal levels preclude a diagnosis of pancreatic insufficiency, but low levels are sometimes present in other forms of steatorrhea.

Pancreatic Enzymes[6, 168, 169]

Serum Amylase.   This enzyme is extremely important in the diagnosis of pancreatitis. Amylase will rise acutely in pancreatitis and fall to normal in 48 hours. The actual values, however, do not correlate with the extent of pancreatic damage. Normal values are 40 to 150 units per dl. Amylase may be elevated from intestinal obstruction and inflammation of the ovaries.[72, 114, 116]

Urine Amylase. This measurement is also useful in diagnosing pancreatitis. Amylase is easily cleared by the kidney and will often remain elevated once the serum values have returned to normal. However, one should always establish that the patient has good renal function before measuring an accurate urine amylase. Normal values are 1200 to 7200 units per 24 hours.

Amylase-Creatinine Clearance. This test is thought to be extremely reliable in diagnosing acute pancreatitis. An elevated value is abnormal, as tubular reabsorption of amylase is thought to be inhibited in pancreatitis. A normal ratio

$$C_{am}/C_{cr} =$$

$$\frac{\text{amylase in urine}}{\text{amylase in serum}} \times \frac{\text{creatinine in serum}}{\text{creatinine in urine}} \times 100$$

is 4 per cent or less.

Amylase Isoenzymes. This can occasionally be useful. There are three major isoenzymes. One of these is pancreatic, and the other two are salivary isoenzymes. Separation of the isoenzymes is sometimes necessary to distinguish between inflammation of these organs, as is demonstrated in mumps infection.

Serum Lipase. There is controversy in the literature about the value of this test, for small quantities of the enzyme are contributed by the small intestine. Certain investigators believe that the serum lipase remains elevated longer than the serum amylase in patients with pancreatitis. Normal levels are 20 to 136 IU per liter in urine and 0.06 to 0.87 Bunch Emerson unit in the serum.

Methemalbumin. This test is occasionally used to differentiate between hemorrhagic and edematous pancreatitis. In hemorrhagic pancreatitis, hemoglobin is broken down to heme plus globin by trypsin or elastase. The heme is oxidized to hematin and absorbed to combine with albumin, thus forming methemalbumin. It is important to note that this is a nonspecific test,

since one can see elevated methemalbumin with a ruptured ectopic pregnancy, intraperitoneal bleeding, intestinal obstruction, and intravascular hemolysis.

Phospholipase A in serum is increased in acute pancreatitis.

Secretin-Pancreozymin Test (Direct Test)

This is a very valuable test, although the wide range of normal values often makes the results difficult to interpret. Patients are kept NPO and are then sedated prior to the test (with Valium or Nembutal). A double-lumen duodenal tube (one tube at each end of the duodenum) is inserted, and resting duodenal fluid is collected. Twenty minutes later, 2 units per kilogram of secretin are given intravenously. Three 10-minute collections of duodenal fluid are taken. Pancreozymin is then given in an intravenous dose of 2 to 3 units per kilogram. Three more 10-minute collections of duodenal fluid are obtained. Normal values, shown in Table 15–2, exhibit a very wide range.

Bz-Ty-PABA Test

Many of the tests for pancreatic function are quite cumbersome, often requiring duodenal intubation. N-Benzoyl-L-tyrosyl-p-aminobenzoic acid (Bz-Ty-PABA) is cleaved by pancreatic chymotrypsin to Bz-Ty and PABA. PABA is absorbed in the gastrointestinal tract and excreted in the urine. Thus, the concentration of PABA in the urine indirectly reflects intraluminal chymotrypsin activity and pancreatic function. This test implies normal renal function. In normal subjects, 6-hour urinary excretion ranges between 60 and 87 per cent, averaging 70 per cent, whereas in pancreatic insufficiency, values range from 19 to 50 per cent, averaging 37 per cent.

Miscellaneous Tests

The listed x-ray studies (Table 15–1) are useful in different instances, and all are helpful to some degree. Endoscopic retrograde cannulation of the pancreas (ERCP) can provide direct visualization of the pan-

Table 15–2 Pancreatic Function After Secretin-Pancreozymin Tests[55, 90, 167, 168]

	BIRTH	24 HOURS AFTER FEEDINGS	1 WEEK	1 MONTH	NORMAL	CYSTIC FIBROSIS	PANCREATIC INSUFFICIENCY
Volume ml/kg/50 min							
Premature	4.4 (4–15)	5.9 (1.5–9.8)	8.2 (1.6–16.8)	8.96 (3.4–18.7)	3.9 (1.8–81)	0.3–2.7	1.8–3.9
Term	5.39 (1.6–9.7)	3.29 (9.6–80)	4.3 (9.6–10.4)				
HCO$_3^-$ mEq/L/50 min					0.19 (.08–.37)	.001–.04	.008–.19
Trypsin µg/kg/50 min							
Premature	60 (0–482)	43.1 (1.6–148)	233.3 (5–660)	196.1 (.9–660)	765 (215–2100)	0–450	.9–320
Term	66.1 (1.2–350)	26.3 (5–67.8)	96.6 (5–230)				
Lipase IU/kg/50 min							
Premature	77.4 (3–343)	65.9 (2.4–209)	328.8 (7.2–1249)	283.6 (11–730)	1464 (350–5000)	0–270	0–68
Term	143.9 (2.2–785)	31.7 (4.9–67.4)	39.9 (6.2–125)				
Chymotrypsin µg/kg/50 min					860 (252–1900)	0–126	0–105
Amylase IU/kg/50 min							
Premature	0.88 (0–3.6)	0.62 (0.2–1.4)	2.07 (0.2–8.2)	1.67 (0–4.6)	665 (160–2150)	0–117	0–31
Term	3.20 (0.1–9.8)	0.38 (0.2–0.5)	1.29 (0.1–3.0)				
Carboxypeptidase A IU/kg/50 min					724 (141–2480)	0–204	0–149

creas. However, it should never be attempted in a patient with acute pancreatitis, and it may indeed induce pancreatitis.

The selenomethionine scanning test can be done if one suspects pancreatic insufficiency or a pseudocyst. Selenomethionine is selected because of its preferential uptake by the pancreas. This test should be done if less invasive methods yield only equivocal results.

Ultrasonography is of value in determining size and consistency of the pancreas in investigations of acute pancreatitis, pseudocyst, and abscess.

CONGENITAL ANOMALIES

Congenital anomalies of the pancreas are uncommon, and the cause is usually unknown. It is conceivable that maternal stress or infection could cause maturation arrest or altered development, although this has never been documented. The following are the more common congenital anomalies of the pancreas encountered in infancy.

AGENESIS OF THE PANCREAS

Agenesis of the pancreas is usually associated with agenesis of the gallbladder and with intrauterine growth retardation.[92] It is not totally incompatible with life, for survival to 26 months has been reported in an infant treated with Pregestimil and insulin.[66]

Congenital absence of the islets of Langerhans in a normal-sized pancreas has also been reported in an infant with intrauterine growth retardation. In this instance, the endocrine function of the gland seems to be intimately associated with intrauterine growth.[35]

ABERRANT PANCREAS

Ectopic pancreatic tissue is rarely responsible for any well-defined symptom complex and is usually discovered as an incidental finding.[30, 155]

Incidence. It is estimated to occur in approximately 2 per cent of the population and occurs twice as often in males as in females.[108a]

Etiology. This developmental error occurs before or during rotation of the ventral pancreatic buds, with small buds of tissue being grafted to various locations in the alimentary tract away from the pancreas.

Pathology. Ninety per cent of ectopic tissue is located in the antrum of the stomach; it occurs with less frequency in the duodenum or jejunum and lies near the embryologic site of development of the pancreas. Rarely, ectopic tissues may be found in the spleen umbilicus, gallbladder, or esophagus or in a Meckel's diverticulum. In the stomach it appears as a small (1 to 2 cm) nodule with an umbilicated center and ducts opening to its surface. Tissue may be of three types: (1) typical pancreatic tissue with acini, ducts, and islets, (2) tissue with many acini but few ducts and no islet cells, and (3) tissue of predominantly ducts with few acini and no islet cells.[108a]

Symptoms. There may be either no symptoms or intermittent pain or vomiting. Rarely, the ectopic tissue ulcerates to cause bleeding.

Diagnosis. Endoscopic examination will visualize the nodule, and radiologic studies will show a prepyloric nodule with a central filling defect.

Treatment. Simple surgical excision is curative in some patients but symptoms are not always relieved in others.[72a]

ANNULAR PANCREAS

Annular pancreas is the most common cause of extrinsic duodenal obstruction in infancy.[105]

Incidence. Annular pancreas is responsible for 10 to 30 per cent of all cases of duodenal obstruction. In some instances it is combined with duodenal stenosis or atresia. It is more common in males than in females and has also been described in siblings.

Etiology. If one ventral bud becomes attached to the duodenum or rotates around it, it partially or completely encircles the area to create this anomaly. Another theory suggests a basic duodenal lesion with the pancreas actually growing into an empty space surrounding a constricted duodenum. Complete obstruction is present in 53 to 83 per cent of cases.[133]

Pathology. The anulus measures 1 to 1.5 mm in width and contains both islet cells and ducts. It often penetrates the duodenal wall and encircles the second portion of the duodenum distal to the ampulla of Vater. Less often, it is located above the ampulla. When it compresses the common bile duct or the pancreatic duct, it may cause acute pancreatitis. One study cites a 29 per cent association with Down's syndrome and a 20 per cent incidence of congenital heart disease, 60 per cent of which are tetralogy of Fallot.

Symptoms. The lesion, if incomplete, may cause no symptoms or a relatively late

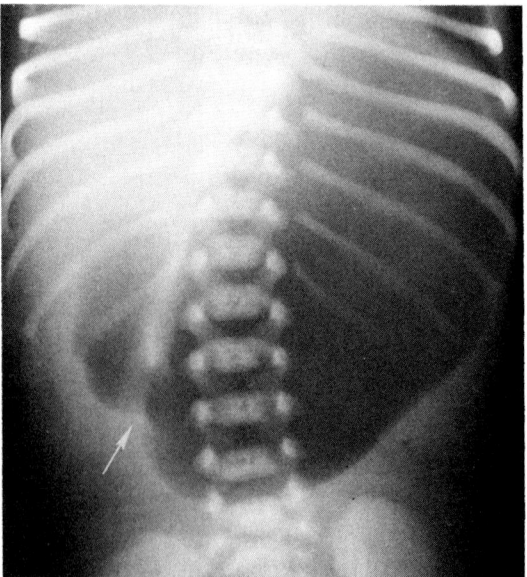

Figure 15–2 "Double bubble" sign of duodenal obstruction caused by annular pancreas.

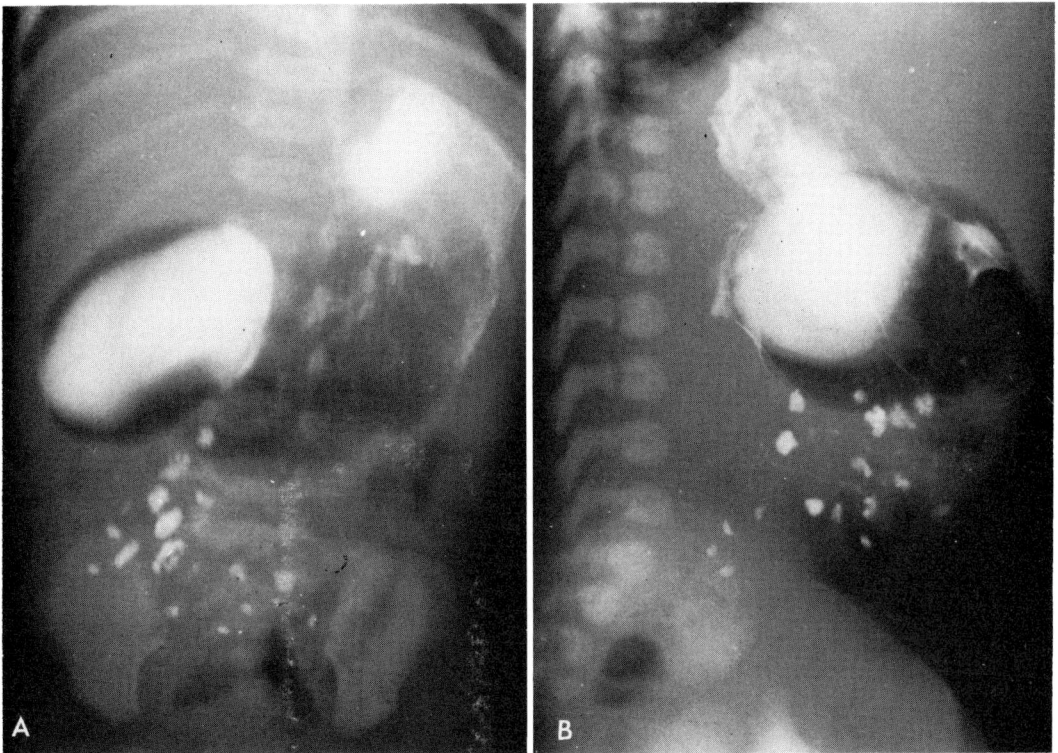

Figure 15–3 Duodenal stenosis with annular pancreas. A newborn male presented with bilious vomiting. Frontal *(A)* and lateral *(B)* views from a barium upper gastrointestinal series show markedly dilated duodenal bulb and only small flecks of contrast and air in the bowel distal to that point. Duodenal stenosis associated with annular pancreas was found at surgery. (Courtesy of Richard Markowitz, M.D.)

onset of intermittent abdominal pain, nausea, and vomiting. In infancy the symptoms are those of partial or complete duodenal obstruction with postprandial and, later, continuous bilious vomiting. The epigastrium is distended, and peristaltic waves move across the upper abdomen from the left upper quadrant toward or across the midline.

Diagnosis. The lesion must be differentiated from duodenal atresia or stenosis and, in some instances, from pyloric outlet obstruction. If the duodenum is completely obstructed, plain films of the abdomen show the "double bubble" sign produced by air in the dilated proximal duodenum superimposed upon that in the dilated stomach (Fig. 15–2). In about one third of babies there is no air-fluid level in the duodenum, and extrinsic compression is confirmed only by contrast studies showing a smooth compression or narrowing of the right side of the second duodenum (Fig. 15–3).

Complications. Pancreatitis or jaundice or both may result from ductal obstruction. Hyperinsulinism is a rare complication. If duodenal lesions are present, the rate of associated anomalies is similar.

Treatment. Because of the proximity of the anulus to the biliary and pancreatic ducts and its intimate connection to the duodenum, duodenojejunostomy is the treatment of choice.

DUPLICATIONS OF THE PANCREATIC DUCTS

This anomaly is extremely rare, only seven cases having been reported by 1972.

Etiology. The origin is similar to that of other duplications, most likely being a carrying along of predestined duodenal or gastric mucosal cells during the budding process, in which the pancreatic ducts form the primitive foregut.

Pathology. These cysts contain a layer of smooth muscle and are lined by gastric or duodenal mucosa. They lie at the juncture of the body and tail over the head of the pancreas and communicate with the pancreatic ducts or perforate into the pancreas to cause pancreatitis and ascites.

Symptoms. In the reported cases the onset of symptoms has been variable from infancy to adult life. All patients had abdominal pain and, at some time, an epigastric mass. Irritability, recurrent abdominal pain, and reluctance to eat were the usual complaints. One infant was explored for a cause of ascites several times before the duplication was identified.

Diagnosis. Radiologic examination is usually negative, and the diagnosis has been made only at surgery after one or more operations. Ultrasonography should now prove of assistance in defining the mass.

Treatment. Excision of the cyst and Roux-en-Y jejunostomy are the surgical procedures that have been employed.

Congenital Pancreatic Cysts

These cysts are extremely rare and difficult to diagnose, for they may lose their epithelial lining after prolonged intraluminal pressure or after secondary infection. They may be multiple or single, unilocular or multilocular. Occasionally they are associated with polycystic disease of the liver, kidneys, or spleen.

The cysts are usually localized to the body or tail of the pancreas, contain some pancreatic tissue, and are lined by epithelium. The inner cloudy yellow fluid does not necessarily contain enzymes. These cysts seldom produce symptoms unless they attain a size to displace or compress the stomach or colon, or when they cause vomiting or constipation. Treatment is simple excision of the cyst.

Retention Cysts of the Pancreas

These lesions resemble congenital cysts but contain cloudy fluid with high enzyme concentrations. They result from chronic obstruction of the ductal system. Simple excision is not always possible because of potential fistula development. Internal drainage by anastomosis of the cyst wall to the posterior stomach wall is the preferred treatment.

INHERITED DISORDERS OF PANCREATIC FUNCTION

A variety of disorders of the pancreas have been described — some of isolated enzyme deficiencies and others of multisystem involvement.

Cystic Fibrosis

More than 95 per cent of all children with pancreatic insufficiency have cystic fibrosis. It is a chronic, debilitating disease affecting the pancreas, lungs, liver, intestine, exocrine glands, and many other systems. There is an enormous literature on the subject, but as yet neither the basic defect nor the cure has been ascertained.[138-143]

Incidence and Inheritance. Cystic fibrosis is the most common genetic disease known to man. It is inherited as an autosomal recessive trait, with an incidence between 1 in 1000 and 1 in 2000 live Caucasian births. Transmission from mother to daughter has been observed.[64] Therefore, 5 per cent of the population are carriers of the disease, indicating a survival advantage that is as yet unknown. The disease is rarer among other populations, with an incidence in blacks in Washington, D.C. estimated at 1 in 17,000.[84]

Numerous attempts have been made to identify the heterozygote state without consistent success. Cultures of white blood cells and skin fibroblasts have shown metachromasia in specimens from patients and parents, but this may also occur in Gaucher's, Marfan's and Hurler's diseases. Sera from patients and parents do contain an abnormal euglobulin that inhibits normal rhythmic motility of tracheal epithelial cilia.[25] Plasma from patients will inhibit jejunal uptake of a glucose analog, and that from parents has an intermediate effect. Skin fibroblasts from both groups contain increased amounts of calcium. Fibroblast stimulation by Tamm-Horsfall glycoprotein has recently been considered successful in identifying the carrier. The sweat test is not appropriate for detecting carriers because of the wide range of normal values, the change in electrolyte secretion with age, and the variations with pulmonary disease.

Etiology. The abnormality of exocrine secretions, the electrolyte abnormalities of the eccrine sweat glands, and the abnormal physicochemical properties of mucus cannot be tied into one unifying hypothesis. A recent implication of selenium deficiency in the etiology has not been substantiated.[67] Investigators have attempted to implicate abnormal calcium metabolism, abnormal electrolyte transport, changes in permeability of ductal epithelium, and defects in autonomic control of secretion as etiologic factors. Skin cultures do contain enhanced UDPG-galactose glycoprotein galactosyl transferase activity, which may, in turn, explain enhanced glycoprotein secretion, increased calcium in secretions, and ductal obstruction.[42, 76, 122] The one consistent abnormality remains an increased secretion of sodium and chloride by the sweat glands. Genetically, it has also been associated with celiac disease.[48]

Pathology. Although the pathologic changes are widespread, this discussion will be limited to the gastrointestinal tract.

PANCREAS. Pancreatic insufficiency is present in about 89 per cent of affected infants at birth and in 90 per cent by the end of the first year. Recent evidence indicates that the pancreas shows either a lack of maturation of exocrine tissue or the persistence of a fetal pattern.[95] The pancreatic ducts become plugged with viscid eosinophilic material, which causes distal obstruction and proximal ductal dilatation. In young infants, the pancreas appears edematous with some subcapsular hemorrhage. Eventually it becomes firm and lobulated and appears gray or white as the acinar epithelium becomes atrophic, parenchymal cells disappear, and fibrosis and inflamma-tory changes progress. The islets of Langerhans remain intact.

LIVER. Liver involvement occurs in about 30 per cent of patients, with focal biliary cirrhosis being found as early as the third day of life. The usual changes in infancy are mild periportal fibrosis, focal bile duct proliferation, and moderate inflammation. In long-standing disease, the bile ducts are plugged with inspissated eosinophilic material and are surrounded by fibrosis, inflammatory reaction, and biliary proliferation.

GALLBLADDER. Twenty to 30 per cent of patients have abnormalities, varying from microgallbladder to cholelithiasis. The organ is lined with tall columnar epithelium and does not usually show inflammatory change. There is increased staining of mucocarmine-positive cells. The bile is white and viscous.

PORTAL SYSTEM. Portal hypertension and hypersplenism may develop as a result of biliary cirrhosis.

INTESTINE. Small bowel biopsy specimens appear smooth and mucoid, but a normal villous pattern is present when the overlying mucus is removed. Microscopically the villi are slender and the epithelial surface is normal. Characteristically there are increased numbers of goblet cells among the epithelial cells, and Brunner's glands may be dilated and filled with inspissated, acidophilic material (Fig. 15–4). These changes are present even within the appendiceal lumen. Jejunal IgA production is tripled.[40]

Rectal biopsy reveals inspissated secretions within dilated rectal glands and increased numbers of goblet cells upon the epithelial surface (Fig. 15–5).[112]

Symptoms. Cystic fibrosis can present clinically in many different ways.[83] Fifteen per cent of patients present with neonatal intestinal obstruction, known as meconium ileus. These patients have the worst prognosis.[103] It is thought that the absence of pancreatic enzymes and abnormal intestinal mucus secretion cause obstruction of the bowel by thick, tenacious meconium.[6, 161] The abdomen becomes increasingly distended, with concurrent vomiting, and the

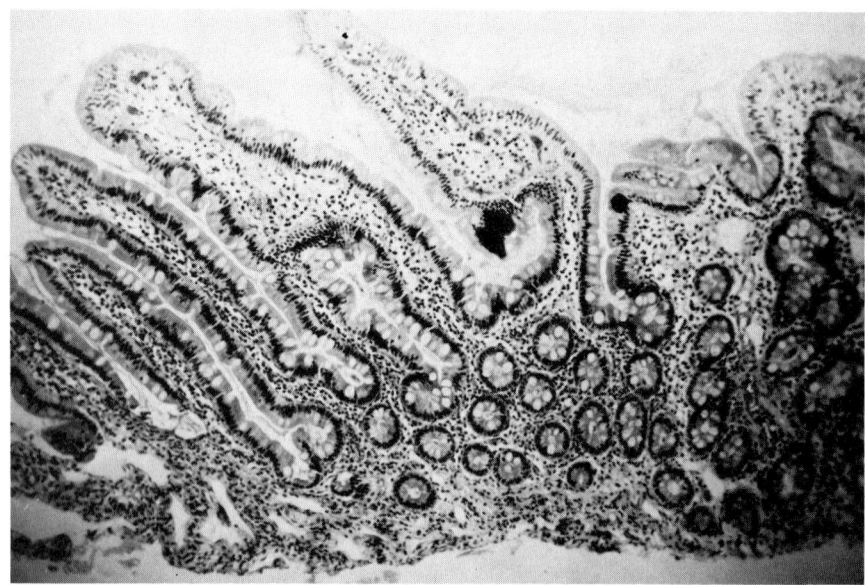

Figure 15–4 Small bowel biopsy of patient with cystic fibrosis. There is an increase of goblet cells in the surface epithelial layer.

course can be complicated by meconium peritonitis. Not all infants with meconium ileus have cystic fibrosis.[140]

Many others present with failure to thrive, salty sweat, bulky malodorous stools with oil droplets, and repeated respiratory infections. Despite a healthy appetite, they show no weight gain and become seriously malnourished, with muscle wasting and abdominal distention. Untreated, they devel-

op pot belly and rectal prolapse (Fig. 15–6).

Clubbing is thought to be related to increased levels of circulating prostaglandins F and E.[23a, 91]

Malnutrition is for the most part due to fat malabsorption, because pancreatic lipase is the enzyme that is most deficient. This is compounded by the depletion of bile acids as the result of increased fecal loss-

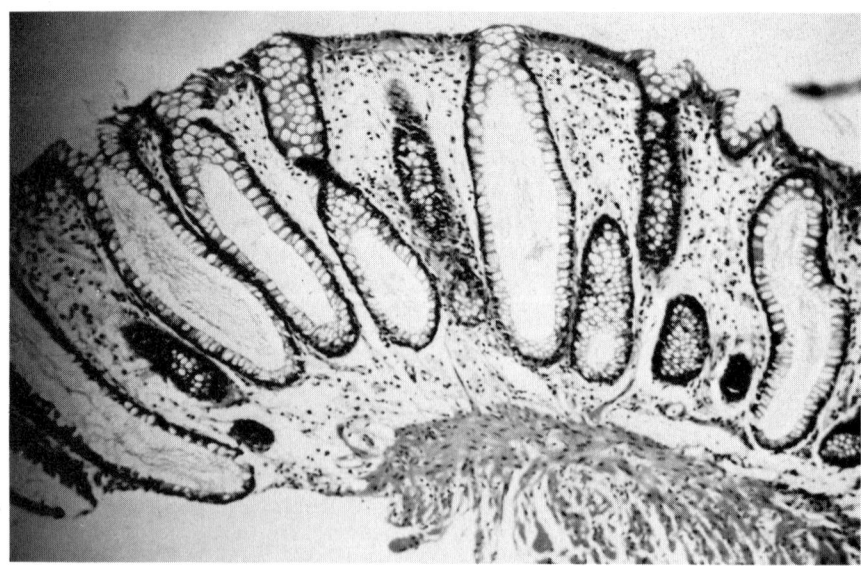

Figure 15–5 Rectal biopsy from patient with cystic fibrosis. Note the increase in goblet cells and dilation of the crypts.

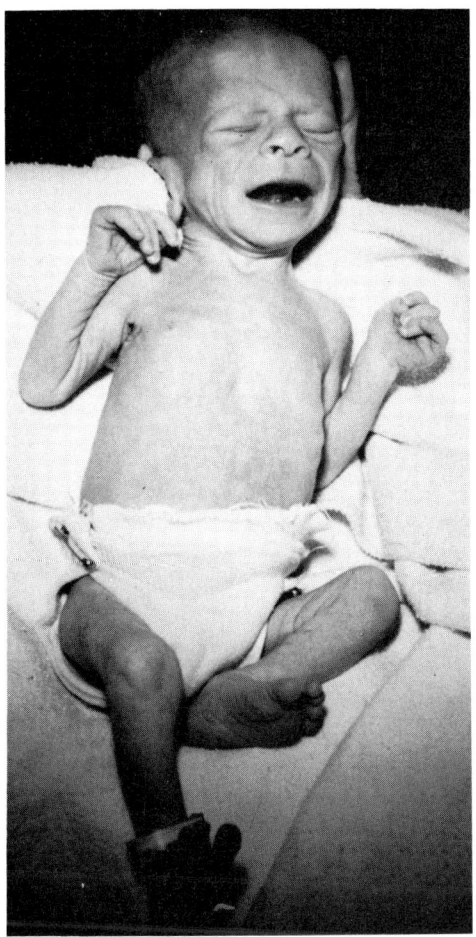

Figure 15–6 Twelve week old male infant with cystic fibrosis. Malnutrition is evident in the wasting of the arms and legs and facial fat.

es.[129, 153, 162, 163] Deficiencies of the fat-soluble vitamins are intimately associated with fat malabsorption. Hypoprothrombinemia from vitamin K deficiency causes a hemorrhagic diathesis, which in some infants is the first manifestation of the disease. Vitamin A deficiency leads to xerophthalmia, which may superficially resemble cataracts. Vitamin D deficiency, however, is unusual, and rickets is rare, perhaps in part because of the selective absorption of vitamin D through the lymphatics without the need for esterification.[68] Tetany, however, may result from hypocalcemia due to saponification of intraluminal calcium by unabsorbed fats. Vitamin E deficiency may be obvious as neonatal hemolytic anemia, with abnormal red cell hemolysis tests, and as the "brown bowel syndrome," consisting of ceroid deposition in the serosa and muscularis of the intestine. Vitamin B_{12} deficiency and malabsorption seem directly related to pancreatic enzyme deficiency, since they are corrected by the administration of pancreatic enzymes.[158]

Hypoproteinemia and edema may be the first symptoms of this disease and result from protein malabsorption (Fig. 15–7).[10] They are particularly apparent in infants who are breast-fed or who are taking soy formula. More unusual single symptoms are persistent neonatal jaundice and/or hepatomegaly or increased intracranial pressure

Figure 15–7 Five month old infant with periorbital edema and hypoproteinemia.

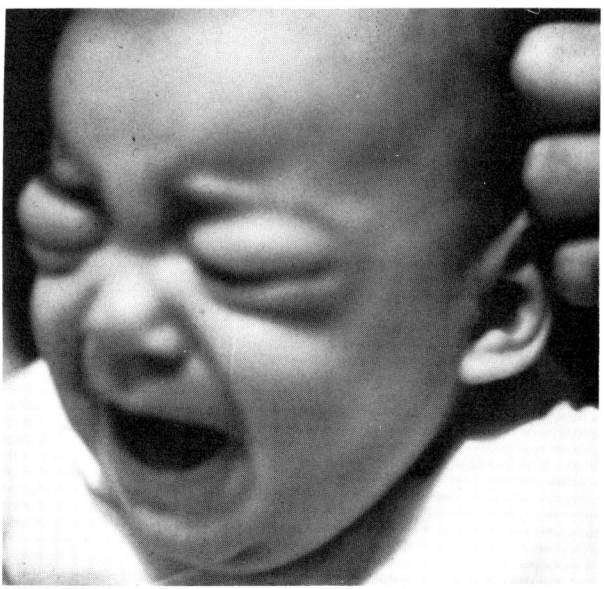

attributed to increased venous pressure and pulmonary disease.[78] Hyperelectrolytemia and metabolic alkalosis may develop in warm weather in breast-fed infants.[12]

In older infants and children, a "meconium ileus equivalent" syndrome produces symptoms of recurrent abdominal pain, intermittent intestinal obstruction, or pain simulating appendicitis.[101, 113] Abnormal intestinal mucus and decreased motility contribute to the development of fecal impactions in the terminal ileum, cecum, and ascending colon. A less liquid stool reaches the terminal ileum, and putty-like material accumulates in these regions. Fecal masses are palpable in the right lower quadrant. Obstruction may also be caused by the stool masses acting as a lead point for an ileoileal or ileocecal intussusception.

Since 15 to 20 per cent of patients have normal or partially normal pancreatic function, they do not require enzyme replacement. However, this group is prone to develop acute pancreatitis, the etiology of which is unknown.

Episodic arthritis has recently been described.[110]

Diagnosis. The prenatal diagnosis of cystic fibrosis is strongly (although not absolutely) suggested by an absence of an arginine esterase activity in mid-trimester amniotic fluid.[161a]

Every child with intermittent or constant diarrhea, regardless of growth rate or respiratory symptoms, should be screened for cystic fibrosis by means of a sweat test. The pilocarpine iontophoresis sweat test is 98 per cent reliable, except in neonates. At least 50 mg of sweat is needed for an adequate analysis, and the neonate does not often produce this quantity. A sweat chloride measurement of 60 mEq/L or more is diagnostic of the disease. However, an infant with edema had a normal sweat test that became abnormal after edema subsided.[98] If sweat is inadequate, stool trypsin and chymotrypsin can be measured. Most infant stools contain trypsin in a dilution of 1:100, but, as transit time decreases in older children, the enzyme is degraded by colonic bacteria and is no longer present.

Much has been written about the meconium strip test to detect increased albumin content in infants with cystic fibrosis, but the test has not gained wide acceptance owing to a relatively high rate of false negative and false positive results.[47, 128, 130] Increased lactase activity in meconium has identified infants with cystic fibrosis in some screening programs.[12b]

One can directly measure pancreatic secretion with the secretin-pancreozymin test.[58] Lipase is absent or present in only small amounts; the other enzymes are variably affected and may selectively diminish over the years. Lingual lipase provided by unaffected lingual glands aids in fat digestion in both stomach and duodenum.[1] Water and bicarbonate production is severely impaired, even in those with relatively normal enzyme activity.

Three-day stool collections for fat and nitrogen will reveal extremely high fat values, with 30 gm in a collection being fairly typical. The nitrogen content may or may not be increased, although in some cases it exceeds several grams. The level of serum carotene is well below 20 μg per dl and reflects impaired fat absorption. Interestingly, xylose absorption is increased.[135]

Radiologic examination of the chest often reveals early changes of hyperinflation or irregular aeration. In some, there is a pneumothorax. The later changes of fibrosis — patchy atelectasis and pneumonitis — develop with time. Examination of the small bowel shows nonspecific changes associated with malabsorption: dilatation of loops of bowel and loss of a normal small bowel mucosal pattern. The barium enema often shows a shaggy and nodular appearance caused by dilatation of glands and adherence of stool to the colonic wall (Fig. 15–8). This may be referred to as a chrysanthemum effect. In those with meconium ileus or its equivalent, a three-way film of the abdomen must be obtained to determine the degree of obstruction and the presence or absence of free intraperitoneal air. A barium enema will demonstrate the filling defects in the cecum and ascending colon.

Treatment. The hallmark of therapy is pancreatic enzyme replacement.[49] There

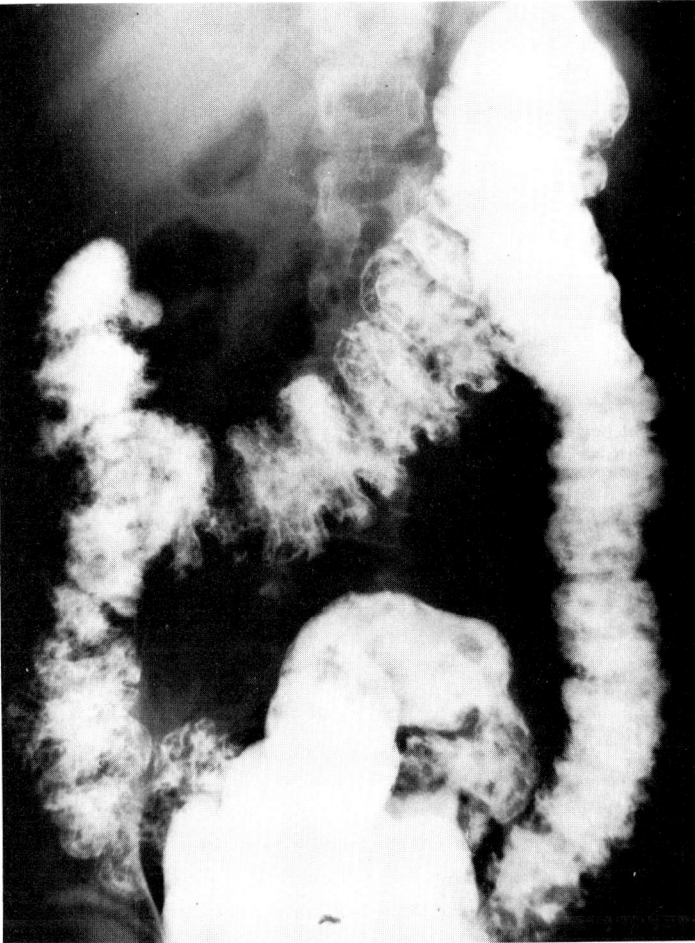

Figure 15–8 Cystic fibrosis in a boy with recurrent episodes of lower abdominal pain and occasional benzidine-positive stools. Barium enema demonstrates a rather striking abnormality in the appearance of the colon, which has a very shaggy and somewhat nodular marginal pattern. This appearance results in part from adherence of the tenacious stool to the colon wall and in part from adherence of mounds of viscous mucus to the mouths of mucous glands.

are numerous products on the market, with Cotazym (each capsule digesting 17 gm fat) and Viokase (same lipolytic but more proteolytic activity) being the most popular. Recently Pancrease, composed of enteric-coated granules, has been used in older children to reduce the number of tablets and to increase the efficiency of digestion. These tablets are taken prior to meals and the dosage titrated by stool consistency and degree of steatorrhea. In some refractory cases, hourly administration of enzyme is required. Recently, the addition of cimetidine to decrease gastric acidity has improved effectiveness of the supplements, since lipase is inactivated in an acid pH.[16, 32] However, its use has been related with a meconium ileus equivalent in one child.[105a]

One must institute a low-fat, high-calorie diet providing 200 calories per kg for infants and 150 to 200 calories per kg for older children. Formulae containing medium-chain triglycerides, such as Pregestimil, are usually given, but even here enzyme supplementation may be required for optimal absorption.[18, 39] As fat intake increases with expansion of the diet in older children, so does the degree of steatorrhea. A low-fat diet with medium-chain triglyceride supplementation is recommended.[96] Intralipid infusion has been employed to raise essential free fatty acid levels.[4] Water-soluble vitamins should be added to the diet in double the recommended dosage. It is essential to establish a good nutritional intake early in the course to assure normal growth.

Lactose intolerance has been demonstrated in 25 per cent of children with cystic fibrosis, and some infants may be intolerant to sucrose as well.[7] Interestingly, lactase has been reported to be increased in the stools of neonates with cystic fibrosis. Iron absorption is increased in pancreatic insufficiency states, and iron supplementation should be avoided.

All infections should be treated promptly and cultures and sensitivities of the predominant organism should be obtained, since *Staphylococcus* and *Pseudomonas* rapidly develop resistance to conventional antibiotics.

Treatment of meconium ileus or its equivalent is determined by the degree of obstruction. A three-way film of the abdomen will demonstrate obstruction, and a barium enema will outline the filling defects in the colon and cecum and will reduce an intussusception, if present. Complete obstruction must be treated surgically, but incomplete obstruction is managed medically with pancreatic enzymes and acetylcysteine given orally and by enema to break up the fecal impactions. Gastrografin enemas are also successful. Small and large intestinal radiographic patterns remain abnormal (Figs. 15–9 and 15–10).

Complications. The complications of the disease are multiple, with respiratory infections, pulmonary fibrosis, and cor pulmonale the most urgent medical problems. Nasal polyps develop as a result of abnormal mucus formation and often obstruct the nares. Rectal prolapse develops in 20 to 25 per cent of infants, and the prolapse often becomes incarcerated.[85] It is caused by the passage of massive, bulky stools in babies who have lost ischiorectal fat and musculature. It is a condition more easily prevented than treated. Manual replacement of the prolapse and softening of the stools along with improved nutritional status will prevent frequent recurrences.

The most serious gastrointestinal complication that may develop at an early age (2 per cent) is portal hypertension due to focal biliary cirrhosis. Treatment is symptomatic, and bleeds are managed medically for as long as possible. Portacaval shunts have been performed, but the overall prognosis has not been greatly improved because of the severe pulmonary disease in most patients.[137]

Gastroesophageal reflux, leading to esophagitis, bleeding, and even stricture, may

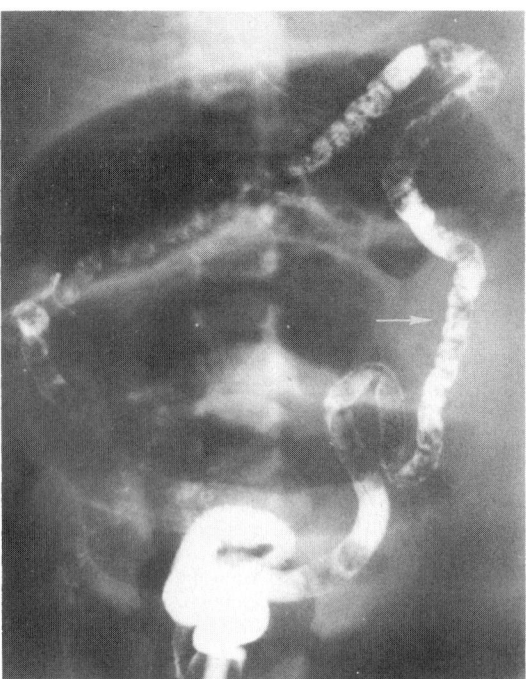

Figure 15–9 Barium enema in a patient with meconium ileus. Note pellets of meconium in colon (*arrow*) and air-filled dilated loops of small bowel.

be due to flattening of the diaphragm and disruption of normal anatomic relationships of the lower esophageal sphincter.[12a]

Duodenal ulcer is attributed to the lack of buffering of acid secretions in the duodenum, and normal and increased incidences have been reported. Frequent feedings and antacids are the usual therapy.

Hyperuricemia is a recently noted complication and is attributed to purine contamination of enzyme preparations.[29] Abnormal glucose responses may be related to impaired insulin and gastric inhibitory polypeptide responsiveness.

Aspermia has been reported in males and associated with absence of the vas deferens. This seems to be an associated congenital anomaly rather than a secondary phenomenon. Fertility has not been compromised in females of childbearing age.

Glycosuria has been noted in only 1 per cent of patients, although abnormal glucose tolerance tests are more prevalent. Twenty-six of 130 patients in Schwachman's series had diabetes mellitus, with onset after the tenth year in most. However, it developed in one infant at 18 months. Half the patients

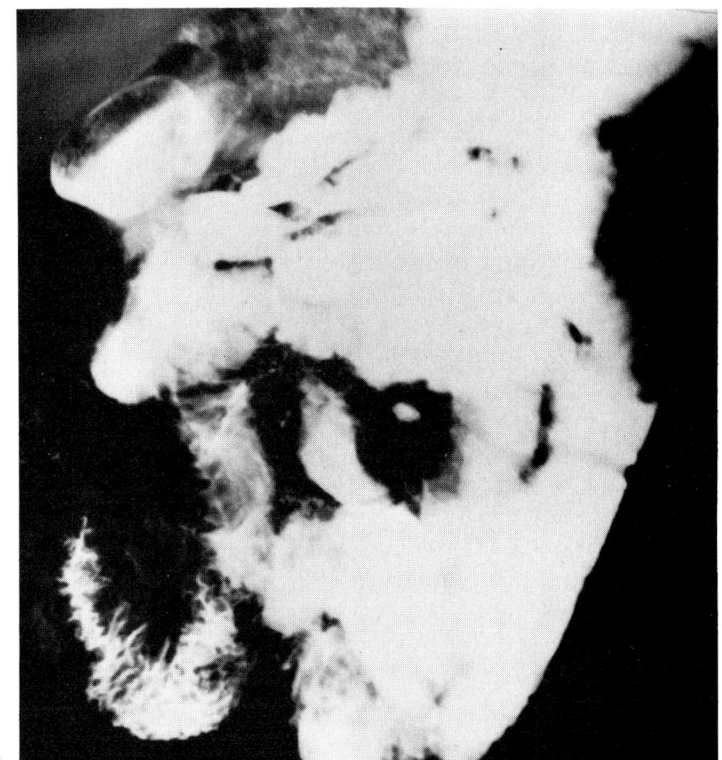

Figure 15–10 A, Cystic fibrosis in a 1 year old boy who had had surgery in the neonatal period for meconium ileus. Small bowel series demonstrates loss of the normal pattern with irregular dilation and some suggestion of thickened valvulae conniventes seen near the left flank. The mucosal pattern of the ileum in the right lower quadrant is very coarse and irregular. B, Small bowel examination in a 4 year old patient shows irregular dilatation of loops with segmentation and flocculation of barium.

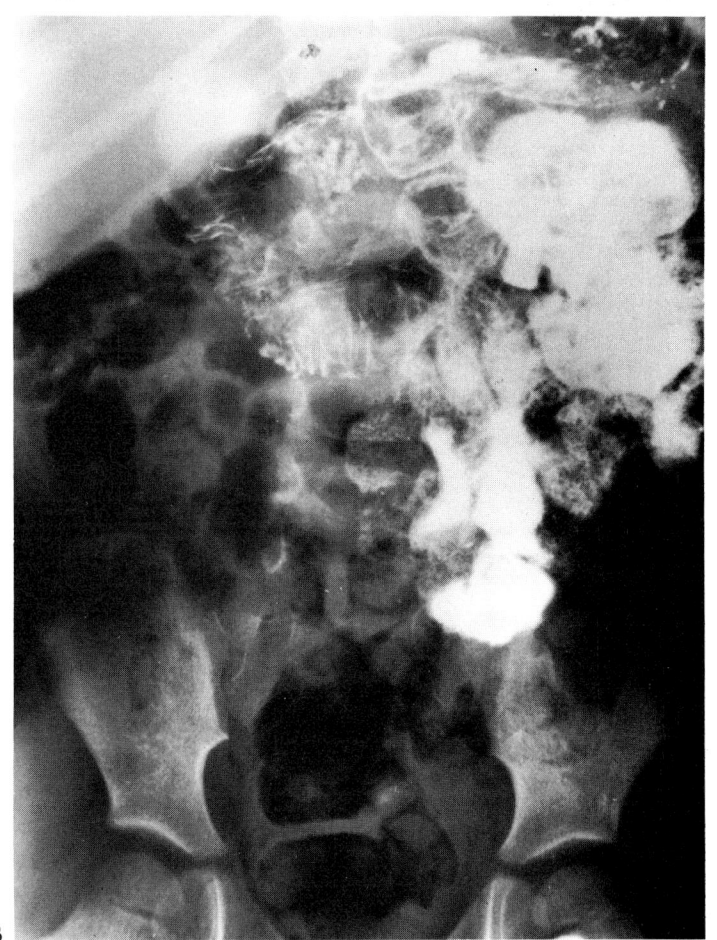

403

had a family history of diabetes and none had ketoacidosis, neuropathy, or nephropathy. Long-standing disease predisposes to the development of amyloidosis.[127]

Prognosis. The prognosis has greatly improved since diagnosis is made early and therapy instituted promptly.[34, 145] Pulmonary complications remain the limiting factor. More than three quarters of patients reach 20 years or more, and a classification system for the statistical prediction of survival is available.[81] In general, those with meconium ileus in infancy have the poorest prognosis, and those with no pulmonary disease and only pancreatic insufficiency, the best. Good nutrition and adequate enzyme replacement permit near-normal growth and development. With early treatment, pulmonary aerosols, and antibiotic therapy, pulmonary disease may be fairly well controlled.

SIDEROBLASTIC ANEMIA AND PANCREATIC INSUFFICIENCY (PEARSON'S SYNDROME)

A new syndrome of refractory sideroblastic anemia and pancreatic insufficiency was recently described by Pearson et al. in four patients.[117] Since then, several new cases have been recognized.

Etiology. The etiology of the disease is as yet unknown.

Pathology. Transfusion-dependent macrocytic anemia and variable degrees of neutropenia and thrombocytopenia are peripheral hematologic manifestations, with bone marrow showing normal cellularity but vacuolization of erythroid and myeloid precursors, hemosiderosis, and ringed sideroblasts. Bone marrow cultures show abnormal erythroid and myeloid progenitor cell growth. At autopsy, the pancreas is fibrotic and atrophic. Several patients also had splenic hypoplasia and hepatic dysfunction.

Symptoms. One of the original four patients had clinical malabsorption. All were anemic, having 5 to 9 gm per dl of hemoglobin by six to ten weeks of age. Half of the original patients were small for term, but growth failure and diarrhea were present in all by one year of age.

Differential Diagnosis. This syndrome must be differentiated from copper deficiency, chloramphenicol therapy, cystic fibrosis, and the Schwachman syndrome.

Diagnosis. The hematologic diagnosis is established by peripheral blood and bone marrow examination. Pancreatic insufficiency is documented by steatorrhea and/or pancreatic secretory tests, which demonstrate decreased water and bicarbonate secretion and, often, normal pancreatic enzymes.

Treatment. Hematologic agents and vitamin therapy are unsuccessful, and patients require transfusion for anemia. Pancreatic enzyme replacement is used to correct malabsorption.

Prognosis. Two of the four original patients died at 26 and 29 months, while the others experienced spontaneous improvement.

PANCREATIC INSUFFICIENCY AND BONE MARROW DYSFUNCTION (SHWACHMAN'S SYNDROME)

Pancreatic insufficiency and bone marrow dysfunction were first described by Shwachman et al. in 1964. Since that time, nearly 100 cases have been reported, and this condition is considered to be the second most common form of pancreatic insufficiency in childhood. Features common to most patients are diarrhea, failure to thrive, neutropenia, bone marrow hypoplasia, elevation of fetal hemoglobin, and inconstant galactosuria.

Inheritance. There is a familial incidence in this disease; three siblings in one family have been affected. It is most likely an inherited lesion with variable penetrance. Both sexes have been affected.[1b, 147]

Pathology. The pancreatic tissue is replaced by fatty tissue. Grossly, the pancreas may appear atrophic or may have fatty lobulations. Pancreatic ducts are present and patent. Microscopic examination shows fatty replacement of the pancreatic exocrine tissue. The remaining glands are shrunken, and the cells have pyknotic nuclei and no secretory granules. The lumens of the glands are small. Periductal fibrosis is prominent. The islets of Langerhans are intact. This is undoubtedly the same congenital hypoplasia of the exocrine pancreas as that described by Bodian.[17]

Early portal fibrosis may be present in the liver.

Neutropenia may become apparent between the first day of life and the fifth year. It may be cyclic and may not be noted during intercurrent infection. The neutrophils that are present show a maturation arrest, with increased band forms and minimal segmentation. Bone marrow aspirates are hypocellular, although in some patients marrow proliferative activity is normal.[134] In some cases there is fibrosis and fat deposition in the marrow. Thrombocytopenia occurs in varying degrees and is due to decreased platelet production. Mild refractory anemia may develop for the same reason. The percentage of fetal hemoglobin is elevated, as it may be in other types of aplastic anemia.

Bone age is retarded, and sometimes a dissociation between the osseous centers in the hands and wrists is noted; the centers of the fingers and metacarpals correspond to standards for the age, but those of the carpals are delayed by a year or more. Bone lesions resembling metaphyseal dysostosis are present in the femur, tibia, or ribs in 10 to 15 per cent of patients.

Symptoms. The symptoms develop when the child is between two months and one year of age. Hepatomegaly may be present early but resolves with age.[2a] Most affected infants pass loose, frequently oily, greenish yellow stools 5 to 12 times a day. They continue gaining weight for the first few months after the onset of symptoms, but then weight gain ceases and weight loss ensues. Increases in both height and weight become severely retarded. The stools become malodorous and may contain mucus. In some of the infants, eczematoid rashes may develop between the sixth week and the fifth month. The appetite is ravenous, and even as the infants become malnourished and marasmic, they remain alert. Later, as solid foods are added

to the diet, the stools become bulky and frothy and pale. The abdomen is distended and rather dull to percussion. Dilated loops of bowel are visualized or palpated in the abdomen. There is no evidence of intraperitoneal fluid.

Hematologic findings are neutropenia (95 per cent), anemia (50 per cent), thrombocytopenia (70 per cent), and, rarely, erythroleukemia.[2a]

There may or may not be a history of frequent respiratory infections, but there are reduced thoracic gas volume and chest wall compliance. Some infants may show severe dwarfism, with growth retardation most evident in older children.

Developmental and/or intellectual retardation is present in 85 per cent. Hypotonia, deafness, and retinitis are less frequent findings.

Dental abnormalities, dysmorphic features, renal dysfunction, and an ichthyotic maculopapular rash may develop.

Diagnosis. The diagnosis may be suspected in an infant with diarrhea, anemia, peripheral neutropenia, and absence of trypsin in the stools. The white blood count is low, but this may be cyclic, and frequent determinations must be made. Neutrophil counts vary from 4 to 13 per cent of the white blood cells in the peripheral smears and total counts are less than 1500 per cubic millimeter. Thrombocytopenia, mild anemia, and elevated fetal hemoglobin are characteristic blood findings. Metaphyseal dysostosis of the femur, tibia, or ribs is contributory evidence. Intermittent galactosuria is noted in some patients (urines should be screened with Clinitest rather than the usual Clinistix). Steatorrhea is documented by increased 72-hour fecal fat. The sweat electrolytes are normal. The blood sugar responses to glucose and tolbutamide are normal. The definitive diagnostic test is measurement of pancreatic enzymes, preferably by means of the pancreozymin-secretin test. Hepatic dysfunction may also be present.[20]

Treatment. The treatment of pancreatic insufficiency is with pancreatic enzymes such as pancrelipase (Cotazym) or timed-release Pancrease. The dosage depends on the severity of the symptoms and the degree of steatorrhea. The anemia in some infants may respond to folic acid or to vitamin B_{12}. Vigorous early treatment of any infection is imperative.

Prognosis. Most of the children remain small and thin even when they receive adequate therapy. Some of them after several years no longer have gross steatorrhea or require pancreatic enzyme supplementation, despite some degree of pancreatic insufficiency. Nine of 36 children reported in one series died in infancy; in most of them the cause of death was infection. In some of the survivors the metaphyseal dysostosis produced coxa vara and abnormalities in gait. Diabetes mellitus may be a late complication.

VARIANTS OF THE SHWACHMAN SYNDROME

The disease is apparently one of variable penetrance, for siblings of a propositus may have neutropenia with mild or no pancreatic insufficiency. One patient has been described who had had pancreatic insufficiency and anemia since birth, frequent respiratory infections, and low serum immunoglobulins.[69] In another variant there is chronic liver disease, pancreatic insufficiency, and recurrent respiratory infection but normal hematologic findings.[55] One of our own patients had selective IgA deficiency.

ENTEROKINASE DEFICIENCY

Enterokinase, an enzyme secreted by the duodenal mucosa, activates the proteolytic pancreatic enzymes as they are secreted into the duodenum. Enterokinase catalyzes the conversion of trypsinogen to trypsin. In turn, trypsin aids in the conversion of chymotrypsinogen. Its deficiency was first described in 1969. The symptoms and laboratory findings associated with this defect resemble those of trypsinogen deficiency.[59, 63, 89, 156]

Incidence. Only five patients have been reported since this disease was first described.

Pathology and Pathophysiology. In the absence of enterokinase, there are deficiencies of trypsin, chymotrypsin, and carboxypeptidase. Small amounts of trypsin noted in the duodenal juice of one patient were thought to result from the autoactivation of trypsinogen. Haworth et al.[63] noted trypsin concentration to be less after stimulation than before and found a trypsin inhibitor substance in the stimulated specimen. Histologic study of the duodenal mucosa and disaccharidase assays from two infants were normal; biopsy from a six-and-one-half-year-old-boy showed broadening and blunting of the villi with a moderate infiltrate of lymphocytes and plasma cells in the lamina propria. Lactase activity was absent and that of sucrase and maltase was normal. Liver biopsy from the same patient revealed fatty metamorphosis but no evidence of fibrosis.

After pancreatic stimulation tests, volume, bicarbonate, and the enzymes lipase and amylase respond normally. However, trypsin, chymotrypsin, and carboxypeptidase usually are not detected until their zymogens are incubated with normal duodenal mucosa or porcine enterokinase.

Symptoms. Symptoms include diarrhea, failure to thrive, anemia, and steatorrhea during the first few months of life. The stools are malodorous and may be watery or bulky. Clinically, these babies cannot be distinguished from those with other malabsorption syndromes, for they have loss of subcutaneous tissue, abdominal distention, and even anorexia. They may show some improvement with a gluten-free diet but soon relapse. Hepatomegaly develops as malnutrition progresses, but the spleen is not enlarged. Lactose intolerance, hypoproteinemia, and edema are associated findings.

Diagnosis. The difficulty in diagnosis lies in distinguishing this enzyme deficiency from trypsinogen deficiency. In the latter, the addition of trypsin to the duodenal juice will activate chymotrypsinogen and procarboxypeptidase, but not trypsinogen. Enterokinase deficiency is documented by duodenal intubation studies with the finding of absent or low levels of trypsin, chymotrypsin, and carboxypeptidase and the appearance of these enzymes after the addition of enterokinase.

Treatment. The treatment is that for pancreatic insufficiency, with dietary supplementation by pancreatic enzymes.

Prognosis. Subnormal growth and development may result in the untreated case, as evidenced by the patient of Haworth et al., in whom diagnosis was not made and treatment not begun until he was six and one half years of age. After treatment is instituted there is impressive increase in weight and height.

TRYPSINOGEN DEFICIENCY

Trypsinogen is a pancreatic zymogen that depends upon intestinal enterokinase for its activation to trypsin.[106, 160] Trypsin then converts more of the proenzyme into trypsin and, as noted previously, activates procarboxypeptidase and chymotrypsinogen to their active forms. Its deficiency results actually in deficiency of three proteolytic enzymes.

Incidence. This deficiency was first described in 1965.[160] Townes et al. suggest an incidence of 1 in 10,000. The mode of inheritance has not yet been determined.

Pathology and Pathogenesis. Because of the absence of trypsinogen, the other pancreatic proteolytic enzymes are therefore deficient. This causes malabsorption of protein and resulting hypoproteinemia and edema. Two patients had anemia that was unresponsive to iron therapy and unaccompanied by any abnormalities of the peripheral blood smear. Neutropenia of 5 per cent was found in one. Bone marrow aspirates are slightly hypocellular.

Symptoms. In one patient, failure to gain weight was noted at one month of age. At five weeks, she began to vomit intermittently. Her mother reported that she had a consistently good appetite and passed only two or three formed yellow stools per day. At five months, generalized edema developed and she was hospitalized for this and for failure to gain weight. In two other patients, the histories were similar, but edema developed at eight weeks. Both patients had anemia. Depigmentation of the hair was present in one child.

Diagnosis. Protein-losing enteropathy is not present, and liver function is normal. This disease must be differentiated from enterokinase deficiency.[121]

The 72-hour stool fat is elevated, fat constituting more than half the stool dry weight. Protein excretion may reach 60 per cent of ingested nitrogen, and is decreased when protein hydrolysate is fed. Pancreatic stimulation tests are abnormal only in the absence of trypsinogen, trypsin, carboxypeptidase and chymotrypsin. The addition of bovine trypsin will demonstrate the presence of procarboxypeptidase and chymotrypsin, but not of trypsinogen.

Treatment. Protein hydrolysate formula with pancreatic enzyme supplementation is the only available treatment.

LIPASE DEFICIENCY

Only a few cases of this deficiency have been reported, but Sheldon in 1964 described two families in which siblings were affected.[124] In these the disease was considered congenital; in one patient it followed varicella infection.[43, 144]

Symptoms. In all the congenital cases the stools were offensive from the time of birth and were described as resembling melted butter or containing orange oil droplets that solidified on standing. Oily soiling of the diapers or pants occurred between defecations. Most of the children were somewhat small, but severe growth retardation was not noted. There were no signs of anemia or of abdominal distention.

Diagnosis. Fat absorption measured 68 to 70 per cent, although duodenal lipase was absent or reduced by more than half the normal amount. Trypsin and amylase were somewhat decreased. Intestinal lipase was normal.

Treatment. Large doses of pancreatic extract are required to provide adequate lipase. A low-fat diet is also helpful in controlling the steatorrhea and oil seepage.

PROTEOLYTIC AND LIPOLYTIC
DEFICIENCY OF THE PANCREAS

In 1969 Townes reported the association of proteolytic and lipolytic deficiency of the exocrine pancreas in a girl with severe growth retardation, psychomotor retardation, anemia, and imperforate anus.[159]

Symptoms. The infant was born of an uncomplicated pregnancy and delivery and was noted at birth to have an imperforate anus, type III. This was treated by transverse colostomy. She gained weight poorly, and severe anemia developed. The bone marrow revealed decreased erythropoiesis. At six months of age, edema developed, and at one year, diarrhea. Recurrent episodes of diarrhea and edema continued until the fourth year, when duodenal intubation studies showed absence of proteolytic enzymes and lipase. The amylase was normal. Sixty-seven per cent of ingested fat was excreted in the stool.

Treatment. A diet high in protein hydrolysate, low in fat, and supplemented by pancreatic enzymes provided adequate nutrition for good growth in this patient.

AMYLASE DEFICIENCY

This enzyme deficiency has been reported in only two patients with symptoms of starch intolerance.[97] Because of its rarity, it is mentioned only for completeness. A physiologic amylase deficiency can be induced in premature and young infants by feeding diets high in starch, because of relatively low amylase levels.[94] Diarrhea, the major symptom, is alleviated by lightening the starch load.

OTHER SYNDROMES WITH
PANCREATIC INSUFFICIENCY

Cutis laxa and pancreatic insufficiency are associated lesions.[82] The Johanson-Blizzard syndrome includes deafness, hypoplasia or aplasia of the alae nasi, microcephaly, absent permanent teeth, hypothyroidism, and mental retardation along with pancreatic insufficiency. Variations have been reported, with nasal deformity a fairly consistent anomaly.[136, 160a] Grand et al. reported a similar patient with XXY karyotype.[51]

HEREDITARY PANCREATITIS

Hereditary pancreatitis is thought to be a major cause of pancreatitis in children and must be considered in the differential diagnosis of recurrent abdominal pain in childhood.[125, 148]

Incidence. Since the disease was first described in 1952, several hundred cases have been reported in the literature. All patients have been white, and there is no predilection for sex.[77, 100]

Inheritance. The defect is inherited as an autosomal dominant gene with incomplete penetrance, and several affected kindred have lived in close regional proximity.

Etiology. The etiology is unknown, although many patients have had congenital malformations of the ductal system or stenosis of the sphincter of Oddi. It has been linked with hyperthyroidism and hyperlipoproteinemia.

Pathology. Grossly, the pancreas resembles that of patients with cystic fibrosis. There is induration with dilatation of major and minor ducts, extensive interstitial fibrosis, and loss of acinar tissue with preservation of islet cells. There is an inconstant aminoaciduria, with lysine and cystine found in those from American families and taurine in those from English ones. Other aminoacidurias consist of lysine, cystine, and arginine or histidine or lysine. One kindred had hemorrhagic phenomena and elevated sweat electrolytes without cystic fibrosis. Loss of pancreatic function occurs initially in the tail or body of the pancreas.

Symptoms. The typical history is one of recurrent pain beginning in childhood, although a few date symptoms to infancy. Attacks in infants may be precipitated by excessively large meals. The attacks last two to seven days, occurring every two to three weeks or only every few years. At onset the pain is epigastric but later involves the entire abdomen and extends into the back. Nausea and vomiting may require hospitalization for correction of dehydration and electrolyte imbalance. Spontaneous recovery is evident after four to six days. The symptoms improve with age, and, indeed, the number of attacks decreases with time.

Diagnosis. The more usual causes of pancreatitis must be first considered, but the diagnosis is suggested by a family history of recurrent abdominal pain in three relatives. During an attack, pancreatic enzymes are elevated in the serum and there is leukocytosis and hypochloremic alkalosis. In long-standing disease, there is evidence of pancreatic insufficiency. A morphine-neostigmine provocative test will reveal subtotal ductal obstruction by the development of pain and increased serum enzymes after their injection. Calcifications in the head of the pancreas develop in more than 50 per cent of patients by adolescence and differ from the parenchymal calcifica-

tions of cystic fibrosis (Fig. 15–11). The small intestinal mucosa is normal, although decreased lactase and alkaline phosphatase have been reported in four patients.

Treatment. Treatment for the acute attack is as for acute pancreatitis.

Complications. Diabetes is not a problem in the young patient, and its overall incidence is probably not greater than in the normal population. Portal or splenic vein thromboses have been reported, usually in individuals over 20 years of age.[102] The incidence of carcinoma is increased, particularly in those with pancreatic calcifications. In one report of 54 patients, eight died of pancreatic carcinoma and five of other intra-abdominal tumors.

Prognosis. If the disease is treated promptly during acute attacks and complications are dealt with, the patient has a nearly normal life expectancy. There is speculation that those with calcifications of the pancreas have an increased risk of developing carcinoma.

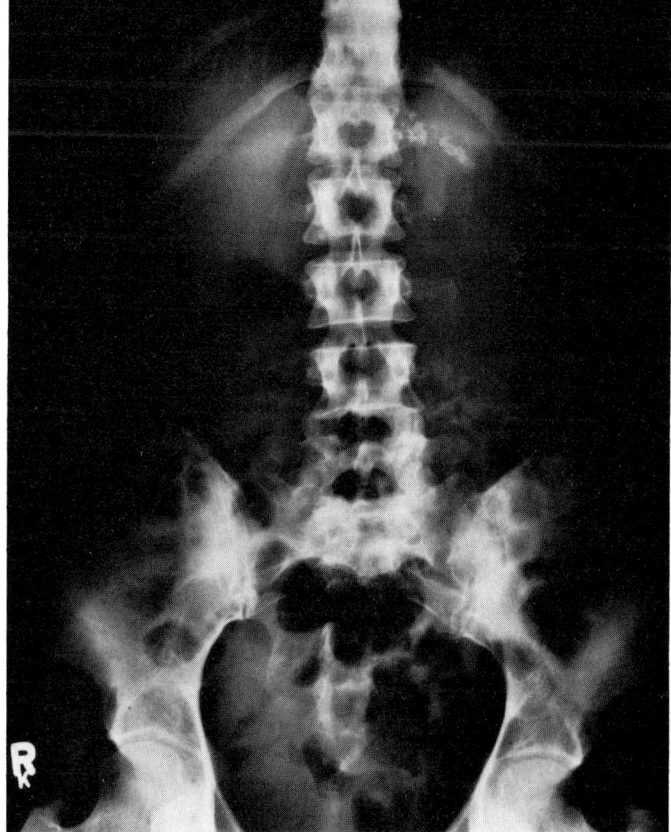

Figure 15–11 Abdominal x-ray of a patient with hereditary pancreatitis. The pancreatic calcifications are seen as large rounded concretions suggesting intraductal obstruction. (From Kattwinkel, J., Lapey, A., di Sant'Agnese, P. A., and Edwards, W.: Hereditary pancreatitis: three new kindreds and a critical review of the literature. Pediatrics, *51*:55, 1973.)

ACQUIRED DISEASES OF THE PANCREAS

ACUTE PANCREATITIS

Although acute inflammatory disease of the pancreas is unusual in infancy, it must always be considered in the differential diagnosis when vomiting and abdominal distention develop in an infant.[22, 86, 108, 149, 150]

Incidence. The incidence is approximately 1 in 500,000 children.

Pathogenesis and Pathology. The cause of acute pancreatitis is not identified in a quarter to two thirds of patients. In some it is definitely related to a congenital anomaly of the ducts, such as stenosis or hypertrophy of the sphincter of Oddi, to impaction of the pancreatic duct by gallstones, or to obstruction of the duct by an annular pancreas or choledochal cyst.[2, 5] It has been associated with systemic or endocrine disorders, among them hyperparathyroidism, polyarteritis, systemic lupus erythematosus, cystic fibrosis (in 15 per cent of patients without total enzyme deficiency), peptic ulcer, malnutrition, uremia, hypercholesterolemia, and deficiencies of vitamins A and D.[13] *Ascaris* migration from the duodenum up into the pancreatic ducts can cause obstruction and pancreatitis. Blunt trauma and the battered child syndrome are increasingly recognized causes of pancreatitis as well as of duodenal or jejunal hematoma, and here, fistula may become a complication.[50, 104, 152] When the disorder follows surgical procedures in the upper abdomen, it is related to local injury of the pancreatic ducts or of the pancreas itself. In some, drug-induced pancreatitis follows ingestion of steroids, indomethacin, azathioprine (Imuran), chlorothiazides, salicylates, isoniazid, 6-mercaptopurine, anticoagulants, alcohol, and valproic acid (Table 15–3).[11, 65, 71, 75, 109, 116b]

Steroid-induced pancreatitis in children has received the greatest attention. It occurs twice as often in boys as in girls, and it usually follows a change in dosage in either an upward or a downward direction. Pancreatic focal changes are found in patients taking steroids who do not have clinical pancreatitis. Those with symptoms have epithelioid proliferation of the ducts, inspissated secretions, and dilated atrophic acini.

An infectious origin is thought likely in infants with pancreatitis because gram-negative organisms are isolated from nearly two thirds of affected infants. Acute hemorrhagic pancreatitis has been described in children with acute encephalopathy and other visceral changes (liver and kidney) resembling Reye's syndrome. This disease occurs with viral infection by a number of agents: adenovirus, rubella virus, reovirus, echovirus 8, and coxsackievirus B4.[19, 33, 69a] The incidence of pancreatitis during the course of mumps infection may be as high as 15 per cent. Fasting, followed by refeeding, may precipitate pancreatitis. In one study, convalescent titers indicated infection with *Mycoplasma pneumoniae* in one third of patients with acute pancreatitis,[44a]

Table 15–3 Etiology of Pancreatitis in Childhood[42, 149]

Idiopathic	Mumps, coxsackie B, rubella virus; Reye's syndrome
Trauma	Blunt injury; battered child syndrome
Hereditary	
Drugs and toxins	Steroids, chlorothiazide, L-asparaginase
Hyperlipoproteinemia	Types 1 and 4
Hypercalcemia	
Structural abnormality of pancreatic ducts	
Gallstones	
Ascaris lumbricoides	
Choledochal cyst	
Cystic fibrosis	
Diabetes mellitus	
Malnutrition	
Alcoholism	

and similar rises in titer have been reported in children.[115a]

Islet cell necrosis may be a part of the hemolytic-uremic syndrome.[22a]

Whatever the cause of the pancreatitis, the mechanism that is triggered seems to be the same. Trypsin activates trypsinogen beyond the capacity of pancreatic trypsin inhibitor substance to inhibit it. The other proteolytic enzymes are then activated, and the end effect is autodigestion of the gland.[123] There is dispute over the actual mechanism of autodigestion, for many studies show trypsin is not elevated in the pancreatic juice in pancreatitis. Free lipase causes fat necrosis in the surrounding tissue, and amylase is released to become elevated in the blood. The basic pathologic changes are proteolytic destruction of pancreatic tissue, necrosis of blood vessels causing hemorrhage,[155a] fat necrosis, and inflammation. Ascitic fluid in experimental pancreatitis is toxic to the lungs.[22b]

There are two general types of pancreatitis: interstitial and hemorrhagic. Interstitial pancreatitis is characterized by edema, inflammation, exudate, proliferation of fibroblasts, and deposition of collagen within the acini. Necrosis is not marked, and there are only isolated areas of fat necrosis. The disease is mild and of only two or three days' duration. Hemorrhagic pancreatitis, on the other hand, is severe, and the entire pancreas or large areas of it become necrotic and hemorrhagic. The normal architecture is completely lost, and the pancreas is swollen. The ducts, acini, stroma, and blood vessels are all involved. After healing, there is fibrosis about the ducts and dilatation of ducts and acini. Jaundice and elevation of the serum bilirubin are due to spasm of the sphincter of Oddi. Ascites and pleural effusions often develop during the acute attack. Fat necrosis of bone marrow is reported in 10.4 per cent of cases of acute or subacute pancreatitis. There are endosteal erosion and cortical destruction followed by periosteal new bone formation. Intramedullary calcification follows later. The lesions are best seen in the short bones of the hands and feet.

Symptoms. There is always abdominal pain, although it may vary greatly in character, being mild or excruciating and constant or intermittent. Unlike the adult, the infant cannot describe the typical radiation of pain into his back.[131] If he can point to the site of the pain, he will point to the epigastric or periumbilical region. Nausea and vomiting are present, but vomiting does not relieve the pain as it does that of gastric or duodenal obstruction. The majority of patients have fever and leukocytosis. In children who are recovering from mumps, vomiting, epigastric tenderness, and generalized abdominal pain develop suddenly and fever reappears. Shock is the major cause of death during the just few hours of illness and is due to plasma volume losses of 30 to 40 percent.[22b]

The infant appears acutely ill and assumes a position of comfort lying on his side with his knees flexed. The abdomen is distended and tender to palpation, but it is not rigid. Bowel sounds, present early, disappear as ileus develops.[131] Jaundice is often present, and shock can rapidly supervene. Cullen's sign, blue discoloration around the umbilicus, or Grey Turner's sign, around the flanks, accompanies hemorrhagic pancreatitis and ascites. Pleural effusion produces respiratory embarrassment; if it is tapped, the pleural fluid contains a high amylase content.

The PO_2 is decreased in half the patients, and severe pulmonary problems develop in 10 per cent. (Phospholipase A is increased in blood and pulmonary change, and surfactant is altered.) Patients with hemorrhagic pancreatitis will often present with hypotension due to kallikrein and phospholipase release from the pancreas, which act to release histamine from mast cells. Hypocalcemia may be associated with hypomagnesemia owing to dilution and hyperglucagonemia.[22b]

Diagnosis. The symptoms suggest peritonitis, peptic ulcer, intestinal obstruction, or perforation. Abdominal films reveal ileus or a distended loop of bowel near the pancreas, termed the sentinel loop, in 30 per cent of cases. Absence of gas in the transverse colon is sometimes noted. Exam-

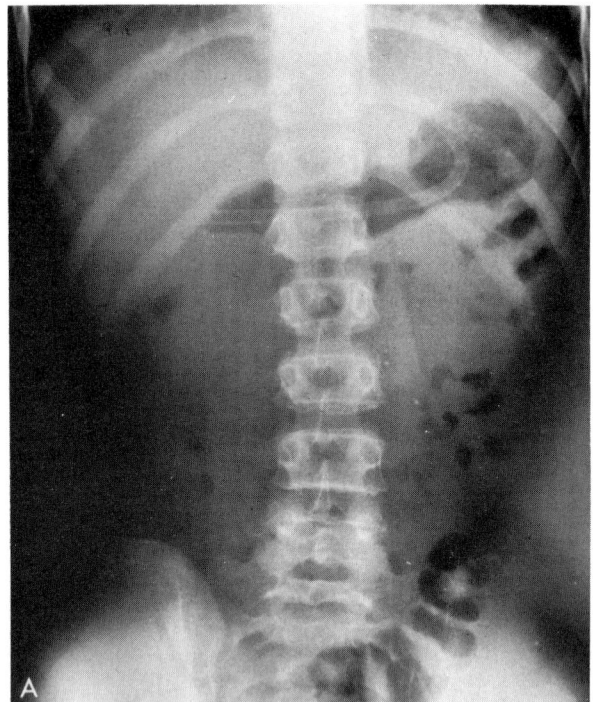

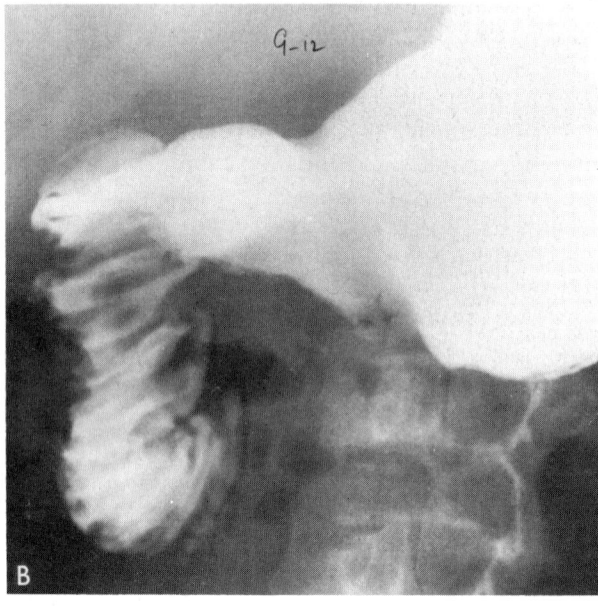

Figure 15–12 After suffering a blow to the upper mid abdomen, this young girl was brought to the hospital because of vomiting and increasing pain. On examination some signs of peritoneal involvement were found, and the serum amylase was elevated. *A*, Plain film shows a nasogastric tube in place and a smooth impression along the inferior aspect of the greater curvature of the stomach. *B*, Spot film from an upper gastrointestinal series shows thickening and irregularity of the mucosal folds in the postbulbar duodenum, transient delay in passage of barium through the duodenum, and an extrinsic pressure defect on the inferior portion of the gastric antrum. These findings resulted from pancreatic and peripancreatic edema which gradually subsided over a period of days of medical management.

ination of the upper gastrointestinal tract with barium shows the stomach to be displaced anteriorly and the duodenal loop widened by edematous pancreas. The duodenum appears normal, dilated, or even narrowed (Fig. 15–12). Ultrasonography will reveal changes in size and consistency of the pancreas.[27]

Serum amylase is greatly elevated within several hours after the onset of symptoms and returns to normal within several days. In children with mumps, the amylase is elevated first because of parotid involvement; it then declines and rises a second time as the pancreas is involved by the disease. Normal serum amylase levels are between 80 and 150 Somogyi units, and the increase in amylase is not directly proportional to the severity of the disease. The serum amylase is elevated in some other conditions, such as penetrating duodenal ulcer, intestinal obstruction, and gallbladder disease, after opiate medication, and, since some amylase is contributed by the liver, in hepatitis. The urinary amylase value remains elevated for at least a week after an attack of pancreatitis and can be used to document the disease after serum values have fallen. The normal urinary level is 300 units per hour to 7000 units per 24 hours. The serum lipase is elevated at about 24 hours and reaches peak levels on the second or third day. The level remains high for about ten days. The normal level is 0.06 to 0.87 unit. Amylase-creatinine ratios greater than 6.5 indicate pancreatitis.[53, 93]

An elevation of serum ribonuclease three to four days after the patient has stabilized indicates necrosis.[161b]

Hyperglycemia is sometimes present during the acute stage, but some infants have hypoglycemia and 15 per cent have glycosuria. Hypocalcemia is a frequent accompaniment of pancreatitis; it is due to binding of calcium in areas of fat necrosis.[8a] Hyperlipemia arises from several factors: decreased plasma lipoprotein lipase activity, increase in serum glycerides, and absorption of fat from peritoneal fat necrosis. Bone lesions are noted three to six weeks after acute pancreatitis, and radiologic studies show increased periosteal reaction with lytic lesions in the tarsal and short bones.[79, 111] They are estimated to occur in 10 per cent of patients and are due to thrombosis of the end arteries.[22b] Polyarthritis and cutaneous nodules also occur.[47a]

Intravascular coagulation is due to a hypercoagulation state with increased Factor 8 and fibrinogen.

In the central nervous system, demyelination has been noted.

Treatment. Medical therapy is aimed at elimination of all factors that stimulate pancreatic secretion.[3] Nasogastric suction removes the stimulus of hydrochloric acid and helps to decompress the gastrointestinal tract. Nothing is given by mouth. Anticholinergics, e.g., atropine or propantheline bromide, help diminish vagal stimulation, although they enhance ileus if it is present.

Cimetidine has been used to decrease gastric secretion but statistically has not proved effective.[19a] Intravenous fluids containing adequate calcium replacement are continued until the amylase level falls and signs of active disease have lessened. Some physicians give antibiotics even though the pancreatic exudate is usually sterile; we do not recommend their use unless there is a positive blood culture. Meperidine is used for pain.

Trasylol, an inhibitor of kallikrein, has been advocated to combat the shock in pancreatitis, but its success has not been impressive. Theoretically, trypsin forms kallikrein from its pancreatic precursor and kallikrein in turn acts upon an alpha$_2$ globulin of plasma to release a hypotensive polypeptide resembling bradykinin. Inhibition of this last step theoretically should prevent shock.

After peristalsis has returned, the patient is without pain or tenderness and enzymes are normal. Antacids and a low-fat diet are given for several weeks, and then diet is increased gradually.

Complications. Coagulation abnormalities of disseminated intravascular coagulation are presumed due to the release of proteolytic enzymes from the inflamed pancreas. Proteolytic activity has been found in the serum of one patient with disseminated intravascular coagulation, and pulmonary microthrombi have been induced in experimental animals after trypsin infusion.

An unusual complication is jejunal infarction, in which fat necrosis leads to thrombosis of the mesenteric arteries or veins.[52] Venous thrombosis is more common than arterial.

When there is ascites, pancreatitis can be diagnosed by measurement of amylase in the ascitic fluid. Surgical drainage of the pancreas may be required to eliminate the ascites and prevent further peritoneal irritation.

Pleural effusion is usually left-sided and is a complication in 8 per cent of children with pancreatitis. Amylase content also is elevated in this effusion fluid, which may be hemorrhagic. Pericardial effusions are rare.

Subcutaneous fat necrosis results from

increased blood pancreatic enzymes and appears as raised, red, tender nodules over pressure points. Pancreatic pseudocyst is discussed later in the chapter. Pancreatic insufficiency and diabetes are late complications.

Evidence of hepatic or renal disease is a complication with a poor prognosis; in one review of 18 infants, 14 died and 11 of them had evidence of hepatic or renal disease.

Prognosis. The mortality in infants with this disease is high, as seen from the figures just given. Mumps pancreatitis is mild, lasting only a few days, and is rarely fatal.

PANCREATITIS AND THE HYPERLIPOPROTEINEMIAS

Pancreatitis associated with these diseases is diagnosed as described under acute pancreatitis. Five different types of hyperlipemia are differentiated by the lipoprotein carriers of cholesterol and triglycerides. Types II and IV are the most common, although types I and II are those of import to the pediatrician.[13, 41]

Type I

Type I, familial hyperchylomicronemia, or fat-induced hyperlipemia, is characterized by elevated chylomicrons in the fasting state.

Inheritance. It is assumed that these patients are homozygous for a rare mutant gene, since some of the parents have a mild hyperlipemia and a decreased postheparin lipolytic activity (PHLA).

Etiology and Pathogenesis. This is probably due to a deficiency of lipoprotein lipase. This enzyme, located in the capillary walls, clears exogenous triglyceride bound to chylomicrons. Activated by heparin, it is measured by postheparin lipolytic activity. When the enzyme is deficient, PHLA is reduced and foam cells fill the reticuloendothelial system.

Symptoms. Infants who are otherwise healthy begin having episodes of colic and increasing abdominal distention. There is hepatosplenomegaly. Papular xanthomas appear on the skin and about the mouth and sometimes resemble pustules. The retinal vessels appear white. Older children have severe recurrent attacks of abdominal pain simulating acute pancreatitis or even acute abdomen.

Diagnosis. Suspicion of hyperlipemia is aroused when blood is drawn and the serum is grossly lipemic. Electrophoresis shows a dense chylomicron band, decreased alpha and beta lipoproteins, and a slightly decreased or increased prebeta band. Triglycerides are greatly increased over a normal maximum of 180 mg per dl, and the cholesterol is normal. The glycerol-cholesterol ratio is greater than 8:1. The oral glucose tolerance is normal.

Treatment. Since this glyceride excess is directly related to dietary fat, the treatment is a low-fat diet. This lowers the lipid level, decreases the frequency and intensity of abdominal pain, and reduces the size of xanthomas.

Type II

Type II, familial hyperbetalipoproteinemia, or familial hypercholesterolemia, is characterized primarily by xanthomas and increased serum cholesterol and beta-lipoproteins.

Inheritance. This is of an autosomal dominant type. Heterozygotes have a moderately abnormal lipoprotein pattern and xanthomas.

Etiology and Pathogenesis. The primary cause of the disease is not known, although it is thought probable that the genes governing lipoprotein synthesis are affected. Secondary forms are seen with hypothyroidism, obstructive liver disease, nephrosis, hyperglobulinemias, idiopathic hypercalcemia, and acute intermittent porphyria.

Symptoms. Xanthomas are rarely present at birth, but they appear during infancy on tendons of the hands and feet, particularly the Achilles tendon. Tuberous xanthomas involve the elbows and knees. Vascular involvement of the aortic valve, endocardium, or coronary arteries can be fatal in childhood. Arcus senilis is visible after several years.

Diagnosis. The serum is clear, but there

are increased levels of cholesterol and beta-lipoproteins. Triglyceride levels are usually normal but sometimes rise as high as 500 mg per dl. The prebeta-lipoprotein levels are normal or slightly elevated, and their concentration rises with age and increases in dietary triglycerides. The glucose tolerance and uric acid are normal.

Treatment. A low-fat diet must be instituted as early as possible to decrease the cholesterol and fatty acid content of the blood and to forestall atherosclerosis. Cholestyramine, beta-sitosterol, D-thyroxine, and chlorphenoxyisobutyric acid all have been used with variable success.

Type III

Type III hyperlipemia is termed floating beta, or broad beta, disease and is of little concern to the pediatrician for it is manifest in early adult life or later. The etiology is unknown, but there is a broad beta band that overlaps into the prebeta region on electrophoresis. The beta-lipoproteins are abnormal, and the cholesterol and tricylcerides are increased. The serum is turbid, and if chylomicrons are present, there is an additional creamy layer. The disease is inherited as an autosomal recessive and can be induced by carbohydrate. It causes tendon, palmar, and periorbital xanthomas, lipemia retinalis, and infiltration of the bone marrow by foam cells. Most patients have carbohydrate intolerance, increased uric acid, and arteriosclerosis. The treatment is weight reduction and a diet low in cholesterol and saturated fats.

Type IV

Type IV, hyperprebetalipoproteinemia, or carbohydrate-induced hyperlipemia, is seen in older patients and is usually secondary to other diseases such as diabetes, obesity, pancreatitis, nephrosis, hyperthyroidism, estrogen administration, Niemann-Pick disease, and hyperglobulinemias. It is thought to be due to excess glyceride release or the formation of anomalous lipoproteins. Inherited as an autosomal dominant, it is usually associated with a family history of diabetes. Affected persons have

xanthomas, lipemia retinalis, foam cells in the reticuloendothelial system and marrow, and recurrent attacks of abdominal pain. The prebetalipoprotein levels and serum triglycerides are elevated, and the alpha- and beta-lipoproteins are decreased. The cholesterol is normal or slightly increased, and the serum is turbid. There is no creamy layer because there are no chylomicrons. The treatment is a low-fat diet.

Type V

Type V, hyperprebetalipoproteinemia and hyperchylomicronemia, has its onset between adolescence and midadult life, with recurrent abdominal pain and xanthomas of the knees, shoulders, buttocks, and back. There are sometimes hepatosplenomegaly and lipemia retinalis. In addition to the chemical abnormalities by which it is named, there are elevated triglycerides and uric acid, normal or elevated cholesterol, and abnormal glucose tolerance. The serum is turbid with a creamy layer. The treatment is weight reduction and dietary restriction of fats and carbohydrates.

PANCREATIC TRAUMA

Blunt abdominal trauma, particularly that caused by bicycle injury or the "battered child syndrome," is responsible for increasing numbers of cases of pancreatic injury.[50]

Incidence. Pancreatic trauma or secondary pseudocyst formation is responsible for 4 per cent of blunt abdominal injuries that require surgery. It is twice as common in boys as in girls.

Etiology and Pathology. In high blunt abdominal trauma there is compression of the pancreas against the vertebrae; in the most severe type, this may cause transection of the pancreas at the junction of its head and body. Otherwise, the result is contusion and release of enzymes into the lesser sac leading to the development of a pancreatic pseudocyst. This is composed of a fibrous capsule containing inflammatory cells, calcium, and cholesterol and often lined with granulation tissue. There is no true endothelial lining. Acute pancreatitis develops

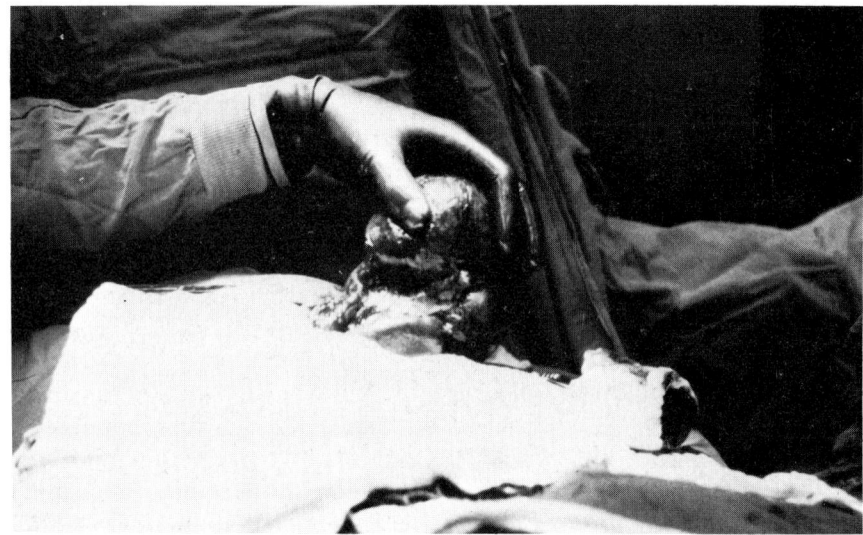

Figure 15–13   Pancreatic pseudocyst, which developed 2 weeks after abdominal trauma.

in up to half the infants and children with these injuries.

Symptoms. Symptoms develop slowly, and it may be difficult for the parent to recall a specific fall or injury hours or days earlier in the eventful life of a toddler or baby that correlates with the present illness. The toddler in whom transection of the pancreas occurs when he falls over a toy bucket or truck may not become sick until eight hours later, when vomiting, crying, abdominal distention, and tenderness develop.

Like the infant with acute pancreatitis, the baby cannot describe the characteristics of the pancreatic pain. In most there is only diffuse abdominal pain and tenderness; in a few, dyspnea is the only complaint. One infant had only transitory diarrhea and abdominal distention for six days before his demise. As the illness progresses a mass becomes palpable in the epigastrium.

Diagnosis. Radiologic examination of the upper gastrointestinal tract characteristically shows anterior and upward displacement of the stomach and widening of the duodenal loop. This finding cannot always differentiate pseudocyst from retroperitoneal tumor or gastric duplication cyst. Urinary or serum amylase may be elevated or, if the cyst develops slowly, may not be (Fig. 15–13). Angiography may show occlusion of the pancreatic vessels.

Treatment. If the pancreas has been transected, a distal pancreatectomy may be necessary. Such surgery is not always followed by diabetes or pancreatic insufficiency. Surgical procedures used include excision, marsupialization of the pseudocyst, and Roux-en-Y cystojejunostomy with internal drainage.

Complications. Occasionally, there is recurrence of the cyst. In some infants, a diabetic blood sugar curve develops, although this is more common in those with pseudocyst from pancreatitis.

PANCREATIC PSEUDOCYST

The pseudocyst is a complication of acute pancreatitis, of hereditary pancreatitis,[45] or of trauma and develops any time from 24 hours to 4 years after the initial insult. In one third of children presenting with pseudocyst, the original cause is undetermined.[17, 120, 164]

Pathology. These are false cysts with no epithelial lining. Instead there is fibrous or granulation tissue. The cysts measure from several millimeters to a size that fills the abdomen, masquerading as ascites. They are filled with pancreatic secretions (Fig. 15–13), blood, tissue, fluid, and debris.

Symptoms. Trauma or pancreatitis precedes the appearance of a pseudocyst. In addition to abdominal pain and tenderness, a visible epigastric mass or generalized abdominal enlargement is the prime symptom. If the pseudocyst becomes infected, there is sepsis with fluctuating high fever, a very high white blood cell count, and an increase in abdominal pain. Nausea, vomiting, or jaundice may result. A slow leak in the peritoneum causes chronic pancreatic ascites. Rupture into the thorax results in pleural effusion or chylothorax. The cyst may fistulize to the colon.[26]

Diagnosis. Prolonged elevation of serum and urinary amylase and of serum lipase after pancreatitis indicates pseudocyst formation. On the other hand, a cyst can develop in the presence of normal enzyme levels, particularly when it develops slowly. It is unknown why there is increased renal clearance of amylase. Radiologic examination of the upper gastrointestinal tract shows widening of the duodenal loop with elevation of the stomach and depression of the ligament of Treitz like that seen in acute pancreatitis. If gas is present in the region of the pseudocyst in "soap bubble" appearance, the diagnosis of abscess is certain. In such instances, blood cultures are usually positive. Ultrasonography and CAT scanning have improved the ability to follow cyst size and consistency.

Treatment. Large pseudocysts should be drained or marsupialized. Immediate drainage is indicated if abscess is present. Rupture of a pseudocyst carries a mortality of 50 per cent. If the capsule is fibrous, drainage is accomplished through a cystenterostomy. Small cysts often resolve spontaneously with medical management.

PANCREATIC INSUFFICIENCY FROM INTRAUTERINE VIRAL INFECTION

Pancreatic insufficiency may follow intrauterine viral infection, particularly that from the rubella virus.[21, 36, 73]

Pathology. The congenital rubella syndrome was thought at first to include cataracts, perceptive deafness, central nervous system damage, cleft palate, and cardiac anomalies. A great deal more was learned after the pandemic of the mid-1960's, and congenital glaucoma, purpura, cephalitis, hepatitis, myocarditis, chorioretinitis, interstitial nephritis, osteitis, and spontaneous bone fractures were added to the list. Many of these children grew poorly, but this was attributed in the past to the basic disease and the cardiac abnormalities. It was only in 1972 that published data appeared to document interstitial pancreatitis as another element of the rubella syndrome. Necropsy studies of an infant with this syndrome who died at three and one-half months of age of cardiac arrest revealed a grossly normal pancreas, but one with extensive lymphocytic infiltration of interstitial and periglandular tissue in the head and tail of the pancreas. The virus may be recovered from cultures of the pancreatic tissue.

Several authors have independently reported the association of diabetes mellitus and the rubella syndrome.[44] This led Johnson and Tudor[73] to hypothesize that in utero rubella infection can affect islet cell development. However, damage to the islet cells has not been found in necropsy studies, and diabetes has not developed in our 12-year-old patient with the congenital rubella syndrome and pancreatic insufficiency.

Symptoms. These infants are typically microcephalic at birth. The stigmata of the rubella syndrome may overshadow gastrointestinal symptoms, with cardiac failure and evidence of brain damage and cataracts being most prominent. Other infants may present less marked symptoms, with diarrhea and failure to thrive the predominant complications (Fig. 15–14).

Diagnosis. Any infant with failure to thrive or digestive disorders, and with other signs suggestive of intrauterine viral infection, should be tested for assessment of pancreatic function: serum carotene, fecal fat, and intubation studies should be included.

Treatment. These infants respond well to enzyme therapy.

Prognosis. In our first patient, the response was encouraging. Growth has been normal over the past five years, and consecutive testing has demonstrated that he has outgrown or spontaneously recovered from

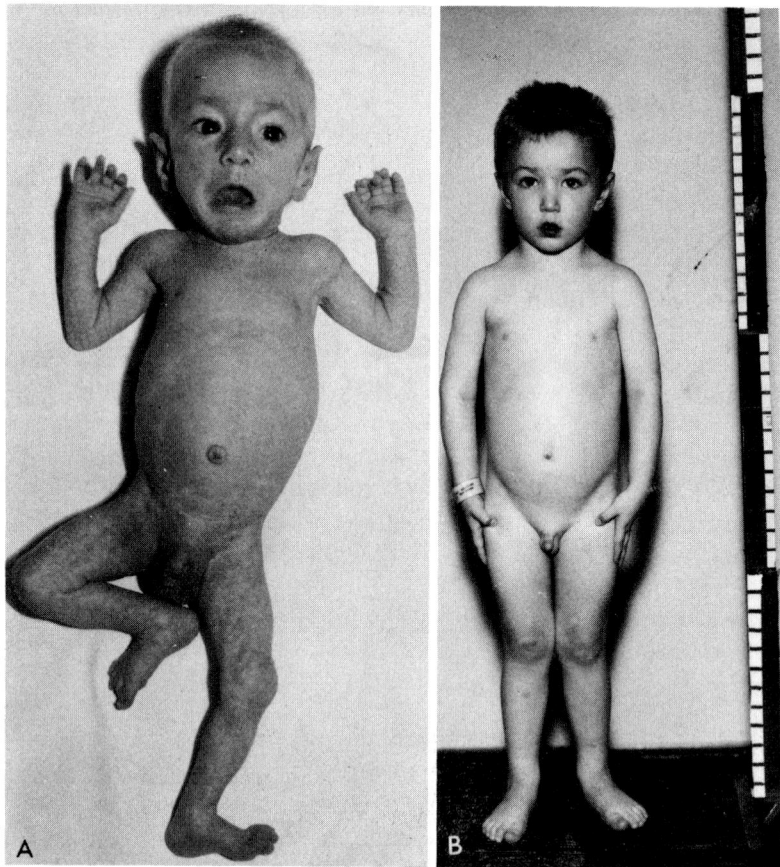

Figure 15–14   *A,* Infant P. S. at 6 weeks born to a mother exposed to rubella during pregnancy. He was found to have pancreatic insufficiency and was treated with pancreatic extract. *B,* Same patient at 3½ years of age: nutrition is considerably improved and he has reached the twenty-fifth percentile for both height and weight.

the pancreatic lesion. Diabetes has not developed. In more severely affected infants, the ultimate prognosis is governed by the central nervous system and cardiac defects.

PANCREATITIS, DIABETES, MALABSORPTION, AND IMMUNOGLOBULIN A DEFICIENCY

All or some of these disorders can be associated.[118] A patient has been reported with pancreatitis, malabsorption, diabetes, and immunoglobulin A deficiency in whom diabetes preceded the abdominal pain and steatorrhea by a year. Pancreatitis is more common in persons with diabetes, particularly juvenile diabetes, than in normal populations. Small bowel villous atrophy and gluten sensitivity occur in diabetic adults,

and conversely there seems to be an increased incidence of diabetes in children with celiac disease. Immunoglobulin A deficiency alone is associated with malabsorption in some patients. Just how or why all these factors are interrelated is not clear.

PANCREATIC INSUFFICIENCY AND MALNUTRITION

Pancreatic insufficiency develops in protein-calorie malnutrition and is reflected in a diminution of enzymes with relatively normal volume and bicarbonate secretion.[9, 62] It has been reported in kwashiorkor, in severe forms of malabsorption, and in chronic small bowel diarrhea. Recovery of pancreatic function has been noted as early as four days after the initiation of treatment in infants with kwashiorkor.[28] In marasmic infants with protein-calorie malnutrition, full return of pancreatic function may require several months, even after an excellent clinical response has been noted. Some studies indicate that these patients have fibrotic changes in the pancreas, and recovery may never be complete. Lipase is the most severely affected of the enzymes and the last to return. Pancreatic insufficiency secondary to celiac disease often requires several months of pancreatic replacement therapy after initiation of a gluten-free diet and is probably secondary to some degree of enterokinase deficiency.[88]

Animal experiments on rats, malnourished *in utero*, show that if the newborn is provided a proper diet, abnormal pancreatic function returns in 13 to 19 weeks and is associated with a return to near-normal growth curves. However, chronic calcific pancreatitis has been reported with celiac disease.[119]

TUMORS OF THE PANCREAS

Tumors of the pancreas are extremely rare in childhood, with peak incidence during adolescence.[54, 74, 99, 107] When they do occur, they are of two types, functioning and nonfunctioning, and can often be differentiated by the cell type from which they arise (Table 15–4). Islet cell tumors are the most common, but there are few data on the relative frequencies of the other types of tumors to be described below.

FUNCTIONING PANCREATIC TUMORS

More common than the nonfunctioning tumors, these are of the beta islet cell or nonbeta islet cell types. Most are adenomas, although some may be adenocarcinomas.

Beta Islet Cell Tumors

These tumors are small and nonpalpable but cause severe hypoglycemia, convulsions, growth retardation, and, eventually, profound mental retardation.[154, 165]

Incidence. In 1971, a total of nine cases

Table 15–4 Tumors of the Pancreas

ENDOCRINE CELL
Beta Cell
    Nesidioblastosis
    Islet cell adenoma
    Hyperplasia of the islets
    Hypertrophy of the islets
    Islet cell adenocarcinoma
Non-Beta Cell (Zollinger-Ellison syndrome)
    Adenoma
    Hypertrophy
    Adenocarcinoma

EXOCRINE CELL
Cystic Tumors
    Cystadenoma
    Cystadenocarcinoma
Solid Tumors
    Adenoma
    Adenocarcinoma
Others:
    Neurofibrosarcoma
    Hemangioendothelioma
    Fibrosarcoma
    Papillary epithelial neoplasm

were reported in the literature and in 1978, 32 patients were reported from one center over a ten-year period. Islet cell hyperplasia causes approximately 62 per cent of all cases of hypoglycemia; benign adenomas, 37 per cent, and adenocarcinomas, 1 per cent.

Etiology. The etiology is unknown, although some infants have relatives with multiple adenomatosis. A genetic basis cannot be excluded.[157]

Pathology. A classification of lesions has been presented by Thomas et al.[157]: (1) *nesidioblastosis* — multiple neoislet formation from ductal epithelium; (2) *islet cell adenoma* — focal tumorous nodule of islet cells; (3) *nesidioblastoma* — an adenoma derived from ductal epithelium; (4) *hyperplasia of the islets*; and (5) *hypertrophy of the islets*.

Adenomas most often arise in the body of the pancreas but may also arise from the head or tail. Their size varies from 5 mm to 0.5×1 cm, and often they cannot be palpated at the time of surgery.[83a] They may be multiple, with as many as eight being found in one patient. Microscopically, they consist of cords of islet cells containing beta granules, and the majority are encapsulated. Three per cent are aberrant in location, being situated in the wall of the duodenum or stomach, the spleen, a Meckel's diverticulum, or the retroperitoneum.

Symptoms. The classic diagnostic triad of Whipple includes (1) hypoglycemia after fasting or exertion; (2) fasting blood sugar below 50 mg per dl; and (3) relief of symptoms by oral or intravenous glucose. In neonates, blood sugar is considered abnormal if it falls below 30 mg per dl, and in premature infants, below 20 mg per dl. The babies are normal in size and born of a term pregnancy, unlike the premature or low birth weight infants with transient hypoglycemia. Cyanosis, apnea, and a shock-like state characterize hypoglycemia in young infants, whereas older ones have sweating and tachycardia. All exhibit twitching, clonic movements, and seizures that become increasingly severe. Oral feedings and intravenous administration of glucose are only temporizing measures in controlling the hypoglycemia. As the disease progresses, both linear and head circumference growth are impaired and severe brain damage results from repeated episodes of hypoglycemia.[24]

Diagnosis. The diagnosis must be suspected in a term infant with seizures and low blood sugar levels that cannot be controlled by oral feedings. If hypoglycemia persists for more than two weeks, it must be thoroughly investigated for causes such as glycogen storage disease, fructose intolerance, galactosemia, liver disease, and hyperinsulinism. Confirmation of the disease may be extremely difficult, for serum insulin levels may be elevated only intermittently and a normal insulin value does not preclude the diagnosis. Insulinomas release excessive insulin continuously, unaffected by stimulation. Islet cell hyperplasia produces excessive insulin only in response to stimulation. Intravenous tolbutamide stimulates insulin release and causes a greater fall in blood glucose than occurs in normal controls. This is not specific for adenoma, as some infants with idiopathic hypoglycemia or leucine sensitivity also show an exaggerated response. Furthermore, leucine sensitivity may be associated with islet cell tumor. Epinephrine and glucagon promote a normal hypoglycemia, although hypoglycemia may be produced in children with tumor. The insulin-glucose ratio has been considered of value in the diagnosis of insulinoma, with normal values of zero when the blood glucose is 20 mg per dl. Using a corrected formula

$$\left(\text{insulin } \frac{(\text{uU/ml} \times 100}{\text{glucose (mg/dl)} - 20}\right)$$

values of 100 to 1000 indicate tumor. Calcium infusion, using 10 mg Ca^{++} per kg, proves a sensitive test for the diagnosis of tumor, causing hypoglycemia in those with adenoma but not in those with functional hypoglycemia or islet cell hyperplasia. Since hyperinsulinism is associated with low levels of fatty acids and increased beta-hydroxy-butyrate, normal values of these exclude hyperinsulinism.

Localization of occult tumors has been facilitated by percutaneous portal venography and selective portal vein blood samplings for immunoreactive insulin.[80] Angiography has not been helpful in identifying adenomas.

Treatment. Immediate therapy is directed at preservation of serum glucose levels to prevent brain damage. Critically ill infants are given intravenous glucose as required and frequent feedings with low-leucine formula. Hypoglycemia is usually not responsive to insulin antagonism by steroids or glucagon. Insulin secretion may be suppressed by epinephrine or diazoxide. Diazoxide is given orally in increasing dosage up to 15 mg per kg per day in four divided doses, but those with insulinoma may show only transient improvement. If therapy is ineffective, islet cells may be destroyed by surgery or streptozocin. Surgical inspection and palpation of the entire gland are essential, and if no tumor is palpable, resection of 75 per cent or more of the pancreas is advisable.[126] Blood sugar must be monitored during the procedure, since a hyperglycemic response occurs within minutes of removing the tumor.

Complications. Postoperative blood sugar levels may reach as high as 1000 mg per dl, and insulin control is required for days to weeks. Thereafter, the blood sugar returns to normal. Pseudocyst may be a late complication.

Prognosis. This varies with the type of tumor: Islet cell tumors tend to be multicentric, and ectopic tumors may cause a recurrence of symptoms. Probably more than half the patients are cured, but sequelae of seizures and mental retardation depend upon the degree and duration of early hypoglycemia. Diabetes is a complication of near-total pancreatectomy.

Nonbeta Islet Cell Tumors

These tumors produce gastrin to cause the Zollinger-Ellison syndrome of recurrent peptic ulceration, gastric hypersecretion, and diarrhea.[38] The tumors are represented by adenoma, hyperplasia, or adenocarcinoma and cause symptoms through production of gastrin. Although the tumor has been reported in approximately 20 children, it has not yet been described in infants.[37] Only 10 per cent of tumors in the adult are malignant, but the potential in children is greater. The ulcers are most often located in the jejunum but may occur in the stomach and duodenum and are usually multiple. Treatment consists of removal of all gastric parietal cells by total resection of the stomach. Palliative medical management has recently been reported using cimetidine.

Exocrine Pancreatic Tumors

The exocrine pancreatic tumors are usually nonfunctional and occur less often than endocrine tumors. They may be cystic or solid, with solid adenomas being so small as to be detected only at autopsy.[46] The benign cystic adenoma, or *cystadenoma*, is the most common of this type and presents as a steadily enlarging epigastric or left upper quadrant mass.[57] Most are found in the tail of the pancreas. Radiologic examination may show widening of the duodenal sweep and, sometimes, displacement of the duodenum. *Benign hemangioendothelioma* involves the head of the pancreas to cause an obstructive-type jaundice as well as a palpable epigastric mass.[23] Partial resection of the pancreas and, at times, pancreaticoduode-

nectomy are required for removal of these tumors.

Adenocarcinoma and undifferentiated carcinoma are the second most frequent malignant tumors after islet cell carcinoma. These solid, nonfunctioning tumors arise from the head of the pancreas and are palpated as a cystic or solid mass. In infancy they cause anorexia and weight loss rather than the typical pain and biliary tract obstruction seen in adults. Less frequent presentations are incomplete or complete duodenal obstruction.

Other tumors are myxoid variants of neurofibrosarcoma, fibrosarcoma, and embryonal rhabdomyosarcoma. These tumors metastasize to liver and portal, mesenteric, periaortic, and perihilar lymph nodes. Locally, they extend to lungs, spleen, and kidneys. Pressure upon, or extension to, the duodenum may cause mucosal ulceration and upper gastrointestinal hemorrhage. Pancreaticoduodenectomy has been performed successfully in some young infants.

REFERENCES

1. Abrams, C., Hamosh, M., Hubbard, V. S., Datta, S., and Hamosh, P.: Cystic fibrosis; Compensatory role of lingual lipase in gastric and duodenal fat digestion. Pediatr. Res. 16:155A, 1982.
1a. Adrian, T. E., McKiernan, J., Johnstone, D. I., Hiller, E., Vyas, H., Sarson, D. L., and Bloom, S. R.: Hormonal abnormalities of the pancreas and gut in cystic fibrosis. Gastroenterology 79:460, 1980.
1b. Aggett, P. J., Cavanaugh, N. P. C., Matthew, D. J., Pincott, J. R., Sutcliffe, J., and Harries, J. T.: Schwachman's syndrome: A review of 21 cases. Arch. Dis. Child. 55:331, 1980.
2. Agrawal, R., and Brodmarkel, J. R.: Choledochal cyst prevention as pancreatitis. Am. J. Gastroenterol. 71:408, 1979.
3. Aldrete, J., Jiminez, H., and Halpern, N.: Evaluation and treatment of acute and chronic pancreatitis. A review of 380 cases. Ann. Surg. 191:664, 1980.
4. Allue, X., and Sanjurjo, P.: Triglyceride levels after intralipid infusion in children with cystic fibrosis. Pediatrics 61:924, 1977.
5. Altman, M., Halls, J., Douglas, A., and Renuer, I. G.: Choledochal cyst presenting as acute pancreatitis. Am. J. Gastroenterol. 70:514, 1978.
6. Antonowicz, I., Ishida, S., and Schwachman, H.: Studies in meconium in cystic fibrosis: the activities of alpha-D-mannosidase, beta-

glucuronidase, beta-D-fucosidase, acid and alkaline phosphatase Biol. Neonate *34*:225, 1978.

7. Antonowicz, I., Reddy, U., Khaw, K., and Schwachman, H.: Lactase deficiency in patients with cystic fibrosis. Pediatrics *42*:492, 1968.

8. Arvanitakis, C., and Cooke, A. R.: Diagnostic tests of exocrine pancreatic function and disease. Gastroenterology 74(1):932, 1978.

8a. Balart, L. A., and Ferrante, W. A.: Pathophysiology of acute and chronic pancreatitis. Ann. Intern. Med. *142*:113, 1982.

9. Barbezat, G. O., and Hansen, J. D. L.: The exocrine pancreas and protein-calorie malnutrition. Pediatrics *42*:77, 1968.

10. Bass, H. N., and Miller, A. A.: Cystic fibrosis presenting with anemia and hypoproteinemia in twins. Pediatrics 59:126, 1977.

11. Batalden, P. B., van Dyne, B. J., and Cloyd, J: Pancreatitis associated with valproic acid therapy. Pediatrics *64*:520, 1979.

12. Beckerman, R. C., and Taussig, L.: Hypoelectrolytemia and metabolic alkalosis in infants with cystic fibrosis. Pediatrics *63*:580, 1979.

12a. Bendig, D. W., Seilheimer, D. K., Wagner, M. L., Ferry, G. D., and Harrison, G. M.: Complications of gastroesophageal reflux in patients with cystic fibrosis. J. Pediatr. *100*: 536, 1982.

12b. Berry, H., Kellogg, F. W., Lichstein, S., and Ingberg, R.: Elevated meconium lactase activity: Its use as a screening test for cystic fibrosis. Am. J. Dis. Child. *134*:930, 1980.

13. Betro, M. G.: The hyperlipoproteinemias: a review. N. Z. Med. J. 75:131, 1972.

14. Bodian, M., Sheldon, W., and Lightwood, R.: Congenital hypoplasia of the pancreas. Acta Paediatr. Scand. 52:282, 1964.

15. Bonin, A., Roy, C., Lasalle, R., Weber, A., and Morin, C.: Fecal chymotrypsin: a reliable index of pancreatic function in children. J. Pediatr. 83:594, 1973.

16. Boyle, B. J., Long,W. B., Balistreri, W., Widzer, S. J., and Huang, N.: Effect of cimetidine and pancreatic enzymes on serum and fecal bile acids and fact absorption in cystic fibrosis. Gastroenterology 78:950, 1980.

17. Bradley, E. L., Gonzalez, A. C., and Clements, J. L.: Acute pancreatic pseudocysts: Incidence and implications. Ann. Surg. *184*:734,.1976.

18. Bradley, J. A., Azon, T. B., and Hill, G.: Natural element diet for retarded growth in a patient with cystic fibrosis. Br. Med. J. *1*:167, 1979.

19. Branski, D., Lebenthal, E., Faden, H., Hatch, T., and Krasner, J.: Reovirus type infection in a suckling mouse: the effect on pancreatic structure and enzyme content. Pediatr. Res. *14*:8, 1980.

19a. Broe, P. J., Zinner, M. J., and Cameron, J. L.: A clinical trial of cimetidine in acute pancreatitis. Surg. Gynecol. Obstet. *154*:13, 1982.

20. Brueton, M. J., Mavromichalis, J., Goodchild, M. C., and Anderson, C. M.: Hepatic dysfunction in association with pancreatic insufficiency and cyclical neutropenia. Arch. Dis. Child. 52:76, 1977.

21. Bunnell, C. E., and Monif, G. R. C.: Interstitial pancreatitis in the congenital rubella syndrome. J. Pediatr. *80*:465, 1972.

22. Buntain, W., Wood, J., and Woolley, M.: Pancreatitis in childhood. J. Pediatr. Surg. *13*:143, 1978.

22a. Burns, J., Berman, E. R., Fagre, J., Shikes, R., and Lum, G.: Pancreatic islet cell necrosis: Association with hemolytic-uremic syndrome. J. Pediatr. *100*:582, 1982.

22b. Carey, L. C.: Extra-abdominal manifestations of acute pancreatitis. Surgery 86:337, 1979.

23. Chappell, J.: Benign hemangioendothelioma of the head of the pancreas treated by pancreaticoduodenectomy. J. Pediatr. Surg. 8:431, 1973.

23a. Chase, H. P., and Dupont, J.: Abnormal levels of prostaglandins and fatty acids in blood of children with cystic fibrosis. Lancet 2:236, 1978.

24. Chase, H. P., Marlow, R. A., Dabiere, C. S., and Welch, N. N.: Hypoglycemia and brain development. Pediatrics 52:513, 1973.

25. Cohen, L. F., di Sant'Agnese, P. A., Taylor, A., et al.: Inhibition of mucociliary clearance in cystic fibrosis. J. Pediatr. 90:579, 1977.

26. Cooney, D. R., Jacobowitz, I., Telander, R. L., and Allen, J. E.: Pancreaticocolonic fistula: A complication of pancreatic pseudocysts in childhood. J. Pediatr. Surg. *13*:492, 1978.

27. Cox, K. L., Ament, M. E., Sample, W. Y., Sarti, D. A., O'Donnell, M., and Byrne, W. J.: Ultrasonic and biochemical diagnosis of pancreatitis. J. Pediatr. 96:407, 1980.

28. Danus, O., Urbina, A. M., Valenzuela, I., et al.: The effect of refeeding on pancreatic exocrine function in marasmic infants. J. Pediatr. 77:334, 1970.

29. Davidson, G., Hassel, F., Crozier, D., et al.: Iatrogenic hyperuricemia in children with cystic fibrosis. J. Pediatr. 93:976, 1978.

30. DeCastro-Barbosa, J. J., Dockerty, M. B., and Waugh, J. M.: Pancreatic heterotopia. Surg. Gynecol. Obstet. 82:527, 1946.

31. Delachaume-Salem, E., and Sarles, H.: Normal human pancreatic secretion as a function of age. Arch. Fr. Mal. App. Dig. 59:135, 1970.

32. DiMagno, E. P., Malagelada, J. R., Go, U. L. W., and Moertel, C. G.: Fate of orally ingested enzymes in pancreatic insufficiency. N. Engl. J. Med. 296:1318, 1977.

33. Dipietro, C., Delguercio, M. J., Paolino, G. B., Barbi, M., Ferrante, P., and Chiumello, G.: Type 1 diabetes and coxsackie virus infection. Helv. Paedr. Acta 34:561, 1980.

34. di Sant'Agnese, P. A.; Cystic fibrosis in adults. Am. J. Med. 66:121, 1979.

35. Dodge, J. A., and Laurence, K. M.: Congenital absence of islets of Langerhans. Arch. Dis. Child. 52:411, 1977.

36. Donowitz, M., and Gryboski, J. D.: Pancreatic insufficiency and the congenital rubella syndrome. J. Pediatr. 87:241, 1975.

37. Drake, D. P., Macker, A. G., and Atwell, J. D.: Zollinger-Ellison syndrome in a child: medical treatment with cimetidine. Arch. Dis. Child. 55:226, 1980.

38. Dunnick, N. R., Doppman, J., Mills, S., and McCarthy, D.: Computed tomographic de-

tection of non-beta pancreatic islet cell tumors. Radiology 135:117, 1980.

39. Durie, P., Newth, C., Forstner, G., and Gall, D. G.: Malabsorption of medium chain triglycerides in infants with cystic fibrosis: correction with pancreatic enzyme supplements. J. Pediatr. 96:862, 1980.

40. Falchuk, Z. M., and Taussig, L. M.: Jejunal immunoglobulin A synthesis in cystic fibrosis Pediatr. Res. 6:374, 1972.

41. Farmer, R., Winkelman, E. I., Brown, H. B., and Lewis, L.: Hyperlipoproteinemia and pancreatitis. Am. J. Med. 54:161, 1973.

42. Feigal, R. J., and Shapiro, B.: Altered intracellular calcium in fibroblasts from patients with cystic fibrosis and heterozygotes. Pediatr. Res. 13:764, 1979.

43. Figarella, C., DeCaro, A., Leupold, D., and Poley, J.: Congenital pancreatic lipase deficiency. J. Pediatr. 96:412, 1980.

44. Forrest, J. M., Menser, M. A., and Burgess, J. A.: High frequency of diabetes mellitus in young adults with congenital rubella. Lancet 2:332, 1971.

44a. Freeman, R., and McMahon, M. J.: Acute pancreatitis and serologic evidence of infection with *Mycoplasma pneumoniae*. Gut 19:367, 1978.

45. Fried, A. M., and Selke, A. C.: Pseudocyst formation in hereditary pancreatitis. J. Pediatr. 93:950, 1978.

46. Gauderer, M., Stanley, C., Baker, L., and Bishop, H.: Pancreatic adenomas in infants and children. J. Pediatr. Surg. 13:591, 1980.

47. Gibson, L.: Screening of newborns for cystic fibrosis. Am. J. Dis. Child. 134:925, 1980.

47a. Golubuff, N., Cram, R., Ramgotra, B., Singh, A., and Wilkinson, G. W.: Polyarthritis and bone lesions complicating traumatic pancreatitis in two children. Can. Med. Assoc. J. 118:924, 1978.

48. Goodchild, M., Nelson, R., and Anderson, C.: Cystic fibrosis and celiac disease: report of two cases. Arch. Dis. Child. 48:684, 1973.

49. Graham, D. Y.: Enzyme replacement therapy of exocrine pancreatic insufficiency in man. N. Engl. J. Med. 296:1314, 1977.

50. Graham, J., Pokany, W., Matlox, K., and Jordan, G.: Surgical management of acute pancreatic injuries in children. J. Pediatr. Surg. 13:683, 1978.

51. Grand, R. J., Rosen, S. W, di Sant'Agnese, P. A., and Kirkham, W. R.: Unusual case of XXY Klinefelter's syndrome with pancreatic insufficiency, hypothyroidism, deafness, chronic lung disease, dwarfism, and microcephaly. Am. J. Med. 41:478, 1966.

52. Griffiths, R. W., and Brown, P. W.: Jejunal infarction as a complication of pancreatitis. Gastroenterology 58:709, 1970.

53. Grosberg, S. J., Wapnick, S., Purow, E., and Purow, J. R.: Specificity of serum amylase and amylase creatinine clearance ratio in the diagnosis of acute and chronic pancreatitis. Am. J. Gastroenterol. 72:41, 1979.

54. Grosfeld, J., Clatworthy, W., and Hamoudi, A. B.: Pancreatic malignancy in children. Arch. Surg. 101:370, 1970.

55. Gryboski, J. D.: Gastrointestinal Problems in the Infant. Ed. 1. Philadelphia, W. B. Saunders Company, 1975, pp. 456–489.

56. Gryboski, J.: Congenital disorders of absorption. *In* Lebenthal, E. (ed.): Textbook of Gastroenterology and Nutrition in Infancy. New York, Raven Press, 1981, pp. 931–959.

57. Gundersen, A. E., and Janis, J.: Pancreatic cystadenoma in childhood. J. Pediatr. Surg. 4:478, 1969.

58. Hadorn, B., Johansen, P. G., and Anderson, C. M.: Pancreozymin-secretin test of exocrine pancreatic function in cystic fibrosis and the significance of the result for the pathogenesis of the disease. Can. Med. Assoc. J. 98:377, 1968.

59. Hadorn, B., Tarlow, M. J., Lloyd, J. K., and Wolff, O. H.: Intestinal enterokinase deficiency. Lancet 1:812, 1969.

60. Hadorn, B., Zoppi, G., Shmerling, D. H., Prader, A., McIntyre, I., and Anderson, C. M.: Quantitative assessment of exocrine pancreatic function in infants and children. J. Pediatr. 73:39, 1968.

61. Hamoudi, A. B., Misugi, K., Grosfeld, J. L., and Reiner, C. B.: Papillary epithelial neoplasm of the pancreas in a child. Cancer 26:1126, 1970.

62. Hatch, T. F., Lebenthal, E., Krasner, J., and Bronski, D.: Effect of postnatal malnutrition on pancreatic zymogen enzymes in the rat. Am. J. Clin. Nutr. 32:1224, 1979.

63. Haworth, J. C., Gourley, B., Hadorn, B, and Sumida, C.: Malabsorption and growth failure due to intestinal enterokinase deficiency. J. Pediatr. 78:481, 1971.

64. Herrod, H., and Spick, A.: Mother and daughter with cystic fibrosis. J. Pediatr. 91:276, 1977.

65. Hillemeier, A. C., and Gryboski, J. D.: Acute pancreatitis. *In* Rothstein, P. (ed.): *Pediatric Intensive Care*. In press.

66. Howard, C., Go, V., Infante, A. J., Perrault, J., Gerich, J. and Haymond, M. W.: Long term survival in a case of functional agenesis. J. Pediatr. 97:786, 1980.

67. Hubbard, V. S., Barbero, G., and Chase, H.: Selenium and cystic fibrosis. J. Pediatr. 96:421, 1980.

68. Hubbard, V. S., Farrell, P. M., and di Sant'Agnese, P. A.: 25-hydroxycholecalciferol levels in patients with cystic fibrosis. J. Pediatr. 94:84, 1979.

69. Hudson, E. H., and Aldor, T.: Pancreatic insufficiency and neutropenia with associated immunoglobulin deficit. Arch. Intern. Med. 125:314, 1970.

69a. Imbrie, C. W., Ferguson, J. C., and Sommerville, R. G.: Coxsackie and mumps virus infection in a prospective study of acute pancreatitis. Gut 18:53, 1977.

70. Imrie, J. R., Fagan, D. G., and Sturgess, J. M.: Quantitative evaluation of the development of the exocrine pancreas in cystic fibrosis and control infants. Am. J. Pathol. 95:697, 1979.

71. Isenberg, J. N.: Pancreatitis, amylase clearance and aziothioprine. J. Pediatr. 93:1043, 1978.

72. Jam, I., Shoham, M., Wolf, R. O., and Mishkin, S.:

Elevated serum amylase activity in the absence of clinical pancreatic or salivary gland disease. Am. J. Gastroenterol. 70:480, 1978.

72a. Jochimsen, P. R., Shirazi, S., and Lewis, J.: Symptomatic ectopic pancreas relieved by surgical excision. Surg. Gynecol. Obstet. 153:49, 1981.

73. Johnson, G. H., and Tudor, R. B.: Diabetes mellitus and congenital rubella infection. Am. J. Dis. Child. 120:453, 1970.

74. Jones, P. G., and Campbell, P. E.: Tumours of Infancy and Childhood. Blackwell Scientific Publications. Philadelphia, Lippincott, 1976, Chap. 20.

75. Jordan, S. C., and Ament, M.: Pancreatitis in children and adolescents. J. Pediatr. 91:211, 1977.

76. Katz, S.: Calcium and sodium transport processes in patients with cystic fibrosis. A specific decrease in Mg^{2+} dependent, Ca^{2+} adenosine triphosphatase activity in erythrocyte membranes from cystic fibrosis patients. Pediatr. Res. 12:1033, 1978.

77. Kattwinkel, J., Lapey, A., di Sant'Agnese, P. A., and Edwards, W.: Hereditary pancreatitis. Pediatrics 51:55, 1973.

78. Katznelson, D.: Increased intracranial pressure in cystic fibrosis. Acta Paedr. Scand. 67:607, 1978.

79. Keating, J., Shackelford, G, Shackelford, P., and Ternberg, J.: Pancreatitis and osteolytic lesions. J. Pediatr. 81:350, 1972.

80. Kirkland, J., Ben-Menachem, T., Akhtar, M., Marshall, R., and Dudrick, S.: Islet cell tumor in a neonate: Diagnosis by selective angiography and histological findings. Pediatrics 61:790, 1978.

81. Knoke, J., Stern, R., Doershuk, C., Boat, T., and Matthews, L.: Cystic fibrosis: the prognosis for 5 year survival. Pediatr. Res. 12:676, 1978.

82. Kocoshis, S. A., McGuire, J. S., Arulananthan K., Flynn, F. J., and Gryboski, J. D.: Congenital cutis laxa associated with exocrine pancreatic insufficiency. J. Clin. Gastroenterol. 3:69, 1981.

83. Kopel, F. B.: Gastrointestinal manifestations of cystic fibrosis. Gastroenterology 62:483, 1972.

83a. Kramer, J., Bell, M., de Schryver, K., Bower, R., Ternberg, J., and White, N.; Clinical and histologic indications for extensive pancreatic resection in nesidioblastosis. Am. J. Surg. 143:116, 1982.

84. Kulczycki, L.: Incidence of cystic fibrosis in black children — revisited. J. Pediatr. 92:855, 1978.

85. Kulczycki, L. L., and Schwachman, H.: Studies in cystic fibrosis of the pancreas: Occurrence of rectal prolapse. N. Engl. J. Med. 259:409, 1958.

86. Lebenthal, E., and George, D. E.: Pancreatic diseases. In Lebenthal, E. (ed.): Textbook of Gastroenterology and Nutrition in Infancy. New York, Raven Press, 1981, pp. 1037–1055.

87. Lebenthal, E.: Pancreatic function and disease in infancy and childhood. Adv. Pediatr. 25:223, 1978.

88. Lebenthal, E., Antonowicz, I., and Schwachman, H.: The interrelationship of enterokinase and trypsin activities in intractable diarrhea of infancy, celiac disease, and intravenous hyperalimentation. Pediatrics 56:585, 1975.

89. Lebenthal, E., Antonowicz, I., and Schwachman, H.: Enterokinase and trypsin activities in pancreatic insufficiency and diseases of the small intestine. Gastroenterology 70:508, 1976.

90. Lebenthal, E., and Schwachman, H.: The pancreas — Development, adaption and malfunction in infancy and childhood. Clin. Gastroenterol. 6:397, 1977.

91. Lemen, R. J., Gates, A. J., Mathe, A. A., Waring, W. W., Hyman, R. L., and Kadowitz, P. D.: Relationship among digital clubbing, disease severity, and serum prostaglandins F_2 and E concentrations in cystic fibrosis patients. Am. Rev. Respir. Dis. 111:639, 1978.

92. Lemons, J. A., Ridenour, R., and Orsini, E.: Congenital absence of the pancreas and intrauterine growth retardation. Pediatrics 64:255, 1979.

93. Levitt, M., Johnson, S., Ellis, C., and Engel, R. R.: Influence of amylase assay technique on renal clearance of amylase:creatine ratio. Gastroenterology 72:1260, 1977.

94. Lilibridge, C., and Townes, P. L.: Physiologic deficiency of pancreatic amylase in infancy. A factor in iatrogenic diarrhea. J. Pediatr. 82:279, 1973.

95. Lippe, B., Sperling, M., and Dooley, R.: Pancreatic alpha and beta cell functions in cystic fibrosis. J. Pediatr. 90:751, 1977.

96. Lloyd-Still, J. D.: Oral fatty acid supplementation in cystic fibrosis. Pediatrics 64:50, 1979.

97. Lowe, C. U., and May, C. D.: Selective pancreatic deficiency: absent amylase, diminished trypsin and normal lipase. Am. J. Dis. Child. 82:459, 1951.

98. MacLean, W., and Tripp, W.: Cystic fibrosis with edema and falsely negative sweat test. J. Pediatr. 83:86, 1973.

99. Mah, P. T., Loo, D. C., and Tock, E P. C.: Pancreatic acinar cell carcinoma in childhood. Am. J. Dis. Child. 128:101, 1974.

100. Malik, S A., Vankley, H., and Knight, W. A., Jr.: Inherited defect in hereditary pancreatitis. Am. J. Dig. Dis. 22:999, 1977.

101. Matseshe, J. W., Go, V. L., and DiMagno, E. P.: Meconium ileus equivalent complicating cystic fibrosis in postneonatal children and young adults. Gastroenterology 72:732, 1977.

102. McElroy, R., and Christiansen, P. A.: Hereditary pancreatitis in a kinship associated with portal vein thrombosis. Am. J. Med. 52:228, 1972.

103. McPartlin, J. F., Dickson, J. A. S., and Swain, V. A. J.: Meconium ileus: immediate and long term survival. Arch. Dis. Child 47:207, 1972.

104. Meier, D., Graivier, L., Votteler, T., et al.: Blunt

trauma to the pancreas in children. South. Med. J. 71:895, 1978.

105. Merrill, J. R., and Raffensperger, J. G.: Pediatric annular pancreas: twenty years' experience. J. Pediatr. Surg. 11:921, 1976.

105a. Mitchell, E. A., White, P. R., and Elliot, R. B.: Meconium ileus equivalent in a child with cystic fibrosis taking cimetidine. N.Z. Med. J. 92:155, 1980.

106. Morris, M. D., and Fisher, D. A.: Trypsinogen deficiency disease. Am. J. Dis. Child. 114:203, 1967.

107. Moynan, R. W., Neerhout, R. C., and Johnson, T. S.: Pancreatic carcinoma in childhood. J. Pediatr. 65:711, 1964.

108. Myren, J.: Review: Acute pancreatitis. Scand. J. Gastroenterol. 12:513, 1977.

108a. Nakao, T., Yanoh, K., and Itoh, A.: Aberrant pancreas in Japan: Review of the literature and report of 12 surgical cases. Med. J. Osaka Univ. 30:57, 1980.

109. Nakashima, Y., and Howard, J. M.: Drug induced pancreatitis. Surg. Gynecol. Obstet. 145:65, 1977.

110. Neuman, A., and Ansell, B.: Episodic arthritis in children with cystic fibrosis. J. Pediatr. 94:594, 1979.

111. Neuer, F., Roberts, F., and McCarthy, V.: Osteolytic lesions following traumatic pancreatitis. Am. J. Dis. Child. 131:738, 1977.

112. Neutra, M. R., and Trier, J. S.: Rectal mucosa in cystic fibrosis. Morphologic features before and after short term organ culture. Gastroenterology 75:701, 1978.

113. Niwayama, G., and Vadakan, V. V.: Intestinal obstruction associated with fibrocystic disease of the pancreas. Tohoku J. Exp. Med. 104:289, 1971.

114. Notham, M., and Callow, A. D.: Investigations on the origin of amylase in serum and urine. Gastroenterology 60:82, 1971.

115. Nousia-Arvanitakis, S., Arvanitakis, C., Desai, N., et al.: Diagnosis of exocrine pancreatic insufficiency by the sympathetic peptide N-benzoyl-L-tyrosyl-p-aminobenzoic acid. J. Pediatr. 92:734, 1978.

115a. Odera, G., and Kraut, J.: Rising antibody titer to *Mycoplasma pneumoniae* in acute pancreatitis. Pediatrics 66:305, 1980.

116. Otsuki, M., Saeki, S., Yuu, H., Maeda, M., and Baba, S.: Electrophoretic pattern of amylase isoenzymes in serums and urine of normal persons. Clin. Chem. 22:439, 1976.

116a. Park, R., and Grand, R.: Gastrointestinal manifestations of cystic fibrosis: A review. Gastroenterology 81:1143, 1981.

116b. Parker, P. H., Helinek, G. L., Ghishan, F. K. and Greene, H. L.: Recurrent pancreatitis induced by valproic acid. A review of the literature. Gastroenterology 80:826, 1981.

117. Pearson, H., Lobel, J., Kocoshis, S., Naiman, J., Windmiller, J., Lammi, A., Hoffman, R., and Marsh, J.: A new syndrome of refractory sideroblastic anemia with vacuolization of marrow precursors and exocrine pancreatic dysfunction. J. Pediatr. 95:976, 1979.

118. Penny, R., Thompson, P., Polmar, S., and Schultze, R.: Pancreatitis, malabsorption and IgA deficiency in a child with diabetes. J. Pediatr. 78:512, 1971.

119. Pitchumoni, C. S., Thomas, E., Balthazur, E., and Sherling, B.: Chronic calcific pancreatitis in association with celiac disease. Am. J. Gastroenterol. 68:358, 1978.

120. Pokorny, W., Raffensperger, J., and Harberg, F.: Pancreatic pseudocysts in children. Surg. Gynecol. Obstet. 181:182, 1980.

121. Polonovski, C., and Bier, H.: Pseudotrypsinogen deficiency due to a lack of intestinal enterokinase. Acta Paedr. Scand. 59:458, 1970.

122. Rao, G. J. S., Spells, G., and Nadler, H.: Enhanced UDP galactose: glycoprotein galactosyltransferase activity in cultivated skin fibroblasts from patients with cystic fibrosis and its possible relationship to the pathogenesis of the disease. Pediatr. Res. 11:981, 1977.

123. Renner, I. G., Rinkerknecht, H., and Douglas, A. P.: Profiles of pure pancreatic secretions in patients with acute pancreatitis: the possible role of proteolytic enzymes in pathogenesis. Gastroenterology 75:1090, 1978.

124. Rey, J., Frezel, J., Ryper, P., and Lanny, M.: L'absence congénitale de lipase pancréatique. Arch. Fr. Pediatr. 23:5, 1966.

125. Riccardi, V. M., Shih, V. E., Holmes, L. B., and Nardi, G. L.: Hereditary pancreatitis: Nonspecificity of aminoaciduria and diagnosis of occult disease. Arch. Intern. Med. 135:822, 1975.

126. Rich, R., Dehner, L., Okinaga, K., Deeb, L. C., et al.: Surgical management of islet cell adenoma in infancy. Surgery 84:519, 1978.

127. Ristow, S., Condemi, J., Stuard, D., et al.: Systemic amyloidosis in cystic fibrosis. Am. J. Dis. Child. 131:586, 1977.

128. Robinson, P. G., and Elliot R. B.: Cystic fibrosis screening in the newborn. Arch. Dis. Child. 54:301, 1976.

129. Roller, R., and Kern, F., Jr.: Minimal bile acid malabsorption and normal bile acid breath tests in cystic fibrosis and acquired pancreatic insufficiency. Gastroenterology 72:661, 1977.

130. Rosenstein, B. J., and Langbaum, T. S.: Incidence of meconium abnormalities in newborn infants with cystic fibrosis. Am. J. Dis. Child. 134:72, 1980.

131. Rubin, S. Z., and Ein, S. H.: The unusual presentation of pancreatitis in infancy. J. Pediatr. Surg. 14:146, 1979.

132. Sacher, M., Kobsa, A., and Shmerling, D. H.: PABA screening test for exocrine pancreatic function in infants and children. Arch. Dis. Child. 53:639, 1978.

133. Salonen, I.: Congenital duodenal obstruction. Acta Paediatr. Scand. (Suppl.) 272:786, 1978.

134. Saunders, E. F., Gall, G., and Freedman, M.: Granulopoiesis in Shwachman's syndrome. Pediatrics 64:515, 1979.

135. Schaad, U., Kraemer, R., Gaze, H., and Hadorn, B.: One hour blood xylose in cystic fibrosis. Arch. Dis. Child. 53:756, 1978.

136. Schussheim, A., Choi, S., and Silverberg, M.: Exocrine pancreatic insufficiency with congenital anomalies. J. Pediatr. 89:782, 1976.

137. Schuster, S., Schwachman, H., Toyama, W., Rubino, A., and Khaw, K.: The management of portal hypertension in cystic fibrosis. J. Pediatr. Surg. 12:201, 1977.

138. Shwachman, H.: Cystic fibrosis. *In* Lebenthal,

E. (ed.): Textbook of Gastroenterology and Nutrition in Infancy. New York, Raven Press, 1981, pp. 1027–1036.

139. Shwachman, H., Diamond, L., Oski, F., and Khaw, K.: The syndrome of pancreatic insufficiency and bone marrow dysfunction. J. Pediatr. 65:645, 1964.

140. Shwachman, H., and Holsclaw, D.: Complications of cystic fibrosis. Editorial. N. Engl. J. Med. 281:500, 1969.

141. Shwachman, H., and Holsclaw, D.: Examination of the appendix at laparotomy as a diagnostic clue in cystic fibrosis. N. Engl. J. Med. 286:1300, 1972.

142. Shwachman, H., Kulczycki, L., and Khaw, K. T.: Studies in cystic fibrosis: A report of 65 patients over 17 years of age. Pediatrics 36:689, 1965.

143. Shwachman, H., Redmond, A., and Khaw, K. T.: Studies of cystic fibrosis: report of 130 patients diagnosed under 3 months of age over a 20 year period. Pediatrics 46:335, 1970.

144. Sheldon, W.: Congenital pancreatic lipase deficiency. Arch. Dis. Child. 39:268, 1964.

145. Shepherd, R., Cooksley, W., and Cooke, W.: Improved clinical status following nutritional therapy in cystic fibrosis. J. Pediatr. 97:351, 1980.

146. Shigemoto, H., Endo, S., Isomoto, T., Sano, K., and Taguchi, K.: Neonatal meconium obstruction in the ileum without mucoviscidosis. J. Pediatr. Surg. 13:475, 1978.

147. Shmerling, D. H., Prader, A., Hitzy, W. H, Giedon, A., Hadorn, B., and Kuhni, M.: The syndrome of exocrine pancreatic insufficiency, neutropenia, metaphyseal dysostosis and dwarfism. Helv. Paediatr. Acta 24:547, 1969.

148. Sibert, J. R.: Hereditary pancreatitis in England and Wales. J. Med. Genet. 15:189, 1978.

149. Sibert, J. R.: Pancreatitis in childhood. Postgrad. Med. J. 55:171, 1979.

150. Sibert, J. R.: Pancreatitis in children: A study in the North of England. Arch. Dis. Child. 50:443,.1975.

151. Singh, M., and Webster, P.: Neurohormonal control of pancreatic secretion — A review. Gastroenterology 74:294, 1978.

152. Slovis, T. L., Berdon, W. D., Haller, J. O., Baker, D. H., and Rosen, L.: Pancreatitis and the battered child syndrome: report of two cases with skeletal involvement. Am. J. Roentgenol. Radium Ther. Nucl. Med. 125:456, 1975.

153. Smalley, C., Brown, G., Parkes, M. E. T., Tease, H., Brookes, V., and Anderson, C.: Reduction of bile acid loss in cystic fibrosis by dietary means. Arch. Dis. Child. 53:477, 1978.

154. Stanley, C. A., and Baker, L.: Hyperinsulinism in infants and children. Adv. Pediatr. 23:315, 1976.

155. Strobel, C. T., Smith, L. E., Fonkalsrud, E. W., and Isenberg, J. N.: Ectopic pancreatic tissue in the gastric antrum. J. Pediatr. 92:586, 1978.

155a. Stroud, W. H., Cullom, J. W., and Anderson, M. C.: Hemorrhagic complications of severe pancreatitis. Surgery 90:657, 1981.

156. Tarlow, M. J., Hadorn, B., Arthurton, M. W., and Lloyd, J. K.: Intestinal enterokinase deficiency. Arch. Dis. Child. 45:651, 1970.

157. Thomas, C. G., Jr., Underwood, L. E., Carney, C. N., Dolcourt, J. L., and Whitt, J.: Neonatal and infantile hypoglycemia due to insulin excess. Ann. Surg. 185:505, 1977.

158. Toskes, P. P., Hansen, J., Cerda, J., and Deren, J. J.: Vitamin B_{12} malabsorption in chronic pancreatic insufficiency. N. Engl. J. Med. 284:627, 1971.

159. Townes, P. P.: Proteolytic and lipolytic deficiency of the exocrine pancreas. J. Pediatr. 75:221, 1969.

160. Townes, P. L., Bryson, M., and Miller, G.: Further observations on trypsinogen deficiency disease: report of a second case. J. Pediatr. 71:220, 1967.

160a. Townes, P. L., and White, M.: Identity of two syndromes. Am. J. Dis. Child, 135:248, 1981.

161. Venugopal, S., and Shandling, B.: Meconium ileus: laparotomy without resection, anastomosis or enterostomy. J. Pediatr. Surg. 14:715, 1979.

161a. Walsh, M. J., and Nadeer, H.: Methylumbelliferyl guanidinobenzoate — Reactive proteases in human amniotic fluid: Promising marker for the intrauterine detection of cystic fibrosis. Am. J. Obstet. Gynecol. 137:978, 1980.

161b. Warshaw, A. L., and Lee, K. H.: Serum ribonuclease elevations and pancreatic necrosis in acute pancreatitis. Surgery 86:227, 1979.

162. Watkins, J., Tercyak, A., Szczepanik, P., and Klein, P.: Bile salt kinetics in cystic fibrosis: influence of pancreatic enzyme replacement. Gastroenterology 73:1023, 1979.

163. Weber, A., Roy, C., Chartraud, L., Lepage, G., Dufour, O., Morin, C., and Lasalle, R.: Relationship between bile acid malabsorption and pancreatic insufficiency in cystic fibrosis. Gut 17:295, 1976.

164. Winship, D., et al.: Pancreatitis: Pancreatic pseudocysts and their complications. Gastroenterology 73:593, 1977.

165. Wolsdorf, J. I., and Senior, B.: Insulinoma. Pediatrics 64:496, 1979.

166. Wood, R. E.: Cystic fibrosis: Diagnosis, treatment and prognosis. South. Med. J. 72:189, 1979.

167. Wood, R. E., Boat, T. F., and Doershuk, C. F.: state of the art — Cystic fibrosis. Am. Rev. Respir. Dis. 113:844, 1976.

168. Zoppi, G., Andreotti, G., Panjo-Ferrara, F., Njal, D. M., and Baburro, D.: Exocrine pancreas function in premature and full term neonates. Pediatr. Res. 6:880, 1972.

169. Zoppi, G., Shmerling, H., Gaburro, D., and Prader, A.: The electrolyte and protein contents and outputs in duodenal juice after pancreozymin and secretin stimulation in normal children and children with cystic fibrosis. Acta Paediatr. Scand. 59:692, 1970.

Chapter Sixteen

DISEASES OF THE SMALL INTESTINE

The small intestine is the major site of intestinal transport and absorption of nutrients. During fetal life it lengthens and differentiates from a primitive gut into a small bowel approximately 250 cm in length. Figure 16–1, a modification from Arey,[5] illustrates developmental progression.

Embryology. The small intestine arises from the fetal midgut, when during the third and fourth weeks of gestation it protrudes into the vitelline sac.[21a, 62] There it elongates and rotates counterclockwise about the superior mesenteric artery. At about ten weeks, after the duodenum and splenic flexure of the colon have been fixed by mesenteric bands, the small intestine returns to the abdomen to complete a 270 degree counterclockwise rotation and to continue to grow in length and thickness, elongating 1000 fold between 5 and 40 weeks of gestation. At birth, intestinal length is approximately three times the crown to heel length of the infant, and up to two years of age a rough approximation can be made by multiplying this length by five or six.[115, 139] In premature infants, measurements of the small bowel have varied between 160 and 240 cm. Intestinal length is increased, however, in infants with prune belly.[101]

During the first few months of development, the intestinal epithelium is composed of inner and outer epithelium and central mesenchyme. The primitive intestinal epithelium forms in a cylindric shape and is filled with glycogen. It proliferates and becomes pseudostratified to occlude the duodenal lumen, which is later re-established by dissolution and vacuolization of the cells. By the 17-mm embryonic stage (five to six weeks), the lumen is patent and smooth, and by the 19- to 23-mm stage (seven to eight weeks), mesenchymal clusters are noted and villi begin to form. By 10 to 11 weeks, villi are obvious in the proximal small bowel, and crypts with Paneth cells are noted at 12 weeks. Changes progress caudad, although total occlusion of the lumen never occurs beyond the duodenum. By the 24-mm stage, villi are present in the jejunum, less developed in the proximal ileum, and still absent from the distal small bowel. By the 78-mm stage, villi cover the entire small bowel and at three months are present even in the colon. Colonic villi later disappear.

The musculature too develops in a craniocaudal fashion in the small bowel, contrary to caudocranial development in the colon, with circular muscle present in the proximal duodenum in the 10-mm fetus. By the 21-mm stage, this extends throughout the small bowel. Longitudinal muscle first appears at this time and is complete in the 30-mm stage.[60]

At seven weeks, neuroblasts are present in the midgut, with Auerbach's plexus noted at nine weeks and Meissner's plexus

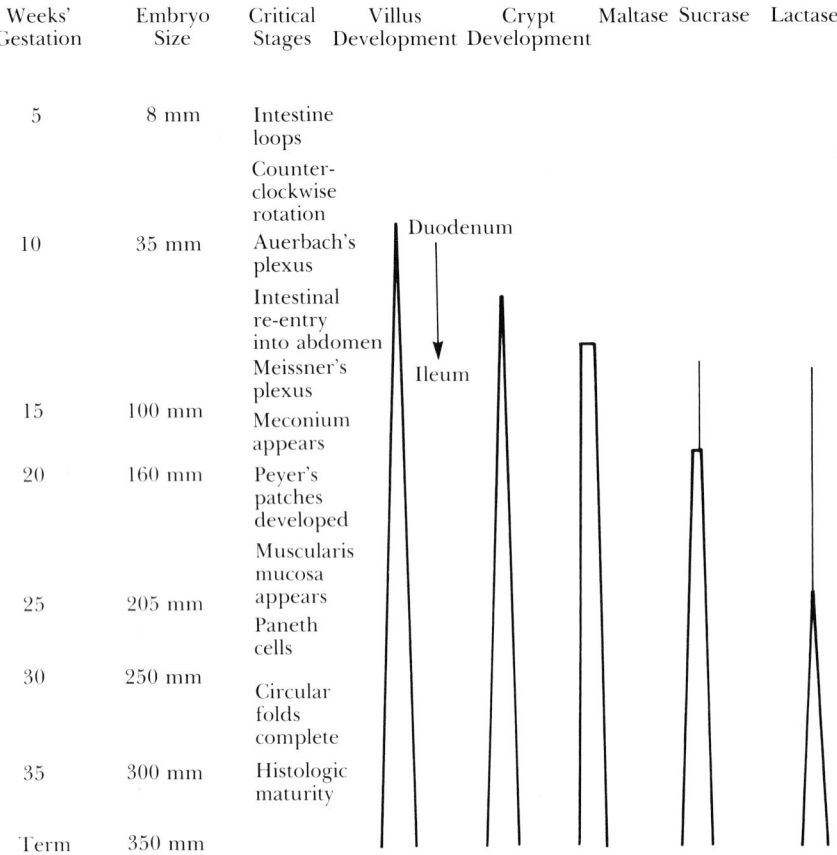

Weeks' Gestation	Embryo Size	Critical Stages	Villus Development	Crypt Development	Maltase	Sucrase	Lactase
5	8 mm	Intestine loops					
		Counter-clockwise rotation					
10	35 mm	Auerbach's plexus					
		Intestinal re-entry into abdomen Meissner's plexus					
15	100 mm	Meconium appears					
20	160 mm	Peyer's patches developed					
		Muscularis mucosa appears					
25	205 mm	Paneth cells					
30	250 mm	Circular folds complete					
35	300 mm	Histologic maturity					
Term	350 mm						

Figure 16–1 Development of the small intestine through gestation.

at 13 weeks — a time when peristalsis is first observed.

Lymphocytes are apparent at 15 weeks and Peyer's patches at 20 weeks. The latter increase throughout gestation until 20 years of age. As villi attain their shape, mucosal epithelial cells become columnar and by eight to ten weeks have demonstrable microvilli. Between 10 and 20 weeks, the absorptive cells contain glycogen and meconium corpuscles, which may be lysosomes and which, although they decrease in number, are still present at term. Enteroendocrine cells are identified between 9 and 12 weeks and mast cells by 15 weeks. In intestinal biopsies of neonates, immunoglobulin-containing cells are not noted before 12 days of age. IgA and IgM cells appear at 12 days and IgG cells at two weeks.[109] Before one month of age, the predominant cells are of the IgM type, but thereafter IgA cells increase. There seems to be no difference in duodenal concentra-tions of immunoglobulins between 2-week-old infants and 19-year-olds.[95]

The small bowel epithelial differentiation remains a dynamic process throughout life, for humans, like all vertebrates, have increased small intestinal surface area through the development of the villous epithelial projections into the intestinal lumen. The histologic organization of the intestinal epithelium is summarized in Figure 16–2. In a span of six days, the epithelial cells arise by proliferation in the crypt, migrate up the villus, and are extruded into the intestinal lumen. As noted, DNA synthesis is restricted to the crypt, with protein synthesis persisting as the cells migrate upward. Absorptive capacity is maximal in the mature villous epithelial cell.

Motility. Peristalsis has been detected as early as 11 weeks in distressed fetuses. Very little is actually known about transit time through the infant small bowel, but studies using carmine red markers indicate

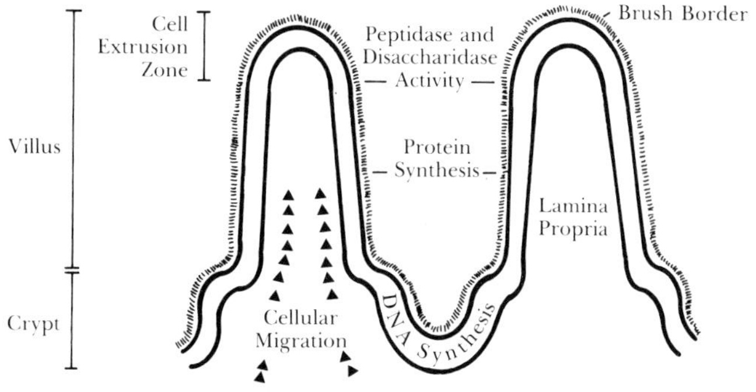

Figure 16–2 Histologic organization of small intestinal epithelium.

mouth-to-anus transit time to be 13.4 ± 4.4 hours in the normal infant three to five days old. Other studies, however, have noted transit times of three to ten hours, with longer transit times recorded for breast-fed infants and increased transit in infants subjected to phototherapy.[68, 128] The motor contribution of the small bowel provides both mixing and propulsion of the bolus, with radiographic studies showing segmentation and peristalsis. Manometric studies record a number of types of pressure waves in the adult, but there are essentially no data available from the infant.[29] Type I waves are 3- to 8-second pressure peaks, usually occurring in groups of two to four after feedings and associated with segmentation. Type III waves are baseline increases in pressure, lasting one to two minutes and associated with propulsion. Type II waves are rare and noted as prolonged pressure peaks. Type IV waves are 0.5 to 1 second long, confined to the terminal ileum, and probably associated with propulsion. An electrical slow wave, continuous with that of the stomach, is considered to be the pacemaker for other waves and moves as a ring caudad. Electrical spike waves appear with small bowel contractions.

Intestinal motility in the infant is difficult to assess because of the presence of complex waves that increase after feedings.[9] Peristalsis is affected by a number of factors. Hormones such as prostaglandins, released during peristalsis, affect contraction of circular and longitudinal muscles; ephedrine suppresses contractions, and kinins and 5-OH-tryptamine stimulate them. Drugs such as neostigmine augment propulsive motility, but morphine delays motility by in-

creasing intraluminal pressure without propulsion. Fever and hyperthyroidism increase the frequency of the slow waves, but hypothyroidism decreases it.

LESIONS OF THE DUODENUM

INTRINSIC CONGENITAL LESIONS

Duodenal Atresia or Stenosis

The duodenal atresias present as high gastrointestinal obstruction, and symptoms vary according to the completeness and site of the lesion.[56, 60, 129, 175]

Incidence. A ten-year survey by the American Academy of Pediatrics Surgical Section revealed 503 cases of duodenal atresia, in which females numbered slightly more than half. The incidence varies from 1 in 9000 to 1 in 40,000 births.

Etiology. The lesion is most likely caused by a persistence of the proliferative stage of gut development and a defect in vacuolization and recanalization that occurs between the fifth and tenth fetal weeks. The extremely high incidence of other embryonic anomalies supports its early embryonic origin. In the 15-mm embryo (37 days), vacuoles coalesce to form first two channels: the larger one on the greater, and the smaller one on the lesser, curvature. Two small openings develop in the region of the hepatopancreatic duct. In the 18-mm embryo, the two channels fuse into one, and one opening into the ampulla obliterates. It is speculated that the rare intraluminal duodenal diverticulum represents a remnant of one of the channels. Unlike more distal atresias, there is little evidence for an intra-

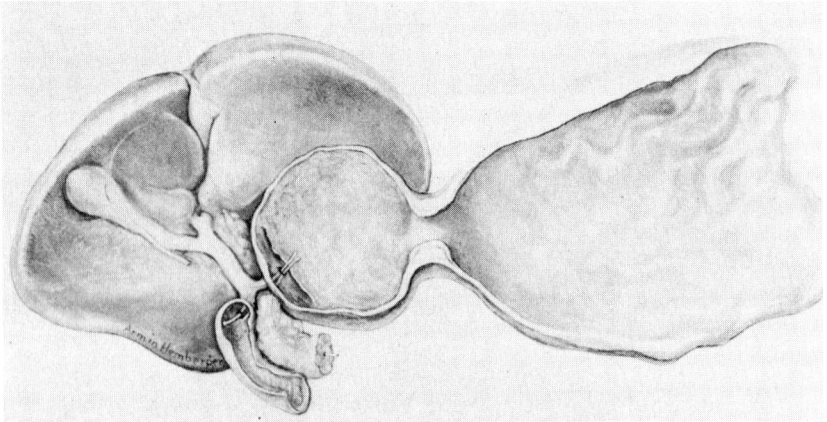

Figure 16–3 Artist's representation of duodenal atresia. The common duct is bifurcated, so that it enters both superior and inferior segments. (Illustration by A. Hemberger, Yale University School of Medicine Collection.)

uterine vascular accident, as this was found in only 1 of 60 cases examined by Nixon and Tawes.[105] Extragastrointestinal tract anomalies occur in nearly 60 per cent of affected infants, with 27 to 30 per cent having Down's syndrome.[125] In one family, four siblings were affected, suggesting an autosomal recessive type of inheritance.

Pathology. Of the intrinsic lesions, atresia constitutes 40 to 60 per cent; web, 35 to 45 per cent, and stenosis, 7 to 20 per cent.

Fewer than half the lesions are supra-ampullary, and the others are infra-ampullary (Fig. 16–3). Occasionally the duodenal atresias are multiple. Gastric diaphragm has been associated with duodenal atresia, but lesions below the ligament of Treitz are extremely unusual.

Nearly all diaphragms attach at the level of, or a few millimeters from, the ampulla of Vater. They are thin, contain little or no muscle, and are lined proximally and dis-

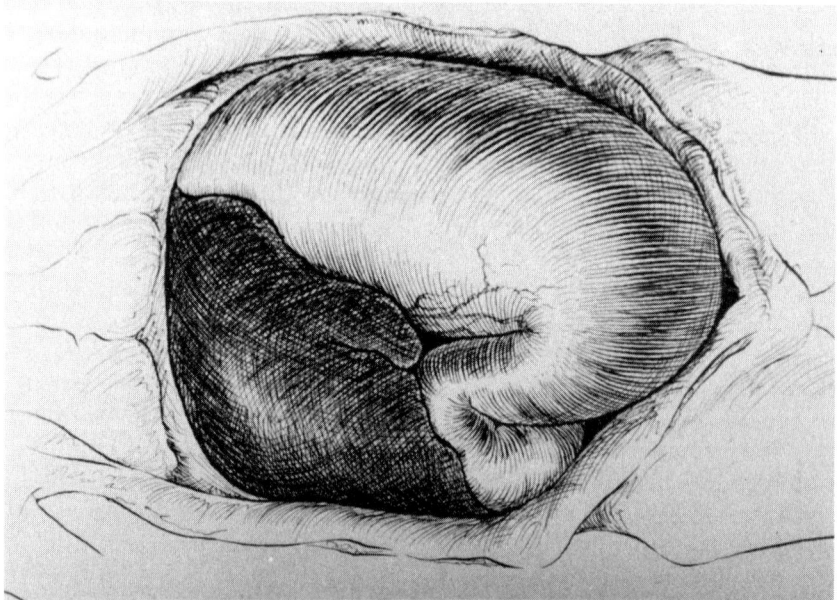

Figure 16–4 Drawing of duodenal atresia in an infant, demonstrating the degree of gastric dilation that develops as a result of duodenal obstruction. (Illustration by A. Hemberger, Yale University School of Medicine Collection.)

tally by duodenal mucosa. Rarely, bile ducts open on the upper or lower surface. The luminal aperture varies from 1 to 10 mm, and the sac may contain old food and concretions. Depending upon the size of the aperture, obstruction varies from complete to partial. In cases with significant obstruction, the stomach and first portion of the duodenum are dilated and occasionally perforate (Fig. 16–4). Associated gastrointestinal anomalies are, in order of frequency: anorectal, esophageal, ileal, multiple atresias, jejunal, and colonic as well as nonrotation with extrinsic duodenal bands, annular pancreas, and anomalies of common duct and gallbladder (Fig. 16–3).[124, 147] Less frequent are omphalocele and renal and pulmonary malformations. If the infant has tracheoesophageal fistula, it is of the atresia with distal fistula type (Table 16–1).

Symptoms. More than half the infants with duodenal atresia are born prematurely, as are 56 per cent of those with multiple atresias (Fig. 16–5). One quarter to one half of the mothers had hydramnios. Those with complete obstruction vomit during the first 24 hours of life, but in those with an incomplete diaphragm or stenosis the onset of symptoms is delayed for days to years. Duodenal lesions cause epigastric distention, pain, and vomiting. Since 30 to 50 per cent of the lesions lie above the ampulla, bilious vomiting, although frequent, is not a prerequisite for diagnosis. Whether the lesion is atresia or stenosis, nearly half the infants pass meconium, which is often gray, green, and mucoid rather than dark and tarry.

Those with milder forms of obstruction often have a history of poor feeding and

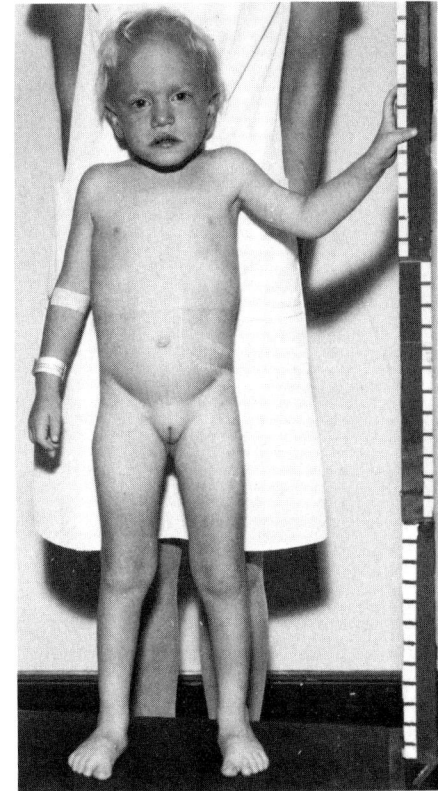

Figure 16–5 This four-year-old girl was operated on as a premature infant for correction of duodenal atresia. She remained below the third percentile for height and weight and had moderate developmental retardation. The white hair and peculiar facies suggested a chromosomal or metabolic defect, but none could be determined.

frequent bouts of vomiting. Older patients describe intermittent abdominal pain, which is worse upon awakening and is not relieved by food or antacid.

Differential Diagnosis. High lesions require differentiation from gastric outlet obstruction.

Diagnosis. A yield of more than 10 ml of gastric juice from the infant stomach is strongly suggestive of upper gastrointestinal obstruction. Supra-ampullary duodenal atresia resembles pyloric stenosis, but flat and lateral erect films of the abdomen will differentiate the two by showing massive distention of both stomach and proximal duodenum. The "double bubble" contour seen in lateral films is characteristic of duodenal atresia (Fig. 16–6). If the obstruction

Table 16–1 Anomalies Associated with Duodenal Atresia

Down's syndrome, 27–30%
Esophageal atresia, 13%
Annular pancreas, 33%
Less common: Imperforate anus
                        Megacolon
                        Omphalocele
                        Biliary malformation
                        Renal malformation
                        Lung malformation

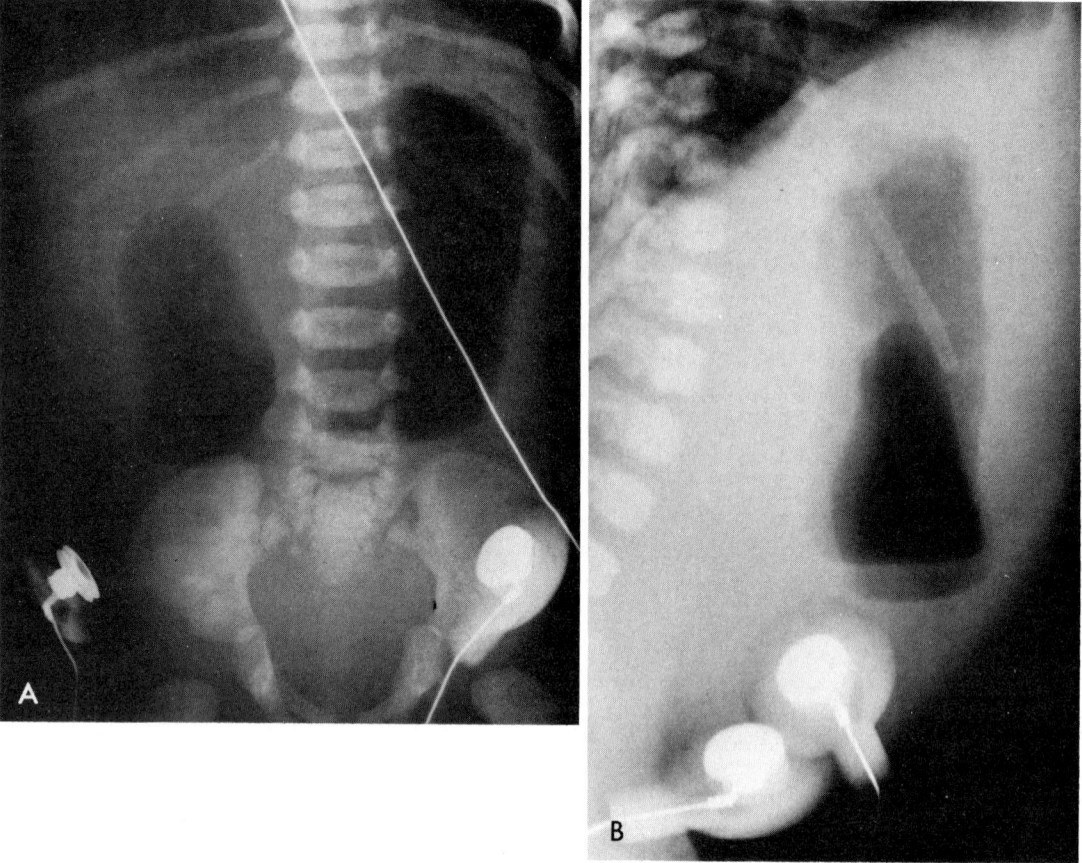

Figure 16–6 Duodenal atresia. A neonate with trisomy 21 was seen for vomiting. Frontal (*A*) and lateral (*B*) erect radiographs show dilatation of stomach and duodenal bulb ("double bubble" sign) as well as fluid-air levels. Patient had complete duodenal atresia. Note the abnormal configuration of the bony pelvis associated with Down's syndrome. (Courtesy of Richard Markowitz, M.D.)

is complete, there is no air distal to it; in cases with stenosis or a wide-aperture diaphragm, however, there is some air in the small bowel and the degree of gastric and duodenal distention is less. Upper gastrointestinal studies, performed only if there is not complete obstruction, will define the rounded cutoff of a diaphragm and perhaps a prolapsed or wind-sock lesion. If barium passes through the aperture, the distal wall of the diaphragm may be outlined. Demonstration of an annular pancreas does not preclude intrinsic obstruction, since the two may coexist.

Endoscopy may be performed to determine the nature of the obstruction in older children with incomplete lesions; in one instance we were successful in dilating the aperture and relieving symptoms for six months.

Treatment. Surgical correction remains the definitive therapy, and simple excision of a diaphragm is often possible. Many lesions require an end-to-end or oblique duodenoduodenostomy or a duodenojejunostomy. Failures do occur and are attributed to anastomosis distal to the actual origin of the diaphragm or to the presence of multiple atresias.[117, 124] Resection of the duodenum is to be avoided because of the proximity of the biliary and pancreatic ducts. In recent studies, the use of a transanastomotic feeding tube has nearly doubled the survival rate.

Complications. Many of the complications associated with duodenal atresia are actually those of prematurity or of other serious congenital anomalies.

Mortality. The overall mortality rate has decreased from 36 per cent to close to 20 per cent.

THE WIND SOCK WEB

The wind sock web or diaphragm is unique in that it represents a ballooning web that has the configuration of an airport wind sock.[126a] Although the origin of the web is stationary, the lead point is pushed distally by peristalsis, and the actual site of obstruction is difficult to localize (seeming distal to where it actually is). As in the more typical duodenal web, the onset of symptoms depends upon the size of the aperture; those that are imperforate or have small apertures cause early upper gastrointestinal obstruction, and those with larger apertures cause only intermittent postprandial vomiting or bloating. The incidence of associated congenital anomalies is similar to or higher than in the simple duodenal atresias. Rowe and associates reported ten infants with wind sock web, nine of whom had multiple congenital anomalies (six, incomplete ro-

tation of the bowel; three, situs inversus; five, second obstructing lesion of the bowel; and three, Down's syndrome). Other anomalies were hypoplastic kidneys, cardiac septal defects, coarctation of the aorta, omphalocele, imperforate anus, Hirschsprung's disease, accessory spleen, and genitourinary and osseous malformation.

To avoid the pitfalls in diagnosis and treatment of this lesion, air contrast radiographic studies are often required (Fig. 16–7). A catheter should be threaded through the pylorus to the point of obstruction, and a marker stitch placed at the point of invagination of the bowel (site of origin of web). The duodenum should be incised longitudinally, and the web incised. At the time of surgery, patency should be established to the bowel above and below the diaphragm.

Congenital Hypertrophic Stenosis of the Duodenum

This extremely rare disorder is indistinguishable clinically from pyloric stenosis.[68]

Incidence. It has been reported in only two infants.

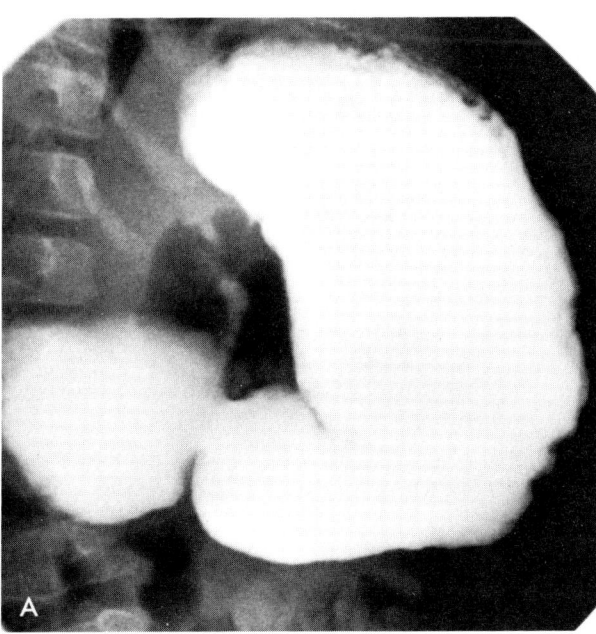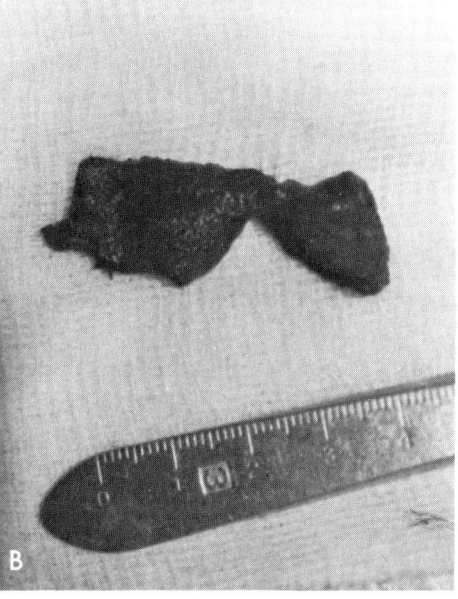

Figure 16–7   A, Radiologic examination of a 6-month-old infant with recurrent vomiting, more marked for solids than for liquids. The duodenal bulb and proximal duodenum are distended, and a small trickle of barium is seen passing through the duodenum. *B,* Resected duodenal wind sock web from the same patient.

Etiology. The cause is unknown.

Pathology. There is hypertrophy of the muscularis of the proximal duodenum.

Symptoms. The symptoms are those of gastric outlet obstruction and develop after the first weeks of life. Vomiting is at first intermittent but becomes continuous and increases in intensity until it is projectile. The vomitus contains digested or undigested formula or gastric contents and does not contain bile. Gastric peristaltic waves are visible in the left upper quadrant, and the abdomen is scaphoid below the umbilicus. The bowel sounds are normal. An olive-like mass may be palpated in the epigastrium or right upper quadrant.

Diagnosis. Radiologic examination of the abdomen shows a large, dilated stomach in the flat film, and barium examination demonstrates a narrowed first portion of the duodenum and delayed gastric emptying.

Treatment. As in pyloric stenosis, myotomy (duodenomyotomy) is curative.

Hypertrophy of Brunner's Glands

An extremely rare cause of duodenal obstruction and bleeding is congenital hypertrophy of Brunner's glands, which produces radiologic findings resembling one or more polyps. In some patients, it has been considered a response to gastric hypersecretion. Biopsy of the lesion will determine the origin, and surgical removal is curative.[137]

Gastric Heterotopia in the Small Bowel

Heterotopic gastric tissue in the small bowel is often asymptomatic and is found only incidentally at surgery or at autopsy. In a few cases it causes partial intestinal obstruction, chronic gastrointestinal blood loss, or acute hemorrhage.[28, 104]

Incidence. In one autopsy survey of 150 patients, none had ectopic tissue below the ligament of Treitz, but 1.4 per cent had gastric tissue in the duodenum. Fourteen cases have been described with heterotopic tissue in the jejunum or ileum.

Etiology and Pathology. Congenital gastric heterotopia occurs most often within the esophagus, duodenum, vitelline duct remnants, or Meckel's diverticulum. The secondary or acquired type, on the other hand, is found in jejunum or ileum and is considered to represent gastric metaplasia arising in areas of inflammation undergoing mucosal regeneration. The tissue resembles gastric pyloric glands with mucus-secreting cells and contains few or no parietal or chief cells. True congenital or ectopic tissue resembles a polyp or rugosal mass, measuring 1.5 to 7 cm in length and containing gastric glands, parietal cells, and chief cells.

Symptoms. Lesions in the duodenum are often asymptomatic, although a few cause gastrointestinal bleeding. Those within the small bowel below the duodenum cause chronic, incomplete small bowel obstruction either because of ulceration and stricture formation or because the heterotopic tissue serves as a lead point for small bowel intussusception. Two infants, 11- and 12-months old, had acute gastrointestinal hemorrhage, and two other patients had recurrent melena and anemia.

Diagnosis. The diagnosis is usually made only at the time of surgery. In a few cases, radiologic examination shows a polypoid lesion in the duodenum, but lesions within the small bowel are usually not visualized. It is often only the complications of stricture or intussusception that are evident. The technetium scan is of value in detecting gastric mucosa and may prove of value in the diagnosis of this lesion as well as of Meckel's diverticulum.

Treatment. Resection of the affected segment is curative.

PANCREATIC HETEROTOPIA

This lesion is less common, often presenting as a polypoid, small bowel lesion causing small bowel obstruction. Diagnosis is made at operation, and resection is curative.[3b]

EXTRINSIC DUODENAL LESIONS

Annular Pancreas

Although this anomaly of the pancreas is sometimes associated with pancreatitis or hyperinsulinism, it most often causes obstruction of the duodenum. It is therefore discussed here[68, 118] as well as in Chapter 15.

Incidence. Annular pancreas is the most common cause of extrinsic duodenal obstruction in infancy and accounts for 10 to 30 per cent of all duodenal obstructions. It is more common in males than in females, and in a few instances it has been reported in siblings.[103]

Symptoms. The lesion, which is discussed in detail elsewhere, may cause symptoms resembling those of duodenal atresia: complete upper gastrointestinal obstruction or chronic abdominal pain and vomiting.

Diagnosis. The radiologic examination may show the "double bubble" sign of complete atresia or may show a smooth compression or narrowing of the right side of the second portion of the duodenum (Fig. 16–8).

Treatment. The treatment is duodenojejunostomy and examination of the distal duodenum for additional intrinsic atresias or webs.

Congenital Preduodenal Portal Vein

This is one of the more unusual causes of extrinsic duodenal obstruction and may be confused with a diaphragm or extrinsic band.

Incidence. The disease is being recognized with increasing frequency; 54 cases were reported by 1980 as compared with 43 in 1978.[47, 58, 86]

Etiology and Pathogenesis. The anomalous portal vein causes straightening of the proximal duodenal curve and superior and medial displacement of the proximal duodenum. Actually, an anterior position of the portal vein in the free edge of lesser omentum or in its relation to the duodenum is extremely rare, and that obstruction is usually due to other causes. In one group, 70 per cent had malrotation; 28 per cent, situs inversus; and 23 per cent, an annular pancreas. Biliary atresia is an associated anomaly in one sixth of patients.

Symptoms. Symptoms develop between the second day and several months of life. The babies become uncomfortable as they feed, and the epigastrium is distended. At

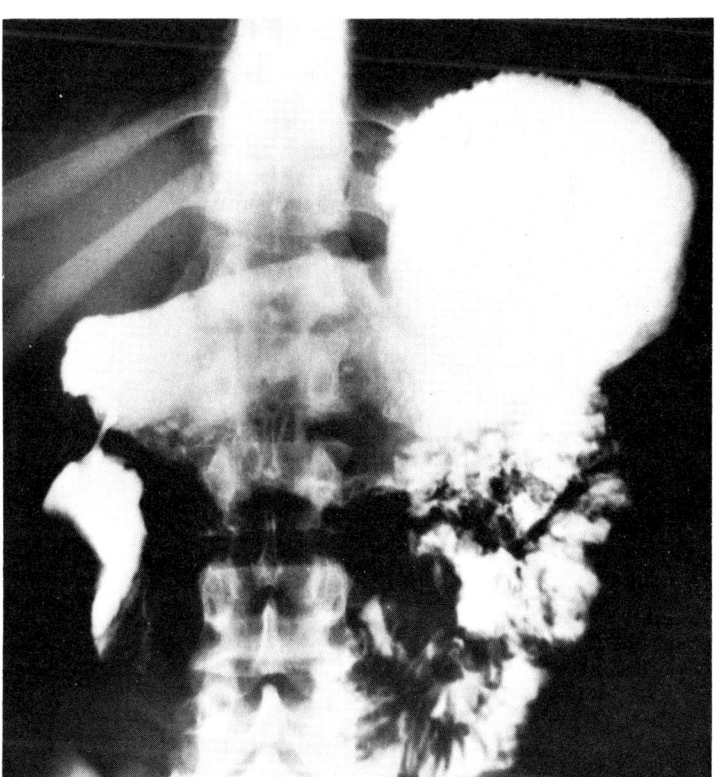

Figure 16–8 Annular pancreas in a patient presenting with vomiting. A short, markedly narrowed segment of descending duodenum is seen. The diagnosis was confirmed at the time of surgery at which time a bypass operation was performed.

first, they vomit only after feedings but later vomit at any time, and eventually the vomitus contains bile and occasionally blood. Peristaltic waves are visible in the left epigastrium. The bowel sounds are normal, and the abdomen below is not distended.

Diagnosis. Plain films of the abdomen show a dilated stomach and large proximal duodenum, which in the lateral view suggests a "double bubble" effect. Barium examination shows the dilated stomach, large duodenal bulb, straightening of the normal duodenal curve, and superior and medial displacement of the proximal duodenum.

Treatment. Gastrojejunostomy provides drainage of the gastric contents into the small bowel without disrupting duodenal structures.

Superior Mesenteric Artery Compression of the Duodenum

This form of vascular compression of the duodenum involves the distal or third part of the organ and causes near-total obstruction.[2, 113]

Incidence. Although the total incidence is unknown, in burn patients it approximates 1 per cent, and the incidence is undoubtedly higher in infants in body casts. The largest reported series contains 20 patients.

Etiology and Pathogenesis. Superior mesenteric artery compression takes either an acute or a chronic form. The acute form, termed the cast syndrome, also includes gastric dilatation and occurs in children placed in body casts, usually for scoliosis. In the absence of casting, the disorder can be precipitated by exaggerated lordosis or by severe weight loss as in dieting athletes, anorectics, or burn patients; it may also occur in patients maintained for long periods in the recumbent position. Normally, retroperitoneal fat lies between the superior mesenteric artery and the root of the mesentery to keep the vessel from pressing against the aorta and spine. After weight loss, hyperextension, or casting, the duodenum may be compressed. At operation, obstruction is usually found to be caused by a retroperitoneal attachment of the mesentery. The chronic form produces

less obstruction and is caused by tension upon the artery, often by duplication cysts of the distal small bowel. Other factors may be a high, tight insertion of the ligament of Treitz or an abnormal angulation of the artery.

Symptoms. Epigastric pain, postprandial vomiting, and intermittent epigastric obstruction are characteristic of this type of obstruction. The onset may be sudden, as with complete obstruction, or chronic and intermittent, with symptoms persisting for weeks to years. The infants limit their intake and are relieved by lying in the prone position.

The physical examination is often unremarkable during asymptomatic periods, but during the attack of pain there is epigastric distention and visible peristaltic waves over the left upper quadrant. The vomiting may cause severe electrolyte imbalances and malnutrition.

Diagnosis. The diagnosis is readily suspected in a child with a body cast. Many children with chronic symptoms have had multiple "negative" radiologic studies. The postprandial pain may suggest small bowel disease, pancreatitis, or superior mesenteric insufficiency. Radiologic examination is best performed when the patient is symptomatic. The most helpful radiologic sign is a line of obstruction in the third portion of the duodenum that passes toward the right lower quadrant (Fig. 16–9). The stomach and proximal duodenum are dilated, and barium passage through the area of obstruction is delayed. The fluoroscopist may note churning of the barium and reverse peristalsis in this area. The obstruction may be diminished by changing the patient's position from supine to lateral or prone.

Complications. Gastric perforation may result from acute obstruction.

Treatment. Body casts must be opened to relieve the intra-abdominal compression. Continuous nasogastric suction and positioning the patient in the prone position are often sufficient to relieve symptoms. If obstruction persists, surgical correction is indicated. A controversy exists as to the procedure of choice for this lesion: duodenojejunostomy, mobilization of the ligament of Treitz, or gastrojejunostomy.

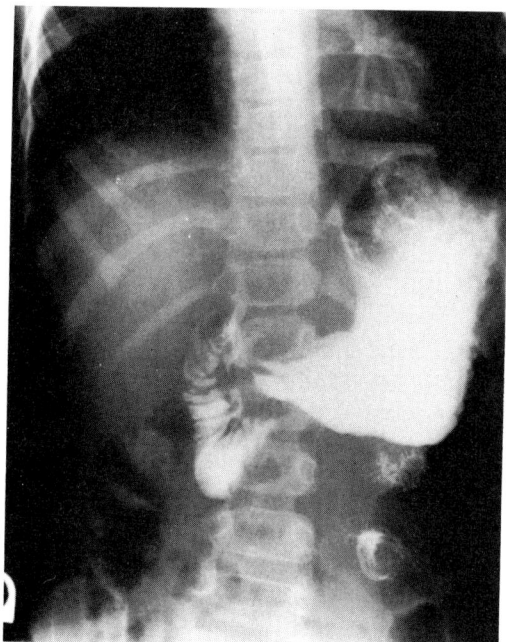

Figure 16–9 This six-year-old female entered the hospital because of recurrent episodes of vomiting since two years of age. Attacks occurred about once every two months and lasted for four or five days. They began with an uneasy, churning feeling in the stomach and continued with vomiting, first of food, then of gastric contents, and finally of bile. Severe electrolyte imbalances had necessitated numerous hospitalizations. Upper gastrointestinal study obtained at the time of admission and when she was symptomatic showed obstruction of the duodenum with the line of cut-off of barium extending from the left upper to the right lower quadrants. Gastric atony and marked delay in the passage of barium from the stomach were noted. A small amount of barium in the region of the ligament of Treitz indicated that the obstruction was not a total one. Surgical exploration revealed obstruction of the duodenum by a fibrous band from the mesentery of the superior mesenteric artery.

SMALL BOWEL DISORDERS

Congenital Lesions

Duplication Cyst or Enterocystomas

The manifestations of the abdominal enteric duplications are related to their location and type.

Incidence. The incidence of all gastrointestinal duplications in infants varies from 0.025 per cent to 1 per cent.[17] The lesions are most common in the ileum and next most common in the esophagus; only 5 to 7 per cent involve the duodenum and in 1978, 63 cases had been accumulated in the litera-

ture.[39] In most series, boys have been affected more often than girls, but in 23 children studied by Grosfeld et al.[65] the lesion was twice as common in girls. A triple duplication involving esophagus, duodenum, and ileum has been described.[136]

Etiology. The theories about the cause are the same as those described for esophageal duplications. Favara et al.[49] suggest a fetal vascular accident as an etiologic factor, since in four patients they found atretic areas of bowel close to the duplications.

Pathology. Duodenal duplication cysts lie within the first or second portion and on the anterior pancreatic side of the organ.[39] They are not mobile and are nearly always noncommunicating. Those in the jejunum or ileum are located on the mesenteric side of the intestine and are mobile. The cysts are cystic or tubular and appear as thin-walled, pale masses that possess an outer wall of smooth muscle and share a common blood supply and intestinal wall with the adjacent bowel (Fig. 16–10A. Heterotopia is unusual, and most cysts are lined by epithelium similar to that of the region whose wall they share. The few that are lined by gastric epithelium are complicated by peptic ulceration. Most of these cysts in the small bowel are noncommunicating and tend to enlarge as they amass secretions. They may be submucosal, intramuscular, or subserosal, measuring 1 to 12 cm. Those that communicate are tubular, and the communication is proximal, distal, or at both ends (Fig. 16–10B). Cysts with only a proximal communication dilate distally to cause volvulus or intrinsic obstruction. Smaller cysts may serve as a lead point for intussusception.[65] Rarely, a duplication of the duodenum may resemble a double gallbladder.[183]

Bleeding results from marginal ulceration of the intestinal mucosa near the site of a communication or from pressure necrosis of the mucosa overlying a large tense cyst.

Symptoms. Although some cysts remain totally asymptomatic throughout life, most of them cause complete or partial intestinal obstruction at some time. Symptoms are usually apparent after the first few days of life and are well defined by the third month. Intermittent vomiting after feeding be-

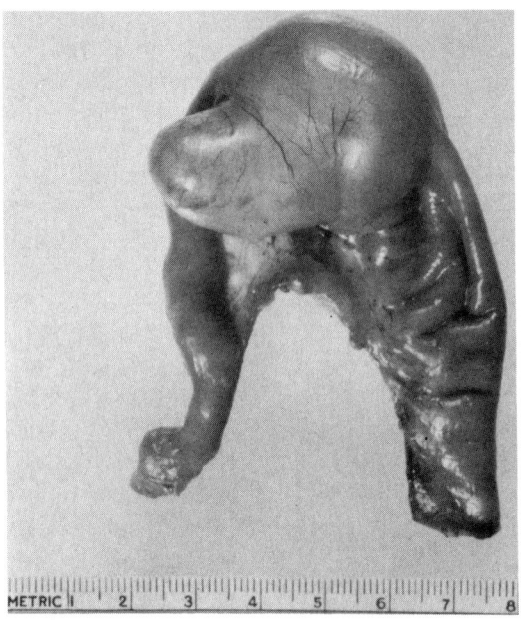

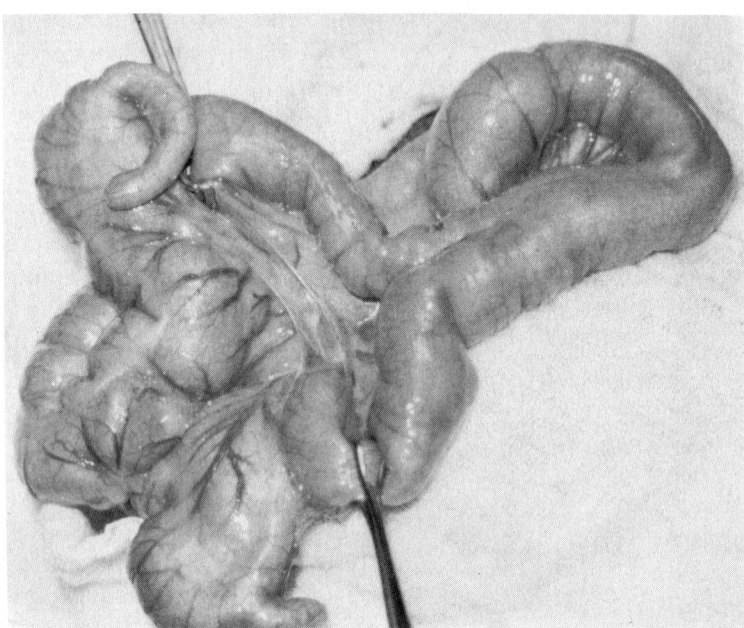

Figure 16–10 A, Noncommunicating duplication cyst of the small bowel. *B,* Long, tubular duplication of the ileum. Cecum and appendix are at upper left. (Courtesy of L. Pickett, M.D.)

comes more and more frequent until oral intake can no longer be retained. As the cyst distends it eventually compresses the intestinal lumen and causes complete obstruction. The vomitus is bile-stained except when the cyst lies in the first portion of the duodenum, in which case the vomitus is gastric in character.[145] Epigastric distention and a palpable mass in the right upper quadrant are the typical physical findings of duodenal duplication cysts. Acute pancreatitis is an unusual form of presentation, occurring when the duplication lies within the pancreas.[176]

Lower small intestinal obstruction is caused by cysts of the jejunum or ileum. There is generalized abdominal distention with bilious or fecal vomiting, and the bowel sounds are either hyperactive or alternate with periods of quiet. A movable mass is palpable in only half of these patients.

Pain and bleeding are caused by peptic ulceration of the intestinal mucosa, torsion of the cyst, or ischemic change in the mucosa overlying the cyst. Volvulus or intussusception are signaled by the sudden development of an acute abdomen.

Diagnosis. Duodenal duplication cysts are often confused with pyloric stenosis, although the cyst is softer to palpation than is the pyloric olive. If it compresses the common bile duct and causes jaundice, it is confused with a choledochal cyst. Right hydronephrosis or a renal tumor is ruled out by pyelography. The cysts lower in the small bowel mimic malrotation, stenosis, diaphragm, tumor, appendiceal abscess, or Meckel's diverticulum.

Radiologic examination of the upper gastrointestinal tract will often show a duodenal duplication as an intramural mass within the first or second duodenum. However, the examination may be entirely normal. Cholecystography in one child suggested a double gallbladder, which proved at surgery to be a duodenal duplication arising from a mass in the vicinity of the common bile duct. Lesions beyond the duodenum are difficult to visualize because they only rarely fill with barium. Scout films of the abdomen will show, if the cyst is of significant size, a mass displacing the abdominal viscera. If the cyst lies in the ileum or near the ileocecal valve, the barium enema examination will show bowel displacement by an extrinsic mass. A duplication in this area that fills with barium cannot be differentiated from Meckel's diverticulum with certainty.

If the lesion arises in the small bowel and extends up through the diaphragm, it is best seen in the lateral chest film as a posterior mediastinal soft tissue density.

A radiologic diagnosis of small bowel duplication cannot be made in nearly half the cases.

Isotope pertechnetate scanning will help to confirm the diagnosis if the cyst contains gastric mucosa, but it will not differentiate it from a Meckel's diverticulum. Echograms are not yet diagnostic in our experience and are used to corroborate other findings suggesting a cystic lesion.

Treatment. Segmental resection of the involved area of bowel with end-to-end anastomosis is the treatment of choice. Simple excision of the cyst is usually impossible because of its mesenteric location and proximity to the vascular supply of the involved segment. Cysts of the duodenum lie in close proximity to the biliary and pancreatic ducts and are treated by creation of a window in the common wall. If the enteric duplications are long and tubular and unresectable for some anatomic reason, they are partially resected, and some form of internal drainage is established between the bowel and remaining cyst. Stripping of gastric mucosa prevents future hemorrhagic complications.

Complications. Complications within the cyst are ulceration with perforation or hemorrhage. Those secondary to it are obstruction, volvulus, or intussusception. Recurrent pancreatitis from a duodenal duplication is a rare but possible complication, as is jaundice from biliary compression.

Intestinal Atresias and Stenosis

Although atresia literally means a lack of perforation, current discussions of the atresias include the congenital stenoses and diaphragms.

Incidence. These anomalies are estimated to occur in 1 of every 20,000 live births. A ten-year survey by the American Academy of Pediatrics Surgical Section revealed 619 cases of jejunal or ileal atresia, which were divided equally between the sexes. In the Lake St. John region of Quebec, ten cases of hereditary multiple atresias lying between the stomach and rectum were found in a ten-year period, and multiple atresias constitute 15 per cent of the lesions.[44]

Inheritance. Small bowel atresias are not usually considered to be genetically transmitted. As just noted, however, there are scattered reports of familial jejunal or ileal atresias, which probably have an autosomal recessive type of inheritance.[35]

Associated Anomalies. The incidence of anomalies outside the gastrointestinal tract is minimal in infants with jejunal or ileal atresia, but it reaches 60 per cent in those with duodenal atresia.

Etiology. Lesions involving the lower small bowel are attributed to a fetal accident occurring after the formation of bowel lumen.[105, 155a] The presence of bile droplets and epithelial cells in meconium indicates that the obstruction developed after the third month of gestation and the presence of lanugo hairs indicates that it developed after the sixth month. The vascular accidents are due most often to prenatal volvulus and less often to incarceration of a fetal physiologic umbilical hernia, intussusception, omphalomesenteric duct, or local perforation.[64, 107] The volvulus is most often localized to the part of bowel distal to the atresia, and nearly one tenth of infants with prenatal volvulus have had cystic fibrosis. Ileal atresia and fistula to the umbilicus have followed amniocentesis at 18 weeks.[121] Experimentally, temporary hypoxia leads to necrotizing enterocolitis changes, whereas local ischemia causes stenosis.[158a]

A viral etiology cannot be entirely dismissed, for jejunal atresia has been reported in twin premature female infants with congenital rubella syndrome.[48]

Pathology. In the jejunum and ileum, atresia is far more common than stenosis, and 38 per cent of patients have multiple atresias (Fig. 16–11). The lesions lie mostly in the proximal jejunum and distal ileum, less often in the distal jejunum, and least often in the proximal ileum, although in one study they were three times more frequent in the midgut than in the proximal or distal end. Wedge defects in the mesentery are common. In one series of 24 infants with jejunal atresia, only 3 had simple obstruction, 5 had other gastrointestinal lesions, 7 had multiple atresias, and 9 had a Christmas-tree or apple-peel deformity.

The atresias are classified in four types. Type I is the diaphragm in which the small bowel wall retains its continuity; in some cases the small bowel is divided by multiple septa. This type is the most common. In type II the atretic areas form long cords, and in type III the bowel ends in a sausage-like blind sac that is separated from the next segment. Type IV, the "apple-peel small bowel," is discussed in the next section.[63, 64, 146] Multiple atresias or septa may extend from stomach to rectum.[72, 123]

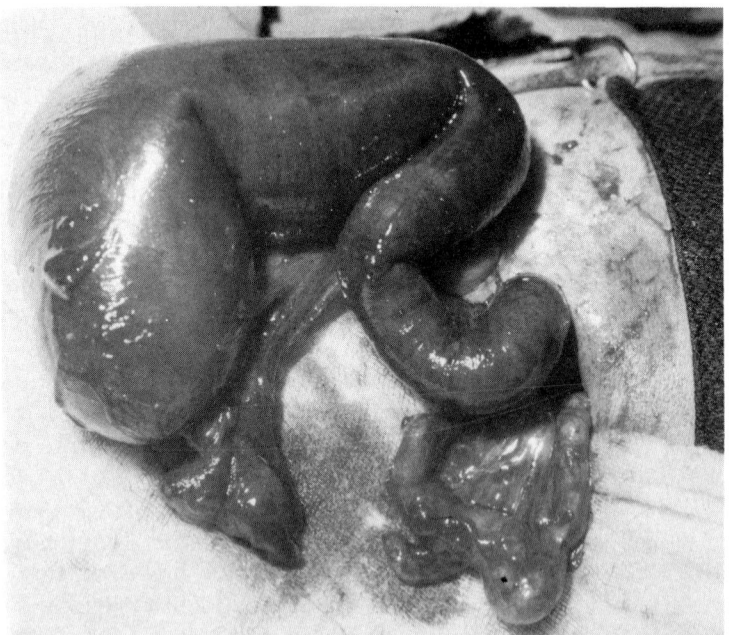

Figure 16–11 Type I, or diaphragm-type, atresia in the mid small bowel. Note massive dilation of intestine above the level of obstruction. (Courtesy of L. Pickett, M.D.)

Symptoms. Prematurity is a factor in infants with small bowel atresias; 25 per cent of those with ileal atresia, 38 per cent of those with jejunal atresia, 54 per cent of those with duodenal atresia, and 56 per cent of those with multiple atresias are premature.

Babies with lesions below the duodenum become symptomatic at or after 24 hours. The vomitus is bilious or fecal, and there is generalized abdominal distention. Most of these babies do not pass meconium before operation, but those who do pass normal meconium.

If abdominal distention is present at the time of birth, one must suspect meconium ileus or peritonitis, for these are often associated with jejunal or ileal atresia. Jaundice may occur with jejunal atresia, and although there is an indirect hyperbilirubinemia, its cause is unknown. There is no evidence of hemolytic disease.

Small bowel stenoses do not always produce obstructive symptoms; sometimes they cause a chronic intractable diarrhea by creating a blind-loop syndrome and bacterial overgrowth.

Diagnosis. Lower intestinal atresias must be differentiated from duplication cysts, meconium ileus, and intestinal infarction; again, plain film of the abdomen is nearly diagnostic. Dilated air-filled loops of bowel extend to the level of atresia, and there is total absence of air below that site (Fig. 16–12). One should hesitate in performing barium enema, for in some cases the distal segment opens freely into the peritoneum. Contrast studies with water-soluble materials show the unused or "micro-" colon and define a low ileal atresia if contrast material is refluxed through the ileocecal valve. Intra-abdominal calcifications indicate a meconium peritonitis, and restriction of bowel shadows to the right upper quadrant suggests intrauterine peritonitis. Small bowel examination with barium is contraindicated in cases of complete obstruction.

Treatment. Simple excision of a diaphragm is adequate therapy for lesions in the jejunum or ileum.[63] Treatment of stenoses in the jejunum or ileum consists of enterostomy or limited resection with end-to-end anastomosis. Side-to-side anastomoses are too often complicated by a blind-loop syndrome. More extensive resections with end-to-end anastomoses are performed for the other types of atresia. There is evidence that the widely dilated bowel proximal to the atresia does not readily adjust to decompression and establish motility, and so proximal resection of the dilated bowel is often undertaken. If this is not possible, as in jejunal lesions, a tapering jejunoplasty may be used. Intraluminal catheters are to be avoided because of the danger of erosion.

Complications. All types of atresia carry the immediate risk of pneumonia, peritonitis, sepsis, and disruption of the anastomosis. Postoperative volvulus, infarction, and functional obstruction sometimes develop. One must always bear in mind that recurrent obstruction may be due to atresia at another site that was overlooked. Obstruction developing a week to several years after surgery is most often the result of adhesions.

The short bowel syndrome is a complication of significant intestinal resection.

Prognosis. In general, the more distal the atresia, the better the prognosis; one study reports a 100 per cent survival in distal atresias in good-risk infants and a 60 per cent survival in poor-risk ones. Survival in jejunal atresia is 50 per cent without proximal small bowel resection and 65 per cent with resection. Proximal small bowel resection does not seem to affect an overall survival rate of 63 per cent in infants with ileal atresia. Those with multiple atresias often require repeated operations.[67a]

Apple-Peel Small Bowel or Type IV Atresia

This type of atresia is discussed separately because it is typically familial and associated with errors in fixation.[40]

Incidence. Fewer than a dozen cases are reported in the literature.

Etiology and Pathology. The lesion derives from either an intrauterine vascular accident or a primary developmental error.

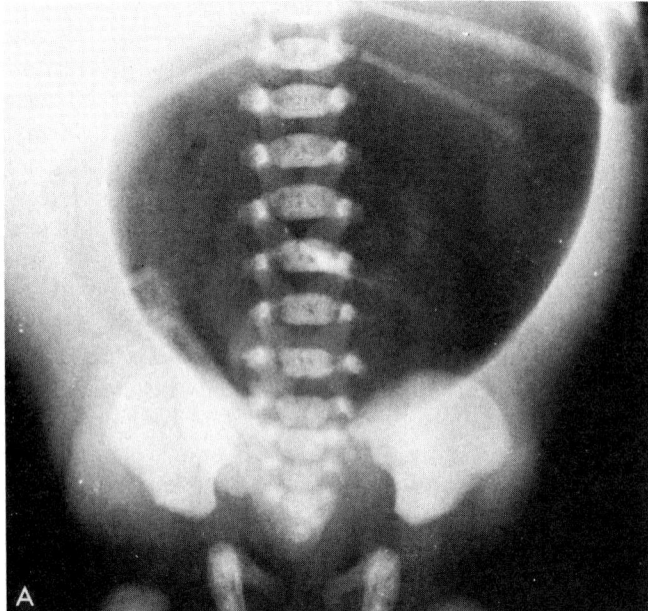

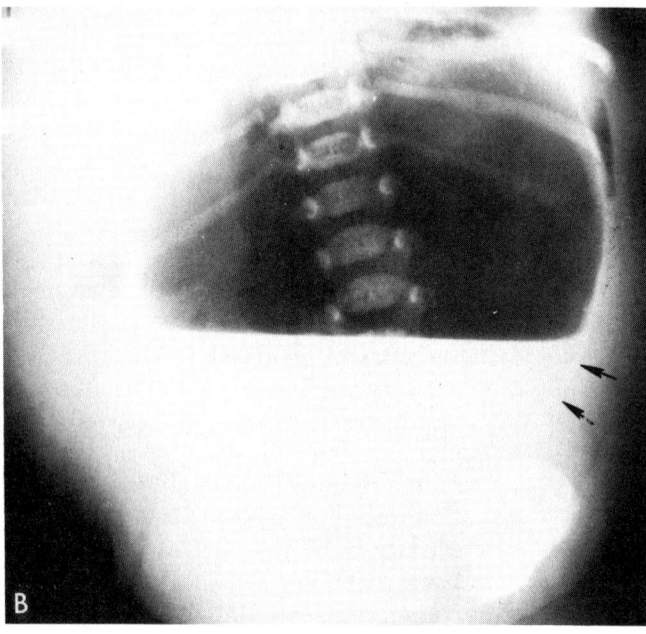

Figure 16–12 Jejunal atresia in a one-day-old infant with progressive abdominal distention. *A*, The KUB demonstrates a large, gas-filled structure in the mid abdomen. On other films, the gas-filled stomach and duodenal bulb were seen to be normal. On inspection of the original films a thin line of calcification was seen surrounding the gas-filled area. The lucent area was found at surgery to be a hugely dilated loop of jejunum immediately proximal to the segment of atresia. The atretic and massively dilated segments of bowel were resected and the ends were connected with an end-to-side anastomosis. *B*, Erect film of the abdomen showing a large air-fluid level in the dilated loop. A faint rim of calcification is indicated by the arrows.

A large portion of proximal intestine is missing because of duodenal and jejunal atresia, and there is malfixation of the remaining small bowel and ascending colon. The proximal small bowel is dusky or blue, and the distal bowel contains meconium. The area of atresia is compatible with an intrauterine volvulus that produces obstruction of the superior mesenteric artery. The distal small bowel lies to the right of an unfixed cecum and twists along a marginal artery derived from the inferior mesenteric artery (Fig. 16–13). The configuration of small bowel about this artery resembles a hanging apple peel, a Maypole, or a Christmas tree, all of which are names given to it.

Symptoms. All of the infants are born prematurely and have symptoms and clinical findings identical to those of duodenal atresia.

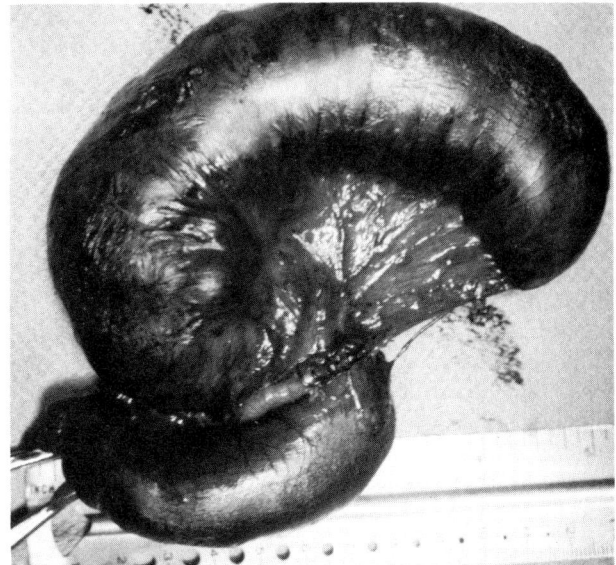

Figure 16–13 Apple-peel small bowel. The distal small bowel lies to the right of an unfixed cecum. (Courtesy of R. Touloukian, M.D.)

Diagnosis. Radiologic studies cannot distinguish this anomaly from duodenal atresia of the simple type. The diagnosis is made at surgery.

Treatment. The atretic bowel is resected, good proximal and distal bowel is anastomosed, and a feeding tube is threaded through a gastrostomy into the distal small bowel.

Prognosis. Malabsorption on the basis of a relative vascular insufficiency in the remaining small bowel is a common postoperative complication and is best treated by a formula containing medium-chain triglycerides, such as Pregestimil. The combination of prematurity, a high incidence of postoperative infection, and anastomotic leakage because of the poor vascular supply contributes to a high mortality.

Errors in Rotation and Fixation of the Gut

Errors in rotation of either the duodenum or the cecum occur during their developmental counterclockwise rotation. Malrotation results in abnormal mesenteric fixations of the small intestine and cecum and obstructive bands. Volvulus or obstruction caused by knotting or twisting of the bowel is present in nearly three quarters of patients with malrotation.[151]

Incidence. These defects are not uncommon, although an exact incidence is not known. They are twice as common in boys as in girls and in rare instances are familial.[162] In the neonate they are associated with diaphragmatic abnormalities and mesenteraxial volvulus.

Etiology. The failures in rotation occur at different times in the normal embryologic process. Two counterclockwise rotations take place, one of the duodenum and the other of the cecum. The gastrointestinal tract of the one-month or 5-mm embryo is a straight tube divided into a primitive foregut, which ends just beyond the pylorus; a midgut, which ends just beyond the later-formed ileocecal valve; and a hindgut, which forms most of the colon and rectum. As rotation begins, the duodenum rotates 90 degrees and downward to the right and lies to the right of the superior mesenteric artery. The small intestine and the right and transverse colon extend into the umbilical cord as they are displaced somewhat by the growing liver. The mesentery attaches lower foregut and upper hindgut close together to the posterior abdominal wall. The midgut is supported by the duodenocolic isthmus. By eight weeks the developing embryo measures 25 mm, and the third part of the duodenum has rotated to 180 degrees under the superior mesenteric artery. By 11 weeks, in the 40-mm embryo, the small intestine returns to the left side of the abdomen and is followed by the cecum and colon. It pushes the fourth part of the duodenum and proximal jejunum to the left of the superior mesenteric artery and cephalad and causes the duodenum to rotate to 270 degrees. The cecocolic loop then moves through the left and right upper quadrants to its final position in the right lower quadrant and completes its own 270 degree rotation about the superior mesenteric artery axis. Its mesentery fuses with the posterior parietal peritoneum, and it becomes fixed permanently.

Pathology

CONGENITAL PERITONEAL BANDS. Congenital peritoneal bands produce extrinsic obstruction of the duodenum and are classified into four types. In type I the cecum lies in the right upper quadrant, and bands extend from it across the descending duodenum to the right paravertebral gutter (Fig. 16–14). In type II the position of the colon is normal, and bands extend from its hepatic flexure across the descending duodenum. Type III bands represent a hypertrophied hepatoduodenal ligament and cross the junction of the first and second portions of the duodenum. They are unassociated with other gastrointestinal anomalies. Type IV bands coexist with an incompletely rotated duodenum and a normally rotated colon. The duodenum lies to the right of the midline, and dense bands bind it to the paravertebral fascia and obstruct the distal duodenum.

ROTATIONAL ANOMALIES. Nonrotation of the midgut results from failure of rotation after the midgut has re-entered the abdomen and sometimes coexists with omphalocele or posterolateral diaphragmatic her-

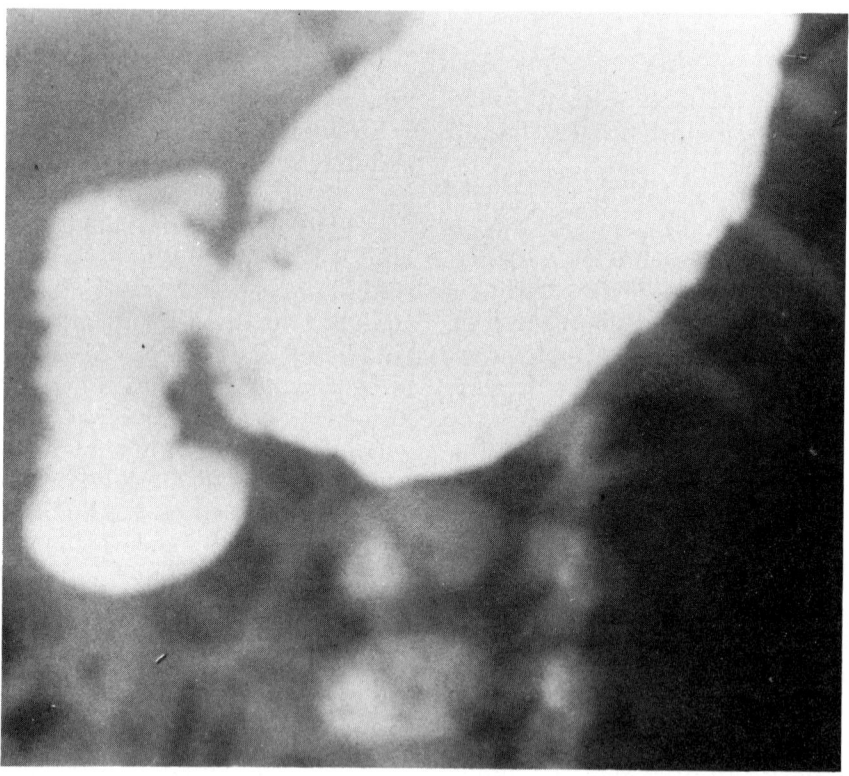

Figure 16–14 Five-day-old infant with midgut volvulus. There was a history of bile-stained vomiting from birth, but a meconium stool was passed on the second day of life. Upper gastrointestinal series demonstrates complete obstruction to the flow of barium at the junction of the third and fourth duodenum. At surgery, a 270-degree clockwise volvulus was found. The entire colon with the exception of the hepatic flexure was on a mesentery, and the lateral peritoneum at the hepatic flexure was stretched over the duodenum, causing the obstruction.

nia.[141] The mesentery of the midgut attaches only in the region of the superior mesenteric vessels and lacks its usual broad posterior anchor. The duodenum extends downward from the pylorus to the right of the superior mesenteric artery and continues into the jejunum out along the direction of the vessels (Fig. 16–15). The small bowel lies to the right and the cecum to the left of the midline. The ascending colon extends inward and attaches to the vessels, duodenum, or jejunum. Volvulus is a hazard if the midgut is not stabilized.

Incomplete duodenal rotation is due to failure of the duodenum to pass behind the superior mesenteric artery and attain its retroperitoneal position. Instead, there is kinking of the duodenum and peritoneal bands pass between it and the first portion of jejunum, causing some degree of obstruction. Volvulus develops if there is a stalklike attachment at the duodenojejunal junction (Fig. 16–16).

Failure of complete rotation of the cecum is the most common form of malrotation and has a familial incidence and an autosomal recessive type of inheritance. The cecum lies in the right upper quadrant or in the midline. The base of the small bowel mesentery is short, and the entire small bowel and right colon are extremely susceptible to volvulus. Extrinsic adhesive bands pass from the colon to the right abdominal wall

and are continuous with the ligament of Treitz. These often cause partial duodenal obstruction. Other variations of cecal malrotation include an inverted cecum, retroperitoneal cecum, internal hernia to the paraduodenal foramen of Winslow, and the anomaly of liver and colon in the right abdomen.

Reversed rotation occurs when the distal midgut re-enters the abdomen first and rotates clockwise to 90 degrees. The cecum rotates behind the superior mesenteric artery, and the transverse colon lies behind the duodenum and artery rather than anterior to them.

Anomalous fixation of the mesentery results if the jejunum fails to pass beneath the superior mesenteric artery. The normal attachment of the small bowel from the left upper to the right lower quadrant fails, and the mesentery is attached in only a small area above the artery. Because of free twisting of the mesentery, volvulus is common. If there is fusion of the posterior parietal peritoneum over the bowel, a paraduodenal hernia develops.

Malrotation with congenital short or undifferentiated intestine has been reported in five patients.[74] It is attributed to defective elongation of the bowel, which normally takes place between nine and ten weeks. Two of three infants had no other anomalies, but one had sirenomelus. Severe diar-

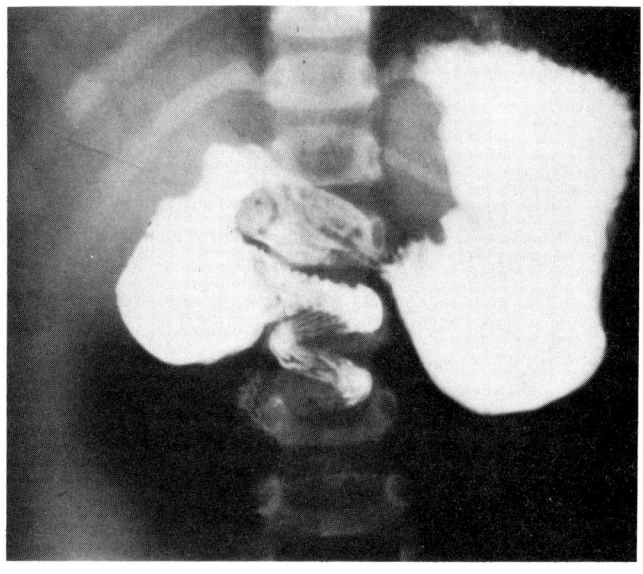

Figure 16–15 Upper gastrointestinal examination of a three-year-old boy who had been operated on nine months earlier for duodenal obstruction. A duodenal band was freed, and he was well for one month. Then chronic diarrhea developed, but radiologic examination and laboratory studies all were normal. Six months later intermittent vomiting developed, and a repeat examination of the upper gastrointestinal tract showed the duodenum to be greatly dilated and to extend just to the right of the vertebrae. Some kinking was noted in the anomalous origin of the proximal jejunum. Surgical exploration revealed obstructive peritoneal bands and an incomplete rotation of the duodenum.

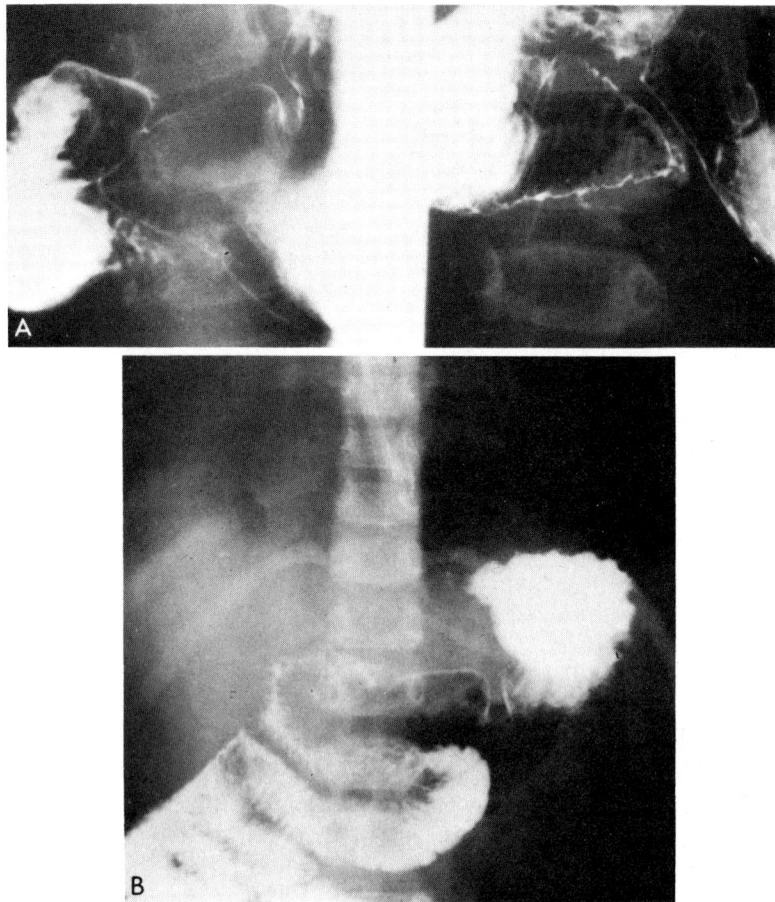

Figure 16–16   P.S., a four-year-old boy, has been operated on at two years of age for lysis of duodenal bands causing duodenal obstruction. At four years of age, chronic diarrhea and vomiting of increasing intensity developed. Radiologic examination of the upper gastrointestinal tract showed *(A)* an incomplete rotation of the duodenum and *(B)* partial duodenal obstruction with a greatly dilated second portion of the duodenum.

rhea and bilious or fecal vomiting were the major symptoms. Two patients had cecal and appendiceal agenesis as well as short, undifferentiated small and large bowels. Two adults had malrotation with cecal and appendiceal agenesis.

Symptoms.   Symptoms are the result of duodenal obstruction or of the complications — volvulus or incarceration of bowel.[24, 144]

Nearly half the infants have symptoms during the first week of life. Bilious vomiting is characteristic of this type of obstruction, and nearly one quarter of babies with duodenal obstruction have projectile vomiting. The presence and type of abdominal distention depends upon the site of the obstruction; epigastric distention is most apparent in those with duodenal bands. A few babies pass blood in their stools; this symptom is most often associated with volvulus. Severe, generalized abdominal distention followed by vascular collapse represents acute volvulus, and in some cases vascular collapse develops so rapidly that few abdominal symptoms precede it. Jaundice is reported in 29 per cent of infants with malrotation who are under one month of age.

Those whose symptoms appear later have cyclic vomiting and intermittent abdominal pain. A few have constipation or a malabsorption syndrome caused by lymphatic obstruction or intermittent volvulus. Chronic diarrhea without steatorrhea can result from a blind-loop syndrome and intestinal stasis with bacterial overgrowth.

Diagnosis.   Plain films of the abdomen

show multiple, dilated, air-filled loops of small bowel.[140] Duodenal obstruction is demonstrated as an air-filled duodenal bulb that contains a fluid level or even as a "double bubble" sign. If the baby has been vomiting, the plain film will not always show dilatation of the duodenum. A barium enema will permit identification of the cecum and demonstrate the degree of rotation of the large bowel. The upper gastrointestinal study will define the site of obstruction and the location of the duodenojejunal junction and jejunum (Figs. 16–14 to 16–17).

Treatment. Obviously, the treatment depends upon the anomaly and consists of surgical transection of bands, release of volvulus, or repositioning of the duodenum or cecum. Appendectomy should be performed at the time of surgery. The reoperation rate is slightly lower if malrotation is corrected without fixation of the mesentery than if the mesentery is fixed. Both groups have a similar survival (84 or 85 per cent). Vascular compromise of the twisted bowel is an indication for resection.[148] Parents of children with uncorrected malrotation must be warned of the position of the cecum in the event of appendicitis. The recurrence of obstructive symptoms after surgery suggests development of adhesions or a band that was missed during the first operation.

Prognosis. The mortality in the neonate is 80 per cent if there is evidence of hemorrhage and necrosis.

Small Bowel Diverticula

Small intestinal diverticulosis is extremely rare in infancy and childhood, with two cases of diffuse small bowel disease reported by 1977.[34]

Etiology. Some diverticula are congenital, but others develop secondary to defects

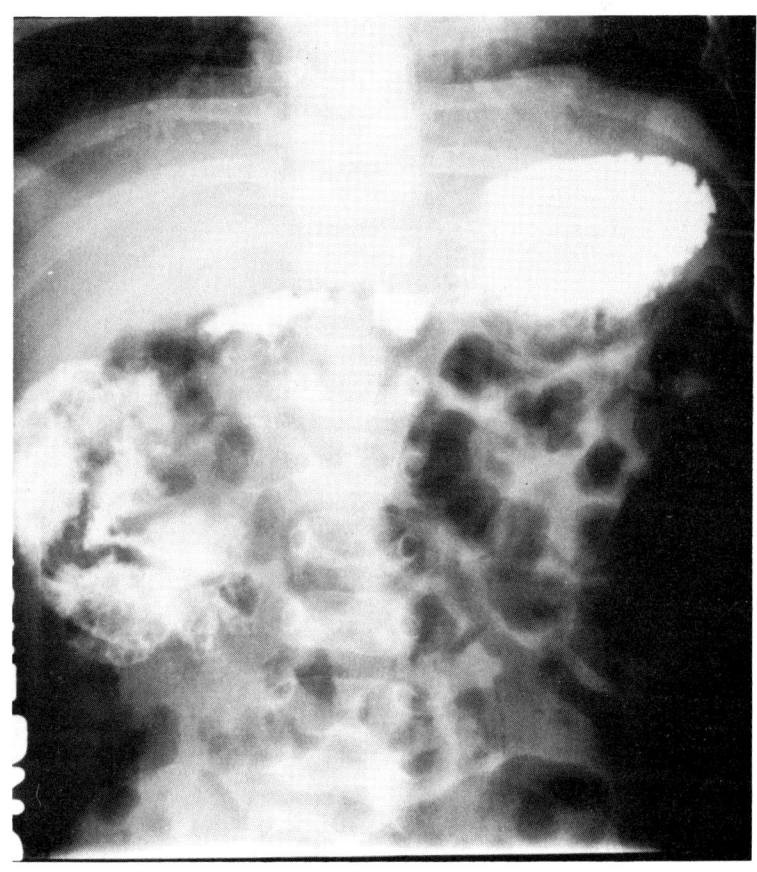

Figure 16–17 Upper gastrointestinal series demonstrating malrotation in a six-month-old boy. The ligament of Treitz is not well demonstrated but is situated to the right of the spine, and proximal small bowel loops are in the right abdomen rather than at the normal location on the left side.

in the adjacent mesentery. Pseudodiverticula associated with Crohn's disease must be differentiated. In one reported infant, diffuse small intestinal diverticula were associated with Noonan's syndrome.

Pathology. In diffuse disease, the diverticula are true congenital ones, extending from the duodenum to the terminal ileum. In one infant there was an associated incomplete rotation of the cecum. Occasionally, small bowel diverticula cluster in the terminal ileum. Solitary duodenal diverticulum arises from the medial wall of the descending duodenum. The diverticula arise from the mesenteric border of the bowel and contain all layers of bowel wall. Not only may they serve as sites for lodgment of foreign bodies, but they may become inflamed to cause perforation or hemorrhage.

Symptoms. There may be no symptoms for years, or they may develop in early infancy. Often, there is some degree of postprandial discomfort, pain, and abdominal distention. Anemia, secondary to malabsorption or chronic gastrointestinal blood loss, may be the only manifestation of the disease. One patient we have seen with this disorder had relatives with megaesophagus and megaduodenum.

Diagnosis. Confirmation is by radiologic examination of the small bowel (Fig. 16–18).

Treatment. Symptoms are treated as for those of a blind-loop syndrome, with broad-spectrum antibiotics and the additional precaution of avoidance of pits in the diet. If symptoms are progressive and disabling and the lesions are localized, segmental resection may be necessary.

Familial Absence of Villi

Described in one patient in 1975,[68] this entity was reported in five more infants in 1978.[36] Characterized by chronic diarrhea from birth, the disease affects both sexes but with a 2:1 preponderance of males to females. In five of the six patients a similar lethal illness had occurred in a sibling, and in two families the parents were related. A fatal disorder of villous atrophy and tubulo-interstitial renal disease has been described in first cousins and may be a similar disease.[43a]

Pathophysiology. Fecal volumes repre-

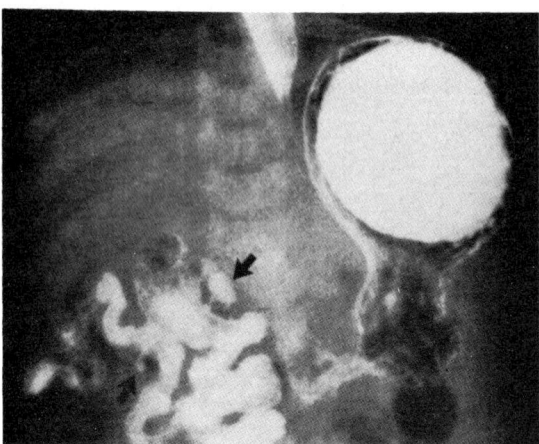

Figure 16–18 Multiple diverticula of the small intestine in an infant. (From Cumming, W. A., and Simpson, J. S.: Intestinal diverticulosis in Noonan's syndrome. Br. J. Radiol. 50:64, 1977, with permission.)

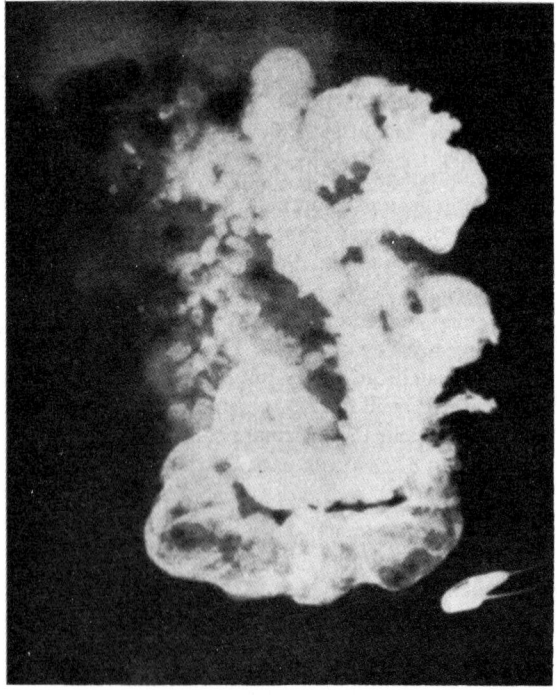

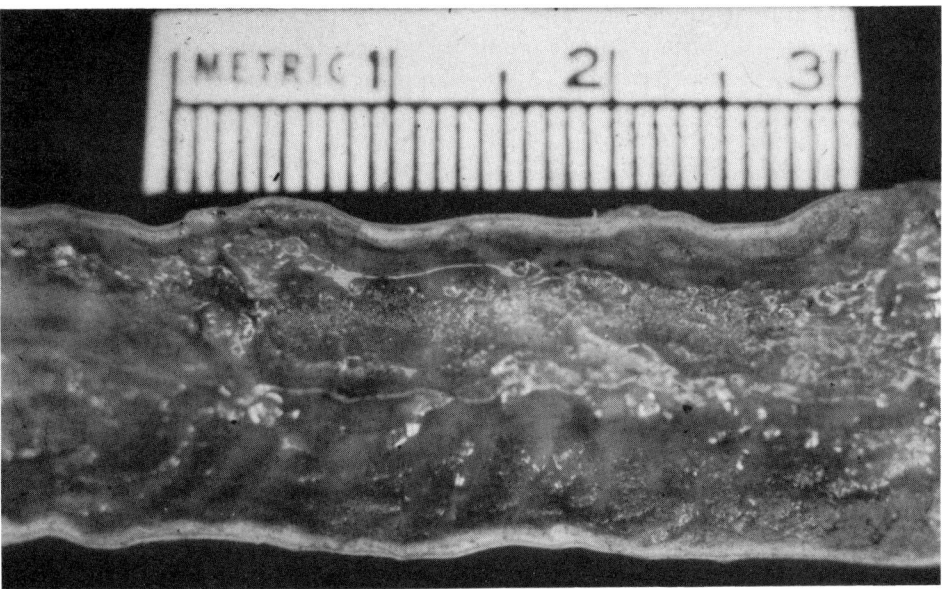

Figure 16–19 R. M., a 10-week-old infant with chronic diarrhea refractory to all therapy, who died two weeks later. The small bowel shows complete absence of villi except in a few scattered areas where there are wartlike clusters of villi.

sented 100 to 200 ml per kg, and the stools contained increased concentrations of Na^+, K^+, and CL^-. Bile salt concentrations in the duodenum were low. Disaccharide, monosaccharide, and vitamin B_{12} absorptions were abnormal. Enteric protein losses were not increased. Small intestinal histology showed total villous atrophy, hypoplastic crypts, and normal or decreased numbers of cells in the lamina propria. Although the small intestine was normal in position and length, it appeared paper-thin (Fig. 16–19). Electronmicroscopic examination showed absent or disturbed brush border, round to oval dense inclusions in the apical cytoplasm of the enterocyte, and an abnormal matrix. Crypt cells, in contrast, were well preserved.

Symptoms. All infants were full-term neonates weighing 2.5 to 3.6 kg. Diarrhea was noted during transitional stooling, and all subsequent stools were watery and foul-smelling. No dietary measures were successful in controlling the diarrhea.

Prognosis. Five of the six infants died, but the survivor showed progressive improvement in small bowel histology at 36 months.

CONGENITAL MOTOR ABNORMALITIES

Intestinal pseudo-obstruction is discussed elsewhere, but congenital motor disorders are described in this section.

Absence of Intestinal Musculature

Mechanical obstruction of the gastrointestinal tract caused by an absence of small intestinal musculature is a disorder that is correctable in only a very few infants.[46, 85, 98a, 149]

Incidence. Fewer than a dozen cases have been reported in the literature.

Etiology. The etiology is unknown, although the defect must be related to a failure of appearance of the anlage of gastrointestinal musculature, which normally develops in the 11- to 13-mm embryo. Genetic factors may be operative, for siblings of some of the babies died in infancy of intestinal obstruction.

Pathology. Congenital absence of duodenal musculature described in one infant was characterized by a grossly normal duodenum, which histologically contained ganglion cells but no musculature. The distal half of the stomach was thickened and hypertrophied, and it and the jejunum contained normal musculature. Another patient had a 30-cm segment of ileum that contained no musculature and was greatly dilated. In the other patients, the lesions were diffuse and the small bowel resembled a string of sausage, having dilated paper-thin areas with short lengths of normal intestine interspersed. The dilated areas contained only mucosa and serosa; the normal areas contained normal intestine. One infant had a local deficiency of circular musculature in the small bowel.

Symptoms. Duodenal lesions simulate duodenal atresia, with a history of maternal hydramnios, vomiting within the first few hours of life, epigastric distention and peristaltic waves in the left upper quadrant. Meconium may be passed. Absence of musculature lower in the small bowel causes symptoms of low intestinal obstruction. These babies are normal at birth but pass no meconium. During the first 36 hours of life, the abdomen becomes distended and the infants vomit bilious and then fecal material. The bowel sounds are variable.

Diagnosis. Plain films of the abdomen show the duodenal lesion, a dilated gas-filled stomach, and gas in the proximal duodenum. Films in those with lower lesions show dilated small bowel loops scattered throughout the abdomen.

Treatment. Treatment of the duodenal lesion necessitates near-total resection of the duodenum with preservation of a small posterior flap to permit entry of the pancreatic and bile ducts and anastomosis of the jejunum to this flap. Single, isolated amuscular segments can be resected, but in most cases extensive lengths of small bowel are involved, and resection is either not feasible or not successful.

Prognosis. Survival has followed surgical treatment of duodenal lesions and of single segmental ones, but more extensive disease is uniformly fatal.

Absence of Peristalsis

This disease affects premature infants and causes a severe functional intestinal obstruction.[132, 142]

Incidence. Approximately a dozen cases have been reported in the literature, all of them in males.

Etiology and Pathogenesis. There is no satisfactory explanation for this absence of peristalsis because the intramural ganglion cells are histologically normal in structure and in number.

Symptoms. In half the infants, distention develops during the first few days of life and no meconium is passed. The remainder pass meconium normally and do not become symptomatic until four to ten days of age. In those, abdominal distention is less severe and the abdomen is soft. Bilious vomiting develops and persists, leading to dehydration. The bowel sounds are hypoactive or absent.

Diagnosis. In most cases, the preoperative diagnosis is low intestinal obstruction most likely due to Hirschsprung's disease, but at operation, the small bowel is distended and no site of obstruction can be determined.

Treatment. The operative procedures used include proximal decompression of the bowel by exteriorization, enterostomy, and flushing of the distal bowel.

Prognosis. None of these methods of treatment is successful, since 84 per cent of affected infants have died between one and seven days of age. In one survivor, spontaneous peristalsis appeared on day eight.

ACQUIRED DISEASES OF THE SMALL BOWEL

Acquired lesions to be discussed are those that are not considered to be congenital in nature. Some are due to trauma or infection, but for others there is as yet no identifiable etiology. Because of the dramatic recent rise in traumatic lesions, these are discussed first.

Duodenal and Jejunal Trauma

As the incidence of the "battered child syndrome" increases, intestinal hematomas are seen with increasing frequency.[59] Older children relate their symptoms to a definite trauma, such as a bicycle mishap or a fall, but in the infant there is often no history of trauma available. It is only when the results of the injury, such as hematoma, hemoperitoneum, or pancreatitis develop that the illness is recognized.[14, 55, 150, 182]

Etiology. Blunt, rather than sharp, trauma causes most of the severe intra-abdominal injuries of children, and injury is most often to the upper abdomen. If the injury is unexpected and there is little anticipatory muscle guarding, the blow is received full-force by the duodenum. This organ is more susceptible to injury than any other mobile part of the intestine, for it is fixed in both its first portion, to the retroperitoneum, and its last portion, at the ligament of Treitz. It lies across the vertebral column, which is an unyielding surface. Being essentially closed at the pylorus and angulated at the ligament of Treitz, it is occasionally subjected to a blowout injury.

Pathology. A hematoma originates in the subserosal vessels along the mesenteric border or in the arteries and veins in the muscular and subserosal layers. Duodenal lesions are most often located in the posterior wall of the second duodenum but may extend distally through the third duodenum. Jejunal hematomas are usually proximal. An isolated injury is unusual, and other organs are also affected. The pancreas, which lies directly behind the duodenum, is most often traumatized, although liver, colon, small intestine, stomach, vena cava, kidney, and biliary tract trauma also occur. Partial intestinal obstruction develops early as the hematoma enlarges with blood. Later obstruction results from liquefaction of the hematoma and its absorption of water. The bowel injury itself causes a paralytic ileus, which further contributes to obstructive symptoms. Rarely, the jejunum perforates at its point of fixation at the ligament of Treitz.

Symptoms. There is a symptom-free period between the time of injury and the development of pain, which ranges from several minutes up to eight days. The abdominal pain is either epigastric or periumbilical and may be constant or colicky. Bile-tinged vomitus is a constant finding as well as a moderate temperature elevation and

tachycardia. The abdomen is tender over the site of the hematoma, usually in the right upper quadrant or epigastrium, but a mass is usually not palpated. If the hematoma ruptures and dissects into the small bowel mesentery and retroperitoneum, pain and tenderness in the right lower quadrant mimic appendicitis. Very rarely, persistent vomiting in the absence of any positive physical findings may be the presenting complaint.

Duodenal or jejunal perforation present acutely, with peritoneal signs and shock.

Diagnosis. A significant fall in hemoglobin is often present. If the patient is unconscious or has signs of peritoneal irritation, peritoneal lavage should be performed, and if there is evidence of bleeding, he should undergo immediate exploratory laparotomy. If the physical findings are equivocal, chest and abdominal radiographs should be taken to look for free air and serum amylase levels drawn to determine pancreatic injury. If there is no evidence of perforation, cautious barium examination of the upper gastrointestinal tract may be performed. The hematoma appears as an intramural filling defect in the second portion of the duodenum (Figs. 16–20 to 16–22). There are thickened folds proximally and a coiled-spring appearance distally.

Treatment. Medical management for hematoma is decompression with nasogastric suction and bowel rest until the hematoma resolves, usually in 10 to 12 days. Its progress may be monitored by ultrasound. Nutritional support is provided by hyperalimentation. Perforation demands a wide exploration of the duodenum for multiple lesions, and repair is usually possible with suture closure.

Prognosis. Hematomas resolve completely after several weeks. The immediate mortality of blunt duodenal injuries is 11 per cent, with most deaths related to late operation for perforation.

Complications. The major complications develop 7 to 14 days after injury and include rupture of the hematoma with peritonitis, pancreatitis, and complete small bowel obstruction due to liquefaction and expansion of the hematoma. The first is

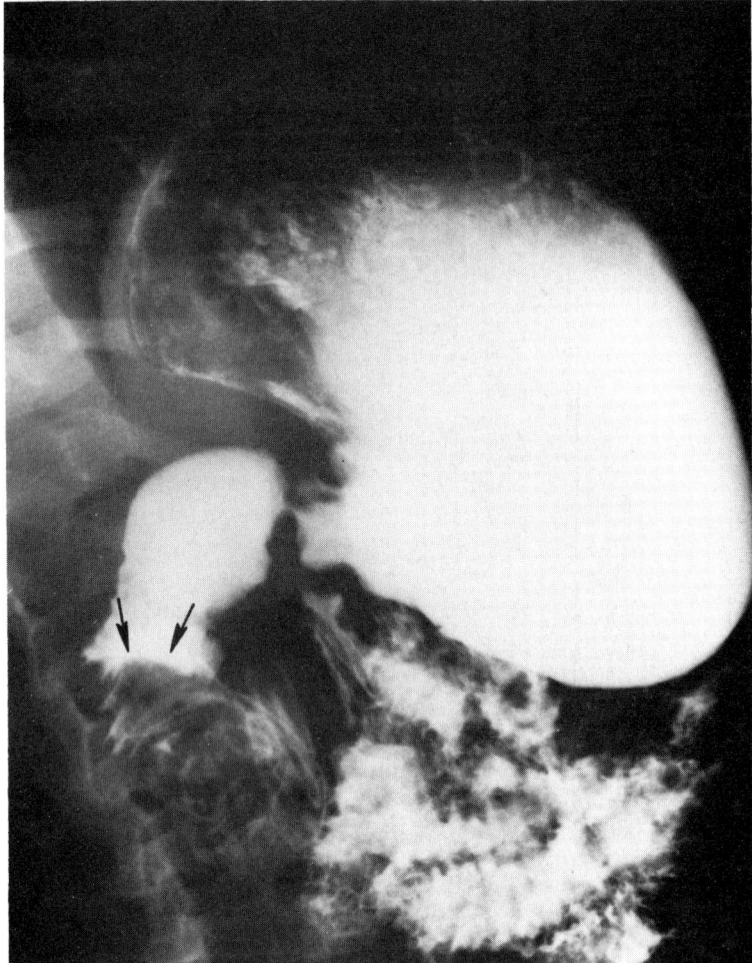

Figure 16–20 Traumatic duodenal hematoma in a three-year-old infant admitted with vomiting, lethargy, and multiple bruises. She was initially suspected of having meningococcal meningitis because of the bruises and petechiae, but a history of parental abuse was later obtained. Because of persistent vomiting, an upper gastrointestinal series was performed. It showed some distention of the stomach and proximal duodenum, with partial obstruction in the descending duodenum (arrows). The finding is consistent with an intramural hematoma. Signs of obstruction persisted for two weeks, and then surgery was performed and an intramural hematoma evacuated. Evidence of pancreatitis was also seen at surgery.

heralded by an increase in abdominal pain and vomiting and is diagnosed by a rise in amylase level. The second is typified by signs of obstruction.

Acute Jejunitis

Acute segmental obstructing jejunitis has been reported in a three-year-old child who experienced the sudden onset of cramping abdominal pain and vomiting.[80] Her illness persisted for six weeks and finally precipitated radiologic examination, which revealed an area of narrowing in the proximal jejunum measuring 0.5 cm in length. Laparotomy revealed three zones of jejunal inflammation, the longest of which measured 10 cm. The largest of the lesions was resected, and microscopic examination revealed

polymorphonuclear infiltration of the mucosa, edema of the submucosa, and leakage of red blood cells. Cultures of stool and mesenteric lymph nodes were negative, but a blood culture obtained after surgery grew *Klebsiella pneumoniae*. She improved after gentamicin therapy. We have encountered another patient of similar age with exquisite tenderness in the left upper quadrant and radiologic changes of jejunitis with several areas suggestive of stricture (Fig. 16–23). Small bowel biopsy was similar to that described above, and jejunal cultures revealed no abnormal numbers or types of bacteria. The patient was maintained on parenteral hyperalimentation and became asymptomatic within two weeks. Radiologic examination one month later was entirely normal. It should be stressed that this disorder should

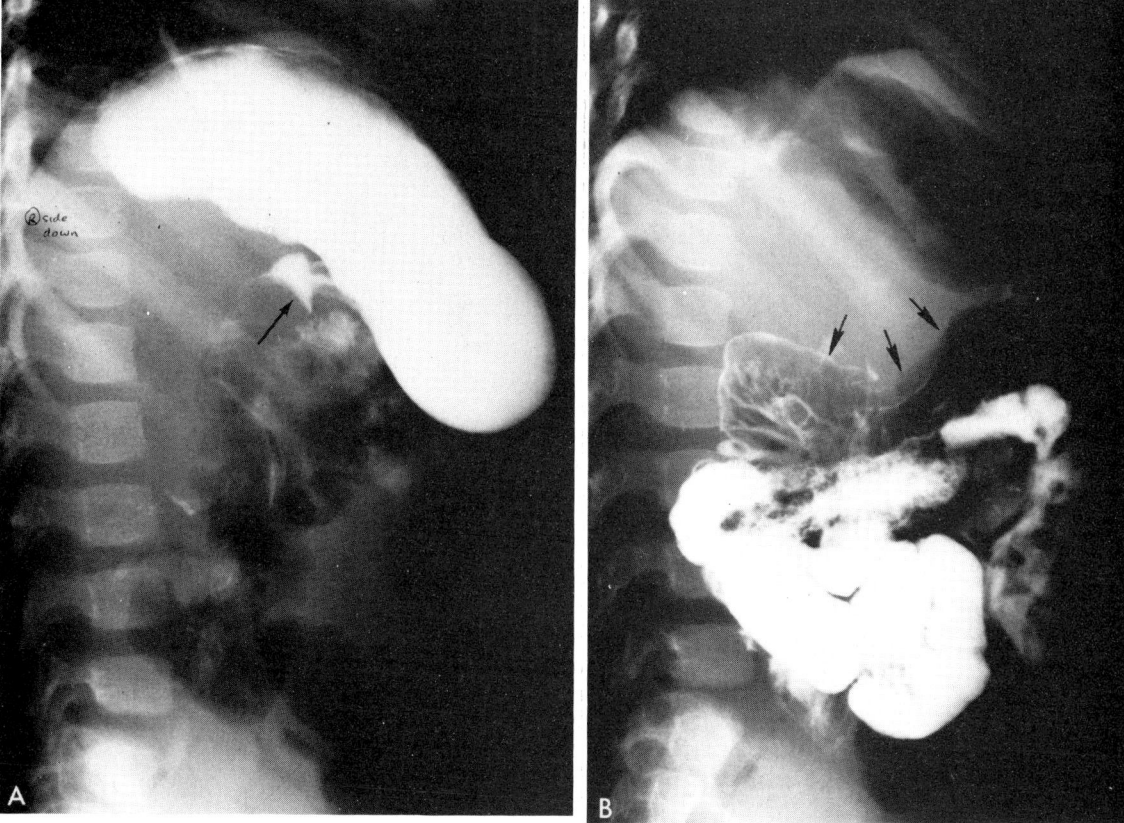

Figure 16–21 Duodenal intramural hematoma and traumatic pancreatitis in a battered child. This patient was seen in the emergency room because of abdominal pain and vomiting and had a past history of parental abuse. She was admitted for observation and had a transiently elevated lipase. She improved over a period of ten days of medical management. *A,* Upper gastrointestinal series on the second hospital day demonstrated partial obstruction by a mass immediately beyond the duodenal bulb (arrows). *B,* Later films demonstrated passage of barium beyond the partial obstruction. There is anterior and inferior displacement of small bowel in the region of the head of the pancreas (arrows).

be treated medically with every effort to support the patient while resolution occurs.

Gastrojejunocolic Fistula

This complication of surgery has been reported in four infants after pyloroplasty, after erosion by a gastrostomy tube, or after umbilical catheterization.[53] It is characterized by the sudden development of massive diarrhea and peritonitis and has been universally lethal.

Gastroduodenal Intussusception

Obstruction of the midportion of the stomach in a child should arouse immediate suspicion of gastroduodenal intussusception.

Incidence. Over 60 cases have been reported, but only three were in children, of whom all were female.[4, 81]

Etiology and Pathogenesis. The majority of reported cases were associated with gastric tumors, all but one of which were benign. A polyp or, less often, an adenoma or leiomyoma serves as the lead point and is carried by peristalsis into the duodenum. Part of the gastric mucosa invaginates along with the polyp.

Symptoms. The lesion presents as gastric obstruction. The youngest patient, 23 months old, was always a poor eater and was fretful during the month prior to the acute illness. She had a three-day history of vague

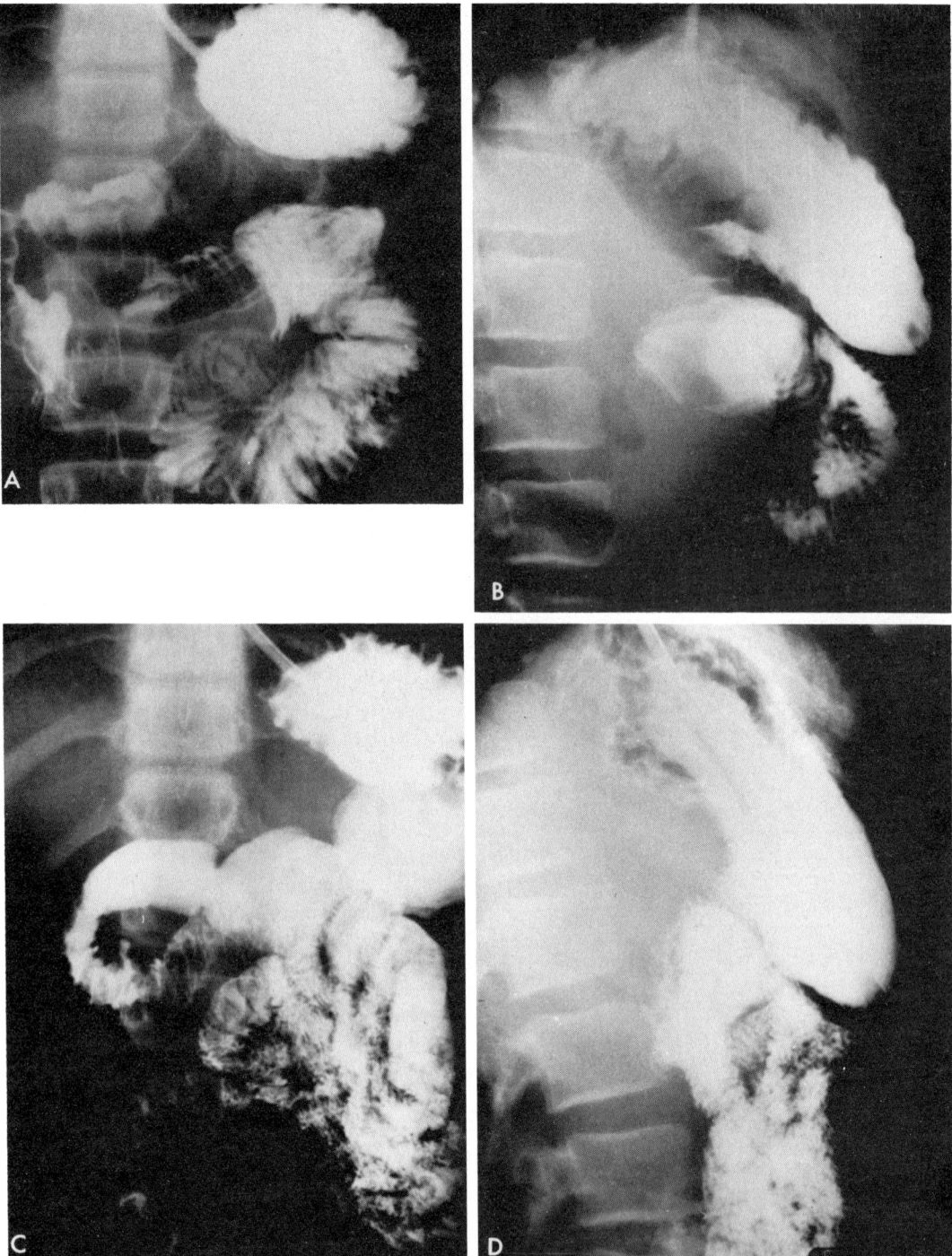

Figure 16–22 Duodenal hematoma. A young teenage male sustained blunt trauma to the epigastrium, which was followed by dull abdominal pain, vomiting, and a drop in hematocrit. *A*, Frontal view of upper gastrointestinal series shows marked irregular narrowing of the second and third portions of duodenum as well as mass effect in distal duodenum. *B*, Lateral view shows displacement of bowel anteriorly by large retroperitoneal mass consisting of a large retroperitoneal hematoma and edematous pancreas. Several weeks following conservative medical management, a repeat upper gastrointestinal series *(C* and *D)* shows return to normal configuration. The small projection extending superiorly from the third portion of duodenum in *C* may be a small diverticulum versus a healing confined perforation. (Courtesy of Richard Markowitz, M.D.)

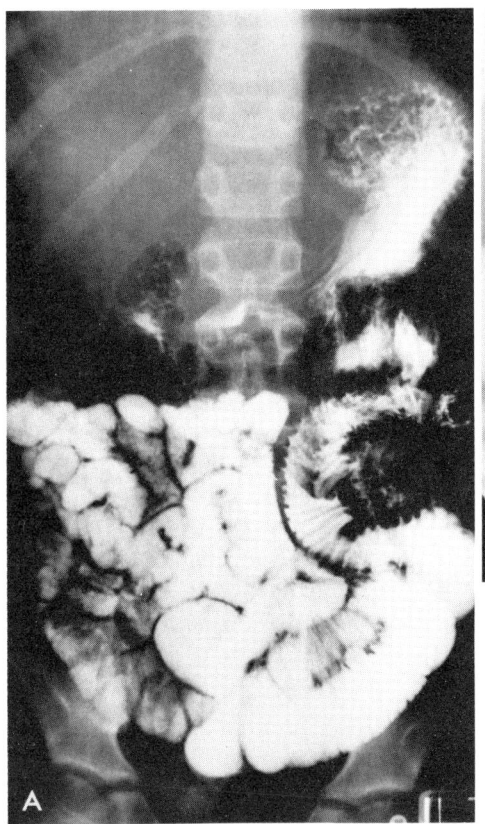

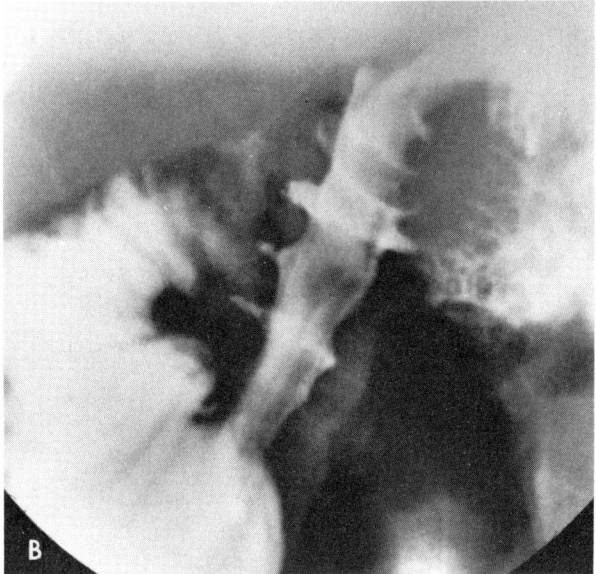

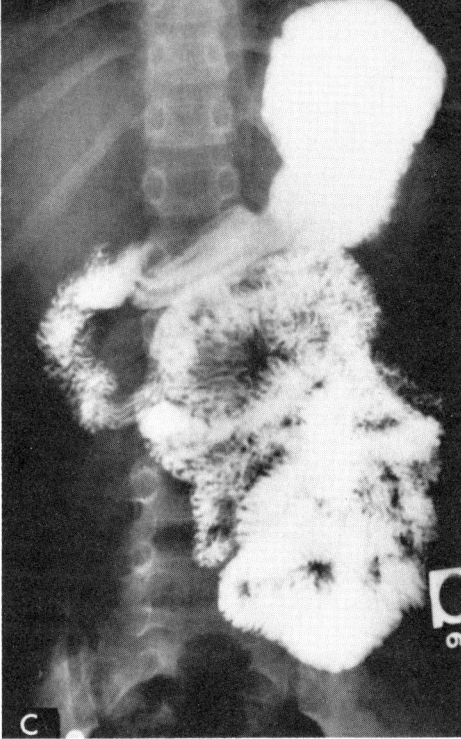

Figure 16–23 Patient with three-week history of fever and exquisite left upper quadrant pain and tenderness. *A*, Note picket-fence appearance of left upper quadrant jejunal loop and narrowed jejunal loop. *B*, Same study showing narrowed, spiculated loop of jejunum. *C*, Study repeated two weeks later.

abdominal pain and vomiting that increased until she could retain no food. Each of the two older girls had a long history of vague epigastric pain and emesis, with an inconstant mass palpated in the epigastrium or periumbilical area.

Diagnosis. Radiologic examination of the upper gastrointestinal tract shows an abrupt cutoff in the midportion of the stomach, narrowing of the body of the stomach, converging axial striations of stomach and duodenum running parallel to the long axis of the organs, a central filling defect in the duodenum, and a coiled-spring appearance in the duodenum.

Treatment. Operative reduction of the intussusception and removal of the gastric polyp are performed immediately.

Complication. Perforation of the duodenum has followed this type of intussusception.

Prognosis. Complete recovery is the rule.

Eosinophilic Gastroenteritis and Chronic Allergic Gastroenteropathy

Eosinophilic gastroenteritis is a disease of varied presentations, with a presumed, although unproved, relation to allergy. The stomach, the small bowel, and, recently, the esophagus are found to be involved.

Incidence. The incidence is unknown, but this is probably the same "chronic allergic enteropathy" related to milk and described in children. Since one group was reported, small series of six or seven patients and isolated case reports have followed.[70, 93]

Etiology. Although systemic signs of allergy such as asthma, rhinitis, and urticaria are present in 50 to 80 per cent of patients, some individuals show absolutely normal immunologic studies and normal reagenic hypersensitivity and lymphocyte transformation studies.[88] A few patients improve with the elimination of milk or other allergens from the diet, but a number do not.[23] Recently, eosinophilic gastroenteritis has been related directly to the use of gold therapy for the treatment of rheumatoid arthritis.[98]

Pathophysiology. In 1961, Ureles et al.[164] classified the disease into two types. Class I consisted of diffuse infiltration of the intestinal wall and class II a circumscribed accumulation forming a granuloma. In 1979, Klein et al.[93] amended the description of class I into three types:

Class I, type 1. Mucosal involvement causing blood loss, protein-losing enteropathy, pain, vomiting, diarrhea, and malabsorption.

Class I, type 2. Involvement of the muscle layer causing obstructive symptoms.

Class I, type 3. Submucosal infiltration causing eosinophilic ascites.

Eosinophilic diseases of the intestine are classified in Table 16–2. Caldwell et al.,[23] who have performed the major immunologic studies in these patients first noted a marked increase in symptoms and in serum

Table 16–2 Eosinophilic Gastroenteritis and Allergic Diseases of the Intestine*

I. Eosinophilic gastroenteritis: Six months to adult life
  A. Pathologic criteria:
    1. Eosinophilic infiltration of bowel wall
    2. Increased peripheral blood eosinophils
    3. Symptoms after ingestion of specific foods
  B. Clinical picture:
    1. Mucosal disease
      a. Iron deficiency anemia
      b. Increased fecal blood loss
      c. Enteric protein loss
      d. Malabsorption
    2. Muscle layer disease
      a. Pyloric obstruction
      b. Small bowel obstruction
      c. Localized polypoid lesion
    3. Serosal disease
      a. Eosinophilic ascites
II. Allergic gastroenteritis
  A. Milk allergy: One week to 16 months
    1. Clinical signs similar to mucosal eosinophilic disease
    2. Chronic diarrhea
    3. Rectal bleeding
    4. Heiner's syndrome
    5. Anaphylaxis, urticaria, angioedema
  B. Soy allergy—same
III. Food allergy with systemic reactions: One month to adult
  A. Anaphylaxis

---

*Adapted from Greenberger, M., and Gryboski, J.: Allergic disorders of the intestine and eosinophilic gastroenteritis. *In* Sleisenger, M., and Fordtran, J. (eds.): Gastrointestinal Disease. Philadelphia, W. B. Saunders Company, 1978.

IgE after challenge with foods that were classic offenders. In later studies of seven patients, however, they found no evidence of systemic allergic response and suggested the disease may be due to an intraintestinal localization of antigen, which in some patients may not be food. One infant has been described with disseminated eosinophilic infiltration of the intestine, lymph nodes, kidneys, liver, and portal tracts, who died at 4 days of age from perforation of the ileum.[103a]

Peripheral eosinophilia varies between 13 and 85 per cent. Serum immunoglobulins A, G, and M are often normal, but IgE may be extremely high, measuring 400 to 3000 ng per ml.

Intestinal biopsies have shown, in some adults, flattening of the intestinal villi, with preservation of columnar epithelium and marked eosinophilic infiltration of the lamina propria by eosinophils. Multiple biopsies may vary from normal or minimally changed villi to severely diseased ones. In children, Katz et al.[91] reported intestinal changes similar to those in the adult but stressed the diagnostic value of gastric biopsies even in the radiologically normal stomach. Gastric biopsies were consistently abnormal, showing necrosis and regeneration of surface and glandular epithelium, eosinophilic infiltrate and abscess aggregation, and neutrophilic infiltration and exudation (Fig. 16–24). Biopsies revert to normal in children who are in clinical remission. Esophageal and colonic involvement is extremely rare, as is infiltration of bladder and pancreas.[41]

Symptoms. The patients of Waldman were two months to two and one-half years

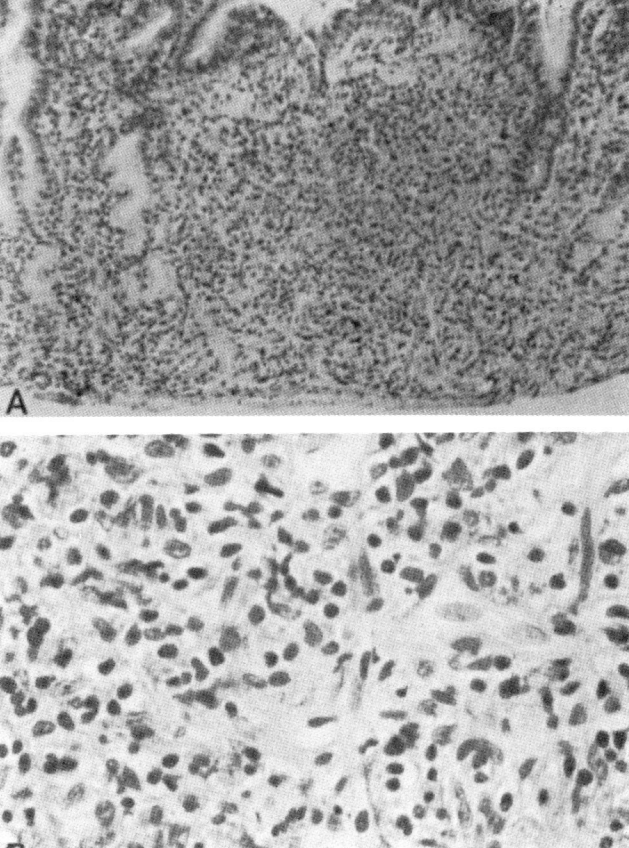

Figure 16–24 A, Biopsy of gastric mucosa (×54) showing necrosis of the glands and replacement with inflammatory exudate (including eosinophils). B, Inflammation extends into lamina propria (×135). (From Katz et al.: Gastroenterology 73: 707, 1977, with permission.)

of age, and those of Katz et al. were six months to ten years.[91, 166, 167] Most children had the diffuse infiltrative mucosal disease. There were often specific food intolerances, specifically to milk, soy, or wheat products, which caused abdominal pain or diarrhea. Edema, often fluctuating in severity, was present in the younger children for up to two years. The majority had evidence of growth retardation, despite dietary restriction and improvement of symptoms. A few had lymphadenopathy or hepatomegaly.

In older children and adults, the obstructive or muscular form is reported to constitute half of all cases, and in these patients the symptoms are those of upper gastrointestinal or small bowel obstruction. Symptoms of the serosal form are discussed in another section under eosinophilic peritonitis.

Differential Diagnosis. A heavy parasitic intestinal invasion must be differentiated from this disease. Localized distal lesions may resemble ileocolitis.[73, 155]

Diagnosis. The peripheral blood work is remarkable for eosinophilia and a normal erythrocyte sedimentation rate. The stools contain occult blood, and serum or stool or both often contain precipitins to milk. Abnormalities in the serum IgE were discussed earlier. Hypoalbuminemia is common and may be severe. Radiologic examination of the upper gastrointestinal tract shows mucosal edema and dilatation and flocculation of barium in the small intestine, with a normal stomach.[156] One patient had an antral polyp. Studies of the obstructive form show antral and pyloric narrowing and rigidity. Studies for enteric protein loss show increased losses, increased albumin synthesis, and decreased half-life. Gastric and small bowel biopsies are diagnostic.

Treatment. Dietary elimination of the offending antigen produced a cessation or reduction of symptoms in the milk-allergic patients in particular but produced no response in others, who required systemic steroid therapy for short seven- to ten-day courses or for months. The use of oral disodium cromoglycate in food allergy and its success in several patients with this disease

may avert the use of steroids and promote growth.

Prognosis. Although the disease persists, requiring the aforementioned control measures, in a few cases it has been fatal.

Eosinophilic Granuloma

Eosinophilic granulomas are mentioned in order to differentiate them from eosinophilic enteritis. They exist as polypoid lesions at or near the pylorus or in the small bowel or colon, where they may cause upper gastrointestinal obstruction, intussusception, or diffuse abdominal or right lower quadrant pain. They do not recur after surgical excision.[100]

Nodular Lymphoid Hyperplasia of the Small Bowel

Although nodular lymphoid hyperplasia of the small bowel does occur with isolated IgA deficiency and with acquired hypogammaglobulinemia, it is most often described in association with dysgammaglobulinemia in which all immunoglobulin levels are depressed. Rarely, it is seen in the presence of normal immunoglobulins.[98b]

Incidence. Since its original description in 1966, the disease has been reported in fewer than 100 patients; we have seen the lesion in ten children.[31, 77]

Etiology and Pathogenesis. Cellular immune function by definition is intact, as the follicles of lymphoid tissue appear to contain T cells. Small bowel biopsy shows diminished or absent plasma cells in the lamina propria and enhanced mitotic activity in the large germinal centers of the lymphoid follicles. The follicles are often so large that they distort villous morphology.

Symptoms. Poor appetite, diarrhea and/or colic develop during the first year of life. Associated symptoms are recurrent respiratory infections, fever, abdominal pain, giardiasis, and growth retardation. Lactose and glucose intolerances are obvious by history.

Diagnosis. The diagnosis of nodular lymphoid hyperplasia of the small bowel, also known as black dot disease, is a radiologic one.[82] The appearance of the bowel is unlike that of any other disease. The mucosal nodules are small, measuring 1 to 3 mm in diameter, and are uniformly distributed throughout the small bowel and even into the cecum and ascending colon. They are most readily identified in the ileum (Fig. 16–25). Small bowel biopsy will show the aforementioned changes. Laboratory studies document malabsorption, and 72-hour fecal fat measurements show steatorrhea.[71] The diagnosis must be made carefully, for lymphoid polyps have also been reported in familial polyposis.[67]

Treatment. Tetracycline or other broad-spectrum antibiotics often relieve the gastrointestinal symptoms — a response suggesting the presence of bacterial overgrowth. Giardiasis and lactose intolerance must be investigated and treated appropriately. Replacement of the deficient globulins, by administration of immune globulin for IgG and fresh frozen plasma for IgA, is often followed by dramatic improvement in symptoms, although there is concern that their long-term use may lead to the development of sensitivities.

Prognosis. The long-term prognosis is guarded, for in nearly one third of the original patients, lymphoma or carcinoma has developed somewhere in the gastrointestinal tract.

Benign Lymphoid Hyperplasia of the Terminal Ileum

Benign lymphoid hyperplasia of the terminal ileum is a finding considered by a few to represent disease and by most, to represent a normal anatomic finding because of its frequent demonstration in asymptomatic children.[25, 52] Although most often seen in adolescents, it is also described in infancy and in the elderly.

Pathology. Hyperplastic lymphoid tissue in the terminal ileum forms discrete polypoid lesions that measure 0.1 to 0.3 cm in diameter. The hyperplastic tissue often extends to the mucosal layer of the polyp to form a secondary polyp. Germinal centers are prominent, and eosinophils are often present. Some polyps are pedunculated.[108, 138]

Symptoms. These lesions may be entirely asymptomatic, but in some children they cause recurrent right lower quadrant pain and diarrhea. Vomiting is infrequent.

Diagnosis. The diagnosis is a radiologic one, best made by barium enema and retrograde filling of the terminal ileum, showing

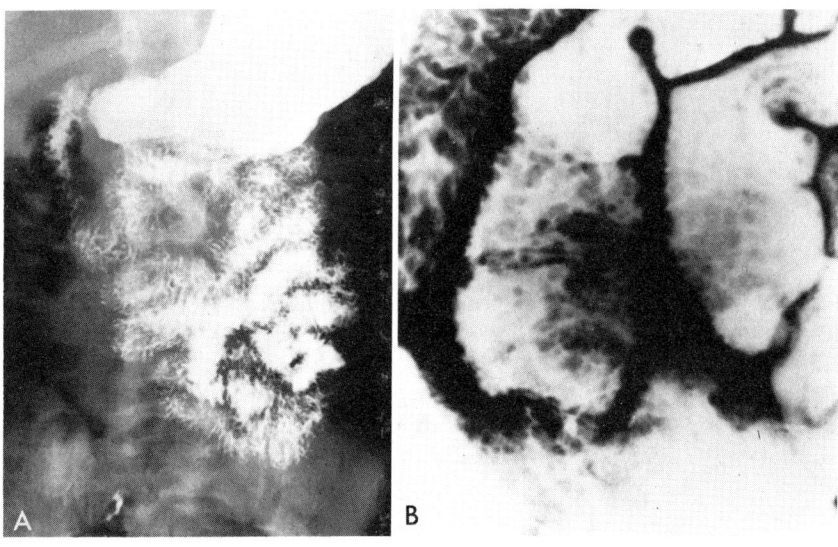

Figure 16–25 Diffuse nodular lymphoid hyperplasia of the small bowel in a boy with dysgammaglobulinemia. This child had had chronic diarrhea, recurrent ear and respiratory infections, and growth retardation since the age of six months. *A*, Generalized coarsening of the mucosal pattern was seen throughout the entire small bowel. *B*, Compression spot film shows the small nodular pattern of the filling defects.

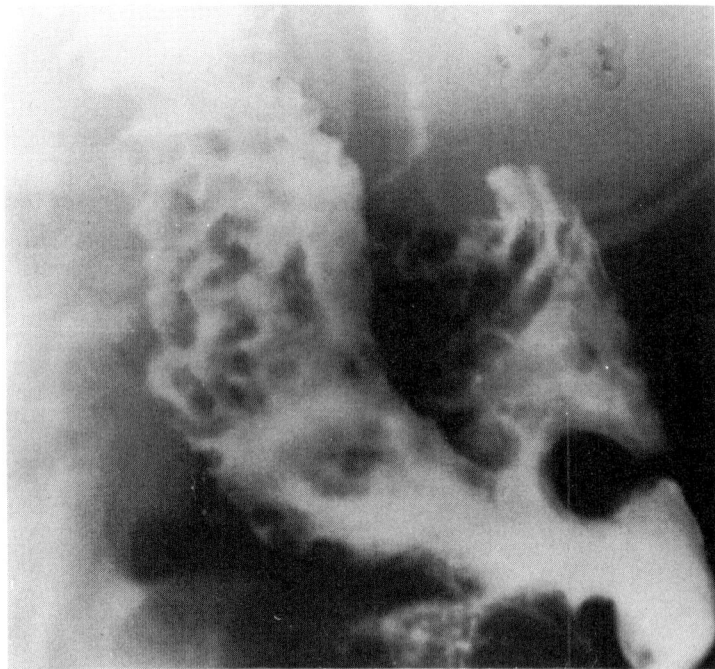

Figure 16–26 Lymphoid hyperplasia of the terminal ileum demonstrated by barium enema. The irregular filling defects in the distal small bowel are seen as a normal phenomenon.

multiple nodular filling defects of varied size (Fig. 16–26). The disorder often cannot be differentiated from the early stages of regional enteritis.

Regional Enteritis (Crohn's Disease)

There is a paucity of information on regional enteritis in infancy, and it is not thoroughly established that this is the same disease as exists in older children and adults.[76, 102]

Incidence. The incidence in large series seems to be increasing in general and increasing specifically in younger children. In most experiences, 3 to 4 per cent of patients are under 11 years of age at the time of diagnosis, but approximately 10 per cent of our pediatric patients date their symptoms or are diagnosed before five years of age. Our youngest patient had florid disease at 18 months.[69] In 1971, Miller and Larsen summarized existing case reports of regional enteritis in infancy and added six of their own to accumulate a total of 12.[102]

Etiology. The etiology remains unknown,[158] but genetics must play a role, for there is a positive family history of Crohn's disease or ulcerative colitis in 25 per cent of patients.[69] In older children and adults, the disease is more common in those of Jewish heritage, but this does not hold true for infants and young children. The incidence is increased significantly in those with Turner's syndrome.[6] An infectious etiology cannot be dismissed, for tuberculosis and certain animal diseases caused by *Mycobacterium* resemble regional enteritis. Other bacteria, such as atypical *Mycobacterium* and cell wall–defective *Pseudomonas*, have been suggested but have not proved to be factors in the disease. Since the original reports of transmission of granulomatous lesions to experimental animals from filtrates of Crohn's disease tissue, a viral agent has been sought.[11] Similar viral particles have been identified in tissues from varied patients, and cytotoxic factors have been isolated from the serum of patients with both Crohn's disease and ulcerative colitis. Abnormalities in delayed hypersensitivity, occasionally noted IgA deficiency, peripheral T and B-cell function, and antibody-dependent cytotoxicity are only a few of the immunologic aberrations noted. Increased incidences of circulating antibodies to milk and other food antigens have been observed, and perhaps these are secondary to mucosal damage. It is presumed that those with a genetic predisposition for the disease suffer an insult to the bowel that sets up an immune reaction which to all effect recovers. A later insult causes repeated cellular damage and activates cytotoxic mechanisms that perpetuates the disease.

Pathology. The disease in infancy fulfills the pathologic description of regional enteritis in the adult, being acute or chronic, transmural and segmental, and involving small or large bowel or both.[32] Involvement is fairly consistent in the ileum and variable in the jejunum and colon. Ulceration, polypoid change, stenosis, and stiffening and kinking of the distal ileum with evidence of proximal progression are all present. Granuloma formation, however, is usually absent. The early histologic changes are hyperplasia of the perilymphatic histiocytes, round cell infiltration of the lymph nodes, and dilatation of the lymphatics. The mucosal ulceration is localized or diffuse, but the lamina propria is infiltrated by round cells.

Deep fissures extend through the submucosa and into the muscularis. As the disease becomes chronic, the mesentery thickens and becomes edematous and infiltrated by fat; the mesenteric lymph nodes enlarge, and loops of bowel adhere together because of dense peritoneal adhesions. The entire bowel wall is thickened.

Symptoms. In infancy, the onset has been described as early as the second day of life. An acute onset is characterized by intestinal obstruction that develops suddenly in an otherwise well baby. A chronic onset is typified by increasing abdominal distention, anorexia, and feeding difficulties. Diarrhea appears and becomes progressively severe, with steatorrhea developing in those with extensive small bowel disease. Blood does not appear in the stool until days or weeks later. Weight loss, growth arrest, and edema are the consequences of longstanding enteric protein loss and malnutrition.

Physical examination shows abdominal

Table 16–3 Differential Diagnosis of Enteritis and Enterocolitis

	NECROTIZING ENTEROCOLITIS	PSEUDOMEMBRANOUS ENTEROCOLITIS	ILEAL ULCER	REGIONAL ENTERITIS
Past history	Neonatal anoxia Prematurity Exchange transfusion	Antibiotics Intussusception Hirschsprung's disease	None	None
Age of onset	First weeks	10 days to 1 year	Several months	Any age but usually older infants
Etiology	Vascular accident	Staphylococci, fungi in some Postoperative Above obstruction After antibiotics	None in infants Vitamin K in adults	None
Area involved	Terminal ileum Right colon	All colon ±Small bowel	Ileum	Ileum ±Right colon ±Jejunum
Symptoms				
Lethargy	++++	+	–	±
Distention	++++	++++	–	++
Diarrhea	++ to ++++	++++	–	++
Gross blood in stool	++	++	++	+eventually
Diagnosis	Radiologic	Sigmoidoscopic	Laparotomy	Usually at laparotomy

distention and some guarding with palpation of the right lower quadrant. If the bowel disease is long-standing, loops of thickened ileum are palpable. Bowel sounds tend to be hyperactive, but if there is obstruction, they cluster in peristaltic rushes with silent periods between them.

Diagnosis. The diagnosis is so rare that other causes must first be sought. Infectious enteritis as with *Campylobacter, Yersinia, Shigella,* and *Salmonella* infections must be excluded, as these can yield similar clinical findings on sigmoidoscopic and radiologic examinations. Ischemia, necrotizing enterocolitis, and lymphosarcoma of the terminal ileum must also be ruled out. One patient, two years of age, referred for Crohn's disease, actually had a retroperitoneal fibrosarcoma that had occluded the vascular supply

to the right colon. Anemia, increased erythrocyte sedimentation rate, reversal of the albumin-globulin ratio, and abnormal vitamin B_{12} absorption — all findings typical for the older child or adult — are not consistently present in the infant (Table 16–3).

Radiologic examination must begin with barium studies of the colon, which usually demonstrate disease of the distal ileu. Antegrade studies will clarify ileal disease and define the extent of small bowel involvement. The more typical changes of regional enteritis are shown in Figures 16–27 to 16–30, and the disease in older children is discussed in detail elsewhere.[69]

Treatment. Steroids have proved of questionable benefit in treatment of the disease in infants. Azulfidine has been ef-

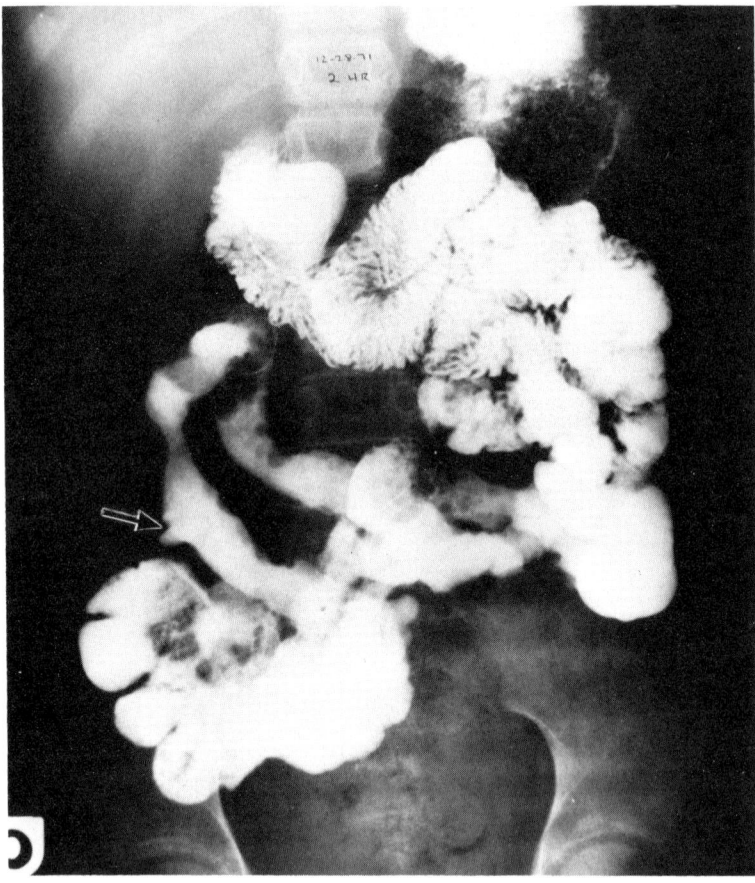

Figure 16–27 Regional enteritis presenting weight loss and finger clubbing. The proximal jejunum is normal radiologically but there is marked involvement of the distal jejunum and ileum, with partial stricture formation, extensive loss of normal mucosal pattern, and at least one deep ulcer indicated by the arrow. Separation of loops of bowel results from rather marked thickening of the wall, perhaps associated with some surrounding inflammatory reaction.

fective in treating those with colonic disease. During the acute illness, parenteral hyperalimentation will provide nutritional support and perhaps in itself is therapeutic. Surgical intervention is reserved for the treatment of intestinal obstruction and consists usually of ileal resection.

Prognosis. The mortality is high: Seven of the 12 reported infants died but at that time were without the benefit of hyperalimentation. The remaining five were asymptomatic 4 to 18 months later, but long-term follow-up is not available. It is now recognized that young adults with Crohn's disease are at risk for developing right colonic or small bowel carcinoma or lymphosarcoma. No figures are available for those who have recovered from the disease in infancy.

Pseudomembranous Enterocolitis

This inflammatory disease of the bowel, characterized by pseudomembrane formation, is well recognized and has recently been associated with antibiotic therapy and overgrowth of *Clostridium difficile*.[19, 163]

Incidence. Although the incidence is not known, the disease is more common in males than in females.

Etiology. Pseudomembranous colitis develops in severely debilitated patients after surgical procedures, intestinal obstruction, antibiotic therapy, or renal failure. It is a complication of clindamycin, lincomycin, ampicillin, penicillin, and broad-spectrum antibiotic therapy. *Staphylococcus aureus* and fungi have been isolated from the stools of some patients, and *Clostridium difficile*

Figure 16–28 Regional enteritis in a boy with a recent history of abdominal pain and diarrhea. *A,* Rather marked mucosal edema is seen throughout the entire small bowel and there is a suggestion of some involvement of the great distal portion of the greater curvature of the stomach.

Illustration continued on following page

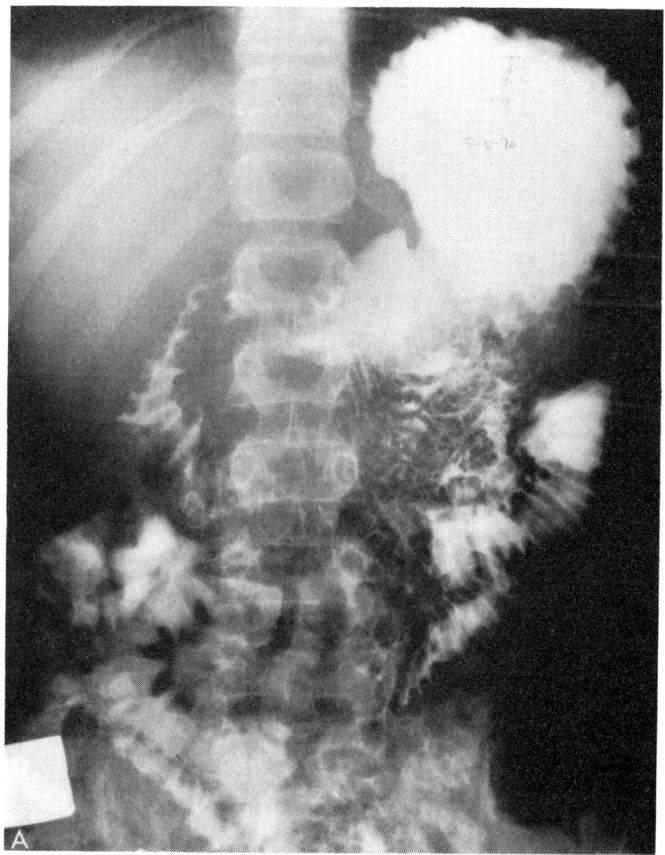

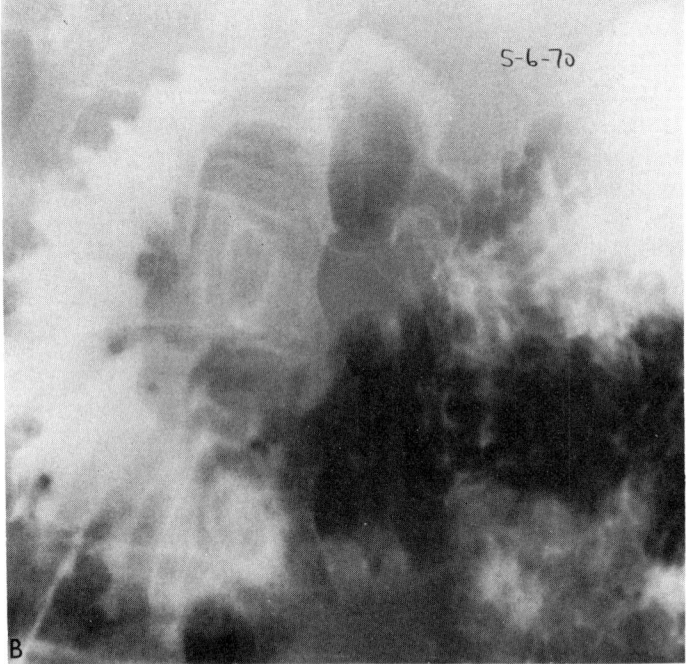

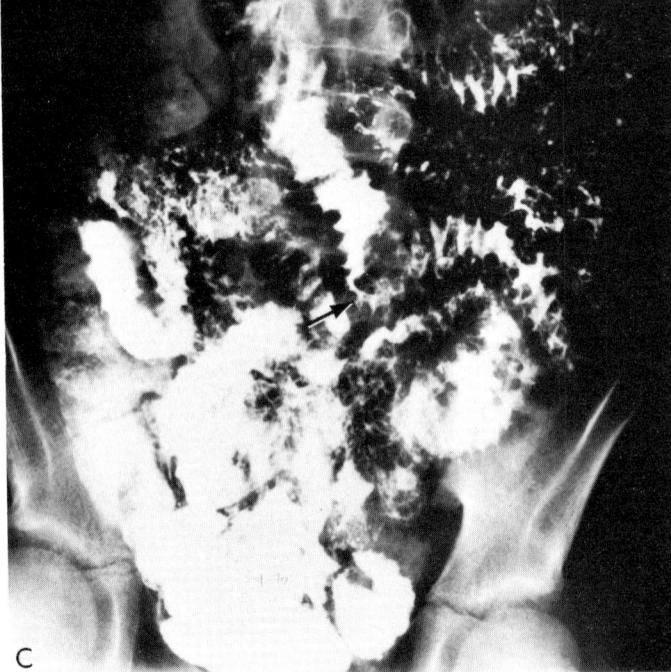

Figure 16–28 Continued B, Spot film of the duodenum better illustrating the rather striking mucosal changes. *C*, Late film in the small bowel series demonstrating similar changes in the mucosa and some suggestion of segmental narrowing (arrow).

toxin has been identified in the stools of many others. Because of the frequent association with intestinal obstruction, it has been hypothesized that a toxic substance may be released from the dilated proximal bowel to cause mucosal pseudomembrane formation. No single cause has yet been identified in all cases of this disease. Clinical characteristics are noted in Table 16–3.

Pathology. The small and large bowel are affected in two thirds of patients and only the colon in one third. The patchy pseudomembrane appears as raised yellow or yellow-green plaques and in some areas

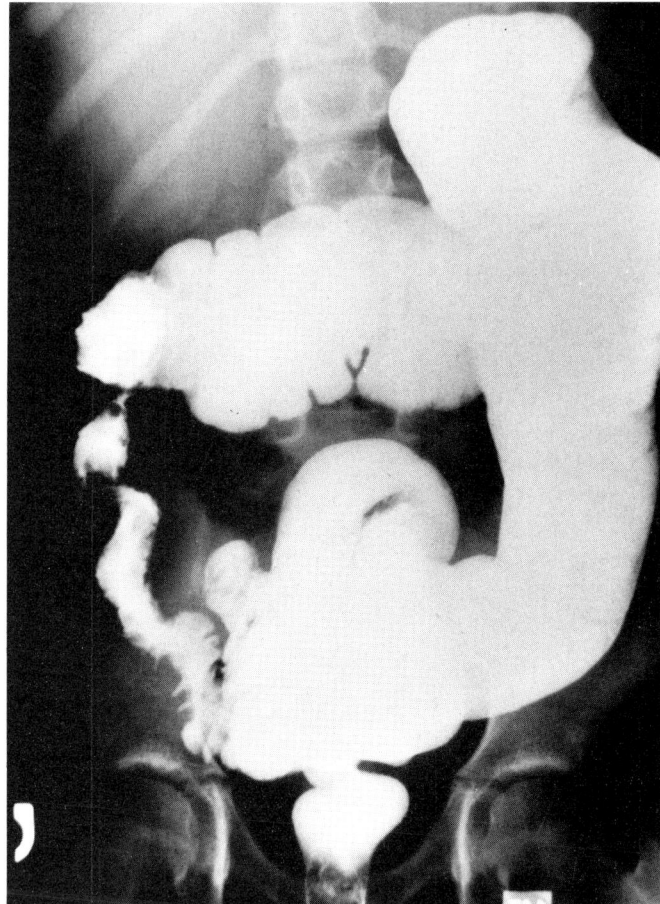

Figure 16-29 Crohn's disease in a girl with crampy abdominal pain. Barium enema shows shortening of the ascending colon, with a stenotic area just below the hepatic flexure and contraction of the cecum. Ulceration can be seen as irregularity of the wall of the distal ileum and the proximal colon.

is confluent. The mucosa below the membrane varies from normal to ulcerated. The earliest microscopic changes are vascular, as the arterioles, venules, and capillaries in the lamina propria and submucosa dilate. The submucosa becomes edematous and filled with macrophages. Mucous glands of the rectal mucosa increase in number. The pseudomembrane itself is composed of mucus, fibrin, blood, and inflammatory cells and sloughs to reveal an ulcerated, pyogenic base. The mesenteric lymph nodes are enlarged.

In cases in which the disease is associated with intestinal obstruction, the pseudomembrane lies proximal to, rather than distal to, the obstruction.

Symptoms. This form of enterocolitis has been described in infants between ten days and one year of age as well as in older children and adults. There is often a history of intussusception, Hirschsprung's disease,

colonic obstruction, or a course of antibiotic therapy. Only rarely does the disorder develop in a well infant.

The onset is abrupt, with high fever, abdominal distention, vomiting, and diarrhea. The stools are foul-smelling and vary in color from yellow to green. Although blood is sometimes present in the stool, it is not constant. Severe fluid losses result from outpouring of plasma, water, and electrolytes into the bowel lumen and lead to shock and renal failure. Abdominal tenderness is marked, and the bowel sounds are hypo- or hyperactive. The leukocyte count is elevated and may reach as high as 20,000. Death may result within 24 to 72 hours.

Diagnosis. There is difficulty in distinguishing the disease from necrotizing enterocolitis, bacillary dysentery, and intestinal ischemia. The diagnosis is best made by stool culture and examination for *Clostridium difficile* toxin and by sigmoidoscopy,

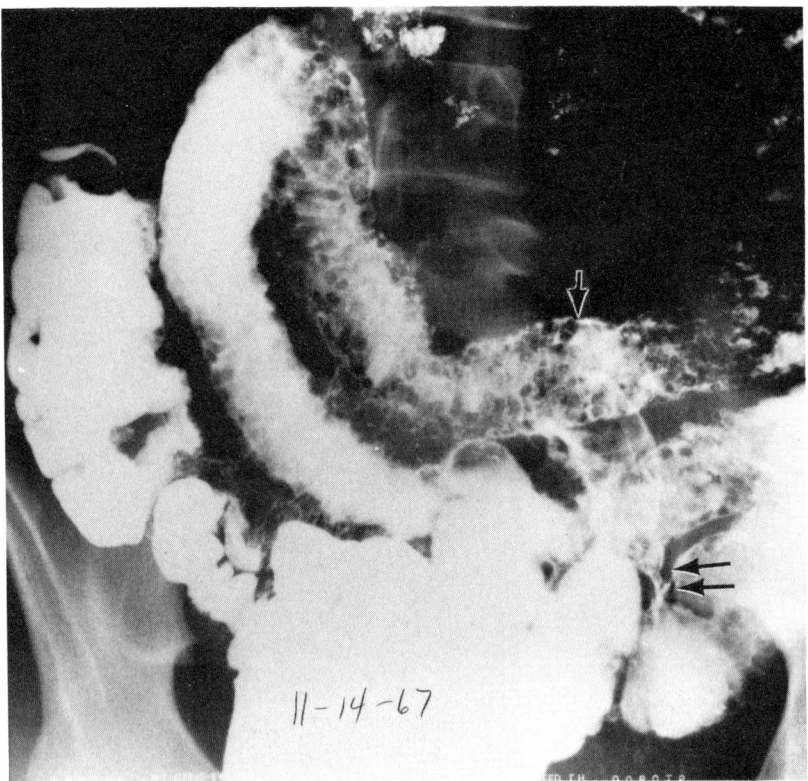

Figure 16–30 A patient with regional enteritis with weight loss and abdominal pain. A film from the small bowel series demonstrates a distinctly abnormal loop of small bowel with obliteration of normal mucosal pattern and a somewhat nodular appearance. Longitudinal tracks of barium seen along portions of the margin of the bowel wall represent confluent ulceration which has undermined the mucosal surface (single arrow), and a stenotic area in another portion of bowel is indicated by double arrows.

which will reveal the typical pseudomembrane. Flat films of the abdomen show dilated small bowel loops and perhaps some mild to moderate dilatation of the colon. Changes in the colon are nonspecific and range from normal studies to those resembling ulcerative colitis. Smears of the stool may show an abundance of staphylococci or fungi.

Treatment. Initial treatment is supportive to combat vascular collapse and to replace lost electrolytes, blood, and plasma. If pathogens or toxin are present in the stool, appropriate antibiotic therapy must be instituted. As noted elsewhere, the treatment for *Clostridium difficile* is vancomycin, metronidazole, or bacitracin given orally.

Diagnosis. The mortality for the untreated patient varies between 50 and 75 per cent. Correction of shock and establishment of adequate urinary flow with a gradual decrease in diarrhea are encouraging prog-

nostic signs and are apparent within 48 to 72 hours.

Primary Nonspecific Small Bowel Ulceration

Nonspecific ulceration of the small bowel is an unusual disease of older infants, causing rectal bleeding or abdominal pain or both.

Incidence. Well over 200 cases have been reported, but only 5 per cent have been in children, and of these, a few were infants.[1, 18, 66, 72, 154]

Etiology. The etiology is essentially unknown, although vascular and central nervous system diseases, infection, and malnutrition have been implicated. Small bowel ulcerations have been associated with the Zollinger-Ellison syndrome, enteric-coated potassium tablets, and acquired hypogammaglobulinemia. Rarely, small bowel ulcerations are a complication of celiac disease.[10]

Pathology. The ulcerations are usually single and are found with twice the frequency in the ileum as in the jejunum. Most, sharply demarcated and punched-out, lie on the antimesenteric border, but some extend about the entire circumference of the bowel lumen. Multiple ulcerations involving a short segment of bowel are much more unusual and are located in the jejunum or distal duodenum. Microscopically, the ulcers appear to be acute and have little inflammatory reaction.

Symptoms. Acute rectal bleeding may be the first and only manifestation of such an ulcer. Some children, however, have recurrent or persistent periumbilical pain and anemia for months to years before the correct diagnosis is established. Longstanding ulcers may cause chronic small bowel obstruction with pain, intermittent diarrhea, and vomiting. There are no consistent physical findings, for the abdomen is soft and the bowel sounds usually are normal; there may be mild periumbilical or right lower quadrant tenderness, but guarding and rebound are absent. The stools are positive for occult blood.

Diagnosis. Barium examination of the small bowel seldom reveals the ulcer, and laparotomy is the definitive diagnostic tool.

Complications. Hemorrhage, perforation of the small bowel, and obstruction are the major complications.

Treatment. In most cases, segmental resection of the involved bowel is curative.

Prognosis. Most children recover uneventfully, although in a few, ulcers recur. Biannual examination of the stool for occult blood should be continued for several years after operation.

Pneumatosis Cystoides Intestinalis

This extremely rare disease is characterized by bullous emphysema of the intestine.[94]

Etiology. The disease can be either primary or secondary, associated with other gastrointestinal diseases such as vascular occlusion, Whipple's disease, necrotizing enterocolitis, scleroderma, peptic ulcer, pyloric stenosis, leukemia, or chronic pulmonary disease.[57] Several theories about its cause have been suggested. Gas-producing organisms may penetrate the serosa or submucosa to form the air-filled cysts, or alterations of the H^+ content may cause gas production in the lymphatics and absorption of gas into the mucosa. The gas content of the cysts varies from 5 to 16 per cent oxygen, from 80 to 90 per cent nitrogen, and from 0.3 to 4 per cent carbon dioxide. The most acceptable theory, however, is a mechanical one, which proposes obstruction followed by perforation or ulceration of the mucosa with extravasation of gas into the tissues.

In patients with pulmonary disease, alveolar rupture is followed by pneumomediastinum and downward dissection of air along the vascular channels through the mesentery and into the bowel wall.

Pathology. The primary lesions are most common in the jejunum and next most common in the ileocecal region or colon. Those associated with pyloric stenosis involve the small bowel; those associated with diarrheal diseases involve the right colon. When there is left-sided involvement of the colon, it usually follows sigmoidoscopy. Grossly, the cysts appear as blebs or polyps that vary in size from several millimeters to several centimeters, are shiny, and have a spongy feel. Clusters of blebs line the submucosa or subserosa and extend into the mesentery. The overlying mucosa is often hemorrhagic.

Symptoms. The disease has been reported in infants as young as two weeks. A history of chronic respiratory disease preceding the onset of diarrhea suggests the diagnosis. Diarrhea is the most common symptom, but if the mucosa overlying the blebs is hemorrhagic, rectal bleeding may be the first sign of disease. Rarely, a large cyst obstructs the lumen of the bowel and causes intestinal obstruction. Pneumoperitoneum is more common in subserosal lesions of the small bowel than of the colon, but if it occurs, it causes abdominal distention, rigidity, and respiratory distress. In young patients, leakage of the cysts is accompanied by ulceration, necrosis, perforation, and even death. Malabsorption results if the entire small bowel is involved. The physical examination is remarkable because occasionally crepitant abdominal masses can be palpated.

Diagnosis. Palpation of such masses or visualization by sigmoidoscopy of small glistening blebs under the rectal mucosa strongly suggests the diagnosis. It is confirmed by radiologic examination of both chest and abdomen. The chest film may show a pneumomediastinum, and plain abdominal films show gas-filled cysts as radiolucent areas or grape-like clusters. A barium enema delineates their location.

Complications. The major complications are obstruction, hemorrhage, and perforation.

Treatment. The cysts usually resolve with time and with treatment of any primary disease present. Resection of an involved area is indicated only in the presence of complications.

Protein-Losing Enteropathy

Hypoproteinemia will complicate a number of primary disorders of the small bowel. For many, this reduction in serum proteins is a reflection of malnutrition, maldigestion, or malabsorption. In others, serum proteins are reduced because of leakage through the bowel wall, and the term "protein-losing enteropathy" is *not* a diagnosis but a symptom.[159, 166, 167]

Protein loss occurs under conditions of increased mucosal permeability or reduced lymphatic flow or both. The major anatomic, inflammatory, and lymphatic lesions are noted in Table 16–4. In the majority of these conditions, excessive protein loss is transient, but in a few, losses are not correctable. Enteric protein loss is less selective than renal losses as in the nephrotic syndrome, in which one sees preferential loss of small molecular weight proteins.

When synthesis fails to meet losses, serum protein levels fall, with the greatest reductions noted in proteins having the longest half-lives: albumin and gamma globulins. Near-normal levels are noted for those with shorter half-lives, such as alpha$_2$-macroglobulin and fibrinogen. Other serum factors are lost as well, including lipids, calcium, and trace minerals. Lymphocyte losses are a hallmark of conditions caused by lymphatic obstruction.

The major symptoms are those of the

Table 16–4   Established Causes of Protein-Losing Enteropathy

Anatomic lesions	Hirschsprung's disease
	Enteric fistula/stricture
	Malnutrition
	Diverticulosis
	Congenital lymphatic abnormalities
	Lymphangiectasia
Inflammatory disorders	Gluten-sensitive enteropathy
	Milk/soy-induced enteropathy
	Hypertrophic gastritis/enteritis (Menetrier's disease)
	Acute transient gastroenteropathy
	Whipple's disease
	Granulomatous enterocolitis (Crohn's disease)
	Lymphoma/lymphosarcoma
	Vasculitis
	Immunodeficiency
	Graft-versus-host disease
	Radiation enteritis
	Parasitic infestation
	Abdominal tuberculosis
	Pancreatitis
	Retroperitoneal tumors
	Retroperitoneal fibrosis
Increased lymphatic pressure	Constrictive pericarditis
	Right heart failure
	Portal hypertension

primary condition, with diarrhea and peripheral edema being obvious manifestations. Even macular edema and blindness have been reported. Despite increased fecal losses of immunoglobulin, systemic infection is rare because of enhanced immunoglobulin synthesis.

Intestinal Lymphangiectasia

This disease, first described in 1961 by Waldmann et al., is characterized by excessive gastrointestinal protein loss and dilatation of the submucosal lymphatics of the small intestine.[166] It has been variously named idiopathic hypoalbuminemia, hypercatabolic hypoproteinemia, and protein-losing enteropathy.

Incidence. Well over 100 cases have been reported, and 15 have been identified in a review of 14 years' experience at a children's hospital unit.[165]

Etiology and Pathogenesis. In most infants, the disease is presumed to be congenital, for it is frequently associated with other congenital lymphatic abnormalities such as lymphedema of one or more extremities, with agenesis of the inguinal, pelvic, or retroperitoneal lymph nodes, or with the angio-osteohypertrophy syndrome of cutaneous hemangiomas, varicose veins, and hypertrophy of soft tissue and bone. The lymphatics may be obstructed at any level of the bowel; therefore, involvement may be either generalized or restricted to the lamina propria or, alternatively, the mesenteric surface. The acquired form is caused by constrictive pericarditis, congestive heart failure, or obstruction of lymphatic drainage from retroperitoneal fibrosis, malrotation, or regional enteritis. It has been associated with immunoglobulin A deficiency, hypobetalipoproteinemia, and the Turner and Noonan syndromes. A transient form has also been reported.[105a]

Pathophysiology. The clinical manifestations are dependent upon rupture of dilated lymphatics into the bowel lumen to cause enteric losses of lymph contents: protein, fat, and lymphocytes. The normal albumin synthesis of 200 mg per kg per day is unable to keep pace with losses that may

approach as much as 10 gm of albumin per day in the infant.

Chylomicrons in the lamina propria and lipid droplets in the lymphatic endothelium testify to the fat losses, which measure as high as 30 gm per day.

Pathology. The intestinal mucosa appears pale, and the villi, normal or edematous. The bowel wall is edematous, and the serosal surface is engorged and dusky. The lumen is narrowed, and the valvulae conniventes are swollen. Microscopically, the lymphatics of the lamina propria and submucosa are dilated and the tips of the villi are swollen. Lipid-filled foamy macrophages fill some of the dilated lymphatics and invade the lamina propria and submucosa (Fig. 16–31). The epithelial cells of the villi and crypts are normal except for those at the villus tip, which contain lipid droplets in their bases. Electron microscopic studies show that the lymphatic endothelial cells of the intestinal mucosa contain prominent ultracellular filaments, and that the surrounding basal lamina, supporting cells, and collagen fibers are more prominent than in normal tissue.[68] There are abundant chylomicrons in the epithelial intracellular peg areas, in the extracellular spaces of the lamina propria, and in the lumens of the lymphatics. Lipid droplets fill the lymphatic endothelial cells. Leakage of other proteins and lymphocytes causes hypogammaglobulinemia, depression of transport proteins, and lymphopenia. T-cell responses are diminished and lymphocyte transformation impaired.[172]

Symptoms. The onset of symptoms may occur at any time from birth to adult life. At birth, a few babies have evidence of lymphedema of an extremity, but in most cases the physical examination is normal. During the first few months, there is a gradual onset of abdominal distention and a decrease in appetite and weight gain. Between two months and two years of age, the abdomen becomes markedly distended and the stools are noted to be malodorous, bulky, pale, and occasionally diarrheal. Only later in the course of the illness does the infant vomit or seem to have abdominal pain.

Nearly half the patients develop chylous

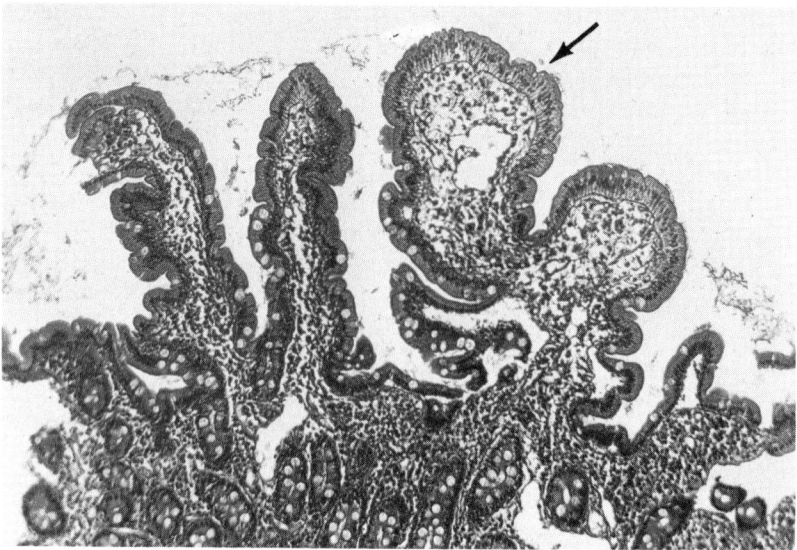

Figure 16–31 Small bowel biopsies from a patient with intestinal protein loss. Jejunal biopsy demonstrates dilated lymphatics in one villus (arrow), with normal-appearing adjacent villi.

effusions. In approximately 20 per cent, the peripheral edema that develops is asymmetric. The edema may be pitting or nonpitting and is usually associated with ascites (Fig. 16–32). Tetany and deficiencies of the fat-soluble vitamins result from malabsorption. Since the immunoglobulins are low, there is an increased susceptibility to infection as well as to tuberculosis and reticuloendothelial malignancies.

A few babies remain well nourished and have only mild gastrointestinal symptoms,

although they eventually develop all of the features associated with hypoproteinemia.

Diagnosis. The disease must be considered in any child with edema who has no evidence of cardiac, renal, or liver disease. The typical hematologic changes are low serum albumin, immunoglobulins, decreased ceruloplasmin, transferrin, and protein-bound iodine (PBI). There is peripheral lymphopenia and an extremely low erythrocyte sedimentation rate. The serum cholesterol is decreased, the xylose toler-

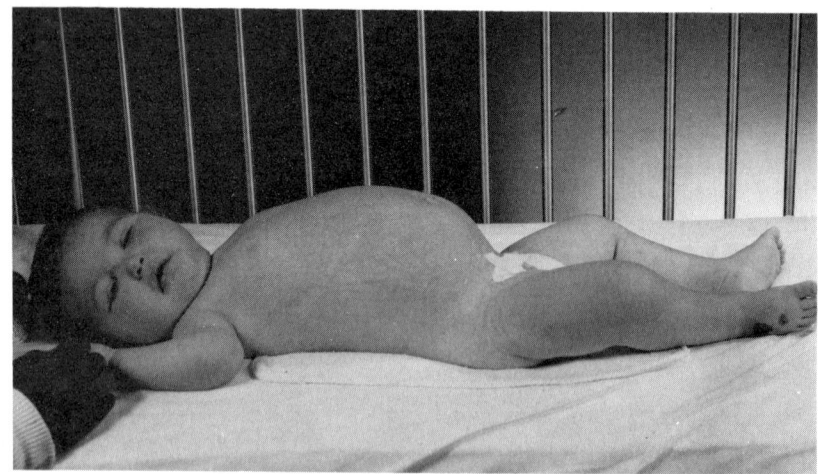

Figure 16–32 A ten-month-old infant with intestinal lymphangiectasia, total-body edema and ascites, and bilateral pleural effusions.

ance abnormal, and the quantitative fecal fat markedly increased. Lymphocytes are present in the stool. The lymphocyte loss leads to a particular depletion of the T cells, which results in abnormal delayed hypersensitivity reactions.

In 20 per cent of patients in whom the disease spares the lamina propria, x-rays are normal.[42] Radiologic examination of the gastrointestinal tract usually shows a normal colon and an abnormal small bowel (Fig. 16–33). The small intestine is of normal diameter or only minimally dilated, but the mucosal folds are symmetrically thickened. The barium is not particularly segmented,

but it is diluted in the distal small bowel by increased secretions. Infrequently, there are tiny dot-like lucencies. Endoscopy will further identify the thickened mucosal folds, but the small bowel biopsy is most essential to the diagnosis. Lymphangiography will determine lymphatic abnormalities, but since the dye is injected into the lymphatics of the foot or lower leg, such studies may be deferred to a later age, when they are more easily performed. Lymphangiography is not without hazard, for the peanut oil used as the vehicle may obstruct existing lymphatics and cause increased abdominal pain and lymphatic obstruction. In

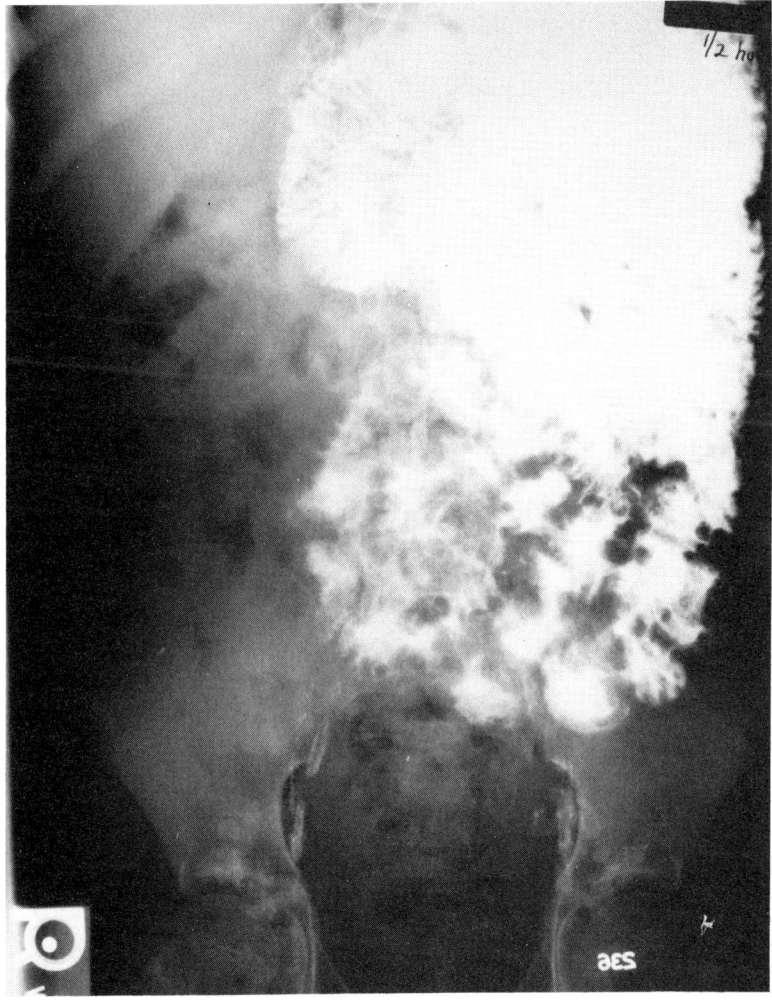

Figure 16–33 The small bowel in intestinal lymphangiectasia. Examination using nonflocculating barium shows coarse mucosal folds and dilution and stippling of barium throughout the lower jejunum and ileum. (From Caplan, D., Herskovic, T., and Gryboski, J. D.: Angio-osteohypertrophy syndrome with protein-losing enteropathy. J. Pediatr. *74*:119, 1969.)

a few studies, the dye has been visualized to pass from lymphatics into the intestinal lumen.

Albumin studies show a rapid degeneration of labeled albumin and normal or increased albumin synthesis. Herskovic et al. showed that injected iodine-131 had a prolonged half-life in a lymphedematous extremity and concluded that there is local trapping of albumin.[77a] Both chromium-51 and iodine-125 albumin are excellent vehicles to measure enteric protein loss, but neither is commercially available at this time. Radiolabeled albumin is restricted to those patients without evidence of significant gastrointestinal bleeding. The Cr-51 label is ideal, for it is not absorbed or secreted by the gut in any significant fashion. The usual dose is 30 uCi of chromium-51 albumin delivered intravenously, with stools and urine collected separately for 96 hours. An aliquot of homogenized stool is assayed in a scintillation counter with an aliquot of the original solution as a standard. Urine contamination of the stool must be avoided, as some label is excreted in the urine. Normally, less than 0.7 per cent of the injected label will appear in the stool, but in patients with this disease, excretion varies from 3 to 35 per cent. With a half-life of only five days, the label subsequently becomes bound to other proteins. I-125 albumin is less satisfactory because the label is reabsorbed after it is rapidly degraded in the gut.

Measurements of alpha$_1$-antitrypsin clearance are now currently the most feasible means of documenting enteric protein loss.[15, 33, 55a, 79] Clearance is also increased in the presence of blood loss. Using the formula:

$$\text{Clearance ml/24 hours} = \frac{\text{alpha}_1\text{-antitrypsin}}{\text{mg/gm}}$$
$$\times \frac{\text{daily stool weight}}{\text{serum concentration mg/dl}}$$

Hill et al.[79] found that normal subjects excreted less than 12.5 ml per day.

Treatment. Although spontaneous remissions are occasionally reported, medical therapy is universally initiated, with the aim of reducing the load delivered to the lymphatics. As a result, high-protein, low-fat diets are utilized, with long-chain fat replaced by medium-chain triglycerides, which are absorbed directly into the portal vein, bypassing the lymphatic route.[106] Although such diets reduce the complications of the disease, they should not be considered curative. Fat-soluble vitamins also should be supplemented. On rare occasions, venous alimentation is necessary to reverse the patient's catabolic state. Steroids have resulted in improvement in a few patients.[54]

When the disease is restricted to a short segment of bowel, a limited surgical resection may be considered. In conditions secondary to constrictive pericarditis or surgically correctable obstructions, the appropriate surgical procedure will lead to rapid resolution of the lymphatic leaks.

Lymphagiectasia of the Colon

Lymphangiectasia of the colon has been reported in several adults but warrants brief mention, for it is surgically correctable. The lesion is localized to the rectosigmoid region, where the mucosa appears studded with translucent elevations that exude clear fluid when incised. Histologic examination shows mucosal and submucosal edema, and dilated lymphatic channels in the submucosa and muscularis.

The major symptoms are watery mucoid diarrhea, edema, weakness, and a potassium depletion syndrome.

Hypoproteinemia and hypokalemia are the major chemical aberrations, and steatorrhea is variable. Barium examination of the colon shows segmental narrowing or polypoid changes suggestive of granulomatous colitis. Surgical resection of the diseased area is curative.

The Short Bowel Syndrome

In 1957, Pilling and Cresson[110] first reported the survival of a neonate following extensive intestinal resection. By 1965, the world literature consisted of but six cases. Now the numbers total in the hundreds owing to improvements in acute care and particularly to the development of techniques for prolonged venous alimentation.[94a]

The short bowel syndrome is defined as a residual small intestine less than 75 cm in length from the ligament of Treitz to the cecum. This is in contrast to a normal length of 250 to 270 cm in the term neonate. The small intestine elongates most rapidly until the child attains a body length of 60 cm, when it measures 325 cm, remaining relatively constant after the child attains a height of 100 cm. In general, the small intestinal length nearly triples from birth to puberty.

In the vast majority of infants, short bowel syndrome follows massive bowel resection for enteric atresias, volvulus, enterocolitis, or mesenteric vascular infarction. A congenital short bowel syndrome has also been described.[109a] Although there are no firm rules on the necessary length of residual bowel required for survival, Wilmore's[177, 178] experience with infants suggests a minimum of 15 cm when the ileocecal valve is preserved, and 40 cm when it has been resected.

Pathology and Pathophysiology. The bowel that remains undergoes morphologic and physiologic change in order to compensate for areas that have been removed.[119, 120] Not only is the absorptive area diminished, but regions of possible endocrine function are severely affected.[13] The nutritional complications of the syndrome obviously vary with the location and extent of resection; Table 16–5 summarizes the anticipated malabsorption from key nutrients.[174] Owing to the specificity of its role in bile acid and vitamin B_{12} absorption, every effort is made to preserve the ileum. The survival of these infants is dependent upon the morphologic and functional adaptation of the residual bowel with the additional long-term promise of elongation not seen in the adult.[43, 160, 161] In the presence of adequate nutrition, the adaptive response is one of hyperplasia with increased cellular proliferation and migration.[111] Intestinal diameter, villus height, and crypt depth therefore increase. Functional adaptation is noted with increases in nutrient, water, and electrolyte transport per centimeter of small intestine.[75] The specific activity of some mucosal enzymes (Na^+-K^+-ATPase, enterokinase, and

Table 16–5 Complications of Small Bowel Resection

Jejunum	Gastric hypersecretion
	Disaccharide intolerance
	Decreased secretin and cholecystokinin
	Decreased pancreatic secretions
	Decreased biliary secretions
	Impaired vitamin absorption (folate)
	Impaired iron, calcium, and magnesium absorption
	Protein malabsorption
	Zinc deficiency
	Steatorrhea
Ileum (distal)	Impaired vitamin B_{12} absorption
	Impaired bile salt absorption
	Bile salt depletion leads to fat malabsorption, vitamin malabsorption, cholelithiasis, colonic diarrhea and impaired water absorption, hyperoxaluria, and renal calculi
	Gastric hypersecretion

peptide hydrolases) has been shown to increase, although the brush border disaccharidases and glycolytic enzymes are usually decreased secondary to net loss of surface area.[99, 116] Lactose intolerance, therefore, is universal and long-lasting. Villous hypertrophy in the distal small bowel is greater after resection of the proximal small bowel than it is in the proximal bowel if the distal segment has been resected. That villous hypertrophy is noted in the segment distal to jejunal atresia in infants operated on shortly after birth suggests that work hypertrophy develops *in utero*.

The rate and degree of mucosal hypertrophy can be controlled, in part, by several factors.[16] Foremost is nutrient exposure.[179] In the absence of enteric delivery of nutrient, mucosal atrophy ensues. This is noted in the rat even when caloric balance is preserved by intravenous means or when non-nutrient bulk is delivered orally. A role for pancreatic and biliary secretions in optimal mucosal adaptation is suggested by complex animal data. As such secretion is dependent upon oral feedings, the true significance in humans is obscure. A third factor in the adaptive response is the trophic effect of the enteric hormone system. Most studies have focused upon gastrin, since an acute increase in gastrin levels follows small bowel resection and causes gastric hypersecretion and mucosal hypertrophy.[152, 180] Gastric hypersecretion probably contributes to diarrhea and causes intestinal ulceration.[22, 134] High fasting gastrin levels that increase sharply after a test meal indicate that the etiology is hypersecretion rather than diminished catabolism.[87] The predominant form of circulating hormone is big gastrin rather than big, big gastrin, which occurs in the fasting state of normal individuals. In the rat, exogenous pentagastrin has been shown to increase small bowel DNA synthesis. The role of other hormones such as secretin, cholecystokinin, glucagon, and vasoactive intestinal polypeptide is obscured by the reduction in the hormone levels after resection.[3]

Adaptation is impaired by prolonged fasting, ischemia, stricture or fistula formation, increased gastric acidity, rapid motility, or the development of retroperitoneal fibrosis.[97]

Resections of up to 25 per cent of the proximal small bowel do not significantly affect growth or nitrogen excretion, but those of 75 per cent are followed by negative nitrogen balance as well as impaired folate, carotene, iron, vitamin, calcium, and magnesium absorption. Resections of the distal small bowel are more often associated with weight loss, malabsorption, gastric hypersecretion, and rapid transit as well as vitamin B_{12} and bile salt malabsorption. Loss of the ileocecal valve decreases transit time and permits bacterial proliferation. Small bowel overgrowth is initially with yeast and later with coliforms as the pH begins to rise. Anaerobic overgrowth is rarely reported.

Symptoms. Infants who were in good nutritional status before operation fare better than those who were severely malnourished. Postoperative diarrheal stools are usually of an acid pH because of disaccharide or monosaccharide malabsorption. The transit time may be as short as 15 minutes. If the diarrhea is excessive, there is anal excoriation and the infant becomes dehydrated and acidotic. Prolonged malabsorption and the infant becomes dehydrated and acidotic. Prolonged malabsorption of fats and proteins leads to anemia and

edema. Tetany or frank seizures result from malabsorption of calcium or magnesium or both. Diarrhea persists for weeks to months and tends to improve as bowel absorptive capacities increase.[90] Vitamin D deficiency rickets may be a late complication.[160a]

Treatment. The nutritional management of these infants must be individualized within the general guidelines discussed in Chapter 9.[50, 157] Medications are reserved for specific complications. Thus, gastric hypersecretion is treated by antacids or, most specifically, by cimetidine.[30] Diarrhea from unabsorbed bile acids is treated by cholestyramine, Amphojel, or Pepto-Bismol, all of which bind bile acids. Treatment of bacterial overgrowth may require broad-spectrum antibiotics.

Increased transit has been treated with a multitude of medications. The derivatives of opium and haloperidol may decrease stool frequency, but third-space fluid losses may preclude their use. The efficacy of anticholinergics is questionable. Interposition of a "reversed segment" of gut to promote antiperistalsis and slow transit is a surgical option, but one with which we have had little experience.[168]

Prognosis. Wilmore reviewed 50 cases of small bowel resection in infants two months of age or younger to determine factors that correlate with survival.[177] All but one infant with more than 35 cm of small bowel survived; half of those with 15 to 25 cm of small bowel and an intact ileocecal valve survived; and none with less than 15 cm of small bowel or less than 40 cm and excision of the ileocecal valve survived. The mean birth weight of survivors was 3.1 kg, and of nonsurvivors, 2.3 kg. A later complication of ileal resection is the development of oxalate renal calculi. A 1979 survey of 15 infants who underwent massive resection, but who had the benefit of long-term hyperalimentation, has shown that two died before one year of age, but that by one year, 12 of the 13 survivors were taking oral feedings and demonstrated compensatory adaptation of the gut. None, however, had less than 25 cm of remaining small bowel. Survival has been reported in a 3300-gm infant with only 12 cm of intestine and an ileocecal valve remaining after resection for malrotation and volvulus.[84a]

BILE ACID METABOLISM

Bile acids are the end products of cholesterol degradation. Bile acids are present in the fetal gallbladder between 14 and 16 weeks of gestation, with chenodeoxycholic acid being found early, and cholic acid, later. The bile acids are excreted as taurine or glycine conjugates into the intestinal lumen. In the fetus, taurine conjugates predominate and some bile acids are present as sulfates.[127]

In the term neonate, bile acid synthesis and pool size are half that of the adult when calculated according to surface area, and are even less in premature infants.[170, 171] Meconium and stools of the newborn contain predominantly cholic and chenodeoxycholic acids and lesser amounts of deoxycholic and lithocholic acids.[21] After the first meconium passage, secondary bile acids are no longer present in the stool but reappear in the stool at five days. Bile acids measured in cord and infant serum decrease sharply following a brief rise shortly after birth[153] and rise throughout the first year, suggesting a transplacental passage of maternal bile acids. Bile acids are mainly conjugated with taurine through the first year of life, but later the ratio of glycine to taurine conjugates approaches the adult ratio of 3:1. Deoxycholate, the major of the secondary bile acids, may be absent during the first year of life, and lithocholic acid is present only in small quantities.[130, 135]

Some bile acids are reabsorbed in the small bowel, but most undergo active reabsorption in the terminal ileum, from which they are returned to the liver through the portal vein.[37] This enterohepatic circulation functions to maintain the bile acid pool. Since the function of bile acids is to form micelles with cholesterol and phospholipid in order to increase their solubility and facilitate the action of cholesterol esterase, they must be present in adequate concentration to be effective in fat digestion (2 to 4 mM/L). Conditions that decrease bile acid pool size result in malabsorption of fat.

DISORDERS OF BILE ACID METABOLISM

The majority of bile acid disorders are secondary to terminal ileal disease or to lesions causing bacterial overgrowth. Those related to specific liver diseases are discussed in Chapter Fourteen. Several disorders have been reported as primary ones and will be described in this section, but it is not certain that these were not due to enteric disease with bile acid loss and subsequent depletion of the bile acid pool.

Bile Acid Deficiency

A syndrome of bile acid deficiency suggesting a possible defect in synthesis was described in a three-month-old infant with chronic diarrhea and steatorrhea.[112] Pancreatic and small bowel function was normal, but intraluminal bile acids were decreased. Improvement followed treatment with oral bile acid supplementation.

Primary Bile Acid Malabsorption

Primary bile acid malabsorption was described in a two-day-old infant who developed watery diarrhea and steatorrhea.[78] Investigation of bile acid metabolism at one year showed a significantly increased fecal excretion and minimal postprandial rise in duodenal bile acids with decreased pool size, suggesting a basic defect in bile acid absorption.

The Blind-Loop Syndrome

The blind-loop syndrome is caused by intestinal stasis due to obstruction, diverticula, or motor abnormalities of the small bowel.[8, 27] Its hallmark is proliferation of small intestinal bacteria. Although it is occasionally asymptomatic, its major manifestations are diarrhea and steatorrhea, vitamin B_{12} malabsorption, weight loss, and anemia.

Etiology and Pathogenesis. Motor disorders of the small bowel and anatomic obstruction serve to create reservoirs for the proliferation of enteric flora.[61] The causes

Table 16–6   Causes of Bacterial
Overgrowth in Children

Functional	Achlorhydria
	Hypoperistalsis
	Pseudo-obstruction
	Postgastroenteritis
	Protein-calorie malnutrition
	Tropical sprue
	Scleroderma
Anatomic	Small bowel diverticula
	Stricture or stenosis
	Crohn's disease
	Tumor
	Error of rotation or fixation
	Billroth II gastrojejunostomy
	Enteroenteric anastomosis or fistula

are summarized in Table 16–6. Normally, the small bowel contains few bacteria because of the antibacterial action of gastric acid and the peristaltic action causing relatively rapid transit through the gut. The proximal small bowel normally contains only 10^3 to 10^4 organisms per ml, and these are predominantly streptococci, staphylococci, diphtheroids, and fungi. It is only in the distal small bowel that coliforms make their appearance; and in the terminal ileum, bacterial counts rise to 10^5 to 10^8 organisms per ml. In situations of stasis and bacterial overgrowth, numbers exceed 10^5, usually ranging between 10^6 and 10^{11} per ml. Coliforms now predominate as well as the anaerobes, bacteroides, bifidobacteria, and clostridia.

Malabsorption is associated with a number of mechanisms. The anaerobes and coliforms are capable of deconjugating bile salts, causing conjugated bile salts necessary for micelle formation and fat digestion to fall below a critical level. Bile acids are increased in the serum owing to accumulations of free acids. The organisms also compete for vitamin B_{12} by binding the vitamin to their cell surfaces.[173] A number of cellular functions are decreased — production of brush border enzymes (especially lactase), mucosal uptake of amino acids and sugars, and even intracellular enzyme function. Although the mucosal damage is usually attributed to the unconjugated bile acids, there is now evidence to show that bacterial enzymes from *Bacteroides, Clostridium,*

and *Streptococcus* may contribute to these abnormalities.[89, 122] Other pathologic changes include enteric blood and protein loss.

Studies of small intestinal histology show patchy changes of blunted, widened villi. Mononuclear cells within the lamina propria are increased, shedding of cells at the tip of the villus is increased, and there is often a mucobacterial exudate.

The diarrhea is the result of increased osmolarity and secretion within the small bowel and stimulation of colonic cyclic AMP by hydroxylated fatty acids and deconjugated bile acids. Water content of the stool is quadrupled, rising from 10.7 to 40.9 per cent, and sodium is similarly affected, rising from 10.8 to 44.8 mEq/L. Total bile acids rise from 16 to 41 μmol/24 hr.

Symptoms.   This complication may develop in a baby who has had correction of an intestinal anomaly or disordered intestinal peristalsis. Some infants are anorectic and vomit, but others have recurrent colicky abdominal pain and abdominal distention. The stools are loose or pale and malodorous. Weight loss and pallor become obvious as symptoms persist.

Diagnosis.   The hydrogen breath test using lactulose has been developed as a tool for the diagnosis of small intestinal bacterial overgrowth. The test uses the inability of lactase to be degraded before it enters the colon: Therefore an early rise in breath hydrogen occurs if bacterial overgrowth is present.

Malabsorption of fat is documented by increased 72-hour fecal fat and of vitamin B_{12} by the Schilling test. Results are abnormal in the presence of intrinsic factor, but administration of broad-spectrum antibiotics is corrective. Small intestinal bacterial overgrowth can be documented only by quantitative cultures, showing numbers greater than 10^6 per ml.

Radiologic examination of the small intestine will document anatomic abnormalities or abnormal peristalsis.

Treatment.   Surgical correction of any anatomic lesions is required. A course of four to six weeks of therapy with broad-spectrum antibiotics is usually sufficient to combat overgrowth and relieve symptoms.

BILE ACIDS IN ILEAL DISEASE OR RESECTION

Since the ileum absorbs more than 80 per cent of the bile acids that enter the intestine, disease or resection of this vital region results in significant fecal losses, increased hepatic synthesis, and a decrease in the total circulating pool of bile acids.[26, 38] Hofman and Poley[84] termed the resultant watery diarrhea "cholereic enteropathy," for the free and dehydroxylated bile acids stimulate colonic secretion and inhibit water and electrolyte absorption.[84]

Eventually, hepatic synthesis cannot keep pace with enteric losses and intraluminal bile acids are no longer sufficient for micellarization; at this point, the watery, diarrheal stools become steatorrheal.

Lester[96] has shown that ileal transport of bile acids is not well developed in the infant until eight months of age, and it has been shown that a number of instances of intractable diarrhea of infancy have been associated with increased fecal losses of bile acids.[7]

Long-term complications of ileal disease include the development of gallstones due to decreased solubility of cholesterol. In adults it is estimated that 25 per cent of patients with ileal resection will develop cholelithiasis, and this has been described even in the infant. Hyperoxaluria leading to the development of renal calculi results from increased colonic absorption of oxalate. Not only do bile acids render the colon more permeable to oxalate, but the concentrations of oxalate are increased because it is no longer bound to calcium that earlier has been saponified by unabsorbed fat.

Diagnosis. Bile acids in the stools may be measured most accurately by gas-liquid chromatography, but this is esentially a laboratory research procedure. Commercial kits are available to measure total bile acid levels, although they will not differentiate individual acids. A rapid test is the measurement of $^{14}CO_2$ present in breath samples after the ingestion of ^{14}C-glycine–labeled bile glycocholate. Increased activity at two or four hours is diagnostic. This form of malabsorption can be differentiated from that due to the bacterial overgrowth syndromes by the finding of increased amounts of label in the stool.

Treatment. The treatment depends upon the status of the bile acid pool. Early in the disease, when the pool is normal and watery diarrhea is prominent, bile acid–binding agents such as Amphojel, Pepto-Bismol, or cholestyramine are often effective. It must be recognized that cholestyramine decreases fat absorption, but the steatorrhea is often mild. When bile acid levels are insufficient for fat digestion, administration of bile salts will decrease steatorrhea but will probably precipitate diarrhea. The diet should be relatively low in fat and oxalate and should be supplemented with medium-chain triglycerides.

TUMORS OF THE SMALL BOWEL

The small bowel is the least common site for tumor development within the gastrointestinal tract. Aside from those associated with genetic disorders such as the polyposes or von Recklinghausen's disease, fewer than two dozen cases have been reported.

Benign tumors are asymptomatic until they cause either obstruction or gastrointestinal bleeding. Adenoma, leiomyoma, and lipoma have not been reported in infants.

VON RECKLINGHAUSEN'S DISEASE

The diagnosis of this disease in infancy is not difficult when the typical multiple café-au-lait spots are present over the skin.[20] Pigmentation in the infant is usually minimal and does not become evident until three or more years of age. This is a disease of multiple neurofibromas of peripheral nerves, skeletal lesions, subcutaneous nodules, and, often, retardation of mental and linear growth as well as sexual retardation. It is closely related to the multiple endocrine syndromes.

Incidence. The disease occurs in about

1 in every 2000 or 3000 live births. Neurofibromas constitute 6 per cent of all benign small bowel tumors.

Etiology. The disease is of a dominant type inheritance, and mothers, fathers, and other siblings may also be affected. Hereditary neurofibromas have a multiple-cell origin, with the tumor stimulus either affecting many cells simultaneously or affecting only one of several cells and altering the growth pattern of adjacent cells.[51]

Pathology. The skin lesions are macular, with abnormal deposits of melanin in the basal epithelial layers. Neurofibromas involve the peripheral nerves, especially the eighth cranial nerve, the vagus, the roots of the spinal nerves, or the sympathetic chain. They may involve any area of the gastrointestinal tract but most often are found in the small bowel, where they arise from the muscularis or the submucosa. They may be single, as in the duodenum, or multiple, as in the jejunum or ileum. The tumors contain an overgrowth of Schwann cells, some mast cells, and increased collagen and reticulin and are penetrated by nerve fibers. As they enlarge, the overlying mucosa tends to ulcerate, with resultant hemorrhage or occult blood loss and hypochromic, microcytic anemia. The polypoid nature of the tumor

may lead to small bowel obstruction because of its size or because of intussusception. Intestinal perforation has occurred in a few patients, and in 13 to 29 per cent of cases, the tumor has undergone malignant transformation.

Intrathoracic meningocele is an infrequent associated anomaly.

Symptoms. The diagnosis is usually made by recognition of the typical pigmentation (Fig. 16–34). A bathing-trunk nevus may be present at birth, and the typical café-au-lait spots may develop later. Crowe et al. state that six or more spots 1.5 cm in diameter are presumptive evidence,[33a] but fewer lesions are significant in the young child. Axillary freckling is also typical. Subcutaneous nodules were noted in one six-month-old infant, but these usually do not appear until puberty. Symptoms attributed to neurofibromas are chronic diarrhea, cramping abdominal pain, rectal bleeding, and melena. Submucosal lesions in the upper esophagus cause dysphagia. Many children suffer mental and growth retardation. One of our own patients had flatulence and lactose intolerance.

Diagnosis. It is important to differentiate this disorder from tuberous sclerosis, in which adenoma sebaceum, mental retar-

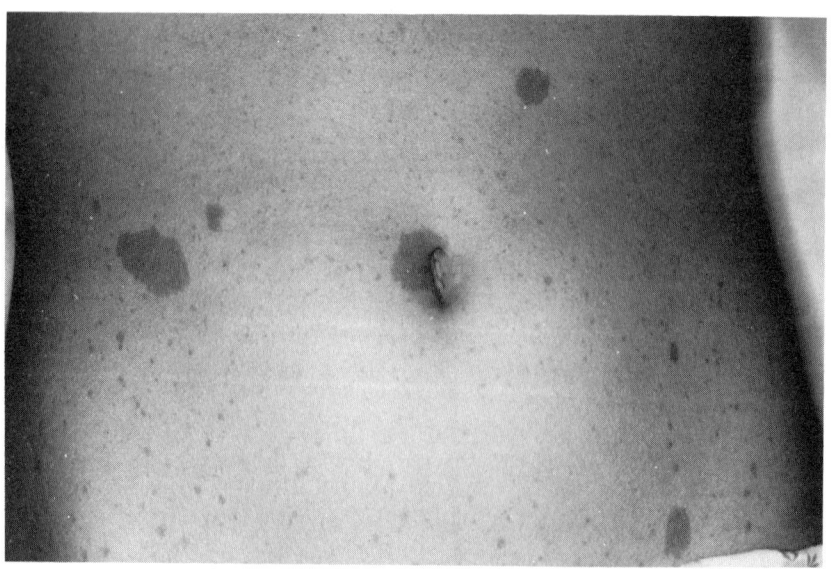

Figure 16–34 Abdominal café-au-lait spots of von Recklinghausen's disease. (Courtesy of Sidney Hurwitz, M.D.)

dation, and depigmented nevi are the manifestations. The cutaneous and subcutaneous lesions are rather characteristic, and a family history of the disease supports the diagnosis. Radiologic examination of the small bowel is unrewarding in most cases but rarely may show small, variably sized, round, intraluminal filling defects. Urinary catecholamines are normal.

Treatment. There is no treatment for the disease, but if intestinal neurofibromas are identified, they should be removed owing to their malignant potential.

Prognosis. The prognosis is discouraging, for 69 per cent of children born with stigmata of the disease have one or more peripheral nerve tumors by 20 years. Bone disease develops in more than half; 19 per cent have brain tumors before 12 years; and other types of malignant tumors develop in 15 per cent.

MALIGNANT TUMORS OF THE SMALL BOWEL

Malignant small bowel tumors are extremely rare, but whenever a small bowel radiograph reveals "abnormal small bowel folds," the issue of potential tumor presence arises. In Table 16–7, the differential diagnosis of such a radiologic finding is presented. As noted, any microbial agent capable of

Table 16–7 Differential Diagnosis of "Abnormal Small Bowel Folds"

Microbial enteritis (enteroinvasive)
  Salmonella, Shigella, Yersinia
  Whipple's disease
  Tropical sprue, tuberculosis
Inflammatory
  Crohn's enteritis
  Protein-induced enteropathy
  Eosinophilic gastroenteropathy
  Necrotizing enterocolitis
Submucosal edema/hemorrhage
  Hypoproteinemia
  Vasculitis (Henoch-Schönlein purpura)
  Intramural hematoma
  Mesenteric vein thrombosis
Tumors
  Leiomyosarcoma
  Lymphoma
  Retroperitoneal mass

invading the mucosal surface can induce an abnormality on x-ray. All of the inflammatory enteropathies can produce similar findings.

Most small bowel tumors are nonepithelial. Burkitt's lymphoma may present simply as an abdominal mass, while others are even more insidious, eventually showing a pattern of extrinsic small bowel obstruction. Congenital leiomyosarcoma has been reported in several neonates, causing intestinal obstruction in one and perforation and abscess in another.[45, 126] A total of 15 cases in children has been reported by 1981.[3a] Long-term follow-up was not available. These tumors may involve stomach, duodenum, or terminal ileum and even colon, causing vague symptoms of early satiety and pain or more definite symptoms of bleeding or obstruction.[143] As in adults, the duration of symptoms prior to diagnosis may be many months to more than one year. Calcification of the tumor mass may be noted.[3a]

Lymphoma of the small bowel is generally in the category of lymphosarcoma when it develops in the infant.[133] The presentation will often mimic celiac disease, with diarrhea, impaired growth, and malabsorption or protein-losing enteropathy. Intestinal blood loss and fever may also be seen. The small bowel lesions are bizarre and can mimic diffuse infiltrative disease, regional enteritis, or hemorrhage into the small bowel. The usual radiographic feature, however, is one of multiple nodular deformities of an extended segment of bowel. Invasion of the mesentery may displace the bowel, and retroperitoneal extension may develop. The small bowel biopsy may show villous blunting with nonspecific round cell infiltration of the lamina propria.

An embryonic mesenchymal jejunal tumor causing intestinal perforation was removed from a three-day-old female infant, who was well five and one-half years later. An angiosarcoma was removed from the small bowel of one infant in whom abdominal distention and a large abdominal mass were noted at birth.

Therapy of these tumors consists of surgical excision, abdominal irradiation, and chemotherapy with mustards, cyclophosphamide, vincristine, 6-mercaptopurine, and steroids. More than half the patients die within the first year of their disease, and the overall survival is less than 10 per cent. Graft-versus-host reactions may follow blood transfusion in children treated with immunosuppressive agents.[181]

Retroperitoneal tumors may involve the small bowel either by direct invasion or by compromising the vascular supply to a region of bowel. The intravenous pyelogram and computerized tomographic techniques will facilitate the diagnosis.

REFERENCES

1. Alexander, W. J.: Ulceration of the small bowel. Ann. R. Coll. Surg. Engl. 60:225, 1978.
2. Altman, D., and Puranik, S.: Superior mesenteric artery syndrome in children. Am. J. Roentgenol. Radium Ther. Nucl. Med. 118:104, 1973.
3. Altman, G. G.: Influence of bile and pancreatic secretions on the size of intestinal villi in the rat. Am. J. Anat. 132:167, 1971.
3a. Angerpointer, F. A., Wertz, H., Haas, R. J., and Hecker, W. C.: Intestinal leiomyosarcoma in childhood. J. Pediatr. Surg. 16:491, 1981.
3b. Anseline, P., Grundfest, S., Carey, W., and Weiss, R.: Pancreatic heterotopia, a rare cause of bowel obstruction. Surgery 90:110, 1981.
4. Apfelberg, D. B., Glickman, M., and Tang, T. T.: Gastroduodenal intussusception in a child. Surgery 69:736, 1971.
5. Arey, L. B.: Developmental Anatomy. Philadelphia, W. B. Saunders Company, 1974.
6. Arulananthem, K., Kramer, M., and Gryboski, J. D.: The association of inflammatory bowel disease and x-chromosome abnormality. Pediatrics 60:63, 1980.
7. Balistreri, W., Partin, J. C., and Schybert, W. K.: Bile acid malabsorption. A consequence of terminal ileal dysfunction in protracted diarrhea of infancy. J. Pediatr. 90:21, 1977.
8. Banwell, J. B., Kistler, L., Gianella, R., Weber, F., Jr., Lieber, A., and Powell, D.: Small intestinal bacterial overgrowth syndrome. Gastroenterology 80:834, 1981.
9. Barbero, G. K., Kim, I. C., and Davis, J.: Duodenal motility patterns in infants and children. Pediatrics 22:1054, 1958.
10. Bayless, T., Kapelowitz, R., Shelley, W., Balinger, W., and Hendrix, T.: Intestinal ulceration — a complication of celiac disease. N. Engl. J. Med. 276:996, 1967.
11. Beeken, W. L.: Transmissable agents in inflammatory bowel disease: 1980. Med. Clin. North Am. 64:1021, 1980.
12. Bennington, J. L., and Huber, S. L.: The embryologic significance of undifferentiated intestinal tract. J. Pediatr. 64:735, 1964.
13. Benson, C. D., Lloyd, J. R., and Krabbenhoft, K.

L.: The surgical and metabolic aspects of small bowel resection in the newborn. J. Pediatr. Surg. 2:227, 1967.
14. Berger, P. E., and Kuhn, J. P.: Blunt abdominal trauma in childhood. Am. J. Roentgenol. 126:105, 1980.
15. Bernier, J. J., Florent, C., and Desmazures, C.: Diagnosis of protein-losing enteropathy by gastrointestinal clearance of alpha-1-antitrypsin. Lancet 2:763, 1978.
16. Bohane, T. D., Haka-Ikse, K., Biggar, W. D., Hamilton, J. R., and Gall, D. G.: A clinical study of young infants after surgical resection. J. Pediatr. 94:552, 1979.
17. Bower, R., Sieber, W., and Kiesewetter, W.: Alimentary tract duplications in children. Ann. Surg. 188:689, 1978.
18. Boydstun, J., Jr., Gaffey, T., and Bartholemew, L.: Clinicopathologic study of nonspecific ulcers of the small intestine. Dig. Dis. Sci. 26:911, 1981.
19. Brandborg, L. L.: Other infectious, inflammatory and miscellaneous diseases. In Sleisenger, M., and Fordtran, J., (eds.): Gastrointestinal Disease. Philadelphia, W. B. Saunders Company, 1978.
20. Brasfeld, R. D., and das Gupta, T. K.: Von Recklinghausen's disease: a clinicopathologic study. Ann. Surg. 175:86, 1972.
21. Bruetow, M. J., Berger, H. M., Brown, G. A., Ablett, L., et al.: Duodenal bile acid conjugation patterns and dietary amino acids in the newborn. Gut 19:95, 1978.
21a. Bustamante, S., and Koldovsky, O.: Synopsis of development of the main morphologic structures of the human gastrointestinal tract. In Lebenthal, E. (ed.): Textbook of Gastroenterology and Nutrition in Infancy. New York, Raven Press, 1981, p. 49.
22. Buxon, B.: Small bowel resection and gastric acid hypersecretion. Gut 15:229, 1974.
23. Caldwell, J. H., Mekhjian, H. S., Hurtubise, P. E., and Beman, M.: Eosinophilic gastroenteritis with obstruction: immunologic studies of seven patients. Gastroenterology 74:825, 1978.
24. Campbell, J. B.: Neonatal gastric volvulus. Am. J. Radiol. 132:723, 1979.
25. Capitanio, M. A., and Kirkpatrick, J. H.: Lymphoid hyperplasia of the colon in children. Radiology 94:322, 1970.
26. Challacombe, D. N., Brown, G. A., and Edkins, S.: Duodenal bile acids in infants with protracted diarrhea. Arch. Dis. Child. 54:131, 1979.
27. Challacombe, D., Richardson, J., Edkins, S., and Hay, I.: Ileal blind loop in childhood. Am. J. Dis. Child. 128:719, 1974.
28. Chandrakamol, B.: Gastric heterotopia in the ileum causing hemorrhage. J. Pediatr. Surg. 13:484, 1980.
29. Christenssen, J. (ed.): Gastrointestinal Motility. New York, Raven Press, 1980.
30. Cortot, A., Fleming, C. R., and Malagelada, J. R.: Improved nutrient absorption after cimetidine in short bowel syndrome with gastric hypersecretion. N. Engl. J. Med. 300:79, 1979.
31. Crabbe, P. A., and Heremans, J. F.: Selective IgA

deficiency with steatorrhea. Am. J. Med. 42:319, 1967.

32. Crohn, B. B., and Yarnis, H.: Regional Ileitis. Ed. 2. New York, Grune & Stratton, 1958.

33. Crossley, J. R., and Elliott, R. B.: Simple method for diagnosing protein-losing enteropathies. Br. Med. J. 1:428, 1977.

33a. Crowe, F. W., Schull, W. J., and Neel, J.: A Clinical, Pathologic and Genetic Study of Multiple Neurofibromatosis. Springfield, Ill., Charles C Thomas, 1956.

34. Cumming, W. A., and Simpson, J. S.: Intestinal diverticulosis in Noonan's syndrome. Br. J. Radiol. 50:64, 1977.

35. Daum, F., and Silverberg, M.: Effect of congenital anomalies of the gastrointestinal tract upon infant nutrition. *In* Lebenthal, E. (ed.): Textbook of Gastroenterology and Nutrition in Infancy. New York, Raven Press, 1981, p. 921.

36. Davidson, G. P., Cutz, E., Hamilton, J. R., and Gall, G.: Familial enteropathy: a syndrome of protracted diarrhea from birth, failure to thrive and hypoplastic villus atrophy. Gastroenterology 75:783, 1978.

37. deBelle, R. C., Vaupshas, V., Vitullo, B. B., Haber, L. R., Shaffer, E., Machee, G. G. Owen H., Little, J. M., and Lester R.: Intestinal absorption of bile salts: immature development in the neonate. J. Pediatr. 94:472, 1979.

38. Demers, L. M., and Lloyd-Still, J. D.: Serum bile acid levels in protracted diarrhea of infancy. Am. J. Dis. Child. 132:1001, 1978.

39. Diard, F., Artuad, J., Bondonny, J., and Guibert, F.: Duodenal duplication in the neonate. Ann Radiol. 21:557, 1978.

40. Dickson, J. A. S.: Apple peel small bowel: an uncommon variant of duodenal jejunal atresia. J. Pediatr. Surg. 5:595, 1970.

41. Dobbins, J. W., Sheahan, D. G., and Behar, J.: Eosinophilic gastroenteritis with esophageal involvement. Gastroenterology 72:1312, 1977.

42. Donzell, F., Norberto, L., Marigo, A., Barbato, A., Tapparello, G., Basso, G., and Zacchello, G.: Primary intestinal lymphangiectasia —comparison between endoscopic and radiologic findings. Helv. Paediatr. Acta 35:169, 1980.

43. Dowling, R. M., and Booth, C. C.: Functional compensation after small bowel resection in man. Lancet 2:146, 1966.

43a. Ellis, D., Fischer, S. E., Smith W. I., and Jaffe, R.: Familial occurrence of renal and intestinal diseases associated with tissue autoantibodies. Am. J. Dis. Child. 136:323, 1982.

44. el-Shafie, M., and Rickham, P. P.: Multiple intestinal atresias. J. Pediatr. Surg. 5:655, 1970.

45. el-Shafie, M., Spitz, L., and Ikeda, S.: Malignant tumors of the small bowel in neonates presenting with perforation. J. Pediatr. Surg. 6:62, 1971.

46. Emmanuel, B., Gault, J., and Sanson, J.: Neonatal obstruction due to absence of intestinal musculature: a new entity. J. Pediatr. Surg. 2:332, 1967.

47. Esscher, T.: Preduodenal portal vein — a cause of intestinal obstruction. J. Pediatr. Surg. 15:609, 1980.

48. Esterly, J. R., and Talbert, J. L.: Jejunal atresia in twins with presumed congenital rubella. Lancet 1:1028, 1969.

49. Favara, B. E., Franciosi, R. A., and Akers, D. R.: Enteric duplications: thirty seven cases: a vascular theory of pathogenesis. Am. J. Dis. Child. 122:501, 1971.

50. Feldman, F. J., Dowling, R. H., MacNaughton, J., and Peters, T. J.: Effect of oral versus intravenous nutrition on intestinal adaptation after small bowel resection. Gastroenterology 70:712, 1976.

51. Fialkow, P., Sagebiel, R., Gartler, S., and Rimoin, D.: Multiple cell origin of hereditary neurofibromas. N. Engl. J. Med. 284:298, 1971.

52. Fieber, S. S., and Schaeffer, H. J.: Lymphoid hyperplasia of the terminal ileum — clinical entity? Gastroenterology 50:83, 1966.

53. Firor, H.: Gastrojejunocolic fistula in an infant. J. Pediatr. Surg. 5:450, 1970.

54. Fleisher, T. A., Strober, W., Muchmae, A., Broder, S., Krawitt, E., and Waldman, T. A.: Corticosteroid-responsive intestinal lymphangiectasia. N. Engl. J. Med. 300:605, 1979.

55. Flint, L., McCoy, M., Richardson, J. D., and Polk, H., Jr.: Duodenal injury: analysis of common misconceptions in diagnosis and treatment. Ann. Surg. 191:697, 1980.

55a. Florent, C., L'Hirondel, C., Desmazures, C., Aymes, C., and Bernier, J.: Intestinal clearance of α-1-antitrypsin. Gastroenterology 81:777, 1981.

56. Fonkalsrud, E. W., De Lorimier, A. A., and Hays, M.: Congenital atresia and stenosis of the duodenum. Pediatrics 43:79, 1969.

57. Galal, O., Osse, G., Weigel, W., and Gahr, M.: Pneumatosis intestinalis in children with leukemia. Eur. J. Pediatr. 137:91, 1981.

58. Georgaccopulo, P., and Vigi, V.: Duodenal obstruction due to a preduodenal portal vein in a newborn. J. Pediatr. Surg. 15:339, 1980.

59. Gornall, P., Ahmed, S., Jollyes, A., and Cohen, S.: Intra-abdominal injuries in the battered baby syndrome. Arch. Dis. Child. 47:211, 1972.

60. Gourevitch, A.: Duodenal atresia in the newborn. Ann. R. Coll. Surg. Engl. 48:141, 1971.

61. Gracey, M.: The contaminated small bowel syndrome: pathogenesis, diagnosis and treatment. Am. J. Clin. Nutr. 32:234, 1979.

62. Grand, R., Watkins, J., and Torti, F.: Development of the human gastrointestinal tract. Gastroenterology 70:790, 1976.

63. Grosfeld, J., Ballantine, T., and Shoemaker, R.: Operative management of intestinal atresia and stenosis based on pathological findings. J. Pediatr. Surg. 14:369, 1979.

64. Grosfeld, J., and Clatworthy, H. W., Jr.: The nature of ileal atresia due to intrauterine intussusception. Arch. Surg. 100:714, 1970.

65. Grosfeld, J., O'Neill, J., and Clatworthy, H. W., Jr.: Enteric duplications in infancy and childhood. Ann. Surg. 172:83, 1970.

66. Grosfeld, J., Schiller, M., Weinberger, M., and Clatworthy, H. W., Jr.: Primary non-specific ileal ulcers in children. Am. J. Dis. Child. 120:447, 1970.

67. Gruenberg, J., and Mackman, S.: Multiple lym-

phoid polyps in familial polyposis. Ann. Surg. *175*:552, 1972.

68. Gryboski, J. D.: Gastrointestinal Problems in the Infant. Ed. 1. Philadelphia, W. B. Saunders Company, 1975.

69. Gryboski, J. D., and Hillemeier, C.: Inflammatory bowel disease in children. Med. Clin. North Am., *64*:1185, 1980.

70. Gryboski, J. D.: Gastrointestinal function in the infant and young child. Clin. Gastrenterol. 6:253, 1977.

71. Gryboski, J. D., Self, T. W., Clemett, A., and Hirscovic, T.: Selective immunoglobulin A deficiency and intestinal nodular lymphoid hyperplasia: correction of diarrhea with antibiotics and plasma. Pediatrics *42*:833, 1968.

72. Guttman, F. M., Brown, P., Garance, P. H., Blanchard, H., Collin, P., Dallaire, L., Desjardins, J. G., and Perrault, G.: Multiple atresias and a new syndrome of multiple atresias involving the gastrointestinal tract from stomach to rectum. J. Pediatr. Surg. 8:633, 1973.

73. Haberkern, C., Christie, D., and Has, J.: Eosinophilic gastroenteritis presenting as ileocolitis. Gastroenterology 74:896, 1978.

74. Hamilton, J. R., Reilly, B. J., and Morecki, R.: Short small intestine associated with malrotation: a newly described congenital cause of intestinal malabsorption. Gastroenterology 56:125, 1969.

75. Hanson, W. R., Osborne, J. W., and Sharp, J. G.: Compensation by the residual intestine after intestinal resection in the rat. Gastroenterology 72:692, 1977.

76. Harrison, H. E., Spear, G. S., and Dorst, J. P.: Chronic idiopathic ileitis in infancy. J. Pediatr. 78:538, 1971.

77. Hermans, P. E., Huizenga, K. A., Hoffman, H., Brown, A. L., and Markowitz, H.: Dysgammaglobulinemia associated with nodular lymphoid hyperplasia of the small intestine. Am. J. Med. *40*:78, 1966.

77a. Herskovic, T., Winauer, S., Goldsmith, R., Kelin, R., and Zamchek, N.: Hypoproteinemia in intestinal lymphangiectasia. Pediatrics *40*:345, 1967.

78. Heubi, J., Balistreri, W., Partin, J., Schubert, W., and McGraw, C.: Refractory infantile diarrhea due to primary bile acid malabsorption. J. Pediatr. *94*:546, 1979.

79. Hill, R. E., Hercz, A., Corey, M. L., and Gilday, D. L.: Fecal clearance of alpha-1-antitrypsin: a reliable measure of enteric protein loss in children. J. Pediatr. 99:416, 1981.

80. Hirschberger, M., Rosental, E., and Thaler, M.: Segmental obstructing acute jejunitis in a child. Gastroenterology 73:166, 1977.

81. Hobb, W. H., and Cohen, S. E.: Gastroduodenal invagination due to submucous lipoma of the stomach. Am. J. Surg. *71*:505, 1946.

82. Hodgson, J. R., Hoffman, H. N., and Huizenga, K. A.: Roentgenologic features of lymphoid hyperplasia of the small intestine associated with dysgammaglobulinemia. Radiology 88:883, 1967.

83. Hofmann, A.: The chemistry of intraluminal digestion. Mayo Clin. Proc. *48*:617, 1973.

84. Hofmann, A., and Poley, J. R.: Role of bile acid malabsorption in the pathogenesis of diarrhea and steatorrhea in patients with ileal resection. Gastroenterology 62:918, 1972.

84a. Holt, D., Easa, D., Shim, W., and Suzuki, M.: Survival after massive small intestinal resection in a neonate. Am. J. Dis. Child. *136*:79, 1982.

85. Humphry, A., Mancer, K., and Stephens, C.: Obstructive circular muscle defect in the small bowel in a one year old. J. Pediatr. Surg. *15*:197, 1980.

86. Johnson, F.: Congenital preduodenal portal vein. Am. J. Roentgenol. *112*:93, 1971.

87. Johnson, L. R., Litchtenberger, L. M., Copeland, E. M., et al.: Action of gastrin on gastrointestinal structure and function. Gastroenterology 68:1184, 1975.

88. Jona, J. Z., Belin, R. P., and Burke, J. A.: Eosinophilic infiltration of the gastrointestinal tract in children. Am. J. Dis. Child. *130*:1136, 1976.

88a. Jonas, A., and Diver-Haber, A.: Stool output and composition in the chronic nonspecific diarrhea syndrome. Arch. Dis. Child. *157*:35, 1982.

89. Jonas, A., Krishran, C., and Forstner, G.: Pathogenesis of mucosal injury in the blind loop syndrome: release of disaccharidases from brush border membranes by extracts of bacteria obtained from intestinal blind loops in rats. Gastroenterology 75:791, 1978.

90. Kajiwara, T., Tamura, K., and Suzuki, T.: Follow up study of gastric response after resection of the jejunum and ileum. Ann Surg. *186*:694, 1977.

91. Katz, A. J., Goldman, H., and Grand, R.: Gastric mucosal biopsy in eosinophilic gastroenteritis. Gastroenterology 73:705, 1977.

92. Khan, W. K., and Kennedy, R.: Non-specific ulceration of the small bowel in children. J. Pediatr. Surg. 7:70, 1972.

93. Klein, N. C., Hargrove, R. L., Sleisenger, M. H., et al.: Eosinophilic gastroenteritis. Medicine 49:299, 1970.

94. Kleinman, P. K., Brill, P. W., and Winchester, P.: Pneumatosis intestinalis. Am. J. Dis. Child. *134*:1149, 1980.

94a. Klish, W. J., and Putnam, T. C.: The short gut. Am. J. Dis. Child. *135*:1056, 1981.

95. Lebenthal, E., Clark, B. A., and Kim, O.: Immunoglobulin concentrations in duodenal fluid of infants and children. Am. J. Dis. Child. *134*:834, 1980.

96. Lester, R.: Bile acid metabolism in the fetus and newborn. *In* Development of Mammalian Absorptive Process. Ciba Foundation Symposium 70. New York, Excerpta Medica, 1979.

97. Levine G., Deren, J., and Yezdimir, E.: Small bowel resection: oral intake is the stimulus for hyperplasia. Am. J. Dig. Dis. *21*:542, 1976.

98. Martin, D. M., Goldman, J. A., Gilliam, J., and Nasrallah, S. M.: Gold induced eosinophilic enterocolitis: response to oral cromolyn sodium. Gastroenterology *80*:1567, 1981.

98a. Mathe, J. C., Khairallah, S., Phat Vuong, N., Bacon-Gibod, L., Rey, A., and Costril, J.:

Segmental dilatation of the ileum in a neonate. Nouv. Presse Med. *11*:265, 1982.

98b. Matuchansky, C., Duprey, F., Briaud, M., Babin, P., Touchara, G., Bloch, P., Lenormand, Y., and Morichaubeauchant, M.: Diffuse nodular lymphoid hyperplasia of the adult small intestine without detectable systemic or digestive immunodeficiency. Gastroenterol. Clin. Biol. *6*:235, 1982.

99. McCarthy, D., and Kim, Y.: Changes in sucrase, enterokinase and peptide hydrolase after intestinal resection. J. Clin. Invest. *52*:942, 1973.

100. McGreevy, P., Doberneck, R., McLeay, J. M., and Miller, F.: Recurrent eosinophilic infiltrate of the ileum causing intussusception in a 2 year old child. Surgery *61*:280, 1967.

101. Miller, M.: Prune belly syndrome. Am. J. Dis. Child. *134*:1182, 1980.

102. Miller, R. C., and Larsen, E.: Regional enteritis in early infancy. Am. J. Dis. Child. *122*:301, 1971.

103. Montgomery, R. C., Poindexter, M. H., Hall, G., and Leigh, J. E.: Report of a case of annular pancreas of the newborn in the two consecutive siblings. Pediatrics *48*:148, 1971.

103a. Murray, S. M., and Woods, C. J.: Disseminated eosinophilic infiltration of a newborn infant with perforation of the terminal ileum and bile duct obstruction. Arch. Dis. Child. *56*:66, 1981.

104. Nawaz, K., Graham, D., Fechnerm, R. E., and Eiband, J. M.: Gastric heterotopia in the ileum with ulceration and chronic bleeding. Gastroenterology *66*:113, 1974.

105. Nixon, H. H., and Tawes, R.: Etiology and treatment of small intestinal atresia analysis of a series of 127 jejunoileal atresias and comparison with 62 duodenal atresias. Surgery *69*:41, 1971.

105a. Orbeck, H., Larsen, T., and Honig, T.: Transient intestinal lymphangiectasia. Acta Paediatr. Scand. *67*:677, 1978.

106. Ockner, R., Pittman, J. P., and Yager, J. L.: Differences in intestinal absorption of saturated and unsaturated long chain fatty acids. Gastroenterology *62*:981, 1972.

107. Okmian, L. G., and Kovamees, A.: Jejunal atresia with intestinal atresia. Strangulation of the intestine in the extra-embryonic coelom of the belly stalks. Acta Paediatr. *53*:65, 1964.

108. Patel, V. K., and Awen, C. F.: Benign lymphoid polyposis of the ileum: three cases and a review of the literature. Can. J. Surg. *14*:402, 1971.

109. Perkkio, M., and Savilahri, E.: Time of appearance of immunoglobulin containing cells of the intestinal mucosa of neonatal intestine. Pediatr. Res. *14*:953, 1980.

109a. Pellergin, D., and Bertin, P.: Primary postnatal volvulus of the small intestine. Ann. Chir. Int. *13*:83, 1972.

110. Pilling, G. P., and Cresson, S. L.: Massive resection of the small intestine in the neonatal period. Pediatrics *19*:940, 1957.

111. Porus, R. L.: Epithelial hyperplasia following massive small bowel resection in man. Gastroenterology *48*:753, 1965.

112. Powell, G., Jones, A., and Richardson, J.: A new

113. syndrome of bile acid deficiency: a possible synthetic defect. J. Pediatr. *83*:758, 1973.

113. Puranik, S. P., Keiser, R., and Gilbert, M.: Arteriomesenteric duodenal compression in children. Am. J. Surg. *124*:334, 1972.

114. Reid, I. S.: Biliary tract abnormalities associated with duodenal atresia. Arch. Dis. Child. *48*:952, 1973.

115. Reiquam, C., Allen, R., and Akers, D.: Normal and abnormal small bowel lengths. Am. J. Dis. Child. *109*:447, 1965.

116. Richards, A. J., Condon, J. R., and Mallinson, C. N.: Lactose intolerance following extensive small intestinal resection. Br. J. Surg. *58*:493, 1971.

117. Richardson, E. R., and Martin, L. W.: Pitfalls in the surgical management of the incomplete duodenal diaphragm. J. Pediatr. Surg. *4*:303, 1969.

118. Rickham, P. P.: Annular pancreas in the newborn. Arch. Dis. Child. *29*:80, 1954.

119. Rickham, P. P.: Massive small intestinal resection in newborn infants. Ann. R. Coll. Surg. Engl. *41*:480, 1967.

120. Rickham, P. P., Irving, I., and Shmerling, D. H.: Long-term results following extensive small intestinal resection in the neonatal period. Prog. Pediatr. Surg. *10*:65, 1977.

121. Rickwood, A. M. K.: Ileal atresia and fistula due to amniocentesis. J. Pediatr. *91*:312, 1978.

122. Riepe, S., Goldstein, J., and Alpers, D. H.: Effect of secreted bacteroides proteases on human intestinal brush border hydrolases. Clin. Invest. *66*:314, 1980.

123. Rittenhouse, E. A., Beckwith, J. B., Chappel, J. S., and Bill, A.: Multiple septa of the small bowel: description of an unusual case with review of the literature and consideration of the etiology. Surgery *71*:371, 1972.

124. Rosselo, P.: Congenital duodenal atresia associated with separate duodenal diaphragm. J. Pediatr. Surg. *13*:441, 1978.

125. Rossi, E., and Moser, H.: Genetic abnormalities of pancreatic and intestinal function. *In* Lebenthal, E. (ed.): Textbook of Gastroenterology and Nutrition in Infancy. New York, Raven Press, 1981.

126. Roth, D., and Farinacci, C. J.: Jejunal leiomyosarcoma in a newborn. Cancer *3*:1039, 1940.

126a. Rowe, M., Buckner, D., and Clatworthy, H., Jr.: Windsock web of the duodenum. Am. J. Surg. *116*:444, 1968.

127. Roy, C., and Weber, A.: Clinical implications of bile acids in Paediatrics. Clin. Gastroenterol. *6*:377, 1977.

128. Rubaltelli, F., and Largajolli, G.: Effect of light exposure on gut transit time in jaundiced newborns. Acta Pediatr. Scand. *62*:146, 1973.

129. Salonen, I. S.: Congenital duodenal obstruction. Acta Paediatr. Scand. (Suppl.) 272, 1978.

130. Sandberg, D.: Bile acid concentrations in serum during infancy and childhood. Pediatr. Res. *4*:262, 1970.

131. Sandheimer, J., and Hamilton, J. R.: Intestinal function in congenital heart disease. J. Pediatr. *92*:572, 1978.

132. Scher, W. K., and Girandy, B. R.: Functional intestinal obstruction in newborn infants

with morphologically normal gastrointestinal tracts. Surgery 53:357, 1963.

133. Schey, W. L., White, H., Conway, J., and Kidd, J.: Lymphosarcoma in children. Am. J. Roentgenol. Radium Ther. Nucl. Med. 117:59, 1973.

134. Scully, J. M., Lynch, F. J., Passaro, E., and Dudgeon, D. L.: Serum gastrin concentrations in infants with short gut syndrome. J. Pediatr. Surg. 11:315, 1976.

135. Sharp, H., Peller, J., Carey, J. B., and Krivit, W.: Primary and secondary bile acids in meconium. Pediatr. Res. 5:274, 1971.

136. Sherman, N., Morrow, D., and Asch, M.: A triple duplication of the alimentary tract. J. Pediatr. Surg. 13:187, 1978.

137. Shiori, T., Ishikawa, N., Hanori, Y., Nomura, H., Goto, H., Ando, S., and Tsuboi, K.: A case of duodenal polyp in a 5 month old infant. Jpn. J. Pediatr. Surg. Med. 3:735, 1971.

138. Sibenga, M. S., Karacadag, S., Capitano, M., and Kirkpatrick, J.: Benign lymphoid hyperplasia of the gut in children. 70th Annual Meeting of the American Gastroenterology Association. Washington, D. C., May 1969.

139. Siebert, J.: Small intestine length in infants and children. Am. J. Dis. Child. 134:593, 1980.

140. Simpson, A., Leonidas, J. C., Krasna, I., Becker, J., and Schneider, K.: Roentgen diagnosis of midgut malrotation: value of an upper gastrointestinal radiographic study. J. Pediatr. Surg. 7:243, 1972.

141. Snyder, W. H., Jr., and Chaffin, L.: Embryology and pathology of the intestinal tract: presentation of 40 cases of malrotation. Ann Surg. 140:368, 1954.

142. Solomon, J.: Functional intestinal obstruction in the neonate. Proc. Pediatr. Surg. Cong. Melbourne 1:38, 1970.

143. Solomons, N. W., Wagonfeld, J. B., Thomson, S., et al.: Leiomyosarcoma of the duodenum in a 10 year old boy. Pediatr. J. Surg. 268:73, 1976.

144. Soper, R. T., and Selke, A.: Congenital extrinsic obstruction of the duodenojejunal junction. J. Pediatr. Surg. 5:437, 1970.

145. Soper, R. T., and Selke, A.: Duplication cyst of the duodenum: case report of discussion. Surgery 68:562, 1970.

146. Spencer, R.: The various patterns of intestinal atresia. Surgery 64:661, 1968.

147. Spitz, L., Ali, M., and Brereton, R. J.: Combined esophageal and duodenal atresia: experience of 18 patients. J. Pediatr. Surg. 16:4, 1981.

148. Stauffer, U. G., and Herrmann, P.: Comparison of late results in patients with corrected intestinal malrotation with and without fixation of the mesentery. J. Pediatr. Surg. 15:9, 1980.

149. Steiner, D. H., Maxwell, J. G., Rasmussen, B. L., and Jones, R.: Segmental absence of intestinal musculature. Am. J. Surg. 118:964, 1969.

150. Stewart, D., Byrd, C., and Schuster, S.: Intramural hematomas of the alimentary tract in children. Surgery 69:673, 1971.

151. Stewart, D., Colodny, A., and Daggett, W. C.: Malrotation of the bowel in infants and

children. 15 year review. Surgery 79:716, 1976.

152. Straus, E., Gerson, C. D., and Yalow, R.: Hypersecretion of gastrin associated with the short bowel syndrome. Gastroenterology 66:175, 1974.

153. Suchy, F., Balistreri, W., Heubi, J., Searey, J., and Levin, R.: Physiologic cholestasis: elevations of the primary serum bile acid concentrations in normal infants. Gastroenterology 80:1037, 1981.

154. Sunaryo, F., Boyle, J., Ziegler, M., and Heyman, S.: Primary non-specific ulceration as a cause of massive rectal bleeding. Pediatrics 68:247, 1981.

155. Tedesco, F., Huckaby, C., Hamby-Allen, M., and Ewing, G.: Eosinophilic ileocolitis: expanding spectrum of eosinophilic gastroenteritis. Dig. Dis. Sci. 26:943, 1981.

155a. Teja, K., Schnatterly, P., and Shaw, A.: Multiple intestinal atresias: Pathology and pathogenesis. J. Pediatr. Surg. 16:194, 1981.

156. Teele, R. L., Katz, A. J., Goldman, H., and Kettell, T.: Radiographic features of eosinophilic gastroenteritis (allergic gastroenteropathy) of childhood. Am. J. Radiol. 132:575, 1979.

157. Tepias, J., MacLean, W., Kolbach, S., and Sherman, D.: Total management of short gut secondary to midgut volvulus without prolonged total parenteral alimentation. J. Pediatr. Surg. 13:622, 1978.

158. Thayer, W. R., Jr.: Inflammatory bowel disease: where are the frontiers? Med. Clin. North Am. 64:1221, 1980.

158a. Tibhoel, D., Van Nie, C., and Molenaar, J.: The effects of temporary general hypoxia and local ischemia on the development of the intestines. J. Pediatr. Surg. 15:57, 1980.

159. Tift, W. L.: Protein losing enteropathies. In Harries, J. T. (ed.): Essentials of Pediatric Gastroenterology. London, Churchill Livingstone, 1977.

160. Touloukian, R.: Antenatal intestinal adaptation with experimental jejunoileal atresia. J. Pediatr. Surg. 13:468, 1978.

160a. Touloukian, R. J., and Gertner, J. M.: Vitamin D deficiency rickets as a late complication of the short gut syndrome. J. Pediatr. Surg. 16:230, 1981.

161. Touloukian, R. J., and Wright, H.: Intrauterine villus hypertrophy with jejunoileal atresia. J. Pediatr. Surg. 8:779, 1973.

162. Townes, P., Wunderlich, R. C., and Gerbasi, M. J.: Familial occurrence of malrotation of the intestine. J. Pediatr. 60:555, 1962.

163. Tully, T. E., and Feinberg, S. B.: Those other types of enterocolitis. Am. J. Roentgenol. Radium Ther. Nucl. Med. 121:291, 1974.

164. Ureles, A. L., Alschebaja, T., Locro, D., et al.: Idiopathic eosinophilic infiltration of the gastrointestinal tract, diffuse and circumscribed. Am. J. Med. 30:899, 1961.

165. Vardy, P., Lebenthal, E., and Shwachman, H.: Intestinal lymphangiectasia: a reappraisal. Pediatrics 55:842, 1975.

166. Waldman, T. A.: Protein losing enteropathy. Gastroenterology 50:422, 1966.

167. Waldman, T. A., and Schwab, P. J.: IgG metabolism in hypogammaglobulinemia: stud-

ies in patients with defective gamma globulin synthesis, gastrointestinal blood loss, or both. J. Clin. Invest. *44*:1523, 1965.

168. Warden, M. J., and Wesley, J.: Small bowel reversal procedure for treatment of the "short gut" baby. J. Pediatr. Surg. *13*:321, 1978.

169. Wathen, L. M., Osborne, J. W., and Loven, D. P.: Effect of two intestinal resections separated by time on cell proliferation in the rat small intestine. Gastroenterology *80*:1535, 1981.

170. Watkins, J.: Role of bile acids in the development of the enterohepatic circulation. Lebenthal, E. (ed.): Textbook of Gastroenterology and Nutrition in Infancy. New York, Raven Press, 1981, p. 167.

171. Watkins, J., Szczpanik, P., Gould, J. B., Klein, D. D., and Lester, R.: Bile salt metabolism in the premature infant. Gastroenterology *69*:706, 1978.

172. Weiden, D. I., Blaese, R. M., Strober, W., Block, J. B., and Waldman, T. A.: Impaired lymphocyte transformation in intestinal lymphangiectasia. Evidence for at least two functionally distinct lymphocyte populations in man. J. Clin. Invest. *51*:1319, 1972.

173. Welkos, S. L., Toskes, P. P., Baer, H., and Smith, G.: Importance of anaerobic bacteria in the cobalamin malabsorption of the experimental rat blind loop syndrome. Gastroenterology *77*:572, 1979.

174. Weser, E.: Short bowel syndrome. Gastroenterology *77*:572, 1979.

175. Wesley, J. R., and Mahour, G. H.: Congenital intrinsic duodenal obstruction: a 25 year review. Surgery *82*:716, 1977.

176. Williams, W. H., and Hendren, W. H.: Intrapancreatic duodenal duplication causing pancreatitis in a child. Surgery *69*:708, 1971.

177. Wilmore, D. W.: Factors correlating with a successful outcome following extensive intestinal resection in newborn infants. J. Pediatr. *80*:88, 1972.

178. Wilmore, D. W., Dudrick, S. J., Daly, J. M., and Vans, H. M.: The role of nutrition in the adaptation of the small intestine after massive intestinal resection. Surg. Gynecol. Obstet. *132*:673, 1971.

179. Winawer, S. J., Broitman, S. D., Wolochow, A., et al.: Successful management of massive small bowel resection based on assessment of absorption defects and nutritional needs. J. Med. *274*:72, 1966.

180. Winborn, W. B., Seeling, L. L., Nakayama, H., et al.: Hyperplasia of the gastric glands after small bowel resection in the rat. Gastroenterology *66*:384, 1974.

181. Woods, W., and Lubin, B.: Fatal graft versus host disease following a blood transfusion in a child with neuroblastoma. Pediatrics *67*:217, 1981.

182. Woolley, M., Mahour, G. H., and Sloan, T.: Duodenal hematoma in infancy and childhood: changing etiology and treatment. Am. J. Surg. *136*:8, 1978.

183. Wrenn, E. J., and Favara, B. E.: Duodenal duplication presenting as a double gallbladder. Surgery *63*:859, 1971.

Chapter Seventeen

THE COLON, RECTUM, AND ANUS

The colon is divided into two portions, each with a different derivation and function. The proximal portion, extending from the cecum to the midtransverse colon, is derived from the embryonic midgut and receives its vascular supply from the superior mesenteric artery. The distal portion, containing the remainder of the transverse, the sigmoid, and the descending colon, is derived from the hindgut and receives its vascular supply from the inferior mesenteric artery. The proximal colon functions to absorb more than 90 per cent of sodium and chloride and variable amounts of bicarbonate and 80 per cent or more of the water entering the cecum.[16] Absorption is by electrogenic Na^+ absorption and both active and neutral Cl^-/HCO_3 exchange. Absorption is greatest in the proximal colon and declines caudally. It is inhibited by glycine and taurine conjugates of bile acids and drugs that stimulate cyclic AMP and is impaired if large volumes of water are delivered to the cecum and overcome its absorptive capacity. The colon is thought to secrete small quantities of potassium because stool contains more potassium than does ileostomy fluid. Mineralocorticoids increase colonic potassium losses. Intraluminal chloride is essential for bicarbonate excretion, because the colon replaces absorbed chloride with potassium. Some glucose, amino acids, short-chain fatty acids, and vitamins are absorbed slowly and in small quantity. Although urea is not absorbed, its end-product, ammonia, is. The distal colon functions primarily as a reservoir.

ANATOMY

Some of the characteristic colonic structures are the haustra, or sacculations, separated by the plicae semilunares and extending transversely from the taeniae coli. The latter are three longitudinal bands that develop in the tenth or eleventh week of fetal life and extend from the cecum to the tip of the rectum. The serosa is covered by fatty appendices epiploicae. The ileum joins the colon at the ileocecal valve, which prevents retrograde reflux of fecal material. After birth, the cecum, with the appendix at its apex, enlarges laterally to form a pouch so that the base of the appendix eventually lies medial to it. In most people the ascending colon is fixed retroperitoneally to the posterior abdominal wall; the transverse colon is suspended in the transverse mesocolon; the descending colon is fixed retroperitoneally; and the sigmoid colon has a mesentery that permits a great deal of mobility. The neonatal colon measures approximately 45 cm.

The rectum, relatively straight in infancy, assumes a curve as the sacral concavity develops during the first few years. The lower rectum lies below the peritoneal reflection, a point to be noted when one takes a rectal biopsy. Its lumen contains three shelf-like valves, the valves of Houston, which are not well developed until after the first year. The short anal canal contains the internal and external sphincters. It is attached posteriorly to the sacrum by the coccygeus muscle and is surrounded by the pelvic diaphragm muscles. Internally, anal papillae connect by a narrow membrane to form anal valves. The internal and external hemorrhoidal plexuses lie within the anal canal. Pressures within the anal canal are higher in infants less than 10 hrs of age than in those 10 to 72 hours old. Pressures are lower in those who have passed meconium than in those who have not.[168]

Histologically, the colon shows serosa, longitudinal and circular muscle, submucosa, and mucosa. As early as 12 weeks, neuroblasts are present in the rectum. Neuroblasts continue to mature after birth up to 5 years of age. Preganglionic parasympathetic nerves synapse in the myenteric plexus of Auerbach, which lies on the outer surface of the circular muscle and contains postganglionic fibers that communicate with the submucous plexus of Meissner. The submucosa contains small veins, arteries, and lymphatics and is separated from the mucosa by the muscularis mucosae. The flat mucosa covered by columnar epithelial and goblet cells is penetrated by uniform glands or crypts of Lieberkühn (Fig. 17–1).

MOTOR FUNCTION

Major activities of the colon are mixing and propulsion.[102] Mixing is accomplished by segmentation and the formation of contraction rings into pockets, the haustrae. Propulsion occurs as a mass movement of a contraction that appears proximal to the bolus and propels it caudally in a sequence of large, positive-pressure waves. Colonic

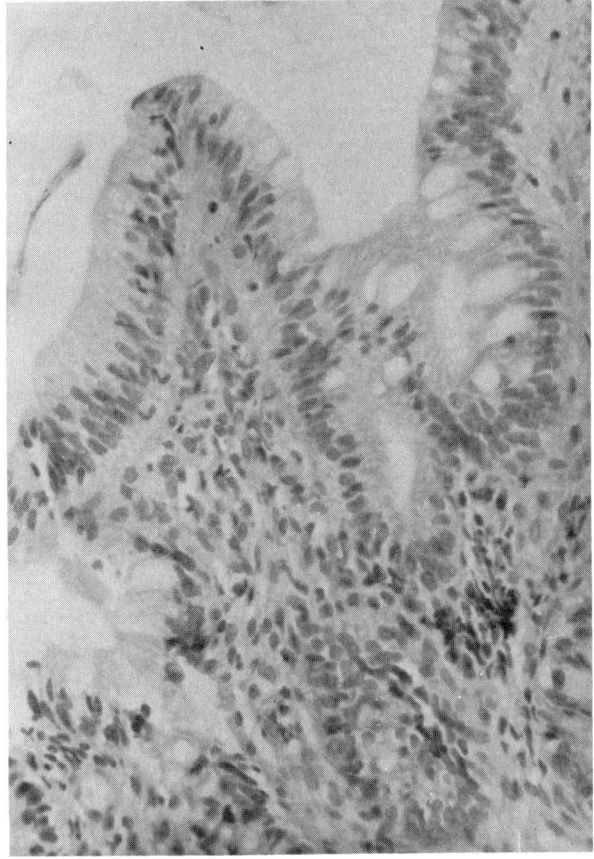

Figure 17–1 Biopsy of normal rectal mucosa to demonstrate the regular arrangement of tall columnar epithelial cells and interspersed goblet cells. The normal lamina propria here contains blood vessels, lymphatics, and round cell infiltrate.

motor activity is slow and variable; it is decreased during sleep and increased during eating or emotional stress, as reflected in the irritable bowel syndrome and colic.[168] Radiologically, antiperistaltic movement is the major finding in the proximal colon: segmentation in the midcolon with ring-like contractions, and strong caudad contractions in the distal colon. Manometric techniques have shown four types of waves. Generally, type I waves are short — only about 5 seconds in duration, are present in the proximal and absent in the distal colon, and are superimposed on type II or III waves. They are probably initiated by the manometric system. Type II waves represent most activity in the descending and sigmoid colon, and in the adult vary in duration between 12 and 120 seconds and in amplitude between 6.5 and 9.7 cm of water. They are sometimes propulsive and sometimes not. Type III waves are of low amplitude — 10 cm of water, and slow, lasting 1 to 4 minutes. Type IV waves are strong propulsive contractions, which have been recorded from patients with ulcerative colitis.

In children, 87 to 91 per cent of waves in the rectosigmoid are 5 cm of water or less in amplitude and 12 seconds or less in duration.[34, 35, 105] In patients with recurrent abdominal pain, in those with irritable bowel, and in a few normal persons the fact that neostigmine (Prostigmin) causes an increase in waves of greater amplitude and duration suggests an autonomic imbalance or increased sensitivity to parasympathetic stimulation. Subcutaneous administration of methacholine (Mecholyl) is followed by relaxation of the phasic action of the distal colon in half the normal population. In some of those with Hirschsprung's disease, this phenomenon is apparent in the normally innervated area and not in the aganglionic segment.

The electrical control activity (ECA) of the colon is irregular compared with that of the proximal intestine and stomach.[159, 193] Three areas of distinct electrical activity are identified. The proximal segment of ascending colon has a low amplitude signal of varying frequency with the major frequency being 4.1 c/min. The second segment includes the proximal transverse to descending or sigmoid colon and has a dominant component in a higher frequency range of 10 c/sec, although low frequency components are also present. The distal segment is characterized by both types of frequency components, with the lower ones dominant. Activity in the proximal and distal colon is not phase locked. Slow waves are therefore present in all segments of colon, increasing in frequency caudally. Spike bursts that are prolonged or periodic may represent muscle release from tonic inhibition from intramural inhibitory nerves.

CONGENITAL ANOMALIES OF THE COLON

Congenital anomalies may involve any segment of the colon but are most often found in the distal large bowel and anus.

GASTRIC HETEROTOPIA IN THE COLON

Gastric heterotopia in the colon may occur with or without an associated congenital intestinal diverticulum.[43]

Incidence. Approximately 10 cases have been reported in the literature to 1980.[36a]

Etiology. The defect is grouped under those abnormalities related to the embryonic ectoendodermal adhesions that result from notochord maldevelopment. Females predominate and in 30 per cent there are associated anomalies, such as Meckel's diverticulum, spina bifida, defective vertebrae, and malrotation of the colon.

Pathology. Gastric tissue is usually located in a congenital diverticulum of the colon but is rarely present as a submucosal nodule. In some patients fibrous bands extend between it and a spina bifida.

Symptoms. These relate to peptic ulceration of the mucosa, with rectal bleeding and abdominal pain manifest at birth or after several years of life.

Treatment. Excision of the diverticulum and/or ectopic tissue is curative.

Duplication Cysts of the Large Bowel

Duplications of the large bowel include also those of the appendix.[72, 131]

Incidence. These account for 16 to 30 per cent of all the enteric duplications. They do not seem to be familial and are twice as frequent in females as in males. Bower et al. in 1978 reported 14 duplications of the appendix, colon, and rectum.[19, 107, 142]

Etiology. The etiology is the same as that of other duplications. The theory that a twinning process occurs when the hindgut divides into two equal parts is supported by the frequent association of duplications of urethra and bladder.[91]

Pathology. The duplications are spherical, tubular, or loop-type and contain mucosal, serosal, and muscle layers. Communicating cysts are more common than noncommunicating ones and usually have only a proximal connection to the colon. Since these cysts do not empty from below, they dilate to become saccular masses filled with stagnant material that serves as a lead point for volvulus. The mucosal lining most often is colonic, but in some cases it is gastric or small intestinal. Bleeding results from autodigestion or ischemia of the intestinal mucosa overlying the cyst. Duplications of the appendix are often associated with bladder anomalies.

These large-bowel cysts are classified into two types: type I is partial and involves only a segment of colon. It can be spherical, tubular, double-barreled, or looped and is sometimes multiple. Only the colon and rectum are involved and other anomalies are rare. Type II duplications tend to involve the entire colon and are double-barreled, having proximal and distal connections. These are often associated with rectovaginal fistula, duplications of the bladder and urethra, and double or imperforate anus.[153] Less usual anomalies are situs inversus, malrotation, pubic separation, omphalocele, and exstrophy of the bladder (Fig. 17–2).

One case of colonic triplication is reported.[70]

Symptoms. The symptoms are multiple and depend in large part upon the type and location of the cyst. The double-barreled duplications are often asymptomatic, for they can empty themselves. In many babies the only finding is palpation of an unexpected abdominal mass. Some have recurrent attacks of abdominal pain and others have rectal bleeding. Lesions in the cecum or ascending colon function as a lead point for intussusception. These cause colicky abdominal pain and rectal bleeding. A sausage-shaped mass is palpated in the right upper quadrant. Cysts in the ascending colon cause pain, progressive abdominal distention, and volvulus. Those more distal in the transverse or sigmoid colon or in the rectum cause tenesmus, chronic constipation, and ultimately, low intestinal obstruction. Rectal duplications are palpated during the rectal examination as posterior soft rectal masses. Very rarely they present as an abdominal mass or as rectal prolapse.[170] The finding of rectovaginal fistula or spina bifida in any infant should initiate an investigation of the colon.[132]

Diagnosis. The diagnostic studies must differentiate teratoma, malrotation volvulus, intussusception, and stenosis of the colon. A plain film of the abdomen shows nonspecific dilatation of small bowel loops or colon proximal to the cyst. A barium enema sometimes fills the communication and outlines the cyst. More often, an extraluminal pressure defect is all that is demonstrated (Fig. 17–2). Rarely the mass reaches such size that it compresses a ureter to cause hydronephrosis or to perforate. Scanning of the abdomen after intravenous injection of technetium 99m pertechnetate will detect these duplications lined by gastric mucosa, but technical difficulties are encountered if they lie in the transverse colon near the stomach.

Treatment. Duplications of the colon are treated by segmental resection. In cases of total colonic duplication, partial resection and establishment of a distal connection between the cyst and colon are the recommended treatment. The rectal duplications are frequently loosely attached and can often be excised through a para-anal approach.

Prognosis. Obviously the prognosis depends upon the type of lesion. If the ileocecal valve is resected, persistent diarrhea is a problem. If cystic remnants remain, they can cause intestinal hemorrhage and perforation.

DUPLICATIONS OF THE ANUS AND GENITOURINARY TRACT

Until 1969, only 57 cases of this anomaly had been reported[22, 40] and patients have been reported sporadically since.[28]

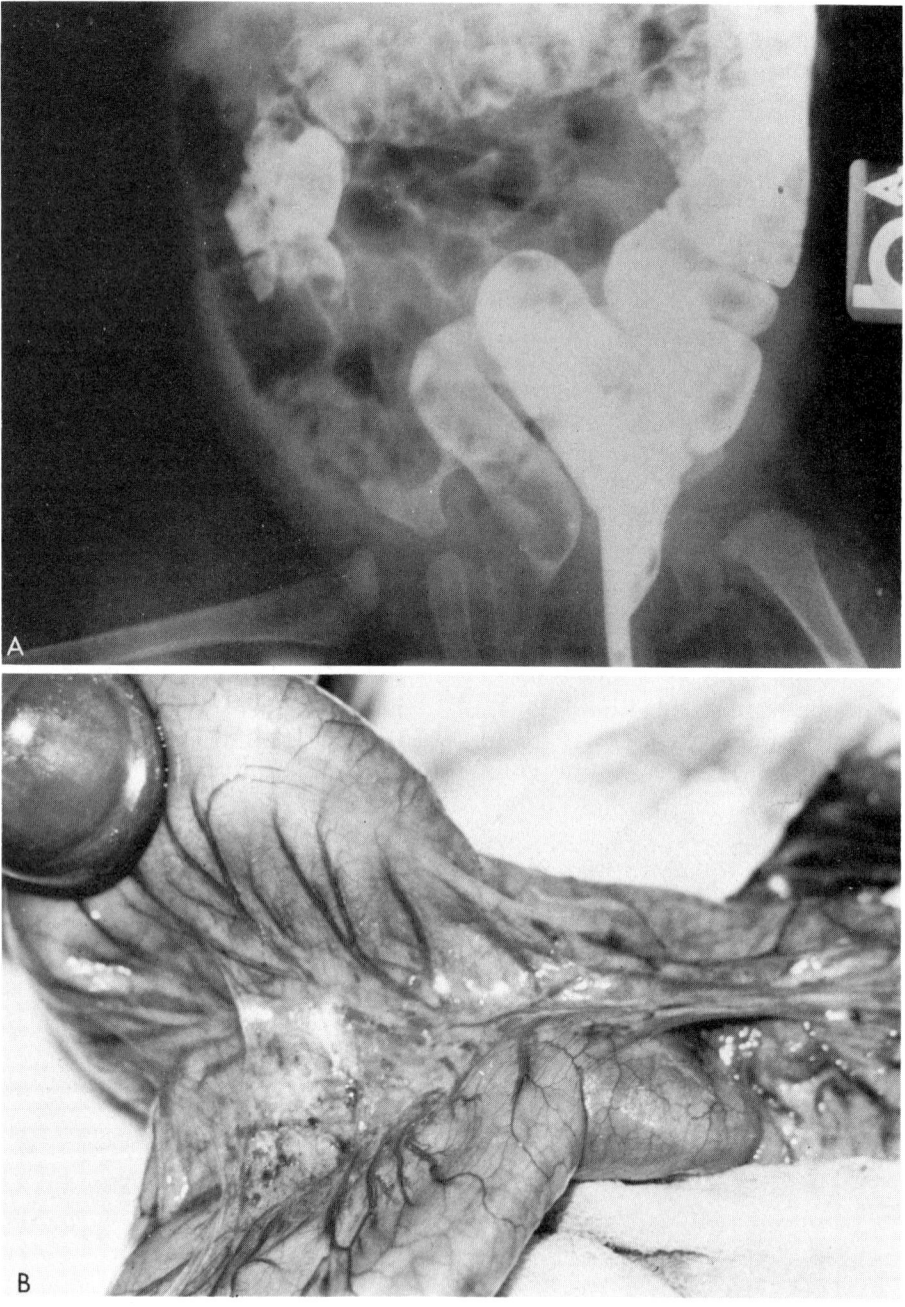

Figure 17–2 A, Duplication of the rectum demonstrated by barium enema study. B, Photograph of the duplication at the time of surgery. (Courtesy of L. Pickett, M.D.) C, Infant with duplication of rectum, anus, vulva, vagina, bladder, and urethra.

Illustration continued on opposite page

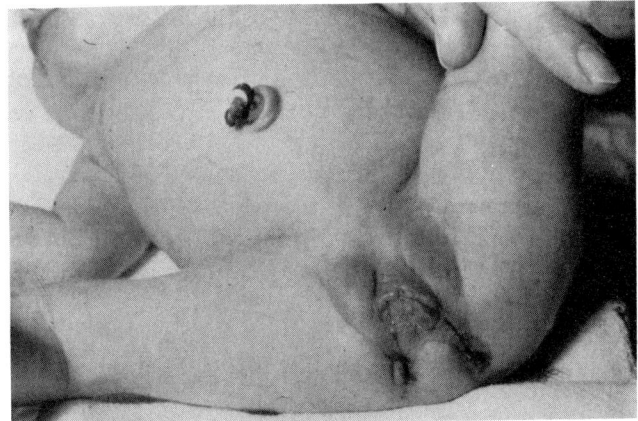

Figure 17–2   Continued

C

These lesions, probably due to a persistence of the cloacal anus, are of three patterns. The most common anomaly is duplication of rectum and colon extending to the cecum, with double anus, vulva, vagina, bladder, and urethra (Fig. 17–2C). In the second type there is a double anus, one of which may be imperforate; a common puborectalis muscle and external sphincter; and two internal sphincters. The genitalia are usually normal. The third and most unusual type consists of a double anus terminating as fistulas or as one normal rectum with a fistula to the vestibule or vagina.[82] There may or may not be duplication of the genitalia and urethra. Anterior sacral meningocele is an associated anomaly.[1] These defects are obvious in the newborn examination, and later the infants pass stool through other than the normal anus. The treatment is anoplasty or vestibuloanal pull-through with transplantation of the fistula. The duplications of the colon are treated as described earlier.

ATRESIA OR STENOSIS OF THE COLON

The colon is the most unusual site of gastrointestinal atresias.

Incidence. This lesion accounts for less than 10 per cent of all bowel atresias. It affects both sexes equally, with an incidence varying from 1 in 20,000 to 1 in 50,000 live births.[62]

Etiology. Recent evidence suggests that this anomaly is caused by a vascular accident late in gestation.[52, 118]

Pathology. Like those in other areas of the bowel, the atresias are most often membranous or fibrous diaphragms within the intestinal lumen, which do not interrupt external bowel continuity. They are sometimes segmental. Occurring anywhere within the colon, half are proximal and half are distal to the sigmoid flexure. Microcolon exists below the area of atresia. Atresia has coexisted with Hirschsprung's disease.[77, 87]

Symptoms. Because the obstruction is low, the symptoms are delayed until after several feedings. Abdominal distention is noted first, and, as this progresses, it is accompanied by vomiting. The vomitus initially contains only formula but becomes bilious or fecal and eventually the infant is unable to tolerate any feedings. The outlines of dilated loops of small bowel and peristaltic waves are seen on the abdomen. The percussion note is tympanitic, and the bowel sounds are hyperactive and periodic. The infant passes no meconium, and there is no material in the rectal ampulla. There are significant water losses into the dilated bowel, which, combined with those from vomiting, lead to marked dehydration. The increasing abdominal distention eventually causes respiratory distress.

Diagnosis. Other causes of low intestinal obstruction, such as Hirschsprung's disease, the anorectal anomalies, and low-lying duplication cysts, must be differentiated from the atresias. Plain films of the abdomen show large dilated loops of small bowel. If the atresia is complete there is no gas in the colon below the level of the lesion. A barium enema will establish the level of the atresia or diaphragm and will demonstrate the unused microcolon below it. It should be remembered that Hirschsprung's disease and anterior sacral meningocele can be associated with this atresia.[164]

Treatment.   The treatment is the same as for the small bowel atresias and depends upon the type of lesion. If the infant is in poor condition, an ileostomy if the lesion is cecal, or a Mikulicz colostomy if the lesion is distal, will decompress the bowel. Only later, after the infant's condition is improved, are resection and primary anastomosis performed. Distal atresia requires colostomy and, later, establishment of continuity. If the atresia is proximal to the splenic flexure, the dilated proximal colon should be resected and an ileotransverse anastomosis performed.[149a]

Prognosis.   The overall mortality is now at 10.5 per cent, with distal atresia requiring less colonic resection than proximal colonic atresia.[149a]

ANORECTAL ANOMALIES

Anorectal anomalies reflect abnormalities in the formation of the anorectal canal or in the location of the anus within the perineum.

Incidence.   The overall incidence is between 1 in 5000 and 1 in 15,000 live births.[158] These anomalies are one and one half times more frequent in males than in females. The high anomaly (the most significant) is present in 50 per cent of affected males and in 19 per cent of affected females. Anal stenosis seems more likely to be familial than other lesions. Winkler and Weinstein suggest that when imperforate anus occurs in siblings it may be of recessive inheritance, with a 25 per cent risk of its occurrence in other siblings.[211] Dominant inheritance has been demonstrated in a mother and two daughters with imperforate

anus and rectovaginal fistula and in a mother and son with anal stenosis.[209] Dominant inheritance is also noted in the syndrome of imperforate anus, triphalangeal thumbs, sensorineural deafness, and bone anomalies.[109, 206b]

Etiology.   The lower gastrointestinal and urogenital tracts are in close proximity as they differentiate between the fifth and eighth weeks of embryonic life. At first there is a large common cloaca, which is closed distally by the cloacal membrane. It is gradually divided by downward growing of the urorectal septum into ventral and dorsal chambers. A cloacal duct communicates between these but closes at the seventh week as the septum continues its growth. The dorsal chamber, destined to become the rectum, grows caudally and posteriorly. The cloacal membrane separates into a ventral urogenital and a dorsal anal membrane. The proctodeum, an invagination of ectoderm, reaches the region of the anal membrane, which opens at eight weeks. The external sphincter, which originates from mesoderm, is not involved in these malformations.

The various malformations develop in relation to the time of maturation arrest. Fistulas between the rectum and lower genitourinary tract result from incomplete formation of the urorectal septum; atresias and stenoses are related to complete or incomplete resolution of the anorectal membrane, and ectopic anus is due to failure of posterior migration of the anus.[118, 200, 204]

Pathology.   The usual classification of these anomalies, proposed by Ladd and Gross, describes four types.[110] Type I represents stenosis of the anus or lower rectum, with both being patent. Type II represents persistence of the anal membrane. In type III, the anus is imperforate and the rectum ends blindly as a pouch a variable distance above it. In type IV the anal canal and lower rectum form a distal pouch and are separated from the blind upper rectal pouch. This classification has been revised; Table 17–1 shows the new suggestions.[129, 157] In most series the old type III anomaly is ten times more common than the others, and 75 per cent of these are associated with fistulas that in the male are rectourethral, rectovesical,

Table 17–1 Anorectal Anomalies: Suggested International Classification[*]

MALE	FEMALE
A. *Low (Translevator)*	
1. At normal anal site (a) anal stenosis (b) covered anus, complete	1. Same (a) same (b) same
2. At perineal site (a) anocutaneous fistula (covered anus, incomplete) (b) anterior perineal anus	2. Same (a) same (b) same
B. *Intermediate*	
1. Anal agenesis (a) without fistula (b) with fistula rectobulbar	1. Same (a) without fistula (b) with fistula rectovestibular rectovaginal, low
2. Anorectal stenosis	2. Same
C. *High (Supralevator)*	
1. Anorectal agenesis (a) without fistula (b) with fistula rectourethral rectovesical	1. Same (a) without fistula (b) with fistula rectovaginal, high rectocloacal rectovesical
2. Rectal atresia	2. Same
D. *Miscellaneous*	
Imperforate anal membrane Cloacal exstrophy Others	

[*]From Santulli, T. V., Kiesewetter, W. B., and Bill, A. H., Jr.: Anorectal anomalies: A suggested classification. J. Pediatr. Surg. 5:281, 1970.

or rectoperineal, and in the female either rectovaginal or rectoperineal.[99] Associated anomalies occur in 28 to 72 per cent of patients and consist of congenital heart disease, esophageal atresia, hydronephrosis, and spinal anomalies, especially anterior meningocele.[124] Aganglionosis, duplications of the rectum and colon, and short colon or small bowel are less frequent anomalies.[49] The internal sphincter is absent in those with high lesions.[99]

Symptoms. Most infants with anorectal anomalies are born at term, and only 6 per cent have a birth weight of less than 2000 gm. The diagnosis is made or suspected during the newborn examination if there is an imperforate anus or a perineal fistula. Meconium may be seen coming from the vagina or urethra. Those infants with only a pinpoint anal perforation will pass tiny dots of meconium. Anal stenosis often is not obvious during the first few days while the baby passes meconium and transitional stools, but as the stool consistency becomes firmer the stools are small and thin. The babies have a great deal of discomfort during defecation. Fecal impaction results and causes abdominal distention and partial or complete intestinal obstruction. The child may be treated for constipation for weeks or months before a good digital examination is performed. In a number of instances, the anus appears anterior in location.[81a, 111a] Anal stenosis has been reported in a syndrome of abnormalities of hands and feet and sensineuronal deafness.[206a]

In babies with a persistent anal membrane, the anus appears normal, and the bulging dark membrane is seen within the anal canal. These infants pass no meconium and, after 24 or more hours, the abdomen becomes distended and they vomit bilious or fecal material. There is no anus in the type III deformity — only an anal dimple of varying degrees of prominence. The skin overlying the external sphincter puckers as the sphincter contracts. If the rectal pouch is low, there is some bulging in the area of the anus as the baby strains. There is usually a fistula with meconium passing through it to the perineum or vagina.[130] Low intestinal obstruction is apparent 24 to 48 hours after birth if the fistula is small, but if it is large there is no obstruction. In the type IV deformity, the anus appears grossly normal; the disorder often is not suspected until intestinal obstruction develops. On digital examination of the rectum the blind anorectal pouch can be palpated. Symptoms of the N-type lesion, stenosis with fistula, are watery diarrhea and little or no urination. Females pass feces through the fistula.[210] High imperforate anus has been associated with congenital short colon and absence of the inferior mesenteric artery.[206a]

Diagnosis. Visual and digital rectal examinations are essential in making the diagnosis. The classic upside-down x-ray study has advantages and disadvantages, but it is not recommended as a diagnostic determinant. It cannot be performed before 24 hours or more after birth — that is, after air has passed through the intestine and outlines the distal pouch. If meconium fills the distal blind segment, air does not reach the terminal end of the sac. If the marker is not placed accurately into the dimple or anus, the films can suggest a longer space between the segments than actually exists. This type of film is most reliable when the lesion is very low.[211]

Air in the bladder represents a rectovesical fistula and suggests a type III lesion. Injection of contrast material into the vagina or urethra confirms the presence of the fistula. The presence of rectal gas extending below the pubococcygeal line is thought to indicate a low lesion, but Winslow et al. have stressed that this is misleading, be-cause in four of their patients with low lesions there was no air below this line.[212] The old technique of examining urine for meconium or epithelial debris cannot be dismissed in establishing the diagnosis of fistula. Urography and cystography are required for all these patients both before and after surgery. Ultrasound scanning may be of help in differentiating high and low imperforate anus.[163]

Treatment. Anal stenosis is treated by repeated dilation, but, if the stenosis is very tight, a plastic procedure followed by dilations is recommended. Persistent anal membrane is simply excised or incised, with suturing of the anal mucosa to skin. If the anus is quite anterior, it may need to be repositioned posteriorly. Some postoperative anal dilations may be necessary. For repair of the type III anomaly, either a perineal or abdominoperineal approach is used, the choice depending upon the depth of the rectal pouch. Some now feel the sacral approach is better. Concern is given to the capacity of the distal bowel segment in high anomalies. Translevator anomalies require only direct perineal repair. In the supralevator type of pouch, the bowel ends above the levator, which itself is abnormal, and an abdominal approach must be used because a perineal approach would destroy any sphincter potential of the muscle.[100, 106] The N-type lesion, with anovestibular or anorectalurethral fistula, entails anterior perineal resection of the fistula.

If there are other severe congenital anomalies, colostomy is performed and the repair is postponed until the infant's condition is improved. The timing of fistula repair varies from center to center and ranges from infancy to 5 years. Louw et al. have abandoned primary abdominoperineal rectoplasty because of the high complication rate and wait three to six months before attempting repair.[119]

Complications. A number of complications can occur: rectal prolapse or stenosis, separation of the anastomosis, urethral injury and stricture, urinary retention and infection, recurrent urinary fistulas, fecal impaction or incontinence, and small bowel obstruction.

Fecal incontinence is one of the most

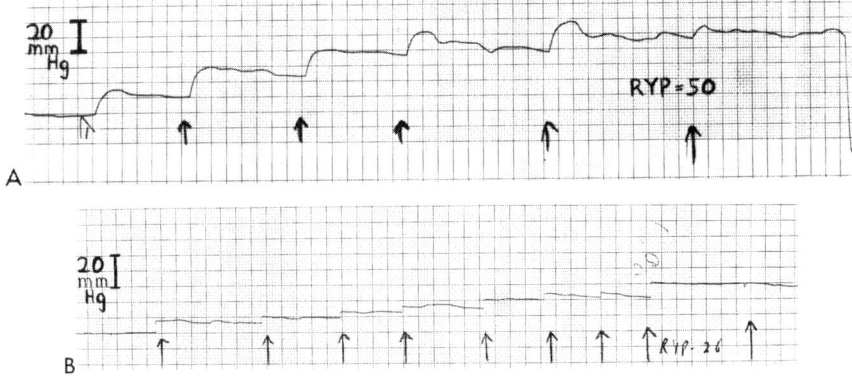

Figure 17–3 Manometric tracings of resting yield pressures and response to distention within the rectum. *A*, Arrows indicate added increments of 0.05 ml of air into the balloon. A stepwise increase in intraluminal pressure is noted after each stage of balloon distention until a plateau is reached and further distention of the balloon produces no increase in pressure. This is termed the resting yield pressure, and in normal subjects it varies between 30 and 57 mm Hg. *B*, The same study in a patient who has had repair of a type III imperforate anus. The rises in pressure after air injection are less marked and the resting yield pressure is only 26 mm Hg.

difficult and most frequent postoperative complications,[101, 172] particularly after the type III repair, with slightly less than half of reported series noting poor results. Fecal retention and soiling have been attributed to damage to the nerve supply during dissection of the blind pouch, disruption of the levator ani muscles, and impaired sensation in the anal canal.[194] Kiesewetter and Turner stress preservation of the puborectalis muscle and its sensory fibers for the development of continence.[100] Others have achieved some success by release of the levator sling or use of autogenous muscle transplantation.[78]

Manometric techniques have been used to study anal sphincter function in children in whom these anomalies have been repaired.[32, 160] Those with type II or very low type III lesions had the best degree of continence and had normal or near-normal results in the studies. Resting sphincter competence was low in those with type III lesions, and these patients showed no internal sphincter response to distention (Fig. 17–3). This is understandable in view of the anatomic dissections necessary in infants with type III deformities that included absence of the internal sphincter.

A radiologic correlation with a poor surgical result is the absence of a demonstrable rectal shelf before defecation.

Prognosis. The prognosis depends directly upon associated anomalies, with a fatal outlook in those having an average of 3.3 anomalies and survival in those with 1.5 or fewer.

VESICOINTESTINAL FISTULA

This term has rather a benign connotation considering the catastrophic anomaly it describes.[58] It occurs in about 1 in 200,000 births and is due to an arrest in development of the urogenital and gastrointestinal systems during the third or fourth week of gestation.[187] There is exstrophy of the bladder and ileocecal portion of the gut, imperforate anus, and absence of the major portion of the colon. Other associated anomalies are omphalocele, phallic abnormalities, vertebral malformations, and bifid uterus. Prematurity is an additional complication.

On the abdominal wall, there is a large area of exposed mucosa with an omphalocele just superior to it. The exposed bladder is bifid and separate from the exposed bowel. A blind, short colon opens through the inferior orifice. Successful treatment has been the creation of an end-ileostomy and closure of the omphalocele with excision or later use of the colon. Cutaneous ureterostomy and cystectomy are performed after

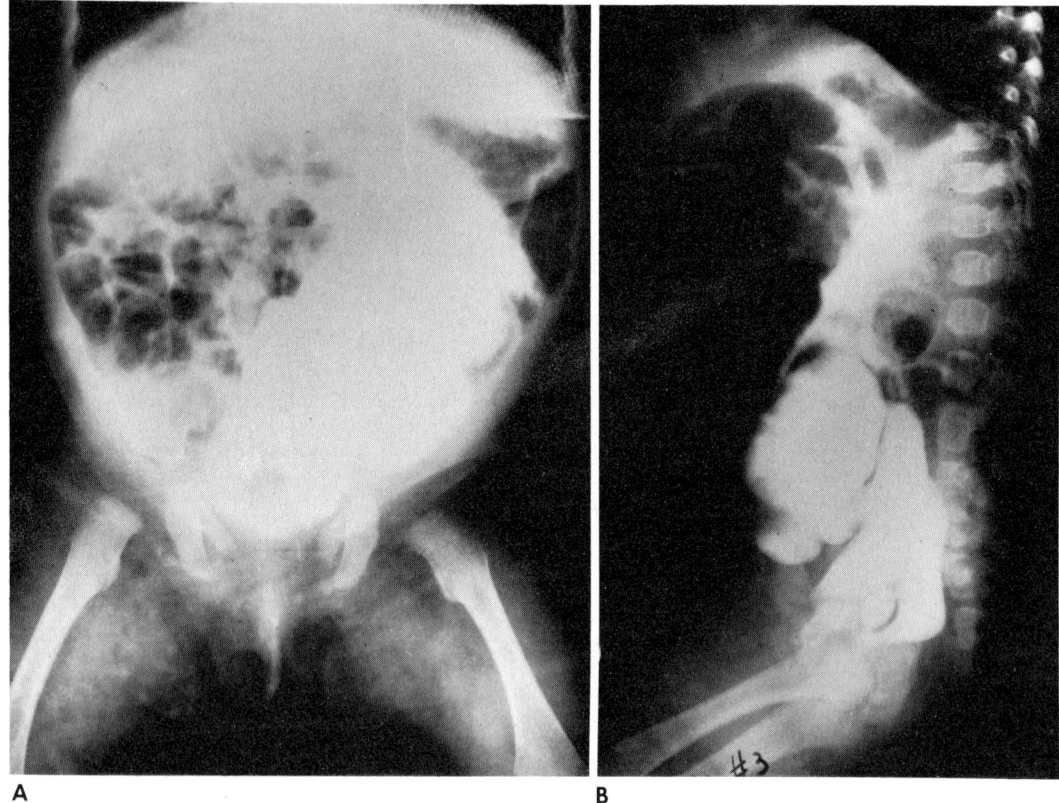

A **B**

Figure 17–4 A, Antegrade pyelogram showing a large hydronephrotic renal mass with dye in sigmoid colon. B, Lateral film of same. (Courtesy of Dr. H. Hochman.) Infant had renal ectopia and fusion of the right to left kidney with the ureter entering the sigmoid.

the infant reaches a weight of 25 pounds. One recent report suggests use of the appendix as a colostomy.[26] Survival approaches 33 per cent.

ABNORMAL ENTRANCE OF URETER INTO SIGMOID

An extremely rare cause of chronic diarrhea in the infant has been detected by intravenous pyelography (Fig. 17–4), showing a fusion of two kidneys and aberrant entry of a ureter into the sigmoid.

MOTOR DISORDERS OF THE COLON AND RECTUM

VOLVULUS OF THE COLON

Volvulus is a form of intestinal obstruction caused by twisting of the bowel upon itself (Fig. 17–5). It involves the cecum, the sigmoid, or the transverse colon.[31]

Volvulus of the Cecum

Etiology. This type of volvulus is associated with errors in rotation that result in excessive cecal mobility.[184]

Pathogenesis. Torsion occurs at a point where the cecum is attached and below which it is unattached. The rotation is clockwise and partial or complete; there may or may not be vascular occlusion. If the torsion is sudden and accompanied by vascular compromise, there is hemorrhagic infarction with gangrene and perforation. If there is no infarction, torsion alone produces a close-loop picture with marked distention of the cecum.

Symptoms. Symptoms develop at any age, with acute pain in the right lower quadrant. This pain is at first colicky but then becomes continuous. If the obstruction

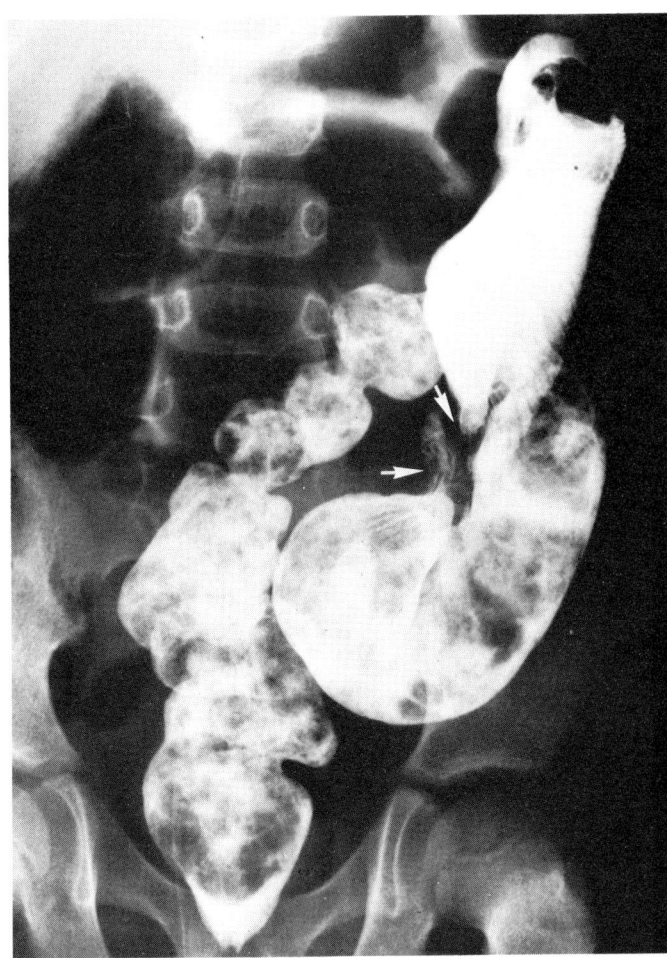

Figure 17–5 Axial torsion volvulus in a child who presented to the emergency room with signs of acute gastrointestinal obstruction. Barium enema was obtained because of dilation of bowel loops. The narrowed segment indicated by arrows is the distal twisted portion of colon, but it did not produce obstruction to flow of the barium. The contrast material passed to the level of the splenic flexure, at which point an obstruction was encountered. The point of obstruction of the splenic flexure is behind the barium in the photograph. The mechanism of this abnormality is a twist along the axis of the bowel.

is intermittent, bouts of abdominal pain recur and are accompanied by distention and tenderness in the right upper or lower quadrant. Children find some relief by assuming a knee-chest position. If there is intestinal necrosis and perforation, signs of shock and peritonitis override those of obstruction.

Diagnosis. The flat film of the abdomen is essential in the differentiation of this disease from others causing intestinal obstruction or peritonitis. Characteristically, an extremely dilated cecum is located in the right or left upper quadrants.

Treatment. Detorsion of the twisted bowel and anchoring of the cecum and right colon in their normal positions is usually curative. Resection of any areas of infarcted bowel is required.

Prognosis. The mortality rate varies between 30 and 60 per cent. If fixation of the bowel is not performed, a recurrence at some future date is likely.

Volvulus of the Sigmoid Colon

Volvulus of this type is most common in patients with a long, redundant sigmoid colon.[8]

Etiology. These long sigmoid loops may be congenital or may develop as the result of prolonged constipation. Shortening of the mesosigmoid or narrowing of the mesenteric attachment so that the proximal and distal sigmoid ends approximate each other is implicated in the pathogenesis.

Pathogenesis. This is essentially the same as in other types of volvulus. Rotation is usually clockwise, although it may be counterclockwise, and often achieves a complete 360-degree circle.

Symptoms. The onset is acute with colicky abdominal pain. The duration of symptoms has varied between several hours and 46 days. There are nausea, vomiting, abdominal distention, constipation, and, infrequently, diarrhea. The abdomen is tympanitic and tender to percussion, and the rectum is empty. Strangulation with infarction is heralded by rectal bleeding and a mucoid discharge, and signs of peritoneal involvement follow within a few hours.

Diagnosis. Flat films of the abdomen show a greatly dilated sigmoid flexure, which extends to the right of the midline and up to the epigastrium. Fluid and air-fluid levels are present, and one sometimes sees the two points of proximal and distal obstruction. The descending colon above the site of obstruction is often quite dilated.

Treatment. If there is no evidence of infarction or peritonitis, a proctoscopic reduction is attempted first. Barium enema is sometimes successful in reducing this type of volvulus. Decompression with a long rectal tube is used in adults but is not recommended in children because of the risk of perforation. If nonsurgical reduction is unsuccessful, detorsion and fixation of the sigmoid and its mesentery, with perhaps sigmoid resection of the redundant bowel, are therapeutic. If there is necrotic bowel, a segmental resection with proximal colostomy is mandatory.

Prognosis. The operative mortality is somewhat more than 20 per cent. Recurrence occurs in 20 to 90 per cent of patients after nonoperative reduction.

Volvulus of the Transverse Colon

This disorder has been reported in only two children, aged two and ten years.

Etiology. It usually follows obstruction in the distal colon that has caused generalized colonic distention or occurs through mesenteric defects.

Symptoms. The symptoms are those of intermittent or chronic constipation with episodes of abdominal distention and tenderness. During the acute attack the abdomen is tender and tympanitic to percussion. Stool may or may not be present in the rectal ampulla.

Diagnosis. Flat film of the abdomen shows dilatation of the cecum and proximal transverse colon, with little or no air in the distal colon. The right hemidiaphragm may be elevated.

Treatment. Detorsion of the volvulus with the appropriate fixation of abnormal mesentery is performed if there is a mesenteric defect. If no defect is identified, the distal colon is examined for any obstructive lesion and a biopsy is obtained to rule out Hirschsprung's disease.

MENINGOMYELOCELE

This topic is mentioned only briefly because nearly two thirds of children with meningomyelocele have fecal incontinence. This is due to paralysis of the levator ani muscles rather than of the anal sphincter.

NEUROLOGIC IMMATURITY

Functional obstruction of the intestine with a clinical picture of Hirschsprung's disease is caused by neurologic immaturity and occurs primarily in premature infants. It is discussed in Chapter 8 under Gastrointestinal Obstruction.

HIRSCHSPRUNG'S DISEASE

Hirschsprung's disease is caused by abnormalities in the pelvic parasympathetic system: absence of ganglion cells from the distal colon, absence of peristalsis in affected areas, and partial intestinal obstruction.[161] Although it usually involves the rectosigmoid, it can involve only a small segment of rectum or it can extend through the entire colon and into the small bowel.[44, 121]

Incidence. Aganglionosis is estimated to occur in 1 in 5000 people in the general population.[147] A survey of American Academy of Pediatrics members revealed 1196 patients in 1979.[188] A review of the world literature in 1981 uncovered 489 cases of long-segment disease in a total of 3124 cases in 46 series. The incidence in siblings of index patients is 7.2 per cent, and the risk is higher for siblings of affected females than of affected males. Those with long-segment disease are more likely to have a family history of Hirschsprung's disease as well as of diabetes, and males predominante 28:1 over females.[24] The typical segmental disease is four times more frequent in boys than in girls, and other congenital anomalies are unusual. Two per cent of patients have a chromosomal anomaly, usually trisomy 21. A few others are reported to have colonic atresia or imperforate anus.[206]

Etiology. Developmentally, the innervation of the intestine proceeds in a craniocaudal direction. At five weeks the vagal trunks reach the esophagus, and the pelvic and preaortic plexuses innervate the rectum. At six weeks, neuroblasts are present in the stomach; at seven weeks they reach the midgut and at eight weeks they reach the proximal colon. By 12 weeks, the neuroblasts extend to the rectum. The myenteric plexus, developing in the stomach at seven weeks, moves caudally between the eighth and twelfth weeks. After this is formed, the longitudinal muscle layer develops. During the third trimester, Auerbach's plexus is better defined than Meissner's plexus, and maturation continues for a month after birth.[171] Any arrest in migration of the parasympathetic nerves must occur around the twelfth week of gestation.[144]

The ganglion cells are particularly sensitive to anoxia, and a clinical picture identical to that of Hirschsprung's disease has been produced in experimental animals by the intra-arterial injection of mercuric chloride and Tyrode's solution.[143] Acquired aganglionosis has been reported twice.[198, 199]

Pathology. Evidence that aganglionosis affects the bowel early lies in the hypertrophy of muscle of the transitional segment and distal part of the normally innervated segment in infants operated on just after birth.

Histologic sections from aganglionic segment show an almost complete absence of ganglion cells.[46] The normal patterns of the myenteric plexus are lost, and bundles of unmyelinated nerve fibers form wavy configurations and weave in and out of adjacent muscle. Large numbers of axons are present. In the superior regions of the aganglionic segments, there may be some ganglion cells but these are abnormal and have no or irregular axons. Histologic techniques confirm the normal adrenergic innervation of the external muscularis but demonstrate pathologic innervation of the muscularis mucosae and the submucous plexus. That there is excessive acetylcholinesterase staining of aganglionic tissue suggests an abnormality in the development of the nervous pathways rather than frank denervation, and acetylcholinesterase levels in the serum as well as tissue are increased.[18, 29, 33, 88, 136] 5-Hydroxytryptamine neurons are absent from aganglionic segments.[155] Occasionally there is neuronal dysplasia.[152]

The involved area is usually limited to a segment beyond the sigmoid and varies in length to involve either the distal rectum or the entire length of rectum and some sigmoid. In 6 to 21 per cent of cases, involvement extends to the cecum and is termed long-segment disease. Occasionally it is segmental in the sigmoid colon, and normal ganglion cells are present in the rectum. Skip aganglionosis has been reported affecting left and right colon with normal transverse colon.[11b] Total aganglionosis is discussed separately. Hirschsprung's disease has occurred in a child with meconium plug syndrome and cystic fibrosis and in another with Waardenburg's syndrome. Pseudodiverticulitis of the appendix may coexist with Hirschsprung's disease to result in appendiceal perforation.[183]

Pathophysiology. Absence of peristalsis in the aganglionic segments results in functional obstruction and partial intestinal obstruction. As the partially obstructed small bowel becomes chronically dilated, there is excessive intraluminal loss of water and electrolytes. Rectal and colonic distention cause obstructive uropathy.[45]

Symptoms. Most of the affected infants are full-term and appear normal at birth, although the disease may occur in premature infants. There is a delay in passage of meconium, and most do not pass stool within the first 24 hours. Ninety-four per cent do pass stool after 24 hours, however. In a rare instance, meconium plug syndrome may herald the disease.[81] Constipation and abdominal distention are the most prominent symptoms and develop in half the babies.[66] Next in frequency are vomiting and diarrhea. In most of 300 infants described in one study by Swenson et al., obstruction appeared during the first or second day of life, and the majority of infants had symptoms by the sixth month.[191] A less acute presentation occurs in the baby with chronic abdominal distention, intermittent diarrhea, and failure to gain weight. The diarrhea is usually of the overflow type. Evacuation is prompted by suppositories or enemas. Infants with the mildest symptoms require some occasional stimulus for evacuation. Eventually these babies have feeding problems and are irritable during feedings or are reluctant to feed. It is not unusual for several episodes of intestinal obstruction to occur before the correct diagnosis is made.

In 17 per cent of 501 patients, diagnosis was not made until after the sixth year.[191] Fecal soiling is not typical of this disease unless only a very short, low segment of rectum is involved. Pitting edema appears in those with severe protein loss.[71] In one infant, the disease presented as peritonitis due to cecal perforation.[4] Another patient presented only rectal bleeding during the first week of life, with negative radiologic studies.

The physical examination shows a somewhat emaciated and dehydrated infant with a greatly distended abdomen. Dilated small bowel loops are easily visualized and palpated in the abdomen. Fecal impaction in the colon feels like a ropy mass that extends down the left side of the abdomen and across the epigastrium. The ampulla is found to be empty on rectal examination in 60 per cent of cases, but a high impaction is often palpable. As the examiner withdraws the finger, a gush of flatus and foul-smelling stool follows.

Diagnosis. This disease must be distinguished from rectal stenosis and the meconium plug syndrome,[112] and in older chil-

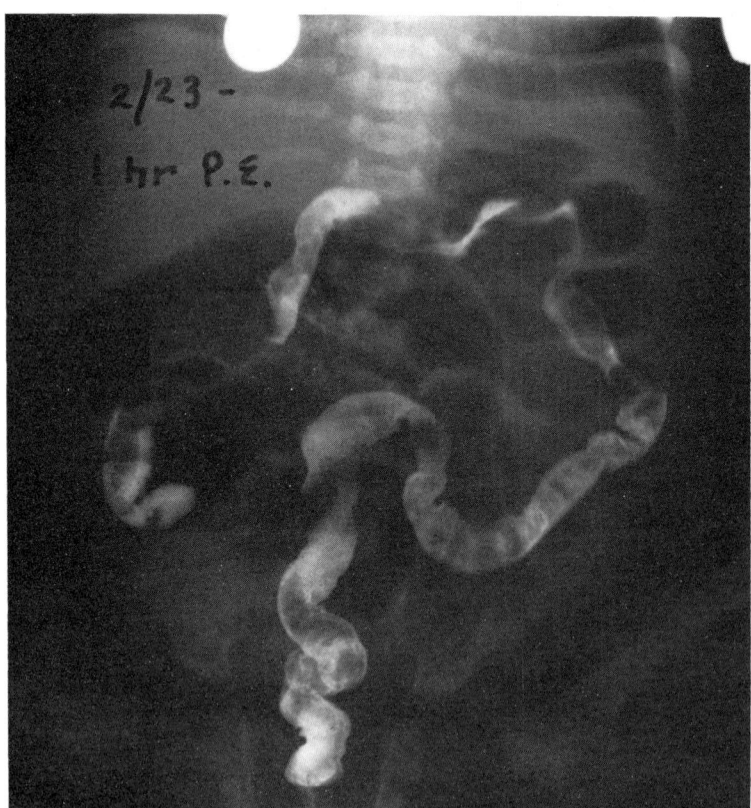

Figure 17–6 One-hour post-evacuation film of infant with total colonic aganglionosis.

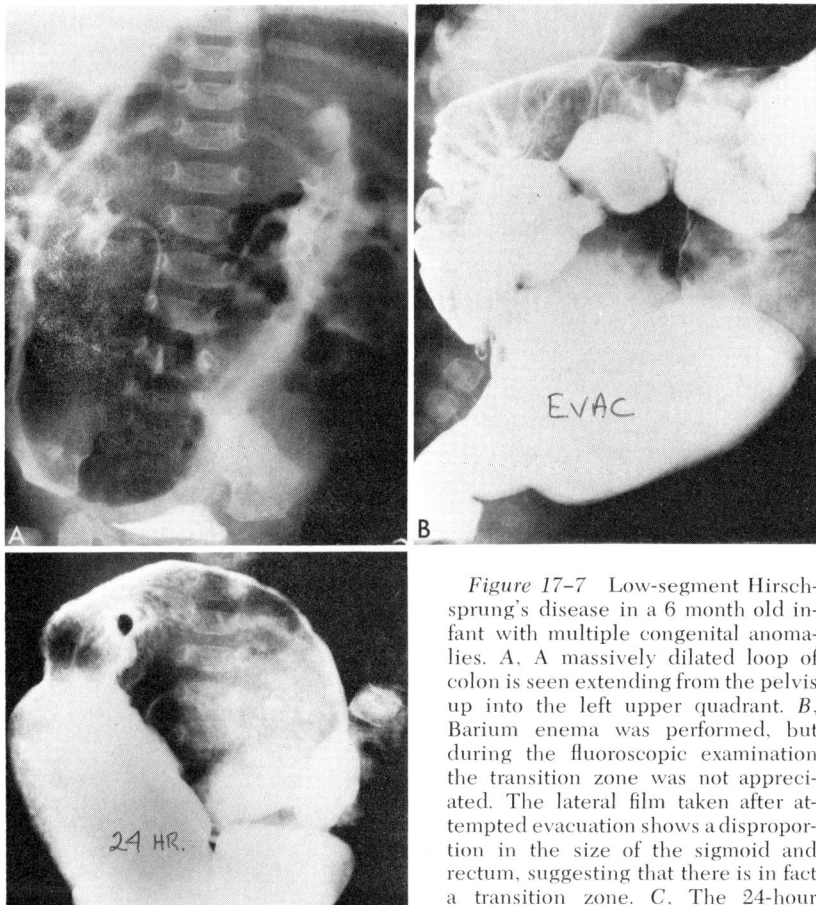

Figure 17–7 Low-segment Hirschsprung's disease in a 6 month old infant with multiple congenital anomalies. *A,* A massively dilated loop of colon is seen extending from the pelvis up into the left upper quadrant. *B,* Barium enema was performed, but during the fluoroscopic examination the transition zone was not appreciated. The lateral film taken after attempted evacuation shows a disproportion in the size of the sigmoid and rectum, suggesting that there is in fact a transition zone. *C,* The 24-hour followup film demonstrates a fairly characteristic pattern of retained barium mixed with fecal contents. The very large barium-containing structure seen on the film is the sigmoid colon. The disease was confirmed at surgery.

dren, from physiologic constipation. Plain films (Fig. 17–6) in the erect position show some gaseous distention of the colon and often an end-point of air. Fluid levels are present in distended loops of bowel. The key diagnostic point in the plain film is the variation in length and degree of distention of the bowel loops. Large loops measuring up to 3 cm in diameter follow the distribution of the transverse and descending colon (Fig. 17–7).

A few words of caution are necessary in the interpretation of the barium enema. Not only is this disease rare in premature infants, but the barium enema is normal early and does not show the characteristic narrowed segment until several weeks or months after birth.[145] In the full-term infant, the enema is difficult to interpret during the first six days of life because there is often a normal transition zone or the characteristic narrowed segment is simply not seen. The enema must be performed with small amounts of barium and with the patient in the Trendelenburg position. The bowel should be only partially filled and no more than 5 or 10 ml of contrast material allowed to run in at any one time. The transition zone is apparent as the barium enters the dilated proximal colon above the narrowed area in the rectosigmoid. Pathognomonic of Hirschsprung's disease is the funnel-shaped dilatation of the colon as it ends in the narrowed length of bowel that characteristically assumes a fishhook shape. Sometimes the narrowed segment is not demonstrated, and only the dilated rectosigmoid and colon are visible.[113] Barium retention for 24 hours or more after the study is one of the most significant findings, and rectal biopsy is mandatory if retention is demonstrated (Figs. 17–8 and 17–9). Meconium plug syndrome can resemble Hirschsprung's disease, and complicating enterocolitis can cause spasm and prevent demon-

stration of the narrowed segment. Rectal stricture resembles the narrowed segment.

The definitive method of diagnosis is rectal biopsy done by suction or deep surgical wedge section. Suction biopsy using a Rubin or Woods tube is simple and can provide adequate samples to rule out at least the diagnosis if ganglion cells are demonstrated. Some recommended taking the biopsy specimen from the valves of Houston, but these are not well developed during the first year of life. A normal hypoganglionic zone exists above the anus, and care must be taken to obtain tissue high enough to assure a normal concentration of ganglion

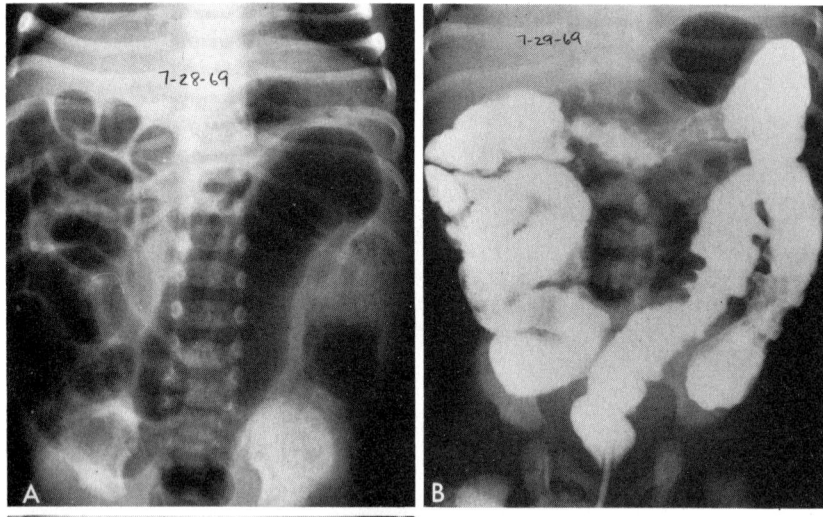

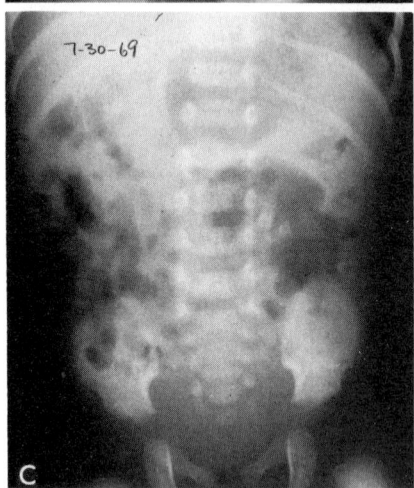

Figure 17–8 Low-segment Hirschsprung's disease is a 3 day old infant with increasing abdominal distention. *A,* Fairly characteristic plain film findings in Hirschsprung's disease, with a large, gas-filled loop of sigmoid extending out of the pelvis toward the left upper quadrant. Distention of small and large bowel is seen also in other areas. *B,* When barium enema was done the following day, the colon distention was no longer apparent and no transition zone was seen. Irregular contraction of the colon has been described in Hirschsprung's disease, and the notching seen in the mid sigmoid may represent this phenomenon. The patient had had several rectal examinations following the plain films the previous day, and this was followed by passage of gas and fecal material. *C,* A 24-hour follow-up film showed complete evacuation of barium. Because of the clinical improvement and the minimal radiologic findings, it was elected to follow the patient medically rather than obtain a biopsy at that time.

Illustration continued on opposite page

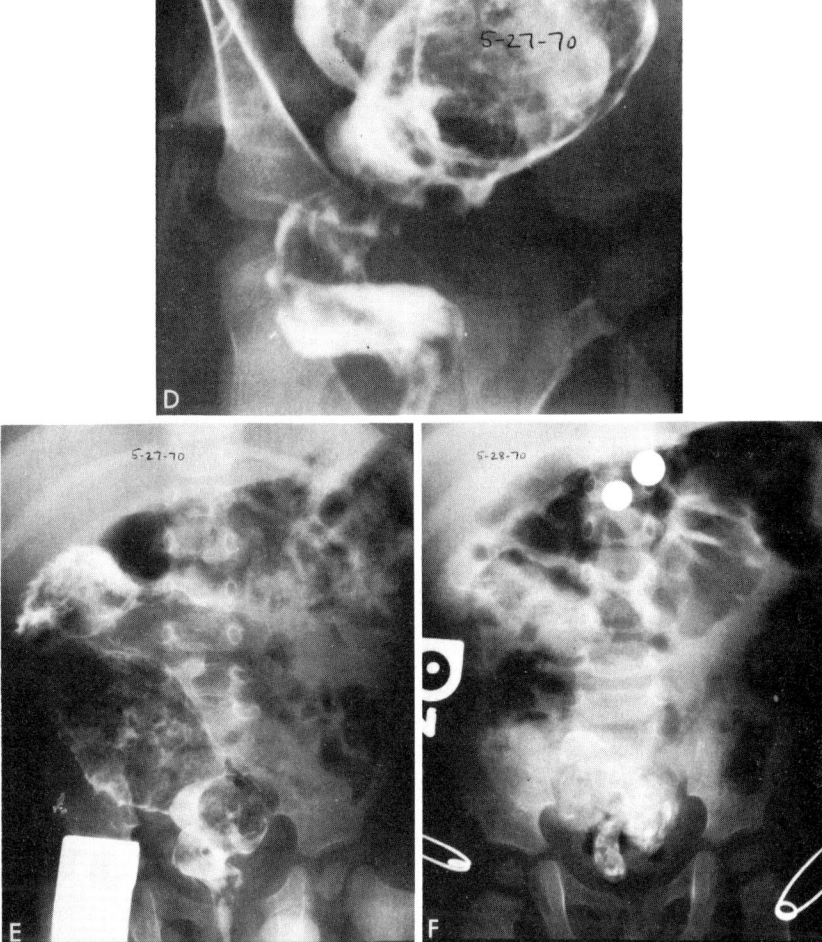

Figure 17–8 Continued D, The patient was studied again 10 months later because of recurrent constipation and abdominal distention. At this time a well-defined transition zone was seen at the rectosigmoid level, as illustrated in the spot film. *E*, The contrast study was halted after the transition zone was noted. The overhead film demonstrates rather significant dilation of the sigmoid colon, which has swung over into the right side of the abdomen, a common finding in low-segment Hirschsprung's disease. *F*, The 24-hour follow-up film shows retention of barium and again demonstrates the transition zone.

This case exemplifies the difficulty that may be encountered in the clinical and radiologic diagnosis of Hirschsprung's disease in early infancy. The rectal examination presumably overcame the functional obstruction and obscured the typical x-ray findings.

cells. Preliminary enemas or digital examinations are omitted as these cause edema and inflammation in the mucosa and submucosa. Ideally, the tube biopsy, with tissue taken 2 cm above the mucocutaneous junction and using suction pressures of 20 to 25 mm of mercury that are maintained for 2 to 3 seconds, will include circular and longitudinal muscle and be satisfactory.[6, 25] If ganglion cells are not seen, surgical biopsy is necessary. Histochemical staining for acetylcholinesterase (AChE) is rather specific. Type A, showing prominent nerve fibers throughout the muscularis mucosa and lamina propria, was consistently positive in Hirschsprung's disease. Type B, with prominent staining only in the muscularis mucosae and adjacent lamina propria, was seen only in males with Hirschsprung's disease who were 1 month old or younger.[86b]

Manometric studies show characteristic changes in the motor responses in Hirschsprung's disease and are now considered an excellent diagnostic tool although false-negative and -positive responses may occur.[64] Most young infants, even premature

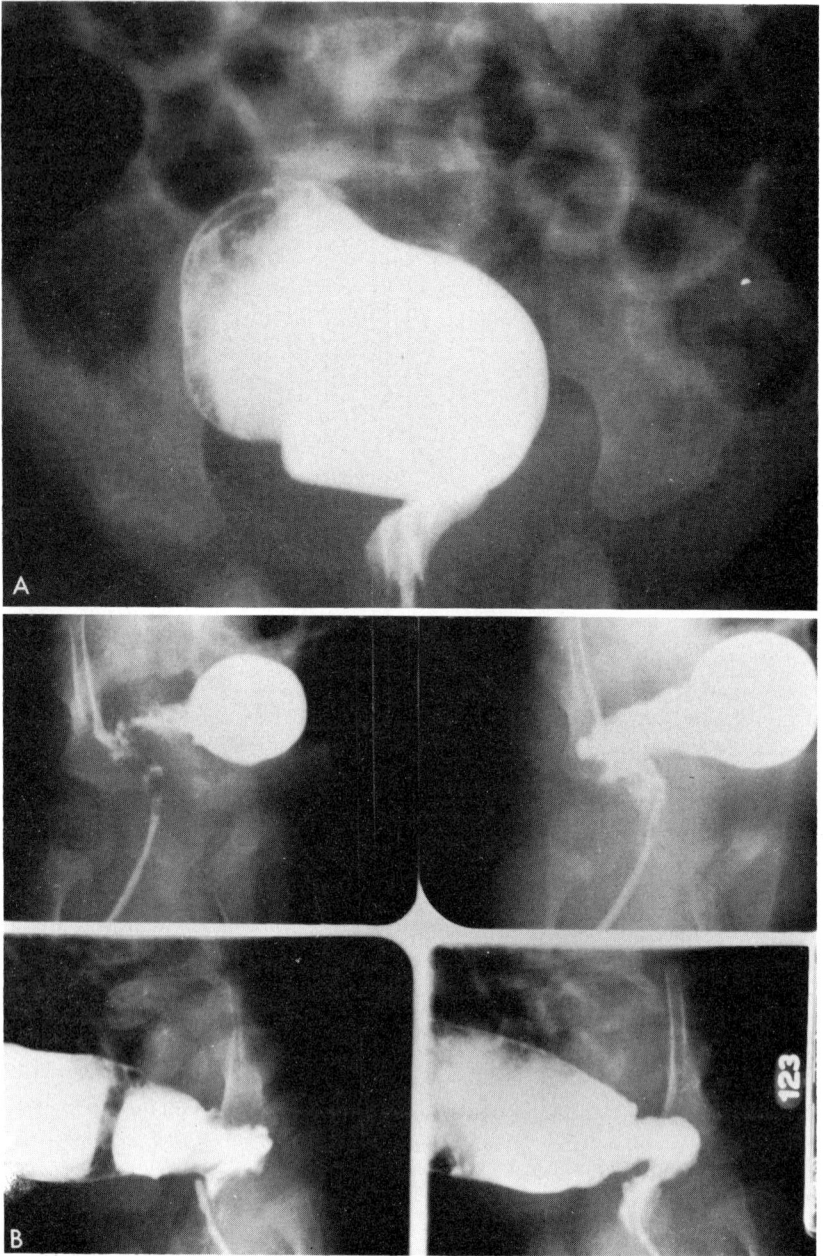

Figure 17–9 Low-segment Hirschsprung's disease in a 2 month old infant with progressive abdominal distention. *A,* A barium saline suspension was instilled through a straight catheter taped to the buttocks without an inflated balloon. A transition from narrow to distended bowel was demonstrated about 5 cm above the anus, and the examination was then discontinued. *B,* Overhead films. Following the fluoroscopic study confirms the transition.

babies, have a satisfactory anorectal reflex.[20, 65, 89, 133] In normal subjects, rectal distention causes relaxation of the internal sphincter and contraction of the external sphincter, whereas it causes contraction of both sphincters in those with agangliono-

sis.[111] Patients with chronic constipation may require great distention of the rectal balloon to elicit a response[137a] (Fig. 17–10). The normal internal sphincter shows intermittent rhythmic contractions at 10 to 13 per minute, whereas the sphincter in the

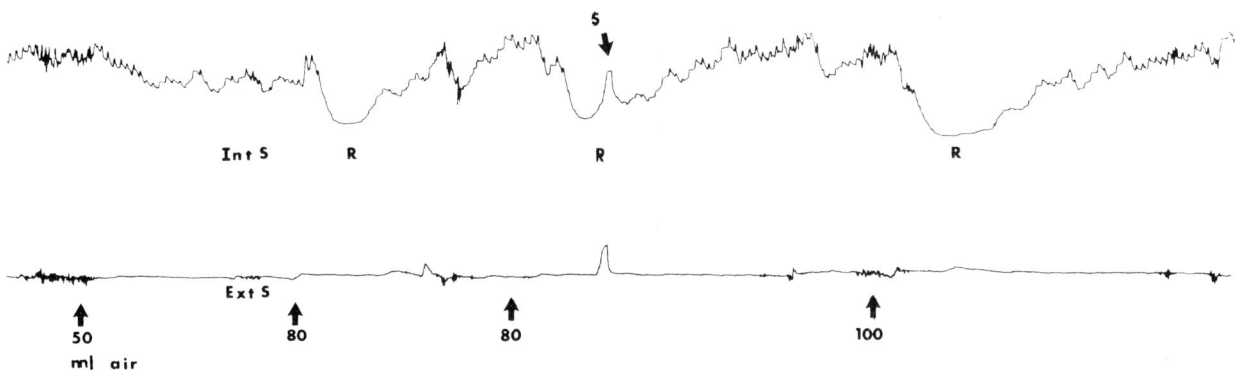

Figure 17–10 Normal anorectal manometry showing relaxation of internal sphincter and contraction of external sphincter with rectal distention.

aganglionic patient shows continuous rhythmic contractions at rates between 5 and 16 per minute.[162] Many neonates, however, do not show rhythmic cycles in the anal canal.[88a]

Treatment. The only definitive treatment is removal of the aganglionic, nonfunctioning segment of bowel.[140] The small infant should be treated by colostomy, with final repair deferred until he or she has reached eight or more months of age. In any surgical procedure, serial sections of the bowel are examined to assure anastomosis of ganglion cell–containing proximal bowel to the rectum, and it is wise to await the final section reading before proceeding to a definitive repair.

After resection of the segment, a number of surgical procedures are available. The original Swenson operation used a low end-to-end anastomosis.[190] Objections to this were postoperative fecal and urinary incontinence in many of the surviving infants. Swenson has since modified his operation by making the anastomosis oblique and adding a partial internal sphincterotomy. The Duhamel procedure retains the rectum, and the proximal bowel is anastomosed to the posterior rectal wall. Sometimes the internal sphincter is damaged and an anterior rectal pouch is formed, which, if it becomes large enough, causes obstruction. The Soave procedure involves removal of the rectal mucosa and suturing of proximal

normal bowel to the denuded rectum.[175, 176] A modified endorectal pull-through with ileal mobilization is used for long segment disease.[96]

Complications. Hydroureter and hydronephrosis are caused by direct pressure upon the ureters by the distended bowel. The Martin pouch repair has been followed by stenosis, ulceration, bacterial overgrowth, and enteric protein loss.[148]

Enemas given to these infants must be isotonic because of the delay in colonic emptying. Water intoxication has resulted from tapwater enemas, and tetany has developed from hypocalcemia produced by phosphate absorption from Fleet enemas.[180]

Cecal perforation is a complication of extreme colonic distention,[182, 197] and volvulus of the transverse colon may occur.[128]

Enterocolitis is the major cause of death in these infants, and it develops in nearly half of them.[15] Its onset occurs typically in infancy, but it can occur at any age, and either before or after surgery. It is directly related to the partial mechanical obstruction and relieved by colostomy. It is present in 15 per cent of patients at the time of diagnosis. Colonic dilatation may compromise the vascular supply and cause mucosal ulcerations, which are a fine site for bacterial invasion of the bowel. Although enteric pathogens have not been isolated from these infants, a hypersensitivity reaction to an antigen produced by intraluminal organisms that invade the submucosa has been suggested as the trigger mechanism for enterocolitis.

The infants usually are in a stable condition either before or after surgery, when suddenly recurrent signs develop of intestinal obstruction with constipation, abdominal distention, and vomiting. After rectal examination, some stool is passed and there is temporary improvement. However, in a short while diarrhea becomes severe enough to cause hypovolemic shock, for there is massive secretion of water and electrolytes into the bowel lumen. In the postoperative child, this form of obstruction must be differentiated from intestinal obstruction due to adhesions, for immediate decompression of the bowel by colostomy is lifesaving. In the unusual case, an older infant who has been mildly constipated since birth may suddenly become febrile, with severe diarrhea and abdominal distention as the first real manifestation of Hirschsprung's disease. Once an infant has had enterocolitis, it can be expected to recur after surgery or after any enteroviral illness. Many children, particularly after the Swenson procedure, have a low-grade enteritis that persists for months to years, causing anal excoriation and poor weight gain.

Mortality. The mortality has varied between 5 and 43 per cent, with the highest figures associated with enteritis.

Prognosis. The outcome was excellent or good in 80 per cent of infants who had the Duhamel procedure and in 92 or more per cent of those who had the Soave procedure.[90, 92, 93, 179] Anorectal reflexes returned 2 to 12 months after surgery in 77 to 84 per cent.[138]

Total Aganglionosis Coli

This type of aganglionosis involves all of the colon and variable lengths of the small bowel and carries with it a significantly greater mortality.[10, 25a, 83, 166]

Incidence. This form accounts for 8 per cent of all cases of Hirschsprung's disease. To 1973, 141 cases had been reported, and I have seen one additional case. The ratio of males to females is about 2.2 to 1, and a family history is present in 21 per cent, suggesting an autosomal recessive form of inheritance.[83, 123] By 1981, 489 cases had been collected.[93]

Pathology. Most often the entire colon and part of the terminal ileum are aganglionic, but in a few instances the disease extends into the jejunum or even into the duodenum, in which case it is incompatible with life.[63] In the usual form the ileal walls are thickened, dilated, and filled with inspissated curds of milk and barium. It tapers abruptly to normal-appearing ileum. Asch et al. found a perforated appendix in two of their nine patients.[10]

Symptoms. In most of the patients, diagnosis was made in the first month, but two patients reported in the literature were 13 years old before diagnosis was made. Vomiting and abdominal distention are the most common presenting symptoms and usually appear during the first four days of life. The vomitus is bilious or fecal and is either continuous or intermittent. Nearly a third of affected infants have constipation or some delay in the passage of meconium. When meconium is passed, it is usually scanty. Those with high involvement do not pass meconium. Diarrhea alone or diarrhea alternating with constipation is a presenting symptom in only 2 to 4 per cent, but becomes more apparent as the disease progresses. The small bowel loops are dilated and peristalsis is visible over the abdominal wall. Fecal masses are palpable throughout the abdomen. The bowel sounds at first are hyperactive but become hypoactive as the infant becomes debilitated. In general, the symptoms are those of incomplete lower intestinal obstruction.

If there is involvement of the jejunum as well as the ileum, the symptoms are those of high intestinal obstruction, with epigastric distention and visible peristaltic waves in the left upper quadrant suggesting duodenal obstruction.[3]

Associated anomalies are Down's syndrome, congenital heart disease, pulmonary hypoplasia or agenesis, and vertebral or rib anomalies. Our patient had syndactyly of the first and second toes and marked incurving of the fifth fingers (Fig. 17–11).

Diagnosis. The diagnosis must differentiate among all the causes of low or even high small bowel obstruction: the atresias,

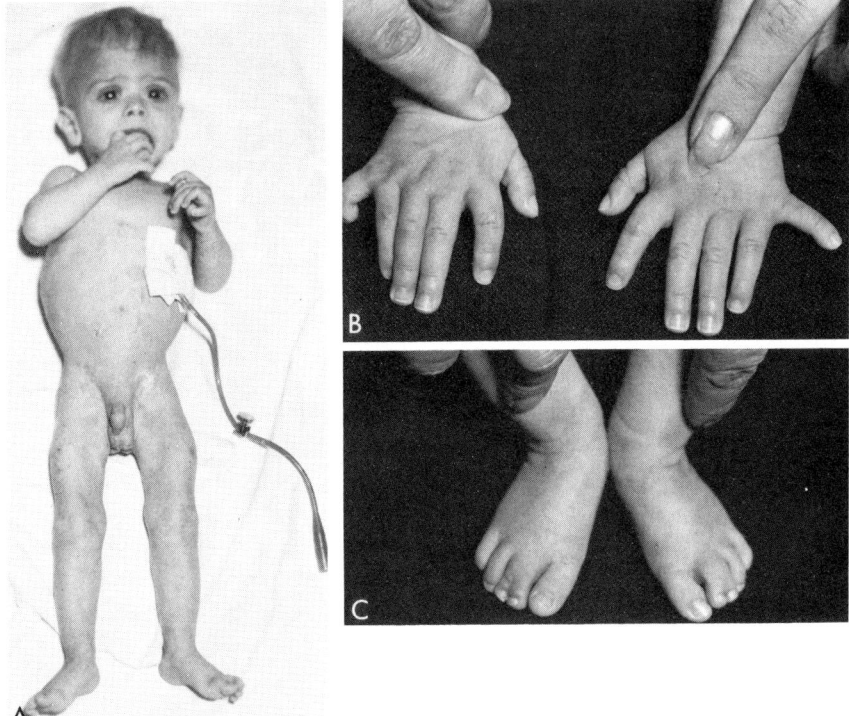

Figure 17–11 A, Infant with total colonic aganglionosis and involvement of lower half of the ileum. B, Note the marked curving of fifth finger. C, Syndactyly of second and third toes in same patient.

stenoses, volvulus or malrotation, and duplication cysts. The radiologic diagnosis is difficult, for plain films of the abdomen show only air-fluid levels in dilated loops of small bowel. Some studies report free intraperitoneal air, flecks of calcium, and intraluminal meconium. There is no true transitional zone, but a false one is seen in the distal colon in 15 per cent of cases. The colon appears normal in 22 per cent, small in 38 per cent, or dilated in 3 per cent of infants. Abnormal contractions in the large bowel appear as transverse folds. In 19 per cent, the colon appears shortened and the cecum malpositioned. Eight per cent have meconium plugs. Colonic stasis is present in 21 per cent but evacuation of barium often is not delayed. Occasionally one sees retrograde filling of the entire small bowel after a barium enema.[27, 135]

The upper gastrointestinal study shows massive gastroesophageal reflux and marked stasis in the small bowel. Barium remains in the intestine for 24 hours or more and in some cases up to one week. Regurgi-

tated fecaliths are seen in the jejunum as ovoid filling defects. The final diagnosis rests upon the absence of ganglion cells in the intestinal biopsy.

Treatment. Ileostomy is lifesaving for the infant with long-segment disease. After several weeks most babies pass fairly firm stools through the ileostomy and have minimal fluid losses. However, some with high ileostomies do lose a great deal of fluid and become severely dehydrated.[116] Enemas into the unused colon provide increased fluid absorption. After the baby is a year old, a long side-to-side ileorectal anastomosis provides internal continuity. It is stressed that any resection of small bowel requires examination of serial sections of tissue for ganglion cells so that the anastomosis is performed with normal small bowel.

Complications. Enterocolitis is a hazard in about 40 per cent of these infants after surgery and is treated as described earlier.

Prognosis. Early overall mortality figures in this disease ranged between 76 and 100 per cent, but now only 10 to 50 per cent (average, 49 per cent) of affected infants will die. The mortality is directly related to the extent of aganglionosis through the small bowel and failure to recognize the disorder. Although bowel movements are frequent after surgery, after 6 months the stools stabilize to an average of 3 to 6/day.[93]

Short-Segment Hirschsprung's Disease

This mild form of the disease is considered separately because it resembles psychogenic megacolon more than Hirschsprung's disease in its classic form and is usually not diagnosed or treated until late infancy or childhood. Aganglionosis involves only a short, low segment of rectum.[204a]

Incidence. Thirty-nine cases were seen in a 14 year period in Israel.[204a] More than two thirds of the patients are male.

Symptoms. The typical symptoms are those of chronic constipation. In older, infants and children there are fecal soiling, bed wetting, and, at times, daytime enuresis. Only 20 per cent of patients have signs of intestinal obstruction in infancy. Most are well nourished and healthy.

Diagnosis. The rectal ampulla is packed full of feces, and digital sphincter tone seems good. Radiologic examination is of little help; the barium enema is usually normal. Manometry demonstrates a lack of relaxation of the internal sphincter in the presence of rectal distention. Rectal biopsy shows aganglionosis in a short segment of rectum.

Treatment. Successful treatment of this disease has been accomplished by anorectal myomectomy.[165]

Megacolon and Intestinal Ganglioneuromatosis

This rare form of neuromatosis has been reported in 21 patients.[139]

Etiology. This is undoubtedly one variant of the neuromatoses since some of the infants have a family history that is positive for von Recklinghausen's disease.

Pathology. There are hyperplasia of the submucous and myenteric plexuses, giant ganglia, and increased acetylcholinesterase. Isolated ganglion cells are present in the lamina propria.

Symptoms. The symptoms resemble those of Hirschsprung's disease, with constipation from infancy, abdominal distention, growth retardation, and repeated episodes of partial low-intestinal obstruction.

Diagnosis. Rectal examination shows firm feces in the ampulla, and rectal biopsy demonstrates a marked increase in ganglion cells and hyperplasia of Meissner's and Auerbach's plexuses. Massive megacolon is seen on barium enema examination, but the colon evacuates normally.

Treatment. The only treatment is symptomatic, with frequent enemas and lubricants to assure colonic evacuation.

Prognosis. The long-term prognosis is not yet known.

Megacystis-Microcolon Syndrome

This disorder represents a form of in-intestinal pseudo-obstruction and is discussed under *Intestinal Obstruction*.[213a]

THE NEONATAL SMALL LEFT COLON SYNDROME (SLCS)

Originally described in 1974 by Davis et al.[36] in infants with evidence of low colonic obstruction, the syndrome was later reported by Stewart et al.[185] in four infants born to diabetic mothers, three of whom required drug management, and later still in infants whose mothers were taking phenothiazines.[53]

Incidence. The incidence of symptomatic disease is not known although 40 per cent of infants born to diabetic mothers have radiologic evidence of a small left colon.[36, 149]

Etiology. The normal neonate has a fall in blood glucose and a rise in glucagon, but the infant of the diabetic mother has exaggerated findings, with high glucagon levels not influenced by intravenous glucose. Since glucagon inhibits gastrointestinal motility, it is proposed that there is a neurohumoral imbalance, in which hypoglycemia-stimulated hyperglucagonemia and increased autonomic activity, in combination with immature ganglion cells, inhibit jejunal and sigmond motor activity.[120] However, some infants actually had a blunted glucagon response.[181] Davis et al. and others have suggested that increased magnesium plays a role.[177]

Pathology. There is an increased ratio of small cells to multipolar ganglion cells in both right and left colonic tissue. The ratio normally is 1:13 but in this disease it is 1:21 to 1:25. The plug contains increased protein and lacks tryptic activity.

Symptoms. There is a maternal history of diabetes, which is usually insulin-dependent. Half the mothers have had toxemia, and many have had polyhydramnios. The infants have respiratory distress, hypoglycemia, cardiomyopathy, cyanosis, persistent fetal circulation, and abdominal distention. They fail to pass meconium.

Differential Diagnosis. Hirschsprung's disease, meconium plug syndrome,[192, 214] and inspissated milk curd syndrome are the major disorders from which SLCS must be distinguished.[30]

Diagnosis. Plain films of the abdomen reveal dilated loops suggesting low colonic obstruction; cecal dilatation may be evident. Barium enema, performed if there is no evidence of perforation, shows a decreased colon caliber from anus to splenic flexure with a transition zone at the splenic flexure; the zone is longer than that seen in Hirschsprung's disease, and the margins of the colon are smooth. Colon proximal to the transition zone is dilated and distended with meconium, but the entire colon fills easily with barium (Fig. 17–12).

In half the patients, a flat film reveals evidence of pneumoperitoneum, indicating perforation, which occurs usually in the cecum or ileum.

Treatment. The water-soluble contrast enema is both diagnostic and therapeutic but must be performed early. Hypaque should be used and Tween 80 in Gastrografin should be avoided. Several enemas may be necessary to relieve the obstruction. Infants who are symptomatic for 24 hours are at risk of perforation.

If perforation is evident on plain film,

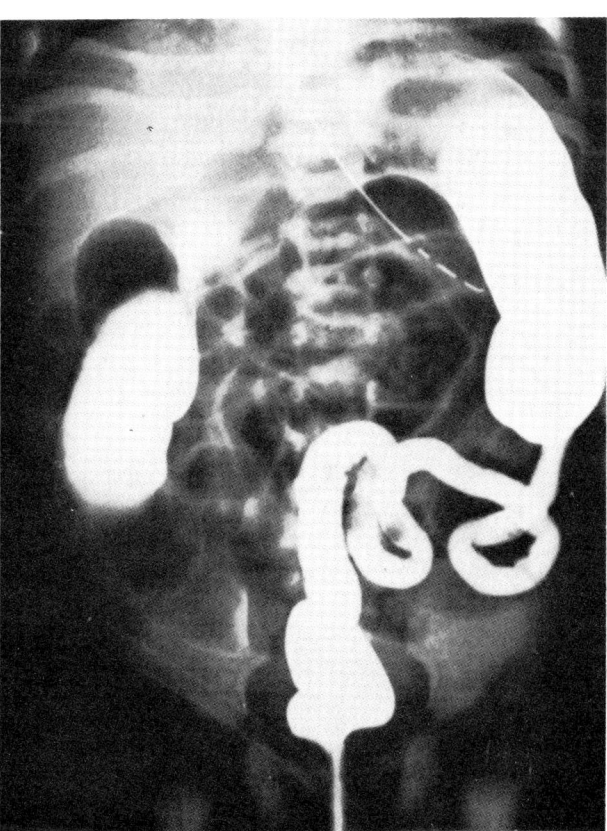

Figure 17–12 Contrast enema examination in SLCS showing transition zone; the colon is smooth-walled and somewhat less redundant than normal.

laparotomy with closure of the perforation or resection of nonviable bowel is undertaken.

Prognosis. In those with perforation the mortality reaches 50 per cent, but, if the disease is treated early, the course should be benign.

GANGLIONEUROFIBROMATOSIS

Ganglioneurofibromatosis of the bowel is an extremely rare disease in which multiple sessile and pedunculated polyps extend through the colon and into the last few centimeters of ileum.

Etiology. The etiology is unknown.

Pathology. Histologic examination of the polyp reveals groups of ganglion cells and nerve fibers above the muscularis within the polyp and in the adjacent colonic mucosa. One type of polyp is neural, and the other contains ganglion cells and nerve fibers and resembles retention or juvenile polyps, although the stalk mucosa also contains clusters of ganglion or nerve cells not present in the typical juvenile polyp.

Symptoms. Recurrent rectal bleeding is the major complaint and is usually not excessive. Blood and mucus are passed with or after the stool.

Treatment. There is no specific treatment for this disorder except segmental resection or ileorectostomy if the symptoms become severe enough to warrant therapy.

THE SYNDROME OF COLONIC DIVERTICULA, NEUROMATOSIS, PHEOCHROMOCYTOMA, AND MEDULLARY CARCINOMA OF THE THYROID

This syndrome has been reported in adolescents and adults and is mentioned because our one patient in whom diagnosis was made at 11 years of age had symptoms by age 2 years.[74] Originally the syndrome included only medullary carcinoma of the thyroid and pheochromocytoma, but it has since been expanded to include colonic diverticula and enteric neuromatosis. The patients have a typical facies, with thickened eyelids, thick lips, a prognathic jaw, and long, slender arms resembling somewhat those of Marfan's syndrome (Fig. 17–13).

Inheritance. An autosomal dominant transmission has been noted in some families, and von Recklinghausen's disease is present in others.

Pathology. Some patients have parathyroid hyperplasia. The medullary carcinoma of the thyroid does not arise from thyroid epithelium but from the same parafollicular cell as that which produces calcitonin, a calcium-lowering substance. It is speculated that the calcitonin present in some of the tumors causes secondary hyperparathyroidism. Prostaglandins are also produced by some of the tumors and likely play a role in producing diarrhea. Pheochromocytomas can be unilateral or bilateral and extra-adrenal. Although the rectal mucosa appears normal, the biopsy specimen resembles that of intestinal ganglioneuromatosis and contains neuromas composed of ganglion cells that are scattered throughout the submucosa and myenteric plexus.

Symptoms. Patients may have only one or two manifestations of the complete syndrome but must be presumed prone to develop others. The case history of our patient demonstrates the course of the disease.

Diagnosis. The typical facies in a patient should arouse immediate suspicion of the diagnosis. Elevation of the serum prostaglandins and calcitonin indicates a secreting tumor. The finding of colonic diverticula should lead to investigation of the thyroid, for such diverticula are not often seen in young people. It is stressed that the thyroid tumor often lies below the sternum and cannot always be palpated in the neck. Because the incidence of thyroid carcinoma is so high in patients with this syndrome, some advocate prophylactic thyroidectomy.

SEGMENTAL DILATATION OF THE COLON

This rare disorder has been reported in 7 cases since 1959.[80a]

Clinically there is constipation from birth, and radiologically there is sigmental dilatation of the colon. This has been observed in a congenital form in the neonate and there is no evidence of muscular hypertrophy. In

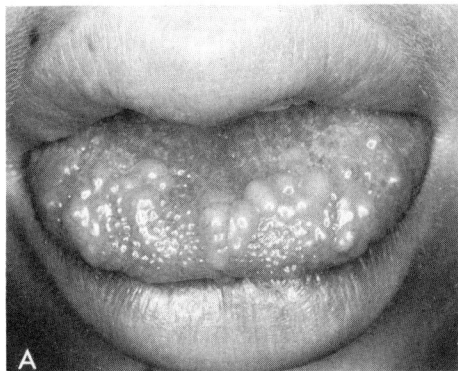

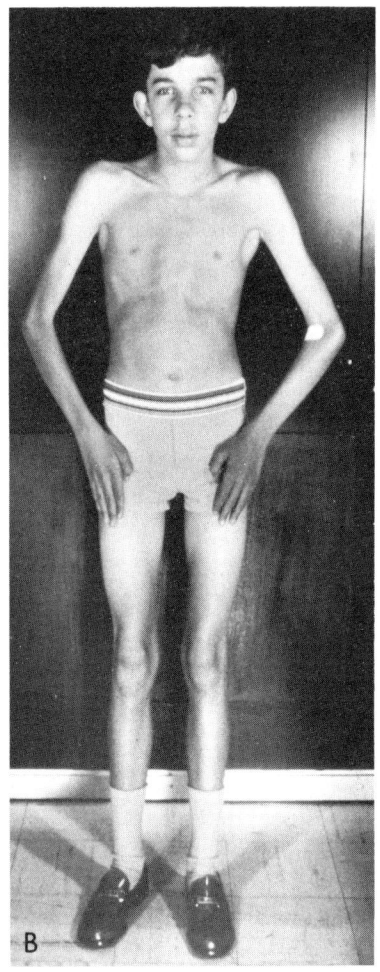

Figure 17–13 A, Tongue lesions in boy with intestinal ganglioneuromatosis, sigmoid diverticula and medullary carcinoma of the thyroid. B, Physical appearance of the same boy. He is 12 years old. All the patients have had a similar facies, with thickened lips, poor dentition and broad bridge of the nose. The long arms suggest Marfan's syndrome. (From Anderson, T., Spackman, T., and Schwartz, S.: Roentgen findings in intestinal ganglioneuromatosis. Radiology, *101*:93, 1971.)

older infants, who presumably have an acquired form, muscle hypertrophy is present. No motility is present in the dilated segment, but colon proximal and distal to it is normal. The dilated segment contains no taenia coli but there are normal submucosal and intermyenteric ganglion cells in all areas. Hypertrophy is of both circular and longitudinal muscle. Depending upon the extent of the lesion, segmental or total resection is required.

ACQUIRED DISEASES OF THE LARGE BOWEL

ACUTE APPENDICITIS

Because the infant cannot tell us of pain in the right lower quadrant, the diagnosis of appendicitis in infants is usually made only after the appendix has perforated and signs of peritonitis prevail.[85, 151, 186] The delay in making the diagnosis is usually due to failure to consider this disease in the infant.[12, 13, 123, 174]

Incidence. Although this is the most common surgical disease of childhood, only 0.4 per cent of affected children are under one year of age, and 1 to 2.9 per cent are under two years old.[73] Appendicitis has been reported even in premature infants.[23, 56]

Etiology. Acute appendicitis is caused by mucosal invasion of bacteria that are present in the appendiceal lumen.[117] Bacterial invasion sometimes occurs through ulcerations in the mucosa but is most often secondary to chronic distention of an appendix obstructed by a fecalith or hyperplastic lymphoid tissue. Pinworms are present in about 7 per cent of all the appendices re-moved, but it is debatable whether they play any role in initiating the disease. In some older children, however, the chronic right lower quadrant pain associated with pinworms in the appendiceal lumen is re-lieved by appendectomy. A higher inci-dence of appendicitis in children with measles has been reported.

The infant appendix is transitional in structure between the conical shape of the fetal appendix and the vermiform type seen in older children. It is less likely to become obstructed, although fecaliths are present in the abdominal films of one third of infants with acute appendicitis.[125]

Pathology and Pathogenesis. Bacteria invade the mucosa, submucosa, and mus-cularis and cause edema, vascular engorge-ment, and hyperplasia of the lymph folli-cles. Eventually, in the untreated patient there is necrosis, thrombosis of vessels, and perforation within 6 to 12 hours. Because the infant omentum is short and does not always reach the lower quadrants, it is not accessible to wall off a perforation.[150] Gen-eralized peritonitis is therefore more com-mon in the infant than is abscess formation. If the inflamed appendix lies near a ureter or near the bladder, it causes pyuria. Organ-isms are mixed aerobes and anaerobes, with *Escherichia coli,* alpha-hemolytic strepto-coccus, gamma-hemolytic streptococcus, group D streptococcus, and *Pseudomonas* predominating of the aerobic group. *Bac-teroides* is the major anaerobe, with gram-positive cocci, *Fusobacterium* and *Clostrid-ium* being lesser isolates.[21]

Symptoms. In the small infant, anorexia and irritability are the first signs of illness.[146] In the premature infant, symptoms mimic necrotizing enterocolitis. Within a few hours the baby begins to vomit and be-comes lethargic. The symptoms then are those of intestinal perforation and peritoni-tis. The baby becomes anxious and is reluc-tant to move about. The abdomen is at first soft, but it becomes distended and moder-ately to quite rigid. Older infants and chil-dren complain first of generalized or periumbilical pain, and after a few hours the

pain is localized to the right lower quadrant. Pain is intermittent at the onset but be-comes constant as it increases in severity. Constipation is the rule, but in a few babies the bowel habits remain normal. If the ap-pendix lies near the sigmoid or the terminal ileum or if it has perforated, there is diar-rhea.

Examination of the abdomen in acute appendicitis shows the bowel sounds to be hypoactive or hyperactive. With perfora-tion, the bowel sounds become hypoactive and absent. There are guarding of the whole abdomen or the right lower quadrant and tenderness to deep palpation with rebound tenderness in the right lower quadrant. In one series, 19 of 40 infants had a palpable mass.[152] The infant assumes a position of comfort with legs flexed. Straightening or lateral rotation of the legs causes pain. The temperature is between 100 and 102°F. in uncomplicated appendicitis. Higher tem-peratures signify perforation.

Diagnosis. This disease must be dif-ferentiated from pyelonephritis, pneumo-nia, and other causes of peritonitis. Chest film, urinalysis, and urine culture will dif-ferentiate the first two. Three-way films of the abdomen are of help if one sees a fecalith, which is present in 28 to 33 per cent of cases of acute appendicitis (Fig. 17–14), scoliosis due to muscle spasm, in-crease in thickness of the lateral abdominal wall, or free intraperitoneal fluid or air. In a few patients, dilated loops of small bowel in the right lower quadrant are the only radio-logic findings to suggest a pathologic condi-tion. Barium enema shows nonfilling of the appendix and irregularities of the mucosal wall.[114]

An appendiceal abscess, which forms in older children, is represented by a right lower quadrant mass with some displace-ment of bowel loops out of the right lower quadrant (Figs. 17–15 and 17–16). Ultraso-nography may define an abscess.

Although the white blood cell count in older children with appendicitis varies be-tween 12,000 and 15,000 per cubic millime-ter, it is low or normal in 40 per cent of babies less than 2 years of age. A white

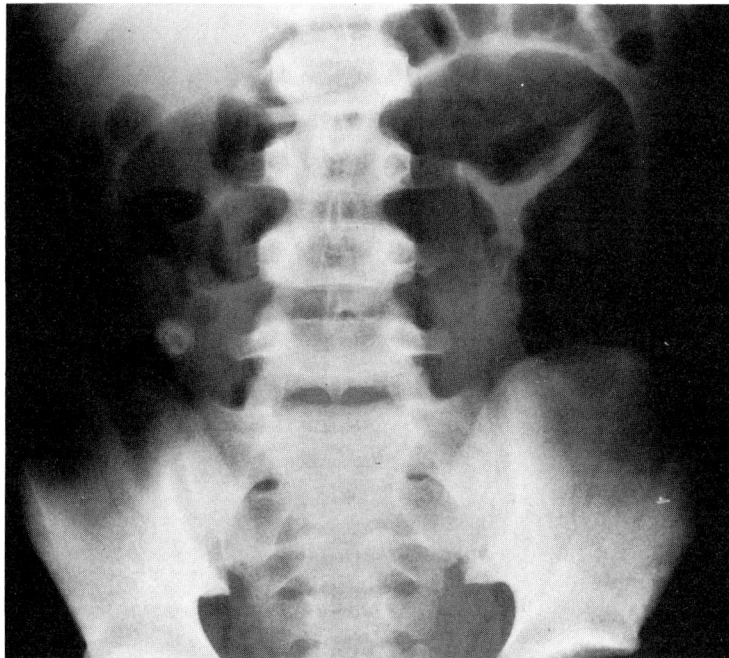

Figure 17–14 Appendicitis and appendicolith in a boy with right lower quadrant pain. The lamellated stone is seen just to the right of the transverse process of the fourth lumbar vertebra.

blood count greater than 20,000 indicates perforation.

Treatment. Once the diagnosis is made, the baby should be kept in a semi-erect position. Broad-spectrum antibiotics, such as ampicillin or clindamycin or a combination of penicillin and kanamycin, are given if perforation is suspected. The treatment is appendectomy.

Complications. The appendix is perforated in 80 to 94 per cent of infants with appendicitis, and more than half these infants have a significant morbidity, with wound infections, pelvic abscesses, wound drainage, and fecal fistulas.[54] Early administration of antibiotics significantly affects abscess formation, for abscess will develop in 20 per cent of those with appendiceal perforation who are given antibiotics after surgery, whereas it occurs in only 1.5 per cent of those given antibiotics before, during, and after surgery. Antibiotics do not affect the development of wound infections, however. These seem to be modified only by delaying closure of the skin and subcutaneous tissue until 3 to 4 days later. Fecal fistulas are treated successfully by hyperalimentation.

Peritoneal drainage seems to prolong the hospitalization by three to four days.[79]

Prognosis. In older children with uncomplicated appendicitis, the mortality is essentially nil, but in infants it is 9.3 per cent because of perforation.

DIFFUSE NODULAR LYMPHOID HYPERPLASIA OF THE COLON

Lymphoid hyperplasia of the colon is of crucial diagnostic importance for it may be misdiagnosed as familial polyposis and result in needless colectomy. Further confusion arises when it appears in a child whose family does have polyposis.

Incidence. Once considered rare, the disease is being recognized commonly with the use of air contrast barium enema studies.

Etiology. Although unknown, many consider the etiology to be an immune or inflammatory reaction of the bowel to some as yet unidentified antigenic stimulus: 20 per cent of our patients were IgA deficient.

Pathology. Yellow-white, smooth, rounded 1 to 2 mm nodules are most numerous in the left colon although they may involve the entire colon. Concentrations range from 1 to 5 to as high as 18 nodules

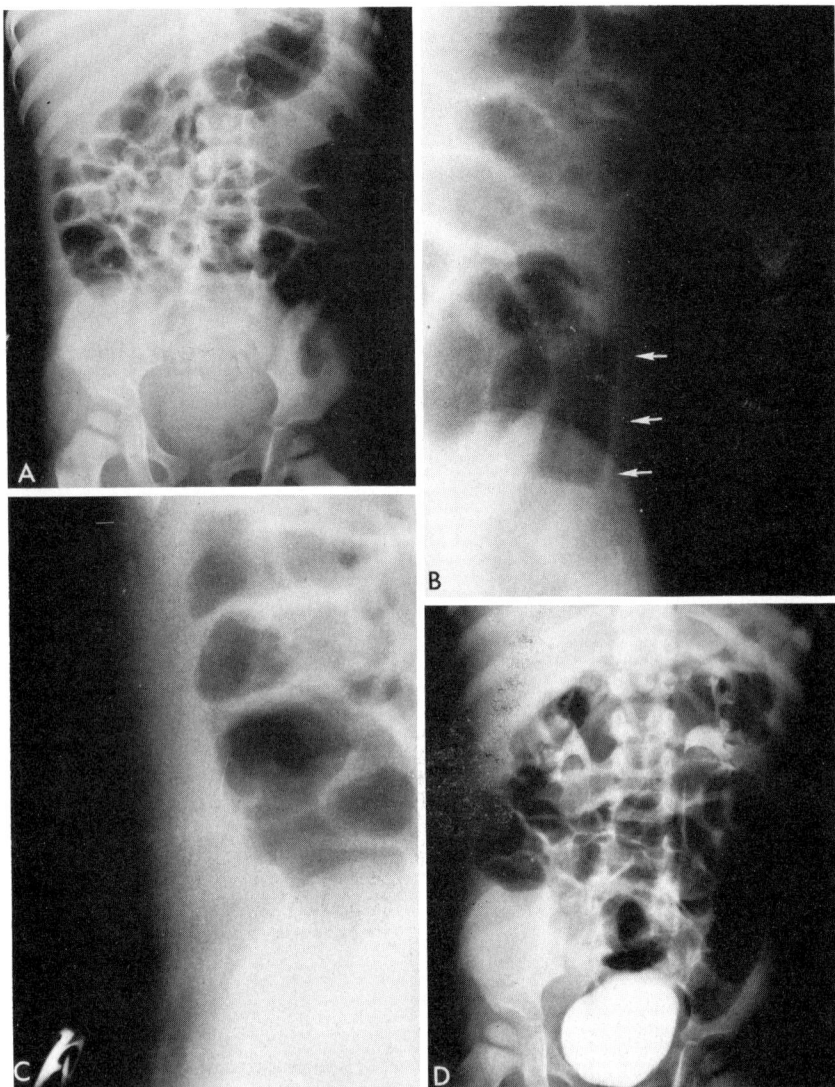

Figure 17–15 Appendiceal abscess in an 18 month old girl who presented to the hospital with right lower quadrant pain and tenderness and an ill-defined mass in the right lower quadrant. *A,* Plain film of the abdomen shows an absence of gas-filled bowel loops in the right lower quadrant, without any discrete mass. *B,* A close-up view of the left side of the abdomen demonstrates a discrete lucent line representing the flank stripe (arrows). There is no displacement of the gas-filled loop of bowel away from the flank stripe, and this represents a normal appearance. *C,* Close-up view of the right side of the abdomen shows a loss of the lucent flank stripe and some displacement medially of the bowel loops. The medial displacement suggests a mass effect. Loss of the flank stripe represents edema of the fat, causing it to take on a water density, and is indicative of an inflammatory process. *D,* Intravenous pyelogram again shows absence of bowel loops in the right lower quadrant and some displacement of the right side of the upper bladder. All of these radiologic findings are indicative of a right lower quadrant inflammatory mass extending into the pelvis.

per square centimeter in the sigmoid and rectum. Very few are umbilicated. Histologically they are identical to those of small bowel lymphoid hyperplasia (Fig. 17–17).

Symptoms. Symptoms appear as early as three months or in adolescence as recurrent abdominal pain or rectal bleeding with or without diarrhea. Many patients have had freckles. Physical findings are minimal except for mild tenderness over the colon. Abdominal distention and malnutrition are rare.

Diagnosis. Radiologically and sigmoidoscopically one cannot always differen-

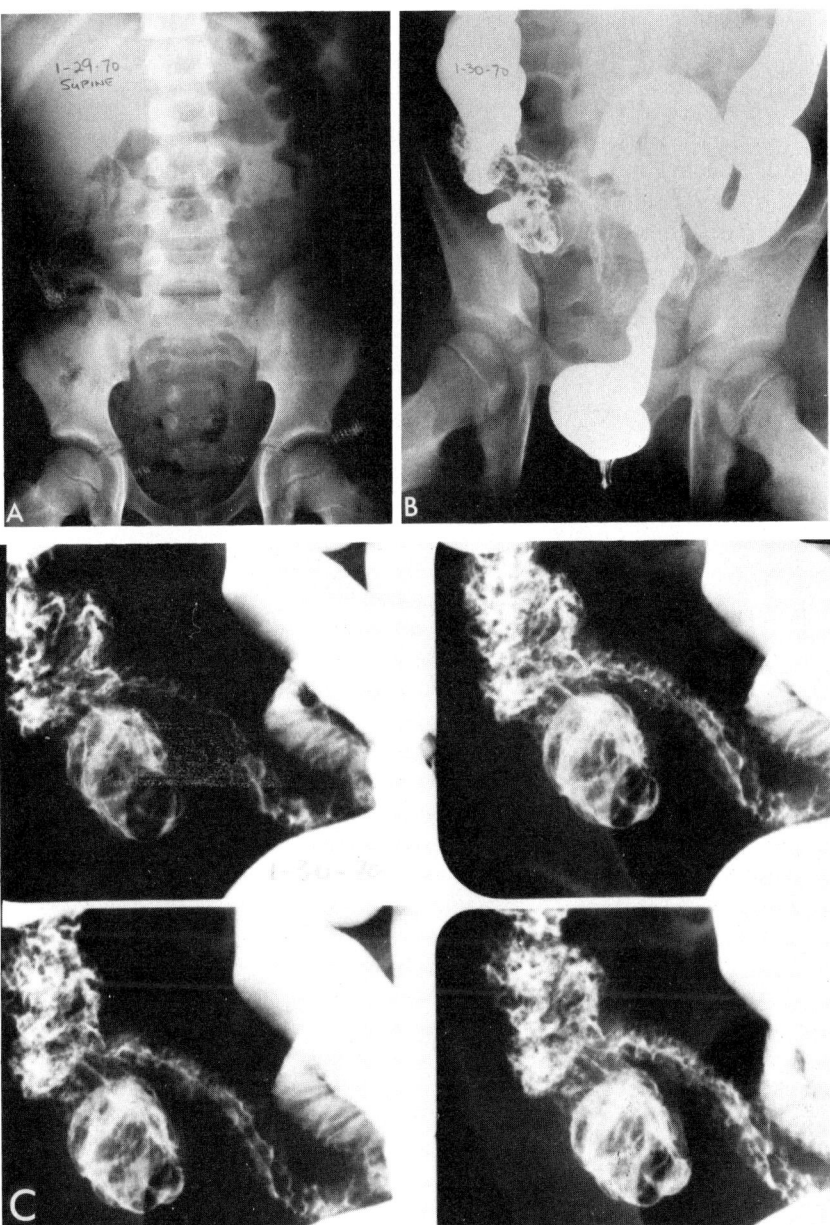

Figure 17–16 Appendiceal abscess in a girl with a 6 weeks' history of abdominal pain, constipation, and vomiting. On physical examination diffuse abdominal tenderness was found, without a discrete palpable mass. *A*, The scout film obtained before the contrast study was essentially normal although mottled shadows were seen extending down into the right side of the pelvis. This can be seen in instances of a distended rectosigmoid or a low-lying cecum but should suggest the possibility of a gas-containing abscess. *B*, Fill-up films from the barium show that the cecum is in a normal position, and the mottled shadows in the right pelvis correspond to a large filling defect that stretches and compresses the terminal ileum and displaces the rectosigmoid. *C*, Spot films of the terminal ileum show no evidence of filling of the appendix and an intrinsically normal mucosal pattern in the terminal ileum. This latter finding speaks against the diagnosis of regional enteritis, which was another of the clinical considerations. Filling of the appendix with barium can be used as evidence against appendicitis; nonfilling may be seen in appendicitis and in normal patients.

tiate this disease from familial polyposis. Central ulcerations are apparent in these pale polyps, but intervening mucosa is normal. Biopsy shows the nodules to be lym-

phoid polyps with large, active germinal centers.

Treatment. Steroids have been used in some patients to decrease symptoms, but

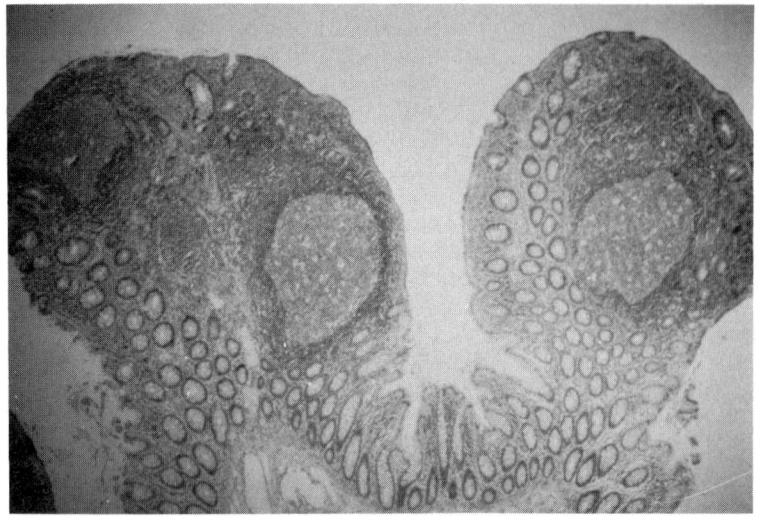

Figure 17–17 Lymphoid polyposis of the colon. Two large colonic polypoid lesions are present and have active germinal centers. The lesions are in the lamina propria, and the colonic epithelium remains relatively intact. (Courtesy of Dr. D. Sheahan.)

the lesions are benign and such therapy is usually not indicated. Hypoallergenic diets also have alleviated symptoms.

Prognosis. The long-term outlook is usually one of resolution of symptoms, although one of our patients later developed ulcerative colitis.

LYMPHOID POLYPS

Lymphoid polyps seem to be a separate entity from lymphoid hyperplasia of the colon.

Incidence. Nearly 50 cases have been reported in the literature, and several children in the same family have been affected.[24a]

Etiology. These polyps are thought to represent perhaps hamartoma or response to inflammation.

Pathology. Lymphoid polyps, though often singular, in children tend to be multiple, with the vast majority limited to the rectum. They are usually sessile but may be pedunculated, measuring a few millimeters to several centimeters. They may occur with one or more juvenile polyps. The lesions are smooth or polypoid, and the surface may be ulcerated with no definite capsule. Larger polyps contain fibrous septa. Lymph follicles within have germinal centers and may contain macrophages but have no definite capsule.

Symptoms. The lesions are noted because of rectal bleeding or prolapse of the polypoid tissue.

Diagnosis. The diagnosis is established by sigmoidoscopy and biopsy. Air contrast barium studies should be performed to determine the number and location of the polyps.

Treatment. Local excision is usually curative.

ULCERATIVE COLITIS

Ulcerative colitis is an inflammatory disease affecting the mucosa of the rectum and the colon. It is extremely rare in infancy and must not be confused with "milk-induced colitis," which is a manifestation of allergy to cow's milk protein.[205]

Incidence. In one 20-year review of ulcerative colitis in children, only eight cases in infants under one year of age were found.[48, 51, 57] In two of these, the symptoms were aggravated or initiated by the addition of milk to the diet. A decade ago, only 3 per cent of our patients had onset of their disease before the age of two and a half years, and now 8 per cent are less than two years of age at onset.[76]

Etiology. A number of hypotheses are proposed to explain the development of ulcerative colitis, but its etiology actually is still unknown.[76, 103] Some favor an infectious origin, since *Entamoeba histolytica*, mycoplasma, and occasionally other organisms have been isolated from a small percentage of patients. Increasing evidence suggests that viruses play a role in the etiology. An allergic origin is supported by many, because a delayed sensitivity type of reaction can be produced in the colon of experimental animals after local instillation of a substance to which they have previously been cutaneously sensitized. Furthermore, sera from a number of patients contain antibodies to normal colonic tissue, and their colonic mucosal cells absorb anticolon antibody.[195, 202] Milk for years has been thought to play a role in producing ulcerative colitis, and in 1961, Truelove's group reported milk-induced exacerbations of colitis as well as an increased incidence of milk protein antibodies in the sera of their patients.[202] A number of possible factors are listed in Table 17–2.

Psychogenic factors, although often identified with the onset of the disease and certainly associated with a number of exacerbations, have not been proved to cause ulcerative colitis.

Heredity undoubtedly plays some role, for there is an increased family incidence, to between 15 and 25 per cent compared with an estimated 1 per cent[86] in the general population. Evidence also exists for similar HLA typings of affected patients in families with inflammatory bowel disease. Colitis has been reported in both members of monozygous twins. It is more common in white than in black populations and in boys than in girls; it is four times more frequent in those of Jewish extraction than in non-Jews.

Since the earliest pathologic changes involve the collagen of the lamina propria, it is suggested that colitis may be one of the collagen diseases.

Immune factors are also included among the etiologic considerations, for lymphocytes from patients have proved cytotoxic for tissue cultures of colonic epithelial cells. Colitis has occurred in some infants born to mothers with ulcerative colitis. We have noted a more than chance association of this disease and Turner's syndrome (Table 17–3).

Pathology. The pathologic changes are those of nonspecific inflammatory disease involving in most cases the rectum, rectosigmoid, and part or all of the remaining colon.[86] Extension into the appendix and terminal ileum is found in 10 per cent of patients. Typically this is a mucosal disease but in its fulminant form it can extend through the full thickness of the bowel. In such cases, toxic megacolon with massive dilatation of the transverse and left colon develops and perforation is impending. During a severe, acute attack there is sloughing of the superficial mucosa and thinning and destruction of the muscle layers. Residual edematous mucosal islands remain in the denuded areas and resemble polyps. True pseudopolyps or inflammatory polyps result from deep ulcerations that extend into the submucosa and undermine the mucosa as they scar. Pseudopolyps adhere to one another through mucosal bridging. Stricture formation is unusual although

Table 17–2   Infectious, Immunologic and Genetic Factors in Inflammatory Bowel Disease

Bacterial Isolates:	*C. difficile* or its toxin *Pseudomonas* variant *Mycoplasma*
Viral Isolates:	Cytomegalovirus in UC, rare in CD
	Small RNA virus from CD
Cytotoxic Agents:	Serum and lymphocytes
	IBD tissue extracts[129a, 135]
	CD, mol wt 27,000
	UC, mol wt 43,000
Immunocytes:	Increased IgA, IgM, and IgG cells in lamina propria[137a]
	Increased lamina propria lymphocytes
	Increased intraepithelial lymphocytes
	? Increased K cell activity
	Decreased suppressor T cell generation
	? Immune complexes react with K cells for antibody-dependent, cell-mediated cytotoxicity
Genetic Factors:	Familial disease often associated with same HLA type
	Increased in Turner's syndrome
	15 to 20% IgA deficiency in CD

Table 17–3 Characteristics of Disease in Ulcerative Colitis
and Crohn's Disease

	CROHN'S DISEASE	ULCERATIVE COLITIS
Site of disease	Small bowel, colon	Colon
	Rarely, any site from mouth to anus	"Backwash to ileum" rare
	Skip areas	Continuous
	Usually spares rectum	Rectum involved
Depth of lesion	Transmural, with granulomas	Mucosal
Extraintestinal lesions	+	+
Positive family history	+	+

possible. As the disease progresses, the colon becomes shortened and rigid and its diameter narrows.

Grossly the diseased mucosa appears vascular and deep pink, with a velvety, granular or cobblestoned texture. It is characteristically friable and bleeds readily after gentle wiping with a cotton swab. Diffuse ulcerations resemble petechiae or superficial erosions in their early stages, but later they appear deeper and are arranged in a linear fashion. Exposed submucosa is covered by a mucoid or mucopurulent exudate.

Histologic examination shows destruction of the surface epithelium in some areas and hyperplasia in others. Goblet cells are decreased or lost, and there is enlargement and hyperchromatism of the mucosal cell nuclei. The mucosa and submucosa are edematous with dilated and engorged blood vessels and cellular infiltration. The infiltrate contains some polymorphonuclear cells but mostly lymphocytes, plasma cells, and eosinophils (Fig. 17–18). There is some hyperplasia of the lymphoid follicles. The rectal glands are widely separated, and crypt abscesses are a common but not a diagnostic finding, for they are present in other inflammatory diseases. As the abscesses enlarge they burst and spread under the mucosa. The crypts of Lieberkühn contain Paneth cells and in chronic cases an increased number of Kulchitsky cells. Rectal and perianal fistulas are uncommon.

Symptoms. Disease in the infant is either mild and short-lived or severe and progressive.[86] The major symptoms in either case are irritability and the passage of blood and mucus in the stool. Diarrhea alone may persist for weeks to months before gross or occult bleeding is noted. In a few cases gross rectal bleeding lasts only one or two days, then disappears only to recur six months to a year later. Usually the stools are loose and contain fresh blood and mucus. Pallor and anemia result from chronic blood loss. Young babies and children do not seem bothered by abdominal pain. If there is a significant enteric loss of protein, pitting edema and ascites appear (Fig. 17–19).

Extracolonic manifestations such as uveitis, erythema nodosum, joint inflammation, and pyoderma gangrenosum are not seen in infants and young children. Malnutrition, dehydration, and electrolyte imbalances are the major complications.

The physical examination shows loss of subcutaneous tissue. The abdomen is scaphoid, although in some babies it can be distended. Gentle palpation elicits tenderness and some guarding over the descending or the entire colon. The bowel sounds are hyperactive. The temperature is normal or mildly elevated in the mild or moderately ill baby and can rise to 104°F. in the severely ill one. Classification of the disease is discussed under treatment.

Diagnosis. In infants the diagnosis is usually delayed until after the diarrhea and rectal bleeding have persisted for some time. Other causes to be ruled out are immunoglobulin deficiency, bacterial or amebic dysentery, milk-protein allergy, granulomatous colitis, nonspecific gastroenteritis, hemolytic-uremic syndrome, blood dyscrasia, and vascular thrombosis.

Sigmoidoscopy with rectal biopsy is the

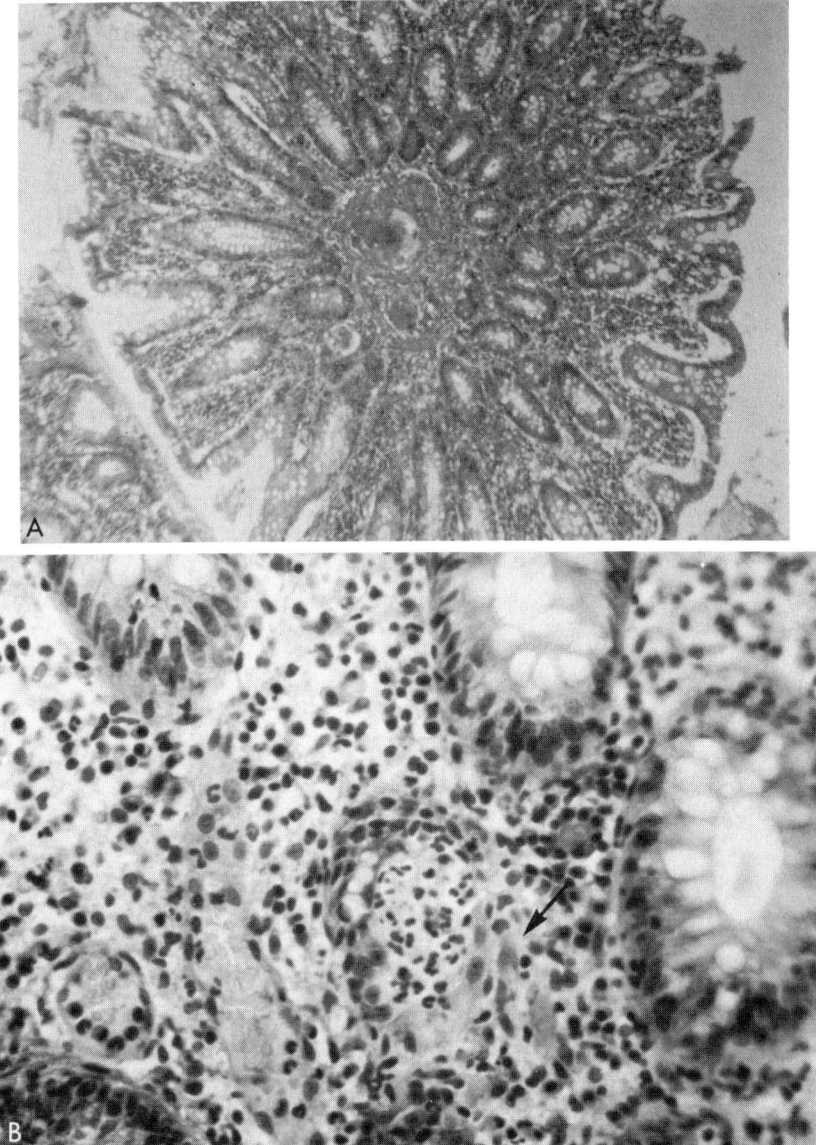

Figure 17–18 A, Rectal biopsy from patient with ulcerative colitis. There is some separation of the rectal crypts and destruction of areas of rectal mucosa. There is a heavy round and polymorphonuclear cellular infiltration of the lamina propria. B, Crypt abscess containing polymorphonuclear cells (arrow).

most important diagnostic study. The bowel lumen contains free blood or mucopurulent exudate. The mucosa is friable or edematous, and there is loss of the normal vascular pattern. Its color varies from deep pink to red, and its consistency is granular, velvety, or cobblestoned. Ulcerations, petechial lesions, and erosions are not always visible. In the acute stages the mucosa is extremely friable, but in the convalescent stages friability is diminished and there is little or no exudate. Since shigellosis and amebiasis can cause similar changes in the rectal mucosa, multiple stools must be examined for bacterial and parasitic pathogens.

Radiologic examination of the colon must be performed at some time during the course of the disease, but we prefer to withhold this study until a patient's condition is stable and bleeding has diminished.

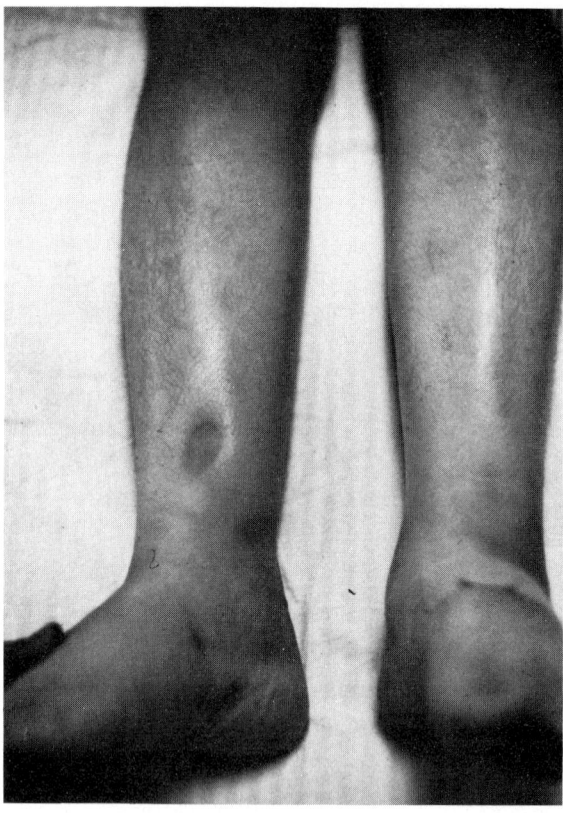

Figure 17–19 Pedal and lower extremity edema in an 8 year old girl with severe ulcerative colitis. She had a 3-month history of diarrhea with blood in the stool. The serum albumin at the time of admission was 1.8 gm per 100 ml.

A three-way film of the abdomen is mandatory in any child with distention in order to rule out toxic megacolon. When a barium enema is scheduled, we prepare the colon with saline enemas. Under no circumstances should castor oil be used, for this can exacerbate the disease. The barium enema is interpreted through both filled and postevacuation studies of the colon. Filled films outline the contour of the bowel and its distensibility and length. Ulcerations are seen as small, fine, saw-tooth spicules involving the mucosa, or as the more ominous "collar-stud" ulcerations that emerge through the serosa and have a small, thin neck (Fig. 17–20). When these subserosal ulcerations become confluent they appear as a double contour — a separate tract of barium that parallels the contour of the colon. Inflammatory polyps or pseudopolyps usually signify longstanding disease (Fig. 17–21). Postevacuation films show abnormal or absent haustrations and a coarse reticular or honeycombed appearance of the

mucosa. Shortening and narrowing of the colon causes a "pipe-stem" appearance. Widening of the retrorectal soft tissue space due to perirectal inflammation and edema, noted on lateral films, is fairly consistent in indicating active rectal disease (Fig. 17–20).

Early in the disease the barium enema may be perfectly normal, even in the presence of significant bleeding. There are certain accepted poor prognostic signs: deep ulcerations, decreased tone, and polyposis. In our experience, deep ulcerations carry the poorest prognosis for recovery under medical management. Pseudopolyposis, on the other hand, is sometimes seen in patients who are in complete clinical remission.

Laboratory findings that correlate with the activity of the disease are leukocytosis, fever, and elevation of the erythrocyte sedimentation rate. Anemia is usually of the hypochromic, microcytic type. Hypoproteinemia with reversal of the albumin-globulin ratio reflects enteric albumin

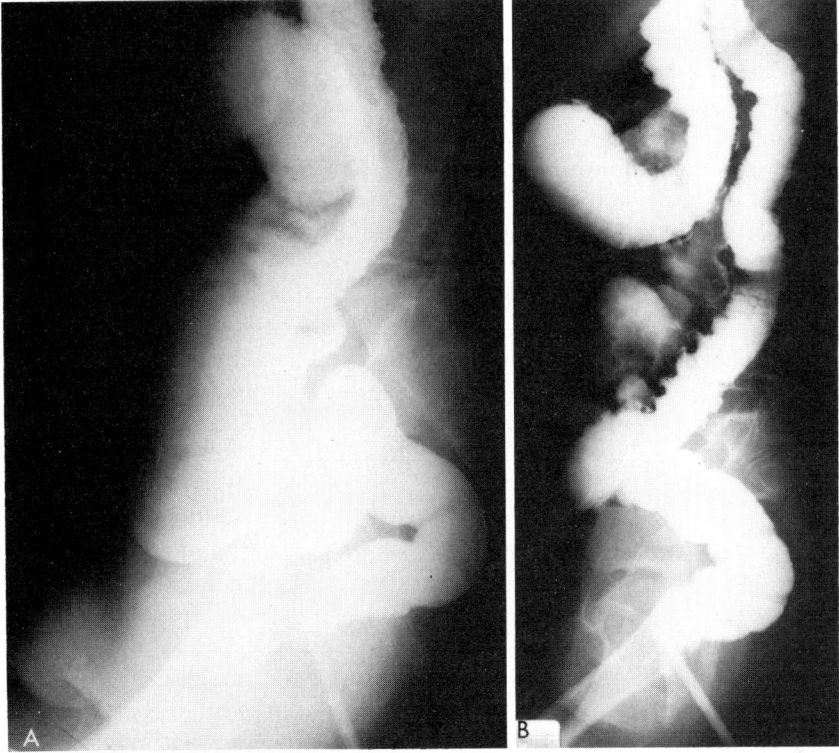

Figure 17–20 *A*, Barium enema in an 11 year old girl with ulcerative colitis. Fine ulcerations in the rectum and sigmoid are not readily apparent, but the feathery appearance of larger ulcerations is visible in the descending colon. Superiorly there are discrete submucosal or "collar-stud" ulcerations. *B*, In this study of a 12 year old girl with ulcerative colitis, fine ulcerations in the rectum cause a sawtooth appearance, and collar-stud ulcerations in the transverse, descending, and sigmoid colon are seen. Areas of double contour are visible. There is widening of the retrorectal soft tissue space.

Figure 17–21 Pseudopolyps in ulcerative colitis. Multiple lucent filling defects are present, and there are small and deep mucosal ulcerations.

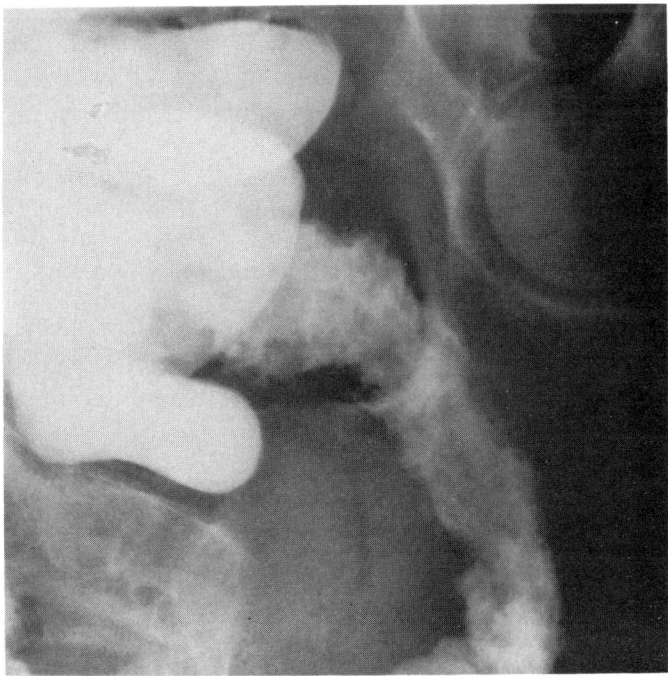

losses. Elevation of the alpha$_2$ globulin often precedes an exacerbation of colitis. The serum carotene is normal or it can be quite low, depending upon the degree of diarrhea and the oral intake of the patient. The lactose tolerance test, abnormal in 40 to 50 per cent of adults with active colitis, is usually normal in young children with the disease. Precipitating antibodies to milk proteins may be present in the stool or in the serum.

Complications. Failure of the inflamed colon to absorb water and electrolytes causes dehydration, hyponatremia, and hypokalemia.

Perforation is the most imminent complication and is of greatest risk during the first attack, particularly in those with involvement of the whole colon. Acute perforation is signaled by tachycardia and an elevation of temperature, abdominal distention, and rigidity. In some cases, perforation is insidious and accompanied only by an increase in abdominal pain. The mortality rate of those in whom perforation is handled conservatively lies between 87 and 100 per cent, and surgical intervention must be immediate.

Acute dilatation or toxic megacolon develops in 1.6 to 3 per cent of patients and accompanies the acute attack in the patient with involvement of the total colon. Hypokalemia, anticholinergic medications, and mechanical distal obstruction all have been considered causative factors, as has local destruction of muscle and nerve endings, but the true etiology remains unknown. The symptoms are those of low intestinal obstruction with severe abdominal distention, decreased or absent bowel sounds, and rapid deterioration of the clinical state. The diagnosis is easily confirmed by a flat film of the abdomen, which shows a greatly dilated transverse colon. Conservative management using large doses of intravenous steroid, nasogastric suction, and a rectal tube is successful in a few cases. This complication carries a mortality rate of 30 per cent and many consider it a surgical emergency. Treatment must be individualized, and, if medical therapy is attempted, the patient must be watched cautiously. Surgical intervention is indicated by progression of the colonic dilatation or by its persistence after 24 hours.

Massive hemorrhage is unusual and occurs in only 1 per cent of cases. Idiopathic thrombocytopenia and Christmas disease have been associated with ulcerative colitis, and thromboembolic phenomena have been reported.

Growth retardation is present during the acute disease, but chronic growth retardation is less marked than that seen with granulomatous bowel disease.

Anorectal fistulas, pericholangitis, erythema nodosum or multiforme, pyoderma gangrenosa, central venous thrombosis, and uveitis are complications of the disease in older children and adults but are extremely unusual in the infant or young child.

Treatment. Treatment is aimed at terminating the acute attack and preventing future relapses. The type of therapy depends upon the severity of the colitis and the physical condition of the patient. Patients with lactose intolerance or zinc deficiency should be treated appropriately by diet or supplementation.[39]

MILD ULCERATIVE COLITIS

Children with sigmoidoscopic changes, normal barium enema, minimal weight loss, and abnormal laboratory findings who are having two to six blood-streaked stools per day often undergo complete remission of symptoms after treatment with Azulfidine. Infant dosage is 125 mg (a quarter tablet) four times a day for the first week. The dosage is increased to 250 mg four times daily in those between one and two years old. Reactions to the drug include nausea, vomiting, urticaria, fever, leukopenia, and agranulocytosis. Nausea and vomiting are relieved by decreasing the dosage. Azulfidine is discontinued if the other side effects appear. Most patients undergo remission during the next few weeks. The drug is continued in therapeutic dosage for one month or until the serum albumin and erythrocyte sedimentation rate have returned to normal. The dosage is then halved and therapy is continued for six months to one year. Small daily doses of Azulfidine have been shown to be more effective than steroids in preventing exacerbation of colitis. Folate supplementation may be necessary, for the drug has reently been shown to decrease its absorption.[61]

MODERATE DISEASE

In moderate disease, significant exudate and friability are noted on sigmoidoscopy, barium enema shows fine ulcerations and some loss of haustrae, mild anemia and hypoproteinemia are present, and more than six loose stools containing blood are passed each day. Prednisone, in dosage of 2 mg per kilogram per day, is indicated. This dosage is continued for at least two weeks and until the laboratory parameters of activity have returned to normal. The dose on alternate days is tapered until after three to four weeks every other day therapy is reached. There is no true generalized steroid schedule, for each child has an individual threshold. Some cannot tolerate alternate-day therapy, and some are controlled on far lower dosages of steroid than others. Advantages of the alternate-day program are less growth retardation and fewer steroid side effects. The ideal dosage is one that will control the disease and yet permit growth. In those with a good response, the steroid dosage is decreased and terminated after eight to ten weeks. The addition of Azulfidine during the tapering period permits easier steroid withdrawal.

Another alternative for treatment is the use of steroid enemas or suppositories that contain 15 to 25 mg of hydrocortisone. These act locally for the most part and avoid systemic steroid effects. They are not satisfactory for the small infant in whom defecation is frequent, for they are expelled too rapidly. Anticholinergics are unpredictable in their effect upon diarrhea. Lomotil will diminish passage of stools when given in dosage of no more than 1 mg three times daily, but it must be used with caution and its routine use in children under two years of age is contraindicated. Fiber is omitted from the diet, as are milk and milk products if there is lactose intolerance or if milk precipitins are present in the serum or stool.

SEVERE ULCERATIVE COLITIS

This is characterized by extreme toxicity, fever usually between 102 and 104°F., and tachycardia. The infants daily pass ten or more diarrheal stools containing blood and mucus and often pass blood alone. Anemia is marked, and usually there is some evidence of edema. Sigmoidoscopy shows a heavy intraluminal exudate and a weeping mucosa. These patients are hospitalized and given intravenous ACTH, ten units every 24 hours or hydrocortisone, 25 to 100 mg every 24 hours. Depending upon clinical condition, the baby is given clear liquids or oral or parenteral hyperalimentation. Transfusion replaces protein as well as blood losses. Treatment is continued for two or more weeks. If at the end of this time there is no improvement, one must consider colectomy. Most patients do undergo remission during this intensive treatment period and are then given prednisone, which is tapered as in moderate disease.

All hospitalized patients are followed by the pediatric surgical team and early in their treatment period are introduced to the team social worker, for most parents feel some sort of guilt or responsibility for their child's illness and most children at some point need help in dealing with a long-term illness. Psychologic tests are given to those who have apparent problems or who are not responding well to medical treatment. This has been extremely helpful in determining perceptual or intelligence difficulties. It is the rare patient who requires a psychiatric referral, and the children and their families function best within the framework of the team.

Intractibility with chronic invalidism and growth retardation is the indication for elective surgery.[203] The operative procedure is total colectomy with ileostomy, for the rectum is almost always involved. Ileoproctostomy is complicated by the risk of hemorrhage from the rectal stump, infection, perforation, and carcinoma and is indicated only in the rare patient in whom the rectum is spared. Endorectal ileal pull-through is a new procedure, but one with inconsistent results.[59]

Without surgery the disease can never be considered cured. The course is intermittent, with periods of well-being punctuated by relapses, or it assumes a chronic form in which mild bleeding and diarrhea persist.

Prognosis. The mild form of the disease in infancy is associated with a good prognosis, but the severe infantile form is progressive and responds poorly to steroids and even to surgery, with half the infants dying during the first few months of treatment. In our experience of three patients in whom the disease developed before the second year, two had severe and one had mild disease. All have responded extremely well and have required steroids only during exacerbations, precipitated usually by upper respiratory infections. They exhibit normal growth and development three to ten years after the initial diagnosis was made.

The mortality during the first attack in adults varies between 3.4 and 10 per cent. Edwards and Truelove correlated the outcome after the first attack with the severity of the disease: 90 per cent of those with mild disease attain remission, whereas only 50 per cent of those with severe disease improve.[42a] Eighty-five per cent of those with only rectal involvement in radiologic studies undergo remission, whereas only 51 per cent of those with total colonic disease do so. Recurrences are more severe in those with total colonic disease. Recurrences in children are particularly precipitated by gastroenteritis, respiratory infection, and severe emotional trauma.

The risk of carcinoma is formidable.[68] Not only is the overall incidence of cancer increased in patients with colitis, but the risk increases yearly. The susceptibility to carcinoma begins between the ages of five and nine years; once the disease has been present for ten years, the incidence is 14.5 per cent. Most cancers develop in the rectum and sigmoid and are extremely virulent; by the time they are diagnosed, they have already metastasized. In some centers, a ten-year duration of disease is considered an indication for prophylactic colectomy. At ten years we institute bi-yearly sigmoidos-

copy and rectal biopsy to look for metaplasia.

MILK-INDUCED COLITIS

Milk-induced colitis is a definite disease of infancy that may be mistaken for ulcerative colitis since it is characterized by the passage of bloody, mucoid, diarrheal stools.

Incidence. Although considered rare, colitic changes may be observed in a number of milk-allergic infants with only occult blood in the stool.

Etiology. The cause is undoubtedly an immune reaction within the colon to milk protein antigen or its derivatives.

Pathology. Grossly, the rectal mucosa is hemorrhagic and friable and may or may not be covered with a mucoid or purulent exudate. Fecal smears contain white blood cells, some eosinophils, and even colonic epithelium. Biopsy taken during the acute stage shows nonspecific proctitis, with edema of the mucosa and submucosa and infiltration of round cells and polymorphonuclear leukocytes, or the changes of acute ulcerative colitis, with destruction of mucosa, marked cellular infiltrate, crypt abscesses, and even destruction of crypts (Fig. 17–22).

Symptoms. The onset may occur at any time between the second day and sixth month of life. The symptoms are those described under milk protein allergy, but diarrheal stools contain more blood and mucus in the stools. The Mitchell-Rubin syndrome of milk-allergic acute gastrointestinal hemorrhage is of similar origin. The babies are critically ill at the time of diagnosis and if challenged with even minute amounts of milk are subject to hypovolemia, shock, and hemorrhage.

Diagnosis. The initial diagnosis must be made on clinical grounds after bacterial causes are ruled out, for sigmoidoscopy cannot differentiate either of these from ulcerative colitis.[68] The barium enema is usually normal. While cultures and bleeding studies are pending, milk elimination is both diagnostic and therapeutic. Within 24 hours, a clinical result is obvious. In our experience, milk precipitin testing of the stool is still of value. Skin testing, RAST-

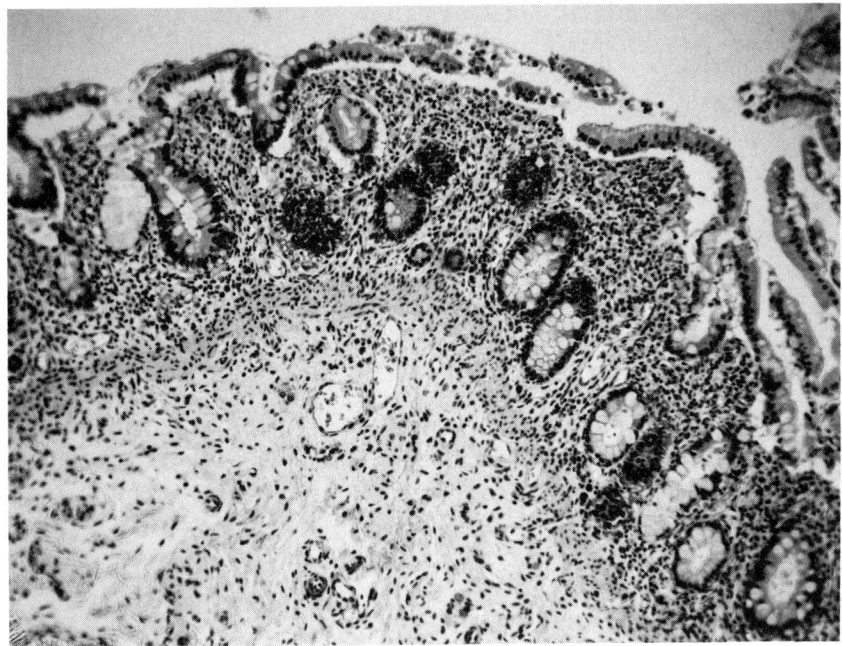

Figure 17–22   The rectal mucosa in milk protein allergy resembles that in ulcerative colitis. There are disruption of the mucosa, separation of the rectal glands, and marked infiltration with inflammatory cells.

specific antimilk IgE, and hemagglutination titers are not especially valuable in establishing the diagnosis. Clinical challenge is to be avoided for at least 6 and probably 12 months.

Treatment. A rigid milk protein–free diet (as well as beef-free initially) is curative. Rectal steroid enemas of 10 to 15 mg of hydrocortisone in 10 ml of saline have been effective in decreasing acute colonic inflammation.

Complications. Anemia and hypoproteinemia are often severe. Electrolyte imbalances may mimic adrenal insufficiency.

Prognosis. Until one year of age, most infants are exquisitely sensitive to milk challenge — some until five or six years of age. At least 15 per cent later will develop respiratory allergic symptoms.

EOSINOPHILIC COLITIS

We have seen eosinophilic colitis in two infants, with onset between two and four weeks of age. In one, the serum gamma globulin was 65 mg/dl with small amounts of IgA and IgM, and in the other, all immunoglobulins were not detectable. Colitis

persisted despite milk elimination, parenteral hyperalimentation, Azulfidine therapy, steroid enemas, and plasma or gamma globulin therapy. The first infant required months of alimentation before recovering and the second expired. The basic defect was not identified, but it was presumed that enteric protein loss contributed to the profound depression of immunoglobulins.

ANTIBIOTIC VASCULITIS

Both penicillin and clindamycin may cause an allergic vasculitis of the colon that must be distinguished from *Clostridium difficile* overgrowth.[189] Cramping and bloody diarrhea resemble symptoms of ulcerative colitis, but sigmoidoscopy is not diagnostic. Barium enema shows characteristic thumb printing changes, often most prominent in the right colon.

TYPHLITIS (ILEOCECAL ULCERATION)

Ileocecal ulceration, at times called typhlitis, is a rare complication in children with neutropenia, vascular ischemia,[80] and pseudo-obstruction, and after renal transplantation.[9, 37, 167, 207]

Etiology. Vascular compromise or disorders that interfere with normal intestinal motility may result in bacterial invasion of the bowel wall and development of mucosal ulcerations. The most commonly associated organism is *Pseudomonas.* In leukemic patients, it is not certain whether the lesion is a complication of the disease itself or of impaired immune responses. Other hematologic disorders with which it has been reported are aplastic anemia, thalassemia, and cyclic neutropenia, in which symptoms recur at three to four week intervals as a result of a periodic failure of myeloid maturation.

Pathology. There is particular involvement of the distal ileum, cecum, appendix, and right colon, with resultant ulceration, local necrosis, and peritonitis.

Symptoms. The usual symptoms are abdominal distention and pain, fever, diarrhea, or vomiting. The right lower quadrant is tender to palpation, and the bowel sounds are decreased or absent. A right lower quadrant mass may be palpated if there is an appendiceal abscess, but if there is free perforation the entire abdomen is rigid. The disease cannot always be differentiated from acute appendicitis.

Diagnosis. Plain films of the abdomen show an absence of bowel gas in the right lower quadrant and some distention of the distal small bowel. Later, a soft tissue mass is evident and small bowel loops are dilated. Barium enema shows a rigid, irregular cecum that has no haustrae. Fistulas may be evident.

Treatment. Surgical resection of the diseased area or loop colostomy is helpful in patients who are in remission. When the syndrome develops in leukemic patients in hematologic relapse, it is usually a fatal terminal complication.

One child with cyclic neutropenia transiently corrected the maturation defect of his neutrophils after infusion of plasma from donors whose granulocyte maturation was stimulated by typhoid vaccine. In a few instances, lithium has been helpful in treating the neutropenia.

COLITIS CYSTICA PROFUNDA

This benign disease is important because its diagnosis is elusive and it carries a high morbidity.

Incidence. Fewer than 50 cases have been reported in the literature.[42]

Etiology. The etiology is unknown, but some consider these lesions to be of congenital or hamartomatous origin. Others believe them to be secondary to mucosal ulceration and destruction of the muscularis. The multiplicity of the lesions and their disappearance after diversion of the fecal flow support an inflammatory origin.

Pathology. The disease occurs in one of three forms. In the first and most common type, there is either a single polypoid lesion or several plaque-like areas localized in the anterior wall of the rectum between 5 and 12 cm from the anal verge. These are sometimes accompanied by submucosal cysts. The second type is localized to one segment of the colon, most often the rectosigmoid, and rarely in the transverse and descending colon. Affected segments contain multiple polypoid or cystic lesions. In the third, or diffuse, type, submucosal cysts are scattered throughout the colon but congregate predominantly in the rectosigmoid. Some of these cases are associated with dysentery or ulcerative colitis, and there are sessile and pedunculated polyps. Histologically, there is a downgrowth of mucous glands into the submucosa. In the localized forms there is interspersion of irregular distorted glands among normal glands, fibrosis, and polymorphonuclear and plasma cell infiltration of the lamina propria. The gland openings are wide and the mucosa is ulcerated or denuded. Some of the cysts become completely filled with mucus and contain no epithelial cells. Despite their extension into the submucosa there is no evidence of malignant change.

Symptoms. The onset is usually in adult life, although a four-year-old child with the disease has been reported. In those with diffuse disease, the symptoms are most often related to associated ulcerative colitis or dysentery. Those with more localized disease have rectal bleeding, rectal prolapse, diarrhea, mucus in the stools, abdominal pain, tenesmus, and weight loss.

Diagnosis. A rectal mass or polyp is palpated during the rectal examination. Sigmoidoscopy does not always show the lesion, or the lesions are misinterpreted as polyp, ulcer, or plaque-like lesion of nonspecific etiology. Barium enema is either negative or shows segmental changes resembling those of colitis.

Treatment. Local excision or resection of the affected segment has been the accepted treatment, but a recent report suggests that a diverting colostomy is followed by regression of the lesions.

COLITIS CYSTICA SUPERFICIALIS

This lesion is mentioned only briefly for it appears in association with pellagra as small superficial cysts in the colon that disappear after treatment of the primary vitamin deficiency.[208]

PNEUMATOSIS CYSTOIDES INTESTINALIS

These emphysematous blebs involving the small bowel or colon are discussed in detail in Chapter 16.[122]

BEHÇET'S DISEASE

Behçet's disease, as originally described, was limited to the triad of ocular inflammation and recurrent oral and genital aphthous ulcerations. These diagnostic criteria have been expanded to include arthritis, colitis, thrombophlebitis, encephalopathy, pancreatitis, peripheral neuropathy, subungual infarctions, and malignant lymphoma.[50, 137]

Incidence. The disease is still considered extremely rare in children.

Etiology. The cause is unknown. Viral and bacterial studies have proved controversial. Five patients have had anticytoplasmic antibodies, and a viral origin is likely.[14]

Symptoms. The usual age of onset is adulthood, but our patient, aged 5, had symptoms at age two years, when superficial ulcerations developed on her tongue and buccal mucosa. A diagnosis of aphthous stomatitis was made, and the ulcers disappeared after four weeks. She was well for three months, and then the ulcerations recurred, this time accompanied by similar lesions in the vagina and about the anus. Recurrences every three to four months were treated with local anesthetic ointments and warm soaks. At five years, there were wedge-shaped grooves in the tongue edges and ulcerations throughout the mouth and perianal region. Changes consistent with colitis developed.

Diagnosis. The diagnosis is primarily clinical. Biopsy specimen of the mucocutaneous lesions shows a nonspecific vasculitis. Early sigmoidoscopy is normal, as is the barium enema. Laboratory studies are usually normal. Our patient had an elevated IgG level. Later, sigmoidoscopy and biopsy specimen resemble ulcerative colitis.[173]

Treatment. Steroids taken systemically sometimes decrease the number of lesions and the pain, but they have not prevented the development of neurologic signs nor uveitis. Improvement followed blood transfusions in two of three patients reported by O'Duffy et al.[141]

Prognosis. The disease is chronic and relapsing. A few patients experience complete remission, but in others encephalitis or colitis may be fatal. Obstruction of the inferior vena cava has been reported.[95]

MALAKOPLAKIA OF THE COLON

This granulomatous disease involves the urinary tract most often but in the past ten years has been reported in the colon as well.[69]

Incidence. Fifteen cases have been reported in the world literature.[94]

Etiology. Viral, bacterial, tubercular, sarcoid, and neoplastic origins have been suggested, but most evidence favors a type of inflammatory process. Electron microscopy has recently shown bacilliform organisms within the macrophages infiltrating the gastrointestinal tract. It is suggested that susceptible patients have an altered immune mechanism.

Pathology. The lesions are sessile polypoid masses 0.3 to 0.4 cm in diameter and usually involve the descending colon, sigmoid, and rectum. They contain normal glandular epithelium but show a dense submucosal infiltration of histiocytes with PAS-positive granular cytoplasm and round or oval laminated Michaelis-Gutmann bodies with a dark center and peripheral halo.[115, 196] The glycolipids of the inclusions are mucopolysaccharide and of bacterial origin. All layers of the bowel are infiltrated by the malakoplakic cells. Bacteria of bacilliform structure lie within these cells.

Symptoms. A number of patients with this disease have had tuberculosis, sarcoidosis, or neoplasm. In the few children reported, symptoms began in early infancy or childhood and became progressively more severe with each recurrence. Episodes of rectal bleeding, recurrent abdominal pain, and anemia were eventually associated with weight loss and edema. Physical examination shows only some tenderness over the descending colon.

Diagnosis. Sigmoidoscopic examination shows sessile polypoid masses throughout the mucosa, and the barium enema shows small polypoid lesions extending through the rectum and sigmoid. These cannot be differentiated from multiple polyposis or granulomatous bowel disease. The diagnosis is confirmed by the biopsy finding of submucosal histiocytic infiltrate and Michaelis-Gutmann bodies. Electron microscopy shows bacteria within the histiocytes.

Treatment. Treatment with broad-spectrum antibiotics has given variable results, but resection of the involved areas of colon and rectum is followed by symptomatic cure.

COLONIC DISEASE AFTER RENAL TRANSPLANTATION

As renal transplantation is performed more and more frequently and with greater success, complications involving other organ systems are being recognized. Colonic disease is reflected in an ischemic type of colitis.

Etiology. It is likely that impaired splanchnic blood flow on the basis of congestive heart failure or hypovolemia after transplant contributes to the insult. Coagulation defects or the hemolytic uremic syndrome may also be implicated, but not all the patients are uremic at the time the disease develops. Coagulase-positive *Staphylococcus aureus* has been isolated from the stools of some patients.

Symptoms. Two to five days after renal transplantation, generalized abdominal pain, fever, and bloody diarrhea develop. The abdomen is distended and the bowel sounds are hyperactive.

Diagnosis. Sigmoidoscopy shows a granular, edematous, and friable mucosa. Barium enema shows a cobblestone appearance of the colonic mucosa with maximal involvement in the descending colon.

Treatment. Treatment consists of vigorous administration of blood, treatment of infection, and correction of electrolyte abnormalities. In some cases, however, bleeding is severe enough to warrant colectomy.

Prognosis. The disease is often self-limited and subsides within several weeks. Depending upon the time of diagnosis and treatment, the mortality varies from zero to greater than 50 per cent.

RADIATION INJURY TO THE BOWEL

Radiation therapy for abdominal, pelvic, and sacral tumors can produce intestinal damage.[67, 201]

Pathogenesis and Pathology. The cause of radiation lesions is twofold: direct injury to the mucosa affecting primarily mitotic cells, and secondary vascular insufficiency from radiation-induced endarteritis.

In experimental animals, the first lesion to appear is cessation of mitoses within the small bowel crypt cells. These become vacuolated and pyknotic, and there is infiltration of the lamina propria by inflammatory cells. Early, the villous epithelial cells appear normal, but as cell replacement fails they become cuboidal and slough. Within 72 hours the villi and crypts are shortened, and the mucosa is atrophic. In the human, these changes, which are accompanied by some degree of malabsorption, return to normal after two weeks. The rectal mucosa, which is easily studied, shows a leukocytic and particularly an eosinophilic infiltration and formation of eosinophilic crypt abscesses. These changes revert to normal after one month. If damage is severe, ulceration, perforation, fistulization, and abnormal regeneration of tissue may be the end results.

Symptoms. Diarrhea typifies the acute stage of intestinal radiation damage and usually subsides when therapy ends. There is some nausea and vomiting and evidence of malabsorption. If there is significant proctitis, tenesmus and rectal bleeding become the most distressing symptoms.

Chronic changes are suggested by the persistence of diarrhea after the termination of treatment. Stricture formation is most common in the rectum or sigmoid, but the strictures usually do not cause obstruction until several years later.

Physical examination reveals the skin changes from irradiation and lower abdominal tenderness. Sigmoidoscopy shows an ulcerated, friable mucosa.

Treatment. The treatment of acute diarrhea is symptomatic, with restriction of fiber in the diet and use of Lomotil or codeine. Antiprostaglandin agents such as salicylate or Imodium provide good symptomatic relief. Late, chronic diarrhea due to stricture often requires resection of involved areas.

CHAGAS' DISEASE

Endemic in South America, Chagas' disease is caused by *Trypanosoma cruzi*, which is transmitted through the bite of the reduviid bug. By the time megacolon has developed it is no longer considered infectious.[41, 213]

Incidence. The disease is most prevalent in Brazil, where an estimated 4 million people are affected. In some areas, up to 25 per cent of the population have a positive complement-fixation test. The disease is not found in Europe, Africa, or Asia and has been reported in only rare instances in North America. Males are affected more often than are females.

Transmission. The infected bug, which lives in the walls or roofs of native huts, bites a small infant, usually on the face, and leaves infected feces near the area. The wound is contaminated as the infant rubs the bite, and this causes a unilateral orbital swelling, Romaña's sign. Neonatal infection is acquired either transplacentally or through the mother's milk.[17]

Pathology. The parasites multiply within the cells of the wound in the manner of leishmania.[55, 104] They liberate a second generation into the blood in eight to ten days. This larger, flagellated form invades smooth and cardiac muscle, the ganglion cells of Auerbach's and Meissner's plexuses, spinal cord, brain, and the sympathetic nervous system. These organisms multiply by binary fission and in three to four days form pseudocysts that rupture to liberate more flagellated forms. In this acute phase, the intestinal smooth muscle and cardiac muscle are primarily affected, with waxy degeneration of muscle cells, lymphocytic infiltration, and granuloma formation with giant cells. In the arteries there is hyaline degeneration and necrosis in both the media and the intima. Chronic megacolon eventually develops after 50 per cent of the ganglion cells have been lost. The entire colon can be involved, but the sigmoid is most often, and the rectum least often, affected.

Symptoms. Local irritation occurs at the site of the bite, accompanied by regional lymphadenopathy. Most infants become febrile, anorectic, and lethargic, but some older children complain only of myalgia. This phase is often self-limited and subsides after several weeks. In some infants it progresses further to generalized edema and hepatosplenomegaly or even to death from meningoencephalitis or myocarditis. The chronic phase develops over the next few years — even as late as 40 years — with cardiac lesions, swelling of the sublingual and submaxillary glands, megacolon, mega-esophagus, megastomach, megaduoden-um, or even megajejunum. Megacolon is the most frequent complication, and the symptoms resemble those of Hirschsprung's disease.

Diagnosis. This disease is to be suspected in any patient with megacolon or meg-aesophagus who has lived in an endemic area. Antibody production begins within the first few weeks of infection, and the precipitation test is positive only during the first few weeks of the disease. A complement-fixation test, the Machado-Guerreiro test, becomes positive later and remains so for the rest of the patient's life.

Complications. The complications of megacolon are large bowel obstruction from fecal retention and sigmoid volvulus.

Treatment. Proctosigmoidectomy is the recommended treatment for this type of megacolon.

Prognosis. The mortality in the acute stage of the disease is between 6 and 10 per cent.

PERIRECTAL ABSCESS

This type of abscess often follows infection of deep perianal fissures or peritonitis.

Incidence. The incidence is not known, although series of 28 and 29 patients have been reported. There is a male predominance of 79 to 90 per cent. The majority of patients are neonates or infants.[108]

Etiology. In 25 per cent of the patients a primary serious illness with immune deficiency and neutropenia occurs. It is felt that diarrheal or hard stools injure the anal canal and promote bacterial invasion, with obstruction of the anal glands. Abscess develops, which may extend through the rectal sphincter to the anus to form fistula-in-ano (18 per cent) or through the musculature of the perirectal sling to form an ischiorectal abscess (17 per cent). In 83 per cent of patients, the abscess is perirectal, which

may be associated with scrotal or gluteal cellulitis. In 75 per cent of patients, only one organism is isolated, with *Staphylococcus aureus* predominating and *Escherichia coli* next. Abscess contents rarely yield *Actinomyces.*

Symptoms. More than half the infants are febrile with leukocytosis and nearly half have pain on defecation or pelvic pain as well as a palpable tender mass noted on rectal examination. The mass seems to be adjacent to the rectum and is fluctuant.

Diagnosis. Barium enema shows an extrinsic pressure defect in the rectum (Fig. 17–23).

Treatment. Some abscesses rupture spontaneously through the rectum: otherwise, surgical incision and drainage are necessary along with antibiotic therapy. Warm soaks provide symptomatic relief and help keep the incision patent and draining.

Prognosis. Complications occur in 42 per cent of patients as fistula-in-ano or recurrent abscesses. In one leukemic patient, gangrene of the anus developed.

RECTAL PERFORATION

Rectal perforation may result from thermometers and presents similar signs and symptoms.[60]

RECTAL PROLAPSE

Prolapse is the abnormal protrusion of tissue that is usually located internally.[84]

Etiology. In infants and young children, the rectal mucosa is redundant and only loosely attached to the muscularis mucosa. The frequent occurrence of prolapse in children under three years of age is related to certain anatomic characteristics: a flat sacrococcygeal curve and nearly vertical rectal axis, a cylindric pelvis, relatively low position of the rectum and Douglas fold, mobility of the sigmoid, and underdeveloped pelvic musculature. During normal growth the pelvis tips, the sacrococcygeal region curves, and the pelvic muscles increase in strength.

During the early period of anatomic sus-

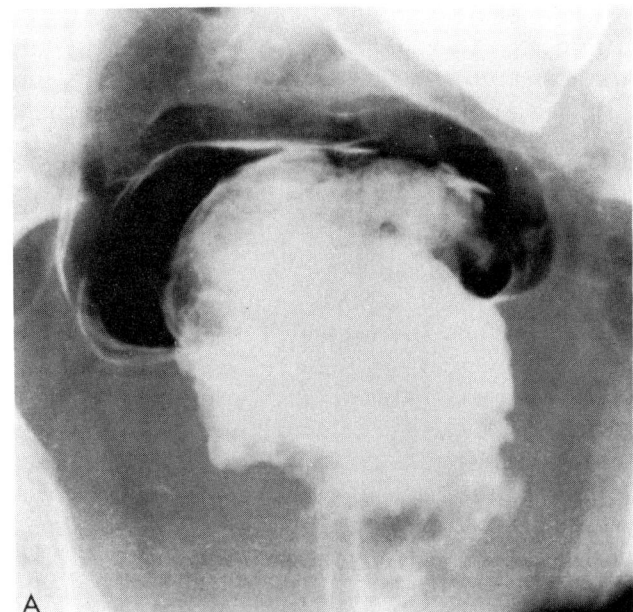

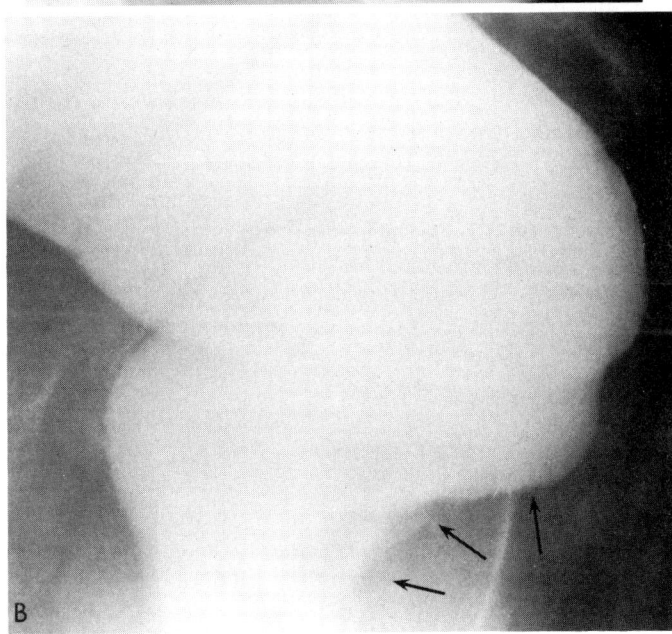

Figure 17–23 Barium enema in a child with pain on defecation and a palpable mass felt during rectal examination. *A*, There is upward and lateral compression on the rectum. *B*, The same extrinsic compression is evident in the lateral views (arrows).

ceptibility to prolapse, a number of factors cause rectal descent, including increased intra-abdominal pressure from coughing, vomiting, or straining and loss of ischiorectal fat from malnutrition. Cystic fibrosis is considered the most common cause of rectal prolapse in children, which reflects not only malnutrition but also the passage of large, bulky stools. Rectal prolapse is a complication of some parasitic infections, such as trichuriasis, and bacterial diarrheas that cause tenesmus, such as shigellosis. Patients with meningomyelocele who have paralysis of the levator or sphincter muscles are prone to rectal prolapse.

Pathology. If the prolapse involves only mucosa, it is termed incomplete; if it involves all the layers of bowel wall, it is termed complete or procidentia.

Symptoms. Rectal prolapse is first noted as the infant defecates and usually reduces itself. However, it tends to recur, and eventually it remains extruded. Rarely, it becomes incarcerated and strangulated. The prolapse measures several centimeters, and its original pink mucosa becomes dark red or violet as it is compressed by the anal sphincter. The smooth mucous surface dries and becomes friable. Blood and mucus pass freely through the prolapse.

Treatment. If the prolapse does not reduce itself, gentle insertion of a lubricated gloved finger into the lumen of the mass usually will reduce it. In some cases, strapping the buttocks between defecations is necessary to maintain reduction. Some recommend the injection of sclerosing agents into the rectal area of prolapse after it is reduced, to prevent recurrence.[97] This seems rather vigorous treatment for a self-limited disorder. The primary treatment of constipation or of the causes of diarrhea and malnutrition that produce the prolapse seems more logical. In the very rare intractable case, excision of the redundant mucosa is indicated. If there is an associated neurologic disorder or paralysis of the levator or sphincter muscles, sigmoidopexy and transabdominal repair may be required to prevent recurrence of the prolapse.

Prognosis. Usually rectal prolapse is no longer a problem after the child reaches the age of three years.

FISSURE-IN-ANO

Fissure-in-ano, the most common cause of rectal bleeding in infants, represents a tear in the anus that extends into the mucocutaneous junction.

Incidence. The lesion is familiar to every pediatrician.[7]

Etiology. This type of fissure most often follows the passage of a hard, sharp, or bulky stool. It sometimes develops after explosive diarrhea. In many babies, however, no cause for the fissure is found.

Pathology. The edges of a fresh fissure are clean and sharp, but if the fissure becomes chronic the edges thicken, become undermined, and tend to pucker. In the young infant the fissures are often multiple and located laterally. In the older infant or child, because of an increased sacrococ-

cygeal curve and increased levator ani muscle pull, the tear is usually posterior.

Symptoms. The onset occurs at any time during infancy and as early as the first day of life. Typically there is blood streaking of the stool or blood in the diaper of an otherwise healthy baby. The blood is bright red and small in amount. Significant bleeding is rare, but it can occur. The baby cries or is uncomfortable before or during defecation.

Examination of the anus will show a small slit in the anal tissue or the "sentinel pile," a tag of edematous skin.

Diagnosis. If the diagnosis is not confirmed by external examination of the anus, the fissure will be visualized through an anoscope.

Treatment. The acute fissure heals quickly with careful cleansing of the anus after defecation. Softening of the stool by increasing the sugar content of the formula or, in some cases, by the addition of mineral oil is indicated. Anal pain and the withholding of stool secondary to it are alleviated by the local application to the fissure of an anesthetic ointment. Fissures that become chronic are treated by cauterization with silver nitrate or by anal dilations.

ANORECTAL ABSCESS

Anorectal or perianal abscesses are not unusual in infancy, but they are particularly significant for nearly half will progress to form a fistula-in-ano.

Etiology. These lesions result from infection of the anal crypts or are the result of a scratch or pinprick that becomes infected.

Pathology. There is redness, heat, and swelling over the perianal region or in the ischiorectal fossa. If the inflammatory process is in the anal ducts that empty into the crypts of Morgagni, the infection spreads into the perianal and perirectal tissue. The lesion, at first firm, later becomes fluctuant. Suppuration eventually leads to the establishment of fistulas from the perianal region into the anus or rectum.

Symptoms. The infant becomes irritable and cries during defecation and may or may not be febrile. Examination of the anus reveals a tender, swollen area near the anus.

Treatment. Warm soaks to the area provide symptomatic relief and localize the abscess. Fluctuation develops late, and the treatment is early incision and drainage. Soaking is continued postoperatively until healing takes place.

FISTULA-IN-ANO

Fistulas in the perianal region are often associated with congenital anomalies of the anorectal canal, but most result from perianal abscess.

Incidence. We have seen only three isolated perianal fistulas over the last ten years in our clinic.

Etiology. The fistula-in-ano is an abnormal connection between the anorectal canal and the perianal skin. In one of our patients the fistula was directly related to the diarrhea of milk protein allergy. It remained closed and silent as long as milk was restricted from the diet and the stools were formed, but it became red and swollen and drained purulent material when the baby took milk products and had an exacérbation of diarrhea.

Symptoms. The diagnosis is made only after the rupture of an apparent perianal boil. Rather than healing after several days of drainage, the lesion continues to drain purulent or fecal material for weeks to months. If the fistulous tract becomes obstructed, there are swelling, redness, and warmth underlying its opening.

Diagnosis. The perianal opening permits passage of a probe into the involved anal crypt or even into the rectum. Radiologic examination of the colon with barium or retrograde injection of dye into the fistula will show the communicating tract.

Treatment. In a few cases the tract will remain closed after drainage and constant cleansing of the area. Complete excision of the fistula or its marsupialization with closure from below is eventually required for cure. Localization of the tract in relation to the anal sphincters is imperative if excision is undertaken.

TUMORS OF THE COLON

Benign Tumors

Polypoid lesions of the colon such as polyps, hemangiomas, lymphoid polyps, and lymphoid hyperplasia are discussed in detail in Chapter 7.

Lipoma and leiomyoma have not been reported in infants and indeed are rare throughout childhood. One benign fibrous hamartoma in the perianal region presented as an enlarging mass.[5] Congenital megaileocolon has been described in association with teratoma.

Malignant Tumors

Colonic sarcoma has been reported in two neonates with small bowel obstruction due to intussusception in one case and perforation in the other.[47] Villous adenoma, although reported in adolescents, has not been described in infants. Villous adenoma is extremely rare.[169]

Carcinoma of the Colon

Colonic carcinoma is also extremely rare in children. When it does occur, it develops predominantly in older children with familial polyposis, ulcerative colitis, or the familial cancer syndrome[2, 38, 134] However, adenocarcinoma has been found in a patient following treatment of Wilms' tumor[156] and has been reported in a nine-month-old infant.[98]

Incidence. Fewer than 200 cases have been reported in children and more than half were in boys.

Pathology. The distribution of the tumor is similar to that in the adult, with half the lesions in the descending and sigmoid colon, 13 per cent in the transverse colon, and 37 per cent in the ascending colon or cecum. The majority are colloid and mucin-producing adenocarcinomas that are extremely malignant and grow rapidly to infiltrate the bowel and metastasize widely throughout the abdomen, even to the ovary. They appear as either polypoid or constricting lesions.

Symptoms. Abdominal pain, accompanied by or followed by changes in bowel habits, is the most frequent complaint. Half the patients vomit; a quarter are constipated; one fifth have weight loss and blood in the stools; and only 8 per cent have diarrhea. The youngest patient described in the literature was a 9-month-old infant whose tumor involved both transverse and descending colon. A few patients had symptoms resembling those of appendicitis: fever, right lower quadrant pain, and tenderness. A mass is palpable in only 5 per cent of patients.

Certain symptoms differentiate lesions of the right and left colon. The right colon is distensible and fluid filled, and therefore its lesions cause anemia or diarrhea rather than obstruction. Lesions of the left colon, which contain firm stool, tend to ulcerate, bleed, and obstruct.

Diagnosis. Rectal and low sigmoid carcinomas are usually seen through the sigmoidoscope. Barium enema will show polypoid or constricting lesions in the colon. Early lesions are not always well demonstrated in the colon when carcinoma is associated with familial polyposis or with long-standing ulcerative colits and pseudopolyposis. Colonoscopy is being used more frequently for the visualization of suspicious lesions, and the diagnosis is confirmed by biopsy.

Treatment. The lesion must be resected whenever possible. 5-Fluorouracil has been used successfully in some children; it acts by blocking the cellular synthesis of DNA and perhaps of RNA. The drug is given in a dosage of 5 to 10 mg per kg for five days and in some cases continued as weekly injections. A second-look operation six months later may permit removal of residual tumor.

Prognosis. Most children are dead one year after the diagnosis of carcinoma of the colon is made, but now, with combined surgery and chemotherapy, there are a few survivors at 38 months.

REFERENCES

1. Aaranson, I.: Anterior sacral meningocele, anal canal duplication cyst and covered anus occurring in one family. J. Pediatr. Surg., 5:559, 1970.
2. Aegis, H., Kahn, E., Silverberg, M., and Daum, F.: Adenocarcinoma of the colon in an adolescent with the familial cancer syndrome. J. Pediatr. 94:632, 1979.
3. Ahmed, S., Cohen, S. J., and Jacobs, S. I.: Total intestinal aganglionosis presenting as duodenal obstruction. Arch. Dis. Child. 46:868, 1971.
4. Ajayi, O. O., Solanke, T. F., Seriki, O., and Bohrer, S.: Hirschsprung's disease in the neonate presenting as cecal perforation. Pediatrics 43:102, 1969.
5. Albukerk, J., Dana, M., and Silverman, J.: A case of fibrous hamartoma of infancy. J. Pediatr. Surg. 14:80, 1980.
6. Andrassy, R. J., Isaacs, H., and Weitzman, J. J.: Rectal suction biopsy for the diagnosis of Hirschsprung's disease. Ann. Surg. 193:419, 1981.
7. Arminski, T. C., and McLean, D. W.: Proctologic problems in infants. JAMA 194:1195, 1965.
8. Arnold, G., and Nance, F. C.: Volvulus of the sigmoid colon. Ann. Surg. 117:527, 1973.
9. Arvanitakis, C., Malek, G., Uehling, D., and Morrissey, J.: Colonic complications after renal transplantation. Gastroenterology 64:533, 1973.
10. Asch, M. J., Weitzman, J. J., Hays, D. M., and Brennan, P.: Total colon aganglionosis. Arch. Surg. 105:74, 1972.
11. Ashcraft, K., and Holder, T.: Congenital megaileocolon with teratoma. J. Pediatr. Surg. 1:178, 1966.
12. Bartlett, R. H., Eraklis, A. J., and Wilkinson, R. H.: Appendicitis in infancy. Surg. Gynecol. Obstet. 13:99, 1970.
13. Bax, N. M., Pearse, R. G., Dommerung, N., and Molenaar, J. C.: Perforation of the appendix in the neonatal period. J. Pediatr. Surg. 15:300, 1980.
14. Berman, L., Trappler, B., and Jenkins, T.: Behçet's syndrome: Family study and the elucidation of a genetic role. Ann. Rheum. Dis. 118:121, 1979.
15. Bill, A. H., Jr., and Chapman, N. D.: The enterocolitis of Hirschsprung's disease. Am. J. Surg. 103:70, 1962.
16. Binder, H.: Colonic secretion. In Johnson, L. (ed.): Physiology of the Gastrointestinal Tract. New York, Raven Press, 1981, p. 1003.
17. Bittencourt, A. L.: Placental infection and congenital transmission of Chagas' disease. Rev. Inst. Med. Trop. São Paulo 5:62, 1963.
18. Boston, V. E., Cywes, S., and Davies, M.: Serum and erythrocyte acetylcholinesterase activity in Hirschsprung's disease. J. Pediatr. Surg. 13:407, 1978.
19. Bower, R., Sieber, W., and Kiesewetter, W.: Alimentary tract duplications in children. Ann. Surg. 188:689, 1978.
20. Bowes, K., and Kling, S.: Anorectal manometry in premature infants. J. Pediatr. Surg. 14:533, 1978.
21. Brook, I.: Bacterial studies of peritoneal cavity and postoperative surgical wound drainage following perforated appendix in children. Ann. Surg. 169:208, 1980.

22. Browne, D.: Some congenital deformities of the rectum, anus, vagina and urethra. Ann. Roy. Coll. Surg. Engl. 8:173, 1951.

23. Bryant, L., Trinkle, K., Noonan, J., and Nighbert, E.: Appendicitis and appendiceal perforation in neonates. Am. Surg. 36:523, 1970.

24. Bugaighis, A. G., and Lister, J.: Incidence of diabetes in families of patients with Hirschsprung's disease. J. Pediatr. Surg. 5:620, 1970.

24a. Byrne, W. J., Jiminez, J. F., Euler, A., and Golladay, E.: Lymphoid polyps (focal lymphoid hyperplasia) of the colon in children. Pediatrics 69:598, 1982.

25. Campbell, P. E., and Noblett, H. R.: Experience with rectal suction biopsy in the diagnosis of Hirschsprung's disease. J. Pediatr. Surg. 4:410, 1969.

25a. Caresky, J., Weber, T., and Grosfeld, J.: Total colonic aganglionosis: Analysis of 16 cases. Am. J. Surg. 143:160, 1982.

26. Castagna, J., and Moore, T.: Use of the appendix as a colon substitute in vesicointestinal exstrophy. J. Pediatr. Surg. 8:331, 1973.

27. Chandler, N. W., and Zwiren, G. T. : Complete reflux of the small bowel in total colon Hirschsprung's disease. Radiology 94:335, 1970.

28. Chatterjee, S. K.: Double termination of the alimentary tract — a second look. J. Pediatr. Surg. 15:623, 1980.

29. Chow, C. W., Chan, W. C., and Yue, P. C.: Histochemical criteria for the diagnosis of Hirschsprung's disease in rectal suction biopsy of acetylcholinesterase activity. J. Pediatr. Surg. 12:675, 1978.

30. Cremin, B. J., Smythe, P., and Cywes, M.: The radiologic appearance of the inspissated milk syndrome. Radiology 43:856, 1970.

31. Cuderman, B. S., Roback, S. A., Weintraub, W. H., and Leonard, A.: Volvulus of the transverse colon. Surgery 69:797, 1971.

32. Cywes, S., Cremin, B. J., and Louw, J. H.: Assessment of continence after treatment for anorectal agenesis: A clinical and radiologic correlation. J. Pediatr. Surg. 6:132, 1971.

33. Dale, G., Bonhaum, J., London, P., Waggert, J., Rangcroft, I., and Snott, D. J.: Diagnostic value of rectal mucosal acetylcholinesterase levels in Hirschsprung's disease. Lancet 1:347, 1979.

34. Davidson, M., and Bauer, C. H.: Studies of colonic motility in children. Pediatrics 21:746, 1958.

35. Davidson, M., Sleisenger, M., Almy, T. P., and Levine, S.: Studies of distal colonic motility in children. I. Non-propulsive patterns in normal children. Pediatrics 17:807, 1956.

36. Davis, W. S., Allen, R. P., Favara, B. E., and Slovis, T. L.: Neonatal small left colon syndrome. Am. J. Roentgenol. Radium Ther. Nucl. Med. 120:322, 1974.

36a. Debas, H. T., Chaun, H., Thomson, F. B., and Soon-Shiong, P.: Functioning heterotopic oxyntic mucosa in the rectum. Gastroenterology 79:1300, 1980.

37. DelFava, R. L., and Cronin, T. G.: Typhlitis complicating leukemia in an adult: Barium enema findings. Am. J. Roentgenol. 129:347, 1977.

38. Donaldson, M., Taylor, P., Rawitscher, R., and Sewell, J., Jr.: Colon carcinoma in childhood. Pediatrics 48:307, 1971.

39. Dronfield, M. W., Malone, J. D. G., and Langman, M. J.: Zinc in ulcerative colitis: A therapeutic trial and report on plasma levels. Gut 18:33, 1977.

40. Durham-Smith, E.: Duplication of the anus and genitourinary tract. Surgery 66:909, 1969.

41. Earlam, R. J.: Gastrointestinal aspects of Chagas' disease. Am. J. Dig. Dis. 17:559, 1972.

42. Ecker, J. A., Williams, R. G., and Clay, K. L.: Pneumatosis cystoides intestinalis — bullous emphysema of the intestine. Am. J. Gastroenterol. 56:125, 1971.

42a. Edwards, H., and Truelove, S. C.: The course and prognosis of ulcerative colitis. Gut 4:299, 1963.

43. Edwards, H.: Congenital diverticulum of intestine with report of case exhibiting heterotopia. Br. J. Surg. 17:7, 1930.

44. Ehrenpreis, T.: Hirschsprung's disease. Am. J. Dig. Dis. 16:1032, 1971.

45. Ehrenpreis, T., Ericcson, N. O., and Lividatis, A.: Anomalies of the urinary tract in patients with Hirschsprung's disease. Kinderheilkd. 8:89, 1970.

46. Ehrenpreis, T., Norberg, K. A., and Wirsen, C.: Sympathetic innervation of the colon in Hirschsprung's disease: A histochemical study. J. Pediatr. Surg. 3:43, 1968.

47. Ein, S., Beck, A. R., and Allen, J. E.: Colon sarcoma in the newborn. J. Pediatr. Surg. 14:455, 1979.

48. Ein, S. H., Lynch, M. J., and Stephens, C. A.: Ulcerative colitis in children under 1 year: A twenty year review. J. Pediatr. Surg. 6:264, 1971.

49. El-Shafie, M.: Congenital short intestine and cystic dilatation of the colon associated with ectopic anus. J. Pediatr. Surg. 6:76, 1971.

50. Empey, D. W.: Rectal and colonic ulcerations in Behçet's disease. Br. J. Surg. 59:173, 1972.

51. Enzer, N. B., and Hijmans, J. C.: Ulcerative colitis beginning in infancy. J. Pediatr. 63:437, 1963.

52. Erskine, J. M.: Colonic stenosis in the newborn: The possible thromboembolic etiology of intestinal stenosis and atresia. J. Pediatr. 5:321, 1970.

53. Falterman, C. G., and Richardson, C. J.: Small left colon syndrome associated with maternal ingestion of psychotropic drugs. J. Pediatr. 97:308, 1980.

54. Fekete, C. N., Ricour, C., Duhamed, J. F., Lecoultre, C., and Pellerin, D.: Enterocutaneous fistulas of the small bowel in children (25 cases). J. Pediatr. Surg. 13:1, 1978.

55. Ferriera-Santos, R., and Carrill, C. F.: Acquired megacolon in Chagas' disease. Proc. Roy. Soc. Med. 54:1047, 1961.

56. Fields, I., and Cole, N.: Acute appendicitis in infants thirty-six months of age or younger. Am. J. Surg. 113:269, 1967.

56a. Fonkalsrud, E. W.: Inflammatory bowel disease of childhood. Surg. Clin. North Am. 61:1125, 1981.

57. Fonkalsrud, E. W., and Barker, W. F.: Ulcerative colitis in infancy. Surgery 54:819, 1963.

58. Fonkalsrud, E. W., and Linde, L.: Successful

management of vesicointestinal fistula. J. Pediatr. Surg. 5:309, 1970.

59. Fonkalsrud, E. W.: Total colectomy and endorectal ileal pull-through with internal ileal reservoir for ulcerative colitis. Surg. Gynecol. Obstet. 150:1, 1980.

60. Frank, J. D., and Brown, S.: Thermometers and rectal perforations in the neonate. Arch. Dis. Child. 53:824, 1978.

61. Franklin, J. L., and Rosenberg, I. H.: Impaired folic acid absorption in inflammatory bowel disease: Effects of salicylazosulfapyridine. Gastroenterology 64:517, 1973.

62. Freeman, N. V.: Congenital atresia and stenosis of the colon. Br. J. Surg. 53:595, 1966.

63. French, R.: Aganglionosis involving the entire colon and a variable length of small bowel. Radiology 90:249, 1968.

64. Frenckner, B.: Anorectal manometry in the diagnosis of Hirschsprung's disease in infants, Acta Paediatr. Scand. 67:187, 1978.

65. Frenckner, B., and Molander. M. L.: Activity of the internal anal sphincter during the first days of life. Acta Paediatr. Scand. 69:73, 1980.

66. Gelband, H., Bonforte, R. J., and Krasna, I.: Hirschsprung's disease in a premature infant. Mt. Sinai J. Med. (N.Y.) 37:112, 1970.

67. Gelfand, M., Tepper, M., Katz, L., Binder, H., Yesner, R., and Flock, M.: Acute irradiation proctitis in man. Gastroenterology 54:401, 1968.

67a. Ginsburg, C. H., and Falchuk, Z. M.: Defective autologous mixed-lymphocyte reaction and suppressor cell generation in patients with inflammatory bowel disease. Gastroenterology 83:1, 1982.

68. Goligher, J. C., De Dombal, F. T., Watts, J. M., and Watkinson, G.: Ulcerative Colitis. Baltimore, The Williams & Wilkins Company, 1969.

69. Gonzales-Angulo, A., Corral, E., Garcia-Torres, R., and Quijano, M.: Malakoplakia of the colon. Gastroenterology 48:383, 1965.

70. Gray, A. W.: Triplication of the large intestine. Arch. Pathol. 30:1215, 1940.

71. Griggin, J. W.: Congenital megacolon (Hirschsprung's disease) associated with hypoproteinemia and edema. J. Pediatr. 59:394, 1961.

72. Grosfeld, J. L., O'Neill, J. A., Jr., and Clatworthy, H. W., Jr.: Enteric duplications in infancy and childhood: An 18 year review. Ann. Surg. 172:83, 1970.

73. Grosfeld, J. L., Weinberger, M., and Clatworthy, H. W., Jr.: Acute appendicitis in the first two years of life. J. Pediatr. Surg. 8:285, 1973.

74. Gryboski, J. D.: Diseases of the colon. In Gryboski, J. D.: Gastrointestinal Problems in the Infant. Philadelphia, W. B. Saunders Company, 1975.

75. Gryboski, J. D., Spiro, H. M., and Gelfand, M.: The anal sphincter in fecal incontinence. Pediatrics 41:750, 1968.

76. Gryboski, J. D., and Hillemeier, A. C.: Inflammatory bowel disease in children. Med. Clin. North Am. 64:1185, 1980.

77. Haffner, J. F., and Shistad, G.: Atresia of the colon combined with Hirschsprung's disease. J.

Pediatr. Surg. 5:560, 1969.

78. Hakehus, L., Gierup, J., Grotte, G., and Jorulf, H.: A new treatment of anal incontinence in children: Free autogenous muscle transplantation. J. Pediatr. Surg. 13:77, 1978.

79. Haller, J. A., Shaker, I. J., Donahoo, J. S., Schnaufer, L., and White, J.: Peritoneal drainage versus nondrainage for generalized peritonitis from ruptured appendicitis in children. Ann. Surg. 117:595, 1973.

80. Hargrove, M. C., Rosato, E. F., Hicks, R. E., and Mullen, J. L.: Cecal necrosis after open-heart operation. Ann. Thorac. Surg. 25:71, 1978.

80a. Helikson, M. A., Schapiro, M., Garfinkel, D., and Shermeta, D. W.: Congenital segmental dilatation of the colon. J. Pediatr. Surg. 17:201, 1982.

81. Hen, J., Dolan, T., and Touloukian, R.: Meconium plug syndrome associated with cystic fibrosis and Hirschsprung's disease. Pediatrics 66:466, 1980.

81a. Hendren, W. H.: Constipation caused by anterior location of the anus and its surgical correction. J. Pediatr. Surg. 13:505, 1978.

82. Hendren, W. H.: Urogenital sinus and anorectal malformation. J. Pediatr. Surg. 15:628, 1980.

83. Herman, R. E., Izant, R. J., Jr., and Bolande, R. P.: Aganglionosis of the intestine in siblings. Surgery 53:664, 1963.

84. Herzog, B.: Rectal prolapse in childhood. Helv. Chir. Acta 37:575, 1970.

85. Holgersen, L. O., and Stanley-Brown, E.: Acute appendicitis with perforation. Am. J. Dis. Child. 122:288, 1971.

86. Holowach, J., and Thurston, D. L.: Chronic ulcerative colitis in children. Pediatrics 48:279, 1956.

86a. Holschneider, A. M., Kellner, E., Streible, P., and Sippel, W. G.: Anorectal motility in infants. J. Pediatr. Surg. 11:151, 1976.

86b. Huntley, C., Schaffner, F., Challa, V., and Lyerly, A.: Histochemical diagnosis of Hirschsprung's disease. Pediatrics 69:755, 1982.

87. Hyde, G. A., Jr., and De Lorimier, A. A.: Colon atresia and Hirschsprung's disease. Surgery 64:976, 1968.

88. Ikawa, H., Yokoyama, J., Morikawa, Y., Hayashi, A., and Katsumata, K. A.: A quantitative study of acetylcholine in Hirschsprung's disease. J. Pediatr. Surg. 15:48, 1980.

89. Iwai, N., Ogita, S., Kida, M., Fufita, Y., and Majima, S.: A clinical and manometric correlation for assessment of postoperative continence in imperforate anus. J. Pediatr. Surg. 14:538, 1979.

90. James, A. E., Jr., Greenfield, J. B., Pfister, R. C., Weber, A. L., Hendren, W. J., and Neuhauser, E. B.: The roentgenologic appearance of post-operative congenital megacolon. Am. J. Roentgenol. 109:351, 1970.

91. Jewell, C. T., Miller, I. D., and Ehrlich, F.: Rectal duplication: An unusual cause for an abdominal mass. Surgery 74:783, 1973.

92. Jordan, F., Coran, A., Weintraub, W., and Wesley, J.: An elevation of the modified endorectal procedure for Hirschsprung's disease. J. Pediatr. Surg. 14:681, 1979.

93. Jordan, F., Coran, A., and Wesley, J.: Modified endorectal procedure for management of a long-segment aganglionosis. Ann. Surg. 194:70, 1981.

94. Joyeuse, R., Lott, J., Michaelis, M., and Gumucio, C. C.: Malakoplakia of the colon and rectum. Surgery 81:189, 1977.

95. Kansu, E., Ozer, F., Akalin, E., Guler, Y., Zileli, T., Tamman, E., Kaplaman, E., and Muftugoglu, E.: Behçet's syndrome with obstruction of the inferior vena cava. Q.J. Med. 41:162, 1972.

96. Kasai, M., Suzuki, H., and Watanabe, K.: Rectal myotomy with colectomy: A new radical operation for Hirschsprung's disease. J. Pediatr. Surg. 6:36, 1971.

97. Kay, N. R. M., and Zachary, R. B.: The treatment of rectal prolapse in children with injections of 30 per cent saline solutions. J. Pediatr. Surg. 5:334, 1970.

98. Kern, N., and White, W. C.: Adenocarcinoma of the colon in a 9 month old infant. Cancer 11:855, 1958.

99. Kiesewetter, W. B., and Nixon, H. H.: Imperforate anus. I. Its surgical anatomy. J. Pediatr. Surg. 2:60, 1967.

100. Kiesewetter, W. B., and Turner, R. C.: Continence after surgery for imperforate anus: A critical analysis and preliminary experience with the sacroperineal pull-through. Ann. Surg. 158:498, 1963.

101. Kiesewetter, W. B., Turner, C. R., and Sieber, W. K.: Imperforate anus: A review of a sixteen year experience with 146 cases. Am. J. Surg. 107:412, 1964.

102. Kim, I. C., and Barbero, G. J.: The pattern of rectosigmoid motility in children. Gastroenterology 45:57, 1963.

103. King, R. C., Lindler, A. E., and Pollard, H. M.: Chronic ulcerative colitis in childhood. Arch. Dis. Child. 34:257, 1959.

104. Koeberle, F.: Chagas' disease and Chagas' syndrome: The pathology of American trypanosomiasis. Adv. Parasitol. 6:63, 1968.

105. Kopel, F. B., Kim, I. C., and Barbero, G. J.: Comparison of rectosigmoid motility in normal children, children with recurrent abdominal pain and children with ulcerative colitis. Pediatrics 39:539, 1967.

106. Kottmeier, P. K., and Dziadiw, R.: The complete release of the levator ani sling in fecal incontinence. J. Pediatr. Surg. 2:111, 1967.

107. Kottra, J. J., and Dodds, W. J.: Duplications of the large bowel. Am. J. Roentgenol. Radium Ther. Nucl. Med. 113:310, 1971.

107a. Kraft, S.: Inflammatory bowel disease. In Immunology of the Gastrointestinal Tract. New York, Churchill Livingstone, 1979, pp. 95–116.

108. Kreiger, R., and Chiesid, M.: Perirectal abscess in childhood. Am. J. Dis. Child. 133:411, 1979.

109. Kurnit, D. M., Steele, M. W., and Pinsky, L.: Autosomal dominant transmission of a syndrome of anal, ear, renal and radial congenital malformations. J. Pediatr. 93:270, 1978.

110. Ladd, W. E., and Gross, R. E.: Congenital malformations of anus and rectum: Report of 162 cases. Am. J. Surg. 23:167, 1935.

111. Lawson, J. O., and Nixon, H. H.: Anal canal pressures in diagnosis of Hirschsprung's disease. J. Pediatr. Surg. 2:544, 1967.

111a. Leape, L., and Ramenofsky, M.: Anterior ectopic anus: A common cause of constipation in children. J. Pediatr. Surg. 23:627, 1978.

111b. LaChadarévian, J., Slim, M., and Akel, S.: Double zonal aganglionosis in long segment Hirschsprung's disease with a "skip area" in transverse colon. J. Pediatr. Surg. 17:195, 1982.

112. Leenders, E., Sieber, W. K., and Kiesewetter, W. B.: Hirschsprung's disease. Surg. Clin. North Am., 50:907, 1970.

113. Leonidas, J. C., Krasna, L., Strauss, L., Becker, J. M., and Schneider, K. M.: Roentgen appearance of the excluded colon after colectomy for infantile Hirschsprung's disease. Am. J. Roentgenol. Radium Ther. Nucl. Med. 112:116, 1971.

114. Lewin, G., Mikity, V., and Winger, W.: Barium enema: An outpatient procedure in the early diagnosis of acute appendicitis. J. Pediatr. 92:451, 1978.

115. Lewin, K., Harell, G., Lee, A., and Crowley, L.: Malakoplakia. An electron microscopic study. Gastroenterology 66:28, 1974.

116. Lister, J.: The control of fluid loss in long segment Hirschsprung's disease. J. Pediatr. Surg. 4:657, 1969.

117. Longino, L. A., Holder, T. M., and Gross, R. E.: Appendicitis in childhood. A study of 1358 cases. Pediatrics 22:238, 1958.

118. Louw, J. H.: Investigations into the etiology of congenital atresia of the colon. Dis. Colon Rectum 7:471, 1964.

119. Louw, J. H., Cywes, S., and Crenin, B. J.: The management of anorectal agenesis. Proc. Pediatr. Surg. Cong. Melbourne. 1:13, 1970.

120. Luycky, A. S., Massi-Benedetti, R., Falorni, F., and Lefebvre, P. J.: Presence of pancreatic glucagon in the portal plasma of human neonates. Diabetologia 8:296, 1972.

120a. MacDermott, R. P., Nash, G. S., Bertovich, M. J., Seiden, M. V., Bragdon, M. J., and Beale, M. G.: Alterations in IgM, IgG and IgA synthesis and secretion by peripheral blood and intestinal mononuclear cells from patients with ulcerative colitis. Gastroenterology 81:844, 1981.

121. MacIver, A. G., and Whitehead, R.: Zonal colonic aganglionosis: Variant of Hirschsprung's disease. Arch. Dis. Child. 47:233, 1972.

122. MacKenzie, E. P.: Pneumatosis intestinalis: Review of the literature and report of 13 cases. Pediatrics 7:537, 1951.

123. Mackinnon, A. E., and Cohen, S. J.: Total intestinal aganglionosis: An autosomal recessive condition? Arch. Dis. Child. 52:898, 1977.

124. Malangon, M. A.: Congenital rectal stenosis: A sign of a presacral condition. Pediatrics 62:584, 1978.

125. Marchildon, M., and Dudgeon, D.: Perforated appendicitis. Ann. Surg. 185:84, 1977.

126. Martin, J. D., and Ward, C. S.: Megacolon associated with volvulus of the transverse colon. Am. J. Surg. 64:412, 1965.

127. Martin, L., Buchino, J., Coultre, C., Ballard, E., and Neblett, W.: Hirschsprung's disease

with skip area. J. Pediatr. Surg. *14*:686, 1979.

128. Massot, P., and Lane, J. L.: Volvulus du colon transverse chez l'infant. Ann. Chir. Infant. *6*:145, 1965.

129. McGill, C., Polk, H., and Canty, T.: The clinical basis for a simplified classification of anorectal agenesis. Surg. Gynecol. Obstet. *146*:177, 1978.

129a. McLaren, L., and Gitnick, G.: Ulcerative colitis and Crohn's disease tissue cytotoxins. Gastroenterology 82:1381, 1982.

130. McGovern, B.: Occult perineal fistula in male infants with imperforate anus. Am. J. Dis. Child. *123*:26, 1972.

131. McPherson, A. G., Trapnell, J. E., and Airth, G. R.: Duplications of the colon. Br. J. Surg. *56*:138, 1969.

132. Mellish, R. W. P., and Koop, C. E.: Clinical manifestations of duplications of the bowel. Pediatrics 27:397, 1961.

133. Meunier, P., Marechal, J., and Mollard, P.: Accuracy of the manometric diagnosis of Hirschsprung's disease. J. Pediatr. Surg. *13*:411, 1980.

133a. Meunier, R., Marechal, J. M., and De Beaujeau, M. J.: Rectoanal pressures and rectal sensitivity studies in chronic childhood constipation. Gastroenterology 77:330, 1979.

134. Middelkamp, J. N., and Haffner, H.: Carcinoma of the colon in children. Pediatrics *32*:558, 1963.

135. Mishlanay, H.: Unusually competent ileo-cecal valve. J. Pediatr. Surg. 6:777, 1971.

135a. Morain, C. O., Prestage, H., Harrison, P., Levi, A., and Tyrrel, D.: Cytopathic effects in cultures inoculated with material from Crohn's disease. Gut 22:823, 1981.

136. Munakata, K., Okabe, I., and Morita, K.: Histologic studies of rectocolic aganglionosis and allied diseases. J. Pediatr. Surg. *13*:67, 1978.

137. Mundy, T. M., and Miller, J. J., III: Behçet's disease presenting as chronic aphthous stomatitis in a child. Pediatrics 62:205, 1978.

138. Nagasaki, A., Ikeda, K., and Suita, S.: Postoperative sequential anorectal manometric study of children with Hirschsprung's disease. J. Pediatr. Surg. *15*:615, 1980.

139. Nezelof, C., Guy-Grand, D., and Thomine, E.: Les megacolons avec hyperplasie des plexus myenteriques. Presse Med. 78:1501, 1970.

140. Nissan, S., and Bar-Maor, J. A.: Changing trends in presentation and management of Hirschsprung's disease. J. Pediatr. Surg. 6:10, 1971.

141. O'Duffy, J. D., Carney, J. A., and Doedhar, S.: Behçet's disease. Ann. Intern. Med. 75:561, 1971.

142. Oeconomopoulos, C. T., and Swenson, O.: Duplications of the gastrointestinal tract. J. Pediatr. *60*:361, 1962.

143. Okamoto, E., Iwasaki, T., Kakutani, T., and Ueda, T.: Selective destruction of the myenteric plexus. J. Pediatr. Surg. 2:444, 1967.

144. Okamoto, E., and Ueda, T.: Embryogenesis of intramural ganglia of the gut and its relation to Hirschsprung's disease. J. Pediatr. Surg. 2:437, 1967.

145. Pace, J. L.: The age of appearance of the haustra of the human colon. J. Anat. *109*:75, 1971.

146. Parsons, J. M., Miscall, B. G., and McSherry, C. K.: Appendicitis in the newborn infant. Surgery 67:841, 1970.

147. Passarge, E.: The genetics of Hirschsprung's disease. Evidence for heterogeneous etiology and a study of sixty-three families. N. Engl. J. Med. *276*:138, 1967.

148. Perrault, J., Stockwell, M., Stephens, C., and Forstner, G.: Malabsorption and pouch ulcerations following the Martin repair for total colonic aganglionosis. J. Pediatr. Surg. *14*:468, 1979.

149. Philippart, A., Reed, J., and Georgeson, K. E.: Neonatal small left colon syndrome. J. Pediatr. Surg. *10*:733, 1975.

149a. Powell, R., and Raffensperger, J.: Congenital colonic atresia. J. Pediatr. Surg. *17*:166, 1982.

150. Puri, P., Boyd, E., Guiney, E., and O'Donnell, B.: Appendix mass in the very young child. J. Pediatr. Surg. *16*:85, 1981.

151. Puri, P., and O'Donnell, B.: Appendicitis in infancy. J. Pediatr. Surg. *13*:173, 1978.

152. Puri, P., Lake, B. D., Nixon, H. H., et al.: Neuronal colonic dysplasia: An unusual association of Hirschsprung's disease. J. Pediatr. Surg. *12*:681, 1978.

153. Ravitch, M. M., and Scott, W. W.: Duplication of the entire colon, bladder and urethra. Surgery *34*:843, 1953.

154. Richards, J. J., Gillam, F. E., and Thomas, J. H.: Perforations of duplicated bowel in children. Arch. Dis. Child. 37:72, 1962.

155. Rogawski, M. A., Goodrich, J. T., Gershon, M. D., Touloukian, R. J.: Hirschsprung's disease: Absence of serotonergic neurons in the aganglionic colon. J. Pediatr. Surg. *13*:608, 1978.

156. Sabio, H., Teja, K., Elkon, D., and Shaw, A.: Adenocarcinoma of the colon following Wilms' tumor. J. Pediatr. 95:424, 1979.

157. Santulli, T. V., Kiesewetter, W. B., and Bill, A. H., Jr.: Anorectal anomalies: A suggested classification. J. Pediatr. Surg. 5:281, 1970.

158. Santulli, T. V., Schullinger, J. N., Kiesewetter, W. B., and Bill, A. H., Jr.: Imperforate anus: A survey from the members of the Surgical Section of the American Academy of Pediatrics. J. Pediatr. Surg. 6:484, 1971.

159. Sarna, S. K., Baradakjian, B., Waterfall, W., Lind, J. F., and Daniel, E. E.: The organization of human colonic electrical control activity. *In* Christensen, J. (ed.): Gastrointestinal Motility. Raven Press, New York, 1980, p. 403.

160. Scharli, A. F., and Kiesewetter, W. B.: Imperforate anus: Anorectosigmoid pressure studies as a quantitative evaluation of postoperative continence. J. Pediatr. Surg. 4:694, 1969.

161. Schey, W. L., and White, H.: Hirschsprung's disease. Am. J. Roentgenol. *112*:105, 1971.

162. Schnaufer, L., Talbert, J., Haller, J. A., Reid, N. C. R., Tobon, F., and Schuster, M.: Differential sphincteric studies in the diagnosis of ano-

rectal disorders of childhood. J. Pediatr. Surg. 2:537, 1967.

163. Schuster, S., and Teele, K.: An analysis of ultrasound scanning as a guide in determination of high or low imperforate anus. J. Pediatr. Surg. 14:789, 1979.

164. Shaker, I., Lanier, V., and Amoury, R.: Congenital anal stenosis with anterior sacral meningocele. J. Pediatr. Surg. 6:177, 1971.

165. Shandline, B., and Desjardins, J. G.: Anal myomectomy for constipation. J. Pediatr. Surg. 4:115, 1969.

166. Shashikant, M., Sane, M. D., and Girdany, B.: Total aganglionosis coli. Radiology 107:397, 1973.

167. Sherman, N., and Woolley, M.: The ileocecal syndrome in acute childhood leukemia. Arch. Surg. 107:39, 1973.

168. Siegel, M., and Lebenthal, E.: Development of gastrointestinal motility and gastric emptying during the fetal and newborn periods. In Lebenthal, E. (ed.): Textbook of Gastroenterology and Nutrition in Infancy. Raven Press, New York, 1981, p. 121.

169. Simpson, J. S., Mancer, J. F., and Adeyem, S. D.: Villous adenoma of the rectum: A rare tumor in childhood. J. Pediatr. 13:513, 1978.

170. Singh, S., and Minor, C. L.: Cystic duplication of the rectum: A case report. J. Pediatr. Surg. 15:205, 1980.

171. Smith, B.: Pre- and postnatal development of the ganglion cells of the rectum and its surgical complications. J. Pediatr. Surg. 3:386, 1968.

172. Smith, E., Tunell, W., and Williams, R. A.: Clinical evaluation of the surgical treatment of anorectal malformations. Ann. Surg. 187:583, 1978.

173. Smith, G., Kime, L., and Pitcher, J. L.: The colitis of Behçet's disease: A separate entity? Am. J. Dig. Dis. 118:987, 1973.

174. Snyder, W. H., and Chaffin, L.: Appendicitis in the first two years of life: Report on 21 cases and review of 477 cases from the literature. Arch. Surg. 64:549, 1952.

175. So, H. B., Schwartz, D., Becker, J., Daum, F., and Schneider, K.: Endorectal "pull through" without preliminary colostomy in neonates with Hirschsprung's disease. J. Pediatr. Surg. 15:470, 1980.

176. Soave, F.: Surgery of rectal anomalies with preservation of the relationship between the colonic muscular sleeve and the puborectalis muscle. J. Pediatr. Surg. 4:705, 1969.

177. Sokal, M., Koenigsberger, M. R., Rose, J., Berdon, W., and Santulli, T.: Neonatal hypermagnesemia and neonatal plug syndrome. N. Engl. J. Med. 286:823, 1972.

178. Soltero-Harrington, L. R., Garcia-Rinaldi, R., and Able, L.: Total aganglionosis of the colon: Recognition and management. J. Pediatr. Surg. 4:330, 1969.

179. Soper, R. T., and Figueroa, P.: Surgical treatment of Hirschsprung's disease: Comparison of modifications of the Duhamel and Soave operations. J. Pediatr. Surg. 6:761, 1971.

180. Sotos, J. F., Finkel, M. A., et al.: Hypocalcemic coma following phosphate enemas. Pediatrics 60:305, 1978.

181. Sperling, M. A., Delamater, P., Phelps, D., et al.: Spontaneous and amino acid stimulated glucagon secretion in the immediate postnatal period. J. Clin. Invest. 53:1159, 1974.

182. Spira, I. A., and Wolf, W. I.: Gangrene and spontaneous perforation of the cecum as a complication of pseudo-obstruction of the colon. Dis. Colon Rectum 19:559, 1976.

183. Srouji, M., Chatten, J., and David, C.: Pseudodiverticulitis of appendix with Hirschsprung's disease. J. Pediatr. 93:988, 1978.

184. Stewart, D. R., Colodny, A. L., and Daggett, W. C.: Malrotation of the bowel in infants and children: A 15 year review. Surgery 79:716, 1976.

185. Stewart, D. R., Nixon, G. W., Johnson, D. G., and Condon, V.: Neonatal small left colon syndrome. Ann. Surg. 186:741, 1979.

186. Stone, H., Sanders, S., and Martin, J. D., Jr.: Perforated appendicitis in children. Surgery 69:673, 1971.

187. Sukarochana, K., and Sieber, W.: Vesicointestinal fissure revisited. J. Pediatr. Surg. 13:713, 1978.

188. Surgical Section of the American Academy of Pediatrics: Hirschsprung's disease. J. Pediatr. Surg. 14:588, 1979.

189. Sweeny, E. C., and Sheahan, J. P.: Clindamycin-associated colonic vasculitis. Br. Med. J. 2:1188, 1979.

190. Swenson, O.: Indications for surgery in the patient with congenital megacolon. Med. Clin. North Am. 48:227, 1964.

191. Swenson, O., Sherman, J., and Fisher, J.: Diagnosis of congenital megacolon: An analysis of 501 patients. J. Pediatr. Surg. 8:587, 1973.

192. Swischuk, L.: Meconium plug syndrome: A cause of neonatal obstruction. Am. J. Roentgenol. Radium Ther. Nucl. Med. 103:339, 1968.

193. Szurszewski, J.: Electrical basis for gastrointestinal motility. In Johnson, L. (ed.): Physiology of the Gastrointestinal tract. Raven Press, New York, 1981, p. 1425.

194. Taylor, I., Duthie, H. L., and Zachary, R. B.: Anal continence following surgery for imperforate anus. J. Pediatr. Surg. 8:497, 1973.

195. Taylor, K. B., and Truelove, S. C.: Circulating antibodies to milk proteins in ulcerative colitis. Br. Med. J. 2:924, 1961.

195a. Telander, R., Smith, S., Marcinek, H., O'Fallon, W. M., Van Heerden, J. A., and Perrault, J.: Surgical treatment of ulcerative colitis in children. Surgery 90:787, 1981.

196. Terner, J. Y., and Lattes, R.: Malakoplakia of the colon and rectoperitoneum. Report of a case with a histochemical study of the Michaelis-Gutmann inclusion bodies. Am. J. Clin. Pathol. 44:20, 1965.

197. Thomson, W. N., Seigler, H. F., and Rice, R. P.: Ileocolonic perforation. Am. J. Roentgenol. 125:723, 1975.

198. Touloukian, R. J., and Duncan, R.: Acquired aganglionic megacolon in a premature infant. Pediatrics 56:459, 1975.

199. Towne, B., Stocker, J., Thompson, H., and Chang, J.: Acquired aganglionosis. J. Pediatr. Surg. 14:688, 1979.

200. Townes, P. L., and Brooks, E. R.: Syndromes of imperforate anus and other anomalies. J. Pediatr. 81:321, 1972.

201. Trier, J., and Browning, T.: Morphologic re-

sponse of the mucosa of the human small intestine to x-ray exposure. J. Clin. Invest. 45:194, 1966.

202. Truelove, S. C.: Ulcerative colitis provoked by milk. Br. Med. J. 1:154, 1961.

203. Trumen, H. J., Valdes-Dapena, A., and Haddad, H.: Indications for surgical intervention in ulcerative colitis in children. Am. J. Dis. Child. 16:641, 1968.

204. Trusler, G. A., Mestel, A. L., and Stephens, C. A.: Colon malformation with imperforate anus. Surgery 45:328, 1959.

204a. Udassin, R., Nissan, S., Lernau, O., and Hod, G.: The mild form of Hirschsprung's disease— 14 years' experience in diagnosis and treatment. Ann. Surg. 194:767, 1981.

205. Valdes-Dapena, M., and Valdes-Dapena, A.: Ulcerative colitis in infants: Report of a case. Gastroenterology 18:315, 1951.

206. Vanhoutte, J. V.: Primary aganglionosis with imperforate anus. J. Pediatr. Surg. 4:468, 1969.

206a. Walpole, I., and Haken, A.: Syndrome of imperforate anus, abnormalities of hands and feet, satyr ears and sensorineural deafness. J. Pediatr. 100:250, 1982.

206b. Vazzadeh, K., Gerami, S., Kalami, P., and Sieber, W.: Congenital short colon with imperforate anus: A definitive surgical cure. J. Pediatr. Surg. 17:198, 1982.

207. Wagner, M. L., Rosenberg, H. S., Fernbach, D. J., and Singleton, E. B.: Typhlitis: A complication of leukemia in childhood. Am. J. Roentgenol. 109:341, 1970.

208. Wayte, D. M., and Helwig, E.: Colitis cystica profunda. Am. J. Clin. Pathol. 48:159, 1967.

209. Weinstein, E. D.: Sex-linked imperforate anus. Pediatrics 35:715, 1965.

210. White, J., Haller, J. A., Scott, J., Dorst, J., and Kramer, S.: N-type anorectal malformations. J. Pediatr. Surg. 23:631, 1978.

211. Winkler, J. W., and Weinstein, E. D.: Imperforate anus and heredity. J. Pediatr. Surg. 5:555, 1970.

212. Winslow, O., Litt, R., and Altman, D.: Imperforate anus from a roentgenologic viewpoint. Am. J. Roentgenol. Radium Ther. Nucl. Med. 85:718, 1961.

213. Woody, N. C., and Woody, H. B.: American trypanosomiasis (Chagas' disease). JAMA 159:676, 1955.

213a. Young, L. W., Yunis, E. J., Girdany, B. R., and Sieber, W. K.: Megacystis-microcolon-intestinal hyperperistalsis syndrome—additional clinical, radiologic, surgical, and histopathologic aspects. Am. J. Roentgenol. 137:749, 1981.

214. Zachary, R. B.: Meconium and fecal plugs in the newborn. Arch. Dis. Child. 32:22, 1957.

ed and is the cause of clinical illness, e.g., staphylococcal food poisoning;

2. The bacterium is ingested, proliferates, and elaborates a toxin within the intestinal lumen, which interacts with the intestinal epithelial surface to produce an abnormal response (toxigenic diarrhea; cholera toxin is the prototype). The causes of secretory diarrhea are listed in Table 18–3.

3. The organism may directly invade and disrupt the epithelial surface, resulting in dysentery and diarrhea, as exemplified by *Shigella*.

4. The organism, although invasive, may not destroy the mucosa but simply penetrate it and establish an inflammatory reaction within the submucosa. Prostaglandins are then released from inflammation sites, which in turn stimulate adenyl cyclase–mediated excessive fluid secretion. Nontyphoid *Salmonella* infections are characteristic of this process.[20, 60, 66, 70, 71]

5. The organism may elaborate a toxin, create an inflammatory response, and produce a pseudomembrane that overlies the mucosal surface, as is seen in *Clostridium difficile* colitis.

6. Lastly, an organism such as *Giardia* may or may not invade the epithelium but simply interfere with fluid and nutrient absorption across the epithelial surface, thereby preventing absorption and perhaps competing for those substrates, causing an osmotic diarrhea effect.[14]

Two factors are important in the expression of clinical illness by any of these mechanisms — number of organisms present and bacterial virulence (Table 18–4). This process can best be illustrated in the context

Table 18–3 Causes of Secretory Diarrhea

Bacterial:	*E. coli*
	Vibrio cholerae
	Shigella
	Clostridium perfringens
	Klebsiella
	Aeromonas
	? *Salmonella*
Tumors:	Ganglioneuroma
	Pancreatic tumors secreting VIP
Partial obstruction of the small bowel	
Bile acid malabsorption	

Table 18–4 Bacterial Virulence Factors

Motility
Adherence to mucosa
Penetration of invasive organisms
Toxin production of enteropathogenic organisms
Resistance to antibiotics

of pathogenesis of disease. For example, an invasive organism, once in contact with an appropriate mucosal surface, may penetrate the epithelium and become free of surface defenses.[57] In contrast, toxigenic bacteria must remain within the lumen but in close proximity to the intestinal surface to facilitate toxin efficacy. Therefore, a larger infective dose of toxigenic bacteria than of invasive bacteria is necessary to achieve the same clinical diarrheal response[14] (Fig. 18–1).

Virulence is then dependent, at least in part, on bacterial penetration of (invasive organisms) or adherence to (toxigenic organisms) the mucosa. The mechanisms by which pathogens become juxtaposed to the intestinal surface are being investigated using intergeneric mating and transmissible plasmid DNA. The composition of the lipopolysaccharide somatic ("O") antigens associated with the bacterial cell wall may determine penetration by *Shigella*, since hybrids retaining properties of invasiveness also retain their virulence. In enterotoxigenic *Escherichia coli*, deletion of the plasmid controlling either toxin production or organism adherence (colonization) renders the organism avirulent. This adherence factor in *E. coli* may reside on the cell wall surface in association with the "K" antigen of the cell envelope. In addition, appendages of microorganisms (such as the "F" microvillus appendage of *E. coli* organisms) may contain receptors or adherence sites that contribute to the capacity of those microorganisms to attach to the intestinal surface.

Motility of bacteria may be another virulence factor. For example, nonmotile *Vibrio cholerae* requires 10^2 greater organisms to establish infection than its motile counterpart, and antiflagellar vaccine rendering organisms immobile affords active and pas-

A.

V cholerae
E coli

B.

Rotavirus

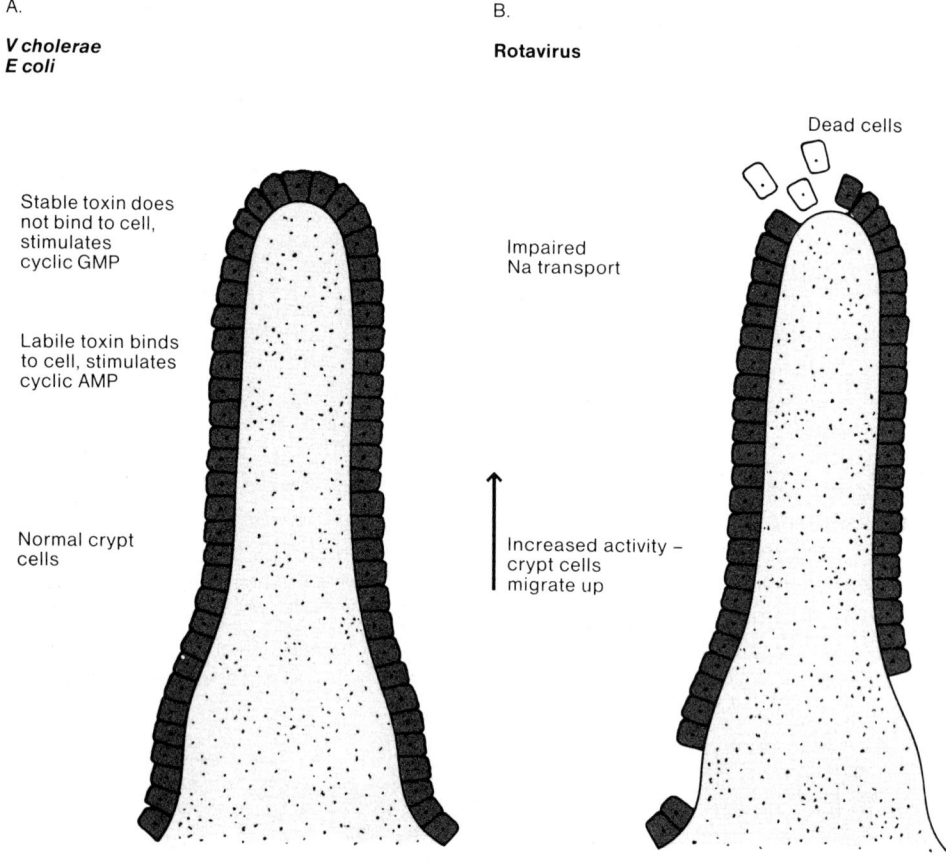

Stable toxin does
not bind to cell,
stimulates
cyclic GMP

Labile toxin binds
to cell, stimulates
cyclic AMP

Normal crypt
cells

Dead cells

Impaired
Na transport

Increased activity –
crypt cells
migrate up

Normal cell morphology. Secretion through
stimulation of AMP and GMP

Damage to cells at tip of villi – immature crypt
cells with decreased ATPase cause malabsorption

Figure 18–1 A, Normal cell morphology. Water and electrolyte secretions are stimulated by cyclic 3',5'-adenosine monophosphate (cyclic AMP) and cyclic, 3',5'-guanosine monophosphate (cyclic GMP). *B,* Cells at tip of villi damaged by rotavirus infection. Epithelial cells are disrupted and replaced by immature crypt cells in which there is defective electrolyte transport. The impaired sodium transport of immature cells combined with the decreased activity of adenosinetriphosphatase (ATPase) contributes to malabsorption.
(From Gryboski, J. D., and Hillemeier, A. C.: Chronic Diarrhea in Children. Current Concepts, 1982. With permission from The Upjohn Company, Kalamazoo, MI.)

sive protection in animal experiments. However, *Shigella*, requiring fewer organisms than any other bacterium for infection, is a nonmotile pathogen. Therefore, motility as a contributory factor may be nonspecific.

Adherence and penetration are, however, only early steps in the infectious process. For example, viral penetration is not necessarily an indication of viral pathogenicity. Since dead influenza virus can readily penetrate intestinal epithelium, viral multiplication and interference with absorptive function must also occur before diarrhea will ensue.

Table 18–5 provides a convenient treatment guide for bacterial diarrhea.

SPECIFIC INFECTIONS

VIBRIO CHOLERAE

Cholera is an acute, violent diarrheal illness that causes profound dehydration and circulatory collapse. Although rare in the United States, it is discussed here because it is the prototype of toxigenic (secretory) diarrhea.[14] It is caused principally by *Vibrio cholerae* or *Vibrio cholerae el Tor.* The

Table 18–5 Antimicrobial Treatment for Bacterial Infections Causing Diarrhea

Organism	Drug	Dosage (Oral Route)	Duration (Days)
Campylobacter	Erythromycin	20–50 mg/kg/day – probably not effective	10
Clostridium difficile	Vancomycin	0.25–2 gm/day	7–14
	Flagyl	25–40 mg/kg/day	7–10
Clostridium perfringens	Penicillin	or self-limited, no treatment	7–10
	Tetracycline antiserum	25–50 mg/kg/day in 4 doses	7–10
E. coli	Neomycin	100 mg/kg/day in 4 divided doses	5
	Colistin	15–20 mg/kg/day in 3–4 doses	5
Klebsiella pneumoniae	Sulfisoxazole	120–150 mg/kg/day	7
	Gentamycin	IV 6–7.5 mg/kg/day in 3 doses	7–10
	Kanamycin	IV 5 mg/kg/day in 2 doses	7–10
Pseudomonas	Gentamycin	IV 6–7.5 mg/kg/day in 3 doses	7–10
	Carbenicillin	IV 400–600 mg/kg/day	7–10
Salmonella	Ampicillin	75–100 mg/kg/day in 4 doses	
	Chloromycetin	50–100 mg/kg/day in 4 doses infants, 25 mg/kg/day	7–14
Shigella	Ampicillin	100 mg/kg/day in 4 doses	5
	Trimethoprim-sulfamethoxazole	40–60 mg sulfa/kg/day in 2 doses	5
V. cholerae	Tetracycline	25–50 mg/kg/day in 4 doses	5–7
	Trimethoprim-sulfamethoxazole	40 mg/kg/day	5–7
Yersinia	Tetracycline	25–50 mg/kg/day in 4 doses	7–14
	Chloramphenicol	50 mg/kg/day in 4 doses	7–14

disease has occurred in epidemic form throughout the Far East: in South Vietnam, India, Pakistan, Thailand, and the Republics of China and the Philippines, and is now found on the Texas Gulf coast.[106a] Although there is no true carrier state, it may be spread by those incubating the disease or convalescing from it via food, drink, or hands contaminated by feces.

Pathology and Pathophysiology. *Vibrio cholerae* is a motile, aerobic, comma-shaped, gram-negative bacillus with a single polar flagellum, whose infectivity is limited to humans. Many organisms (10^6) are required to produce illness, so that attack rates are usually not in excess of 15 per cent. Since the organism is extremely sensitive to acid, most bacteria are destroyed within the stomach. Conversely, achlorhydria or hypochlorhydria is associated with an increased attack rate. With the aid of enzymes elaborated to dissolve mucus (mucinases), the organisms penetrate the small intestinal mucus layer, where they adhere to the epithelium and release endotoxin. The toxin is composed of two subunits, one of which

binds to the cell membrane and activates adenyl cyclase–mediated secretion. Small intestinal secretions are isotonic, with chloride and, often, bicarbonate secretion increased and sodium absorption inhibited. Small intestinal morphology remains normal. In the distal ileum and colon, an aldosterone-mediated sodium exchange adds potassium to the luminal contents and bicarbonate is exchanged for chloride.[15] Average cholera stools contain approximately 125 mEq/L of Na^+, 19 mEq/L of K^+, 47 mEq/L of HCO_3^-, and 94 mEq/L of Cl^-.[93, 152] In adults, water losses can reach 16 liters per day. Glucose absorption remains unaltered. The secretory effect upon the gut persists longer than that elicited by *E. coli*. All of the symptoms can be reproduced by administration of purified toxin. Antibodies against the bacteria, which appear to inhibit its epithelial binding, and antibodies against the toxin are both effective in preventing the disease. There also appear to be genetic differences in susceptibility to cholera.

Symptoms. The incubation period is short, measuring one to three days, and the onset is acute. The diarrheal stools resemble "rice water" and have almost no solid content. Diarrhea persists for four to five days, with major fluid losses occurring during the first 12 hours. The volume of diarrhea decreases after that time. There is little cramping or tenesmus, the major symptoms being due to dehydration and circulatory collapse. Complications are tetany, seizures, coma, anuria, and renal failure.

Diagnosis. The diagnosis is extremely difficult, since the usual media that inhibit growth of enteric nonpathogens also inhibit that of *Vibrio* organisms. If they are subcultured, they ferment lactose slowly and may mistakenly be classified as normal flora.

Treatment. Lifesaving therapy depends on realization of the massive fluid and electrolyte depletion caused by this organism[26] (Table 18–6). Oral isotonic glucose-electrolyte solutions have been shown to decrease sodium losses due to utilization of coupled glucose-Na absorptive processes. Many patients may be successfully treated orally, but others require parenteral fluid therapy. Before it was recognized that sodium losses were less in children than in adults, hydration was accompanied by hypernatremia and seizures.[26, 152] A pediatric fluid solution developed by Gutman et al.,[84] which contains 90 mEq/L of Na^+, 15 mEq/L of K^+, 64 mEq/L of Cl^-, and 45 mEq/L of HCO_3^- (as acetate) with 2 mEq/L each of Ca and Mg and 2000 mg/dl of dextrose is recommended to prevent these complications. Tetracycline results in rapid intraluminal killing of the organisms and, if used early in the disease, will reduce fluid losses by 60 to 65 per cent.

A vaccine is available for those residing in epidemic areas or traveling to areas where the disease is endemic, but full protection cannot be assured.

Prognosis. The illness ends after three to five days. The mortality in untreated patients approximates 50 per cent but in appropriately treated ones is reduced to 3 per cent.

ESCHERICHIA COLI

The enteric pathogenicity of *Escherichia coli*, previously considered to be normal bowel flora, was first suspected in 1923 by Adam[2] and confirmed after the induction of diarrhea in adult volunteers challenged with the organism. No other organism has been the subject of so much controversy during the past decade, for since the identification of its toxin, it has been realized that many of the serotypes considered pathogenic produced no toxin and many not belonging to a recognized serotype were actively toxigenic. Some investigators still hold that well-known serotypes should not be put aside and should still be considered as pathogens. Organisms are now recognized to have one or more of the following properties: toxigenicity, adherence, and invasiveness.

Incidence. The incidence of *E. coli* infection varies widely. It has been incriminated as a cause of traveler's diarrhea[76] and epidemic nursery diarrhea and is most prevalent in third world countries. South has reported frequencies of isolation from stools of infants under two years of age to range from 1 to 23 per cent.[167] She estimates a mortality rate to be just under 10 per 100,000 infants. The disease is more common in infants born in hospitals than in

Table 18–6 Electrolyte Content of Stools in Diarrheal Diseases

ELECTROLYTES	CHOLERA	OTHER BACTERIAL INFECTIONS	ROTAVIRUS
Na^+ mEq/L	101 ± 4	56 ± 11	26.2 ± 3.3
K^+ mEq/L	27 ± 3	25 ± 4	43.5 ± 8
Cl^- mEq/L	92 ± 4	55 ± 11	16.6 ± 2.9
CO_2^- mm/L	32 ± 2	14 ± 4	

those born at home and is virtually nonexistent in breast-fed infants.

Pathology and Pathophysiology. Enteropathogenic *E. coli* (EPEC) appear to consist of two separate and mutually exclusive types of organisms: those that are toxigenic and similar to cholera in pathogenesis, and those that are enteroinvasive, similar to *Shigella*.[37, 149] Some organisms are invasive and produce sepsis, meningitis, or pyelonephritis.[49, 149] Most belong to one of nine antigenic groups of serotypes 1 through 7, 18, and 25. Their invasive properties are probably more marked in infants owing to the lack of bactericidal 19S globulin, which, as a macroglobulin, is not transported across the placenta. Some *E. coli* produce an endotoxin which, upon entering the circulation, causes shock and a Shwartzman-like phenomenon. The enteropathogenic or now "toxigenic" *E. coli* are of particular interest to the gastroenterologist, for they produce infection that may be fatal to the young infant.

The enteropathogenic (EPEC) or toxigenic *E. coli* have a peculiar potential to colonize the proximal jejunum, where they produce both heat-labile and heat-stable toxins. The strains possess fimbriate surface proteins and a colonization factor antigen (CFA). Juxtaposed to the mucosa, they release their enterotoxins, which stimulate intestinal secretion of fluid and electrolytes while causing no morphologic alteration in the intestinal mucosal structure. The more common strains have a heat-labile toxin similar physiologically and antigenically to cholera toxin. This toxin activates secretion by binding to jejunal epithelial cells and stimulating adenyl cyclase–mediated secretion. Although the action is similar to that of *Vibrio cholerae*, secretion is less. Heat-stable toxin stimulates guanylate cyclase, increases cyclic GMP, and causes isotonic secretion. It does not, however, bind to epithelial cells.[186]

The invasive organisms penetrate the mucosa and colonize in the lamina propria, where they are eventually phagocytized by polymorphonuclear leukocytes.[49, 51, 76, 177] In such instances, mucosal changes may resemble those of shigellosis, and symptoms are more like those of colitis.

A new variant of both invasive and toxigenic toxins has been described recently. This adhesive *E. coli* attaches to the surface epithelium but rarely penetrates it.[31a, 136] The lamina propria, however, shows an inflammatory infiltrate of histiocytes rather than bacteria-laden polymorphonuclear cells.

Transmission. The coliforms are excreted directly into the stool, which is the major source of transmission.[38] The infection is passed to other infants by hospital personnel using poor hand-washing techniques. There is some evidence that airborne transmission is possible. During an outbreak, 7 per cent or more of hospital personnel may carry the organism without developing symptoms.[81]

Symptoms. The incubation period varies from as little as 18 hours to as long as 18 days. Some infants carry the organism without clinical disease. Generally, the presentation resembles that of other enteritides with vomiting, diarrhea, and fever. A few infants appear well and have only blood-streaking of their stools, while others have violent diarrhea that progresses to rapid dehydration and vascular collapse. The stools of toxigenic infection are watery and contain no blood or leukocytes. Gastrointestinal hemorrhage, however, has been reported in a six-month-old infant who had no preceding fever or diarrhea. Some clinicians familiar with earlier *E. coli* epidemics describe a characteristic musty odor to the stool of infected infants.

Older infants often have a diarrheal illness that progresses to a malabsorptive syndrome associated with passage of bulky, pale, malodorous stools. Patients with "tourista" note particularly severe postprandial abdominal pain as well as bulky, pale, or loose stools.

The invasive form of infection is comparable to colonic shigellosis and may present similar sigmoidoscopic and radiologic changes. The left shift in the peripheral white blood cell count is, however, lacking.

Intractable diarrhea of infancy and recurrent diarrhea in older children have been associated with *E. coli.* Sepsis may result, and meningitis is assumed to have an enteric origin. In 75 per cent of the infants developing meningitis, the cerebrospinal isolates possess the K, capsular, polysaccharide antigen. In an autopsy study of 28 infants with *E. coli* infection, one quarter were demonstrated to harbor the organism in the lungs.

The disease is felt to be less severe today than when first described — a finding independent of our improved recognition and management. Breast milk appears to afford protection from disease, at least in infants under ten days old, although it does not prevent colonization of *E. coli* containing the "K" antigen.

Diagnosis. Serotyping was begun in order to distinguish enteropathogenic *E. coli* from normal residents of the bowel. It is believed that the toxigenic pathogenicity of the organisms is determined by a nonchromosomal plasmid, which is theoretically transmissible to all *E. coli* strains without regard to serotype. In actuality, some serotypes appear to be carrying this plasmid more frequently or selectively. Typing of *E. coli* with polyvalent antisera and, if positive, with monovalent antisera was one method for identifying early pathogens. Most frequently identified strains were subgroups 026:B6, 055:B5, 086:B7, 0111:B4, 012:B11, 0119:B14, 0124:B17, 0125:B15, 0126:B16, 0127:B8, and 0128:B12. Research laboratories use adrenal cell culture and conjunctival testing for invasive strains, and measurement of secretion in ileal loops for detection of toxigenic ones. Until clinically applicable laboratory methods are available, we will be unable to recognize the role of EPEC in individuals with sporadic diarrhea.[149]

Treatment. Meticulously sterile techniques are required in nurseries to prevent transmission. Affected infants or debilitated patients should be treated with antibiotics and rehydrated. Oral glucose-electrolyte solutions, as in cholera, decrease sodium losses. Multiple resistance to kanamycin, chloramphenicol, and gentamicin has developed.[186] Oral colistin has proved of value. Gentamicin is effective in a dosage of 50 to 100 mg per kg per day given by either the oral or the parenteral route.

Antibiotic therapy is not usually required, as the disease is, as a rule, self-limited. Bismuth subsalicylate has provided symptomatic relief and has been shown to bind toxin.[53] Prophylactic tetracycline has protected adults traveling to areas in which traveler's diarrhea is endemic. Natural immunization develops after repeated exposures to toxigenic *E. coli.*

SHIGELLA

Shigellosis

Shigella diarrhea is often termed bacillary dysentery, for the stools contain blood, mucus, and pus. The organism produces both an exotoxin, which in experimental animals causes injury to both intestine and nervous system, and an enterotoxin, causing fluid secretion. Only a few organisms are required to establish infection, accounting for the ease of person-to-person transmission and food or water fomites contaminated by human fecal material. The neonate may be contaminated directly by the mother during delivery. A few cases of transplacental transmission have been reported.[85] Man is the only natural host, although flies may serve as vectors.

Pathology and Pathogenesis. The *Shigella* group of gram-negative bacilli are nonmotile and nonencapsulated.[61] Four main species cause the majority of disease: *Shigella dysenteriae, S. flexneri, S. sonnei,* and *S. boydii. S. flexneri* was formerly the most frequently identified organism, but now *S. sonnei* and *S. flexneri* are prevalent in developing countries and *S. dysenteriae* is prevalent in Central America. Infections are more frequent in warm months and warm climates. In large cities, *Shigella* is endemic in certain areas and incidence of infection appears directly related to hygienic practices.

The organism proliferates in the jejunum but is noninvasive there.[122] It produces an enterotoxin that causes secretory diarrhea through stimulation of adenyl cyclase.[110] Much like cholera toxin, the toxigenic effects are not additive.[150, 170] Ileal and possibly colonic mucosa are not affected by the toxin. In the colon and at times in the distal ileum, the organism is invasive and releases a toxin that binds to ribosomes and causes cell injury. Microscopically, there are crypt abscesses, edema, submucosal hemorrhage, lymphatic hypertrophy, and necrosis. Occasionally, ulcerations may extend into the muscularis. Although most organisms are only locally invasive, neonatal sepsis has been reported from *S. sonnei*, *S. dysenteriae*, *S. flexneri*, and *S. alkalescens*. Breast-fed infants are protected against the disease.

Symptoms. The disease occurs most often in children under ten years of age, and half of family members are also affected. If the infection is contracted at birth, diarrhea begins as early as two days of age. The incubation period is short, ranging between 24 and 48 hours. Presentations vary from mild (25 per cent) to severe bloody diarrhea or high fever with few gastrointestinal symptoms (25 per cent). Occasionally, a seizure will herald the onset of disease. Many infants progress from one or two days of watery diarrhea to high fever with dysenteric stools and severe abdominal cramping. Vomiting is infrequent. Although dehydration and hyponatremia are common, septicemia and complications are rare.

In younger children, an abrupt rise in body temperature may be associated with prostration and meningismus. Tenesmus and rectal bleeding may simulate symptoms of ulcerative colitis. Straining may be so severe as to cause rectal prolapse. The disease is self-limited, usually lasting two to four days, but may persist for a week or more with convalescence prolonged over several weeks. Extraintestinal complications are unusual.

Diagnosis. The peripheral white cell count is often elevated, but Poh and others have noted that regardless of the total count, there is a predominance of polymorphonuclear cells and their precursor band forms.[57a, 146] Sigmoidoscopy during the dysenteric stage may reveal a red, friable, edematous mucosa covered with petechiae. Stools contain red blood cells and leukocytes. Radiologic examination of the colon varies from normal to a picture consistent with colitis, showing mucosal ulcerations and, in severe cases, collar-stud or rose-thorn ulcerations.

Although the organisms have persisted in fomites for weeks, laboratory growth can be difficult. Cultures must be plated on appropriate media immediately, since a delay of two hours reduces the recovery by half. Carrier media are not recommended, for many inhibit growth of *Shigella*. EMB medium is best; only 25 per cent of 49 strains are recovered from standard media. Hemagglutinin titers showing a rise during, or several weeks after, illness are of help in identifying affected persons in epidemiologic surveys. Serotype identification is useful.

Treatment. The most important aspect of therapy is replacement of fluid and electrolyte losses. Opiates and anionic exchange resins are unnecessary in mild disease. Antibiotics should be restricted to fulminant infections or reserved for young infants or debilitated patients. Ampicillin in dosage of 200 mg per kg per day is the recommended antibiotic, but in some epidemics 90 to 95 per cent of *S. sonnei* strains have been resistant, and 64 per cent are also resistant to streptomycin. Most are still resistant to oral kanamycin, colistin, and trimethoprim-sulfamethoxazole. Trimethoprim is more effective than ampicillin in decreasing stool frequency. Furazolidone has not proved satisfactory.

The organism is usually excreted for one to four weeks by the untreated patient, but in a few the carrier state persists for as long as 17 months. There is evidence that treatment shortens convalescent excretion to as little as two days. Immunity after infection may persist for two years.

Complications. Rectal prolapse is a common complication during the acute illness. More formidable but unusual complications are perforation, peritonitis, osteomyelitis, and disseminated intravascular coagulation. Septicemia and neutropenia have been described in young children.

Prognosis. Although most recover readily, the mortality rate in infants is 16 per cent.

SALMONELLA

Salmonella is the second most prevalent of the bacterial enteritides affecting children. Infection is most common in children under five years of age and has caused epidemic diarrhea in newborn nurseries. More than 1700 serotypes have been identified according to somatic (O) or flagellar (H) antigens, with the most common epidemic-related forms being *typhimurium, heidelberg, enteritidis, newport, montivideo, tennessee, java, bredny, thompson, infantis,* and *choleraesuis* spp. The incidence of infection by *S. typhi* and *S. paratyphi* is decreasing.

The organisms are characterized by invasiveness or by stimulation of a secretory-type diarrhea or by both. Antibodies to the O antigen are located in IgM, and a low level of this immunoglobulin may be related to the development of sepsis.

Transmission. Salmonellae are often transmitted through infected poultry, milk, eggs, and shellfish.[35, 94] Other animals can serve as hosts, e.g., domestic dogs, cats, and turtles.[105] Because of the ease of transmission by infected carriers in the food-handling process and the difficulty in sterilization (organisms grow between 44 and 114°F), food-borne epidemics may occur. Although growth ceases at temperatures below 40°C, the organisms still survive. Refrigeration does not prevent transmission. The human carrier rate is estimated at 2 to 50 per 100, and, according to various studies, 15 to 63 per cent of epidemics are caused by human carriers. Up to 37 per cent of household contacts will have positive stool cultures. The source of some nursery epidemics is an asymptomatic mother. Babies infected before one year of age are more likely to be carriers than are older infants, and some excrete the organism for up to 30 months.

Approximately 10^5 organisms are required to establish infection in the adult. This large number accounts for transmission by contaminated food rather than by person-to-person contact.

Pathogenesis and Pathology. Previous gastric surgery seems to predispose a patient to infection. Once ingested, the salmonellae penetrate the intestinal mucosa, being engulfed by cell membrane invagination. They lodge in and are phagocytized by macrophages of the lamina propria. Some strains predominate in the ileum and colon, but others also invade the jejunum. In cases of mild diarrhea, water absorption may be decreased in jejunum, ileum, and colon, but in severe diarrhea, active secretion occurs. Adenyl cyclase activity is increased and presumably is stimulated by prostaglandins. Indomethacin is able to abolish fluid secretion as well as prostaglandin synthesis. Data indicate that active chloride secretion is stimulated and sodium absorption is decreased. Electrolyte losses are less than in cholera.

The major site of invasion is in the ileum and colon, where the organisms cause ulceration and distortion of the villi and changes resembling those of colitis. There is acute inflammatory and round cell infiltration of the lamina propria. If ileal involvement is severe, there may be transient vitamin B_{12} malabsorption. Early bacteremia may occur and has been particularly associated with *S. typhimurium, S. enteritidis,* and *S. paratyphi*. Cultures of bile are usually negative, although stool cultures are positive. Liver function tests are frequently abnormal.

Symptoms. The incubation period is 12 to 72 hours, averaging 24 to 48 hours, and the course of uncomplicated disease is one week. The infection resembles other enteritides, being associated with fever and watery diarrhea. The stools may or may not contain blood and mucus and occasionally have a "rotten egg" odor. Abdominal cramps, nausea, and fever may be pronounced. The temperature in small infants may be subnormal or elevated. The white blood cell count ranges between 10,000 and 15,000, with a slight predominance of polymorphonuclear leukocytes. The newborn

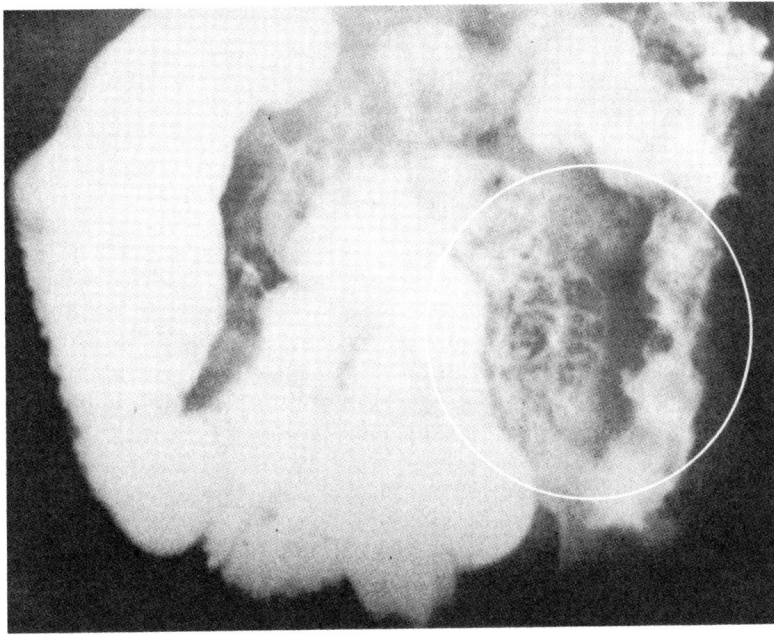

Figure 18–2 This barium enema x-ray film demonstrates mucosal edema in the descending colon of a patient with acute *Salmonella* infection. (From Gryboski, J. D., and Hillemeier, A. C.: Chronic Diarrhea in Children. Current Concepts, 1982. With permission from The Upjohn Company, Kalamazoo, MI.)

infant is more severely affected and is prone to develop sepsis or meningitis signaled only by poor feeding and irritability. Sepsis due to *S. paratyphi* or *S. choleraesuis* is often accompanied by splenomegaly and a fine, pink, maculopapular rash.

Dehydration and acidosis develop in those with severe diarrhea, which, if prolonged, leads to protein-losing enteropathy.

Diagnosis. The organisms are identified after culture on appropriate media. Blood cultures should be obtained from all infected infants to determine the presence of sepsis. Those with central nervous system symptoms must have examination and culture of the spinal fluid. A rise in agglutination titers occurs after four days of illness and is helpful in patients treated with antibiotics before cultures are performed. Radiologic examination of the colon may show significant mucosal edema (Fig. 18–2).

Treatment. Therapy consists of replacement of fluid and electrolytes. The young infant and the debilitated child or the child with hemolytic anemia, particularly sickle cell anemia, should receive antibiotic thera-

py. Ampicillin, 100 mg per kg per day, is the drug of choice, but there are instances in which this is not effective.[106, 138] Chloramphenicol, 25 mg per kg per day (orally), is effective against most organisms. Older infants and children do not require treatment and usually recover within one week. Treatment only prolongs the postconvalescent carrier state. Opiates do not alter fluid secretion but impair peristalsis and may slow shedding of the bacteria.[107]

Complications. Sepsis and meningitis are the most serious complications of infection in the neonate and osteomyelitis in the child with sickle cell anemia. More unusual complications are infection of a subdural hematoma, pneumonia, and metastatic abscess.

Typhoid and Paratyphoid Fever

A parallel severe infection in the older child or adult is usually caused by *Salmonella typhosa* or *S. paratyphi*.[94] Both appear to be exclusive to humans and are transmitted through contaminated feces on hands, on linens, in food, and in water. These enteric fevers represent extension of the infection beyond the intestinal submucosa and lodgment of the organism within the reticuloendothelial system, i.e., bacteremia with secondary infection of liver, spleen, bone marrow, and lymph nodes. The biliary tree is infected and retains the organism long after bacteremia subsides. In the intestine, the Peyer's patches are swollen and necrotic, leaving ovoid ulcers most numerous in terminal ileum and extending upward into the jejunum and distally into the cecum.

Symptoms. The incubation period varies between 10 and 12 days, with fever, cough, and anorexia heralding the onset of the illness. The fever is remitting until the tenth day when it reaches 103 to 105°F. Patients are apathetic and drowsy,[42] and the pulse is disproportionately slow. Abdominal distention, colicky abdominal pain, and diarrhea or constipation become the major complaints. The feces often resemble pea soup. Psychic disorders may be noted. During the second week, the typical rose spots appear over the trunk and abdomen. The spleen is palpable and soft. Salmonella-reactive arthritis has been reported. By four weeks, fever subsides and clinical improvement is noted.

Diagnosis. Leukopenia is common in adults, in contrast to the leukocytosis that may occur in infants. The stools contain occult or gross blood. The organism is recovered from the blood and stool during the first week of illness and from the urine in 20 per cent of patients during the third and fourth weeks. Specific agglutinins rise after seven days and reach peak levels during the third and fourth weeks. Titers of both O and H antigens of greater than 1:160 are probably diagnostic, although a documented rise in titer is the best proof of recent infection.

Treatment. Treatment is the same as for other *Salmonella* infections. Ampicillin is the drug of choice, but resistant organisms do appear. In the 1972 Mexican epidemic, a surprising number of strains were resistant to chloramphenicol, ampicillin, and other antibiotics. Steroids in combination with chloramphenicol have hastened clinical improvement.

Hygienic control measures and the use of vaccines have been effective in reducing the incidence of typhoid fever in the United States. The largest reservoir of infection within our food chain has placed the onus of disease control upon the food industry and the agencies responsible for its regulation.

Complications. The most serious complications are hemorrhage and perforation. Hemorrhage may develop in 20 per cent of patients during the third week of illness, but perforation occurs in only 1 or 2 per cent. Meningitis and thromboembolic disease are early complications. Later ones are gallbladder disease, pyelonephritis, and periostitis. Two per cent of patients become chronic carriers of *S. typhosa* and ultimately require cholecystectomy to eliminate the carrier state.

Edwardsiella Tarda

Edwardsiella tarda is an organism of the Enterobacteriaceae group, which lives primarily in cold-blooded animals but has also been isolated from pigs, cattle, panthers, and human beings.[137a] Infected humans have either lived in tropical climates or have had close contact with pet turtles.

The clinical illness resembles that caused by *Salmonella*, varying from an asymptomatic carrier state to bacteremia. A self-limited, mild diarrhea is the most usual form of presentation. More severely ill patients may have 20 or more stools per day, with or without gross blood and a green membrane covering the rectal mucosa. Perirectal abscess and meningitis have been reported.

Treatment is usually not required except in the very symptomatic patient. The organism is sensitive to broad-spectrum antibiotics except colistin and sulfonamides; amoxicillin or ampicillin is quite effective.

Aeromonas

Aeromonas is an organism that has recently been identified as an enteric pathogen that often causes severe diarrhea. In debilitated hosts it may cause severe disease and even endocarditis.[24a, 77a]

Incidence. The organism has been isolated during diarrheal epidemics in all areas of the world and is most frequently epidemic in the summer months. Although isolated from 0.4 to 10 per cent of asymptomatic individuals, it has been reported in 10 per cent of children seen in hospital situations for treatment of diarrhea. Gracey et al. have found it to be more prevalent than toxigenic *E. coli*, *Salmonella*, *Shigella*, or *Campylobacter*.[77a]

Pathophysiology. This gram-negative motile rod grows aerobically and is a facultative anaerobe. It produces cytolysin, hemolysin, proteolysin, and a cell-rounding factor. One heat-labile enterotoxin is cytotoxic, and a heat-stable "cytotonic" enterotoxin resembles that of *E. coli* and cholera. Its induced secretion however, is not neutralized by cholera antiserum.[27a, 39a] Of 400 strains, *hydrophilia*, *sorbia*, *salmonicida* and *shigelloides* are those most often identified.

The organism has been isolated from drinking water and stool.

Symptoms. Diarrhea is often severe, with watery "rice-water" stools. The disease is usually self-limited and lasts only a few days.

Treatment. In most patients, no therapy is necessary other than fluid and electrolyte replacement. The organism is sensitive to carbenicillin, kanamycin, colistin, sulfamethoxazole and trimethoprim. It is only partially sensitive to ampicillin and streptomycin and is resistant to novobiocin.

STAPHYLOCOCCAL ENTEROCOLITIS

The *Staphylococcus* is associated with two distinct enteral syndromes. Food poisoning is a common entity, which has increased in proportion to the use of processed and canned foods and is related to toxin production. Enterocolitis is usually an opportunistic disease, occurring only in those with a predisposition.[95, 179]

Food Poisoning

Precooked food, usually high in protein, serves as an excellent medium for growth of toxigenic staphylococci. There they elaborate a toxin that is heat-resistant, tasteless, colorless, and odorless. At least four types of enterotoxin have been demonstrated (A through D) with types A and B most often isolated.[119] Milk contaminated with *Staphylococcus* was incriminated in one epidemic, but most pathogenic strains are pigmented, are of the *S. aureus* variety, and are coagulase-positive. Experimentally, the toxin elicits a cholinergic effect, enhancing motility and creating a necrotic, hemorrhagic intestinal mucosa with a marked inflammatory response in both mucosa and muscularis. There may be partial sloughing of the mucosa, lymphoid hyperplasia, and clubbing of the villi.

Symptoms. Symptoms are preceded by a short incubation period of one to seven hours. Individual responsiveness, age, and infective dose determine the severity of the involvement. Nausea, vomiting, colicky midabdominal pain, muscle aching, and headache are most prominent. Diarrhea is relatively mild or absent. The illness is usually self-limited and resolves within 24 hours.

Treatment. Fluid administration is usually all that is necessary. Laxatives are of no benefit.

Diagnosis. Diagnosis is suggested by the commonality of symptoms among those ingesting the toxin or upon identification of the toxin. The disease is best prevented by appropriate storage of material. The bacteria are viable from 4°C (42°F) to 36°C (96.8°F) and toxin production occurs between 18°C (64°F) and 37°C (98°F). Prompt refrigeration or cooking at temperatures greater than 150°F for 12 minutes will reduce the incidence of this disorder.

Enterocolitis

The extremely pathogenic staphylococci of the 1950's and 1960's were VA 80, 52, 52A, and 80:81. These caused severe infections in neonates, including mastitis, pneumonia, enterocolitis, and osteomyelitis. Most organisms were resistant only to penicillin and streptomycin. Since the advent of strict nursery precautions, this type of infection has nearly disappeared. However, since several cases per year are still noted, awareness of the symptoms and prompt diagnosis are essential.

Staphylococcal enteritis develops most often in patients who are debilitated, who have received antibiotics, or who have undergone abdominal surgery. Newborns may be colonized within the nursery unit. The incidence of staphylococcal enteritis has decreased, and most cases of antibiotic-related disease are now caused by toxigenic clostridia. Rarely, *Staphylococcus albus* is implicated.[7]

Symptoms. The infants seem perfectly well until the second or third day of life, when they develop a few pustules on the skin or redness and oozing of the umbilical stump. By the third or fourth day, explosive watery diarrhea occurs. As this progresses, blood is noted in the stool. The infants are febrile and extremely ill. The small intestine is often involved with necrotic change.

Diagnosis. The diagnosis is suspected if Gram stain of the stool contains large numbers of gram-positive cocci. Culture and phage typing confirm the diagnosis.

Treatment. Although most organisms were originally resistant only to penicillin and streptomycin, they are now of phage group III and are resistant to most antibiotics, including methicillin. Appropriate therapy is determined by organism sensitivity.

Campylobacter

Campylobacter, formerly classified as *Vibrio fetus*, has been recognized as a major cause of bovine abortion and diarrhea.[25, 98, 128] Only recently, similar human diseases have been attributed to this pathogen. Enteritis affecting children under five years is usually due to *C. fetus* or *C. jejuni*, whereas that in adults is due to *C. fetus* or *C. intestinalis*.[103, 142, 161, 167, 187]

Pathogenesis. The organism was considered as a related *Vibrio* because of its morphologic similarity as a motile, curved, gram-negative rod. However, the *Campylobacter* species are microaerophilic, non–lactose fermenters and have DNA contacts that differ from other *Vibrio* species. They may be transmitted directly by contaminated foods, poultry and milk being common sources, or by domestic animals, such as dogs.

This illness is very much like shigellosis, progressing from watery diarrhea initially to stools that contain blood and mucus. However, investigations utilizing standard methods have not detected enterotoxins. Invasiveness has been documented in animals, and the organism has been isolated from blood cultures of some humans. Yet, ulceration has been documented in the ileum and colon on x-ray, and villous atrophy has been seen on biopsy. In the bovine disease, invasion has been noted, and it must be suspected in the human variety as well, since bacteremia is not uncommonly seen.

Clinical Findings. The incubation period, estimated as 2 to 11 days, is followed by one to three days of low-grade fever and right lower quadrant abdominal pain, diarrhea, and/or dysentery.[82] In 90 per cent of cases, the stools contain blood and mucus (Table 18–7). These symptoms may occur separately, in combination, or in sequence. Neonates with bloody diarrhea and irritability may not appear severely ill.[2a] The presentation of fever and right lower quadrant abdominal pain has been mistaken for appendicitis or mesenteric adenitis, since the cramping pain is usually periumbilical and the fever is usually mild. The diarrhea is often watery, foul-smelling, and profuse at the onset, with blood-streaking and mucus apparent later. Vomiting is present in one third of patients, but dehydration is unusual. The presence of erythema and a protracted form of the disease may mimic Crohn's ileo-

Table 18–7 Major Symptoms in 37 Children with Campylobacter Enteritis

Symptoms	No. of Patients	%
Fever	32	86
Diarrhea	35	95
Frank blood in stools	34	92
Abdominal pain	22	60
Vomiting	10	30

From Karmali, M. A., and Fleming, P. C.: *Campylobacter* enteritis in children. J. Pediatr. 94:527, 1979.

colitis in some instances. Extension of the infection to bacteremia or sepsis or both has been seen less as more cases of mild diarrhea are diagnosed as being caused by *Campylobacter* organisms. *Campylobacter* is also seen with endocarditis, meningitis, thrombophlebitis, Reiter's syndrome,[121a] and erythema nodosum as well as other systemic syndromes. However, enteritides have been seen in only 35 per cent of those patients with bacteremia, although abdominal pain is present frequently. The majority of nonenteric *Campylobacter* infections are found in older patients with underlying medical conditions, while the peak incidence of those cases associated with enteritis is in patients less than five years of age.[187] Improvement is obvious by one week, but relapses may occur up to a year later. Death is unusual but has occurred in a few infants.[33a]

Diagnosis. *Campylobacter* is a fastidious organism requiring a microaerophilic environment to grow, but even on thioglycolate broth blood agar enhanced by antimicrobials, isolation may require a week. Direct-phase microscopy is reportedly successful. Hemagglutination titers may be helpful if a fourfold rise occurs between acute and convalescent titers or if the patient's serum can be agglutinated by his own isolate. Radiologic examination of the colon and ileum may show changes resembling those of Crohn's disease.[127a] Untreated patients excrete the organism for a median of 26 days and occasionally for 7 weeks.

Therapy. Antibiotics such as streptomycin and tetracycline, and particularly erythromycin (in dosage of 25 to 50 mg/kg/day) for seven to ten days, have been associated with disappearance of the organism from the stool in 48 hours and subsequent clinical improvement. A recent double-blind controlled study, however, has shown no difference in response to erythromycin or to placebo.[2b] However, the physician must be aware of the possibility of recurrences and the risk of bacteremic complications, which may occur despite appropriate therapy.

Gentamicin is preferred if nonenteric sepsis is present, and chloramphenicol may be added or substituted if meningitis is present.

YERSINIA

Since it was first discovered to cause tuberculosis-like infection in animals, the perspective on *Yersinia enterocolitica* infections is changing and its involvement in other conditions is increasingly recognized. It is seen most often in Canada and Belgium. In a prospective study in Montreal (an area considered endemic), *Yersinia* accounted for 181 cases of gastroenteritis in a 15-month period.[46] It may occur in epidemic form, and transmission in milk has been demonstrated.[19, 21] In Europe, most infections are due to types 3 and 9; in the United States, to type 8; and in Canada, to type 3.[17, 130, 180]

Pathogenesis. The organism was originally considered to be *Pasteurella pseudotuberculosis*, since it is a gram-negative, non–lactose fermenting coccobacillus. *Yersinia* infections are accompanied by mucosal ulcerations in the affected areas.[156] The terminal ileum is classically involved, but sigmoidoscopy has demonstrated edematous friable colonic mucosa in adults.[21, 113] The lamina propria is infiltrated by mononuclear cells and by polymorphonuclear leukocytes and epithelioid cells in the ulcerative and necrotic areas. The infection may involve mesenteric lymph nodes. Crypts are dilated in the terminal ileum, but no granulomas are seen (enabling differentiation from Crohn's enteritis). Autopsy studies have shown ulcerations throughout the gastrointestinal tract.

Clinical Findings. Young children present with an acute onset of diarrhea and fever. The illness appears to have a brief prodrome of listlessness, poor appetite, and headache. This is followed by a sudden, acute diarrhea that may contain blood or mucus. Nausea, vomiting, fever of 101° to 104°F or greater, and a target-like rash are seen but may be of only brief duration, particularly in younger children (Fig. 18–3).[46] The enteritis may persist as chronic cyclic diarrhea or abdominal pain. The pain is often in the right lower quadrant and may

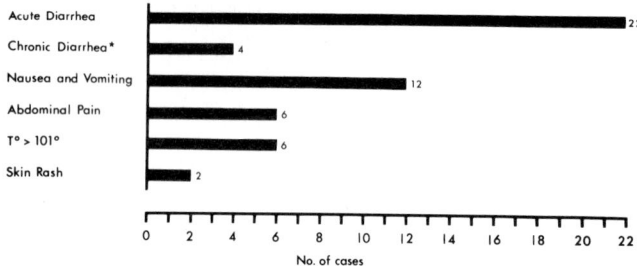

Figure 18–3 Clinical manifestations in *Yersinia* infections in 35 cases. (From Delorme, J., Laverdiere, M., Martineau, B., et al.: Yersiniosis in children. Can. Med. Assoc. J. *10*:283, 1974. Used by permission.)

mimic appendicitis. This may be caused by a terminal ileitis or mesenteric adenitis. Nonsuppurative arthritis has been described but is seen infrequently. Generalized septicemia can occur in debilitated patients and has been described in patients with protein-calorie malnutrition, immunosuppression, and thalassemia. In those who die of perforation with this disease, diffuse lymphadenitis is a prominent finding at autopsy. Persistent erythema and polyarthritis indicate the presence of histocompatibility antigen HL-A27. Typically, the diarrhea subsides in one to two weeks, but it may persist or recur intermittently.

Diagnosis. Clinical suspicion is particularly important in the diagnosis of *Yersinia* infection because the organism is difficult for some laboratories to identify. Successful culture requires stool to be mixed with phosphate-buffered saline and incubated at 40°C for three weeks — conditions that discourage growth of other fecal bacteria. Serotyping may be performed with nonspecific antisomatic rabbit antisera. Recognition of certain clinical parameters helps in identification. Titers of 1:100 or more usually are associated with clinical disease, and peak titers occur after three to four weeks of illness. False negative and false positive results do occur, and there are more than 30 serotypes. The illness is most common in Northern Europe and Canada, particularly during cold months. Leukocytosis and an elevated sedimentation rate are commonly found. Radiologic studies may reveal thickened folds and nodularity early in the course, but later, rectal biopsy shows nonspecific infiltration of the lamina propria with a predominance of mononuclear cells.

Treatment. The value of antibiotics is uncertain at present. Tetracycline and chloramphenicol have been associated with clinical improvement within two to four weeks in an uncontrolled trial. Their effect on the carrier state has not been studied. Aminoglycosides or colistin may be equally effective, but the use of antibiotics should probably be restricted to the fulminant or chronic illness.

PNEUMOCOCCAL DIARRHEA

The pneumococcus, usually considered a respiratory tract pathogen, may cause disease as a result of its frequently associated septicemia. Osteomyelitis, arthritis, and endocarditis are reported complications, but diarrheal diseases are unusual. Diarrhea with blood has been reported in a child from whom pneumococcus was isolated from the stool and not from throat cultures.[135] The course was self-limited, and the patient responded with no therapy.

PSEUDOMONAS DIARRHEA

Although many infants harbor *Pseudomonas aeruginosa* without developing symptoms, others may be severely affected when the organism assumes the role of a virulent pathogen, and these infants may develop colonic stricture.[65, 78] This may occur in young infants or debilitated patients, particularly those who have been treated with long-term antibiotics. In hospitals, the bacterium may thrive in water taps, Isolettes, and instruments. It is also found in children with cystic fibrosis.

Pathology. The organism causes thrombosis of small arteries, tissue infarction, urinary tract infection, sepsis, meningitis, thrombocytopenia, and ulcerative pyoderma. The diarrhea that it causes is explosive, and the stools are green and watery. Paralytic ileus and shock develop, and there may be perforation and peritonitis. Anal stricture has followed *Pseudomonas* infection, sepsis, and diarrhea.

Diagnosis. The organism is easily cultured from the stool.

Treatment. *Pseudomonas* is resistant to the usual antibiotics but is sensitive to gentamicin.

KLEBSIELLA PNEUMONIAE

The group of *Klebsiella-Aerobacter* organisms at times may normally inhabit the mouth and the intestine but have lately been recognized to be pathogens. *Klebsiella pneumoniae* has become one of the frequent causes of hospital infection and sepsis.[147] It has been demonstrated that Indians and Puerto Ricans with tropical sprue harbor the organism within the small intestine.

Pathophysiology. Toxigenic *Klebsiella* species, such as *K. pneumoniae*, have been shown to elaborate both heat-labile and heat-stable toxins,[112] which cause secretion in the same fashion as the toxins of *E. coli*. They may produce structural and malabsorptive changes similar to those that occur in sprue, which may persist in experimentally infected animals for five weeks.

Symptoms. In addition to causing secretory diarrhea, *K. pneumoniae* has caused chronic pulmonary disease, fatal pneumonia, cholangitis, pyelonephritis, peritonitis, epidemic neonatal meningitis, and septicemia. Infants often develop an associated stomatitis consisting of a membrane that covers the buccal mucosa and tongue.

Diagnosis. The diagnosis is established by culture and isolation of the organism. Toxigenicity may be determined by stimulation of the Chinese hamster ovary system or perfusion studies measuring the effect on water transport.

Treatment. Tetracyclines are sometimes effective, but many strains have become resistant to it. Gentamicin therapy is usually successful.

CLOSTRIDIAL INFECTIONS

Botulism

Clostridium botulinum of type A, B, or E is the causative agent in botulism.[80, 119] The disease is contracted by eating food contaminated with either spores or toxin. *C. botulinum* grows anaerobically, and its spores can survive boiling for 22 hours, although the toxin is readily destroyed by boiling for ten minutes. Spores were killed by moist heat at 120°F within ten minutes. Ingestion of the spores alone does not cause disease, for these do not form toxin within the gastrointestinal tract. It is ingestion of the toxin in raw or processed fish, home-canned fruits and vegetables, or cheese that produces symptoms.

Pathophysiology. The botulinus toxin is absorbed from the intestine and acts at the myoneural junction, where it inhibits acetyl choline synthesis.

Symptoms. Nausea, vomiting, and diarrhea develop within one to three hours after ingestion of the toxin. These are followed by weakness, dizziness, and diplopia and finally by paralysis, vagal depression, and tachycardia. Cranial nerve paralysis appears first, and later paralysis becomes generalized to involve the respiratory muscles. In severe cases, death results within two to ten days.

Diagnosis. The diagnosis is established after inoculation into mice of a food extract or serum suspended in saline. The inoculated mice become paralyzed, whereas others injected with specific antiserum do not. The organism may also be cultured directly from the suspected food.

Treatment. Bivalent antiserum is available for infection by types A and B, which are the usual sources of human infection. Antiserum should be administered to all other family members who have eaten the same food. Tracheotomy with use of positive respiratory devices must be performed at the first sign of respiratory weakness.

There have been encouraging reports concerning the use of guanidine hydrochloride from animal studies, which have indicated that in high dosage it reverses the neuromuscular block and antagonizes the action of the toxin presynaptically. The maximal recommended dosage is 45 mg per kg per day. Side effects are gastric irritation, ileus, distal paresthesias, and fasciculations. Recently, however, failures with the use of guanidine have been reported, and its role as an adjunct in treatment is in some doubt.[29]

Prognosis. Those whose disease is not lethal during the first few days recover after one to two weeks.

Clostridium Perfringens Diarrhea

It is recognized that certain strains of *Clostridium* cause outbreaks of food poisoning.[80] *Clostridium perfringens*, a grampositive, spore-forming rod, has caused a number of epidemic and often near-fatal or fatal enteric infections. The bacterium is widely distributed in soil, water, air, and commercial meat and poultry. Five types are recognized, but only two, types A and C, are known to cause enteritis. Type A strains, some of which elaborate an enterotoxin, cause a self-limited diarrhea. Type C contains strains that cause hemorrhagic, necrotizing jejunitis, intermural gas, bloody diarrhea, shock, and death.

Symptoms. The spectrum of this disease varies from a mild gastroenteritis to gastrointestinal obstruction or severe dysentery.

Diagnosis. The diagnosis is established by anaerobic culture of the organism from the stool.

Treatment. Type C antiserum and penicillin are specific treatment. If there is evidence of necrotic bowel, this must be resected.

Clostridium Welchii Diarrhea

Although *Clostridium welchii* is often associated with gas gangrene, it has been implicated in several epidemics of necrotizing enteritis in Germany and New Guinea and in scattered cases in Uganda.[80] The specific organism has been *C. welchii* type C, which produces a heat-resistant toxin.

Pathology. Loops of jejunum are distended and thickened, with areas of purple discoloration and hemorrhage over the serosal surface. Fibrinous or fibrinopurulent exudate covers affected areas. Mucosal lesions begin in the distal duodenum or upper jejunum. The jejunal walls are edematous and rigid, and separate or confluent necrotic areas are scattered through several feet or throughout the entire jejunum. Scattered areas of ulceration extend into the ileum and in a few cases into the proximal colon. Gas bubbles may be noted in the wall of the jejunum.

Clostridium Difficile Toxin

Recently, a substance producing cytotoxicity in tissue culture was detected in the stools of 4 patients with pseudomembranous enterocolitis, of 9 of 54 patients with antibiotic-related diarrhea, and of several patients with nonantibiotic diarrhea.[9, 10] Fecal extracts of patients led to rheocolitis and death after oral administration to hamsters.[147a] These same stool specimens cause diarrhea when injected into the cecum of the rat. Both the cytotoxicity and the diarrheagenic properties were neutralized by pretreatment with gas gangrene antitoxin. These observations along with other work have led to the conclusion that virtually all cases of antimicrobial agent–associated pseudomembranous colitis and approximately one fifth of the cases of antimicrobial agent–associated diarrhea are caused by a toxin produced by *Clostridium difficile*.[4, 10, 11] Preliminary reports have related the presence of *Clostridium difficile* toxin to symptomatic relapses in patients with chronic inflammatory bowel disease, and these relapses have responded dramatically to oral treatment for this toxin-producing organism. The toxin has also been associated with outbreaks of diarrhea in the newborn nurseries, but one must remain rather skeptical about these reports until the true incidence of the carrier state in asymptomatic individuals is described.[21a, 160a, 183a] The toxin or organism has been isolated in 10 per cent of normal neonates and up to 55 per cent of infants in a neonatal intensive care unit, as well as from other healthy children.[48a, 129b, 169a] In infants *C. difficile* may cause chronic diarrhea without gross bleeding.

At present, treatment for this entity can be

enthusiastically recommended only for the rare child with pseudomembranous enterocolitis or moderate-to-severe *C. difficile*–related diarrhea following antibiotic administration.[62-64] Treatment initially involved the use of oral vancomycin, a drug that is minimally absorbed from the intestinal tract (dosage, 2000 mg/1.73 m²/24 hr).[12a] The prohibitive cost of vancomycin has led to the search for more cost-efficient methods of treatment, and it has been apparent that metronidazole and oral bacitracin may be equally effective in eradicating toxin production.[29a, 173a] Toxin-binding agents such as cholestyramine or Pepto-Bismol are effective in mild disease.

Actinomycosis

Actinomycosis is mentioned briefly, since it may involve not only the skin but also the colon and liver. It usually develops in immunocompromised patients or in those being treated for Hodgkin's disease. The organism is an anaerobic, gram-positive one, which on smear appears as branched filaments. It causes chronic suppurative infections. The presentation is as for appendicitis, through pericecal invasion or as an enlarging right lower quadrant mass. The abscess may perforate the rectum and drain the characteristic "sulfur granules." The organism may be identified and isolated by culture. Massive doses of penicillin (250,000 to 400,000 μ/kg/day) given intravenously for four to six weeks are therapeutic.

VIRAL INFECTIONS

Viruses have long been suspected of causing gastroenteritis; however, their presence in equal proportion in asymptomatic controls has made interpretation difficult.[190] With the transmission of illness to human volunteers in several reported series, suspected viral agents could be more directly implicated. Finally, cell culture, electron microscopy, and serologic studies for specific antibody rise have demonstrated that acute gastroenteritis can be caused by several viruses.[18, 54, 101, 114, 159]

Rotavirus

Rotavirus (formerly infantile gastroenteritis virus or reo-, orbi-, or duovirus) appears to be the most common cause of viral, and in fact all, gastroenteritis, although adeno-, parvo-, and enteroviruses have proved etiologic as well.[87, 129a, 171]

Pathogenesis. The 70-nm rotavirus causes blunting, shortening, and distortion of microvilli within the jejunal mucosa (Fig. 18–4).[160, 165, 172, 175] The viruses are seen within the cytoplasm of the villous epithelium but are not found in the deepened crypts.[16] Studies on animal models have suggested that the mature epithelium of the villus tip is rapidly sloughed and replaced by more immature cells migrating up from the crypt.[43, 160] In the process, brush border oligosaccharidases are decreased and generalized absorption documented by D-xylose administration is diminished.[158, 174] This phenomenon appears to antedate clinical illness and occurs in infected, asymptomatic subjects.[157] The return of function and histologic appearance generally occurs within one to four weeks, but clinical symptoms of lactose malabsorption have been known to persist considerably longer. Infants who have died have had extensive intestinal involvement affecting the entire small intestine through the distal ileum. Current investigations demonstrate an increase in stool electrolytes, although not to the high levels usually noted in secretory diarrhea. Adenyl cyclase does appear to be involved, but glucose-sodium coupled absorption may be affected.[160] Parvoviruses, such as the Norwalk agent (27 nm), create a similar histologic picture with hyperplastic crypts and blunted villi.[108] Inflammation may occur earlier and with a predominant polymorphonuclear cell infiltrate in the lamina propria compared with the round cells seen in rotavirus infection. Delayed gastric emptying is caused by rotavirus. Immunity appears to be short-term IgM- or IgG-mediated, and homologous, preventing reinfection with the same strain but having no effect on other strains or other viruses.

Clinical Findings. Rotavirus infections have been recognized primarily in winter

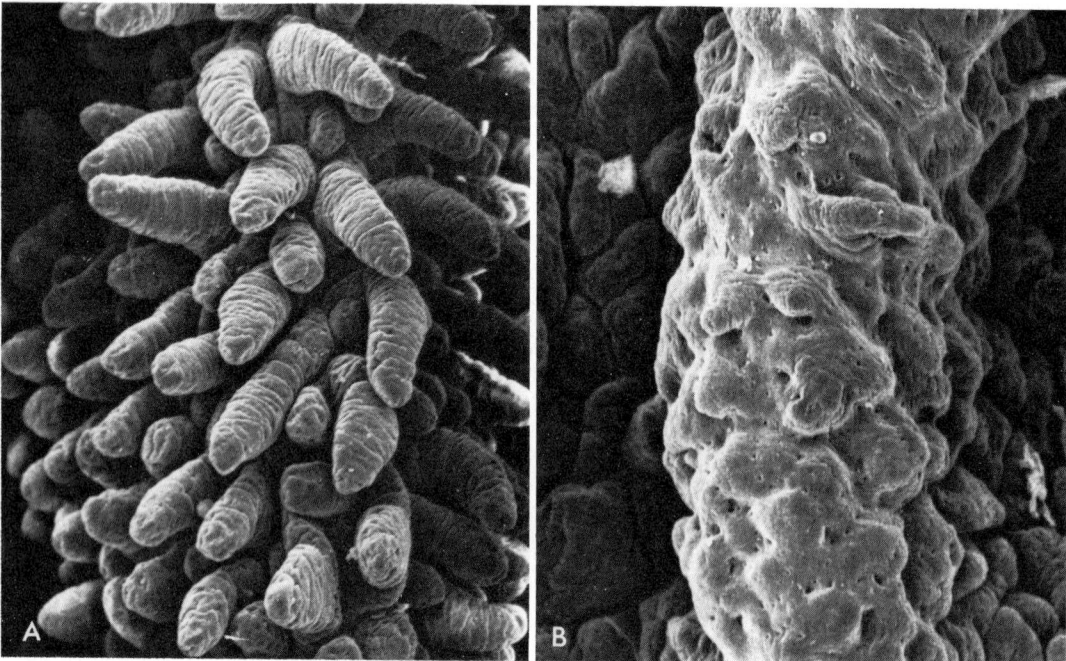

Figure 18–4 Scanning electron micrographs of the distal small intestine. *A*, Section from control showing slender villi. *B*, Section from virally infested pigments at 40 hours. Loss of villi is complete. Crypts appear exposed as pits on the irregular surface. (From Shepherd, R. W., Butler, D. G., Cutz, E. et al.: The mucosal lesion in viral enteritis. Gastroenterology 76:774, 1979. Used by permission.)

and have an incubation period of 48 to 72 hours. A brief period of vomiting is followed by the onset of diarrhea. The stools are characterized as green or yellow, with no obvious blood or mucus, and may number up to ten per day (Table 16–13). Potassium losses are more significant than sodium ones (see Table 18–6). Fever is seen in nearly all of the patients, and respiratory symptoms are present in 20 to 40 per cent. Disease in adults is usually milder, possibly because of an anamnestic response with reinfection. Colostrum and human milk appear to be protective. Excretion of the virus does occur in neonates (30 to 50 per cent) but in excess of the attack rate (8 to 30 per cent). Thus, the disease is seen or at least recognized primarily in the infant and toddler age groups. Although the illness is generally considered benign and self-limited (lasting up to eight days), deaths have been reported. Autopsies performed on these infants revealed that the entire small intestine was infected.

Chronic infection has been noted in children with immunodeficiency.[155a]

Other Viral Agents

The Norwalk agent typifies the parvovirus.[55] The incubation period is 18 to 48 hours with a secondary attack rate of 30 to 50 per cent. It may be contracted through food, swimming exposure, or person-to-person contact.[9a] Symptoms last for an equal period. Vomiting or diarrhea or both may be seen in varying degrees of severity. Low-grade fever, abdominal cramps, myalgias, and headaches may be present as well. Enteroviruses (echoviruses 11, 18, and 14) have been implicated in outbreaks of gastroenteritis occurring in hospital nurseries. Adenoviruses appear to cause diarrhea in 20 per cent of those who develop pharyngoconjunctival fever. These data require confirmation and further investigation.[102]

Diagnosis. Laboratory studies usually demonstrate a white blood cell count and a differential count normal for age. Electrolytes may be abnormal with hypernatremia and metabolic acidosis accompanying dehydration. Fecal electrolytes may yield a mildly elevated stool sodium (20 to 30 mEq/L), but differentiation from a secretory diarrhea is usually possible by specific antibody rise performed on acute and convalescent sera. The results of these tests, however, are of little value in a short, self-limited gastroenteritis. More rapid confirmation may be obtained by electron microscopy, in which 10^5 particles are seen per millimeter of stool suspension. This does not, however, completely separate out the asymptomatic carrier. In effect, the diagnosis is suspected in fall and winter; acute gastroenteritis is confirmed when bacterial stool cultures are negative.

Therapy. No specific therapy is available or necessary; however, adequate hydration must be maintained by enteric or parenteral methods (see Part II). The diminution in disaccharidase levels suggests that carbohydrates, particularly lactose, should be avoided initially.[95a] Aspirin has been effective in reducing acute fluid losses of childhood gastroenteritis.[24] Pepto-Bismol has been equally effective.[171a]

PARASITIC INFECTIONS

The parasitic diseases of the intestine are often complicated by poor socioeconomic conditions, equally poor hygiene, and malnutrition. These same conditions probably predispose to the infections themselves.

The parasites can be grouped as either protozoa or helminths. Table 18–8 provides a guide for treatment.

PROTOZOAL INFECTIONS

GIARDIASIS

This flagellate was first described by Leeuwenhoek in his own stool in 1681. Although *Giardia lamblia* inhabits the small bowel of many healthy subjects, there is considerable evidence to indicate that in some individuals it functions as a pathogen to cause symptoms resembling those of cholecystitis, duodenal ulcer, dysentery, or even the celiac syndrome.[80]

Incidence. A worldwide incidence is estimated at 10 per cent and that in the United States at 7.2 per cent, but in institutions it occurs in 2 to 50 per cent of patients.[1, 22] It has been implicated in diarrheal epidemics of newborn nurseries and day-care centers, and it has caused diarrhea at ski resorts through water contaminated by beaver and sheep excreta. It is now well recognized as one of the causes of traveler's diarrhea. Its highest incidence is in individuals with immunoglobulin deficiencies and in those of blood group type A.[9, 169]

Etiology. Humans were originally considered the major reservoir, but *Giardia* is

Table 18–8 Treatment of the Common Parasitic Infections

	DRUG	DOSAGE
Ameba	Metronidazole	25–30 mg/kg/day × 7 days
Ascaris	Mebendazole	100 mg bid × 3 to 5 days
	Piperazine citrate	50–75 mg/kg (max 3–4 gm) (1 dose) for 2 days
	Pyrantel pamoate	10 mg/kg (1 dose)
Enterobius	Pyrantel pamoate	10 mg/kg in 1 dose
	Pyrvinium pamoate	5 mg/kg in 1 dose
	Piperazine citrate	50 mg/kg/day × 7 days
Giardia	Metronidazole	25–30 mg/kg/day × 7 days in 3 divided doses
	Furoxone	6 mg/kg/day × 7 days
Hookworm	Mebendazole	100 mg bid × 3 days
	Pyrantel pamoate	10 mg/kg (max 1 gm for 1 dose)
Strongyloides	Thiabendazole	25 mg/kg bid × 2 days
	Pyrvinium pamoate	5 mg/kg (max 250 mg) × 1 dose, repeat in 2 weeks
Trichiuris	Mebendazole	100 mg bid × 3 days

now believed to be a pathogen for beavers, rats, mice, and beagle pups. *Giardia lamblia* is particularly common in areas of poverty and poor hygiene. Transmission is by ingestion of the multinucleated cysts (through water or contact with feces); the cysts remain viable for weeks in a moist alkaline environment where the temperature exceeds 10° C. The cysts are resistant to acid to a pH 1.5 but are rapidly destroyed by drying. The organisms multiply by binary fission and excyst in the small intestine as pear-shaped flagellated trophozoites. Some then attach to enterocytes of the intestinal mucosa by means of their ventral suckers, and others pass distally to encyst in distal small bowel and colon. Some cysts, which pass farther, excyst in the distal small bowel and colon and are excreted in the feces.

In addition to age, hypoacidity, malnutrition, bacterial overgrowth, and recent exposure to the agent (e.g., transients in an epidemic area) predispose to infection. This may lower the threshold dose from greater than 100 cysts to tenfold less.

Pathology and Pathophysiology. Experimentally, passive immunity in giardiasis is transferred to suckled offspring through the maternal lymphocytes of breast milk. The pathogenesis has been attributed to (1) direct mucosal injury, (2) elaboration of toxin, (3) deconjugation of bile acids by the organism or by associated bacterial overgrowth, which then activates adenyl cyclase, and (4) competition with the host for nutrients or establishment of a mechanical barrier to absorption. The appearance of the small intestinal mucosa varies from normal to scattered areas of subtotal villous atrophy with loss of nuclear polarity and vacuolization of surface epithelial cells and infiltration of the lamina propria by plasma cells, lymphocytes, and polymorphonuclear leukocytes. Crypt mitosis is increased. Experimentally, invasion is limited to the proximal small bowel with organism preference in the unstirred layers near the epithelium (Fig. 18–5).[140, 141] The organisms attach and release, through suction by their ventrolateral flange, to microvilli along edges of

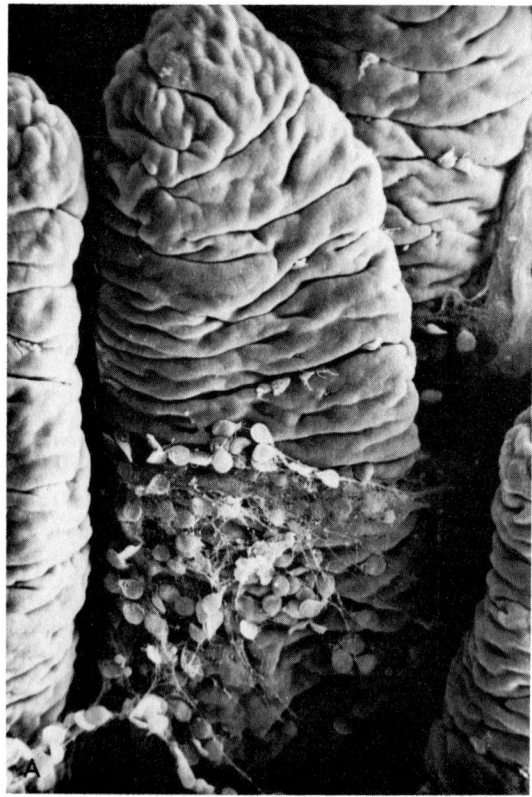
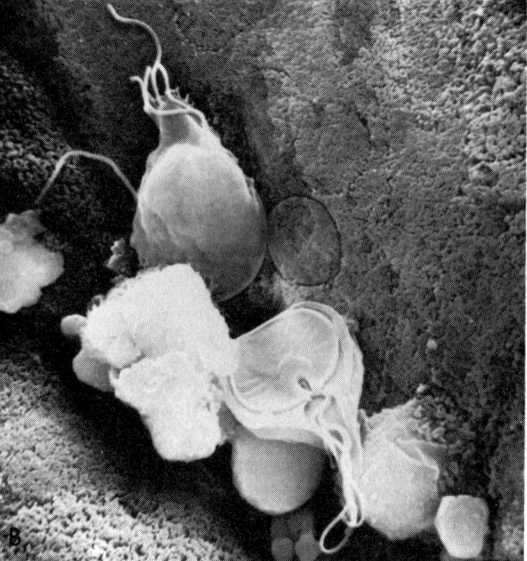

Figure 18–5A and B Scanning electron micrographs of villi in mouse jejunum. *Giardia* trophozoites adhere to microvillous surfaces near bases of villi, wedge into furrows, or lie in mucus. (From Owen, R. L., Nemanic, P. C., and Stevens, D. P.: Ultrastructural observations on *Giardia* in a murine model. Gastroenterology 76:757, 1979. Used by permission.)

Table 18-9 Frequency of Symptoms (%) in Epidemic Giardiasis

	MOORE ET AL. (56 CASES)	WALZER ET AL. (32 CASES)
Loose stools	93	72 (diarrhea)
Increased number of stools	88	72 (diarrhea)
Malaise	80	88
Abdominal cramps	77	59
Foul-smelling stools	75	52
Weight loss	73	NS°
Abdominal bloating	63	NS°
Decreased appetite	60	56
Nausea	59	59
Greasy stools	55	52
Vomiting	NS°	34
Disappearance of symptoms with treatment	97†	100‡

°NS = not stated.
†About 25% suffered recurrence symptoms, but all responded to a second or third course of treatment.
‡Relapse rate not stated.
From Burke, J. A.: Giardiasis in childhood. Am. J. Dis. Child. *129*:1308, 1975, with data from Moore, G. T., Cross, W. M., McGuire, D., et al.: Epidemic giardiasis at a ski resort. N. Engl. J. Med. *281*:402, 1969, and Walzer, P. D., Wolfe, M. S., Schultz, M. G.: Giardiasis in travelers. J. Infect. Dis. *24*:235, 1971.

Peyer's patch follicles and wedge into crypts. They do not attach to the mucosa in asymptomatic individuals. Tissue invasion occurs only in symptomatic ones and is often associated with increases in IgM and IgG. There are increased numbers of intraluminal lymphocytes, particularly during the period of clearance of trophozoites. A mucoid pseudomembrane has been identified that may contribute to the malabsorption.[146a]

In significant infections, there is enough damage to the epithelial cells to cause decreased lactase activity and occasionally malabsorption of sucrose, fat, protein, and fat-soluble vitamins. Vitamin B_{12} deficiency has been reported, and there is evidence of bile salt deconjugation and bacterial overgrowth.[37] The incubation period is two to ten days. Untreated disease may persist for 12 weeks.

Symptoms. The clinical symptoms vary from acute, limited diarrhea to chronic diarrhea. In young infants a watery, malodorous diarrhea may be intermittent or continuous and is associated with poor weight gain. Older infants and young children may show a celiac picture with marked abdominal distention, weight loss, and steatorrhea. Fever is unusual. Others note abdominal cramping for several days followed by diarrhea. More unusual symptoms are anorexia or epigastric pain and vomiting (Table 18–9). Very rarely, *Giardia* may cause a blood-tinged, mucoid diarrhea. An odor of hydrogen sulfide has been noted in the stools of some children.

Diagnosis. Eosinophilia is present in fewer than 20 per cent of patients.[36] The excretion of cysts in the stool is variable, and at best the yield approximates 40 per cent. Every patient with unexplained chronic diarrhea should be examined for the presence of *Giardia*. Duodenal aspirate yields the organism in 90 per cent (when centrifuged at 500 rpm for five minutes) and a touch mucosal impression preparation of biopsy tissue in 95 per cent.[100, 148] Examination of biopsy tissue requires a trained observer who will patiently examine multiple secretions. A gelatin-weighted capsule on a string, passed into the small intestine and retrieved after four hours, has shown the organism adhering to mucus on the string. Previous radiologic studies with barium decrease the population of organisms, and a search for *Giardia* should be undertaken before x-rays are performed.

The stool pH is often acid, and lactose intolerance is demonstrated. Radiologic examination of the upper gastrointestinal tract shows changes localized to duodenum and proximal jejunum (Fig. 18–6). In the duodenum there is spasm and thickening of the

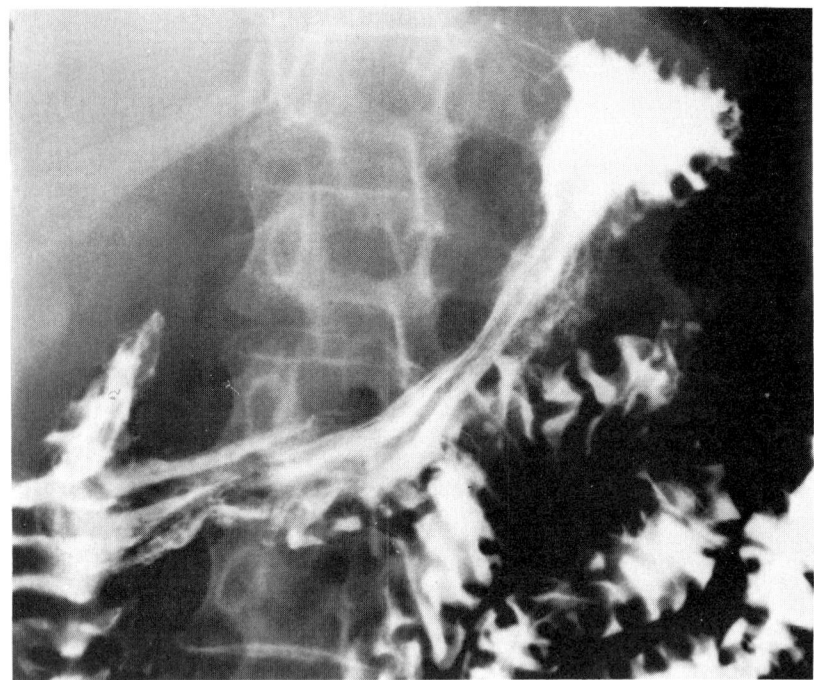

Figure 18–6   Characteristic thickening of the duodenal and jejunal folds in giardiasis.

mucosal folds. In the jejunum there is increased secretion, some fermentation and segregation of barium, and extremely rapid transit.

Evaluation of the immunologic status is indicated in all patients with giardiasis.

Treatment.   Ninety-seven to 100 per cent of patients respond to adequate doses of metronidazole (20 to 30 mg/kg/day in two divided doses). Furoxone has proved effective and is available in a liquid preparation. The dosage is 6 mg per kg per day in four divided doses for seven to ten days. Quinacrine has been an effective treatment for years but causes abdominal pain and is poorly tolerated.

Dientamoeba Fragilis

Dientamoeba occurs in most areas of the world in an incidence of 1.4 to 1.9 per cent. In American Indians, in patients in mental institutions, and in missionary groups, the incidence has been reported to be between 19 and 47 per cent.[168]

In its natural life cycle the organism is considered to have only a trophozoite form, inasmuch as a cyst form has never been identified. Structurally, it seems to be most closely related to the flagellates. Transmission through pinworm ova has been postulated. Although the organism may live for 24 to 48 hours, survival time outside of the body is probably short and stools should be examined immediately.

Symptoms.   The presentation may be that of acute diarrhea or of chronic abdominal pain. In a recent review of infestation, 91 per cent of 35 children reported from California were symptomatic. Other symptoms are anorexia, fever, pallor, flatulence, or constipation. Sixty per cent of patients lived in or had traveled to a foreign country before onset of their symptoms.

Diagnosis.   Peripheral eosinophilia ranges from 6 to 50 per cent. Stools contain red blood cells, white blood cells, eosinophils, macrophages, and Charcot-Leyden crystals. Diagnosis is confirmed by identification of the organism in the stool.

Treatment.   Metronidazole, 250 mg three times daily for seven days, or in infants, 25 to 30 mg/kg/day, has been curative.

AMEBIASIS

Of the many different species of amebae found in humans, only *Entamoeba histolytica* is clearly pathogenic, although we have seen a child with chronic diarrhea that was directly related to *E. bucheri*.

Amebiasis is caused by infestation with *Entamoeba histolytica*.[118] This protozoan causes primary disease in the large bowel but also invades the ileum, liver, lungs, brain, and pericardium.[50]

Incidence. Amebiasis has its highest incidence in tropical and subtropical regions, but estimates of its frequency in the United States are as high as 10 per cent. Transmission is from person to person through fecal contamination of food, hands, or water.[118, 145]

Etiology. *E. histolytica* takes either of two forms: the active trophozoite, which has fine nuclear detail, a central karyosome, and clear cytoplasm and which characteristically ingests red blood cells; and the cyst, which has eight nuclei. Amebae larger than 17 μ in diameter are seen in dysentery whereas those of 12 to 17 μ diameter are seen most often in chronic amebiasis.[72] The organisms are ingested in cyst form and pass unchanged to the lower small bowel, where they excyst to form eight trophozoites.[115] These multiply by binary fission, some invade the colon, while others are passed in the feces to become available for ingestion by a subsequent host. Trophozoites may be excreted in the stool but do not survive in acid gastric pH after ingestion.

Pathology. The cecum, ascending colon, and rectosigmoid are the most common sites of amebic invasion. In the submucosa and mucosa they form the typical flask-shaped ulcers (Fig. 18–7). They secrete cytolytic enzymes that aid in tissue destruction. The ulcers have irregular, undermined edges and the intervening mucosa is usually intact, although it can appear friable. Cobblestoning of the mucosa, seen in the adult, is usually not present in children. Microscopically, there is necrosis of the mucosa with edema and round cell infiltration. Sigmoidoscopic and microscopic changes are sometimes difficult to differentiate from those of ulcerative colitis, and identification

of the amebae in section is the only characteristic finding.

In infants and debilitated persons, the organisms and ulcerations penetrate the muscularis and serosa to cause perforation and peritonitis. The colon perforates most often in the cecum or in the rectosigmoid, and both perforations can develop simultaneously. The incidence of perforation in adults is between 10 and 30 per cent and rises to 75 per cent in children. The peritoneal fluid in these cases is serous and contains amebae. Half of those in whom perforation occurs have negative stool examination for parasites. Perforations of the ileum and the appendix have also been reported in infants.[184]

Symptoms. Most babies have some history of diarrhea, fever, and vomiting.[73] The stools are semi-solid and frothy or watery and contain bright red blood and mucus. Constipation sometimes alternates with diarrhea. In the very acute form there is colicky abdominal pain, tenesmus, and abdominal distention. The stools are continuous and watery and contain no blood. The bowel sounds are hyperactive. Fluid losses are significant, and the babies are acidotic and toxic. Fever and hepatosplenomegaly are major symptoms in a few babies, and diarrhea is a minor complaint. Even a celiac syndrome has been described in amebiasis, in which there is chronic, foul-smelling, bulky diarrhea, foul flatus, abdominal distention, and marked malnutrition.

The white blood cell count is variable and ranges from mildly elevated to as high as 30,000. Anemia is of the hypochromic, microcytic type.

Diagnosis. Sigmoidoscopy shows a hyperemic mucosa with hemorrhage and shallow or deep discrete ulcerations. The mucosa between ulcers appears normal. The mucosa can at times appear identical to that of ulcerative colitis. Feces or material obtained directly must be examined while warm. Use of cotton swabs will result in trophozoite adherence. Active, motile amebae that are swimming about and engulfing red blood cells are diagnostic of amebic disease. Stools that have cooled contain largely cyst forms. An abundance of mono-

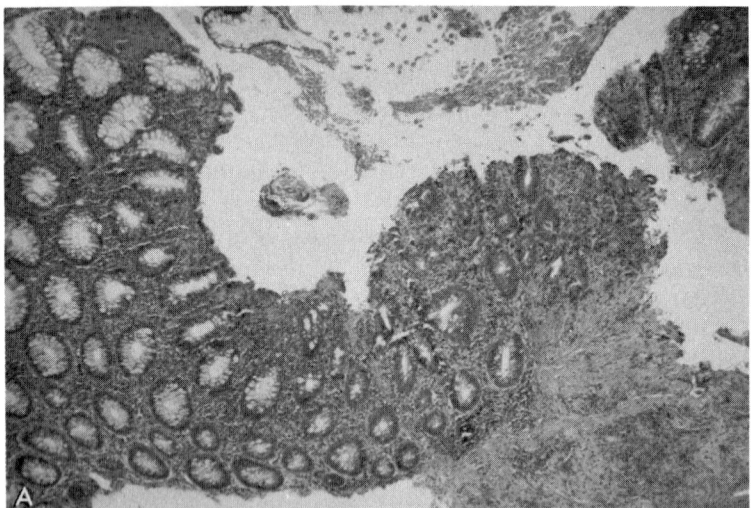

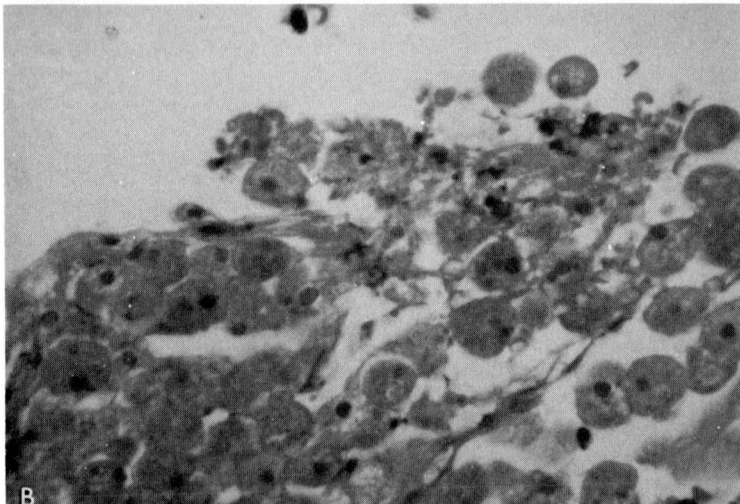

Figure 18–7 A, Typical flask-shaped amebic ulceration of the colon, with tissue necrosis, some destruction of crypts and marked inflammatory infiltrate. *B, Entamoeba histolytica* in the exudate of the same ulcer. (Courtesy of Daniel Sheahan, M.D.)

nuclear cells in the exudate differentiates this type of dysentery from that of *Shigella*, in which polymorphonuclear cells predominate. Unfortunately, trophozoites are not often identified in acutely ill infants. Serologic tests are not always positive during the active disease or in that localized to the intestine, but they are positive in 90 per cent of patients with hepatic involvement. Routine screening of single specimens can be performed using agar gel diffusion or cellulose acetate diffusion. With these and more sensitive hemagglutination, complement fixation, and immunoelectrophoresis tests, 60 to 90 per cent of cases of amebic dysentery will be detected. It is interesting that one infant with bloody diarrhea and repeatedly negative stool examinations re-

sponded after treatment was initiated when the parasite was identified only in her mother's stool.

Treatment. The current treatment of choice is metronidazole (Flagyl), 50 mg per kg per day for seven to ten days. Erythromycin, diiodohydroxyquin (Diodoquin), and other drugs have been used in the past, but metronidazole therapy is rapid and causes few serious side effects.

Complications. Amebic perforation of the colon can develop at any time.[29] It may be sudden or may be preceded by a picture identical to that of toxic megacolon or ulcerative colitis. The abdomen becomes distended and tense, bowel sounds decrease or disappear, and the area of liver dullness is obliterated. Dyspnea is severe enough to suggest pneumonitis. Abdominal tenderness is not always present, and its absence often leads to unnecessary delay in establishing the diagnosis.

Liver abscess develops in about 5 per cent of cases of amebic dysentery. The amebae travel through the portal system to the right lobe of the liver, where they cause necrosis and parenchymal degeneration with very little inflammatory reaction. Parasites are present in the stool in only half of patients with liver abscess. Although the symptoms are sometimes those of hepatitis, more often there is no jaundice but only fever, vomiting, and tenderness over the liver. Hepatomegaly, weight loss, and cough from diaphragmatic irritation develop. Radiologic examination shows elevation of the right dome of the diaphragm and obliteration of the cardiophrenic and costophrenic angles. The abscess is filled with thick, chocolate-like material, and amebae are contained in its wall. Until recently, combined treatment with chloroquine and emetine was preferred, but emetine is cardiotoxic and not without hazard. Niridazole and metronidazole are now used successfully with few side effects. Aspiration of the abscess is not recommended unless the abscess causes severe pain or dyspnea.

COCCIDIOSIS

Intestinal coccidiosis must be considered among the rare causes of chronic diarrhea in infancy.[124]

Epidemiology. Coccidia are found primarily in southeast Asia, South America, and Africa but also occur in warm regions of the United States. The micellular parasite exists in the intestinal tract of domestic animals, where it reproduces both sexually and asexually. Asexual trophozoites divide to release merozoites, which invade the mucosal cells and again divide, or which mature into females (macrogametes) or males (microgametes). After it is fertilized, the zygote matures into an oocyst. This releases sporozoites that reinvade the mucosal cells and repeat the cycle.

Pathogenesis. Changes within the small intestine are patchy shortening of villi, in-

creased depth of crypts, and cellular infiltration of the lamina propria by inflammatory cells and eosinophils. Electron microscopy shows the organisms in cytoplasmic vacuoles of cells. There may or may not be hepatic involvement.

Symptoms. Although in adults the disease is usually self-limited, in children it may cause prolonged secretory diarrhea. In older children, the major symptoms are steatorrhea and eosinophilia.

Diagnosis. The diagnosis is best made by identification of the merozoites or schizonts in intestinal tissue.

Treatment. Improvement has followed administration of combined pyrimethamine and sulfadiazine for seven weeks.[124]

ROUNDWORM OR NEMATODE INFECTIONS

STRONGYLOIDIASIS

Strongyloides is a round, thread-like worm measuring about 2.5 mm in length, which produces symptoms through its inhabitation of the upper small bowel. It is common in the tropics and the Far East and is also endemic in the southern United States. We are recognizing it with increasing frequency, as it is being carried into this country by veterans returning from the Far East.[23, 39, 104, 131]

The cycle begins with a rhabditiform larva that is discharged from the bowel. In the soil the larva changes into a free-living adult or into a filariform larva, which is infective for humans and which penetrates the skin or even the oral mucosa. The larva passes through the blood stream into the lungs, where the adolescent female is fertilized and deposits her eggs in the bronchial epithelium. Some larvae, male and female, pass directly up the trachea to the pharynx and are swallowed. In these cases, the females are fertilized within the gastrointestinal tract and burrow under the mucosa to lay their eggs, which eventually develop into the rhabditiform larvae. Autoinfection occurs through the anal skin.

Pathology. During migration there are some tissue hemorrhage and mechanical irritation in areas contacted by the larvae. Local tissue reactions consist of pseudotubercles and granulomas. Intestinal ulceration is present in severe cases.

Symptoms. The skin penetrated by the larvae becomes red and pruritic. In many individuals the infection is so light there are no symptoms. Cough, dyspnea, and patchy pneumonia are caused by the larval migration through the lungs and persist for two to three weeks. Invasion of the upper small bowel is signaled by abdominal pain, nausea, and vomiting. A malabsorption syndrome or protein-losing enteropathy or obstruction is associated with heavy infestation.[183] One 12-month-old boy presented with green, watery diarrhea of 6 to 12 stools per day for two months. He had no evidence of malabsorption or of sugar intolerance, although examination of the small bowel revealed a malabsorptive pattern. Stools were consistently negative for ova and parasites until the seventh specimen, which showed rhabditiform larvae.

Diagnosis. Difficulties are encountered in confirming the diagnosis, for only small numbers of larvae are excreted and concentrated specimens must be examined. The radiographic findings in the gastrointestinal tract vary. Some studies are perfectly normal, whereas others show a nonspecific inflammatory disease of the proximal small bowel with duodenal dilatation and thickened mucosal folds. In more advanced cases, nodular intramural defects are produced by granulomas. Effacement of the mucosal pattern due to fibrosis and rigidity of the duodenal and gastric walls is a late finding. The lower small bowel shows mucosal thickening and dilatation. Changes in the colon are unusual and simulate ulcerative or granulomatous colitis. Reflux of barium into the biliary tract may be seen during study of the duodenum. A peripheral eosinophilia is present.

All individuals who are found to harbor strongyloides organisms should be treated because of the pathogenic potential of this parasite. The drug of choice is thiabendazole; the dose is 25 mg per kg of body weight twice daily for two days. A single course of treatment may fail in 10 to 20 per cent of cases, and a second course of treat-

ment is indicated in these instances. As in other parasitic disorders, immunodeficient patients may be prone to massive infections and may prove extremely difficult to treat. A second drug of choice is pyrvinium pamoate in one dose of 5 mg per kg repeated after two weeks.

Complications. Decreased host resistance or treatment with corticosteroids can lead to an overwhelming and fatal infection.

ASCARIASIS

Ascaris is the largest intestinal roundworm found in human beings; adult worms measure 20 to 40 cm in length. The extremely fertile female lays about 200,000 eggs per day. Ascaris is found throughout the United States but is most common in Appalachia and the South. It is contracted by ingestion of the embryonated egg in food or from contaminated hands. Covered by a thick shell, the eggs are particularly resistant to drying and may remain viable and infective for months to years. They hatch in the duodenum; the liberated larva invades the intestinal wall and travels through the venous system and liver to the lungs, where it remains for about ten days. It then travels up the pharynx, is swallowed, and develops into an adult worm in the small intestine (Fig. 18–8). After two to two and a half months, mature worms mate and females then lay eggs to repeat the cycle.

Symptoms. Usually the adult worms cause few or no gastrointestinal symptoms, and pulmonary complications are more obvious. Infants with a heavy infestation have severe bronchopneumonia (Loeffler syndrome) as the larvae migrate through the lungs, and hemorrhagic foci may be established in the kidneys and brain. Lighter infestations are more typical, with some diarrhea, weight loss, and colicky abdominal pain. Heavy infestation within the intestine may cause mucosal inflammation and diarrhea, volvulus, intussusception, or intestinal obstruction. Some cases present only when the mother notes the passage by the child of a pencil-sized fleshy worm.

Neonatal ascariasis has been reported in

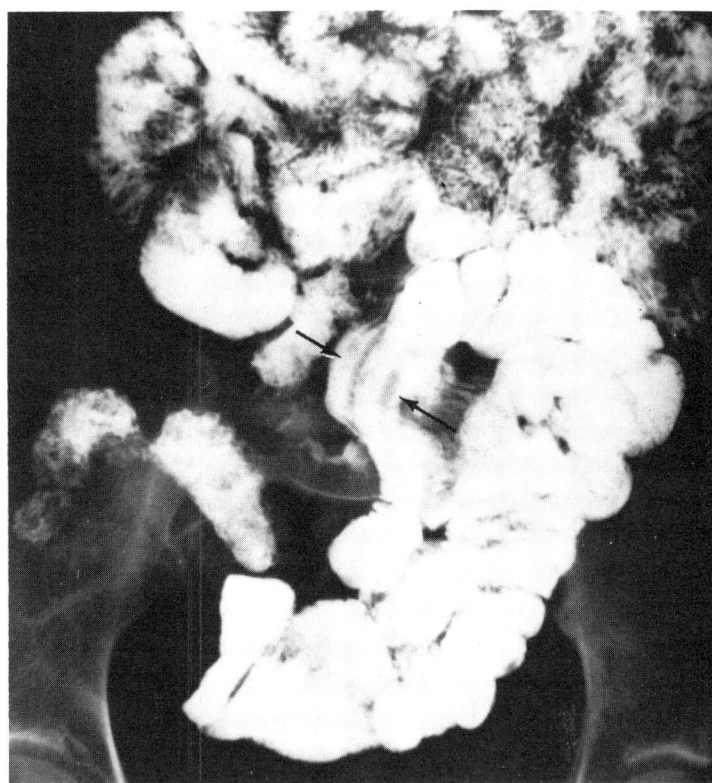

Figure 18–8 Small bowel ascariasis in a patient being evaluated for the suspected pelvic mass. Several worms are outlined by barium in the small bowel (arrows).

an infant born of a mother with intestinal and placental infection.[31]

Diagnosis. The typical eggs are found within the stool. Radiologically the worms digest barium so that their intestine is outlined (see Figure 18–8).

Treatment. The preferred treatment is mebendazole, 100 mg twice daily for three to five consecutive days. Alternative therapies are pyrantel pamoate, 10 mg per kg in one dose not to exceed 1 gm; piperazine, 50 to 75 mg per kg not to exceed 4 gm and given in a single dose for two days, or thiabendazole, 25 mg per kg twice a day for two days.

Complications. Ascaris can migrate up the pancreatic or biliary and hepatic ducts to cause pancreatitis or hepatitis. The worms have been known to obstruct the appendiceal lumen and cause appendicitis or to migrate up the esophagus and cause airway obstruction.

HOOKWORM DISEASE

The adult hookworms *Ancylostoma duodenale* and *Necator americanus* are the

ones that cause disease in humans. Measuring 7.5 to 13 mm in length, they lodge in the small intestine to cause a blood loss of 0.02 to 0.2 ml per day for each worm. The distribution of hookworm is worldwide, although tropical and semitropical climates are most suitable for its development. The ova survive in a cool, moist environment for several weeks but are extremely susceptible to drying. Within a few days they change into the rhabditiform larvae and then into the filariform larvae that penetrate the skin, are carried to the lungs, enter the alveoli, ascend to the pharynx, and are swallowed. After three to four weeks the larvae mature into the adult form in the small bowel, where females mate and lay several thousand eggs per day. Disease produced by *Ancylostoma* is more serious and more difficult to treat than that due to *Necator*. *Necator*, however, is the major hookworm found in the United States.

Symptoms. The skin is red, edematous, and pruritic in the area invaded by the larvae. These lesions are seen most often on the feet and between the toes. Cough is prominent during pulmonary transit, and, as the hookworm migrates through the small intestine, it causes epigastric pain, tenderness, vomiting, and diarrhea. Usually about six weeks after entry into the body adult hookworms mature to cause blood loss and anemia. The anemia may reach such proportions as to cause cardiac failure. With chronic infestations there are malnutrition and edema.

In infants, hookworm infestation has been reported as early as three weeks of age. Tarry stools containing some frank red blood and even gastrointestinal hemorrhage are caused by this parasite.[92]

Diagnosis. Hookworm eggs are detected in fecal smears, but the two types, *Ancylostoma* and *Necator,* are not distinguishable in most laboratories. Charcot-Leyden crystals are present in the stool. The stools contain gross or occult blood. The white cell count is elevated, with an eosinophilia that reaches to 15 or even 30 per cent. The anemia is hypochromic and microcytic. Small bowel mucosal changes and malabsorption are rare. A skin test is of use in screening populations for *Necator* infestation and uses an extract of larva as antigen.

Treatment. The current treatment is mebendazole, 100 mg twice daily for three days. Next in favor is pyrantel pamoate[74] in a dosage of 10 mg per kg (maximum of 1 gm) in one dose.

CAPILLARIASIS

Intestinal capillariasis, reported from the Philippine Islands, is a diarrheal disease associated with malabsorption of fats and carbohydrates and protein-losing enteropathy.[143] The *Capillaria philippinensis* measures only 3 to 4 mm in length. Its hosts are shellfish, and the disease is contracted by ingestion of raw shellfish or by swimming in infected waters.

Pathology. After ingestion, the eggs mature in the small bowel and the worms invade the mucosa and lamina propria. The jejunum is most severely affected, with blunted villi, round cell infiltrate in the lamina propria, and congestion of the blood vessels.

Symptoms. The clinical manifestations are chronic or fulminating diarrhea, vague abdominal pain, muscle wasting, edema, and anorexia.

Diagnosis. The diagnosis is made by demonstration of the eggs in the stool. The serum carotene, calcium, potassium, and proteins are decreased and the xylose tolerance test is abnormal. Protein loss is documented by radioisotope studies and malabsorption by quantitative fecal fat determinations. Radiologic studies of the small bowel show thickened mucosal folds and dilution of barium in those with edema. Changes noted in the absence of edema are nodularity and fragmentation of barium. The duodenum is usually spared.

Treatment. Prolonged mebendazole therapy is the only treatment.

Prognosis. In untreated patients the mortality rate is as high as 35 per cent.

ENTEROBIASIS

Enterobius vermicularis, or the pinworm, is a tiny roundworm measuring 2 to 12 mm in length. It is the most common parasitic infection of children, with incidences of 40 per cent cited in school-age groups. Adult worms live in the cecum and colon, and at night the female migrates to the perianal area and lays her eggs. Embryos develop into infective larvae a few hours after hatching. After the eggs are ingested by autoinoculation or contact with toys handled by contaminated fingers, the larvae are released and mature within a month.[80]

Symptoms. The common symptom is pruritus ani, which is most marked at night and which can cause utter misery. Adult worms that migrate into the vagina and even into the fallopian tubes cause vaginitis and salpingitis. Meatitis occurs in boys with pinworm infection. Many investigators state unequivocally that pinworms do not cause abdominal pain, but we have seen this direct relationship in at least three children, in whom the pain was completely relieved after eradication of the worm. If the pinworms invade the appendix, they sometimes cause symptoms resembling those of appendicitis.

Diagnosis. Eosinophilia is not constant but can be as high as 12 per cent. Eggs are not always present in stool samples, and the best method of diagnosis is the pinworm swab applied to the perianal area before the child rises in the morning. This is a swab covered by cellophane tape to which the eggs adhere; they are then identified by examination of the tape under the microscope.

Treatment. There is a strong likelihood that other members of the family are also infected, and the entire family should be treated. Pyrantel, in one dose of 10 mg per kg or in suspension, 1 ml per 4.5 kg (not over 1 gm) is now the recommended treatment, for there is no staining associated with the medication. Side effects are nausea, vomiting, drowsiness, and elevation of the SGOT. Pyrvinium pamoate (Povan) in a dosage of 5 mg per kg in one dose is effective, but the drug is red and can stain clothing and teeth. The side effects are red stool, vomiting, and cramping or diarrhea. Another dose should be given after two weeks. Piperazine (Antepar) has been standard therapy for pinworm for years but requires daily treatment at 50 mg per kg per day for seven days. Side effects are neurotoxicity, vomiting, and diarrhea. Its use is contraindicated if the patient is taking phenothiazines. During treatment, children should be bathed daily and their nails should be cut very short.

TRICHURIASIS

Trichuris trichiura, the 4-cm whipworm, is most common in the South but is seen in the northern United States; it is estimated that over 2 million Americans are affected.[80] Children are the most frequently affected hosts in conditions of poor hygiene. Ova ingested in water, dirt, or contaminated food hatch in the duodenum and migrate to the cecum, where they can live up to five years in the untreated host. In heavy infestation they inhabit the entire colon. Hemorrhage and inflammation develop at the points of attachment of the worms. Isotope studies show that each worm ingests 0.005 ml of blood a day, an amount that becomes significant in cases of heavy infestation, in which 800 worms will cause anemia. In heavy infestation, one sees through the sig-

moidoscope a rectal wall covered with waving white threads so numerous that the mucosa is nearly obliterated from view.

Diagnosis. The typical barrel-shaped eggs are identified in the stool.

Symptoms. The majority of infected individuals are asymptomatic. Those heavily infected show diarrhea, tenesmus, anemia, eosinophilia, weight loss, and abdominal distention. If the tenesmus is severe, rectal prolapse occurs.

Treatment. Asymptomatic or mild infections often are not treated. Children with symptoms are given mebendazole, 100 mg twice a day for three days, with an 80 per cent cure rate reported for each course of therapy. Hexylresorcinol 0.2 per cent enemas are effective in rapid cleansing of the worms from the colon.

CESTODE OR TAPEWORM INFECTION

Infestation by meat or fish tapeworm is the most common type of human cestode infection.

TAENIA SAGINATA

The beef tapeworm measures 5 to 10 meters and has about 1000 proglottids, each of which has 15 to 30 lateral uterine branches.[80] The proglottids are motile after their discharge in the stool. The scolex has four suckers but no hooklets. The eggs are ovoid with a hexacanth embryo and are covered with a striated shell. Gravid proglottids in soil are ingested by cattle and the eggs released in the intestine. Liberated embryos invade the intestinal wall and pass through the blood vessels to striated muscle, where they encyst to the cysticercus stage. This is ingested in undercooked meat and develops into the tapeworm, which matures in about two months in the human intestine.

Symptoms. There is usually vague abdominal pain, nausea, increased appetite, and weight loss. Mothers sometimes note a motile proglottid in the child's stool. Very rarely, segments become impacted in the appendiceal lumen and cause appendicitis.

Diagnosis. Diagnosis is confirmed by identification of the ova or proglottid.

Treatment. The treatment is niclosamide, 500 mg (1 tablet, ground up), given to the infant in the fasting state. Late breakfast is given. Quinacrine (Atabrine) is not preferred because of the high incidence of vomiting that accompanies its use. It is given in four 200-mg doses, ten minutes apart, followed in two hours by a saline purge. Stools should be examined again at 6 to 12 weeks. Niclosamide has a 90 per cent, and quinacrine a 75 per cent, cure rate.

TAENIA SOLIUM

The pork tapeworm measures about 3 meters long and has a scolex with rostellum and hooklets. Gravid proglottids contain 8 to 12 lateral branchings. The cycle resembles that of the beef tapeworm, but the pig is the intermediate host. Rarely, cysticercosis develops in the human through autoinfection and at the larval stage the worm lodges in the eye or brain. Gastrointestinal symptoms are the same as those caused by *T. saginata,* but the passed proglottids are nonmotile. Quinacrine (Atabrine) is the recommended treatment. It is thought by some that niclosamide causes the release into the intestine of large numbers of eggs that might penetrate the mucosa and lead to cysticercosis.

DIPHYLLOBOTHRIUM LATUM

The fish tapeworm measures 5 to 10 meters in length and possesses 3000 to 4000 proglottids. The proglottids contain operculate eggs, from which ciliated embryos develop in fresh water into the cyclops stage. The larvae encyst and are ingested by a freshwater fish in which it migrates to muscle. Gefilte fish is one of the best-known sources of this disease in human beings. Ingested larvae develop into the adult form in the human intestine in about three weeks.

Symptoms. Most infections are asymptomatic or produce only slight abdominal discomfort. There is sometimes mild diarrhea. Anemia is often present and is of the macrocytic type, for the worms have a high requirement for vitamin B_{12}, folic acid, and intrinsic factor.

Diagnosis. The diagnosis is made by finding a typical proglottid.

Treatment. Niclosamide, in one dose as described for *T. saginata,* is effective.

HYMENOLEPIS NANA

The dwarf tapeworm is the most common tapeworm in the United States and is particularly prevalent in the South. Humans are the main host, although rats and mice can be infected. After the egg is ingested, the oncosphere is freed from it in the small bowel and enters a villus, where it develops into the cerocyst. This form erupts into the intestinal lumen and in two weeks matures to the adult, which measures about 2 cm and has more than 100 proglottids. Eggs from the proglottids are infective as soon as they are released.

Symptoms. Most infections are asymptomatic, but in heavy infestation there is diarrhea and abdominal pain.

Diagnosis. Mild eosinophilia is common, but the diagnosis is made by finding the eggs in the feces.

Treatment. The treatment is with niclosamide, as for *T. saginata.* Because the larval forms are developing in the villi while the adult forms are in the intestinal lumen, the drug, which acts against the adult form, must be used daily for five days and is 90 per cent effective.

MISCELLANEOUS PARASITIC INFECTIONS

Other cestode infections have been reported to affect the gastrointestinal tract of children.

Mesocystoides is indigenous to the Orient and Africa, but in four instances children in the United States (Texas, Missouri, Ohio, and New Jersey) have contracted the parasite.[83] Complaints were epigastric pain and diarrhea. The stools were mushy and contained actively moving proglottids. The adult cestode lives in the gastrointestinal tracts of skunks, foxes, opossums, and dogs and cats, with the life cycle requiring first an arthropod and next, mice, snakes, lizards, or birds as intermediate hosts. The tapeworm may be confused with *Hymenolepis* or *Dipylidium* but is characterized by a medial genital pore and a parauterine organ containing eggs. Treatment is with quinacrine or niclosamide.

Nematode infestations may be caused by *Toxocara cati* and *T. canis* (7 to 12 cm), and in children these usually cause visceral larva migrans with hepatomegaly, pulmonary infiltrates, eosinophilia, and orbital involvement.[181] In some instances, disease has proceeded beyond the larval to the adult stage, even in infants. The worm may be grossly confused with ascaris but has arrow-shaped cervical alae. Treatment is with mebendazole.

FUNGAL INFECTIONS

HISTOPLASMOSIS

Histoplasmosis is a worldwide fungal infection, which in the United states occurs most frequently in central and south central locations. *Histoplasma capsulatum* is a small yeast at body temperature but transforms into mold form in nature or in cooler areas. It is grown in the soil and is transmitted to human beings by inhalation of spores. Large flocks of starlings have been implicated as carriers in the South. The portal of entry is through the lung, and the organism causes mild, self-limiting pneumonia. Very rarely, it leads to a chronic calcifying disease that may resemble tuberculosis. In a few instances, a patient may develop a disseminated form that involves the reticuloendothelial system and particularly the liver, spleen, and lymph nodes.[34] The majority of the population living within endemic areas have evidence of previous infection, as demonstrated by a positive skin test.

Pathology. Although the organism has been found to enter the gastrointestinal tract directly in animals, its route in humans is probably through the reticuloendothelial system from the lungs.[6] It causes changes resembling those of granulomatous enterocolitis with enlarged mesenteric lymph nodes and extensive enteritis.[166] Colonic involvement resembles that of ulcerative colitis. Intestinal ulcerations are small and superficial, and the submucosa is thickened with an infiltrate of mononuclear cells within the lamina propria. There are noncaseating granulomas in addition to giant cells and macrophages.

Symptoms. The symptoms in young children are rather nonspecific, with diarrhea, abdominal pain, cough, hepatosplenomegaly, adenopathy, anemia, and leukopenia.[75, 96] There have been associated pustular, vesicular, or gangrenous skin lesions. Protein-losing enteropathy has been reported in association with gastrointestinal histoplasmosis, and occasionally bowel perforation has occurred.[55]

Diagnosis. Radiologic examination shows the gastrointestinal tract to resemble granulomatous enterocolitis. In the colon there are cobblestoning and pseudopolyp formation. A rise in complement-fixation titers during illness and a fall during convalescence are strongly suggestive of the diagnosis. Titers should be drawn before the skin test is placed so the test will not interfere.[42] A positive skin test simply indicates a sensitivity to *Histoplasma*, but there is some degree of cross reaction with *Coccidioides*, poliomyelitis virus, and some other agents. As in tuberculosis, a negative skin test may occur with overwhelming infection. A definitive diagnosis is made by identification of the organism within the tissue and culture of the organism.

Treatment. The treatment of choice is intravenous amphotericin B for at least 12 weeks beginning with a dosage of 5 to 10 mg per kg per day initially, increasing to 35 mg per kg per day. Serum potassium levels and renal function should be monitored carefully. In less severe forms, triple sulfonamides to a blood level of 10 to 12 mg per dl have proved helpful.

CANDIDA ENTERITIS

Candida albicans is considered a regular inhabitant of the infant's oropharynx and possibly the intestinal tract in the early neonatal period. Thrush is not unusual, developing after exposure to the flora of the mother's vaginal canal. Indeed most infants by one year have positive skin tests to *Candida,* indicating immunity after previous infection. Under certain circumstances, such as severe debilitation, prolonged antibiotic therapy, immunoglobulin deficiencies, transfer factor deficiency, and hypoparathyroidism, *Candida* may become a pathogen.[52]

Pathophysiology. *Candida albicans* has been isolated from gastric and small bowel secretions in children with viral gastroenteritis. Its significance has not been defined. However, within the small intestine of some children, the organism develops the capacity to invade tissue and to cause fulminant and even fatal enteritis. Its presence in the small bowel has been associated with lactase deficiency.[116, 117]

Symptoms. Most affected infants have associated oral or cutaneous moniliasis. There is usually a monilial rash in the perianal area. Diarrhea becomes increasingly severe and is often accompanied by vomiting.[116, 117]

Diagnosis. The presence of mycelia in stool specimens is considered to indicate invasive *Candida albicans.* Yeast forms are not significant. Serologic testing using precipitin or agglutination methods is helpful but not diagnostic of invasive *Candida.*[99]

Treatment. Oral nystatin in a dosage of 100,000 units four times daily for seven to ten days will result in improvement in 80 per cent of patients. Continuation of a lactose-free diet for several weeks will aid further in controlling the diarrhea. Otherwise, amphotericin B in a dosage of 0.25 to 1 mg per kg per day must be administered for several weeks with strict attention to monitoring renal function.

MUCORMYCOSIS

Mucor is an organism of the family Mucoraceae and of the class Phycomycetes. Its entry into the body is by ingestion of fomites or by hematogenous dissemination. Within the intestine it causes a rapidly expanding lesion that is ulcerating, necrotic, and crater-like. There are surrounding perivascular inflammation, thrombosis, necrosis, and granulomas infiltrated with multinucleated giant cells. The organisms are identified by Gomori methenamine silver stains but may be seen with hematoxylineosin. Other sites affected are lung, nasal cavities and sinuses, brain, and heart.

Eighty patients have been reported, 38 per cent being children, 17 of whom were less than one year old. Lesions occurred in the stomach in 59 per cent, the small bowel in 24 per cent, and the colon in 53 per cent. Malnutrition and prematurity as well as diabetes and leukemia seemed to be predisposing illnesses. The youngest patient was a premature infant who developed cyanosis and respiratory distress followed by abdominal distention and evidence of perforation. Amphotericin B is the only known therapy.

PROBABLY INFECTIOUS DIARRHEAS

WHIPPLE'S DISEASE

Incidence. Whipple's disease is a systemic disorder with malabsorption in addition to symptoms of the skin, joints, pleura, heart, and central nervous system. Onset is generally noted in the fourth and fifth decades of life, but, rarely, infants, young children, and adolescents are reported. A male predominance is apparent.[7] Approximately 500 cases have now been reported in the literature.

Etiology. This condition is believed to be the result of an infectious agent, although such an agent has never been cultured. Several patients have lived within 2000 feet of each other and 19 lived within a 20 mile area.[46a] Jejunal biopsy and electron microscopy demonstrate large, foamy macrophages in the lamina propria containing PAS-positive cytoplasmic granules. Similar cells are noted in other involved tissue. Thrombocytosis and circulating immune complexes are often present.[139]

In 1961, Yardley and Hendrix described a rod-shaped organism about half the size of

Escherichia coli, both intracellularly and in the lamina propria and smooth muscle of the lamina propria.[189] The presence of this organism has been confirmed repeatedly, even in patients without diarrhea and malabsorption. Despite many efforts, no organism is isolated consistently in culture,[47] although *Corynebacterium anaerobium*, a *Hemophilus* species, and an atypical hemolytic streptococcus have been isolated from some patients. Forty per cent of cases are associated with the HLA-B27 gene.[46a]

Symptoms. The diarrhea is watery and foul, often accompanied by fever, anorexia, and lymphadenopathy. Abdominal distention and cramping pain are common. Increased enteric protein loss may lead to edema. Arthritis, a common complication in the adult, has not been reported in children. Steatorrhea may be significant owing to both villous and lymphatic disease.

Diagnosis. Standard radiographic and laboratory studies fail to discriminate Whipple's from any other jejunal enteropathy. The small bowel biopsy is thus definitive, though normal children may have a few PAS-positive macrophages. Immunofluorescent studies also may be performed to confirm the antigenic specificity of the PAS-positive granules. Foamy PAS-negative macrophages also are seen in the small bowel of children with chronic granulomatous disease.

Treatment. The use of antibiotics has been confirmed for clinical and histologic recovery. Penicillin, tetracycline, and Bactrim have been utilized. By 12 weeks, intramucosal bacillary bodies disappear.[118a] With infection, there may be a rise, followed by a fall, in antibody titer to *H. influenzae* B.[118a] Recurrences are seen, often years after successful treatment.

TROPICAL SPRUE

Tropical sprue is the most common malabsorptive disease of the tropics. It is endemic in some tropical and subtropical regions, but at times it appears in epidemic form.[125, 133, 134] It causes abnormalities of small bowel morphology and secondary mucosal brush border enzyme damage. Folate

and vitamin B_{12} deficiencies result, which become progressively worse unless treated. It is endemic in Puerto Rico, Hispaniola, and Cuba but not in other West Indies islands. It has been recognized in the Far East and Middle East.[134]

Incidence. Tropical sprue is seldom seen in young infants and children, but it has been reported in an infant of seven months. It affects the lighter races more often than the darker ones. Parents and siblings both may have the disease. It is more common in males and in those with blood type O.[64]

Etiology. The cause is not known, but because of its sporadic epidemic form it has been thought to be of infectious origin. Neither viral nor bacterial agents have been isolated from throat, stool, or blood cultures, but jejunal aspirates have shown an increased colony count of coliform organisms such as *Klebsiella pneumoniae*, *Enterobacter cloacae*, and *Escherichia coli*.[111] These produce an enterotoxin that causes secretion of fluid and electrolytes.

Pathology and Pathophysiology. The typical hematologic changes are megaloblastic anemia and a megaloblastic bone marrow. Thrombocytopenia is found in nearly two thirds of patients. The urine contains increased amounts of methylmalonic acid. Five to 30 per cent of patients have a histamine-fast achlorhydria associated with gastritis or atrophic gastritis.

The morphologic alterations of the small bowel develop only after several months of illness and resemble those of celiac disease but differ in that the mucosa is not entirely flat and the disease involves the terminal ileum.[13] Abnormalities of the jejunum are more severe than those of the ileum at first, but later the entire small intestine is equally involved. There are blunting of the villi with lengthening of the crypts, infiltration of the lamina propria by plasma cells and eosinophils, and abnormal maturation of the epithelial cells. In general, the degree of biopsy abnormality correlates with the severity of the disease. Immunologic changes and intestinal hormone aberrations may be present.[13a, 148a]

There is malabsorption of fat, xylose, and

fat-soluble vitamins.[153, 154] The disaccharidases are decreased to cause secondary lactose and sucrose intolerance. Serum proteins and calcium are low in one third of the patients. As in celiac disease, faulty absorption of water and electrolytes is present.

Symptoms. Tropical sprue may develop weeks to months after a visit to a tropical zone. Typically, the onset is during travel, as acute explosive diarrhea and fever that, within a week, subsides into a chronic form. At the time of diagnosis most children are malnourished and are below the third percentiles for height and weight. Symptoms resemble those of celiac disease. There may be intermittent bouts of mild diarrhea over several months until finally one continuous severe attack elicits alarm. The stools are bulky, pale, and malodorous. The baby complains of abdominal pain and becomes anorectic as folate malabsorption takes its toll. Severe glossitis at six months further decreases oral intake, and the baby becomes anemic and hypoproteinemic. Tetany and convulsions can result from hypocalcemia. A bronzy type of hyperpigmentation appears first over the head, neck, and chest and later over the entire body. Late in the disease there is edema.

A gluten-free diet is followed by little or no symptomatic response. After enteric pathogens are excluded, hematologic and vitamin states are investigated.

Diagnosis. There is a peripheral macrocytosis and megaloblastic bone marrow. The serum folate and vitamin B_{12} levels are reduced, and serum proteins, calcium, and cholesterol are low in one third of the patients. Steatorrhea, an abnormal xylose tolerance test, and vitamin A malabsorption all reflect the malabsorptive disease. Disaccharidase tolerance tests are abnormal. Radiologic examination of the small bowel shows a malabsorptive pattern. Small bowel biopsy shows the changes of tropical sprue[10] and staining with oil-red-O reveals an abnormal lipid distribution, which is considered typical for sprue. Anaerobic culture of a small bowel aspirate for enteric pathogens is indicated and may show bacterial overgrowth.

Treatment. Improvement in symptoms and in laboratory findings follows treatment with folic acid, vitamin B_{12}, and the tetracyclines. The most rapid improvement follows treatment with all three simultaneously. Folic acid, 1 to 2 mg three times daily, vitamin B_{12}, 30 μg per day, and tetracycline in the appropriate dosage for weight are given for 1 or 2 weeks and then continued in lesser dosages for several months.

CHRONIC NONSPECIFIC DIARRHEA SYNDROME
(Irritable Colon of Childhood)

Chronic nonspecific diarrhea (CNSD) is one of the most common causes of prolonged diarrhea in childhood. It may be part of a spectrum of motility disorders that includes colic in infancy and spastic colitis in adulthood.[44, 45, 125]

Pathogenesis. These patients may not have diarrhea by strict quantitative definition (that is, 200 ml of fecal water per m^2 of body surface area per day) but they do have loose to watery stools of increased number,

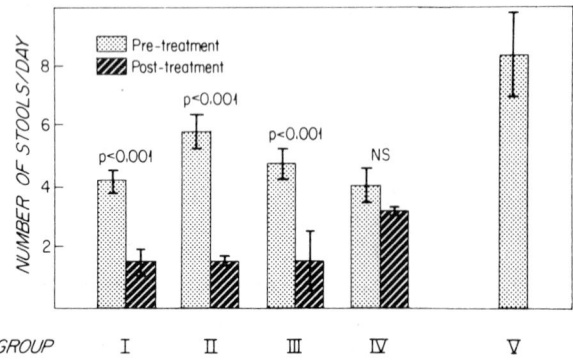

Figure 18–9 Response to dietary management. Stool frequency at time of presentation (pretreatment, dotted bar), and on recommended diet (treatment, slashed bar). (From Cohen, S. A., Hendricks, K., Mathis, R., Laramee, S., and Walker, W. A.: Chronic nonspecific diarrhea: Dietary relationships. Pediatrics *64*:402, 1979.)

which should serve to classify this as a diarrheal syndrome. The patients have a decreased mouth to anus transit time that normalizes frequently with an increase in dietary fat intake (Fig. 18–9). The mechanism whereby dietary fat is effective appears related to a direct or indirect (via stimulation of gastric inhibitory polypeptide or glucagon) effect on gastric emptying. This suggests that gastric emptying is a primary determinant of intestinal motility or that this stimulates the gastrocolic reflux, which also may be a factor in dumping syndromes.

Clinical Course. The patients with CNSD are 6 to 54 months of age and are usually well otherwise.[120, 126] There is no evidence of malabsorption or enteric infection, but a small percentage of patients may have failure to gain weight or actual weight loss secondary to an inadequate caloric intake. A careful dietary history will reveal that many of these patients will have a low fat intake with carbohydrate as their primary source of calories. Retrospectively, many patients will reveal that they suffered from some initial precipitating illness accompanied by diarrhea, but that their diarrhea persisted despite milk (and often wheat) restriction by their physicians (thus reducing their primary source of fat intake).[60, 120, 126] On occasion, the same condition may result from a zealous, unsupervised parental restriction of fat done as prophylaxis for obesity or hyperlipemia.[32, 33] This syndrome has been described in the past as a benign and self-limited illness that may persist after toilet training but becomes less obvious to the parent who is no longer faced with seeing or cleaning diarrheal diapers.

Diagnosis. CNSD previously was an illness diagnosed by exclusion that often resolved at the time the child was placed on a diet for fecal fat collection. Enteric infections are not present, and laboratory specimens are of little value. However, the diagnosis can be made on clinical criteria with a dietary history that demonstrates a low-fat intake in an otherwise well child. The stool pattern classically consists of firmer stools in the morning with lessened consistency during the remainder of the day. A family history may indicate others with functional bowel disorders. In those with possible malabsorption or failure to thrive, a fecal fat collection should be obtained and may resolve the problem.

Therapy. The recognition of nutritional factors as pathogenetic or exacerbating the illness has focused attention upon dietary treatment of the disorder. The fat in the diet should be increased temporarily to a recommended level of 4 to 6 g of fat per day per kilogram of body weight.[162] Because of coronary risk factors, polyunsaturated fats are preferred. Since we are not completely certain of the etiologic role of elevated carbohydrates in the diet (often given as liquids), these may be restricted as well. CNSD patients returning to their previous diets may have re-exacerbation of symptoms, which should once again respond to the above measures. Of note is the successful use of a similar diet in a patient with increased ileostomy output. Metamucil and high-fiber food have been used successfully by others to normalize the stools in these patients.

While symptomatic improvement on an increased fat intake may be considered one of the diagnostic criteria for CNSD, some patients, often older toddlers, will not respond to these measures. For these patients, anionic exchange resins such as cholestyramine or Amphojel have been successful. However, these drugs should not be used for prolonged periods since they bind nutrients and other medications. Antibiotics and metronidazole have been used empirically in these patients, particularly because the diagnosis of infectious agents such as *Giardia* has been so difficult. However, as stated earlier, no enteric infection has been found in conjunction with this illness, and dietary modifications have largely replaced this mode of therapy.

HYPERCALORIC DIARRHEA

Hypercaloric diarrhea is one of the more frequent causes of loose stools in an otherwise normal infant. We warn mothers that if infants take in excess of a calculated 160 calories per kilogram, there is a strong likelihood that they will have diarrhea. Often mothers mistakenly interpret a strong sucking urge as hunger and overfeed their babies. Decreasing the caloric intake by substitution of sugar water or fruit juice or offering a pacifier to the infant whose sucking urge has not been satisfied is sufficient to solve the problem.

WELL WATER DIARRHEA

Infants sometimes have diarrhea when visiting some locale where a well provides the water supply.[30] The high concentrations of nitrates or sulfates in well water may be the cause, and the substitution of bottled water is curative. Well water containing more than 400 mg per liter of sulfate should not be given to infants.

DIETARY DIARRHEA

One's daily food intake contains substances that affect intestinal motility and absorption. Dietary fiber is now being consumed specifically for its hydroscopic properties, which increase stool volume and intestinal transit.

Liquids are osmotically active as they enter the stomach but are usually admixed with gastric and intestinal secretions until they are absorbed. Once absorbed, their obligate free water exits the intestinal lumen via solvent drag. Thus, even pineapple juice with an osmolality of approximately 900 mOsm per liter usually has little effect on fecal content. The exception is when juices or other liquids are ingested in such large quantities that they overwhelm normal absorptive processes in the jejunum and thus contribute to an increased water load that the colon must filter. This effect is enhanced by liquids served cold, since the lower temperature stimulates the gastrocolic reflex and decreases transit time within the intestine.

Food additives and substitutes have been documented to cause clinical diarrhea as

well. Sorbitol is used as a sweetener in dietetic products and in some pharmaceuticals (a vitamin C preparation in Australia).[79] As a poorly absorbable, osmotically active substance, it has caused watery stools in adults as well as children. However, young children appear particularly susceptible to the osmotic action of sorbitol since they are more likely to consume the 0.5 mg per kg of body weight that appears to be the threshold dose for diarrhea.

A popular drink, Kool-Aid, has dioctyl sodium sulfosuccinate added in its manufacture. This is used as a stabilizer in the product, but exists in pharmaceutical form as a stool softener (Colace).

ANTIBIOTIC-ASSOCIATED DIARRHEA

Antibiotic usage is often accompanied by gastrointestinal side effects, including nausea, vomiting, diarrhea, or abdominal pain.[12] Approximately 10 to 20 per cent of patients on ampicillin have an increased frequency in bowel movements.[163, 173] This is far more common than pseudomembranous colitis (described elsewhere), which is more severe and related to the production of *Clostridium difficile* toxin.[60, 144]

Pathogenesis. Although antibiotics cause a quantitative alteration in the intestinal microflora, the mechanism by which this results in diarrhea is still speculative.[178] The suppression of anaerobic bacteria with an increase in other organisms is clear, but neither *Staphylococcus* nor *Candida* can be implicated. One possibility is that an organism (or organisms) similar to *C. difficile* may produce a toxin that stimulates cyclic AMP intestinal secretion without inducing an inflammatory reaction. Perhaps the same toxin is produced in a wider segment of those taking antibiotics, but differences in host susceptibility account for the presence or absence of diarrheal symptoms. Another possibility is that the antibiotic may suppress bacterial dehydroxylation of primary bile acids, allowing them to remain at high concentrations in soluble phase and stimulate the cyclic AMP system once again.[89] This remains speculative, although neomycin has been shown to alter the bile acid metabolism by decreasing or totally inhibiting bile acid dehydroxylation in both humans and experimental animals.[90] Neomycin as well as other antibiotics decreased the lactose actively in hamsters. This may be sufficient to cause the diarrhea and may result from a direct effect on the mucosa or by creating a bacterial overgrowth in the small intestine.[86]

Clinical Course. The nonpseudomembranous diarrhea induced by antibiotics may begin shortly after this initial administration, with a peak in the number of stools per day at four to five days. Broad-spectrum antibiotics have a greater propensity to cause the diarrhea, with 10 to 20 per cent of patients on ampicillin and 10 to 50 per cent of patients on tetracycline affected.[4]

Studies in adults show no correlation with dosage or route of administration.[144] However, one study in a pediatric population demonstrated a positive correlation of the oral dose of ampicillin and the number of stools per day in children under three years of age. It also demonstrated that patients receiving three times as much ampicillin intravenously had fewer stools than those on oral administration. It is unproved that either atopic or immunodeficient patients are more susceptible to antibiotic-induced diarrhea.

Diagnosis. The diagnosis is entirely clinical. However, if blood or mucosal tissue appears in the stools or the patients begin to deteriorate, a work-up for pseudomembranous colitis should be undertaken.

Treatment. The treatment is largely supportive. The medication may be withdrawn if another antibiotic or intravenous administration can be substituted. This obviously must be weighed against the patient's underlying illness. Lactobacillus has been previously recommended for concomitant administration in order to repopulate the intestine with lactose-fermenting organisms.[3, 77] However, no adequate study has proved its effectiveness except in very large doses (3 g q.i.d.). Lack of response to discontinuing the medication should cause one once again to re-evaluate the diagnosis. Depending upon whether the lactose or the bile acid hypothesis is thought etiologic,

one could initiate therapy with a lactose-free diet or cholestyramine, respectively.

DIARRHEA SECONDARY TO LAXATIVE ABUSE

Laxative abuse has been seen in adults, especially in association with depression, personality disorders, and anorexia nervosa. It is included here because of its recent description in children.[40, 59, 137]

Pathogenesis. The diarrheal mechanism depends upon the type of laxative used. Purgatives (for example, magnesium sulfate or hydroxide, lactulose) are poorly absorbable compounds that exert an intraluminal osmotic effect decreasing water absorption. They may also stimulate release of cholecystokinin, which increases intestinal secretion and motility. Ricinoleic acid, the active component in castor oil, is hydroxylated by colonic bacteria and in that form stimulates cyclic AMP induced diarrhea. Dioctyl sodium sulfosuccinate (Colace) inhibits water absorption in the jejunum as well as the colon and may induce the latter effect by cyclic AMP medication.[155] Alkaloids of plants such as *Podophyllum* act similarly and also stimulate motor activity. Cathartics like bisacodyl (Ducolax), oxyphenisatin, and phenolphthalein require biliary excretion before they induce secretion within the intestine. Bulk laxatives such as psyllium seeds (Metamucil) exert a hydroscopic effect retaining water within the intestine, but their partial degradation to hydroxy fatty acids also may serve to stimulate cyclic AMP.

Whether anthroquinones (e.g., senna, cascara) stimulate intestinal secretion is as yet uncertain, but their hydrolytic products in the colon increase colonic peristalsis. These alkaloids are the only agents known to create distinct pathologic findings: mucosal inflammation and pigmentation (melanosis coli), muscularis mucosae hypertrophy, and atrophy of the outer muscle with loss of neurons of the myenteric plexus. This loss may result in escalation of the laxative doses as patients attempt to compensate for diminished effectiveness of lesser doses.

Clinical Course. The patients with laxative abuse have chronic diarrhea often accompanied by hypokalemia (caused by anion exchange and by increased aldosterone secretion to compensate for total body sodium losses). Serum calcium may be diminished and tetany may be present as well. Intestinal protein and fat loss may be present but mild.

Diagnosis. The diagnosis is difficult primarily because of the surreptitious nature of the abuse. Stool osmolality or electrolytes or both may be elevated, depending upon the agent. If phenolphthalein is utilized, alkalinization of the stool will render it pink. A stool sample also may be sent for analysis of senna alkaloids. Serum electrolytes, calcium, and pH levels would indicate the severity of the illness. Radiologic findings of an ahaustral colon with an enlarged cecum and abnormal terminal ileum may be present with the senna alkaloids, but the picture also may be confused by similarity to inflammatory bowel disease. All too frequently, the diagnosis becomes dependent upon spy-type investigations as one searches the patient's belongings. These searches should be done with at least one witness present to avoid legal problems.

Treatment. The treatment usually involves extensive psychiatric counseling of the abuser; for children, social welfare agencies may be required to prevent recurrence of this or other manifestations of child abuse.[56]

SUMMARY

This chapter focused primarily on those conditions characterized by diarrhea. An attempt was made to categorize these conditions into the conceptual models discussed in Chapter 5. Other entities in which diarrhea is one facet of the illness are discussed in the appropriate chapters: inflammation (Crohn's and ulcerative colitis); immunologic (combined variable immunodeficiencies, Wiskott-Aldrich syndrome, and thymic dysplasia); carbohydrate malabsorption (lactose and sucrose intolerances); fat malabsorption (enterokinase deficiency, intract-

able diarrhea of infancy, and so on); and congenital abnormalities (Hirschsprung's disease).

Therapy in acute diarrheal states is based upon replacement of water and solute losses to prevent dehydration. Treatment of chronic diarrhea depends upon the recognition of the underlying cause for the abnormality as well as prevention of dehydration.[8, 97, 127] In infants with marginal dietary intakes, it is especially important to recognize the steatorrhea and diarrhea that occur, to avert the cycle of intractable diarrhea and malnutrition.

REFERENCES

1. Ackers, J. O.: Giardiasis: Basic parasitology. Trans. R. Soc. Trop. Med. Hyg. 74:427, 1980.
2. Adam, A.: Über die Biologie der Dyspepsi coli und ihre Beziehungen zur Pathogenese der Dyspepsi und Intoxikation. db. Kindh. 101:295, 1923.
2a. Anders, B. J., Lauer, B. A., and Paisley, J. W.: Campylobacter gastroenteritis in neonates. Am. J. Dis. Child. 135:900, 1981.
2b. Anders, B., Lauer, B. A., Paisley, J. W., and Retter, L. B.: Double-blind placebo-controlled trial of erythromycin for treatment of Campylobacter. Lancet 1:131, 1982.
3. Anonymous: Bacid, Lactinex and yogurt. Med. Lett. Drug Ther. 14:59, 1972.
4. Anonymous: Antibiotic diarrhea. Br. Med. J. 4:243, 1975.
5. Aust, C. H., and Smith, E. B.: Whipple's disease in a 3 month old infant. Am. J. Clin. Pathol. 37:66, 1962.
6. Bank, S., Trey, C., Gans, I., Marks, I. N., and Groll, A.: Histoplasmosis of the small bowel with "giant" intestinal villi and secondary protein losing enteropathy. Am. J. Med. 39:492, 1965.
7. Barber, M. A.: Milk poisoning due to a type of *Staphylococcus albus* occurring in the udder of a healthy cow. Phillips J. Sci. 9:515, 1914.
8. Barbezat, G. O.: Stimulation of intestinal secretion by polypeptide hormones. Scand. J. Gastroenterol. 88 (Suppl.) 22, 1972.
9. Barnes, G. L., and Kay, R.: Blood groups in giardiasis. Lancet 1:808, 1977.
9a. Baron, R., Murphy, F., Greenberg, H., Davis, C., Bregman, D., Gary, G., Hughes, J., and Schonberger, C.: Norwalk gastrointestinal illness. Am. J. Epidemiol. 115:163, 1982.
10. Bartlett, J. G., Chang, T. W., Gorwith, M., et al.: Antibiotic associated pseudomembranous colitis due to toxin-producing clostridium. N. Engl. J. Med. 298:531, 1978.
11. Bartlett, J. G., Moon, N., Chang, T. V., et al.: Role of *Clostridium difficile* in antibiotic asso-

ciated pseudomembranous colitis. Gastro-enterology 75:778, 1978.

12. Bass, J. W., Crowley, D. M., Stelle, R. W., et al.: Adverse reactions of orally administered ampicillin. J. Pediatr., 83:106, 1973.

12a. Batts, D. H., Martin, D., Holmes, R., Silva, J., and Fekety, R.: Treatment of antibiotic-associated *Clostridium difficile* diarrhea with vancomycin. J. Pediatr. 97:151, 1980.

13. Bayless, T. M., Swanson, V., and Wheby, M. S.: Jejunal histology and clinical status in tropical sprue and other chronic diarrheal disorders. Am. J. Clin. Nutr. 24:112, 1971.

13a. Besterman, H. S.: Gut hormones in tropical malabsorption. Br. Med. J. 2:1252, 1979.

14. Binder, H., and Powell, D. M.: Bacterial enterotoxins and diarrhea. Am. J. Clin. Nutr. 23:1582, 1970.

15. Binder, H.: Net fluid and electrolyte secretion: The pathophysiological basis of diarrhea. Viewpoints Dig. Dis. 12:2, 1980.

16. Bishop, R. F., Davidson, G. P., and Holmes, T. H.: Virus particles in epithelial cells of duodenal mucosa from children with acute nonbacterial gastroenteritis. Lancet 2:1281, 1973.

17. Bisset, M. L.: *Yersinia enterocolitica* isolates from humans in California, 1968–1975. J. Clin. Microbiol. 4:137, 1976.

18. Blacklow, N. R., Echeveria, P., and Smith, D. H.: Serological studies with reovirus-like enteritis agent. Infect. Immun. 13:1563, 1976.

19. Block, R. E., Jackson, R. J., Tsai, T., et al.: Epidemic *Yersinia enterocolitica* infection due to contaminated chocolate milk. N. Engl. J. Med. 298:76, 1978.

20. Bohnhoff, M., Miller, C. P., and Martin, W. R.: Resistance of the mouse's intestinal tract to experimental *Salmonella* infection I. Factors which interfere with the initiation of infection by oral inoculation. J. Exp. Med. 120:805, 1964.

21. Bradford, W. D., Noce, P. S., Gutman, G. T., et al.: Pathologic features of enteric infection with *Yersinia enterocolitica*. Arch. Pathol. 98:17, 1974.

21a. Brook, I.: *Clostridium difficile* and diarrhea. Pediatrics 65:1154, 1980.

22. Burke, J. A.: Giardiasis in childhood. Am. J. Dis. Child. 129:1304, 1975.

23. Burke, J. A.: Strongyloidiasis in childhood. Am. J. Dis. Child. 132:1130, 1978.

24. Burke, V., Gracey, M., Suharyono, S., and Sienoto, M. D.: Reduction by aspirin of intestinal fluid loss in acute childhood gastroenteritis. Lancet 1:1329, 1980.

24a. Burke, V., Robinson, J., Berry, R. J., and Gracey, M.: Detection of enterotoxins of *Aeromonas hydrophilia* by a suckling mouse test. Med. Microbiol. 14:401, 1981.

25. Cadranel, S., Rodesch, P., Butzler, J. P., and Dekeyser, P.: Enteritis due to "related Vibrio" in children. Am. J. Dis. Child. 126:152, 1973.

26. Carpenter, C. C. J.: Treatment of cholera: tradition and authority versus science, reason and humanity. Johns Hopkins Med. J. 139:153, 1976.

27. Carpenter, C. C. J., Monda, A., Sock, R. B., et al.: Clinical studies in cholera. Bull. Johns Hopkins Hosp. 118:174, 1966.

27a. Champsaur, H., Andremont, A., Mathieu, D., Rottman, E., and Auzepy, P.: Cholera-like illness due to *Aeromonas sobria*. J. Infect. Dis. 145:248, 1982.

28. Chandra, R. K.: Immunological aspects of human milk. Nutr. Rev. 36:265, 1978.

29. Chen, W. J., Chen, K. M., and Lin, M.: Colon perforation in amebiasis. Arch. Surg. 103:676, 1971.

29a. Cherry, R., Portnoy, D., Jabbari, M., Daly, D., Kinnear, D., and Goresky, C.: Metronidazole: An alternative therapy for antibiotic-associated colitis. Gastroenterology 82:849, 1982.

30. Chien, L., Robertson, H., and Gerrard, J. W.: Infantile gastroenteritis due to water with high sulfate content. Can. Med. Assoc. J. 99:102, 1968.

31. Chu, W., Chen, P., Huang, C., and Hsu, C.: Neonatal ascariasis. J. Pediatr. 81:783, 1972.

31a. Clausen, C., and Christie, D.: Chronic diarrhea in infants caused by adherent enteropathogenic *E. coli*. J. Pediatr. 100:358, 1982.

32. Cohen, S. A., Hendricks, K. M., Eastham, E. J., et al.: Chronic nonspecific diarrhea: A complication of dietary fat restriction. Am. J. Dis. Child. 133:490, 1979.

33. Cohen, S. A., Hendricks, K. M., Mathis, R. K., et al.: Chronic nonspecific diarrhea: dietary relationships. Pediatrics 64:402, 1979.

33a. Colgan, T., Lambert, J. R., Newman, A., and Luk, S. C.: Campylobacter jejunienterocolitis; A clinicopathologic study. Arch. Pathol. Lab. Med. 104:571, 1980.

34. Collins, D. C.: Histoplasmosis and the gastroenterologist. Am. J. Gastroenterol. 27:251, 1957.

35. Collins, R. N., Treger, M. D., Goldsby, J. B., Boring, J. R., III, Coohon, D. B., and Barr, R. N.: Interstate outbreak of *Salmonella* New Brunswick infection traced to powdered milk. J.A.M.A. 203:838, 1968.

36. Conrad, M.: Hematologic manifestations of parasitic infections. Semin. Hematol. 8:267, 1971.

37. Cowen, A. E., and Campbell, C. B.: Giardiasis — a cause of vitamin B_{12} malabsorption. Am. J. Dig. Dis. 18:384, 1973.

38. Cramblett, H. G., Azimi, P., and Haynes, R. E.: The etiology of infectious diarrhea in infancy with special reference to enteropathogenic *E. coli*. Ann. N.Y. Acad. Sci. 176:80, 1971.

39. Cruz, T., Reboucas, G., and Rocha, H.: Fatal strongyloidiasis in patients receiving corticosteroids. N. Engl. J. Med. 275:1093, 1966.

39a. Cumberbatch, N., Gurwith, M., Langston, C., Sack, R. B., and Brunton, J. L.: Cytotoxic enterotoxin produced by *Aeromonas hydrophilia*: Relationship of toxigenic isolates to diarrheal disease. Infect. Immun. 23:829, 1979.

40. Cummings, J. H.: Laxative abuse. Gut 15:758, 1974.

41. Dack, G. M., and Petran, E.: Bacterial activity in different levels of intestine and in isolated

segments of small and large bowel in monkeys and in dogs. J. Infect. Dis. *54*:204, 1934.

42. David, C., and Tolaymat, A.: Typhoid fever: unusual presentation. J. Pediatr. *93*:533, 1978.

43. Davidson, G. P., and Barnes, G. L.: Structural and functional abnormalities of the small intestine in infants and young children with rotavirus enteritis. Acta Paediatr. Scand. *68*:181, 1979.

44. Davidson, M., Sleisenger, M. H., Almy, T. P., and Levine, S. Z.: Studies of distal colonic motility in children. II. Propulsive activity in diarrheal states. Pediatrics *17*:820, 1956.

45. Davidson, M.: Irritable colon in children. *In* Sleisenger, M. H., and Fordtran, J. S., (eds.): Gastrointestinal Disease. Philadelphia, W. B. Saunders Company, 1973, pp. 1289–1295.

46. Delorme, J., Laverdiere, M., Martineau, B., and Lafleur, L.: Yersiniosis in children. Can. Med. Assoc. J. *110*:281, 1974.

46a. Dobbins, W. O., III: Current concepts of Whipple's disease. J. Clin. Gastroenterol. *4*:205, 1982.

47. Dobbins, W. O., III, and Kawanishi, H.: Bacillary characteristics in Whipple's disease: an electron microscopic study. Gastroenterology *80*:1468, 1981.

48. Donaldson, R. M.: Normal bacterial populations of the intestine and their relation to intestinal function. N. Engl. J. Med. *270*:938, 994, 1050, 1964.

48a. Donata, S., and Meyers, M.: *Clostridium difficile* toxin in asymptomatic neonates. J. Pediatr. *100*:431, 1982.

49. DuPont, H., Foronal, S., Hornick, R. B., Snyder, M., Libonati, J. P., Sheahan, D., LaBrec, E., and Kalas, J.: Pathogenesis of *Escherichia coli* diarrhea. N. Engl. J. Med. *285*:773, 1971.

50. Dykes, A. C., Ruebush, T. K., Gorelkin, L., Lushbaugh, W. B., Upshur, J. K., and Cherry, J. D.: Extraintestinal amebiasis in infancy: Report of three patients and epidemiologic investigations of their families. Pediatrics *65*:799, 1980.

51. Echeverria, P., Chang, C. P., and Smith, D.: Enterotoxigenicity and invasive capacity of "enteropathologenic" serotypes of *Escherichia coli*. J. Pediatr. *89*:8, 1976.

52. Eras, P., Goldstein, M. J., and Sherlock, P.: Candida infection of the gastrointestinal tract. Medicine *51*:367, 1972.

53. Ericsson, C. D., Evans, D. G., DuPont, H. L., Evans, D. J., Jr., and Pickering, L. K.: Bismuth subsalicylate inhibits activity of crude toxins of *Escherichia coli* and *Vibrio cholerae*. J. Infect. Dis. *136*:693, 1977.

54. Fallett, S., MacKenzie, C., Middleton, P., et al.: Clinical, laboratory and epidemiologic features of a viral gastroenteritis in infants and children. Pediatrics *60*:217, 1977.

55. Fenner, F., McAuslan, B. R., Minis, C. A., et al.: The Biology of Animal Viruses. Ed. 2. New York, Academic Press, 1974, p. 340.

56. Fleisher, D., and Ament, M. E.: Diarrhea, red diapers, and child abuse. Clin. Pediatr. *17*:820, 1977.

57. Formal, S. B., Genski, P., Giarella, R. A., and Takeuchi, A.: Studies in the pathogenesis of enteric infections due to invasive bacteria. *In* Ciba Symposium on Diarrhea in Childhood. Amsterdam Associated Scientific Publishers, 1976.

57a. Fried, D., Maytal, J., and Hanukoglu, A.: The differential leukocyte count in shigellosis. Infection *10*:13, 1982.

58. Fubura, E. S., and Freter, R.: Protection against enteric bacterial infections by SIgA. J. Immunol. *111*:395, 1973.

59. Gaginella, T. S., and Bass, P.: Laxatives: an update on mechanism of action. Life Sci. *23*:1001, 1978.

60. Gall, D. G., and Hamilton, J. R.: Chronic diarrhea in childhood: A new look at an old problem. Pediatr. Clin. North Am. *21*:1001, 1974.

61. Gemski, P., Jr., Takeuchi, A., Washington, O., et al.: Shigellosis due to *Shigella dysenteriae*. I. Relative importance of mucosal invasion versus toxin production in pathogenesis. J. Infect. Dis. *126*:523, 1972.

62. George, W. L., Sutter, V. L., and Finegold, S. M.: Antimicrobial agent-induced diarrhea — a bacterial disease. J. Infect. Dis. *136*:822, 1977.

63. George, W. L., Rolfe, R. D., and Finegold, S. M.: Therapeutic implications of *Clostridium difficile* toxin during relapse of chronic inflammatory bowel disease. Lancet *1*:381, 1980.

64. George, W. L., Rolfe, R. U., and Finegold, S. M.: Treatment and prevention of antimicrobial agent–induced colitis and diarrhea. Gastroenterology *79*:366, 1980.

65. Geppert, L. J., Baker, H. J., Copple, B., and Pulaski, E.: Pseudomonas infection in infants and children. J. Pediatr. *41*:555, 1952.

66. Giannella, R. A.: Importance of the intestinal inflammatory reaction in Salmonella mediated intestinal secretion. Infect. Immun. *23*:140, 1979.

67. Giannella, R. A., Broitman, S. A., and Zamchek, N.: The gastric barrier to microorganisms in man: in vivo and in vitro studies. Gut *13*:251, 1972.

68. Giannella, R. A., Broitman, S. A., and Zamcheck, N.: Influence of gastric acidity on bacterial and parasitic enteric infections: a perspective. Ann. Intern. Med. 78:271, 1973.

69. Giannella, R. A., Formal, S. B., Darmin, G. S., and Collins, H.: Pathogenesis of salmonellosis: studies of fluid secretion, mucosal invasion and morphologic reaction in the rabbit ileum. J. Clin. Invest. *52*:441, 1973.

70. Giannella, R. A., Gota, R. E., Charney, A. N., et al.: Pathogenesis of salmonella-mediated intestinal fluid secretion: Activation of adenyl glucose and inhibition of indomethacin. Gastroenterology 68:1238, 1975.

71. Giannella, R. A., Ront, W. R., and Formal, S. B.: Effect of indomethacin on intestinal water transport in salmonella infected rhesus monkeys. Infect. Immun. *17*:136, 1977.

72. Goldberg, S., Shales, W., and Mintzer, S.: A clinical report on amebiasis in infants under one year of age. J. Pediatr. *40*:290, 1952.

73. Goldman, M.: Identification and diagnosis of *En-*

tamoeba histolytica. Am. J. Gastroenterol. *41*:362, 1964.

74. Goldsmid, J. M., and Saunders, C. R.: Pyrantel pamoate for human hookworm infection. S. Afr. Med. J. *47*:205, 1973.

75. Goodwin, R. A., Jr., and Des Prez, R.: Pathogenesis and clinical spectrum of histoplasmosis. South. Med. J. *66*:13, 1973.

76. Gorbach, S. L., Kean, B. H., Evans, D. G., et al.: Traveler's diarrhea and toxigenic *E. coli.* N. Engl. J. Med. *792*:933, 1975.

77. Gordon, D., Macreae, J., and Wheaten, D. M.: A lactobacillus preparation for use with antibiotics. Lancet *1*:899, 1957.

77a. Gracey, M., Burke, V., Rockhill, R. C., and Sunoto, S.: *Aeromonas* species as enteric pathogens. Lancet *1*:223, 1982.

78. Greco, R.: Anal stricture following pseudomonas sepsis. J. Pediatr. Surg. *13*:91, 1978.

79. Gryboski, J. D.: Diarrhea from dietetic candies. N. Engl. J. Med. *275*:718, 1966.

80. Gryboski, J. D.: Diarrhea and malabsorptive disorders of the small bowel. *In* Gryboski, J.: Gastrointestinal Problems of the Infant. Philadelphia, W. B. Saunders Company, 1975, pp. 565–684.

81. Gryboski, J. D., and Hillemeier, A. C.: Chronic diarrhea in childhood. Kalamazoo, Mich., Upjohn Company, 1982.

82. Guerrant, R. L., Lahita, R. G., Wiran, W. C., Jr., and Roberts, R.: Campylobacteriosis in man: pathogenic mechanisms and review of 91 blood stream infections. Am. J. Med. *65*:584, 1978.

83. Guiterrez, Y., Buchino, J., and Schubert, W.: Mesocystoides (cestoda) infection in children in the United States. J. Pediatr. *93*:245, 1978.

84. Gutman, R. A., Drutz, D. J., Whalen, G., and Watten, R.: Double blind fluid therapy evaluation in pediatric cholera. Pediatrics *44*:922, 1969.

85. Haltalin, K. C.: Neonatal shigellosis. Am. J. Dis. Child. *114*:602, 1967.

86. Hardison, W. G. M., and Rosenberg, I. H.: The effect of neomycin on bile salt metabolism and fat digestion in man. Lab. Clin. Med. *74*:564, 1969.

87. Heber, J. P., Shelton, S., Nelson, J. D., et al.: Comparison of human rotavirus disease in tropical and temperate setting. Am. J. Dis. Child. *52*:482, 1977.

88. Heyworth, B., and Brown, J.: Jejunal microflora in malnourished Gambian children. Arch. Dis. Child. *50*:29, 1975.

89. Hofmann, A. F.: Bile acids, diarrhea and antibiotics. Data, speculation and a unifying hypothesis. J. Infect. Dis. *135*:5126, 1977.

90. Hofmann, A. F., Bokkenheuser, V., Hirsch, R. L., and Mosbach, E. H.: Experimental cholelithiasis in the rabbit induced by cholestanol feeding: effect of neomycin treatment on bile composition and gallstone formation. J. Lipid Res. *9*:244, 1968.

91. Holgren, J., and Svennerholm, A. M.: Mechanisms of disease and immunity in cholera. A review. J. Infect. Dis. *136*:S105, 1977.

92. Hollander, M., Tabingo, R., and Stankiewick, W.

R.: Successful treatment of massive intestinal hemorrhage due to hookworm infection in a neonate. J. Pediatr. *82*:332, 1973.

93. Hornick, R. B., Music, S. I., Wenzel, R., et al.: The Broad Street pump revisited; response of volunteers to ingested cholera vibrios. Bull. N.Y. Acad. Med. *47*:1181, 1971.

94. Hornick, R. B., Greisman, S. E., Woodward, T. E., DuPont, H., Dawkins, A., and Snyder, M.: Typhoid fever: pathogenesis and immunologic control. N. Engl. J. Med. *283*:739, 1970.

95. Horowitz, M. A.: Specific diagnosis of foodborne disease. Gastroenterology *73*:375, 1977.

95a. Hyam, S. J., Krause, P., and Gleason, P.: Lactose malabsorption following rotavirus infection in young children. J. Pediatr. *99*:916, 1981.

96. Iams, A., Tenen, M., and Flanagan, H. F.: Histoplasmosis in children. Am. J. Dis. Child. *70*:229, 1945.

97. Jaffe, B. M., Kopen, D. F., DeSchryver-Kecskemeti, K., Gingerich, R. L., and Greider, M.: Indomethacin responsive pancreatic cholera. New Engl. J. Med. *297*: 817, 1977.

97a. Jalili, F., Fraley, J. K., Smith, E., Nichols, V., Klein, E., Mintz, A., and Nichols, B.: Malnutrition in infants with acute diarrheal syndrome. J. Pediatr. Gastroenterol. Nutr. *1*:219, 1982.

98. Jones, E. S., Orcutt, M., and Little, R. B.: Vibrios (Vibrio jejuni n. sp.) associated with intestinal disorders of cows and calves. J. Exp. Med. *53*:853, 1931.

99. Jones, S., Brennan, M., and Kundsin, R.: Candida serology: an aid in the diagnosis of deep organ candidiasis. J. Surg. Res. *14*:235, 1973.

100. Kamath, K. R., and Murugasu, R.: A comparative study of four methods for detecting *Giardia lamblia* in children with diarrheal disease and malabsorption. Gastroenterology *66*:16, 1974.

101. Kapikian, A. Z., Kim, H. W., Wyatt, R. G., et al.: Human reovirus-like agent as the major pathogen associated with winter gastroenteritis in hospitalized infants and young children. N. Engl. J. Med. *244*:965, 1976.

102. Kapikian, A. Z., Wyatt, R. G., Dolin, R., et al.: Visualization by immune electron microscopy of a 27 mm particle associated with acute infectious nonbacterial gastroenteritis. J. Virol. *10*:1075, 1972.

103. Karmali, M. A., and Fleming, P. C.: Campylobacter enteritis in children. J. Pediatr. *94*:527, 1979.

104. Katz, M.: Three serious parasitic infections often missed in clinical practice. Postgrad. Med. *58*:149, 1975.

105. Kauffman, A., Feeley, C., and DeWitt, W.: Salmonella excretion by turtles. Public Health Rep. *82*:840, 1967.

106. Kazemi, M., Gumpert, T., and Marks, M.: A controlled trial comparing sulfamethoxazole-trimethoprim, ampicillin and no therapy in the treatment of *Salmonella* gastroenteritis. J. Pediatr. *83*:646, 1973.

106a. Kelly, M. T., Peterson, J. W., Saries, H. E., Jr.,

Romanko, M., Martin, D., and Hafkin, B.: Cholera on the Texas gulf coast. JAMA *247*: 1598, 1982.

107. Kent, T. H., Formal, S. B., and LaBrec, E. H.: Acute enteritis due to *Salmonella typhimurium* in opium-treated guinea pigs. Arch. Pathol. *81*:501, 1966.

108. Kerzner, B., Kelly, M. H., Gall, D. G., Butler, D. G., and Hamilton, J. R.: Transmissible gastroenteritis sodium transport and the intestinal epithelium during the course of viral enteritis. Gastroenterology *72*:457, 1977.

109. Keusch, G. T.: Ecological control of the bacterial diarrheas: A scientific strategy. Am. J. Clin. Nutr. *31*:2208, 1978.

110. Keusch, G., Grady, G., Takeuchi, A., and Sprinz, H.: The pathogenesis of Shigella diarrhea. II. Enterotoxin induced acute enteritis in the rabbit ileum. J. Infect. Dis. *126*:92, 1972.

111. Klipstein, F., Holderman, L., Corino, J., and Moore, W. E.: Enterotoxigenic intestinal bacteria in tropical sprue. Ann. Intern. Med. *79*:632, 1973.

112. Klystem, F. A., and Eugent, R. F.: Purification and properties of *Klebsiella pneumoniae* heat stable enterotoxin. Infect. Immun. *13*:373, 1976.

113. Kohl, S.: *Yersinia enterocolitica* infections in children. Pediatr. Clin. North Am. *26*:433, 1979.

114. Konno, T., Suzuki, H., Imai, A., and Tshida, N.: Reovirus-like agent in acute gastroenteritis in Japanese infants; fecal shedding and serologic response. J. Infect. Dis. *135*:259, 1977.

115. Kotcher, E., Miranda, M., and Garcia de Salgado, V.: Correlation of clinical parasitological and serological data of individuals infected with *Entamoeba histolytica*. Gastroenterology *58*:388, 1970.

116. Kozinn, P. J., and Taschdjian, C. L.: Enteric candidiasis: diagnosis and clinical considerations. Pediatrics *30*:71, 1962.

117. Kozinn, P. J., and Taschdjian, C. L.: Enteric candidiasis: diagnosis and clinical considerations. Pediatrics *42*:1529, 1968.

118. Krogstad, D. J., Spencer, H. C., and Healy, G. R.: Current concepts in parasitology: Amebiasis. N. Engl. J. Med. *298*:262, 1978.

118a. Kwito, A., Shearman, D., McKenzie, P., LaBrooy, J., Rowland, R., and Woodroff, A.: Whipple's disease: A case with circulating immune complexes. Gastroenterology *79*:1318, 1980.

119. Lamanna, C., and Carr, C. J.: The botulinal, tetanal and enterostaphylococcal toxins: a review. Clin. Pharmacol. Therapeut. *8*:286, 1967.

120. Larcher, V. F., Sheperd, R., Francis, D. E. M., and Harries, J. T.: Protracted diarrhea in infancy. Arch. Dis. Child. *52*:597, 1977.

121. Lebenthal, E., and Lee, P. C.: Glucoamylase and disaccharidase activities in normal subjects and in patients with mucosal injury of the small intestine. J. Pediatr. *97*:389, 1980.

121a. Leung, F. Y. K., Littlejohn, G. O., and Bombadier, C.: Reiter's syndrome after *Campylobacter jejuni* enteritis. Arth. Rheum. *23*:948, 1980.

122. Levine, M. M., DuPont, H. L., Formal, S. B., et al.: Pathogenesis of *Shigella dysenteriae* I (Shiga) dysentery. J. Infect. Dis. *127*:261, 1973.

123. L'Hirondel, J.:. La diarrhee commune de la année de la vie. Quest Med. *31*:473, 1978.

124. Liebman, W. M., Thaler, M. M., DeLorimier, A., Brandborg, L. L., and Goodman, J.: Intractable diarrhea of infancy due to intestinal coccidiosis. Gastroenterology *78*:579, 1980.

125. Lindenbaum, J. L.: Tropical enteropathy. Gastroenterology *64*:637, 1973.

126. Lloyd-Still, J. D.: Chronic diarrhea of childhood and the misuse of elimination diets. J. Pediatr. *95*:10, 1979.

127. Lopes, V. M., Reis, D. D., and Cunha, A. B.: Islet-cell adenoma of the pancreas with reversible watery diarrhea and hypokalemia. Am. J. Gastroenterol. *53:17*, 1970.

127a. Loss, R. W., Mangla, J., and Pereira, M.: Campylobacter colitis presenting as inflammatory bowel disease with segmental chronic ulcerations. Gastroenterology *79*:138, 1980.

128. MacFaydean, F., and Stockman, S.: Final Report of the Departmental Committee Appointed by the Board of Agriculture and Fisheries to Inquire into Epizootic Abortion. III. Abortion in Sheep. London, His Majesty's Stationery Office, 1913.

129. MacLean, W. C., Jr., Klein, G. L., Lopez de Romana G., Massa, E., and Graham, G. G.: Transient steatorrhea following episodes of mild diarrhea in early infancy. J. Pediatr. *92*:562, 1978.

129a. Maki, M.: A prospective clinical study of rotavirus diarrhea in young children. Acta Paediatr. *70*:107, 1981.

129b. March, P., Helm, I., Colleen, I., Oberg, M., and Holst, E.: *Clostridium difficile* toxin in faecal specimens of healthy children and children with diarrhea. Acta Paediatr. Scand. *71*:275, 1982.

130. Marks, M. I., Pai, C. H., Lafleur, L., et al.: *Yersinia enterocolitica* gastroenteritis: A prospective study of clinical, bacteriologic and epidemiologic features. J. Pediatr. *96*:26, 1980.

131. Marsden, D. D. (ed.): Intestinal parasites. Clin. Gastroenterol. *7*:1, 1978.

132. Maynell, G. G.: Antibacterial mechanisms of the mouse gut. II. The role of Eh and volatile fatty acids in the normal gut. Br. J. Exp. Pathol. *44*:109, 1963. Cited in Keusch: N. Engl. J. Med. *285*:900, 1971.

133. Mehta, S., Vishwanath, M. V., Khurana, K., and Chuttani, P. N.: Vitamin B_{12} and folic acid status in tropical sprue. Indian J. Med. Res. *59*:265, 1971.

134. Menéndez-Corrada, R.: Current views on tropical sprue and a comparison to nontropical sprue. Med. Clin. North Am. *52*:1367, 1968.

135. Mills, J., Orenstein, W., and Cohen, S.: Enteritis associated with pneumococci. Am. J. Dis. Child. *126*:244, 1973.

136. Moon, H. W., Nagy, B., and Isaacson, R. E.: Intestinal colonization and adhesion by enterotoxigenic *Escherichia coli*: Ultrastructu-

ral observations on adherence to ileal epithelium of the pig. J. Infect. Dis. *136*:5124, 1977.

137. Morris, A. I., and Turnberg, L. A.: Surreptitious laxative abuse. Gastroenterology 77:780, 1979.

137a. Nagel, P., Serritella, A., and Layden, T.: *Edwardsiella tarda* gastroenteritis associated with a pet turtle. Gastroenterology 82:1436, 1982.

138. Nelson, J. D.: Antibiotic therapy for Salmonella syndromes. Am. J. Dis. Child. *135*:1093, 1981.

139. Nuzum, C. T., Sandler, R. S., and Paulk, T.: Thrombocytosis in Whipple's disease. Gastroenterology *80*:1465, 1981.

140. Owen, R. L.: The ultrastructural basis of *Giardia* function. Trans. Royal Soc. Trop. Med. Hyg. 74:429, 1980.

141. Owen, R. L., Nemanic, P. C. and Stevens, D. P.: Ultrastructural observations on *Giardia* in a murine model. I. Intestinal distribution, attachment and relationship to the immune system of *Giardia lamblia*. Gastroenterology 76:757, 1979.

142. Pai, C. H., Sorger, S., Larckman, L., Sinai, R. E., and Marks, M. I.: *Campylobacter* gastroenteritis in children. J. Pediatr. 94:589, 1979.

143. Paolini, G., and Wittenberg, J.: Intestinal capillariasis. Am. J. Roentgenol. Radium Ther. Nucl. Med. *117*:340, 1973.

144. Phillips, J. A., Lovejoy, F. H., Jr., and Matsumiya, Y.: Ampicillin-associated diarrhea. Effect of dosage and route of administration. Pediatrics 58:869, 1976.

145. Pittman, F., El-Hashimi, W., and Pittman, J. C.: Studies of human amebiasis. Gastroenterology 65:581, 1973.

146. Poh, S.: Shigellosis; a clue to early diagnosis. Pediatrics 39:119, 1967.

146a. Poley, J. A., and Rosenfield, S.: Malabsorption in giardiasis: Presence of a luminal barrier (mucoid pseudomembrane). A scanning and transmission electron microscope study. J. J. Pediatr. Gastroenterol. Nutr. *1*:63, 1982.

147. Reber, R. M., Davis, K., Eitzman, D., and Baer, H.: *Klebsiella pneumoniae* in a premature nursery. Letter to the Editor. J. Pediatr. 78:340, 1971.

147a. Rifkin, G., Silva, J., Jr., and Fekety, R.: Gastrointestinal and systemic toxicity of fecal extracts from hamsters with clindamycin-induced colitis. Gastroenterology 74:52, 1978.

148. Rosenthal, P., and Liebman, W. M.: Comparative study of stool examination, duodenal aspiration, and pediatric entero test for giardiasis in children. J. Pediatr. 96:278, 1980.

148a. Ross, I. N., and Mathan, V. I.: Immunologic changes in tropical sprue. Q. J. Med. *50*: 435, 1981.

149. Ross Laboratories Conference: Etiology, pathophysiology and treatment of acute gastroenteritis. Ross Laboratories, Columbus, Ohio, 1978.

150. Rout, W. R., Formal, S. B., and Gianella, R. N.: Pathophysiology of *Shigella* diarrhea in Rhesus monkeys. Gastroenterology 68:270, 1975.

151. Roy, C., and Silverman, A.: Pediatric Clinical Gastroenterology. St. Louis, The C. V. Mosby Company, 1975, pp. 195–197.

152. Sack, D. A., Islam, S., Brown, K. H., Islam, A., Kabir, A. K., Chowdhury, A. M., and Ali, M. A.: Oral therapy in children with cholera; a comparison of sucrose and glucose electrolyte solutions. J. Pediatr. 96:20, 1980.

153. Santiago-Borrero, P. J., and Maldonado, N.: The xylose excretion test in normal children and in pediatric patients with tropical sprue. Pediatrics 48:59, 1971.

154. Santiago-Borrero, P. J., Maldonado, N., and Horta, E.: Tropical sprue in children. J. Pediatr. 76:470, 1970.

155. Saunders, D. R., Sillery, J., and Rachmilewitz, D.: Effect of dioctyl sodium sulfosuccinate on structure and function of rodent and human intestine. Gastroenterology 69:380, 1975.

155a. Saulsbury, F., Winkelstein, J., and Yolken, R.: Chronic rotavirus infection in immunodeficiency. J. Pediatr. 97:61, 1980.

156. Schieven, B. C., and Randall, C.: Enteritis due to *Yersinia enterocolitica*. J. Pediatr. 84:402, 1977.

157. Schreiber, D. S., Blacklow, N. R., and Frier, J. S.: The mucosal lesion of the proximal small intestine in acute infectious nonbacterial gastroenteritis. N. Engl. J. Med. 288:1318, 1973.

158. Schreiber, D. S., Frier, J. S., and Blacklow, N. R.: Recent advances in viral gastroenteritis. Gastroenterology 73:174, 1977.

159. Shepherd, R. W., Butler, D. G., Cutz, E., et al.: The mucosal lesion in viral enteritis. Extent and dynamics of the epithelial response to virus invasion in transmissible gastroenteritis of piglets. Gastroenterology 76:770, 1979.

160. Shepherd, R. W., Gall, D. G.: Butler, D. G., and Hamilton, V. R.: Determinants of diarrhea in viral enteritis: The role of ion transport and epithelial changes in the ileum in transmissible gastroenteritis in piglets. Gastroenterology 76:20, 1979.

160a. Sheretz, R., and Sarubbi, F.: The prevalence of *Clostridium difficile* and toxin in a nursery population. A comparison between patients with necrotizing enterocolitis and an asymptomatic group. J. Pediatr. *100*:435, 1982.

161. Shurow, M. B.: *Campylobacter* enteritis. A "new" disease. Br. Med. J. 2:9, 1977.

162. Simko, V., McCarroll, A. M., Goodman, S., et al.: High fat diet in a short bowel syndrome. Intestinal absorption and gastroenteropancreatic hormone responses. Dig. Dis. Sci. 25:333, 1980.

163. Smith, E. R., and Goulston, S. J. M.: Antibiotic-induced diarrhea. Drugs *10*:329, 1975.

164. Smith, T.: *Spirella* associated with disease of the fetal membranes in cattle (infectious abortion). J. Exp. Med. 28:701, 1918.

165. Snodgrass, D. R., Ferguson, A., Frances, A., et al.: Intestinal morphology and epithelial cell kinetics in lamb rotavirus infections. Gastroenterology 76:477, 1979.

166. Soper, S. T., Siber, D., and Holcomb, G.: Gastrointestinal histoplasmosis in children. J. Pediatr. Surg. 5:40, 1970.

167. South, M. A.: Enteropathogenic *E. coli* disease:

new developments and perspectives. J. Pediatr. 79:1, 1971.

168. Spencer, M. J., Garcia, L. S., and Chapin, M. R.: *Dientamoeba fragilis*, intestinal pathogen in children. Am. J. Dis. Child. *133*:370, 1979.

169. Springer, G. F.: Importance of blood group substances in interactions between man and microbes. Ann. N.Y. Acad. Sci. *169*:134 1970.

169a. Stark, P. L., and Lee, A.: Clostridia isolated from the feces of infants during the first year of life. J. Pediatr. *100*:362, 1982.

170. Steinberg, S. E., Banwell, J. G., Yardley, J. H., Keusch, G. T., and Hendrix, T. R.: Comparison of secretory and histological effects of *Shigella* and cholera enterotoxins in rabbit jejunum. Gastroenterology 62:309, 1975.

171. Steinhoff, M. C.: Rotavirus: the first five years. J. Pediatr. 96:611, 1980.

171a. Steinhoff, M., Douglas, R. G., Jr., Greenberg, H., and Callahan, D.: Bismuth subsalicylate therapy of viral gastroenteritis. Gastroenterology 78:1495, 1980.

172. Tallett, S., Mackenzie, C., Middleton, P., Kerzner, B., and Hamilton, R.: Clinical, laboratory and epidemiologic features of a viral gastroenteritis in infants and children. Pediatrics 60:217, 1977.

173. Tedesco, F. J.: Ampicillin-associated diarrhea, a prospective study. Am. J. Dig. Dis. 20:295, 1975.

173a. Tedesco, F.: Bacitracin therapy in antibiotic-associated pseudomembranous colitis. Dig. Dis. Sci. 25:783, 1980.

174. Torres, P., Rivera, C., and Rodriquez, H.: Intestinal absorptive defects associated with enteric infections in infants. Ann. N.Y. Acad. Sci. *176*:284, 1971.

175. Totterdell, B. M., Chrystie, I. L., and Banatvala, J. E.: Rotavirus infections in a maternity unit. Arch. Dis. Child. *51*:924, 1976.

176. Tulloch, E., Ryan, K., Formal, S., and Franklin, F.: Invasive enteropathic *Escherichia coli* dysentery. Ann. Intern. Med. 79:13, 1973.

177. Ulshen, M. H., and Rollo, J. L.: Pathogenesis of *Escherichia coli* gastroenteritis in man; another mechanism. N. Engl. J. Med. *302*:99, 1980.

178. Valman, H. B., and Wilmers, M. J.: Use of antibiotics in acute gastroenteritis among infants in hospitals. Lancet *1*:1122, 1969.

179. Van Prohaska, J., Jacobson, M., Drake, C., and Tan, T.: Staphylococcus enterotoxin enteritis. Surg. Gynecol. Obstet. *109*:72, 1959.

180. Vantrappen, G., Agg, H. O., Ponette, S., et al.: *Yersinia* enteritis and enterocolitis: Gastroenterological aspects. Gastroenterology 72:220, 1977.

181. Von Reyn, C. F., Roberts, T. M., Owen, R., and Beaver, P. C.: Infection of an infant with an adult *Toxocara cati* (nematode). J. Pediatr. 93:247, 1978.

182. Walker, W. A.: Host defense mechanisms in the gastrointestinal tract. Pediatrics 57:901, 1976.

183. Walker-Smith, J. A., McMillan, B., Middleton, A. W., Robertson, S., and Hopcroft, A.: Strongyloidiasis causing small bowel obstruction in an aboriginal infant. Med. J. Aust. 2:1263, 1969.

183a. Welch, D., and Marks, M.: Is *Clostridium difficile* pathogenic to infants? J. Pediatr. *100*: 393, 1982.

184. Wijesudira, C., and Desilva, C.: Amebic perforation of the intestine in children. Pediatrics 30:937, 1962.

185. Williams, R. C., and Gibbons, R. J.: Inhibition of bacterial adherence by secretory immunoglobulin A: A mechanism of antigen disposal. Science *177*:697, 1972.

186. Williams-Smith, H., and Linggood, M. A.: Observations on the pathogenic properties of the K88 positive, Hly and EmT plasmids of *Escherichia coli* with particular reference to porcine diarrhea. J. Med. Microbiol. 4:467, 1971.

187. Wyatt, R. A., Younoszai, K., Anuras, S., et al.: *Campylobacter fetus* septicemia and hepatitis in a child with agammaglobulinemia. J. Pediatr. 91:441, 1977.

188. Yancey, R. J., and Berry, L. J.: Motility of the pathogen and intestinal immunity of the host in experimental cholera. Adv. Exp. Med. *107*:447, 1978.

189. Yardley, J. H., and Hendrix, T. R.: Combined electron and light microscopy in Whipple's disease. Johns Hopkins Med. J. *109*:80, 1961.

190. Yolken, R. H., Wyatt, R. G., Zissis, G., et al.: Epidemiology of human rotavirus types 1 and 2 as studied by enzyme-linked immunoabsorbent assay. N. Engl. J. Med. 299:1156, 1978.

Chapter Nineteen

INHERITED AND METABOLIC
DISORDERS OF ABSORPTION

Normal intestinal development and function are clearly critical to normal growth and development of the infant.[72, 117] While the emphasis of this chapter will be on disorders of the absorptive capacity of the small intestine, we must appreciate that the small bowel has many other critical functions, including the terminal digestion of nutrients at both the brush border and the intracellular level; the secretion of electrolytes, glycoproteins, hormones, and immunoglobulins; the regulation of protein, carbohydrate, lipid, vitamin and mineral metabolism via receptor; hormonal and enzyme feedback mechanisms; and the propulsion of luminal contents for excretion.[264] Functional distinctions often occur from one segment of bowel to another, and, within a segment, from crypt to villus epithelium.[12, 348]

Injury at any level of this dynamic process can produce significant malabsorption by reduction in surface area.[4, 85] Villus epithelial injury thus is seen in disorders like viral enteritis and gluten-sensitive enteropathy, while impaired crypt epithelial proliferation is the hallmark of radiation enteropathy, protein-calorie malnutrition, and some of the metabolic abnormalities.[308] Several excellent texts offer detailed discussions of the development and function of the absorptive processes, but in this section the major parameters will be discussed briefly under each topic.

INTRACTABLE DIARRHEA OF INFANCY

In 1968, Avery and his associates defined the clinical syndrome of "intractable diarrhea of infancy" as diarrhea of greater than two weeks' duration with an onset prior to three months of age and for which no microbial pathogen is identified. The progressive diarrhea in such infants fails to respond to routine dietary manipulation.[17A, 297]

Incidence. Intractable diarrhea may be the presentation of a number of primary disorders. As a result, incidence figures are difficult to determine. Recent reviews suggest that from four to ten such infants would be treated yearly at pediatric referral units.

Etiology. Protracted diarrhea may be the presentation of a number of primary disorders of the intestinal tract. These conditions, summarized in Table 19–1, share the capacity to develop a secretory diarrhea secondary to inflammation, metabolic error, or hormonally mediated secretion.[281]

In the majority of patients, no such primary disease is identified. Extensive workup will reveal villus injury with nonspecific inflammatory infiltration of the lamina propria of both small and large bowel. The pathogenesis of this "nonspecific enterocolitis" appears to be multifactorial, with a postulated schema depicted in Figure 19–1.

Table 19–1   Primary Disorders Presenting as Intractable Diarrhea

Anatomic Disorders
  Hirschsprung's disease
  Short bowel syndrome
  Lymphangiectasia
  Enteric stricture/malrotation
Inflammatory Disorders
  Infectious enteritis
  Entercolitis
    Necrotizing, ulcerative
    Pseudomembranous
  Protein-induced enteropathy
    gluten, milk, soy
  Eosinophilic gastroenteritis
  Extraintestinal: 1° UTI
Biochemical Disorders
  Acrodermatitis enteropathica
  Abetalipoproteinemia
  Chloride-losing diarrhea
  Pancreatic insufficiency
  Enterokinase deficiency
  Primary bile acid malabsorption
  Sucrase-isomaltase deficiency
Hormonal Disorders
  Adrenal insufficiency
  Thyrotoxicosis
  Neural crest tumors
Primary Immunodeficiency
  Thymic dysplasia
  Wiskott-Aldrich syndrome
  Severe combined immunodeficiency

The initial episode presents as a "routine" gastroenteritis that fails to resolve. Factors that potentially contribute to this failure include the severity of the insult, disaccharidase deficiency, immunodeficiency, primary bile acid malabsorption, and iatrogenic hypocaloric intake. The common pathway of the persistent diarrhea is villus epithelial injury, a process facilitated by inflammation and "therapeutic" fasting.

A secretory diarrheal state then develops secondary to inflammation and the malabsorption of endogenous bile acids and exogenous nutrients. The diarrhea thus becomes self-perpetuating.

Symptoms. The infant has a reduced rate of growth and a variable degree of dehydration. Emesis, fever, edema, and abdominal distention are frequently reported. In Table 19–2, we summarize a number of metabolic and absorptive abnormalities. The role for each of these as a primary or secondary event in nonspecific enterocolitis remains open to debate.

Diagnosis. The diagnostic evaluation of these infants is clearly geared to exclude primary disease states and to determine the severity of the villus injury. Stools are analyzed for polymorphonuclear cells, blood, pH, reducing sugars, and electrolyte content. Multiple specimens are analyzed for bacterial, viral, and parasitic pathogens. Blood studies include serum electrolytes, albumin, and a complete blood count. Urine is collected for culture and determination of electrolyte and and catecholamine levels. A sweat test is routinely performed. Anatomic lesions are excluded by barium enema, upper gastrointestinal series, and small bowel follow-through. Proctoscopy and rectal biopsy are often necessary to exclude a primary colitis or Hirschsprung's disease.

Abnormalities of D-xylose absorption and disaccharide tolerance are presumed, so these assays serve only as baseline evaluations. Confirmation of the degree of steatorrhea is often limited by inadequate fat intake. Lipid absorption studies may be done,

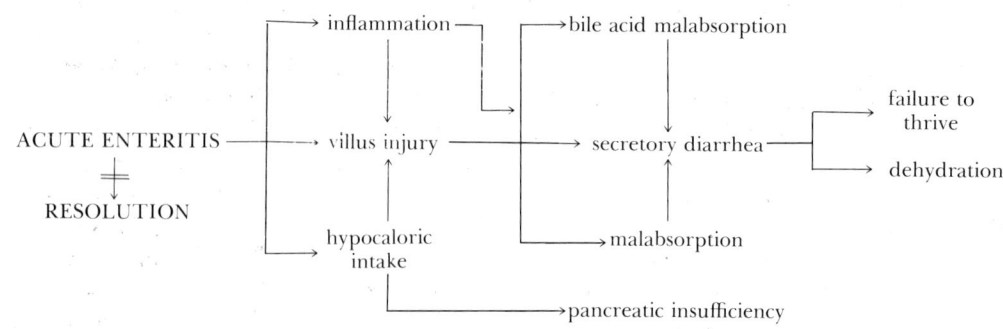

Figure 19–1   Pathophysiology of intractable diarrhea. (Adapted from Sunshine, P., Sinatra, F. R., and Mitchell, C. H.: Intractable diarrhea of infancy. Clin. Gastroenterol. 6:445, 1977.)

Table 19–2 Complications of
Intractable Diarrhea

Malnutrition
Hypoalbuminemia
Disaccharide intolerance
Monosaccharide intolerance
Essential fatty acid deficiency
Protein intolerance
Protein-losing enteropathy
Bile acid deconjugation/malabsorption
Renal tubular acidosis
Acquired immunodeficiency (T-cell)
Bacterial overgrowth
Sepsis

utilizing breath analysis after ingestion of ^{13}C-labeled lipid.

As small bowel biopsy will be "diagnostic" only for abetalipoproteinemia, lymphangiectasia, and Whipple's disease, the timing of jejunal biopsy varies from institution to institution. Demonstration of the flat villus lesion does not establish a "diagnosis," so we generally defer biopsy until dietary challenges can be undertaken. Duodenal intubation for *Giardia*, pancreatic stimulation, or culture is performed on an individual basis. Primary bile acid abnormalities also have been reported.

Treatment. Initial management of these infants addresses dehydration, electrolyte imbalance, and acidosis. Primary disorders receive appropriate specific therapy. Infants with nonspecific enterocolitis generally will require a period of venous alimentation; however, enteric feedings are resumed immediately so as to maximize mucosal regeneration. Feedings are initiated at 20 to 40 Cal/kg/day by continuous intragastric infusion, with fluid and additional caloric and electrolyte needs being met by vein. Enteric feedings are gradually increased; weight gain is generally demonstrated when caloric intakes of 140 to 160 Cal/kg/day are achieved. A number of lactose-free formulas have been suggested with Pregestimil, Portagen, or a modular product utilized in most studies. Lipid is delivered as a 40 to 80 per cent medium-chain triglyceride. When intake of essential fatty acids is delayed or deficiency is apparent at diagnosis, intravenous lipid emulsions are utilized. Supplementation with

trace elements and multivitamins is routine.

When diarrhea persists, anion-binding resins have been proposed to bind bile acids and microbial toxins. Cholestyramine, Amphojel, and Pepto-Bismol have been utilized with mixed success.[11, 12] Cholestyramine acts as a chloride donor, thus hyperchloremic acidosis may develop, especially in those infants who acquire renal tubular bicarbonate wasting. Patients on Pepto-Bismol require monitoring of salicylate levels. Corticosteroids, postulated to induce epithelial maturation, have not been demonstrated to be of long-term value. Prophylactic antibiotics should be avoided.

Prognosis. For the primary conditions listed in Table 19–1, the long-term prognosis is generally independent of the symptom of diarrhea. With nonspecific enterocolitis, mortality has decreased from greater than 40 per cent to 5 to 7 per cent in recent series — an improvement attributed to improved nutritional support. Long-term controlled studies of neurologic function have not been reported, though full recovery of intestinal and developmental capacity should be anticipated.

CARBOHYDRATE DIGESTION AND MALABSORPTION

Carbohydrate provides approximately 50 per cent of the caloric intake in infancy. The form of carbohydrate varies with the feeding regime, with breast milk and cow's milk products containing from 4.3 to 7.0 gm/per dl of lactose. Most meat and soy-base formulas contain equivalent amounts of sucrose and corn syrup solids. Pregestamil contains glucose and a glucose polymer, and Nutramigen contains primarily sucrose. Starches are present not only in infant cereals but also as stabilizers in all the commercial infant foods, in concentrations of 5 to 6 per cent.[196a]

The digestion of starch begins in the mouth with the action of salivary amylase and continues in the small intestine. The contribution of pancreatic amylase is low initially. Although the pancreas has been

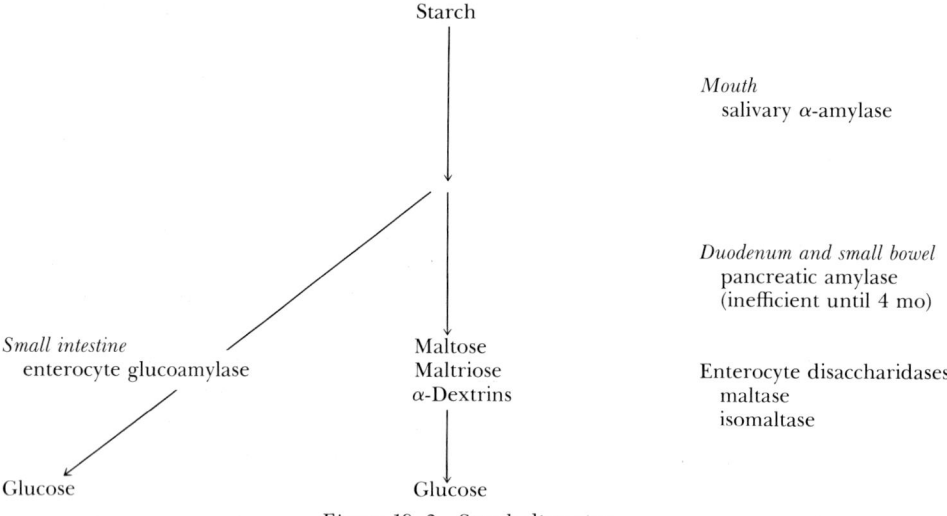

Figure 19–2   Starch digestion.

shown to contain amylase, it does not release it adequately until the infant is about four months of age. Levels in the term infant are 10 per cent of those of the adult, and no amylase has been detected in duodenal secretions of premature infants of from 32 to 34 weeks' gestation. Alpha-amylase has been demonstrated in preterm milk.[172a] The enzyme splits starches at the 1–4 bonds to form oligosaccharides and, when present, does increase in response to feedings. An alternative route for starch digestion is available to the infant in the enzyme glucoamylase, a small intestinal brush border enzyme that removes glucose units from the nonreducing ends of starch[197, 314] (Fig. 19–2).

Figure 19–3 is a summary of the mucosally derived oligosaccharidases responsible for the digestion of dietary carbohydrates.[198] These enzymes are located in the brush border glycocalyx to facilitate hydrolysis of the oligosaccharides to monosaccharides. The enzymes are large glycoproteins with molecular weights of approximately 250,000 daltons and half-lives of 4 to 16 hours. Their substrates, products of hydrolysis and normal levels as a function of age, are described in Tables 19–3 and 19–4.

Reductions in enzyme activity can be primary or acquired. In either case, disaccharidase deficiency is associated with

Table 19–3   Small Intestinal Surface Digestion of Carbohydrates

	MUCOSAL ENZYME	PRODUCTS
Lactose	Lactase	Glucose, galactose
Sucrose	Sucrase	Glucose, fructose
Maltose Maltotriose	Sucrase Glucoamylase	Glucose
α-Dextrins (glucose polymer)	Glucoamylase Isomaltase Sucrase	Oligosaccharide Glucose
Trehalose	Trehalase	Glucose

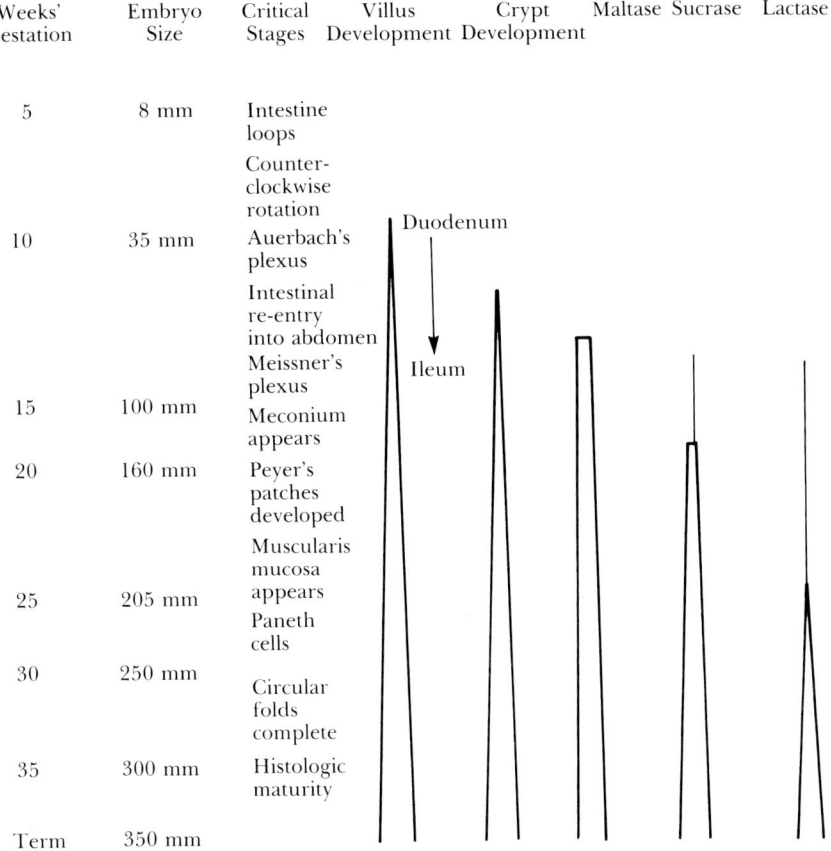

Weeks' Gestation	Embryo Size	Critical Stages	Villus Development	Crypt Development	Maltase	Sucrase	Lactase
5	8 mm	Intestine loops					
10	35 mm	Counter-clockwise rotation					
		Auerbach's plexus					
		Intestinal re-entry into abdomen					
		Meissner's plexus					
15	100 mm	Meconium appears					
20	160 mm	Peyer's patches developed					
		Muscularis mucosa appears					
25	205 mm	Paneth cells					
30	250 mm	Circular folds complete					
35	300 mm	Histologic maturity					
Term	350 mm						

Figure 19–3 Chronologic development of the embryonic small intestine.

an initial osmotic diarrhea, as the nonabsorbed carbohydrate induces an influx of water and electrolyte to produce a volume increase of 150 to 500 per cent and rapid transit through the small bowel. In the colon, not only are sodium and water reabsorption impaired, but also the residual disaccharide is fermented by colonic bacteria into lactic acid, acetic acid, and gas. These change the normally alkaline stool pH to

acid and produce a sour or vinegar-like odor of the stool. Normal stools contain no more than 35 mg of lactic acid, but in disaccharide malabsorption levels reach several grams.

With the exception of lactose, monosaccharide transport is the rate-limiting step in assimilation of carbohydrate. Glucose and galactose are transported into the epithelial cell via a sodium-activated system that is operational against a concentration gra-

Table 19–4 Disaccharidase Activity in the Fetus and Adult

	UNITS/GM PROTEIN			
		Fetus		
ENZYME	3–4 Mo	7–8 Mo	8–9 Mo.	Adult
Maltase	104	235	281	300–1200
Sucrase	40	91	101	70–325
Isomaltase	36	74	85	65–270
Trehalase	11	49	42	–
Lactase	5–9	20	20	39–258
Cellobiase	.88	4.7	4.3	9–21

dient. Fructose is transported separately by a sodium-independent facilitated diffusion.

Studies of intravenously administered disaccharides indicate that maltose is metabolized to carbon dioxide almost as completely as glucose, but lactose and sucrose are poorly oxidized and excreted in the urine.

A simple screening test for the presence of reducing substances in the stool uses the Clinitest tablet. One part of stool is mixed with two parts of water and centrifuged. Fifteen drops of the supernatant are placed in a test tube and a Clinitest tablet added.[182a] After the reaction has subsided, the tube is gently shaken and the color compared with that on the chart. Results are graded from 0 to 4+. Values greater than 1+ in infants over 15 days old suggest sugar malabsorption.[97] If a positive result is obtained, chromatographic or electrophoretic studies reveal the specific sugar responsible for the positive test (Fig. 19–4).[126, 127] Neonates frequently excrete some common oligosaccharides containing glucose, galactose, and fructose.[345a] The hydrogen breath test is now the accepted diagnostic tool. Patients fast for 6 to 8 hours, and breath samples are obtained at 0, 15, 30, 60, 90 and 120 minutes after ingestion of 2 gm per kg of disaccharide (maximum, 50 gm). A rise in hydrogen concentration of 10 or more parts per million over baseline indicates sugar malabsorption.[78a] A rise may not occur in patients in whom colonic flora have been altered by antibiotic therapy[165] or with delayed gastric emptying.

Disaccharide tolerance tests measure the rise in blood glucose after the ingestion of a sugar load. The fasting child drinks the sugar in a dosage of 2 gm per kg dissolved in several ounces of water. Capillary blood samples are taken at 0, 15, 30, 60, 90, and 120 minutes. The blood glucose peak appears between 15 and 60 minutes and is normally 20 mg per dl or more above the fasting level. A rise of less than 20 mg per dl suggests enzyme deficiency.[1] Clinical correlation is demonstrated by explosive diarrhea developing half an hour to 2 hours later. The tolerance test correlates with the patient's symptoms in 80 per cent of cases and with disaccharidase activity in 90 per

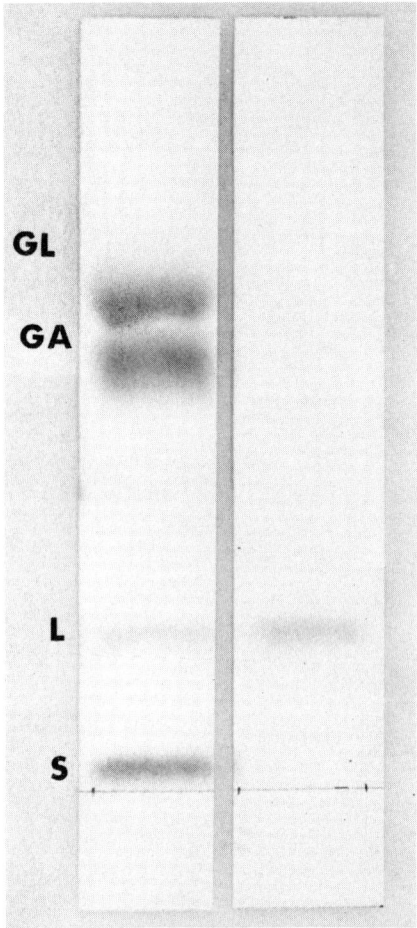

Figure 19–4 High-voltage paper electrophoresis of sugars from stool extract of an infant with lactose intolerance. Strip on the left contains standards, from top to bottom, of glucose, galactose, lactose and sucrose. Strip on the right contains stool extract containing lactose.

cent. An abnormal test must be followed by separate tolerance tests using component monosaccharides.

Direct assay of disaccharidase activity of duodenal or jejunal mucosa obtained through peroral biopsy techniques demonstrates diminished or absent enzyme activity. Despite normal variations of activity, constant ratios between the disaccharidases exist. Maltase activity is three to four times higher than sucrase and isomaltase; lactase, the most variable, is one to four times lower than sucrase or isomaltase.

Radiologic examination of the small bowel of these patients is normal except for rapid transit of barium. This is especially marked when lactose is added to barium given to the patient with lactose intolerance.

Histologically, the intestinal mucosa is usually normal in patients with primary disaccharide intolerance, but partial villous atrophy with normal surface epithelial cells has been noted in a few cases.

Lactase

Lactase is a β-galactosidase with highest activity in the jejunum. While enzyme activity can be demonstrated at 10 weeks of gestation, no significant increase in activity occurs until after 26 weeks of gestation.[17, 60] By 24 weeks, lactase activity is only about 30 per cent that found at term. Three separate lactase enzymes have been demonstrated. Enzyme I hydrolyzes lactose and cellobiose at an optimal pH of 6 and is located in the brush border. Enzyme II hydrolyzes lactose and synthetic substrate at an optimal pH of 4.5 and is lysozomal in location. Enzyme III hydrolyzes only the synthetic substrate at pH 6 and is cytoplasmic in location. Enzyme I is the major hydrolytic enzyme, with Enzyme II assuming increased activity in patients with lactose intolerance.[14, 119]

Under conditions of incomplete hydrolysis, the nonhydrolyzed lactose is fermented by enteric bacteria to produce volatile fatty acids, hydrogen gas, and lactic acid. A metabolic acidosis thus may ensue, even when normal blood sugar "tolerance" is demonstrated. Hydrogen gas production may lead to pneumatosis intestinalis. Breath hydrogen excretion will also be demonstrated, correlating with enteric lactase deficiency.

In the full-term neonate, the tolerance test may seem abnormal if one measures only blood glucose, but, if total reducing sugar is measured, the rise is normal and due to significant amounts of galactose. A normal blood glucose response is present after the first few days of life.

In the premature infant, lactase activity is decreased for two reasons: there is a shorter length of small bowel, and the enzyme does not develop maximally until the end of gestation.[215] Normal lactose tolerance tests have been reported in two-week-old premature infants, and there was no difference in the blood sugar response whether or not lactose had been fed in the diet before the test. However, despite a normal tolerance test, premature infants often develop metabolic acidosis within 15 minutes after loading. Blood pH, serum carbon dioxide, and chloride decrease, and the serum lactate and other organic anions increase. Not all the ingested disaccharide is metabolized, and the rapid formation of lactic acid in the bowel contributes to the acidosis.

Disacchariduria does not always indicate sugar intolerance, for during the first few weeks of life sugars are normally found in the stools and urine of young infants. Lactosuria has been reported in 28 to 50 per cent of full-term infants and in 46 to 65 per cent of premature infants. An acid stool pH and a strongly positive test for reducing sugars in the stool is not unusual during the first week of life. Glucose and galactose as well as lactose are found in the stool at this time. Stools from infants taking breast milk or breast milk–simulated formulas contain more sugar than those from infants taking evaporated milk formulas. Another sugar, lactulose, in which the glucose moiety of lactose has been converted to fructose during the commercial processing of the formula, is present in varying concentrations in formula, and since it is not acted upon by intestinal disaccharidases it often appears in infant urine and stool.

PRIMARY LACTOSE INTOLERANCE

Familial Lactose Intolerance

This is a rare and often fatal disease characterized by vomiting, failure to thrive, dehydration acidosis, disacchariduria, and aminoaciduria.

Incidence. The disease is extremely rare and is described primarily in the European literature.[31, 32, 66, 80, 81, 158]

Etiology. Inheritance is presumed to be of an autosomal recessive type. Parental consanguinity has not been established in any of the families, but siblings and other relatives were also affected. The disease was originally considered due to an intestinal enzyme deficiency, but when lactose tolerance tests were performed the results were normal. One infant studied in greater detail than the others had lactosuria and aminoaciduria after the oral feeding of lactose but not after its intraduodenal administration. Small intestine biopsy has shown normal morphology and disaccharidase activity. It is presumed that some defect localized to the stomach exists, which permits or causes the abnormal transport of lactose into the system.

Symptoms. Vomiting and failure to gain weight develop early in life. Vomiting appears after the first milk feeding or within the first two or three days of life. It follows every feeding and is not projectile. Physical examination is not remarkable early in the disease, although later severe emaciation develops. Renal tubular disease, central nervous system disorders, and convulsions develop, and even subdural hematoma may be noted. Later the vomiting becomes so severe and projectile that the infant is thought to have pyloric stenosis, although radiologic examination is usually normal. Lactosuria and generalized aminoaciduria are present in chromatographic studies of the urine. Sucrose administration is sometimes followed by sucrosuria.

Diagnosis. Pyloric stenosis must be ruled out. The diagnosis is suggested by the presence of lactosuria in the face of a normal lactose tolerance test but normal lactase activity, and disappearance of lactosuria if the sugar is administered into the duodenum.

Treatment. Elimination of lactose from the diet is therapeutic in many of the infants. Unfortunately, not all of them respond, and a number of those reported continued to vomit and eventually died.

Congenital Lactose Intolerance

Congenital lactose intolerance is a far more clear-cut entity. Diarrhea develops shortly after the initiation of milk feedings and varies directly with the lactose content of the formula.[54, 157, 201]

Incidence. An exact incidence is not known, but the disorder is rare, for Lebenthal and Rossi found only one infant with congenital lactase deficiency among 1600 patients with diarrhea who were studied.[196b]

Etiology. An autosomal dominant form of inheritance has been suggested, but four pairs of affected siblings of normal parents demonstrate a recessive type of inheritance. Some siblings or a parent may also have lactose intolerance. This disease is more frequent in males than in females.

Pathology and Pathophysiology. Small bowel biopsy reveals normal intestinal mucosa but diminished or absent lactase activity. Other disaccharidases are normal. There is increased transit and osmotic diarrhea as well as increased gas and fermentative diarrhea.

Symptoms. The infant is apparently well at birth and takes the first few feedings avidly. After one or two lactose feeds he or she becomes irritable, and abdominal distention develops. He passes watery, frothy, explosive stools that smell either sour or like vinegar. Vomiting is sometimes intermittent but is not a prominent part of the symptomatology. The diarrhea varies with the lactose content of the formula and decreases a bit if formula containing lesser quantities of sugar is substituted for the high-lactose formula. Diarrhea ceases if clear liquids are given. If the disease remains untreated, a mild, generalized malabsorption develops, and weight gain ceases. The infant continues to eat ravenously but loses weight until he becomes cachectic (Fig. 19–5). Perianal excoriation is common. Skim milk aggravates symptoms because of its more rapid emptying by the stomach.[200]

Diagnosis. Clinically, the diagnosis should be suspected in an infant in whom diarrhea and abdominal distention develop after the first or second lactose feeds. The diagnosis is suggested by an acid stool pH and strongly positive reducing substances and confirmed by the lactose tolerance test, in which there is a rise of less than 20 mg per dl. The hydrogen breath test is now the best diagnostic tool. Patients fast for six to

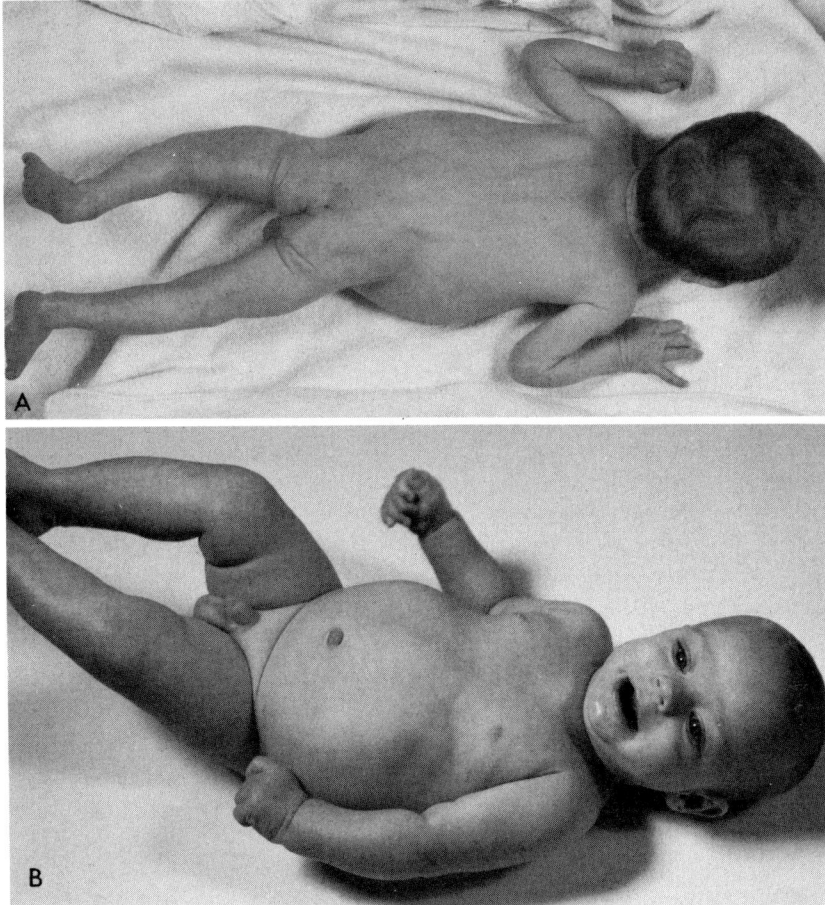

Figure 19–5 A, R. C., infant with lactose intolerance, at the time of diagnosis. At two months of age he was below the third percentile for height and weight. Note the abdominal distention and loss of subcutaneous fat. There is evidence of muscle wasting. *B*, Same infant at four months of age. After six weeks of a lactose-free diet the infant is in the fiftieth percentile for weight and the twenty-fifth for length.

eight hours, and breath samples are obtained at 0, 15, 30, 60, 90, and 120 minutes after ingestion of 2 gm per kg of lactose. A rise of hydrogen concentration of 10 or more parts per million over baseline is diagnostic. The glucose or galactose tolerance tests are followed by a normal rise in blood sugar or hydrogen breath test. Mild malabsorption with steatorrhea is sometimes present due to rapid transit time.

Treatment. A total cure is accomplished by the complete removal of lactose from the diet. After six or more months, many infants can tolerate low lactose diets and show symptoms only when challenged beyond their individual threshold. Some persist in not tolerating even the smallest amount of the sugar, however. It is imperative that any

infant taking this type of lactose-free diet receive adequate calcium and vitamins in formula or by supplementation to provide adequate growth. The elimination of lactose from the diet entails exclusion of milk, milk products, and many tablet or capsule forms of medication that contain lactose as a filler. Unfortunately, the diet is not as simple as it might sound, for milk products are in many unexpected substances. All labels must be studied and, even then, one cannot be entirely certain of the product composition. To be excluded are canned or frozen vegetables or fruits containing lactose; cocoa; Cocomalt; Ovaltine; cakes or mixes containing milk, butter, and margarine; commercial fruit-filled, custard, or cream pies; sherbet; puddings; salad dressings; many cold cuts containing added milk products; instant potatoes; commercial French fries or Corn Curls; cream or dried soups; chocolate or filled candies; and monosodium glutamate extender. A detailed diet is included in the Appendix.

Late-Onset Lactose Intolerance

It seems that ethnic and racial origins are the ultimate determinants of development of lactose intolerance after infancy, with most world populations other than those of northern Caucasian origin affected. Jews, Indians, Orientals, and blacks have incidences ranging between 50 and 90 per cent.[26, 68, 106, 172, 260] Symptoms are absent or minimal before five years of age and increase thereafter. Enzyme deficiencies have been demonstrated in asymptomatic breast-fed infants.[38]

Symptoms. In some older infants and young children, the only symptom may be a distinct aversion to milk. Others present recurrent abdominal pain and flatulence, sometimes simulating appendicitis.[23, 25] Pain often is present for months before the onset of diarrhea. It is interesting that patients drinking skim milk or low-fat products are more symptomatic, because of more rapid gastric emptying.

Diagnosis and treatment are the same as for congenital lactose intolerance.

Secondary Lactose Intolerance

Reductions in brush border lactase activity should be anticipated with any insult to villus epithelial maturity. The greatest sensitivity occurs in infancy. Simultaneous but less pronounced reductions in sucrase, maltase, and glucoamylase also will be seen. As a rule, lactase recovery will be the most delayed.

In Table 19–5 we list the common conditions associated with secondary lactase deficiency. The demonstration of acquired lactose intolerance in infancy is thus a symptom, not a diagnosis. An increased incidence of lactose intolerance also is noted in infants with congenital heart disease and congestive failure.

Table 19–5 Disorders Associated With Secondary Lactase Deficiency

Infection	Viral gastroenteritis
	Bacterial enteritis
	Giardia
Inflammation	Protein-induced enteropathy
	Chronic inflammatory bowel disease
	Immunodeficiency
	Eosinophilic gastroenteritis
	Nonspecific enterocolitis
Reduced Surface Area	Short bowel syndrome
	Malnutrition
	Hypoxia
	Radiation enteritis

Appreciation of the frequency of lactase deficiency in these conditions is critical for the appropriate nutritional management (see Chapter 9).[7] Patients with infectious enteritis alone may demonstrate lactose intolerance for months — those with extensive jejunal resection, for years.[313] With the inflammatory lesions, such as celiac disease, lactase recovery correlates with villus regeneration.

SUCRASE

Sucrase is an α-glucosidase enzyme, with maximal activity in the jejunum, existing in a sucrase-isomaltase complex. Sucrase activity can be demonstrated at the tenth week of gestation and progresses much more rapidly than that of lactase, with 70 per cent of infantile activity achieved by 30 weeks of gestation. Unlike lactase, sucrase activity is inducible by substrate exposure, by steroids, and by T_3.[188]

Sucrose-Isomaltose Intolerance

Patients with this enzyme deficiency are intolerant not only of all products containing table sugar but also of many of the starches. Its recognition and treatment depend upon awareness that more than one enzyme is affected.

Incidence. Well over 100 cases have been reported since this disease was first recognized in 1963. It seems to occur in nearly 10 per cent of Greenland Eskimos, attaining a frequence near 0.2 per cent in North America.[5, 9, 10]

Etiology and Inheritance. There is a consanguinity among the parents of many of the patients. Other siblings often are affected, and inheritance is most likely of the autosomal recessive type. It has been suggested that the homozygous person has symptoms from early infancy whereas the heterozygote is either asymptomatic or acquires symptoms later in childhood. Heterogeneous carriers are estimated as 9 to 63 per cent of the population, averaging perhaps 43 per cent. Several genetic explanations have been offered by Conklin et al:[56A] (1) a "no-sense" defect in which a gene is altered by deletion of synthesized protein or the amino acid linkage is disrupted; (2) unstable messenger RNA; (3) ineffective translocation or insertion of active enzyme into the brush border; (4) a "mid-sense" defect or production of unstable enzyme; and (5) depression of the structural gene. At the moment the most likely cause is deficient but normal enzymatic protein.[183]

Pathology and Pathophysiology. There is an absence of sucrase activity, minimal isomaltase, and low or absent palatinase and dextrinase activities. The overall maltase activity is reduced because of the near-total absence of maltases 3, 4, and 5. Maltase 1 and 2, which normally account for 4 to 29 per cent of the total enzyme function, assume 71 to 98 per cent of maltase activity. Gamma-amylase is reduced to 35 per cent of normal. As in lactose intolerance, the nonabsorbed sugars accumulate in the intestinal lumen, producing first an osmotic and later a fermentative diarrhea. A small amount absorbed into the circulation is not metabolized and is excreted in the urine.

Symptoms. These infants are completely well when taking only milk formula that contains lactose. Explosive, watery, foul-smelling diarrhea follows the introduction of sucrose, dextrins, or starch into the diet. The abdomen is distended and tympanitic. There is a great deal of flatulence and the quantity of stool increases to 300 to 500 gm per day. If solids are withdrawn from the diet and the infant takes only milk or glu-

cose-containing electrolyte solutions, the diarrhea subsides. If, on the other hand, solids and milk are withdrawn and the infant takes sugar water, juices, or soda, the diarrhea persists or increases.

The diarrhea is often erroneously correlated with the ingestion of solids containing wheat or flour and a diagnosis of celiac disease is made. The history does not usually correlate the ingestion of sucrose-containing foods and diarrhea; furthermore, the diarrhea is usually reported as "intermittent." Untreated babies, and especially those taking sucrose-containing formulas, fail to thrive, whereas those raised on milk formula and in whom diagnosis was made late in life have had relatively normal growth.

Diagnosis. The disorder should be suspected in children with acid stools who continue to have diarrhea on a strict, milk-free diet. Because of the associated starch intolerance, celiac disease must be differentiated. This is done by quantitative fecal fat test and by small bowel biopsy. Although villous atrophy is reported in a few patients with sucrose intolerance, most have normal small bowel morphology.[289] There is no steatorrhea. Enzyme assay of the tissue of the small intestine shows the specific reduction in the disaccharidases described above. The stool pH ranges between 4 and 5 if the baby has ingested sucrose and the stool lactic acid is increased to more than 1 gm per day. Since sucrose is not a reducing sugar, Clinitest is of no help in examining the stool sugars, and one must test after acid hydrolysis or refer to chromatographic methods. The breath hydrogen test is abnormal, and oral tolerance tests using sucrose or palatinose are not followed by a rise in blood sugar or glucose. The results of the maltose tolerance test are normal, as are those of the lactose and monosaccharide tolerance tests.

Treatment. Successful dietary treatment entails the elimination of dextrins and starches as well as sucrose. Milk- or carbohydrate-free soy formulas to which glucose is added provide adequate neonatal nutrition. Attempts to induce enzyme development by feeding diets high in sucrose have not been successful in humans. Foods that contain no sucrose include meats, fish, poultry, eggs, vegetable and animal fats, sugar-free carbonated beverages, artificial sweeteners, unprocessed cheeses, and milks. Most vegetables and fruits, pastas, honey, and cereals contain some sucrose, with berries and grapes having a low content. A detailed diet is included in the Appendix.

Prognosis. Symptoms improve with age, although the primary pathologic disorder remains unchanged. The children can gradually tolerate bits of starch from corn or rice as these contain fewer alpha 1–6 bonds than other starches. If partial small intestine villous atrophy is present at the time of diagnosis, it disappears after several months of treatment. A follow-up of children between 5 and 10 years of age shows that many have episodes of abdominal pain and diarrhea. Most could handle starch but if they took fruits containing more than 2 per cent sucrose, they developed diarrhea.[184a]

Secondary Sucrose Intolerance

Although secondary lactose intolerance can occur alone, presumably because lactose is the most sensitive of the disaccharidases, sucrose intolerance of this type is always associated with lactose intolerance.[168, 202] These secondary disaccharidase intolerances, therefore, occur after gastroenteritis, malnutrition, kwashiorkor, small bowel resection, and giardiasis. Both are found in celiac disease, although sucrose intolerance is not usually clinically significant. Moncreiff's syndrome of hiatus hernia, sucrosuria, and mental retardation is discussed in Chapter 11.

LACTULOSE MALABSORPTION

Lactulose is a synthetic sugar formed from lactose in formula by a process of "enolization" in which the molecule is internally arranged to form a beta-galactosido-fructose. Since the human or animal intestine is unable to hydrolyze this carbohydrate, its effect is similar to that of disaccharide intolerance, causing both osmotic and fermentative diarrhea.[126] Indeed

it is now used to soften constipated stools. Lactulose in small concentrations (1 to 2 per cent) is beneficial, for it enhances the development of a bifidus flora and lowers fecal ammonia.[340] In higher concentrations it may cause diarrhea.

TREHALOSE INTOLERANCE

Trehalose intolerance is mentioned for the sake of completeness rather than for practicality, for the major source of this sugar is the young mushroom, which is not a usual dietary provision for the infant.

Incidence. Three cases have been reported in the literature.[34, 216]

Inheritance. The disease has been documented in a father and son, and cousins and an uncle also have symptoms. This pattern suggests an autosomal type of inheritance.

Etiology and Pathophysiology. A deficiency of intestinal trehalase is responsible for the diarrhea that follows ingestion of mushrooms. Trehalase, normally present in intestinal mucosa and in aging mushrooms, hydrolyzes trehalose into glucose. The sugar is a 1-β-glucosido-1-glucoside that occurs in some lower plants and insects but most often in young mushrooms in a concentration of 1.4 per cent. It undergoes conversion to glucose in older mushrooms.

Symptoms. The symptoms are similar to those of other sugar intolerances, with bloating, vomiting, cramping, and watery diarrhea following the ingestion of mushrooms.

Diagnosis. The history is suggestive of trehalose intolerance and the diagnosis is confirmed after a flat trehalose tolerance test using a 50 gm load of the glycoside. In a small bowel biopsy, trehalase activity is absent.

Treatment. Elimination of mushrooms from the diet is curative.

GLUCOAMYLASE

Glucoamylase is a brush border glucosidase with relatively uniform distribution in the small bowel. It acts on dextrins and starch to remove successive glucose units from the nonreducing ends of the molecule. It differs from pancreatic amylase in its mucosal origin, sequential hydrolysis, independence from Cl^- or Ca^{++} ions for activity, and the rapid rate of development in infants in the first few months of life. As a result, its activity is crucial to the tolerance of glucose polymer and starch in the first six months of life.

Like maltase, it is relatively resistant to secondary reduction in villous injury. With severe villous flattening, significant reductions may nonetheless contribute to diarrhea and malabsorption.

GLUCOSE-GALACTOSE MALABSORPTION

This disease presents a clinical picture identical to that of lactose intolerance, for these are the component monosaccharides of lactose.[174]

Incidence. This congenital disorder has been reported in approximately 35 patients since it was first described in 1962.[8, 44, 204, 232-235]

Inheritance and Etiology. Inheritance is probably through autosomal transmission. Many parents of affected infants were cousins to some degree. Either sex is affected, and often there is a history that other siblings have died of diarrhea early in life. There is no report of direct transmission from parent to child. All children have been of Caucasian origin, but the father of one was Oriental. Infrequently lactose intolerance was found in a parent but was considered incidental. Oral glucose tolerance tests in parents have been normal, but jejunal transport studies have revealed abnormalities in glucose transport in several parents and a half-sister. In these the glucose transport was intermediate between normal and patient values, and this seems to be the only method of detecting the heterozygote.

Pathophysiology. The defect in this disease appears to be an inability of the intestinal mucosal cells to transport actively the monosaccharides glucose and galactose.

Only about 8 to 10 per cent of ingested glucose is absorbed by these patients. The morphology of the small intestine mucosa is normal and so are disaccharide and alkaline phosphatase activity and L-alanine and L-leucine transport. Cellular ATPase and sodium are normal.

Crane's theory of sugar transport proposes a mobile carrier common to all actively transported sugars: one that moves hexoses across the cell membrane and is not energy-dependent.[58a, b] In a second site the carrier binds sodium and increases its affinity for substrate. An abnormality in sodium transport would be an attractive suggestion, but both pump ATPase and sodium have been normal when studied. Elsas et al. propose an abnormality at the glucose-binding site of the carrier.[86, 87]

Renal studies have been undertaken to define the intermittent glycosuria that appears in the presence of normal blood sugar. Glomerular filtration rates are normal, and there is no phosphaturia or aminoaciduria. Although maximal tubular reabsorption of glucose is normal, there is a reduced minimal glucose threshold. These data suggest that the kidney and intestine contain different hexose transport systems. In one family there was increased urinary β-aminoisobutyric acid.

Symptoms. The infant is well at birth and takes feedings avidly. Usually diarrhea begins after the first glucose feeding; within the first three days the diarrhea progresses and is accompanied by abdominal distention and flatulence. The stools are explosive, watery, and frothy. Their odor is described as sour. Throughout the illness the infants continue to feed ravenously, but changes to formulas containing sucrose and maltose have no effect upon the diarrhea. Death can occur within the first or second week. Physical examination reveals little other than emaciation, abdominal distention, and rectal and perianal irritation. In a few patients, symptoms are relatively mild, with the passage of soft stools alternating with attacks of "gastroenteritis."

Diagnosis. The stools have a pH of 4 or 5 and give a strongly positive test for reducing substances. Because monosaccharide transport is impaired, these as well as the disaccharides accumulate in the intestinal lumen and cause diarrhea. Monosaccharides and disaccharides are present on chromatographic analysis of the stool. Testing with Clinistix is specific for glucose. Radiologic examination of the gastrointestinal tract is normal except for rapid transit.

All the patients have a slight intermittent glycosuria ranging from 15 to 40 mg per dl, in the absence of aminoaciduria. There is no rise in blood glucose after oral tolerance tests with lactose, glucose, or galactose. There is a significant rise in blood sugar after fructose and a moderate rise after sucrose loading. The sugar content of the stool of normal infants is 0.1 per cent wet weight or less, but in those with monosaccharide malabsorption it rises to 39 per cent after monosaccharide loading.[93]

In older children, an oral sugar load is sometimes followed by a relatively normal rise in blood sugar, and intubation studies are necessary for a definitive diagnosis. In such cases, glucose is always absorbed more slowly than fructose. Xylose absorption may be slightly impaired, and there may be mild steatorrhea.

In acute stages of the disease, the oral fructose tolerance test can be normal and yield extremely high rises in blood sugar. An intravenous tolerance test shows slow removal of fructose from the blood. These tests revert to normal after the infant has had adequate dietary management and has begun to gain weight.

Treatment. Early formulas were prepared to contain casein or casein hydrolysate, butter fat, corn oil, and added fructose and electrolytes. Treatment is now simple; a commercial carbohydrate-free formula composed of a soy or protein hydrolysate base is used, and fructose is added to it in increasing concentrations of 4 to 8 per cent.

Prognosis. Absorption of sugars does not improve with age, but some children can tolerate small amounts of sugar, most likely because of a smaller sugar load in relation to body size and of prolongation of intestinal transit. They still experience flatulence, cramping, and diarrhea after taking small amounts of starch, sugar, or milk.

Secondary Monosaccharide Malabsorption

Intolerance to glucose, galactose, and fructose was first reported in infants in 1966.[159] Diarrhea developed during the first week of life and was associated with pathogenic "*Escherichia coli*" infection in two of the four infants. They tolerated a carbohydrate-free formula and recovered completely one to six months after the initiation of treatment. A similar intolerance has been seen in premature infants and in infants operated on for high intestinal obstruction.[1, 163] An overgrowth of intestinal flora above the area of anastomosis was noted in the latter group. Improperly treated diarrhea may result in first disaccharide and later monosaccharide malabsorption.[203]

In older infants, secondary monosaccharide intolerance can develop during or after infectious gastroenteritis and lasts from several days to weeks. It can be severe enough to cause death if it is not recognized and treated. Hypoglycemia is frequent, and intravenous glucose often is required to maintain the normal blood sugar level. The hypoglycemia often is unresponsive to epinephrine or glucagon, and these infants become hypovolemic after taking small loads of amino acid mixtures. After being diarrhea-free for about two weeks, the infants can usually maintain their blood sugar above 40 mg per dl without intravenous supplementation. Disaccharide intolerance usually precedes the monosaccharide intolerance, and its prompt diagnosis and treatment will prevent this more serious complication.

Whether proliferation of enteric flora produces diarrhea or contributes to sugar malabsorption has been a subject of speculation. Bacterial proliferation seems proportional to the degree of carbohydrate intolerance, with moderate growth in those with lactose intolerance and marked growth in those with monosaccharide intolerance.

DIARRHEA AND DIETETIC CANDIES

Diarrhea develops rapidly in the infant or toddler who ingests large quantities of dietetic candies, soda, or cookies.[122] These products contain sorbitol and mannitol, which are acted upon slowly by oral bacteria and are absorbed by passive transport mechanisms from the gastrointestinal tract. A sufficient quantity of these hexitols produces an osmotic diarrhea. Within two hours after consuming the product the child passes explosive, watery stools, which continue over the next four or so hours. There is usually cramping and abdominal distention. The child recovers and is well until the situation repeats itself. The sugars can be identified in the stools by chromatographic techniques, but a good history is usually adequate in making the diagnosis and providing a solution. Tolerance increases with age.

PROTEIN DIGESTION AND PROTEIN-RELATED DISORDERS

Protein digestion begins in the stomach with the action of pepsin and renin. Pepsin may be identified in the fetal stomach at about 34 weeks' gestation and increases progressively after the 35th week through the second day of life, coincident with gastrin and acid secretion. Pepsin then falls to a level of about one fifteenth that of the adult and increases gradually during the first year. Since it is most effective at a pH of 2 and since acid secretion decreases after the first month and only gradually decreases during the first year, peptic activity remains suboptimal. The protein delivered to the intestine for digestion is both dietary and endogenous, consisting of whole protein, peptides, and amino acids. Eight per cent is absorbed by the time the bolus has passed through the jejunum. In the duodenum, enterokinase (present in the 26-week-old fetus) activates the conversion of trypsinogen to trypsin, which, in turn, activates the other proteolytic proenzymes. Although these are present in the neonate in low concentrations, they increase with feeds and with age. The endopeptidases act upon the inner bonds and the exopeptidases act upon the carboxyl end of the protein. The endopeptidases produce oligopeptides that are hydrolyzed by exopeptidases to small peptides and neutral and basic amino acids.

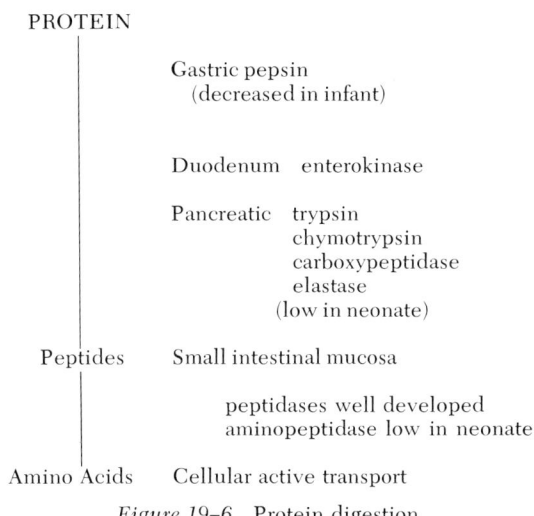

Figure 19–6   Protein digestion.

Within the small intestine the peptidases (except for aminopeptidase) are relatively well developed, being present between 11 and 14 weeks' gestation (Fig. 19–6). Not all exist in the brush border of the enterocyte, for some have been identified in submucosal leukocytes and mast cells. Some di- and tripeptides are hydrolyzed by the brush border enzymes, while others enter the enterocyte and are hydrolyzed within it. Tetra- and larger peptides are hydrolyzed within the brush border. Their end products, amino acids, are transported by several sodium-dependent mechanisms that are well developed during fetal life. They leave the cell to enter the portal system.

Congenital deficiencies of proteolytic enzymes are discussed in Chapter Fifteen.[129, 130, 142, 208, 242, 275, 296]

PROTEIN-INDUCED ENTEROPATHY

In 1880, Dr. S. Gee of St. Bartholomew's Hospital described the "celiac affection"[104] and through the years the "celiac syndrome" came to describe the clinical triad of abdominal distention, malabsorption, and malnutrition. In the majority of children, a sensitivity to gluten — a component of wheat, barley, rye, and malt — has been confirmed, and this condition remains the classic celiac disease.[100] Other children, however, have been demonstrated to have an enteropathy induced by cow's milk or soy bean protein — an important differential, for these are of limited duration, whereas celiac disease is a lifelong entity.

GLUTEN-SENSITIVE ENTEROPATHY (GSE)

Gluten-sensitive enteropathy (GSE) is the term designated to replace "celiac" to underscore the specificity of the dietary protein incriminated and the requirement for histologic enteropathy rather than just clinical disease.[100, 148, 321, 322] GSE is a lifelong disease characterized by the loss of mature villus epithelium in the presence of a gluten-containing diet. In an effort to standardize the diagnostic criteria for GSE, the European Society for Pediatric Gastroenterology developed the Interlaken Criteria in 1970.[327] These criteria, summarized in revised form in Table 19–6, again emphasize the histologic rather than the clinical criteria for diagnosis. Malabsorption is nearly universal in childhood GSE but is not strictly mandated for diagnosis.[335] The "two-year rule" for recurrence of the histologic lesion on reintroduction of gluten is made in an effort to eliminate those rare patients with a transient gluten sensitivity. Recent studies confirm that more than 98 per cent of children with GSE will have mucosal relapse within two years of gluten reintroduction although most show morphologic change within three to six months.

Incidence and Genetics. The incidence of GSE in any population appears to be predominantly a factor of genetic predisposition, though environmental exposure to gluten is obviously mandatory. The highest

Table 19–6 Diagnostic Criteria for Gluten-Sensitive Enteropathy (Celiac Disease)

1. Severely damaged or flat villous lesion
2. Clinical response to gluten elimination
3. Histologic recovery following gluten elimination
4. Histologic recurrence of villous injury within two years of gluten reintroduction

incidence figures are in the west of Ireland, where GSE occurs in 1 of 300 children.[246] The incidence in Switzerland is 1 in 890 while in Sweden it is 1 in 6000.[39, 47] The incidence figures for England and the United States are calculated to be approximately 1 in 3000 births.

The disease is extraordinarily rare in native Africans and Asians. The environmental factor, however, is underscored by a recent report by Nelson, McNeish, and Anderson of GSE in 17 Asian children raised in England by parents from West Pakistan and the Punjab.[229, 250]

There is a familial pattern as parents, siblings, and twins have been affected.[301] At least one pair of identical twins, however, has been discordant.[213, 227] Biopsy specimens of relatives of a confirmed patient, if taken, will show a flat jejunal mucosa in 11 per cent. The incidence in males and females appears to be approximately equal in childhood. It seems to be least frequent in infants who have been breast-fed for 6 months or so.

The search for a genetic predisposition has led to extensive investigation of histocompatibility antigen genes in patients with GSE. These determinations revealed a fourfold increase in the incidence of HLA-B8 types. Nonetheless, 20 to 30 per cent of GSE patients do not bear the HLA-B8 gene, and siblings concordant for HLA-B8 may not demonstrate the disease. A D-locus antigen, HLA-D W3, recently has been shown to have an even higher frequency of occurrence in patients with GSE. A lymphocyte antigen (B1),[184] independent of the HLA system, also has recently been demonstrated in more than 90 per cent of GSE patients studied.[95, 219] Celiac disease may coexist with cystic fibrosis or diabetes.[161, 318]

Etiology. While it has been conclusively demonstrated that the α-gliadin fraction of gluten induces the mucosal injury of GSE, the mechanism remains obscure. Gluten derived from wheat and rye is definitely toxic to the epithelial cells, and the toxicity of gluten derived from barley and oats is presumed but less well substantiated.[282] When gliadin is separated, it is found to be a complex protein rich in glutamine and proline. Several subfractions have been demonstrated to be toxic *in vitro*.[75] Pepsin-trypsin digestion products and subproducts of gluten remain toxic as well as gliadin fractions exposed to pancreatic enzymes. Peptides obtained from *in vitro* mucosal digestion of gluten are also toxic. Fraction 9 of gliadin isolated by column chromatography as well as a subfraction unit is apparently the most toxic to intestinal mucosa. A similar substance has been recovered from exposure of patient duodenal mucosa to gluten. Others have addressed the side-chain structures rather than amino acid sequences and noted that carbohydrase cleavage rendered gliadin nontoxic. There are presently three major, though not necessarily mutually exclusive, hypotheses for this gluten-induced toxicity.[173, 320]

1. *Peptidase Theory.* This theory, first propounded by Frazer et al. in 1959, argues that the lack of an intestinal peptidase results in the accumulation of undigested toxic peptides.[78, 100] This was supported by increases in blood glutamine over normal levels in patients after gluten ingestion. While several studies have confirmed reduced mucosal dipeptidase activity with acute disease, the activity of these enzymes appears to return to normal with mucosal recovery on a gluten-free diet, thus suggesting that the peptidase deficiency is secondary to the epithelial cell damage.[50] Present studies are focusing on the toxicity of highly fractionated pepsin/trypsin digests in healed GSE mucosa.

2. *Altered Epithelial Cell Surfaces (Lectin Theory).* In 1976, Weiser and Douglas suggested that an abnormality of structural glycoprotein or glycolipid at the epithelial cell surface could create a specific receptor for the carbohydrate fraction of gliadin, thus potentiating its toxic effect.[342] Such receptors are generally defined on the basis of binding by specific plant lectins, such as concanavalin A.

The cell surface glycoprotein configuration controlled by the HLA system is regulated, in part, by the glycosyltransferase enzymes that sequence the addition of oligosaccharide side chains to the glycoprotein. When compared with the mature vil-lous epithelial cell, differentiating crypt epithelial cells have altered cell surface lectin binding and elevated levels of glycosyltransferase enzymes. Elevations of galactosyl transferase have been reported in GSE patients and persist into remission. It is thus argued that the patients with GSE have a persistently undifferentiated cell surface that allows gluten or gluten-fragment binding with resultant cellular toxicity.

3. *Immunologic Theory.* The demonstration of antigluten antibody in the serum and intestinal secretions of patients with celiac disease has led to extensive immunologic evaluation in these patients. An immunologic basis is also suggested by the HLA gene compatibility; by "gliadin shock" that develops in celiac children after gluten challenge, which responds favorably to steroids; and by the presence in the serum and stool of wheat or fraction III antibodies and IgD antibodies in higher titer than in normal individuals. Sera from some patients also contain circulating antibodies to small intestinal epithelium, and the incidence decreases after treatment. Similarly, other food antibodies, such as milk, and IgA are increased, and they decrease after therapy.[96, 317] Unfortunately, many of the immunologic phenomena reported are nonspecific and predictable responses to epithelial cell damage and the attendant increase in nonspecific antigen uptake. Immune complexes containing antigluten antibody have been demonstrated in the mucosal epithelium of GSE patients. Following gluten challenge, complement consumption also has been demonstrated.[77, 230] In patients with GSE, alterations in cell-mediated immunity have been suggested primarily by demonstration of gluten-induced release of leukocyte migration inhibitory factor from sensitized lymphocytes. Cell-mediated cytotoxicity studies are under way, focusing on the intraepithelial lymphocyte which may have T-cell effector capacity. Evidence exists for both local cellular and antibody-dependent mitogen-induced cytotoxicity.

Histologic increases in plasma cells and lymphocytes in the lamina propria, and increased intraepithelial lymphocytes have led to a hypothesis presented by Falchuk.[95] Patients with GSE have cell surface proteins coded for by histocompatibility antigen genes and the B-cell GSE gene. These two genes result in formation of a receptor-complex on the epithelial cell to bind gluten. As a result, gluten becomes immunogenic and causes production of antigluten antibody, sensitized lymphocytes, and lymphokines, which, in turn, injure the cell. This is supported by increased immunoglobulin production in the intestine and an increase in endoplasmic reticulum and lymphokine production.

Other etiologic postulates are (1) a reduction in Paneth cells causes or heralds the illness, and decreased mucosal and increased serum lysosome activity have been reported; or (2) a cell membrane defect permits gluten to enter the cell and cause toxicity.

Pathology. Patients with GSE have impaired phytohemagglutination-induced transformation of lymphocytes and decreased lymphoreticular tissue. Many have splenic atrophy. Immunologic studies report varied results: some note a decrease in IgA, an increase in IgM-containing mucosal cells, and increased IgM in intestinal secretions; other note increased IgA synthesis. There is no correlation between serum immunoglobulin levels and the density of small intestinal immunocytes. Both high and low levels of serum IgA are reported, and more than half of patients are deficient in IgM. Most have normal levels of IgE. Abnormal values return to normal after treatment, but an increase in serum IgA has been noted in patients who develop lymphoma. Immunofluorescent studies show fluorescence within the intestinal epithelial cells after staining of jejunal tissue with antigliadin antibody. Gluten-induced damage to the small bowel is most extensive in the duodenum and proximal jejunum. In the more distal bowel, a patchier lesion is noted. If gluten is infused into the ileum of previously treated GSE patients, however, the injury is immediate and localized, confirming that gluten-induced damage is a direct local injury at the site of maximal exposure. It has been appreciated that clini-

cal symptoms correlated more directly with the length of bowel involved than with the severity of the lesion at any given point.

Grossly, or under the dissecting microscope, the normal small bowel mucosa has a pink, velvety appearance due to the finger-like villi that cover it. Normal variants in young children are broader "tongue-like" or "leaf-like" villi. The normal villus to crypt ratio is 4:1. The crypts of Lieberkühn show increased mitotic activity and provide new cells that migrate up the crypts to replace old villous epithelial cells. The mucosal epithelium is replaced every three days, with crypt cells being undifferentiated and containing large amounts of RNA. As they mature, they increase in height and acquire histologically demonstrable enzymes and Paneth and goblet cells. Cells at the tips of the villi are columnar, evenly aligned with basilar nuclei. Each cell has a prominent brush border composed of microvilli and covered by glycocalyx. The lamina propria

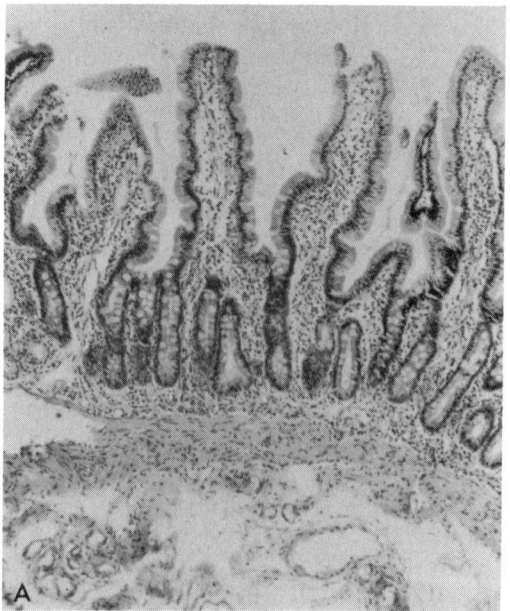

Figure 19–7 Structural abnormalities of gluten-sensitive enteropathy, with comparison with a normal jejunal biopsy. A, Normal jejunal biopsy demonstrating the long, slender villi with neatly arranged columnar surface epithelial cells. The nuclei of these cells are basilar and neatly arranged. Lymphatic channels, capillaries, and some mononuclear cells are present in the lamina propria. Crypts are evident and extend downward between the villi. Villus length is longer than crypt length.

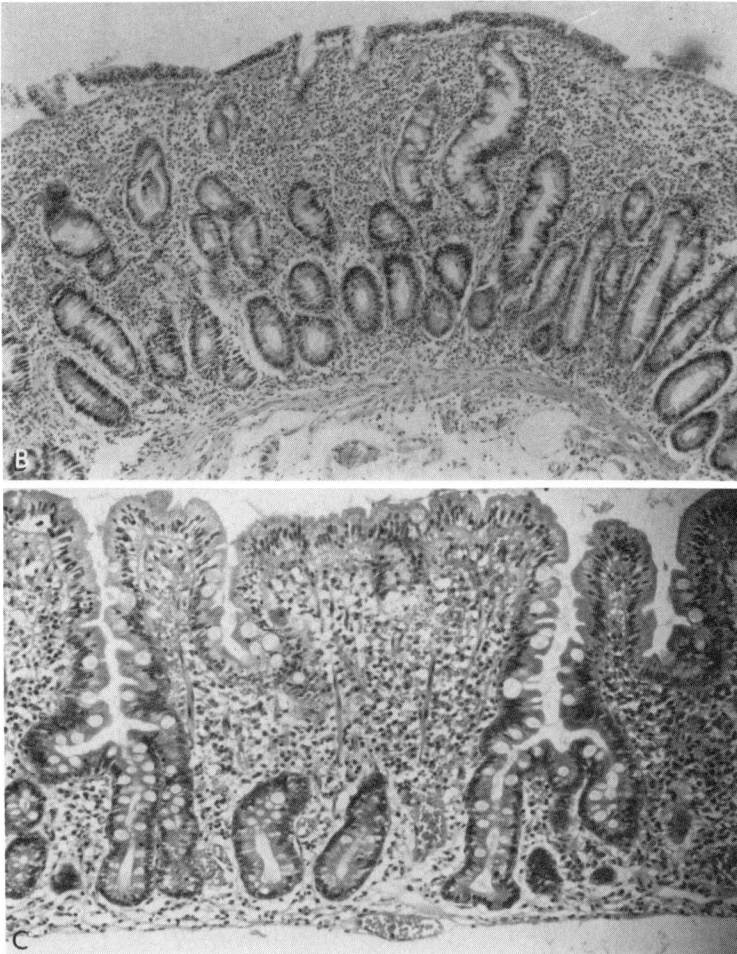

Figure 19–7 Continued B, Severe changes in the jejunal mucosa in GSE: loss of villi and derangement of the surface epithelium. The cells are thinned, degenerating, and infiltrated by mononuclear cells, and their nuclei are irregularly placed. There are an increase of chronic inflammatory cells in the lamina propria and evidence of edema. Crypt epithelial cells are spared. C, Healing jejunum after one month of treatment of celiac disease. There is some return of villi, and healing of the surface epithelium is noted by the reappearance of columnar epithelial cells and a tendency toward basilar alignment of their nuclei. There is less edema and inflammatory reaction in the lamina propria. (Courtesy of Henry Binder, M.D.)

contains occasional lymphocytes and plasma cells.

In celiac disease, small bowel mucosa appears shiny, cobblestoned, and thin. The villi are either flattened or appear as short, thick ridges and the villus:crypt ratio is decreased. Histologic examination shows clubbing and subtotal or total villous atrophy (Fig. 19–7). The crypts are loosely packed and widely separated and appear twice as deep as those in normal mucosa. Their lining cells are immature, with increased mitotic activity. Adult surface cells are degenerative, being irregular and varying from cuboidal to flat; the nuclei are eccentric and the brush border atrophic. Goblet cells and often Paneth cells are decreased. There is a moderate to heavy infiltration of the lamina propria with plasma cells, lymphocytes, and eosinophils and increased intraepithelial lymphocytes. The microvilli are irregular and disorganized and the unicellular lysosomes disrupted. Increased intraluminal DNA indicates increased loss of epithelial cells into the lumen and is termed "exfoliative enteropathy." The earliest changes as noted by electron microscopy occur in the basement membrane of the epithelial cells and in the endothelial cells of blood vessels and connective tissue. The size and number of microvilli are decreased, and there are cellular infiltrates and the deposition of immune complexes.

In previously untreated patients, the small bowel biopsy will demonstrate diffuse moderate to marked villus loss and prominent surface epithelial cell degeneration (Fig. 19–7).[298] Reactive or compensatory crypt hyperplasia will be prominent. The inflammatory cell infiltration of the lamina propria is mixed, with polyps, eosinophils, lymphocytes, plasma cells, and macrophages seen. A significant increase in the intraepithelial lymphocyte population also will be noted. These histologic findings are not unique to GSE, as identical histologic changes may be seen with milk or soy protein-induced enteropathy.

Following the introduction of a gluten-free diet, healing is confirmed, though only in infancy will the bowel return histologically to "normal." Recovery begins at three days, and an increase in cell height is seen after six to ten days. One or two weeks after treatment is begun, symptomatic improvement is noted, but slender villi may not reappear for several months. There is usually some evidence of persistent villus reduction and crypt hyperplasia. The villous epithelial cell degeneration, however, should not persist in adequately treated patients. In some older children and adults the villus region may prove to be resistant to therapy. This refractory lesion is characterized by multiple jejunal ulcers, subepithelial collagen deposition, and vasculitis. In the literature, this complication is referred to as chronic ulcerative jejunitis or collagenous sprue.

In the successfully treated patient, gluten challenge allows for sequential biopsy confirmation of gluten-induced damage. By electron microscopy, Shiner et al. demonstrated cellular infiltration, edema, and endothelial cell hypertrophy appearing within the first 24 hours of challenge.[299, 300] The inflammatory cell response was noted to peak within 96 hours prior to the demonstration of epithelial cell damage. Surface epithelial cell degeneration is reported to precede the development of villus shortening and compensatory crypt cell proliferation.

Pathophysiology. Hypomotility of the bowel and delayed transit are more apparent in older children than in infants. Nonpropulsive type I and propulsive type II waves are reduced. As maximal villus injury occurs at the level of the duodenum and upper jejunum, carbohydrate and protein digestion and absorption may be severely limited as a result of reduced surface area. There is secondary disease in all brush border enzymes, with lactase most severely affected (Table 19–7).[99, 295] Impaired monosaccharide absorption is reflected in abnormal glucose and xylose tolerance tests,[46, 48, 275] but, if these are carried out longer, glucose absorption is actually normal.[96a]

Coincident with mucosal damage are decreases in intestinal hormones: pancreozymin, secretin, gastric inhibitory polypeptide, and cholecystokinin are decreased since these originate from the proximal small bowel. Some, however, have normal enterokinase. Hormones liberated from the distal small bowel, such as pancreatic polypeptides, enteroglucagon, and neurotensin, are normal or increased.

In addition to an osmotic diarrhea, the inflammatory enteritis that develops will lead to secretory diarrhea with excessive loss of electrolytes and protein.[98, 288]

Water and electrolytes are actively secreted into the intestinal lumen rather than absorbed by it. Thus the sodium-dependent active or facilitated diffusion processes are impaired for carbohydrate, amino acids, dipeptides, water-soluble vitamins, and bile salts. The inflamed bowel also has been demonstrated to have reduced permeability to cations. Potassium losses are more severe than those of sodium, and magnesium and calcium malabsorption are reflected by seizures or tetany. Bile acid malabsorption is also seen in patients with GSE, but it is interesting that bacterial overgrowth is rarely a contributory factor. Unabsorbed fatty acids combine with calcium (1 gm fatty acid binding 74 mg of calcium), and secondary hyperparathyroidism increases phosphorus excretion and results in bone reabsorption.

Table 19–7   Enzyme Activity in Intestinal Mucosa of Patients with Celiac Disease

ENZYME	UNTREATED	TREATED	NORMALS
Monoamine oxidase (MAO)	3.8	13.99	–
μg/4 OQ mg protein			
Glutaminase	1.4 ± 0.2	>3.0 if no	6.0 ± 23
μg NH$_3$–N/100 mg		<2.0 if	
		symptoms	
Alkaline phosphatase (mean)	69.2 (16–100)	280 (157–821)	430 (207–790)
Lactase	1.4 (0–3.5)	16.9 (0.8–278)	50 (22–139)
mM/gm protein/min			
	1.49	–	38
Invertase	19.3 (4.6–35)	41.1 (11.6–73.8)	82 (52–129)
mM/gm protein/min			
Isomaltase	13.7 (6.7–23)	31.1 (12.8–71.3)	50 (22–139)
mM/gm protein/min			
Maltase	48.9 (16–70)	121 (11–179)	50 (22–39)
mM/gm protein/min			
Lysosomal enzymes			
hetero-beta-galactosidase	1.08	1.42	1.42
μm/gm protein/min			
β-glucuronidase	1.9	1.9	1.9
Dipeptidases for:			
glycyl-L-leucine	5–160	140–280	–
units/mg N			
glycyl-L-valine	35–150	80–180	–
units/mg N			
L-anyl-L-glutamic acid	0.5–40	22–48	–
units/mg N			
L-valyl-L-glutamic acid	0.5–16	8.20	–
units/mg N			
L-glutamyl-L-valine	0.5–18	12–28	–
units/mg N			
L-alanyl-L-proline	15.6	4–8	–
units/mg N			
L-valyl-L-proline	0.05–2.5	1.2–3.8	–
units/mg N			
L-glutamyl-L-proline	0.5–2.0	1.2–2.6	–
units/mg M			

Calcium is no longer available to bind oxalate in the intestine, and this is absorbed to result in hyperoxaluria.

Abnormal gallbladder function has been noted, and bile acid production may be decreased.[207]

The major cause of steatorrhea is impaired jejunal absorption of fat. Malabsorption may be mild early in the disease, and some infants may have normal fecal fat excretion. Anorexia with decreased intake, however, may offset relatively normal fecal fat values (which if calculated according to grams of fat ingested would actually be increased). Fecal nitrogen is elevated because peptidase deficiencies impair protein absorption. A protein-losing enteropathy in some patients further augments enteric protein losses. Pancreatic function is decreased not only because of decreased hormonal levels but secondary to malnutrition.

Deficiencies of fat-soluble vitamins are noted. Vitamin K malabsorption leads to hypoprothrombinemia. Iron and folic acid malabsorption are reflected in cheilosis, anemia, and a smooth, red tongue in one third of patients. Vitamin B$_{12}$ absorption is usually normal but is impaired in those with extensive ileal disease.

The absorption of folate, iron, and pyridoxine is most avid in the proximal small bowel and thus deficiencies are common in these patients.

Symptoms.   The onset of the disease obviously depends upon the age of the infant at exposure to gluten-containing prod-

Table 19–8   Symptoms of Gluten-Sensitive Enteropathy

	AGE		
	<9 Months	*9–24 Months*	*>3 Years*
FTT	Acute	Gradual	Insidious
Emesis	Prominent	Infrequent	Infrequent
Diarrhea	Severe	Moderate/severe	Moderate
Constipation	Unusual	Occasional	Occasional
Abdominal distention	Occasional	Prominent	Subtle
Abdominal pain	Common	Common	Infrequent
Other	Acute onset	Anorexia	Rickets
	Edema	Hypotonia	Delayed puberty
		Edema	Oral ulcers
		Irritability	Anemia

ucts.[134] In North America, approximately 50 per cent of patients will experience onset before 18 months of age. In a study recently performed in England, in nearly 20 per cent of infants the acute onset of symptoms was directly attributable to the first exposure to gluten. In other children, the latent interval to symptomatology varies from months to years. Diagnosis is enigmatically unusual during adolescence.

As noted in Table 19–8, the presenting symptoms will vary with age and, rarely, short stature may be the only symptom.[119a] It may be associated with congenital heart disease.[55a] Diarrhea is reported in the vast majority of infants, usually as pale, bulky, greasy, and foul-smelling stools occasionally containing oil droplets, with three to five such movements a day. Fulminant diarrhea is unusual and restricted to the infant less than nine months of age. Some infants as early as three to four months of age show growth failure, anorexia, and even constipation. In older patients, constipation is occasionally reported despite the associated steatorrhea: a few have rectal prolapse. Emesis and abdominal pain are prominent in infants and unusual in older children and adults. Anorexia is impressive in its severity and helps to differentiate the disease from cystic fibrosis. The classic physical appearance of failure to thrive, abdominal protuber-

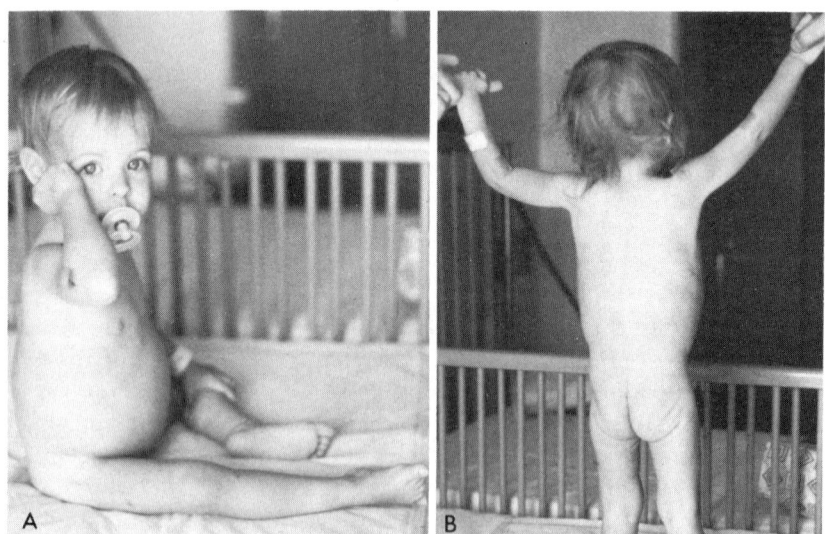

Figure 19–8   Twenty-two-month-old girl with gluten-sensitive enteropathy. *A*, Note the protuberant abdomen and wasted extremities. *B*, Posterior view to show wasting of gluteal musculature. Buttock skin hangs in loose folds.

ance, wasted buttocks and limbs, and hypotonia is encountered in far less than half the infants with GSE (Fig. 19–8). When growth data are available, however, impressive growth arrest following gluten exposure is the rule.

Manifestations of malabsorption may be flagrant. Rickets, anemia, tetany, frank bleeding, and edema may be encountered, and some children have increased nocturnal urination. The tongue is smooth and red, and there may be early bruising and a frank bleeding tendency.

Hypomagnesemia and hypocalcemia are manifest as irritability, tremor, convulsions, tetany, bone pain, and osteomalacia. When vitamin D deficiency is prolonged, there is evidence of rickets. Clubbing of the terminal phalanges is frequent.

Eighty-six per cent of older patients have fingerprint changes consisting of ridge atrophy. These are unusual before five years of age. If present, they return to normal after treatment. In older children delayed puberty and infertility may be a manifestation of otherwise subtle GSE. It is interesting that the passage of red urine following the ingestion of beets (beeturia) is common.[339]

The emotional symptoms of GSE are also most common in infancy. The infant is usually described as irritable, fretful, and clinging. Reduction in appetite is also common. We have seen one infant in whom a tentative diagnosis of childhood schizophrenia was made. The reversal of these emotional components following introduction of a gluten-free diet may be rapid and dramatic.

Complications. The "celiac crisis" is fortunately an unusual presentation or complication of GSE in infancy. These infants have severe diarrhea, often secretory or intractable in nature, with dehydration and hypoproteinemia secondary to the combined insult of malabsorption and protein losing. Immediate volume expansion and electrolyte therapies are indicated. Prolonged venous alimentation may be avoided in such patients by a short course of corticosteroid therapy.[209]

Multiple ulcerations of the jejunum and ileum, occasionally leading to perforation, are rare in childhood.[27] Secondary reductions in disaccharidases, enterokinase, and pancreatic enzyme activity are rapidly reversible with treatment. Hyposplenism also has been reported as a complication of GSE in childhood.[338] Juvenile onset diabetes has been reported with GSE, apparently as a result of an HLA-linked predisposition. Over the course of the last decade, there also has been increasing evidence to suggest that 1 to 10 per cent of patients with GSE are at increased risk for the development of intestinal lymphoma.[24, 139, 169] This complication has not been seen in infancy, and it is not known whether it is the result of inadequate treatment or a reflection of genetically linked predisposition. Hepatitis with elevated alanine, amino transferases, and serum aspartate has been reported in children with active GSE, and has improved after therapy. Hypocitraturia has been noted.[283a]

Diagnosis. The criteria for diagnosis, as cited earlier, are histologic. The small bowel biopsy is mandatory but occasionally may be deferred if the infant is severely malnourished or at increased risk for bleeding. As noted in Table 19–6, page 602, subsequent biopsies are necessary in the presence and absence of gluten to confirm the diagnosis.[226, 283]

In choosing the patients for biopsy, innumerable "malabsorptive screening tests" have been recommended. The best known include the serum D-xylose assay, used to assess upper small bowel surface area.[321] This assay requires obtaining a blood sample 60 minutes following the ingestion of a total dose of 5 gm or a dose of 14.2 gm per square meter of D-xylose as a 10 per cent solution. Blood levels below 20 mg per cent at one to one and a half hours suggest reduced small bowel surface area consistent with GSE. False-negative rates can approximate 10 per cent. Because of delayed motility, the study should be carried out to one and a half or even two hours.

The second screening test is the quantitative 72-hour stool fat determination to confirm steatorrhea, which is present in 80 per cent of infants with GSE. With the severe anorexia, low oral fat intakes may preclude the validity of this test, and oral fat intake always must be calculated.

Other absorption studies include oral carbohydrate tolerance tests performed with both disaccharides and glucose. Carbohydrate tolerance is impaired in the majority of symptomatic infants as a result of diminished brush border surface area. Disacchariduria and generalized aminoaciduria may be noted. Less specific assays include the red cell folate and the reticulin, and determination of serum carotene, serum albumin, calcium, fat-soluble vitamins, and vitamin E levels, all of which commonly will be depressed. The prothrombin time may be prolonged. The vitamin B_{12} level and Schilling test are usually normal in the absence of severe ileal disease. None of these studies should be considered diagnostic.

Anemia is usually microcytic and hypochromic, reflecting iron deficiency, but occasionally one encounters macrocytic anemia due to folic acid deficiency.

Decreased growth hormone and insulin responses follow intravenous tolbutamide. The calcium level is often low and phosphorus elevated. Radiologic changes of rickets may be observed in films of long bones and ribs. The alkaline phosphatase level may be extremely high. In such instances, the 5'-nucleotidase levels should be elevated as these may reflect fatty infiltration of the liver secondary to malnutrition. We have seen one such infant with an alkaline phosphatase value of 2600 units and a 5'-nucleotidase of 25, both of which returned to normal within three weeks of dietary treatment.

Indole metabolism is disturbed, and 5-hydroxy-indoleacetic acid or indole-3-acetic acid is excreted in the urine of the untreated patient. 5-Hydroxytryptamine is increased in the duodenal mucosa.

Skin testing with gluten and its subfractions (B_2) has been undertaken. While patients with GSE often demonstrate positive skin tests, a lack of specificity has been demonstrated in children with other intestinal disorders.[11, 16] A more appealing *in vitro* assay has been proposed by Ashkenazi et al.[13] with evidence of gluten-induced increases in leukocyte migration inhibition factor in patients with GSE.

In vitro incubation of the small bowel biopsy specimen in the presence or absence of gluten also may prove to be of great diagnostic value.[94] In the presence of gluten, epithelial maturity is impaired in this organ culture system.

More sophisticated techniques have proved quite specific for detection of GSE recently. *Organ culture* of small intestinal tissue for 24 to 48 hours in normal subjects shows a significant increase in alkaline phosphatase production (to 350 ± 75).[179] Similar treatment of specimens from patients with acute GSE shows a reversion to normal mucosa and an equivalent rise in the enzyme. GSE tissue grown in the presence of gluten shows no change in morphology, and there is inhibition of alkaline phosphatase production. This effect is not demonstrable in specimens from patients who are in reversion. The *leukocyte migration inhibition factor (LIF) test* using subfractions B_2 and B_3 of fraction III of gluten as mitogens shows that peripheral blood lymphocytes from 95 per cent of patients respond to stimulation by producing increased amounts of LIF.[13] An immunofluorescent blood test has been developed.[326a]

The radiographic contrast studies of the small bowel (Fig. 19–9) often will demonstrate a nonspecific pattern of thickened mucosal folds, dilatation of bowel, and flocculation with segmentation of the barium column.[15, 143] Changes are most pronounced in the duodenum and jejunum. Normal small bowel caliber is about 12 mm at six months and increases to 23.1 ± 1.93 in adults. The disease cannot be excluded by normal small bowel radiography. Colonic dilatation has been reported in patients with constipation.

Differential Diagnosis. The clinical differential is often with cystic fibrosis and milk or soy protein-induced "allergic" enteropathy. Table 19–9 is a clinical summary developed to differentiate these conditions. The histologic differential of the flat villous lesion is much more complex. Table 19–10, adapted from Katz and Grand, reviews the

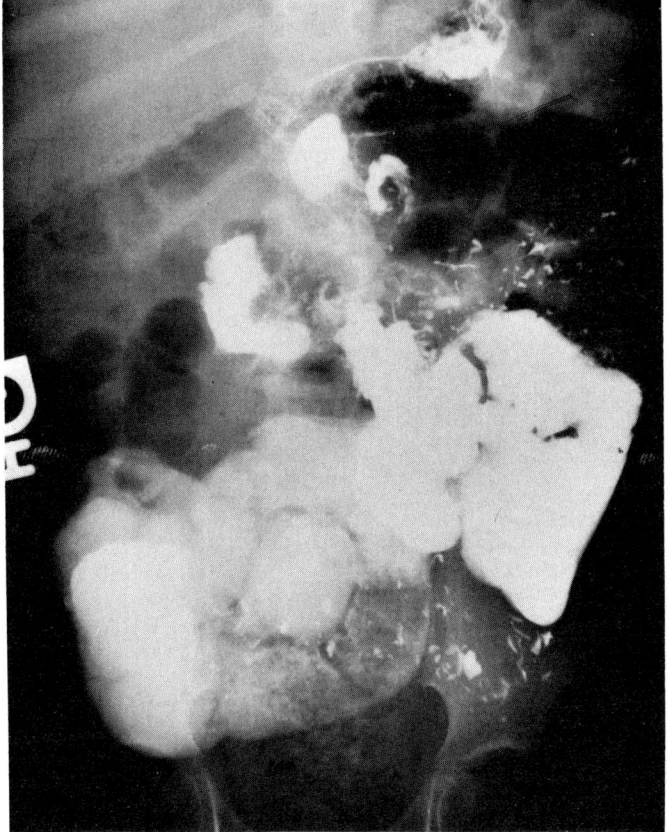

Figure 19-9 In this three-year-old child with a history of bulky stool and failure to thrive, the small bowel series demonstrates a markedly abnormal small bowel pattern with loss of the normal valvulae and mucosal markings, dilation, and dilution of the barium by fluid within the small bowel. The large quantity of stool within the colon is seen distending the rectosigmoid area and can also be seen as mottled lucency near the hepatic flexure.

major considerations that may be histologically indistinguishable from GSE. The most difficult is usually the patient with malnutrition on either a primary or secondary basis. Confirmation of gluten-sensitive enteropathy, therefore, depends upon a positive response to gluten challenge.

Treatment. Treatment of gluten-sensitive enteropathy consists of the immediate and permanent institution of a diet

Table 19–9 Symptoms and Clinical Findings in Celiac Disease, Cystic Fibrosis and Gastrointestinal Allergy

	CELIAC DISEASE	CYSTIC FIBROSIS	GI ALLERGY
Positive family history	Common	Common	Common
Onset	8 months–2 years	95% by 1 year	3–9 months
Respiratory symptoms	Infrequent	Common	Occasional
Appetite	Poor	Excessive	Normal
Stools	Bulky, foul, occasionally liquid	Bulky, foul, oil droplets	Soft, watery, mucoid: occasional blood
Growth	Normal for 8–10 months	Retarded	Variable
Vitamin deficiencies	Unusual	Occasional	Unusual
Calcium deficiency	Frequent	Rare	Occasional
Carotene	Very low	Very low	Low normal
Folate	Very low	Normal	Low normal
Finger clubbing	Frequent	Frequent	Unusual
Lactose intolerance	Frequent	Occasional	Frequent

Table 19–10 Disorders Associated with the Flat Villus Lesion in Infancy

Protein-induced enteropathy
  Gluten, milk, soy

Acute enteritis
  Viral, bacterial, *Giardia*
  Radiation-induced

Chronic enteritis
  Tropical sprue, Whipple's disease
  Intractable enterocolitis
  Immunodeficiency
  Eosinophilic gastroenteritis
  Lymphoma
  Graft-versus-host disease

Malnutrition
  Protein-calorie
  Folate deficiency
  Iron deficiency

free of cereal grains, wheat, rye, barley, oats, and malt.[178, 225] An example of such a diet is included in the Appendix. Lactose intolerance is presumed, so lactose is initially excluded. Infants are routinely treated with vitamin D, iron, and folic acid when such deficiencies can be documented. If the alkaline phosphatase is significantly elevated, calcium therapy as well as vitamin D is initiated. Symptomatic improvement usually is evident within days to several weeks, especially with regard to behavioral manifestations. During treatment, the coefficient of fat absorption will improve by 50 per cent within two weeks and approach normal in three weeks. In infancy, the small bowel biopsy specimen is more likely to show a return to a completely normal state, while that in the older child and adult demonstrates persistent low-grade abnormalities. Those patients not responding to dietary therapy alone may require pancreatic enzyme supplementation or even a short course of steroids.

Dietary indiscretions interfering with recovery are usually subtle as a result of gluten-containing products such as ice cream, prepared meats, candies, peanut butter, ketchup, and other products in which gluten is used as a filler. Any patient with active or partially treated GSE has significant impairment of absorption for most orally ingested medications. Thus patients re-

quiring antibiotics or anticonvulsive therapy should be closely monitored to determine the adequacy of their dosage during the course of active disease.[70] Retarded growth may be the only evidence of dietary indiscretion.[135]

Prognosis. The long-term prognosis of patients with celiac disease is considered excellent. Approximately 25 per cent of patients may suffer from recurrent relapses that interfere with normal growth. It is not appreciated that during late childhood and early adolescence the patients may become clinically tolerant to gluten intake. Examination of a small bowel biopsy specimen, however, shows significant abnormalities despite an absence of clinical symptoms. The dietary treatment of patients with confirmed gluten-sensitive enteropathy is, therefore, a lifelong commitment. Even those assumedly taking a restricted diet may show mucosal abnormalities, and periodic conference with a nutritionist is essential to guarantee accuracy.[56]

COW'S MILK PROTEIN ENTEROPATHY

Despite recent advances in clinical description, the diagnosis of cow's milk protein enteropathy remains controversial. To the query "Have you seen it?" one answers "Of course." "Can you prove it?" "Well ... not really." As true allergy or immediate hypersensitivity is difficult to assess, we will refer to this entity as a sensitivity (clinical criteria) or an enteropathy (histologic criteria).[20, 21, 328]

Incidence. Since the clinical criteria for diagnosis remain obscure, it is no surprise that incidence figures range from 0.3 to 7 per cent of the normal population, rising to 30 per cent in atopic children.[65, 105, 147, 152, 171]

Etiology. The pathogenesis of cow's milk protein enteropathy is not known.[83] As with gluten-sensitive enteropathy, the two major theories are (1) direct protein toxicity, versus (2) altered immunologic response. As cow's milk contains more than 20 antigenic protein components, the distinction has not been and will not be easy.[83, 84] Studies to date suggest that β-lactoglobulin, α-lactalbumin, casein, and bovine serum albumin are most likely to produce clinical symptoms in patients with cow's milk sensitivity, with β-lactoglobulin the most active fraction. Cross sensitivity exists between cow and goat milk proteins.[137, 199] There is evidence on one hand that heating milk modifies its proteins and decreases or eliminates its antigenicity and on the other hand that heating milk increases its anaphylactigenic properties. Some infants tolerate milk boiled 30 minutes but not that boiled 20 minutes. Both intrauterine sensitization and sensitization to the proteins transmitted through breast milk have been postulated.[190]

The mode of milk protein digestion and absorption is not entirely known. Certainly gastric pepsin and pancreatic enzymes form peptides that are then hydrolyzed by intracellular peptidases into their component amino acids. Antigenically active peptides have been prepared from β-lactoglobulin after trypsin hydrolysis, and we have found coproantibodies to pepsin-trypsin peptide digests of casein and β-lactoglobulin. In vivo studies have shown adequate digestion of milk proteins by children with intestinal disease, but inadequate digestion by those with pancreatic insufficiency.[171a]

Innumerable studies have confirmed the development of antibodies to milk proteins in serum, feces, and duodenal secretions in infancy.[334] Antibody levels are highest in children with cow's milk sensitivity, inflammatory bowel disease, celiac disease, and milk aspiration pneumonia. The systemic antibody response is presumably the result of enhanced protein uptake. In a recent study of 46 neonates at six days of age, DeLire et al. demonstrated that all the infants fed cow's milk formulas had circulating antigen IgG antibody complexes in their sera after feedings.[71] This correlates with the original work of Lippard et al. showing infants after their first milk feed developing an antibody response at five days, with high titers appearing between seven and ten days.[205] These persist 20 to 30 days in nor-

mal infants but are higher and more prolonged in allergic infants. Because a similar study in adults demonstrated such complexes only in patients with IgA deficiency, the focus is on the delayed development of secretory IgA antibody in the neonate and delayed IgA production in allergic infants.[59, 316] Ten per cent of our milk-allergic infants under six months of age have extremely low serum IgA, whereas most patients over six months of age have elevated levels. Shiner et al. reported a rise in serum IgE.[299] Enhanced permeability of the neonatal gut to dietary macromolecules is well established. It is our belief, and that of others, that gastroenteritis alone, or particularly in an infant with low intestinal IgA, may predispose to protein sensitization.[140a, 303a, 335b] It is interesting that infants taking feeds with a high protein content have higher immunoglobulin levels than those taking feeds containing less protein.[325a, 354]

The capacity for circulating antigen-antibody complexes to produce tissue damage is more obscure. In support of the concept are the observations of Matthews and Soothill that decreased levels of C3 complement occur following milk ingestion,[221] and the report of Sandberg et al. that in some patients steroid-responsive nephrosis is exacerbated by milk challenge.[284] Neither of these studies has been confirmed. The association of circulating antibodies to cow's milk protein and chronic pulmonary disease in infancy (Heiner's syndrome) is also felt to support an immune complex–mediated cytotoxicity.[21, 71]

In 1975, Shiner et al. proposed that cow's milk sensitivity was mediated by reaginic IgE antibody.[299, 300] In small bowel mucosa, they demonstrated increased IgE immunofluorescence in jejunal plasma cells, mast cell degranulation, and eosinophilic and polymorphonuclear infiltration following milk challenge. IgM and IgG cells increased, but IgA cells did not seem to be involved in early reactions. IgA cells increase in biopsy specimens taken 24 or more hours after challenge, suggesting a later and more sustained response.[223a, 298a] In older children, May and Bock et al. have

Table 19–11   Factors Predisposing to Milk Protein Sensitivity

Family history of allergy
Early exposure to cow's milk proteins
Secretory IgA deficiency
Acute enteritis: infection or gluten-sensitive enteropathy

demonstrated positive skin tests in children with cow's milk sensitivity, but emphasize that confirmation is only achieved with blind challenge.[37, 223] Again, sensitization is felt to occur with enhanced antigen uptake in infancy. Regrettably, skin test positivity is common in asymptomatic children. While the pathophysiology remains obscure, a number of predisposing factors to the development of milk protein sensitivity are proposed. These are listed in Table 19–11.

Symptoms.   The symptoms attributed to cow's milk protein sensitivity have ranged from rash, congestion, and colic to diarrhea, rectal bleeding, emesis, and acute systemic anaphylaxis. Indeed, sudden infant death has been attributed to cow's milk sensitivity. The intolerance of an infant to feeding can reflect many factors, some of which are listed in Table 19–12.

When one focuses on the gastrointestinal manifestations of cow's milk protein sensitivity, three distinct clinical syndromes emerge.[170b, 326b, 335a] The first is acute milk protein–induced enterocolitis.[123] Infants with this disorder are usually two days to four months old and develop severe diarrhea with enteric bleeding within days to weeks after exposure to cow's milk–based formulas or the transition from heat-processed formu-

Table 19–12   Factors in "Formula Intolerance" in Infancy

Dislike/parent expectation
Overfeeding
Bacterial contamination
Disaccharide intolerance
Osmolality
Metabolic imbalance
Chalasia
Pancreatic insufficiency
Type II or immune complex toxicity
Type I or immediate hypersensitivity

la to whole cow's milk.[274b] Abdominal distention and emesis are common findings. The diarrhea and bleeding will resolve rapidly on elimination of cow's milk–based proteins from the diet, though cross reactivity to soy and goat's milk protein may be encountered. This extraordinarily toxic response appears to be a function of immature intestinal (? immune) function, as these infants will generally tolerate milk challenge after one year of age.[349] Isolated gastrointestinal bleeding in excess of 1.8 ml per day has been noted in normal infants exposed to whole cow's milk. Anaphylactic shock is reported, with an incidence from 0 to 33 per cent of cases, and it usually occurs after challenge. Necrotizing enterocolitis and even pneumatosis intestinalis may be seen.[49]

The second and more common clinical syndrome is chronic, often mucoid, diarrhea. While most such infants become symptomatic between four and six weeks of age, onset between two days and six months is seen. A later onset may occur within several weeks of discontinuation of breast feeding. Gastroesophageal reflux and colic may precede the diarrhea, though direct associations with these symptoms are difficult to confirm. With mild symptoms, growth is generally maintained. With severe diarrhea, impaired growth, anemia, hypoproteinemia, and generalized edema may develop.[331, 332, 349] Abdominal distention, muscle wasting, and reduced subcutaneous fat may lead to clinical confusion of the condition with gluten-sensitive enteropathy. Occasionally mothers describe white seedy material or bean-like curds in the stool. Occasionally a wheal-like erythema about the anus is noted. The diversity of the symptoms in these infants is presented in Table 19–13. With failure to appreciate the severity of the process, intractable diarrhea may ensue, with villous atrophy and disaccharide malabsorption.[268]

The third clinical syndrome is noted in infants over six months of age who develop milk protein sensitivity following an episode of acute enteritis. This also may be seen on a transient basis in infants with

Table 19–13 Clinical and Laboratory Findings in Children with Gastrointestinal Milk Allergy*

PATIENT NUMBER	SEX	AGE AT ONSET	SYMPTOMS AT ONSET	CONTINUING† SYMPTOMS	AGE AT DIAGNOSIS	HEMOGLOBIN Gm/Dl	C-V COLLAPSE ON CHALLENGE	GROWTH RETARDATION‡	LATER ALLERGY	AGE OF MILK TOLERANCE	FAMILY HISTORY ALLERGY	FAMILY HISTORY G.I. DISEASE
1	M	2 da	Diarrhea	Diarrhea	4 wk	10.8	+	No	Rhinitis	2 yr	+	Father—blood in stool as infant
2	M	3 wk	Blood in stool	Diarrhea and blood	2 mo	10.2		No	Eczema	1 yr	+	Mother—colitis
3	M	3 da	Diarrhea	Diarrhea	2 wk	8.4		Yes	Eczema, recurring pneumonia	1 yr	−	
4	M	1 wk	Diarrhea	Diarrhea	8 da	9.5	+	Yes	None	8 mo	−	
5	M	3 da	Vomiting	Semi-formed stools	1 mo	8.7	+	Yes	None	5 yr	+	Mother—diarrhea and vomiting from shellfish
6	M	2 wk	Blood, mucus in stool	Diarrhea	2 mo	10.6		No	Rhinitis	3 yr	+	
7	M	4 mo	Colic	Diarrhea	6 mo	10.0		No	Rhinitis, cough	1 yr	+	Sibling had intussusception
8	M	2 mo	Diarrhea, blood, mucus	Diarrhea, blood, mucus	5 mo	10.0		No	None	1 yr	+	
9	M	2 wk	Vomiting	Semi-formed stools	4 wk	16.0		No	None	2 yr	+	
10	M	3 wk	Colic	Semi-formed stools	8 wk	11.0	+	Yes	None	1 yr	−	
11	M	2 da	Vomiting	Diarrhea	6 wk	7.5		Yes	None	3 yr	+	Three siblings—G.I. milk allergy
12	M	7 da	Diarrhea	Semi-formed stools	4 wk	13.0		No	Eczema	1 yr	+	
13	F	5 da	Vomiting	Diarrhea	10 da	10.0		Yes	None	2 yr	−	
14	M	7 wk	Diarrhea, vomiting	Diarrhea	8 wk	7.5	+	Yes	None	1 yr	−	
15	M	3 da	Diarrhea	Diarrhea, blood	3 wk	10.0	+	Yes	Chronic pneumonia	Died at 2 yr	+	
16	M	3 da	Diarrhea	Semi-formed stools	6 mo	9.0		No	None	1 yr	+	
17	M	4 wk	Diarrhea	Diarrhea	2 mo	7.5	+	Yes	Croup	1 yr	−	
18	F	6 wk	Diarrhea	Semi-formed stools	2 yr	10.2		No		Not at 2 yr	+	
19	M	3 wk	Diarrhea	Diarrhea, blood	4 mo	9.6		No	Hives from fruits, chocolate	Not at 2 yr	+	
20	M	3 da	Diarrhea	Diarrhea	2 mo	6.7		Yes		Not at 7 mo	−	
21	M	3 da	Diarrhea	Diarrhea, blood	3 wk	9.8		Yes		Not at 6 mo	+	Mother—G.I. allergy to shellfish; Father—colic as infant

*From Gryboski, J. D.: Gastrointestinal milk allergy. Pediatrics 40:354, 1967.

†Stools from all 21 patients had 2+ to 4+ benzidine reactions. Coagulase-positive staphylococci were present in stools from patients 20 and 21. Patient 20 had a flat lactose tolerance test.

‡Below third percentile in height and weight.

gluten-sensitive enteropathy. Diarrhea remains the prominent symptom, with abdominal distention, reduced appetite, and rash quite frequent. To distinguish this protein-induced phenomenon from acquired lactose deficiency requires a normal lactose tolerance test. However, diarrhea associated with a normal lactose tolerance or breath test may be due to milk protein contamination of the sugar.

Allergy is present in siblings or parents of more than half the infants with any form of gastrointestinal allergy.

Acute, severe gastrointestinal hemorrhage, and even ischemic colitis, have been attributed to milk allergy. Direct exposure of the rectal mucosa to milk in sensitive individuals will result in erythema, inflammation, edema, mucus secretion, and capillary bleeding.

Those with severe symptoms tend to have other allergies later in life, whereas those with only mild reactions do not.

Dermatologic manifestations may occur at any time in relation to diarrhea and consist of urticaria, eczema, and angioedema, with eczema the most common.

Heiner's syndrome of chronic pulmonary disease, wheezing, rhinitis, and recurrent otitis media is associated with the presence of serum precipitins of the IgA and IgG type to milk. Ten per cent of patients have pulmonary hemosiderosis.[146]

Other presumed associated diseases are otitis, sudden infant death syndrome, nephrotic syndrome, and hyperactivity. Abnormalities of gastric function and development of lactobezoar have been related to cow's milk protein intolerance.[187a, 200a]

Diagnosis. To date, no single laboratory test is available to confirm or refute the diagnosis of cow's milk protein sensitivity. As a result, the clinical response to milk challenge is often employed. In 1963, Goldman and his associates established three criteria for the diagnosis of cow's milk protein sensitivity: that the symptoms subside after the elimination of milk from the diet; that they recur within 48 hours after a trial feeding of milk; and that three challenges are positive and similar in clinical expression with symptomatic resolution in the interval between challenges.[113] In practice, the major issue is exclusion of lactose intolerance. Thus, when an infant presents with possible milk protein sensitivity, cow's milk protein is eliminated from the diet. After four to six weeks a lactose tolerance test is performed. If this is normal, a cow's milk challenge is undertaken. The impunity with which this challenge is performed is a function of the infant's age and the severity of the prior enteritis. One can rarely justify re-challenge in infants less than six months of age. If enteric hemorrhage or any question of anaphylaxis was a component of the initial episode, challenge is unconscionable and should be undertaken only after one year of age — even then, only in the hospital setting.

A number of indirect confirmatory studies have been proposed. Serum antibodies often are not present and IgE not elevated. Specific allergo-immunoabsorbent tests are not consistently positive, and skin testing is unreliable.[11] A safe and, in our hands, reliable test has been the examination of the supernatant from a freshly spun stool for the presence of precipitating antibodies (coprantibodies) against cow's milk proteins. Stools are centrifuged for 30 minutes and the clear, colored supernatant is placed in the center well of a micro double-immunodiffusion in agar-gel slide. Milk and 5 to 10 per cent solutions of the milk proteins are placed in the surrounding wells. Plates are incubated at room temperature in a moist chamber and examined at 6, 24 and 48 hours for the development of precipitin bands (Fig. 19–10). While coproantibodies are occasionally noted in normal infants, their presence in the stool allows a presumptive diagnosis and justifies cow's milk elimination.[69, 189] Lymphocyte stimulation by milk and depressed leukocyte chemotaxis have been reported in sensitized patients.[13A, 45]

The role of pre- and postchallenge small bowel biopsy remains controversial.[312] Evidence of villus injury has been reported in acute cow's milk enteropathy. The rapidity with which a reproducible injury is seen following challenge is variable. Routine postchallenge biopsy therefore should re-

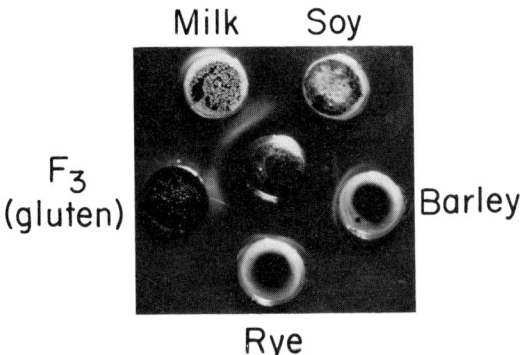

Milk   Soy

F₃
(gluten)   Barley

Rye

Figure 19–10 Agar-in-gel immunodiffusion. Stool supernatant is in the central well, and milk and cereal proteins surround it. Precipitin bands between the supernatant and fraction III, rye, barley, and milk are noted.

main a research tool with limited clinical application. The role of incubation of biopsy specimens *in vitro* with milk antigens is not known. *In vitro* chemotaxis studies suggesting specific inhibition have been reported recently.

Other clinical features noted on milk challenge have been reviewed by Powell, who found consistent peripheral polymorphonuclear leukocytosis and elevation of B_1C globulin as well as fever and increased fecal leukocytes following challenge in infants with cow's milk and soy protein enteritis.[270] Eosinophilia is rarely seen, but anemia is present in 20 to 70 per cent of infants, vitamin K deficiency in 35 to 50 per cent, aminoaciduria in 42 per cent, and elevated alkaline phosphatase in 10 per cent.

The complications of milk protein enteropathy also may be demonstrated: milk steatorrhea, acquired disaccharide intolerance, occult rectal bleeding, protein-losing enteropathy, and hypoalbuminemia. These are secondary manifestations of any number of enteropathies and thus their demonstration does not confirm the diagnosis.

Treatment. Most infants respond to the elimination of cow's milk protein (including beef) from the diet within two to three days. A prolonged recovery should be anticipated in those with established intractable diarrhea; use of a hydrolyzed protein formula, Pregestimil or Nutramigen, is recommended in the early recovery phase since they engender no antibody response.[84a] A trial of a soybean-based formula may be considered in two to four weeks in an effort to reduce formula costs, but intolerance to soy protein is seen in up to 40 per cent of these infants, theoretically due to cross reactivity of major antigens.

The role of medication to allow limited milk protein intake in later childhood is unclear. Success has been reported with oral disodium cromoglycate[101, 187] and cyproheptadine (Periactin) — drugs that block mast cell mediator release or function. Application should be restricted to the rare child with multiple intolerances whose growth is impaired by minimal protein ingestion.[338a]

Prognosis. Tolerance of cow's milk protein is slowly acquired, with most infants tolerating milk-containing products by one to two years of age and whole milk by five years of age. In the presence of a strong family history for atopic disease, persistence of cow's milk protein sensitivity should be anticipated, with acquired intolerance to other dietary proteins all too frequent. In our experience, soy and gluten are the primary forms, but enteropathies related to fish, rice, and chicken have also been described.[327a]

SOY PROTEIN ENTEROPATHY

In the last 15 years, soybean protein has joined gluten and cow's milk as a confirmed cause of villous epithelial injury of the small bowel and even of monosaccharide malabsorption.[110] The condition was originally described by Ament and Rubin,[6] and several series now have been published. The clinical relevance of this condition is the result of the "routine" use of soy formulas in infants after milk allergy has been diagnosed or in those with positive family histories for cow's milk–based formula intolerance, and also the increased use of soy protein as a protein fortification in commercial foodstuffs. The incidence of this condition is a function of the age at which soybean protein–based formulas are introduced, with increased clinical severity in the first two months of life. Soy also will produce allergic proctitis with rectal bleeding.[133]

Etiology. A recent study by Eastham et al. has reinforced the argument that soy protein is every bit as antigenic as cow's milk protein in early infancy, with enhanced uptake suggested by systemic antibody response.[83] The introduction of soy-based formula in the early recovery phase for acute enteritis or milk protein allergy may also predispose to sensitization. The mechanism of villous or colonic injury remains unknown.[345]

Symptoms. The majority of infants will present in the first six weeks of life with persistent diarrhea. As with milk protein, a rare infant will develop fulminant enterocolitis with ulcerative changes on sigmoidoscopy. Abdominal distention, edema, colic, and emesis are not common. Occasionally an infant will manifest recurrent pulmonary disease.

Diagnosis. As most soy-based formulas contain sucrose as the predominant carbohydrate, confusion with congenital sucrose-isomaltase deficiency, hereditary fructose intolerance, and acquired sucrose deficiency must be classified. Precipitins to soy may be detected in the stool. After two to four weeks of stabilization on a diet free of soy protein, one initiates the work-up with a standard sucrose tolerance test. The urine is screened for reducing sugars (fructose) and liver function studies are done if fructose intolerance is suspected. The clinical response to soy protein challenge is monitored for peripheral leukocytosis, increased B_1C globulin, and fecal leukocytes and for fecal precipitins to soy protein. Radiographic bowel contrast studies are of no value. Proctosigmoidoscopy and biopsy are appropriate in those who present with symptoms of enterocolitis. Biopsy specimens should be evaluated for ganglion cells as well as the degree of inflammation so as to exclude Hirschsprung's disease.

Treatment. A soy-free diet is curative, and most infants can tolerate soy after 6 to 12 months' restriction. As soy fortification of food products is so common, routine challenge at 12 to 18 months of age is recommended so as to allow liberalization of the diet where possible.

WHEAT PROTEIN ALLERGY

Wheat protein allergy does not seem to exist alone in infancy but may follow or occur in conjunction with milk or soy allergy. Twenty to forty per cent of our milk allergic infants have developed intolerance to wheat products.[228]

Etiology. Sensitization presumably takes place when wheat is ingested during active cow's milk protein sensitization and wheat proteins penetrate a damaged mucosa.

Symptoms. Either the infant with cow's milk allergy recovers incompletely after elimination of antigen or develops diarrhea several weeks after clinical improvement. Weight loss follows and a regression to pretreatment status. Rickets has even been documented in such children.

Diagnosis. Radiologic examination of the small bowel is normal or may show a mild malabsorptive pattern. Steatorrhea, hypocalcemia, and even hypoalbuminemia are obvious if the disease has persisted for a long time. There may be some mild villous atrophy or normal villous structure, but the lamina propria is infiltrated by round cells and eosinophils. Coproantibodies to wheat and gluten fraction III are present in fresh stool extracts. The serum carotene varies between 25 and 200 μg/dl.

Treatment. Therapy consists of elimination of gluten products from the diet.

Prognosis. Usually the infants can tolerate wheat products within 6 to 12 months and have no further difficulties.

PRIMARY MALABSORPTION SYNDROME OF INFANCY

In 1967, a malabsorption syndrome was reported from Sweden characterized by the early onset of vomiting, diarrhea, and weight loss and associated with intolerance to milk, gluten, or both.[191] Infants with milk intolerance were symptomatic between one and five months and those with gluten intolerance were symptomatic later, between three and ten months. They had radiologic and laboratory evidence of malabsorption and serum precipitins to milk or gluten or both. More than half had subtotal or partial villous atrophy of the small intestine. Stool cultures from more than one third grew either *Staphylococcus* or pathogenic strains of *E. coli*. Gluten intolerance was present in two thirds of the infants with milk intolerance, and several had anaphylactoid reactions after gluten challenge.

Those with milk intolerance responded to dietary management and could tolerate milk after seven to ten months. Those with gluten intolerance required longer to respond — they could not tolerate reintroduction of gluten for months to one year. In both groups, absorption tests became normal at the time patients developed tolerance to the respective proteins. In a long-term follow-up, one third of patients with gluten intolerance had a clinical relapse and abnormal biopsy within six months after return to a normal diet. Serum IgA was elevated, and they developed serum precipitins to gluten and to milk. The remaining two thirds were asymptomatic after restitution of a normal diet; all but one, however, had abnormal small intestinal biopsy examinations. Laboratory studies did not demonstrate malabsorption. Whether this group of patients represents early celiac disease or an allergic response is speculative.[33] As noted in Table 19–10, p. 612, a multitude of causes may contribute to the "flat villus" lesion.[180, 308]

THE OTHER FOOD ALLERGIES?

While acute or chronic enteric sensitivity to gluten, cow's milk, and soy protein is well established, the capacity of other antigenic proteins to induce small bowel disease is unknown. In the absence of objective data, the observations of generations of parents, in-laws, and other "concerned citizens" cannot be ignored. In controlled studies utilizing blind food challenge, Bock et al.[37] and May[223] have confirmed reproducible constitutional symptoms in childhood following ingestion of milk, soy, wheat, corn, nuts, and egg.[37, 168c, 223] The symptoms may or may not suggest localized small intestinal anaphylaxis. Other foods, such as strawberries, may directly induce histamine release without mediation by IgE. In the adult, sensitivity to shellfish is common. In truth, one can argue that it is theoretically possible to develop a systemic anaphylactic response following the ingestion or inhalation of any macromolecular protein to which prior exposure (and sensitization) occurred. When in doubt, dietary elimination is indicated in infancy with a controlled challenge undertaken in the preschool years when the parents first lose the capacity to control intake. Multiple eliminations should be avoided as iatrogenic malnutrition may ensue.

INHERITED AMINO ACID TRANSPORT DISORDERS

Under normal conditions, the cell membranes of intestinal mucosal cells contain at least three distinct active transport systems for protein: one for neutral amino acids (leucine, phenylalanine, and threonine), one for basic amino acids (lysine, arginine, and cystine), and one for proline and hydroxyproline. Separate systems for glycine and for branched-chain amino acids (valine, leucine, and isoleucine) have been proposed. When the normal adult jejunum is perfused with equimolar concentrations of the 18 common dietary amino acids, a consistent pattern of absorption is obtained. Methionine and branched-chain amino acids have the highest rates of absorption.[3] Amino acids with longer side chains or neutral charges have a stronger affinity for the absorption sites and hence more rapid uptake. It now appears that, in normal circumstances, the majority of amino acid absorption occurs as oligopeptide rather than free amino acid.

The specific recognized defects in amino acid transport are summarized in Table 19–14. For the majority, similar defects in renal tubular reabsorption are encountered. As a result, most are classified as aminoacidurias.[291, 292]

Table 19-14 Amino Acid Transport Defects

DISORDER	GUT	KIDNEY	CLINICAL FEATURES
Cystinuria	I. lysine arginine ornithine cystine	cystine lysine arginine ornithine	renal stones, mental retardation
	II. lysine arginine ornithine normal cystine	cystine lysine arginine ornithine	
	III. normal or partially defective lysine and arginine	cystine lysine arginine ornithine	
Hyperdiabasic aminoaciduria (familial protein intolerance)	lysine	lysine dibasic	hepatosplenomegaly, FTT, diarrhea
Hyperdiabasic aminoaciduria with hyperlysinuria and hyperammonemia	lysine	ornithine arginine lysine	mental retardation, FTT, hepatosplenomegaly
Hyperdibasic aminoaciduria with lysine malabsorption	lysine	ornithine arginine lysine	FTT
Iminoglycinuria	normal or impaired	proline OH-proline glycine	rash, photosensitivity, ataxia, short stature
Methione mal- absorption	methionine	—OH—butyric acid	mental retardation, diarrhea, convulsions
Blue diaper syndrome	tryptophan	indican	hypercalcemia nephrocalcinosis

FAMILIAL PROTEIN INTOLERANCE OR HYPERDIBASIC AMINOACIDURIA

Hyperdibasic aminoaciduria, primarily reported from Scandinavia, Japan, and Canada, is also referred to as familial protein intolerance. This disorder is characterized by growth failure, emesis, diarrhea, neutropenia, hepatosplenomegaly, and severe aversion to high-protein foods. Mental retardation is a variable finding.[18, 182, 218, 266, 293]

The Finnish families have displayed increased renal clearance of lysine and moderately increased arginine clearance. French-Canadians had increased clearances of lysine, arginine, and ornithine. Both these and the Finns had impaired intestinal lysing absorption, whereas the Japanese had impaired dibasic acid transport. Malab-sorption of cystine and ornithine has been postulated. Citrulline absorption is normal.

Inheritance. No consistent patterns of inheritance have been established. Consanguinity has been noted in several families; in others, a direct parent-to-child transmission.

Symptoms. Some patients show only hyperdibasic aminoaciduria, but others develop severe disease. Vomiting and diarrhea occur after weaning at some time between 3 and 13 months of age. Although small bowel histology is normal, a number of patients develop a mild steatorrhea. Hepatomegaly is followed later by splenomegaly, and liver biopsy shows round-cell infiltrate of the portal triads and early fibrosis. Some patients are mentally retarded.

Diagnosis. There is postprandial hyperammonemia, and the blood urea nitrogen is low. Urea cycle enzymes were normal in the Finnish and Japanese groups in which they were studied. Blood urea nitrogen and fasting ammonia levels were low, but only the ammonia rose after alanine ingestion. It is of interest that ingestion of alanine and arginine together was followed by a rise in blood urea but not of ammonia. Defective leukocyte and liver glutaminase activity has been described.[303]

Treatment. A low-protein diet often (but not always) is effective in controlling the diarrhea. The diet must be supplemented with arginine, 2 gm per day, to promote growth and nutrition.

CYSTINURIA

In this disorder, dibasic aminoaciduria is associated with one of three defects in the intestinal absorption of the dibasic amino acids. Since cystine is insoluble in urine, some patients develop renal calculi.[51, 241, 280]

Inheritance and Incidence. Inherited in an autosomal recessive or incomplete recessive form, some patients may be heterozygous for two mutations, and some families carry one or more genetic compounds of genotypes I/II. It is the double heterozygotes of types I and II who form calculi. Both males and females are equally affected, with an incidence of 1:40,000 (but perhaps more realistically 1:20,000).

Pathophysiology. In the type I form there is complete absence of active arginine, cystine, and lysine transport in the intestine. Urinary amino acid excretion by heterozygotes is normal. In type II, patients have had active intestinal transport of cystine but not of lysine, and the heterozygotes have increased urinary excretion of all four dibasic amino acids (lysine, cystine, arginine, and ornithine). Recent studies show no difference in intestinal absorption between types I and II. Type III patients have reduced intestinal transport of cystine, lysine, and arginine, and heterozygotes excrete moderate amounts of the four dibasic amino acids.

In the kidney, cystine shares one transport system with the dibasic amino acids, but other systems (one for the dibasics and one for cystine) exist. It is abnormalities in these that account for the three types of disease. No transport defects have been identified in red blood cells, skin fibroblasts, or leukocytes.

Symptoms. There are usually no significant gastrointestinal symptoms. The patients are usually smaller than normal and are otherwise asymptomatic until renal calculi develop between the third and fourth decades. A few show mental retardation or illness. Death is usually from renal failure.

Diagnosis. The diagnosis rests upon a positive urine nitroprusside test and the presence of hexagonal, flat crystals in the urine. Chromatography shows hyperdibasic aminoaciduria and specific increases in cystine.

Treatment. Increasing urinary volumes with water and alkalinization of the urine will help to increase the solubility of cystine. Penicillamine will decrease cystine excretion by thiosulfide exchange but may cause hypersensitivity nephrosis and cannot be recommended in children. Cysteamine recently has been used.[107]

BLUE DIAPER SYNDROME

This disorder is due to impaired tryptophan absorption and is associated with hypercalcemia and nephrocalcinosis.[79] The blue discoloration of the diapers is caused by increased indole excretion in the urine, which results from bacterial action upon the unabsorbed amino acids in the colon.

Reported in two brothers, it is probably inherited in an autosomal recessive form. Tryptophan loading is followed by hypercalcemia.

METHIONINE MALABSORPTION (OASTHOUSE DISEASE)

This disorder derived its name from the peculiar dried celery–like odor of the urine.[160] Presenting symptoms are white hair, edema, hypercapnea, mental retardation, and convulsions. It has been reported in males and male siblings, suggesting a sex-linked inheritance. Urinary amino acids are normal. There is decreased intestinal absorption of methionine, and methionine loading is followed by diarrhea and increased urinary excretion of hydroxyacetic acid, an end-product of bacterial degradation of the unabsorbed amino acid. Other branch-chain keto acids are excreted as well in the urine. Testing with ferric chloride yields a green color in the urine. A low-methionine diet results in improvement of diarrhea, darkening of hair and lessening of the absorptive defect.

LOWE'S SYNDROME

This is an extremely rare, sex-linked disease affecting males, characterized by aminoaciduria, especially of lysine and arginine, mental retardation, glaucoma, cataracts, hypotonia, vitamin D–resistant rickets, renal disease, and choreoathetosis. There is a partial intestinal defect in absorption of lysine and arginine, but cystine absorption is normal. Hepatic complications are noted.

LYSINURIA

Lysine malabsorption includes an aminoaciduria of lysine, arginine, and ornithine.[73, 258, 272, 302] Cystine excretion is normal. Serum amino acids are normal. It is extremely rare, and there is some evidence of consanguinity since maternal and paternal grandmothers of two affected siblings were first cousins. Symptoms are mental and physical retardation. Two affected females had diarrhea and vomiting from birth. Heterozygotes have a slightly abnormal lysine absorption.

Symptoms become milder with age.

LYSINURIA AND HYPERAMMONEMIA

In this disorder, lysine absorption is abnormal as are the absorptions of arginine and ornithine.[41, 259] Plasma levels of lysine and arginine are decreased, and urinary excretion of lysine is increased. Vomiting and diarrhea appear in early infancy but decrease with age. Mental retardation, postprandial coma, seizures, and intermittent hepatosplenomegaly are typical findings.

As in familial protein intolerance, supplementary arginine will prevent hyperammonemia.

IMINOACIDURIA (JOSEPH'S DISEASE)

More than a dozen family pedigrees have been studied.[114] Inheritance is likely of an autosomal recessive type, with some evidence supporting gene mutation. Frequency is estimated at 1:20,000. There has been no direct transmission from parent to child but some parents have been consanguineous. Males and females are affected equally. The classic patient has increased urinary excretion of proline, glycine, and hydroxyproline and normal serum amino acids. Their uptake by leukocytes and skin is normal. Heterozygotes have hyperglycinuria but not hyperiminoaciduria.

After proline loading there is impaired proline absorption but normal glycine and hydroxyproline absorption. A few patients have impaired glycine and iminoacid absorption.

Symptoms develop between 1 and 42 years, with some people being mentally retarded and others seeming perfectly well.

NEUTRAL AMINOACIDURIA (HARTNUP DISEASE)

Hartnup disease has been reported in fewer than 50 patients. Characterized by an aminoaciduria specific for mono-amino-mono carboxylic amino acids with neutral or aromatic side chains, the specific intestinal lesion is defective malabsorption of tryptophan, L-histidine, and phenylalanine.[240, 248]

The classic symptoms of pellagra-like rash, ataxia, and photosensitivity are actually due to nicotinamide deficiency.

The disease is probably inherited as a rare autosomal mutation and is more prevalent in females.

In the bowel, malabsorbed tryptophan is converted to indoles, which are absorbed and excreted in the urine. When tryptophan, histidine, or phenylalanine is given as a dipeptide, absorption is increased.

The patients are usually small, and signs of cerebellar ataxia are predominant as falling attacks. The attacks resolve over a period of four weeks, only to recur. The rash has a glove and stocking distribution. Emotional instability and delirium are additional signs of neurologic disease. Attacks are precipitated by fever, sun, sulfonamides, or stress. Nearly one sixth of patients are retarded.

The symptoms improve with age, but active treatment consists of avoidance of precipitating factors and daily supplementation of the diet with 40 to 250 mg of nicotinamide. Neomycin decreases colonic bacteria and, therefore, indole formation.

FAT DIGESTION — DISORDERS OF FAT METABOLISM

Fat digestion begins in the mouth and continues in the stomach by the action of lingual lipase that functions in the absence of bile salts. This enzyme is present by 26 weeks' gestation and increases after birth to attain adult levels by 17 days. In the stomach, 10 to 30 per cent of ingested fat is hydrolyzed to glycerides (primarily diglycerides) and free fatty acids. In the duodenum, pancreatic lipase and bile salts are relatively low in the neonate, and lower yet in the premature. Fat digestion is facilitated

in the breast-fed infant by bile salt–stimulated lipase and lipoprotein lipase. Through the formation of micelles, insoluble lipids are presented in a more soluble form to the intestinal mucosa, where the micellar aggregates break up. Liberated monoglycerides and free fatty acids are taken up by the cell and resynthesized to triglycerides through the activating (FA-CoA ligase) and the esterifying (acyl-transferase) enzymes, all of which seem to be active in the neonate. Finally, triglyceride droplets are synthesized to lipoprotein particles for transport from the enterocyte, with most lipid being transported as chylomicrons (Fig. 19–11). Tests for the evaluation of fat absorption are discussed later in the chapter.

An isolated co-lipase deficiency has recently been described in two brothers.[117a]

DISORDERS OF MUCOSAL LIPID TRANSPORT

ABETALIPOPROTEINEMIA

In this disorder, the intestinal mucosa is unable to synthesize apolipoprotein B in a form capable of functioning in lipid transport.[290] This defect in triglyceride transport from the villous epithelial cell to the lymphatic system causes defective chylomicron formation, hypocholesteremia, and steator-

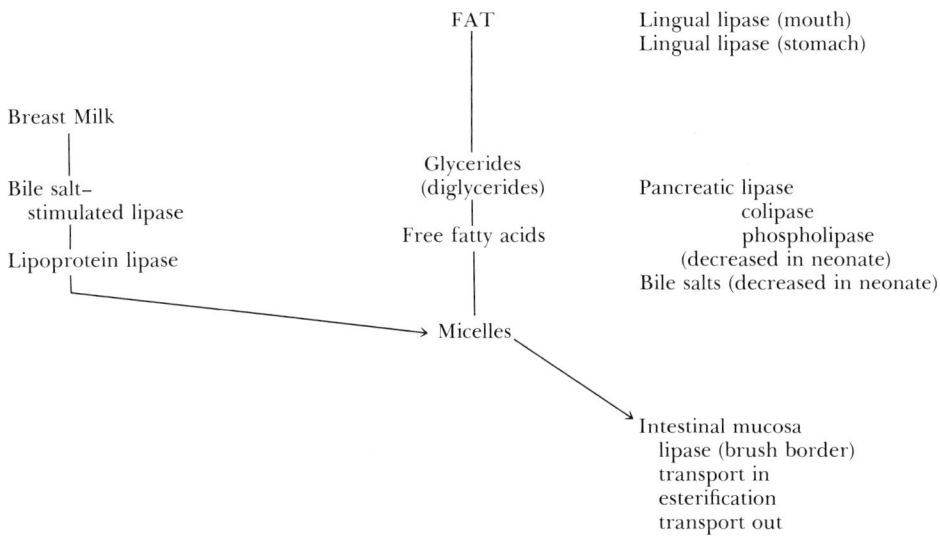

Figure 19–11   Fat digestion.

rhea. It is characterized by a total absence of beta-lipoprotein from the plasma and absent-to-minimal levels of all lipoproteins containing apolipoprotein B (chylomicrons, low and very low density lipoproteins). Acanthrocytes are present in the peripheral blood smear, and additional findings are ataxia, mental retardation, retinitis, and malabsorption.[19, 28] A similar clinical picture without lipoprotein abnormalities has been described.

Incidence. The disease is rare, with fewer than 50 patients reported, one third of which were diagnosed in infancy.

Inheritance. It is transmitted in an autosomal recessive form, associated with a high frequency of parental consanguinity. Many families are of Jewish or Italian extraction. Prenatal diagnosis and detection of heterozygotes are not yet possible.[150] A familial hypobetalipoproteinemia exists in heterozygotes.[9a]

Etiology and Pathophysiology. In the great majority of patients, apolipoprotein B synthesis in the intestine during fat absorption cannot be demonstrated, resulting in an inability of the cell to form chylomicrons and low-density lipoprotein (LDL).[109, 116] The intestinal mucosa is engorged with lipid droplets, even in the fasting state. Normally, triglyceride droplets are surrounded by the endoplasmic reticulum and Golgi apparatus, the cisternae of which contain clusters of chylomicrons. The chylomicrons are synthesized by intestinal mucosa and are added sequentially to the lipid droplet to form a complete chylomicron.[324] In abetalipoproteinemia, the cisternae are empty and large lipid droplets are free in the cytoplasm. Using fluorescent antibody techniques, there is no demonstrable chylomicron apoprotein B (apo B) in the intestinal mucosa or low-density lipoprotein.

Absorption of other nutrients is impaired and steatorrhea is significant.

In the peripheral blood there are milk anemia, slightly increased reticulocyte numbers, and normal or decreased haptoglobins. The acanthrocytes are most obvious in the wet smears and appear as crenated spheres with spiny protrusions (Fig. 19–12). These cells have normal to de-

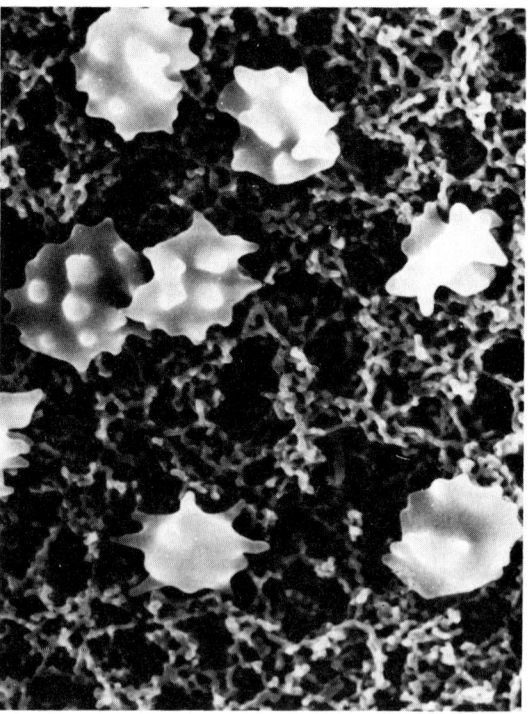

Figure 19–12 Scanning electron microscopy of the acanthocyte from a five-month-old child with abetalipoproteinemia. (Courtesy of Dr. Jean L. Olson, Department of Pathology, The Johns Hopkins University School of Medicine.)

creased survival, normal osmotic and acid fragility, increased susceptibility to trauma, and peroxide hemolysis — the latter being reversed by vitamin E supplementation. The bone marrow is normal. Red blood cell lipids are abnormal, with sphingomyelin increased and lecithin and linoleic acid decreased.

Symptoms. Malodorous diarrhea often develops as early as the first week of life, but some infants only show poor weight gain and linear growth. Eventually, malabsorption becomes obvious. Neurologic manifestations may develop early with areflexia, proprioceptive deficit, and ataxia, progressing to muscle weakness and sensory loss. Mental retardation has been reported, especially in infants from consanguineous families. Visual problems appear after five or more years, caused by pigmented lesions of the retina which progress to retinitis pigmentosa with macular involvement. Blindness is the end result. Many infants were originally diagnosed as having celiac disease until the other manifestations became obvious.

Differential Diagnosis. Celiac disease is the major disorder with which abetalipoproteinemia is confused. Acanthrocytes are not specific for they occur in neonatal jaundice, cholestatic liver disease, and some of the anemias and purpuras.

Diagnosis. The diagnosis is suggested by absence of blood betalipoprotein and low cholesterol, serum lipids, and phospholipids.[287] It is confirmed by small bowel biopsy, showing the villous epithelial cells to be filled with lipid droplets, especially at the tip (Fig. 19–13). Slight reductions in villus height and mild inflammatory cell infiltrate are seen. No lipid is present in macrophages.

Treatment. To date, no treatment regimen has prevented the progression of neurologic impairment and retinitis. Infusion of hyperbetalipoproteinemic serum will ele-

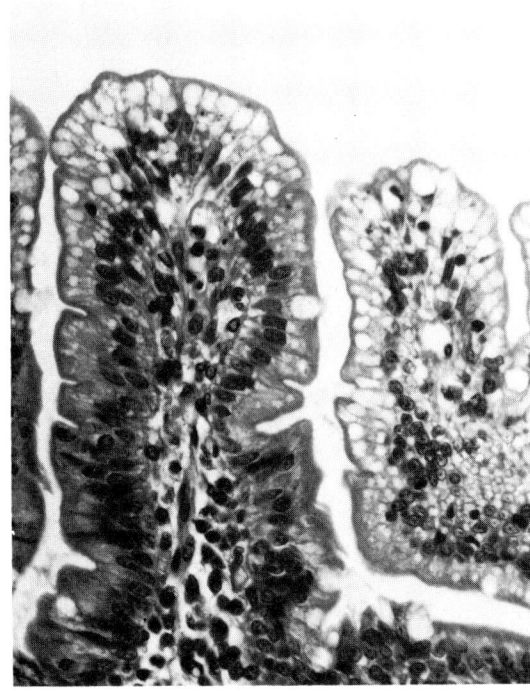

Figure 19–13 Small bowel biopsy from a five-month-old child with abetalipoproteinemia. Note the retention of triglyceride in the mature villous epithelial cells. A modest inflammatory cell infiltration of the lamina propria also is noted in this specimen.

vate betalipoproteins temporarily but with no improvement in clinical status or plasma triglyceride level. Saturated long-chain fat in the diet is reduced, with essential fatty acids provided as linoleic acid. Absorption is intact for medium-chain triglycerides, and improved growth should be anticipated on this regimen. Fat-soluble vitamin supplementation is routine and aggressively undertaken in newly diagnosed patients, especially for vitamin E.[244]

Prognosis. Progressive neurologic and retinal deterioration remains the rule, with death generally in adolescence or the early twenties. Fat absorption increases during childhood, and the children eventually can tolerate some degree of fat. Prenatal diagnosis is not yet possible.

WHITE VILLUS DISEASE

In 1970, Partin and Schubert described an infant with hypobetalipoproteinemia presenting profound diarrhea and marasmus in the first month of life.[261] Steatorrhea with 25 gm of fat in the feces per day was documented. The small bowel biopsy specimen revealed snow white intestinal tissue, with triglyceride storage in the villous epithelial cells but not in the crypts or lamina propria. On lipoprotein electrophoresis, low density lipoprotein (LDL) was reduced and very low-density lipoprotein (VLDL) was absent. Apolipoprotein B was reduced, but the infant failed to demonstrate anemia, acanthrocytosis, or neurologic impairment.

JUVENILE DIABETES MELLITUS

In juvenile diabetes mellitus, Bobo et al. reported increased levels of lipid in the epithelial cells on small bowel biopsy in poorly controlled diabetics.[36] This apparently results from increased endogenous lipid synthesis. Serum levels of cholesterol and triglyceride were mildly elevated, and fecal fats were normal. Villous epithelial development was normal. Associated symptoms included hepatomegaly and abdominal pain.

FAMILIAL CHOLESTEROL ESTER STORAGE DISEASES

Three familial cholesterol ester storage diseases involve the alimentary tract to some degree. In all, there is accumulation of cholesterol, cholesterol esters, and carotene in the viscera. All are extremely rare.

Wolman's Disease

Wolman's disease occurs in early infancy and has been fatal in all of the reported cases.[350]

Inheritance. It is of the autosomal recessive type and several siblings may be affected.

Etiology. The etiology is not known, but an absence of acid lipase activity in the liver and spleen has been found and may explain the accumulation of neutral lipids within swollen lysosomes.

Pathology. The liver and spleen are enlarged and contain deposits of cholesterol and its esters and of triglycerides. Similar deposits also are present in lymph nodes, adrenal glands, and the intestinal mucosa. Lipid storage is within the reticuloendothelial cells of the liver, particularly near the portal areas, and within the epithelial cells of the intestinal mucosa. Grossly the small bowel mucosa appears yellow, greasy, and granular. There are loss of villous structure, mucosal atrophy, and infiltrate of lipid-filled histiocytes in the lamina propria. Calcification and bilateral enlargement of the adrenal glands are considered characteristic of this disease. Foamy histiocytes are found in the thymus and bone marrow and vacuolated lymphocytes in the peripheral blood.

Chemically, the liver contains 3 to 20 times the normal amount of cholesterol but normal phospholipids and glycolipids. One to one and a half per cent of the wet weight of the normal liver is triglyceride or neutral fat, but in infants with this disorder 10 per cent of the wet weight is triglyceride or neutral fat. The spleen contains four to five times the normal amount of cholesterol, and lesser increases are noted in the thymus, lung, and kidney. The gray matter of the brain contains one and a half to two times the normal amount of cholesterol; the amount of cholesterol in the white matter is normal, but there is faulty myelination. Milky ascites may be present.

Symptoms. During the first few weeks of life chronic diarrhea, weight loss, and progressive enlargement of the liver and spleen develop. The infants die of extreme cachexia during the first few months of life. In one infant, development was normal until the fifth month, when vomiting, abdominal distention, weight loss, steatorrhea, and hepatosplenomegaly appeared. She also had alpha- and beta-hypolipoproteinemia. At autopsy there was evidence of lipid storage disease identical to Wolman's disease.

Treatment. None is available.

Cholesterol Ester Storage Disease

This is asymptomatic and characterized only by silent enlargement of the liver and spleen. The serum cholesterol is somewhat elevated, and serum bile acids are increased. Lipoproteins are normal. There is no steatorrhea. Lipid is stored in the liver within the parenchymal cells, and storage vacuoles seem to originate near the bile canaliculi. Biopsy tissue from the small intestine has an orange tint. Lipid is present in the extracellular space and smooth muscle of the lamina propria. The lacteals are filled with vacuoles of stored lipid, and foam cells surround the lacteals. Partin and Schubert postulate a block in lipid transport across the lacteal, although this remains to be proved.[260a] Pulmonary vascular obstruction may develop.

Tangier's Disease

Tangier's disease occurs in relatively healthy persons and is due to an absence of high-density lipoproteins. It is probably inherited in an autosomal recessive form. Lipid (esterified cholesterol), which accumulates in the macrophages, is greatest in tonsils, spleen, and lymph nodes.

Peripheral neuritis, ulcerative colitis, hepatomegaly, and diarrhea all have been encountered in association with this disease. The diagnosis is sometimes made during examination of the throat when huge, lipid-laden tonsils are seen. Biopsy of the large or small intestine will show accumulations of the lipid-containing macrophages in the lamina propria. There is little or no steatorrhea.

VITAMIN MALABSORPTION

Although general vitamin deficiencies may be noted in patients with malabsorption, selective defects in vitamin absorption are rare and to date involve only folic acid and vitamin B_{12}.

FOLIC ACID MALABSORPTION

Isolated folic acid malabsorption is unusual. In five patients reported up to 1973, it was associated with mental retardation or neurologic disease.[195, 196, 212, 285] Currently, folic acid deficiency most often is due to inadequate intake. In 1977, Davidson and Townley reported mucosal abnormalities in four infants with nutritional folic acid deficiency.[67] All were 8 to 11 months old and had been maintained primarily on goat's milk, a diet known to be folate-deficient, for at least six months.

Inheritance. The mode of inheritance of the congenital form of disease is unknown, although two of the infants were siblings. In another family, the parents were first cousins and the father showed an intermediate response after folate loading, suggesting an autosomal recessive mode of inheritance.[88, 277]

Etiology and Pathology. Folic acid constitutes only a minute fraction of the dietary folates, which occur primarily as the oligoglutamyl folates, containing one to six glutamyl residues. These are present in nearly all animal and vegetable foods. Active folate is derived from tetrahydrofolic acid. Humans are unable to synthesize the vitamin and require at least 50 μg per day; more is required if foods are cooked, for the vitamin is heat labile. Most folate is stored in liver, red blood cells, and skin fibroblasts.

Absorption takes place in the proximal two thirds of jejunum to where the vitamin is actively transported after removal of the oligoglutamyl portion. If huge quantities of folate are presented, some is absorbed by simple diffusion.

In folate malabsorption, enzymes required for folate transport also effect histidine degradation to glutamate; after histidine loading,[186] N-formino-L-glutamate (FIGLU), an intermediary, accumulates in the urine.

Because of its critical function in DNA biosynthesis, folic acid is required for normal cellular proliferation. Deficiency produces megaloblastic changes in the epithelial cells, nuclear enlargement, villus blunting, and crypt hypertrophy. The degree of crypt hypertrophy distinguishes these patients from those with villus atrophy secondary to malnutrition. Dietary folate deficiency in rats will produce a similar histologic lesion.

Symptoms. These infants present with pallor, poor weight gain, chronic diarrhea, and lethargy. In a few, the onset is more insidious with malnutrition noted only after 2 to 17 months. Signs of folic acid deficiency such as stomatitis, glossitis, and overt scurvy may develop. Purpura, convulsions, and mental retardation are late sequelae. Several infants have shown mental retardation and relapsing megaloblastic anemia.

Differential Diagnosis. The disorder must be differentiated from vitamin B_{12} deficiency since the peripheral blood smear is identical in both. Small bowel enteropathies must be excluded.

Diagnosis. Analysis of the peripheral smear will reveal macrocytosis, hypersegmented neutrophils, anemia, and, commonly, neutropenia. Megaloblastic precursors will be noted on bone marrow examination. Serum levels of folate reflect folate deficiency, but red blood cell folate reflects the tissue stores more accurately. Serum levels may be low before erythrocyte levels are depleted. Folate and folinic acid absorption are abnormal after oral loading. With prolonged mucosal injury, hypoalbuminemia and hypocalcemia may be found. Small bowel biopsy will reveal the typical morphology.[35] Steatorrhea was not reported in the children studied by Davidson and Townley.[67]

Treatment. Response to oral folate varies, with some patients responding to daily oral doses of 10 mg of pteroylglutamic acid and others requiring up to 40 mg per day. One patient failed to respond to up to 100 mg per day, requiring 15 mg intramuscularly every three to four weeks. Jejunal histology is usually restored after two weeks of therapy. Recently, patients unresponsive to oral folate have improved with intramuscular folinic acid.[269a]

VITAMIN B_{12} MALABSORPTION

The major forms of inherited vitamin malabsorption are for vitamin B_{12} and folic acid — the first absorbed through the distal ileum and the second, through the proximal small bowel.[149] In disorders in which the villous epithelium is abnormal, these vitamins may be malabsorbed. In steatorrhea, a secondary malabsorption of fat-soluble vitamins occurs.

Incidence. Deficiency of vitamin B_{12} is extremely rare in infancy. Fewer than 50 infants have been reported with congenital pernicious anemia, and a small number of children with selective malabsorption of vitamin B_{12} have been described.[99a] In one family, three brothers were affected, suggesting autosomal recessive transmission.[52, 118, 131, 132, 141, 153, 167, 214, 238]

Physiology. Vitamin B_{12}, or extrinsic factor, is a cobalt-containing compound produced in nature solely by microorganisms. Its presence in animal tissue is due to dietary consumption, intestinal absorption, and storage.[239] Because higher plants do not contain this vitamin, the dietary source must be animal foods or products such as milk or eggs.

The process of vitamin B_{12} absorption is complex, proceeding in 4 steps.[57, 121a, 132, 132a, 181, 192] When ingested, vitamin B_{12} is bound to dietary protein and must be freed by proteolytic enzymes. (1) It then binds to intrinsic factor (IF), a glycoprotein secreted by gastric parietal cells. Secretion of IF probably is mediated in part by cyclic nucleo-

tides.[175] (2) In the distal half of the ileum, this vitamin B_{12}/IF complex is specifically absorbed, a process requiring calcium and a pH above 5.8. (3) During absorption the complex attached to the surface of the ileal cell is broken, and vitamin B_{12} detaches to a receptor on the ileal cell surface. It is absorbed within a few hours and actively transported through the cell. Intrinsic factor is disposed of on or in the cell. (4) It then binds to transcobalamin II (TC-II), a transport protein for distribution to body tissues, especially the liver, via the portal circulation. A second binding protein, transcobalamin I (TC-I), appears to act as a storage protein binder. A third binding protein also may be present in the neonate. In the presence of supraphysiologic doses of vitamin B_{12}, modest nonspecific absorption throughout the small bowel may be noted.

Etiology. Deficiency of vitamin B_{12} may develop from dietary deficiency, absence of intrinsic factor, ileal malabsorption, or transplacental transfer of antibody to IF.[112] Table 19–15 summarizes the possible causes in infancy.

The neonate will have serum levels of vitamin B_{12} two to three times higher than those in maternal serum. This transplacental transport against a concentration gradient produces significant hepatic stores of vitamin B_{12}. Thus, a term neonate of a mother with normal B_{12} levels will have sufficient stores for 12 to 18 months. The neonate also has been shown to have normal IF secretion at birth.

Dietary deficiency in early infancy is thus unusual, though breast-fed infants of vitamin B_{12}–deficient mothers have developed profound deficiency. Such cases to date have been secondary to maternal adherence to a strict vegetarian (vegan) diet or untreated maternal pernicious anemia.[151, 193]

Pernicious anemia is, by definition, the result of functional intrinsic factor deficiency. In the adult this is secondary to gastric resection, atrophic gastritis, or the development of antibody to IF or the parietal cell on an autoimmune basis. A rare form of infantile pernicious anemia has been reported, presenting in the first two years of life, with inability to produce IF. It is inherited

Table 19–15 Vitamin B_{12} Malabsorption in Infancy

DISORDER	GASTRIC ACID	INTRINSIC FACTOR	TC-I	TC-II	SERUM B_{12}	MEGALO-BLASTS	OTHER
Nutritional deficiency	+	+	+	+	Low	+	
Congenital pernicious anemia	+	0	+	+	Low	+	
TC-I deficiency	+	+	0	+	Low	0	
TC-II deficiency	+	+	+	0	NL	+	Failure to thrive, diarrhea
Selective ileal defect	+	+	+	+	Low	+	Failure to thrive, proteinuria
Generalized ileal dysfunction/resection	+	+	+	+	Low	+	Diarrhea

as an autosomal recessive condition. The gastric mucosa is histologically normal, and no antibody to either IF or the parietal cell can be demonstrated. Gastric acid production is normal, and a defect in steps 3 or 4 of absorption are postulated. The endocrinopathy often associated with pernicious anemia in later childhood is not seen with this infantile form.

Deficiency of the transport proteins also may be seen. Infants with TC-II deficiency have anemia, growth failure, and diarrhea in the first few weeks of life. Their serum levels of vitamin B_{12} are normal as the defect is in tissue distribution, not absorption. High-dose parenteral B_{12} injections allow normal growth, development, and hematologic recovery. Deficiency of TC-I is also seen. Serum levels of vitamin B_{12} are low; however, unlike all the other conditions, megaloblastic anemia does not develop if dietary intake is maintained.

A selective defect in ileal absorption of vitamin B_{12} also has been described, with symptomatic onset in the first year of life. It is inherited as an autosomal recessive condition; intrinsic factor and transcobalamin levels are normal. An idiopathic proteinuria is frequently present that fails to respond to vitamin B_{12} therapy. These infants otherwise respond nicely to parenteral vitamin B_{12}.

Generalized dysfunction of the ileum is also associated with reduction of vitamin B_{12} absorption. Bile acid malabsorption is usually present as well. The major cause in infancy is ileal resection, though similar reductions may be seen in ileitis, gluten-sensitive enteropathy, or tropical sprue.

With extensive enteropathy, megalobastic anemia is more commonly due to folate deficiency since body stores of folic acid last no more than six months, compared with vitamin B_{12} stores that may last for years.

Vitamin B_{12} malabsorption also may develop as a result of competitive binding with IF. Thus, in bacterial overgrowth, bacteria compete for vitamin B_{12}. In pancreatic insufficiency, vitamin B_{12} may remain bound to dietary protein or to a nondegraded salivary protein called protein R, which has a binding affinity for vitamin B_{12} that is 50 times greater than IF at pH 2.0 and 3 times greater at pH 8.0.[2] Medications such as para-aminosalicylic acid, colchicine, alcohol, and neomycin also interfere with the absorption of vitamin B_{12}.

Symptoms. The most common symptoms are pallor, weakness, listlessness, and failure to thrive. Fever, diarrhea, anorexia, and glossitis also may be seen. As noted, infants with TC-II deficiency are seen earliest, usually before one month of age. Those with congenital pernicious anemia and selective ileal malabsorption generally become symptomatic between 10 and 24 months of age, when neonatal stores are depleted.

The neurologic manifestations of the disease, consisting of paresthesias of the distal extremities and a spastic ataxic weakness of the legs, are not as frequent in childhood as in the adult. When noted, they may become permanent disabilities if not aggressively treated.

Diagnosis. The megaloblastic changes of the peripheral blood smear and bone marrow are identical to those found in folic acid deficiency. As a result, serum levels of vitamin B_{12} are utilized to discriminate these conditions. Vitamin B_{12} may be measured by radioimmunoassay or by a bioassay in which the growth of a microbiologic organism, requiring B_{12} but lacking synthetic ability, is observed in the presence of serum.

The Schilling test is described in detail in Chapter 16. A tracer dose of vitamin B_{12} is given orally, and the urine is analyzed for 24 hours. Normally, when the tracer is accompanied by a large dose of unlabeled vitamin B_{12}, from 15 to 40 per cent of the radioactive label will be excreted in 24 hours. Patients lacking IF or with ileal malabsorption excreted from 0 to 7 per cent of the dose. To exclude specific defects, the test is then repeated sequentially with oral intrinsic factor or following antibiotic treatment for bacterial overgrowth.

Treatment. Conversion of the bone marrow morphology to normal occurs within two days of the initiation of therapy. While therapeutic trials of 5 μg per day may be given to exclude folate deficiency, most patients require 100 μg per month as a parenteral dose. Infants with TC-II deficiency may require 1000 mg per week. If the malabsorption is secondary to fish tapeworm, bacterial overgrowth, or sprue, specific therapy of the primary lesion should suffice.

Mineral Malabsorption

Clinical disease in the human has been reported due to malabsorption of iron, magnesium, zinc, copper chloride, and calcium. Undoubtedly as the metabolism of other minerals is studied, additional malabsorptive studies will be reported.

Trace Metals

Iron

Nutritional Enteropathy

Iron deficiency remains the most common nutritional disturbance in infancy. Surveys of infants aged 6 to 24 months reveal iron-deficiency anemia in 3 to 24 per cent, with an additional 29 to 68 per cent deficient in iron but not anemic. While one thinks primarily of anemia, iron deficiency is a systemic disease, with iron being critical to normal activity of the cytochrome system, catalase, glutathione peroxidase, succinate dehydrogenase, monoamine oxidase, aconitase, and α-glycerophosphate dehydrogenase. The efficiency of iron absorption declines after birth, with some iron probably absorbed by pinocytosis.

The effect of iron deficiency on small bowel morphology and function remains an issue of chickens, eggs, horses, and carts because of the frequency with which a primary condition such as gluten or milk protein enteropathy induces iron deficiency. The only large study in infants was reported by Naiman and associates in 1964.[247] Fourteen infants (mean age = 17 months) with moderate anemia (mean hemoglobin = 5.4 gm per dl) were studied. None had chronic diarrhea, all were on cow's milk, three were at or below the third percentile for height, and four had hypoalbuminemia. Absorption studies revealed that 6 of 14 had impaired xylose absorption, 5 had reduced carotene, and 10 had a flat vitamin A tolerance curve. Mild steatorrhea was noted in 4 and occult blood was found in the stools of 4 of the 14.

Small bowel biopsies in 11 patients revealed villous epithelial injury in 7, though none had true atrophy.[217, 247] Following institution of iron therapy with no other dietary manipulation, repeat biopsy specimens in four patients revealed histologic recovery. No correlation was found between the degree of anemia and the presence of gastrointestinal abnormalities; however, therapeutic restoration of normal serum iron was associated with recovery of absorptive function.

Similar data have been obtained in 26 children aged 4 to 12 years. Two studies in adults found no evidence of jejunal abnormalities in iron deficiency. In a study of five infants with iron deficiency, there was decreased cytochrome oxidase activity in the villous epithelium. Only one of the five infants demonstrated villus flattening.

The argument is thus made that as a result of the iron requirement for DNA synthesis in rapidly proliferating epithelium, marked iron deficiency will impair villus proliferation and absorption. Confirmation requires response to iron in an otherwise unchanged diet. Recovery was documented within four to eight weeks in Naiman's study. As the great majority of infants reported to date were on cow's milk, the role of this protein in the induction of the process remains unknown.

Familial Iron Malabsorption

Incidence. In 1981 the first three cases of selective iron malabsorption were reported in three siblings. They probably represent an inherited defect in transferrin or transferrin receptor protein.[42]

Symptoms. The patients, aged 5 to 15 years, were noted from early infancy to have iron-deficiency anemia refractory to oral iron therapy. They were otherwise in excellent health.

Laboratory Findings. Initial hemoglobin levels ranged from 7.4 to 9 gm per dl and reticulocyte counts from 0.2 to 1.7. Transferrin saturations were 7 to 13 per cent; serum iron, 23 to 49 μg per dl; and serum ferritin, 19 to 28 μg/L. Therapy with iron dextran (Imferon) resulted in a rise of hemoglobin and hematocrit. Values for vitamin A, folic acid, and 72-hour fecal fat were normal.

Treatment. The patients were maintained on 50 mg per month of intramuscular iron.

Acrodermatitis Enteropathica or Primary Zinc Malabsorption

Acrodermatitis is one of the earliest recognized diseases of infancy in which cutaneous and gastrointestinal symptoms are closely associated, and one which is now felt to be due to zinc deficiency. In addition to a primary defect in zinc absorption, a secondary form has been reported in patients with protein-calorie malnutrition and in those receiving prolonged hyperalimentation.[35]

Incidence. First described in 1942, the disease has been reported in both the American and European medical literature.[62]

Inheritance. An autosomal type of inheritance is suggested, for it is certainly familial and in nearly two thirds of cases one or more family members were also affected. Consanguinity was not unusual in the family histories, and females were affected slightly more often than males.[62]

Etiology and Pathogenesis. Although the coincidence of the disease with weaning suggested first an allergic disorder or an abnormality in protein or lipid metabolism, these theories have been dispelled — and zinc malabsorption has been identified as the causative defect. A deficiency of a prostaglandin or an abnormality in the synthesis or function of a zinc-binding ligand is postulated.[90-92] The human fetus has poor zinc reserves and has a high zinc demand during the last trimester. Zinc in amniotic fluid is rather high late in gestation, and the premature and term infants fail to maintain positive zinc balance.

Pathophysiology. Zinc is an essential trace metal involved in protein synthesis and nucleic acid metabolism.[336] It is a component of more than 70 proteins, 40 of which are human enzymes; major examples are alkaline phosphatase, carboxypeptidase, and carbonic anhydrase. Zinc is absorbed through the small intestine, being taken up by the microvillus of the mucosal cell. Inside the cell zinc is affiliated with a number of ligands, one of which is a low molecular weight pancreatic ligand that transports the element to the serosal side of the cell.[164] Zinc leaves the cell bound to albumin. Studies in the rat suggest that this ligand is prostaglandin E_2. The zinc-binding ligand in human breast milk is a picolinic acid. When more zinc than is necessary is absorbed into the cell, metallothioneine is synthesized and binds the residual zinc. With the cell shedding, zinc is returned to the intestinal contents. The intestine seems to be the major route for zinc excretion, with significant quantities present in pancreatic secretions. In cow's milk there is evidence for an inhibitor of zinc absorption.

Within the body, plasma zinc (normal, 68 to 110 μg per dl) is bound to albumin, transferrin, and macroglobulin. Some, bound to amino acids, represents the major fraction excreted through the urine. Zinc is required for cellular growth and is found in highest concentrations in spermatozoa, choroid of the eye, hair, nails, bones, and prostate gland with significant concentrations in the liver, kidney, muscles, and skin. All of these organs therefore are affected by zinc deficiency.

In acrodermatitis, increased susceptibility to infection may be related to abnormal neutrophil and monocyte chemotaxis (corrected *in vitro* by addition of zinc).[343] Thymic atrophy and deficiencies of T and B cells also have been reported. Skin biopsy shows only nonspecific changes such as hyperkeratosis, acanthosis, and chronic inflammation.[274] Electron microscopy has shown virus-like particles in the epidermal cells in one biopsy. Skin zinc normally averages 22 μg per gm of dry weight and is decreased to levels approximating 6.7 μg per gm of dry weight.

The small intestinal morphology is normal in most cases although several patients have had subtotal or focal villous atrophy and one has had an edematous jejunal mucosa with superficial ulcerations.[206] Mucosal epithelial cells have been noted to be cuboidal and to contain large nuclei. Electron microscopy of duodenal and jejunal tissue has shown atypical lysosomal-like structures in the Paneth cells that disappear after zinc therapy. These dense filamentous inclusions are considered *pathognomonic of acrodermatitis*. Measurements of jejunal

zinc are decreased, averaging 77 μg per gm as compared with age-matched control values of 97 μg per gm of dry weight of tissue. These levels increase to 200 to 300 μg per gm of dry weight after treatment.

Specific lesions of the reticuloendothelial system are noted: absence of the thymus; a thymus consisting of epithelial component and only a few thymocytes and Hassall's corpuscles, and absent tonsils or lymphoid germinal centers.

Pancreatic function has been normal in all patients in whom it has been studied.

Acrodermatitis in the presence of normal serum zinc, while rare, has been reported.[103]

Symptoms. The onset is usually coincidental with weaning from the breast. It has, however, been described in breast-fed premature infants who took breast milk low in zinc.[353] Symptoms are usually florid by the ninth month, but a few cases have been clearly identified as early as the first or second week of life. Resumption of breast feeding will induce remission. The disease progresses gradually, although the course is often intermittent. Skin lesions antedate other symptoms and begin as moist or scaling erythematous eruptions, which are either bullous or pustular (Fig. 19–14). They are localized about the mouth and anus and are distributed symmetrically over the buttocks, elbows, hands, and feet, with a particular predilection for the interdigital areas. As the lesions progress they become plaque-like

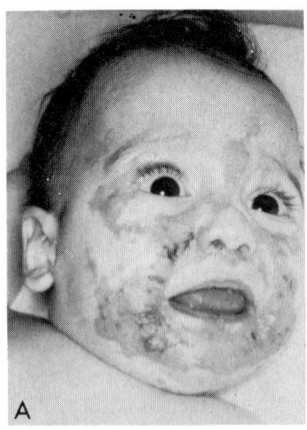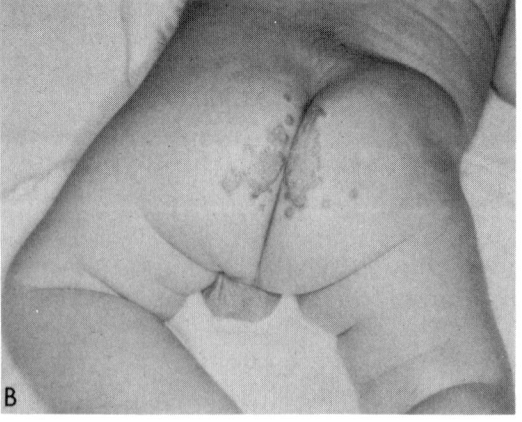

Figure 19–14   Infant with typical lesions of acrodermatitis enteropathica. *A*, Bullous and pustular lesions arise about the mouth. Some are becoming plaque-like. *B*, Perianal region of same infant. (Courtesy of Sidney Hurwitz, M.D., and Irwin Braverman, M.D.)

and scaly and heal without scarring. Nail dystrophy may occur, and more than half of these babies have oral cutaneous moniliasis. In the mouth, there is glossitis and stomatitis and in the eyes, corneal involvement with severe photophobia, micropannus formation, and punctate keratopathy. Alopecia may be total or partial.

Diarrhea occurs shortly after the onset of the skin manifestations, but in a few cases the two occur simultaneously. Ninety-five per cent of affected infants have associated malabsorption, and some seem to have abdominal pain. In older children psychic disturbances, and particularly a schizoid state, are associated with exacerbations. Joint pain, malaise, and growth failure are nonspecific associated symptoms.

Diagnosis. The diagnosis was purely a clinical one until 1974 when zinc deficiency was recognized as the etiologic factor. A low plasma zinc — less than 65 to 70 μg per dl — in association with the cutaneous findings is diagnostic. Diurnal urinary zinc content shows a low zinc level, ranging between 30 and 50 μg per 24 hr as compared with normal values of 100 to 700 μg per 24 hr. One case has been reported with elevated serum and skin zinc and which responded to therapy with 300 mg of zinc sulfate per day. Recently variant acrodermatitis with normal zinc levels is being recognized; it responds to zinc therapy[189a] and is considered to be "zinc-dependent."

Treatment. Initial treatment consists of 10 to 45 mg of zinc per day adjusted to maintain normal serum levels. Since $ZnSO_4$ may be irritating, a solution of zinc acetate containing 13 mg per ml (to provide 1 mg of Zn per ml) is recommended in two to three divided doses administered one or more hours before meals. Remission is maintained using 1 to 2 mg per kg per day of zinc.[243, 249, 256] Isolated IgG hypogammaglobulinemia in this disorder has also been corrected by therapy.[348a]

Prognosis. Although the disease improves after puberty, exacerbations in untreated patients become more frequent and severe, and many die in later childhood. Untreated women who have reached maturity have borne children with a high in-cidence of congenital malformations. Treated children demonstrate catch-up growth, clearing of skin and ocular lesions, and cessation of their diarrhea. A change in emotional status is evident within hours.

Successful treatment with Viokase in a patient with normal zinc levels appears to be the result of the content of picolinic acid (2800 to 3744 μg per day) rather than the content of zinc (1 mg per day).[12]

Primary Hypomagnesemia

The significance of magnesium is demonstrated by its position as the fourth most important cation in the body and the second most important intracellular cation. Most magnesium is stored within the body in bone and muscle, with the rest distributed in soft tissue.[294] Secondary deficiencies are far more common than primary ones and have been reported in association with malabsorptive or endocrine disorders such as celiac disease, short-bowel syndrome, inflammatory bowel disease, neonatal hepatitis, biliary atresia, DiGeorge syndrome, hyperaldosteronism, hyperthyroidism, hypoparathyroidism, chronic renal disease, or transfusion with citrated blood. Intrauterine growth retardation and protein-calorie malnutrition are also associated with hypomagnesemia. Infants born of mothers with celiac disease, hyperparathyroidism, and diabetes mellitus may have significant hypomagnesemia.[237, 251, 263, 310, 323, 351]

A transient magnesium deficiency has been described in neonates who have tetany and, often, normal calcium values. This responds to magnesium therapy for one to several days.

Incidence. Less than a dozen children with this lesion have been reported: two of these were brothers.

Etiology and Pathophysiology. Normal magnesium levels are 1.5 to 2.8 mg per dl or 1.5 mEq per liter. One third of plasma magnesium is bound to protein, and the rest is ultrafilterable. Magnesium activates many of the intracellular enzymes, particularly those requiring ATP for muscle contraction, glycolysis, and coenzyme and protein synthesis. Normal infants absorb 55 to 75 per cent of the ingested cation whereas those with primary hypomagnesemia absorb only 8.8 per cent. Absorption requires both diffusion and active transport. Stromme et al. have shown that patients have the same degree of magnesium malabsorption despite variation in loads and suggest that the defect thus lies in the active transport phase.[310] Milla et al. have provided evidence for a defective carrier-mediated small intestinal transport of magnesium.[237] Intestinal histology is normal, as is Mg-dependent ATPase. Xylose absorption and fecal fat are normal. Electron microscopy shows alteration of the apical part of the cytoplasm of the epithelial cells, dilated endoplasmic reticulum, and mitochondrial swelling, with normal brush border. Renal function is normal, but magnesium excretion is increased in sweat.

Although serum calcium may be low, calcium balance is positive, and oral or intravenous calcium does not correct the disorder. During the period of magnesium deficiency, serum calcium is unresponsive to parathormone but responds normally after magnesium therapy. The hormone does raise magnesium levels slightly and its excretion seems to be inversely related to serum magnesium: increased when the carbon is low and decreased when it is elevated.

Only small amounts of magnesium are excreted through the intestine, and the main route of excretion is through the kidneys. Neonates excrete less than 0.13 or 0.14 mg per kg on the second and third days of life, and up to 1.42 mg per kg by the seventh day.

Symptoms. Affected infants are typically well-nourished, full-term males who are well during the first few days of life. Between five days and six weeks of age, irritability and seizures are noted. Initial attacks are usually mild and consist of eye rolling; in the intervals between attacks the infants are irritable, sleepless, and jumpy. Slowly, generalized seizures appear and increase in intensity and frequency. There are no localized neurologic findings, and the infants sleep after seizing. Trousseau and Chvostek signs are positive. Woodard et al. reported

one infant at two months of age with seizures, diarrhea, edema, and ascites who had hypocalcemia and hypoalbuminemia and an abnormal electroencephalogram showing bilateral temporal spikes.[351] Neither calcium nor albumin therapy relieved the symptoms. Magnesium determinations showed serum levels of 0.1 mg per dl, and seizures ceased after treatment with intramuscular 50 per cent magnesium sulfate (49.3 mg). After four weeks of therapy the serum magnesium was 1.2 mg per dl, and calcium and albumin values returned to normal. Diarrhea ceased and edema resolved. At no time during the illness was fat malabsorption demonstrated.

Differential Diagnosis. This disorder must be differentiated first from hypocalcemia and next from any of the malabsorptive and endocrine diseases producing secondary reductions in magnesium.

Diagnosis. The diagnosis must be suspected in any infant with tetany that does not respond to calcium therapy. Electroencephalographic examination results vary from normal patterns to moderate slow wave or spike activity. Serum magnesium levels are less than 0.5 mg per dl, and magnesium excretion in the urine is minimal. Serum calcium in some way depends upon magnesium, for calcium levels fall when serum magnesium is less than 0.8 mEq per liter or 0.8 mg per dl. Bone age and structure are normal although metaphyseal transverse lines have been reported in some patients. Balance studies after oral ingestion of magnesium 28-chloride show a fecal recovery well above a normal of 30 per cent and urinary excretion below a normal of 10 per cent of the isotope. There is no evidence of other types of malabsorption.

Treatment. In the acute stage of the disease, intramuscular magnesium is administered in a dosage of 3 mEq per liter per day in three divided doses or in an emergency injection of 0.25 to 1 ml of 50 per cent $MgSO_4$ (administered slowly). Serum levels should be determined twice daily for several days. Maintenance therapy is provided as the sulfate, lactate, chloride, or citrate in a dosage of 10 to 20 mg per kg per day. In severe cases, 1.25 ml/kg of 50 per cent

MgSO$_4$ may be needed to maintain magnesium levels. Vitamin D has had no demonstrable effect upon magnesium absorption.

With correction of hypomagnesemia, the serum calcium returns to normal, neurologic status improves, diarrhea ceases, and physical growth progresses. Large doses of magnesium sulfate will induce diarrhea. Hypermagnesemia may produce hypotension and central nervous system depression.

Prognosis. Primary malabsorption of magnesium is a permanent disorder that requires continuous treatment. Secondary deficiencies respond to treatment of the primary disorder.

Menkes' Kinky or Steely Hair Syndrome (SHS)

This inherited disorder of copper absorption and perhaps of increased retention by certain cells, manifests as severe mental retardation, coarse facies, pili torti, temperature instability, scorbutic bone changes, growth retardation, susceptibility to infection, arterial intimal disease, and early death. Milder forms are now being recognized.[270a]

Incidence. Since first reported in 1962, it has been described in approximately 50 patients throughout the world, involving Caucasian, black, and Oriental infants. The frequency in Victoria, Australia, has been estimated at 1:35,000 live births.[61, 63, 64, 111, 236, 344, 347]

Inheritance. SHS is inherited as an X-linked recessive trait affecting male infants. Pili torti occurs occasionally in heterozygotes, but normal hair does not exclude the diagnosis. One black heterozygote female has been reported to have blotchy depigmentation of the skin. A similar syndrome has been reported in mottled mutants of mice with the gene located on the X-chromosome. Serum copper and copper oxidase, low in the homozygote, are normal in the heterozygote.

Pathology and Pathogenesis. Increased maternal retention of copper during pregnancy assures adequate copper supplies to the developing fetus, and there is some evidence of copper absorption by pinocytosis in the neonate. After birth the efficiency of copper absorption seems to decline with age. In SHS there is evidence for prenatal malformation of Purkinje cell dendrites and light electron microscopy of the brain shows diffuse neuronal damage, gliosis, and cystic degeneration. The cord copper and ceruloplasmin are normal at birth and do not decrease until after the first few days of life, findings that probably account for the early normal development of these babies.[29, 30, 220]

The normal individual, after ingestion of ^{64}Cu, has a peak in circulating ^{64}Cu at 40 to 60 minutes, a small secondary peak at 4 hours, and a gradual rise to 32 hours, with 55 per cent whole blood radioactivity in the plasma from 8 to 48 hours.[210, 211] Stool radioactivity by 48 hours totaled 24 per cent of the ingested dose. The major route of copper excretion is through bile into the stool. Patients with SHS have low plasma copper and ceruloplasmin not significantly increased after copper ingestion. Isotope loading studies show no early blood peak, with only 10 per cent of the copper persisting in the circulation. Stool radioactivity approximates 94 per cent. Copper malabsorption is not total, however, with studies showing patients absorbing 10 to 25 per cent of the ingested copper load.[138]

The defect in intestinal absorption of copper may be partially overcome by high doses of copper. Administration of ten times the normal daily requirement combined with L-histidine was followed by the restoration of low-normal copper values in several children. Although copper levels were increased, serum ceruloplasmin did not rise. Lott et al. have suggested that copper absorbed in the presence of histidine is in an abnormal complex with albumin, and that this does not allow its availability for ceruloplasmin synthesis.[208]

Intestinal studies suggest that the defect in absorption is at the level of cellular copper transport, for duodenal and jejunal morphology are normal and studies have shown normal copper uptake by the mucosa. Biopsy specimens contain 50 to 76 mg of copper per gm of dry weight, compared with normal values of 18.5 ± 6.3 mg per gm of dry weight. These data suggest that an abnormal metal-binding protein may be present in the duodenal mucosa or that copper transport to the serosal surface of the cell is abnormal.

Intravenously administered copper is metabolized normally, being followed by rises in serum copper and ceruloplasmin. Apoceruloplasmin, which is copper-free, is normal.

Tissue analyses have produced variable results. Copper has been low or increased in the liver, low or normal in the brain, and increased in skin fibroblasts, amniotic cells, and red blood cells. Unlike patients with nutritional hypocupremia, patients have not had anemia or neutropenia. Urinary excretion of copper, which in the normal averages 0.08 per cent of ingested dose per 24 hr, is increased to eight times the normal rate, suggesting a renal inability to conserve copper.

Copper deficiency is reflected in hair, bone, brain, and blood vessels. Pili torti refers to a microscopic kinking of the hair, which actually appears to the eye as straight, coarse, and extremely brittle (Fig. 19–15). The hair contains excessive amounts of free sulfhydryl groups. Biosynthesis of proteins in the skin, particularly of collagen, is reduced since copper deficiency reduces the cross linking required in the development of mature forms of collagen and elastin. Skeletal changes include the presence of wormian bones within the skull sutures; widening of the metaphyses of ribs and femur, humerus, or radius with the formation of lateral spurs; and osteoporosis. Arterial lesions include tortuosity and elongation of cerebral, visceral, and limb arteries, with fragmentation and reduplication of the internal elastic lamina and thickening of the intima. Total occlusion of the vessels may occur. Generalized copper deficiency is reflected in the unresponsive-

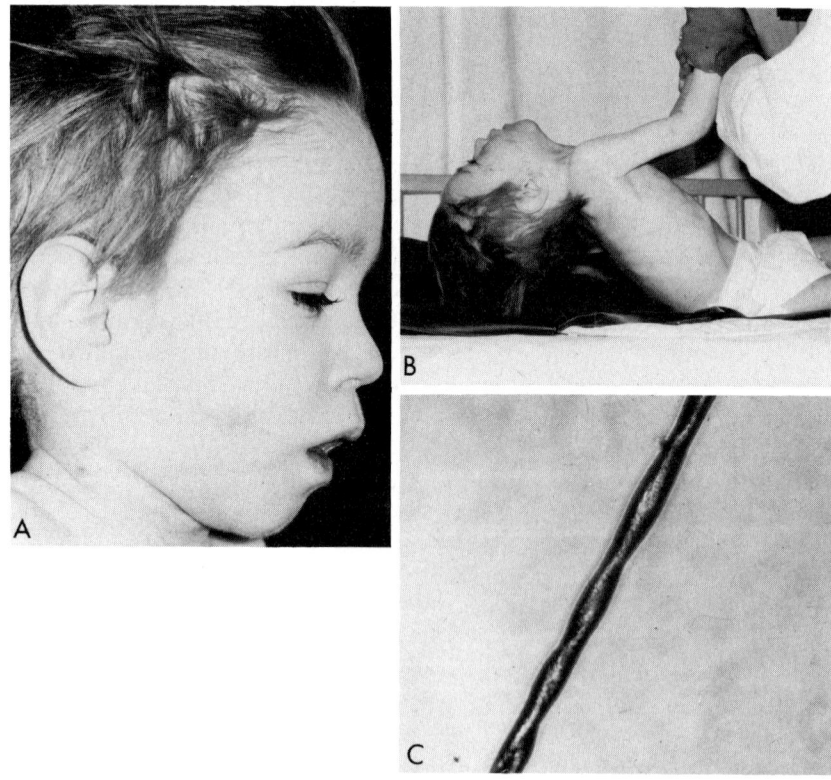

Figure 19–15 A, In this profile view of a baby with Menkes' kinky hair disease, it is evident that the hair does not appear kinky to the naked eye, but rather is straight, dry and has a brittle texture. B, The extreme floppiness and lack of muscle tone are evident as the patient is pulled toward an upright position. C, Microscopic view of the hair demonstrating pili torti. (Courtesy of E. Hsia, M.D., and A. Lucky, M.D.)

ness of copper metalloenzymes. In the brain there is diffuse neuronal damage with cystic degeneration and gliosis.

Symptoms. Since primary fetal hair is not affected and since many infants have little permanent hair before the third month, the disease may go unrecognized before death. Male infants are affected, and many are born prematurely between 36 and 38 weeks' gestation. Others born at term are noted to be small for gestational age. All infants have a typical facies with pudgy cheeks, pallid, rather puffy skin; and horizontal, twisted eyebrows. Well for the first week or two, the infants soon show temperature instability, lethargy, drowsiness, jaundice, and vomiting. Between one and two months of age, lethargy increases and they have difficulty in feeding. Seizures develop early in some and later in others, beginning with myoclonic jerks and blinking and becoming increasingly severe and more difficult to control. Motor development rarely progresses beyond a smile and deteriorates progressively after the first few months, with drooling, crying, increasing lethargy, and failure of visual following. Muscle tone may be flaccid or increased, but deep tendon reflexes are increased and there is bilateral ankle clonus. With acute illness, flaccidity is the rule.

As permanent hair emerges it is sparse, brittle, and dull, often rubbing off on the sheets. The babies eventually become unresponsive and require tube feedings. Most infants reach between the 3rd and 25th percentiles for growing between six and nine months. Their courses are complicated by vomiting, diarrhea that may be accompanied by enteric protein loss, respiratory infections, and subdural hematoma. Pulmonary emphysema has been reported in one patient, and diffuse dilation of the gastrointestinal tract in three others.

Differential Diagnosis. SHS must be differentiated from the variety of central nervous system degenerative disorders.

Diagnosis. A prenatal diagnosis may be made by finding increased copper uptake by cultured amniotic cells.[162] Very low levels of ceruloplasmin and of copper, combined with the typical physical appearance, strongly suggest the diagnosis (Fig. 19–15). Microscopic examination of permanent hair is a relatively simple method of rapid diagnosis and will reveal the characteristic kinking and twisting. Ceruloplasmin and serum copper are normal.

Confirmation is made by copper absorption studies. Normal subjects absorb 30 to 70 per cent of ingested copper, whereas those with SHS have significantly decreased levels. Cultured skin fibroblasts from patients and heterozygotes have an intense metachromasia after staining with toluidine blue. Cells from patients show increased copper uptake and a copper concentration six times normal and are more sensitive than those from controls because of the toxic effects of high copper levels. In a copper-free medium, patient cells release copper less readily than do those from normal subjects. Most copper is bound to a molecule of 10,000 molecular weight.

Fibroblasts of heterozygotes have a twice normal copper concentration.

Treatment. There is evidence that parenteral copper in ten times the normal daily requirement, up to 600 mg per kg per week, in some cases will restore normal serum and liver copper and occasionally restore ceruloplasmin levels.[43, 120] Subcutaneous injections also have been effective in accomplishing the same ends. However, although occasional improvement has been noted in several cases treated up to 12 months, the disease is usually progressive and fatal between 3 and 4 years.

Calcium Malabsorption

Rickets, characterized by osteomalacia, hypocalcemia, and secondary hyperparathyroidism, typically is due to calcium malabsorption secondary to vitamin D deficiency.[311] An autosomal recessive form is probably due to decreased renal synthesis of the physiologically active form, since patients respond to treatment with 1,25-dihydroxyvitamin D.[311] Recently, however, patients with clinical and laboratory evidence of rickets have been described as having normal or increased levels of circulating vitamin D metabolites and failure to respond to pharmacologic levels of vitamin D or 1,25-dihydroxyvitamin D. Such patients are presumed to have a failure of end-organ response. Calcium malabsorption also may develop as a consequence of any jejunal malabsorptive state.[140] Familial absorptive hypercalciuria and renal tubular acidosis have been noted.[166]

Incidence. End-organ unresponsiveness to the active vitamin D derivative is extremely rare; fewer than ten patients have been reported.[22, 40, 108, 267, 276, 304, 352]

Etiology and Pathophysiology. Our current knowledge of vitamin D metabolism encompasses two steps of hydroxylation within the body: first in the liver to 25-hydroxyvitamin D, and next in the kidney to 1,25-dihydroxyvitamin D. Calcium is absorbed by passive diffusion and active transport dependent upon 1,25-dihydroxyvitamin D, for which there are specific intestinal receptors.[144] Vitamin D also has a trophic effect upon the mucosa. Several calcium-binding proteins are found in the microvillous membrane, as well as Ca^{++}-stimulated ATPase, all the synthesis of which is stimulated by vitamin D.[3, 58] Other proteins involved in vitamin D–dependent calcium transport have been isolated from mitochondria or lateral basement membranes.

Calcium uptake by the Golgi body membranes consists of calcium transport followed by binding to the vesicle. The small bowel is the site of absorption while the colon, experimentally, seems to be the site of calcium excretion. Net jejunal calcium absorption, which is depressed with vitamin D–resistant rickets, measures 300 mg per day in control children. Two types of transport defects have been identified in patients: decreased cellular uptake or increased calcium leak, and both were corrected with vitamin D therapy. Lack of intake of the vitamin or reduced synthesis in the absence of sunlight, as occurs sporadically in ghetto children, results in the typical syndrome of vitamin D deficiency rickets. Genetic rickets, type I, is due to decreased synthesis of the renal enzyme required for final hydroxylation, and here the circulating 1,25-dihydroxyvitamin is deficient. Inheritance is autosomal recessive.

A type II vitamin D–dependent rickets exists in which end-organ unresponsiveness is postulated as the cause, and recently, Eil et al.[85a] have demonstrated a failure of end-organ nuclear uptake of $1,25(OH)_2D_3$. In the patient reported, 25-hydroxyvitamin D was normal and the 1,25-dihydroxyvitamin D was increased. In both types, hypocalcemia and secondary hyperparathyroidism are corrected by pharmacologic doses of the vitamin D. More recently a type of rickets has been reported in which circulating 1,25-dihydroxyvitamin D is increased but calcium absorption is decreased, with other absorptive parameters being normal.

Rosen et al. have reported two sisters and described four other children with an autosomal recessive type of rickets with alopecia.[276] Serum 25-hydroxy- and 1,25-dihydroxyvitamin D levels were normal, and the administration of the active D_3 form of vitamin D had no effect. They postulated an absence of receptors in intestine and bone and ultimately treated their patients with elemental phosphorus, a regimen known to increase bone formation in vitamin D–resistant disorders (Table 19–16).

Symptoms. In all patients except the vitamin D–dependent type II children, rickets was present within the first two years. The one older patient developed symptoms in adolescence. Bony deformities consisted of valgus deformities in the proximal third of the legs, bowing of the distal legs, and poor linear growth. Gradual loss of teeth and alopecia were noted after one year in the patients of Rosen et al.[276]

Laboratory Studies. Typically, hypocalcemia, hypophosphaturia, increased alkaline phosphatase, elevated levels of parathyroid hormone, and evidence of secondary hyperparathyroidism are diagnostic of rickets. The differentiation of type depends upon circulating levels of hydroxylated forms of vitamin D and the response to therapy (Table 19–16). Radiologic examinations of bone reveal changes compatible with rickets and osteomalacia.

Differential Diagnosis. The types of primary disease must be differentiated from other causes of calcium malabsorption as a result of small bowel disease.

Treatment. Treatment varies with the

Table 19–16   Vitamin D–Dependent Rickets

TYPE	INHERITANCE	25(OH)D	1,25(OH)$_2$D	DEFECT	TREATMENT
I	Autosomal recessive	Normal	Decreased	Defect in 1-α-hydroxylation of 25(OH)D	1–2 μg/day of 1,25-dihydroxy D$_3$ or 1-hydroxy D$_3$
II		Normal or decreased	Normal or increased	Defective nuclear uptake of 1,25-(OH)$_2$D$_3$	Dose of dihydroxy D$_3$ to 50× normal
Impaired or absent end-organ responsiveness	?Autosomal recessive				Dose of dihydroxy D$_3$ to 50× normal
Alopecia and end-organ unresponsiveness	Autosomal recessive				1-α-(OH)D$_3$ or vitamin D$_2$ or elemental P

degree of end-organ unresponsiveness and varies from pharmacologic doses of vitamin D$_3$ to massive doses of vitamin D$_2$ or elemental phosphorus.

Prognosis. Hypocalcemia and secondary hyperparathyroidism can be reversed by adequate medication in all but the totally refractory patients. In those, elemental phosphorus has increased height, decreased physical deformity, and increased muscle strength.

Familial or Congenital Chloride Diarrhea

This congenital chloride diarrhea, characterized by a marked intestinal loss of chloride and development of systemic alkalosis, was originally termed "congenital alkalosis with diarrhea."[252]

Incidence. The disease was first described in 1945 separately by Darrow[115] and Gamble et al.[102] It is most prevalent in eastern Finland, where it was first appreciated in 1965. Since that time approximately 2 new patients per year are detected and Holmberg et al.[156] have treated 22 patients — the larges series to date. Approximately 20 others have been reported from other countries.

Inheritance. The disease is familial and inherited as an autosomal recessive trait. Families of all the Finnish patients originated from northern or eastern Finland, where

there is an increased incidence of other diseases having autosomal recessive inheritance. Consanguinity has been noted in a number of families. In some reports, females have been affected more often than males, but in others, the sex distribution is essentially equal.

Etiology and Pathology. Originally Darrow suggested the defect lay in intestinal chloride absorption while Gamble et al. postulated that it was one of intestinal chloride excretion.[154, 273] The first view is now considered correct, for intestinal perfusion studies have identified normal sodium absorption with impairment of active chloride and bicarbonate transport in the distal ileum and colon, resulting in fecal chloride loss and osmotic diarrhea (Fig. 19–16). In one patient, the colon was permeable to chloride. Although stool concentrations of sodium and potassium are normal, their losses are increased because of increased stool volumes.[265, 325] Sodium excretion is further increased because its absorption is impaired by the acidity of the intestinal contents secondary to reductions in luminal bicarbonate. The stools thus contain large quantities of sodium and chloride, causing systemic hyponatremia and hypochloremia. The metabolic alterations are present as early as one hour after birth.

Dehydration is at first iso-osmolar. However, as sodium and water absorption through the kidney and intestine increase in

Lumen   Mucosa

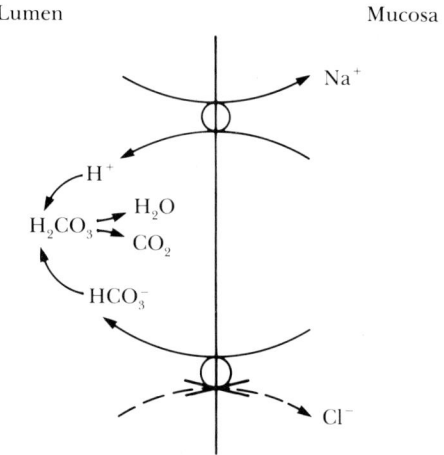

Figure 19–16 Normally, chloride is absorbed actively and passively by the ileal and colonic mucosa. The passive process is by an electrochemical gradient and is usually not required. The active transport is coupled to bicarbonate efflux (HCO_3^- united with hydrogen is converted to H_2CO_3, CO_2, and H_2O, which is then reabsorbed). In chloridorrhea, chloride is not secreted; it simply is not exchanged for bicarbonate and therefore is not actively absorbed. The resultant intraluminal electronegativity obligates positive ions (Na^+, K^+, and H^+) and retains bicarbonate within the serum.

an attempt to compensate, potassium loss occurs.[155] As a result, serum sodium rises to normal but hypochloremia persists, and hypokalemia and metabolic alkalosis appear. Alkalosis results from both increased H^+ excretion and absent HCO_3 secretion.

Untreated or inadequately treated patients develop renal disease and secondary hyperaldosteronism. Pasternack et al. postulate that the primary defect in chloride absorption causes depletion of water and electrolytes, leading to hyperplasia of the juxtaglomerular renal cells and increased renin activity.[262] Increased angiotensin causes angiopathy and secondary aldosteronism. This, in turn, leads to a high urinary excretion of potassium. Renal biopsies show juxtaglomerular hyperplasia and calcification, thickening and hypercellularity of arteriolar and arterial walls, and swelling of their medial layer. In older children the glomeruli are hyalinized. A defect in bile acid–concentrating ability of the gallbladder also has been noted.[21a]

Symptoms. More than half the infants passed no meconium and presumably had intrauterine diarrhea. Diarrhea is often

present on the first day of life but sometimes is not apparent until the baby is several weeks of age. The stools resemble urine and the infants are often though to have polyuria. Abdominal distention and ileus develop. There are growth and motor retardation and hypotonia. Urinary infections are frequent. The infants are hospitalized often for the treatment of severe dehydration, and serum electrolyte levels reveal high bicarbonate and low sodium potassium and chloride. If alkalosis is not present early, it is usually well developed by the time the infant is several weeks to months old. It is interesting that the teeth of these children are particularly resistant to caries.[245]

Differential Diagnosis. This is the only diarrheal disorder associated with hypokalemic, hypochloremic alkalosis. However, we must be aware that alkalosis and secondary chloride-losing diarrhea can develop in infants under 18 months old after bowel surgery, and an acquired form has been described individually and in seven Inuit Eskimos.[176]

Diagnosis. The chloride content of the stool is markedly elevated. In the first few months it ranges between 30 and 100 mEq per liter but later it remains constant at about 150 mEq per liter. Chloride is greater than the sum of potassium and sodium ions (90 mmole per liter). Urinary chloride is negligible or absent, and potassium equals sodium. Hypochloridemia, hypokalemia, and mild hyponatremia develop. As metabolic alkalosis develops there is an increase in urinary potassium and an increase in the potassium:sodium ratio. Urinary aldosterone and plasma renin activity are elevated. The blood pressure is normal. Hyperuricemia, proteinuria, and nephrocalcinosis may be noted.

Treatment. The treatment is with supplemental potassium, 2 to 14 mEq per day in dosage sufficient to maintain plasma electrolytes and pH at normal levels.

Prognosis. Patients treated with only potassium chloride had increased aldosterone levels and renal disease, whereas those treated with sodium chloride and potassium chloride had normal growth and less frequent episodes of dehydration.

IMMUNE COMPETENCE AND IMMUNODEFICIENCY

The host defenses of the small bowel are designed to protect the mucosal epithelial cell surface from the uptake of toxic macromolecules derived either from the external environment (dietary products) or internal milieu (microbial proliferation and metabolism). The host defense system is composed of both nonimmunologic and immunologic factors that seek to prevent antigen binding to the epithelial cell surface (Table 19–17). This binding, especially for microbial species, is highly specific for epithelial cell receptors and is critical to the development of local microbial proliferation and toxicity.[224]

The nonimmunologic factors facilitate the degradation and clearance of antigenic material within the intestinal lumen. Gastric acid and pepsin initiate the destruction of dietary antigens and effectively suppress most microorganisms arising from the oropharynx and respiratory tree. Individuals with reduced gastric acidity are prone to increased small bowel bacterial colonization. Bile acids also appear to suppress microbial proliferation, thus limiting small bowel bacterial overgrowth. Intestinal mucus appears to restrict antigen binding by functioning as a viscous matrix in which antigens are entrapped, thus facilitating intraluminal degradation by proteolytic enzymes of pancreatic and epithelial cell ori-

Table 19–17 Gastrointestinal Host Defense to Prevent Adherence to and Penetration of Epithelial Cell Surface

Nonimmunologic Factors
  Gastric acid
  Bile acids
  Mucus layer
  Proteolytic enzymes
  Peristalsis
  Intact mucosa
  Bacterial flora
  Hepatic filtration

Immunologic Factors
  Secretory antibodies: Dimeric IgA, IgM
  Systemic antibodies: IgG, IgE, IgD
  Cellular immune system: Lymphocytic, macrophages

gin. Normal bowel motility, or peristalsis, produces a mechanical cleansing action, the effectiveness of which is underscored by the bacterial proliferation encountered in blind loop situations. The physical integrity of the intestinal mucosa is also important, because increased antigen uptake is noted when the mucosa is disrupted from immaturity, ulceration, inflammation, or ischemia. When antigen uptake does occur, the reticuloendothelial system of the liver appears to function as an effective filter for antigen in portal blood.

The immunologic factors are uniquely adapted to mucosal surfaces. There is a secretory immunoglobulin system composed primarily of dimeric IgA and polymeric IgM.[41a] These immunoglobulins are synthesized locally and secreted across epithelial cells and in bile. Within the lamina propria, nonsecretory antibodies of the IgG, IgE, and perhaps IgD class respond to antigenic stimulation. The cellular immune system, while less completely understood, is critical with regard to the control of plasma cell immunoglobulin synthesis, macrophage activity, and delayed-type hypersensitivity.

The predominant secretory antibody is secretory IgA. This molecule is synthesized in local plasma cells and is composed of two IgA monomers joined by a J chain. The dimeric IgA is secreted from the plasma cell into the lamina propria and reaches the base of the columnar epithelial cell. There it interacts with secretory component (SC), which is synthesized in the epithelial cell and appears to act as a membrane receptor for dimeric IgA (and IgM). Coupled to SC, dimeric IgA is transported across the epithelial cell and is secreted into the intestinal lumen.[305] It remains bound to SC, which then appears to protect secretory IgA from intraluminal proteolytic degradation by either native enzymes or microbial IgA proteases. Recent studies suggest that hepatic epithelial cells also produce SC and that bile is a major source of intraluminal secretory IgA.

The specificity of the secretory immunoglobulin system results from local immunization initiated by a process of selective antigen uptake. On the mucosal surface, overlying Peyer's patches is a unique cell population referred to as microfold or M cells. These cells lack a brush border and appear to have an affinity for antigen binding and uptake. By the process of pinocytosis, antigens are transported across the M cell to lymphocytes that lie within an invagination of the M cell. These lymphocytes, which appear to be thymus-derived, process the antigen and proceed to the Peyer's patch where they stimulate proliferation of B lymphoblasts to produce plasma cells synthesizing antibody against that specific antigen. This proliferation appears to be under the complex control of other T cells that act to "suppress" or "help" this response. If B lymphoblast proliferation is suppressed, no plasma cell response occurs, specific antibody does not appear, and a state of "tolerance" ensues.

The plasma cells produced in Peyer's patches appear to exit via the lymphatics and reach the circulation through the thoracic duct.[257] The majority of these plasma cells return to the lamina propria where immunoglobulin synthesis ensues, predominantly of the IgA and IgM type. As noted earlier, these immunoglobulins are transported across the epithelial cell by secretory component (SC). Within the lumen, SC appears to remain with dimeric IgA while more easily dissociating from IgM. The secretory immunoglobulins bind to antigen at the luminal brush border, thus preventing antigen adherence, proliferation, and uptake. This process is referred to as immune exclusion.

Some of the plasma cells derived from the intestinal Peyer's patch are distributed via the circulation to other mucosal surfaces, especially the lung (bronchial lymphoid tissue) and the lactating mammary gland. In this fashion, secretory antibodies directed against enteric antigens can be found in respiratory secretions and breast milk as well as other mucosal secretions.

IMMUNODEFICIENCY

Immunodeficiency in infancy can be either primary or secondary. The primary immunodeficiency states result from a failure to produce an effective humoral and/or cellular immune response because of a failure of B- and/or T-lymphocyte differentiation or function. The secondary immunodeficiency states are a result of a reduction in the immune response secondary to acquired alterations in lymphocyte function. Such secondary immunodeficiencies are encountered following malnutrition, radiation or chemotherapy, protein-losing enteropathy, intestinal lymphangiectasia, or malignant lymphoproliferation. The small intestinal consequences of immunodeficiency are protean, and the common manifestations seen with the primary immunodeficiencies are summarized in Table 19–18.[254]

PRIMARY IMMUNODEFICIENCY

Congenital X-Linked Agammaglobulinemia (Bruton's)

Pathophysiology. These patients demonstrate a failure of antibody synthesis with an absence of plasma cells in lymph nodes, bone marrow, spleen, and the intestinal tract. Peyer's patch differentiation is not apparent within the small bowel. Cell-mediated immunity and other T cell–dependent processes, however, are intact. The disease is inherited as an X-linked recessive disorder. The hallmark of this disorder is the development, between 6 and 18 months of age, of recurrent bacterial infection, predominantly with encapsulated pyogenic organisms. Viral infections are usually tolerated well, though persistent rotavirus and ECHO enteritis and chronic hepatitis have been reported. The gastrointestinal manifestations are not prominent in these patients though some will demonstrate severe diarrhea secondary to villus destruction, usually in the setting of bacterial enteritis or because of mucosal invasion by bacteria. The small bowel biopsy of such a patient is demonstrated in Figure 19–17. Giardiasis, steatorrhea, and protein-losing enteropathy have been reported.[255] The lack of intestinal complications in most patients underscores the critical role of cellular immunity at mucosal surfaces. The long-term complications include bronchiectasis and

Table 19–18 Small Bowel Manifestations of Primary Immunodeficiency

| Name | IMMUNODEFICIENCY | | | | GI MANIFESTATIONS | | | | | |
| | B Cell | | | | | | | | | |
	IgA	IgM	IgG	T Cell	Severe Diarrhea	Flat Villus Lesion	Giardia	Bacterial Overgrowth	Candida	Lymphoid Hyperplasia
X-linked agamma-globulinemia	↓	↓	↓	NL	+	+	+	+	+	+/0
Selective IgA deficiency	↓	NL (↑)	NL	NL	++	++	++	+	++	++
Transient hypogamma-globulinemia of infancy	↓	↓	↓	NL	++	+	+	+/0	+/0	+
Common variable agamma-globulinemia	↓	↓	↓	NL/↓	+++	+++	+++	+++	+/0	+++
Thymic hypoplasia	NL↓	NL↓	NL↓	↓	+++	+++	+/0	++	+++	+/0
Severe combined immunodeficiency disease	↓	↓	↓	↓	+++	+++	+/0	++	+++	+/0
Wiskott-Aldrich syndrome	↑	↓	NL	↓	++	++	+/0	++	++	+/0

NL, normal limits.

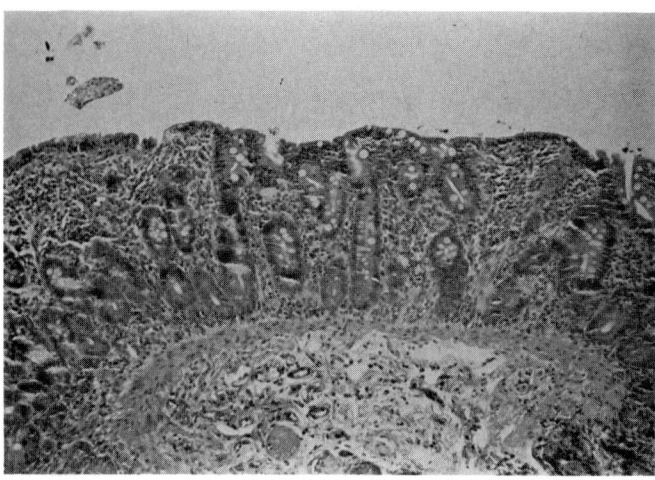

Figure 19–17   Small intestinal biopsy from an 18-month-old white boy with Bruton's type of agammaglobulinemia. The patient had been treated for diarrhea with a milk- and wheat-free diet for one month before admission. Cultures of nose, throat, and stool yielded *Candida albicans*; a course of treatment with nystatin (Mycostatin) eliminated the *Candida* infection but had no effect upon the diarrhea. Small bowel secretions contained no *Giardia* organisms. An empirical course of metronidazole (Flagyl) and substitution of Pregestamil for soy formula were without effect. Culture of the small bowel flora grew *Staphylococcus epidermidis*, and the small intestinal biopsy showed flattening of the villi, distortion of the mucosal cell nuclei, and a heavy infiltration of polymorphonuclear cells within the lamina propria. The child improved dramatically after one week of therapy with ampicillin, as evidenced by dimunition in stool volume and weight gain. A repeat biopsy two weeks later was normal.

the development of autoimmune phenomena.

Another congenital X-linked agammaglobulinemia has been reported that has specific elevation or normal levels of IgM. These patients also have few gastrointestinal manifestations but appear to have a significantly increased risk for the development of malignancy, including lymphomas and tumors of the GI tract.

Diagnosis and Management. Patients with Bruton's agammaglobulinemia are distinguished from those with acquired forms by the age of onset, the positive family history, and the hypoplastic lymphoid tissue, which often includes absence of the adenoids. Immunoglobulin levels will fall with a clearance of maternal antibody in the first few months of life, while delayed hypersensitivity and lymphocyte function studies will be normal for age. The majority of patients appear to do well on gamma globulin injections, if these are initiated prior to the development of irreversible lung disease. All suspected pyogenic infections are treated aggressively with antibiotics; diarrhea, when encountered, may respond to wide-spectrum antibiotics.

Common Variable Immunodeficiency

Pathophysiology. These immunodeficiencies become manifest at any age and are characterized by severe humoral immunodeficiency with variable alterations in T-cell function. Recent studies suggest that some of these patients' B lymphocytes or plasma cells can function normally when cocultured with normal control T lymphocytes, thus suggesting that the humoral immunodeficiency in at least some of these patients is secondary to an abnormal T-cell suppressor activity.[333]

Up to 50 per cent of patients with common variable agammaglobulinemia will demonstrate significant gastrointestinal disease. The most commonly recognized cause of diarrhea and villus injury in these patients is not dietary gluten but *Giardia lamblia*. This flagellated protozoan is usually transmitted indirectly from person to person by contaminated water. Chronic infestation and severe villus damage from *Giardia*, which are distinctly unusual in immunocompetent hosts, becomes the rule. As discussed in Chapter 18, diagnosis from the stools may be difficult, thus mandating the

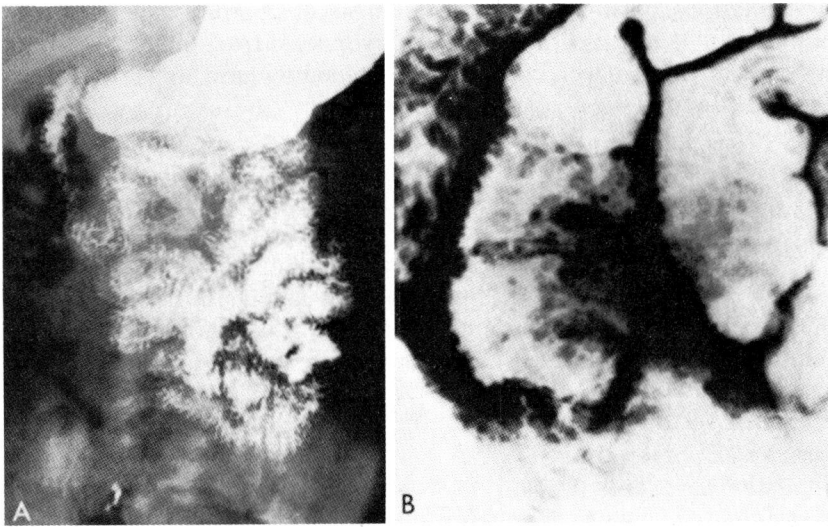

Figure 19–18   Diffuse nodular lymphoid hyperplasia of the small bowel in a boy with dysgammaglobulinemia. This child had had chronic diarrhea, recurrent ear and respiratory infections and growth retardation since the age of 6 months. *A*, Generalized coarsening of the mucosal pattern was seen throughout the entire small bowel. *B*, Compression spot film shows the small nodular pattern of the filling defects.

use of duodenal aspiration or small bowel biopsy for confirmation. Jejunal biopsy results should revert to normal following treatment for *Giardia*, and recurrences are uncommon. Unfortunately, other patients have severe villus injury that does not appear to be related to either gluten or *Giardia lamblia*. These patients, who are often labeled as having hypogammaglobulinemic sprue, may respond to corticosteroid therapy and wide-spectrum antibiotics.

The development of lymphoid nodular hyperplasia is frequent (20 to 60 per cent) in these patients, though rarely is manifested until late adolescence or adulthood. A classic example of the radiographic findings on small bowel follow-through is demonstrated in Figure 19–18. The lymphoid nodules are 1 to 3 millimeters in size and located within the lamina propria. Either the entire bowel or localized areas from duodenum to colon may be involved. This lymphoid hyperplasia also may involve other nonintestinal lymphoid tissue, and the development of hyperplasia appears to require an intact cell-mediated immune system. Indeed, recent reports emphasize that the lymphocytes in these nodular masses are predominantly of T-cell origin. There is some evidence in adults to suggest that nodular lymphoid hyperplasia predisposes to the development of intestinal lymphoma and carcinoma. Rectosigmoid colitis has been reported in this immune disease.[308a]

Additional gastrointestinal manifestations of common variable agammaglobulinemia include the development of atrophic gastritis with pernicious anemia; bacterial overgrowth; lactose intolerance; and destructive ulcerations of the distal small bowel and colon, viral in etiology.

Diagnosis and Management. The diagnosis depends on the demonstration of impaired humoral immunofunction with intact delayed hypersensitivity. Lymph node biopsy specimens reveal reduced cellularity in B cell–dependent areas. Lymphocyte transformation to phytohemagglutinin is depressed in 40 per cent of patients, and other T-cell functions may become abnormal secondary to severe malnutrition. Lymphopenia and even neutropenia may complicate the picture. Regular injection of gammaglobulin is the accepted mode of therapy. Diarrhea refractory to the elimination of lactose and treatment for *Giardia* mandates small bowel culture for bacterial colonization, since the gastrointestinal manifestations of nodular lymphoid hyperplasia in older children and adults often respond to treatment with a wide-spectrum antibiotic such as tetracycline. In many patients, plasma infusions or breast milk treatment have been initiated to control the diarrhea, as gammaglobulin injections will fail to provide significant amounts of IgA. Transfer factor may be of help. Some patients require prolonged peripheral or central hyperalimentation.

Selective IgA Deficiency

Pathophysiology. This deficiency occurs in approximately 1 in 700 individuals and has several forms. The most common is selective failure to elaborate IgA from normal B lymphocytes, apparently due to specific T-cell suppression. Less commonly there is a deficiency of B lymphocytes with IgA surface immunoglobulin. In both circumstances, serum and secretory levels of IgA are diminished. A compensatory increase in secretory IgM may develop and appears to be sufficient in the majority of patients to maintain normal secretory immunologic integrity. Cell-mediated immune functions are generally normal.

Recently two patients with selective deficiency of secretory IgA alone have been reported, apparently as a result of decreased synthesis of secretory component.[309] These patients had normal serum IgA levels and appeared to have intact secretion of IgM, an ironic finding in light of IgM's requirement for secretory component as well. Villus injury and *Candida* enteritis were confirmed in both these patients.

All the gastrointestinal complications cited above for common variable agammaglobulinemia have been reported in patients with selective IgA deficiency, though the frequency and severity are significantly diminished. It is interesting that the flat villus lesions seen in patients with selective IgA deficiency are often gluten-sensitive, unlike those seen with common variable agammaglobulinemia. The nodular lymphoid lesions are rare in infancy but may contribute to diarrhea in older children. An increased incidence of inflammatory bowel disease is suspected in these patients and merits evaluation in symptomatic adolescents.

Diagnosis and Management. The diagnosis requires a demonstration of normal serum IgG and IgM levels, with severe reduction in serum and/or secretory IgA. T-lymphocyte numbers and function are normal. Lymphoid tissue is histologically intact. As the majority of patients are asymptomatic, treatment is obviously individualized. Malabsorption and small bowel injury are managed initially as gluten-sensitive enteropathy, with milk restriction also appropriate in the younger infants. Gamma globulin injections are not an effective, source of IgA. In those patients with severely enteric disease, breast milk feedings have been recommended.

Transient Hypogammaglobulinemia of Infancy

Pathophysiology. These infants demonstrate a prolongation of the physiologic depression in immunoglobulin IgA and/or IgG levels seen in the first six to eight months of life.[319] Spontaneous improvement is the rule, but normal levels may not be achieved for several years. It is important to remember, however, that the capacity to form specific antibodies (isohemagglutinins, antidiphtheria, antitetanus) can be demonstrated in these patients by 6 to 12 months of age. Transient hypogammalobulinemia is often found in relatives of immunodeficient patients, leading Soothill and others to suggest that it may be a manifestation of genetic heterozygosity.[306] The frequency of this syndrome is not known, but we have noted it in approximately 20 per cent of our patients under two years of age who have chronic diarrhea. The intestinal manifestations are variable and incompletely described, with frequent gastroenteritis, including rotavirus. Malabsorption is rare and villus lesions and *Giardia* infections are distinctly uncommon. Nodular lymphoid hyperplasia, however, has been reported.

Diagnosis and Management. Immunoglobulin levels will be uniformly reduced, with IgG levels usually less than 200 mg per dl between six and nine months of age and IgA levels varying from 0 to 6 mg per dl. The IgG levels will remain below normal at one year of age. Peripheral lymphocyte counts are normal, as are T-cell functions. No specific therapy is warranted in these patients with gamma globulin injections restricted to those few patients with recurrent pyogenic infection and low serum IgG. Hypoallergenic diets often lead to improvement in diarrhea.

T-CELL DEFECTS

As noted in Table 19–18, patients with a predominant T-cell immunodeficiency have gastrointestinal manifestations clinically distinguishable from those with predominant B-cell deficiencies. Intractable diarrhea is a common presentation in these infants, occasionally caused by *Shigella,* *Salmonella,* or enteropathic *Escherichia coli.* Unfortunately, the etiology of the diarrhea in the majority of patients is never determined. When these patients receive T-cell reconstitution, a rapid reversal of this diarrhea has been noted. Of note, neither *Giardia* infestation nor lymphoid nodular hyperplasia is common in patients with T-cell defects.

Thymic Hypoplasia (DiGeorge Syndrome)

Pathophysiology. This syndrome is a reflection of a failure of differentiation from the third and fourth pharyngeal pouches *in utero.* As a result, thymic and parathyroid function are absent and cardiovascular abnormalities of the aortic arch are common. Intractable diarrhea develops in infancy, with frequent chronic monilial infections of the mouth, esophagus, and small bowel.

Diagnosis and Management. Neonatal tetany is the usual presentation. Immunologic studies will reveal normal immunoglobulin levels, normal lymphocyte counts, negative skin tests, and abnormal *in vitro* lymphocyte functions. The thymic shadow on chest radiograph will be absent, and lymph node biopsy specimens will reveal lymphocyte depletion in the subcortical or thymic-dependent portions.

Therapy consists of immediate treatment for hypoparathyroidism. Thymus transplant is the treatment of choice with retransplantation often necessary because of rejection.

Severe Combined Immunodeficiency Disease (SCID) (Swiss Type)

Pathophysiology. These syndromes encompass several disorders, all manifesting as depression of both T- and B-cell function. They are inherited as either sex-linked or autosomal recessive disorders with a male to female ratio of 3:1. The basic defect is felt to be a failure of "stem cell" differentiation. The autosomal recessive forms may show a reduction in adenosine deaminase, with ectodermal dysplasia and epiphyseal dysostosis (short-limbed dwarfism), or with generalized hematopoietic hypoplasia (reticular dysgenesis).

Chronic diarrhea with severe malabsorption, chronic hepatitis, and recurrent monilial infections develop in the first six to nine months of life. Small bowel biopsy specimens will reveal villus loss, reduced brush border disaccharidases, crypt abscesses, and absence of plasma cells. Within the lamina propria large vacuolated macrophages are reported, similar to those noted in Whipple's disease and chronic granulomatous disease. Bacterial enteritis is often documented, but specific therapy often fails to produce relief from the diarrhea.

Diagnosis and Management. Severe bacterial, viral, fungal, and protozoal infections will usually begin by six months of age.[346] Rarely, manifestations do not begin until school age. Immunoglobulin levels will be very low, lymphocyte counts will be diminished, and T-cell stimulations will be impaired if not absent. Infections with *Candida, Pneumocystis carinii,* and cytomegalovirus often will be fatal in infancy. Therapy is geared to providing stem cells by either bone marrow or fetal thymus transplant. Patients with adenosine deaminase deficiency have been treated with irradiated red cells as a potential source of enzyme replacement.[269]

Wiskott-Aldrich Syndrome

Pathophysiology. These patients present within the first 12 months with an X-linked recessive immunodeficiency characterized by eczema, thrombocytopenia, and recurrent infection. Inheritance is X-linked recessive. Bloody diarrhea with malabsorption is common in infancy and may be the presenting manifestation. Few small bowel biopsies have been done in these patients, because of the severe thrombocytopenia. Some patients demonstrate reduction in diarrhea on milk or soy protein-free diets, suggesting a protein-induced inflammatory process. Nodular lymphoid hyperplasia and *Giardia* infection commonly are not seen.

Diagnosis and Management. Immunoglobulin levels will vary with age, but generally IgM levels are decreased, IgG levels will vary, and IgA levels will be increased. These patients are not able to produce antibodies to polysaccharide antigen. T-cell function is initially normal but usually decreases dramatically with age. Treatment is directed at specific infections with transfer factor therapy, plasma infusions, and various transplant techniques now being utilized experimentally.

Ataxia-Telangiectasia

This autosomal recessive condition is characterized by telangiectasia, progressive ataxia, and immunodeficiency of T-cell function usually associated with decreased IgA. Gastrointestinal hemorrhage is common, with malabsorption well described only for vitamin B_{12}. An increased risk for intestinal malignancy and lymphoma has been confirmed.

Chronic Mucocutaneous Candidiasis

These patients appear to have a unique failure of T-cell responses to *Candida albicans*, coupled with an associated humoral immune defect, both predisposing to recurrent *Candida* infection. Many patients have an associated endocrinopathy, felt to be autoimmune in nature. *Candida* infection of the skin and mucous membranes begins in the first few years of life. Severe esophageal disease may then develop, with stricture and occasionally perforation over the years. Chronic hepatitis is also common. Gastric

and small bowel monilial infections, though reported, are distinctly unusual.

Graft-Versus-Host Disease

With the ever-expanding use of organ and bone marrow transplantation in childhood, graft-versus-host disease has become a major clinical challenge in pediatric referral hospitals. The disorder arises when immunocompetent cells are given to a histoincompatible immunodeficient host. The major cause is attempted reconstitution by bone marrow, fetal thymus, or fetal liver transplantation. It may also be seen following transfusion, including maternal-fetal transfusions *in utero*.[337]

The primary sites of human graft-versus-host disease are the skin, lymphoid tissue, liver, and gastrointestinal tract. The earliest manifestation is generally rash, usually maculopapular in nature. Skin biopsy remains a major clinical tool for diagnosis. Over the ensuing days, cramping, abdominal pain with diarrhea and melena and hepatic dysfunction may ensue. In chronic graft-versus-host disease, failure to thrive and wasting become prominent. The intestinal lesion is clinically prominent in the esophagus and small bowel. Mucosal villus flattening with ulcerations and a mononuclear infiltration will be seen on biopsy. Rectal involvement also has been confirmed by rectal biopsy. Bleeding, malabsorption, secretory diarrhea, and protein-losing enteropathy may be the clinical manifestations of this inflammation. The treatment of graft-versus-host disease focuses on prevention or early immunosuppression, for little of proved value has been found for established disease.

Systemic Mastocytosis

In addition to its association with peptic ulcer, systemic mastocytosis may be accompanied by severe diarrhea and abdominal pain. Oral disodium cromoglycate may produce a dramatic decrease in diarrhea through its effects upon the mast cell membrane.[210a, 306a]

TUMORS

VASOACTIVE INTESTINAL POLYPEPTIDE (VIP)-SECRETING TUMORS

Ganglioneuroma and Ganglioneuroblastoma

Verner and Morrison first described a syndrome of watery diarrhea and hypokalemia associated with a non-beta islet cell tumor of the pancreas. It has since been associated with pancreatic hyperplasia, bronchogenic carcinoma, pheochromocytoma, and ganglioneuroma or ganglioneuroblastoma. In children, only the latter two tumors have been associated with VIP production and this may well develop as the major hormone causing diarrhea in infants with this tumor.[53, 315]

Incidence. In 1980, Kaplan et al. reported one patient and accumulated seven others from the literature.[177]

Etiology and Pathophysiology. These tumors are derived from the APUD series (amine precursor uptake and decarboxylation), which contain ganglion cells and produce greater than 35 active peptides.[329, 330] Most of the peripheral APUD cells are located in the gastrointestinal tract and pancreas. It is interesting that VIP and norepinephrine effects are antagonistic, the one being a potent vasodilator and the other, a vasoconstrictor. When VIP was first recognized, it was felt that all noninsulin secreting pancreatic tumors or hyperplasia produced this hormone in excess to cause symptoms via its various properties: stimulation of adenylcyclase, stimulation of intestinal motility, inhibition of gastrin-stimulated gastric acid secretion, and vasodilation. However, several patients with similar symptoms have had normal serum VIP but increased levels of prostaglandin E. Of the eight children, four had ganglioneuromas, three had ganglioneuroblastomas, and in one the tumor was not found. Two were in the abdomen, three in the thorax, one in the neck, and one in the thorax and abdomen.[37a]

Symptoms. The ages of the eight patients ranged from six months to seven and a half years. Diarrhea was the major symptom, being often copious and devastating in its effect. It remains unchanged in character despite variation in dietary intake or bowel rest and total parenteral nutrition. As a result, patients often are dehydrated and have severe electrolyte abnormalities. Most often, hypokalemia is seen, with significant loss of potassium and bicarbonate in the feces (with relative sparing of sodium because of colonic ion exchange). Hypo- or hypercalcemia may be seen in half the patients, but hypomagnesemia with tetany may be seen in the face of a normal calcium level. Skin flushing, hypertension, and gastric achlorhydria are also common in this syndrome. Hyperglycemia is present in nearly half of adults. Gallbladder distention is a rare finding. Unfortunately, many of these patients have malabsorption with villous atrophy by the time of presentation. This appears to be due to the severe protein-calorie malnutrition they endure. The malabsorption contributes further to the diarrhea and malnutrition because of the effects on bile acid secretion and inactivation of pancreatic enzymes. Because of their severe secondary malnutrition, two of the three pediatric patients described died of secondary sepsis. Adult patients do equally poorly because of nutritional and electrolyte disruptions and because of the malignant nature of the tumor in 37 per cent.

Diagnosis. The most important diagnostic step is the recognition that the diarrhea is a secretory process. The suggestion is apparent from the continuation of watery stools despite cessation of oral intake. The stools should then be analyzed for osmolality and electrolyte levels. A normal or increased stool sodium level (normal, approximately 10 to 30 mEq per liter), with a high fecal osmolality, confirms a secretory diarrhea. The various causes of secretory diarrhea should be considered. The patient should then be evaluated by means of stool cultures and titers for pathogens (cholera, salmonella, *Shigella, E. coli*) and hormone levels (vasoactive intestinal peptide, gastric inhibitory peptide, pancreatic polypeptide, secretin, prostaglandin, VMA, serotonin, and HIAA). Urinary catecholamines were increased in six of eight children, as were plasma and tissue VIP.

While awaiting those results, one may consider a pancreatic scan that would be sensitive to non-beta islet cell tumors. Selenomethionine (^{75}Se) has been used since methionine is not required for insulin synthesis. Computed tomography will identify paraspinal masses well, and venograms have shown inferior vena cava compression in a few patients.

Treatment. The only completely effective therapy appears to be surgical removal of the tumor or complete pancreatectomy in diffuse non-beta cell islet cell hyperplasia. With removal of the tumor, the diarrhea should cease. Care must be taken during surgery because of the increased catecholamines also found in those children, for there may be hypo- or hypertensive crisis. Indomethacin has been utilized as a temporary measure in a patient with elevated prostaglandins while awaiting surgery. Electrolyte and fluid requirement were reduced and diarrheal volume diminished with this inhibitor of prostaglandin synthesis.

Careful attention to fluid electrolytes and nutritional management is necessary to prevent imbalance and inanition. Parenteral alimentation with adequate protein and caloric delivery should be accompanied by potassium, bicarbonate, calcium, and magnesium replacement as soon as the secretory nature of the diarrhea is recognized. The role of oral glucose-electrolyte solutions has not been established. While such a solution should be of the same benefit as in cholera, the chronicity of this syndrome and long-term needs of the patient make this an impractical alternative. Cholestyramine and nasogastric suction have proved of no value.

THE NEURAL CREST TUMORS

The neural crest tumors are perplexing and fascinating not only because of the spectrum of diseases with which they are associated but also because they undergo changes in malignant potential and can, at times, virtually disappear.

Neuroblastoma

The most common tumor of the neonate and probably of early childhood, neuroblastoma is variable in both its histologic picture and its natural course.[222]

Incidence. In the infant, one third of tumors are neurogenic and one third to one sixth are within the abdomen. Six to seven per cent of all childhood tumors are neuroblastomas. Beckwith and Perrin reviewed autopsies of infants up to three months old who died of other diseases and found 40 times the expected rate of neuroblastoma in situ.[28a] In view of these data, one may estimate that for every 100 known clinical cases there are presumably 4000 tumors in neonates that disappear spontaneously without ever becoming clinically apparent. Most studies reflect a preponderance of males although in a few there seems to be no predilection for sex. A familial tumor has been reported, affecting three individuals in one family, of whom one child had an abnormal number 11 chromosome.[145] Three cases have been reported in association with the fetal alcohol syndrome,[185] and others with Horner's syndrome and heterochromia iridis.[231]

Pathology. A classification has been proposed to include four stages of neuroblastoma: stage I, localized and resectable; stage II, regional and unresectable; stage III, generalized but without bone marrow involvement; and stage IV, generalized with bone or bone marrow involvement. The IV S tumor, a small primary lesion and metastatic disease to liver, skin, or marrow, without bone involvement, is unique to children under one year of age (comprising 10 per cent of total neuroblastomas) and has a 70 per cent survival rate.[89] It is interesting that an E rosette inhibitory factor and increased serum ferritin are present in those with type IV but not with type IV S tumors. The tumor is composed of sympathetic nerve cells that vary in immaturity from sympathogonioma through sympathoblastoma to the most immature neurocystoma. In general, the more differentiated the cell form, the less the malignant potential of the tumor. It tends to undergo spontaneous maturation.[272a] Most of these arise from the adrenal medulla, although derivation from any of the sympathetic ganglia is possible—40 per cent of neonatal tumors derive from sites other than the adrenal.

Grossly, the tumor is nodular and appears encapsulated, varying in color from red or purple (in areas of hemorrhagic necrosis) to yellow. Neuroblastomas are extremely cellular, with the cells arranged in sheets. The nuclei lie peripherally, and rosette forma-

tion is often apparent. Variable degrees of cellular differentiation exist within the same tumor. Metastases occur early and are most frequent in the liver, long bones, skull, meninges, and bone marrow (Fig. 19–19). When they involve the soft tissue of the orbit, they cause unilateral proptosis. Over half of neonatal tumors have metastasized by the time of diagnosis: 65 per cent to liver,

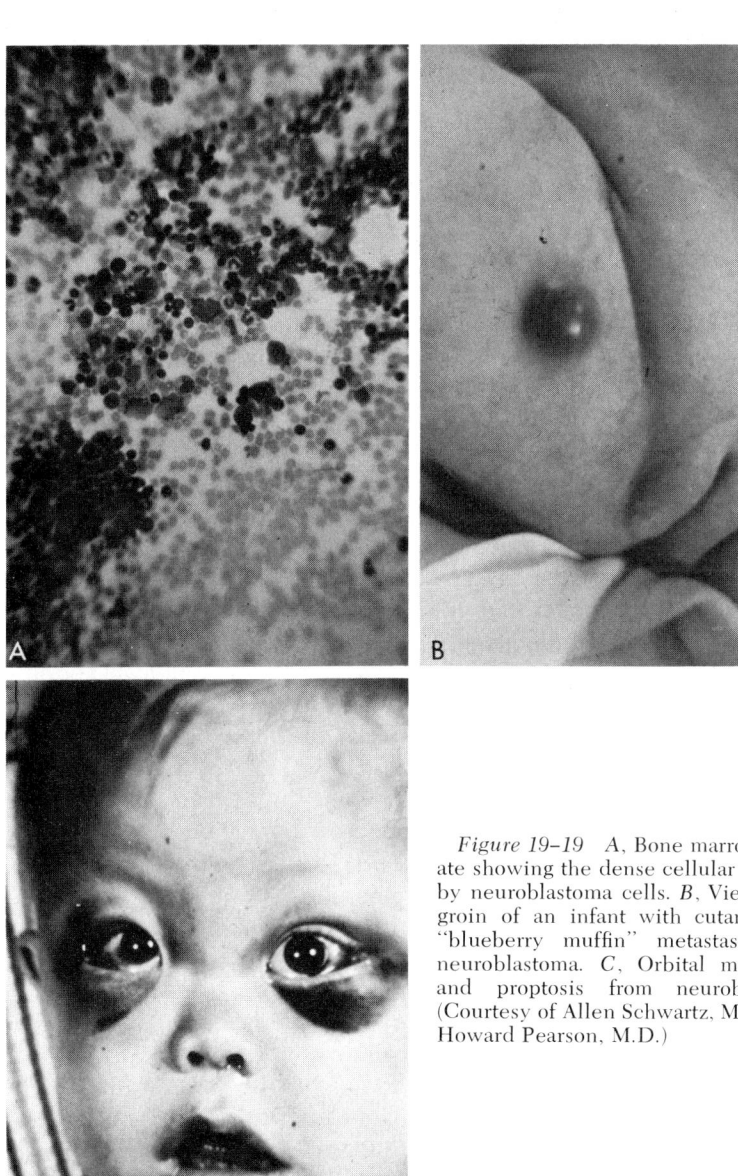

Figure 19–19 *A*, Bone marrow aspirate showing the dense cellular invasion by neuroblastoma cells. *B*, View of the groin of an infant with cutaneous or "blueberry muffin" metastases from neuroblastoma. *C*, Orbital metastases and proptosis from neuroblastoma. (Courtesy of Allen Schwartz, M. D., and Howard Pearson, M.D.)

3 per cent to bone, and 35 per cent to skin in the form of subcutaneous nodules. The lung, bone, and soft tissue are most often affected in older children.

Since many of these tumors show spontaneous disappearance even when associated with metastatic disease, there has been a great deal of interest in the immunologic mechanisms that might be involved. Early studies suggested that the tumors matured to a benign form, but recent evidence indicates that there is actual disappearance of tumor cells rather than transformation or regression. Tumor infiltration by plasma cells or lymphocytes is regarded as evidence of an immune reaction and occurs in tumors that have a good prognosis. That lymphocytes and plasma cells from patients with neuroblastoma have a lethal immune reaction against target cells of tumor in tissue culture suggests that immune reactions are responsible for the spontaneous regression of some tumors. Surgical treatment is in a sense immunologic, for, if a significant amount of tumor tissue is removed, the immune mechanism then can function on the remaining antigenic tissue.

Symptoms. Nearly half the patients are under two years of age, and one third are less than one year old when symptoms first appear. The manifestations of the tumor are protean, and the earliest presentation of the tumor is as abdominal dystocia due to massive metastatic involvement of the liver. Jaundice, hepatomegaly, and a palpable mass in the left upper quadrant of the neonate may lead to an erroneous diagnosis of erythroblastosis fetalis. In young infants progressive abdominal enlargement from hepatic metastases is the most frequent complaint, and in older infants and children unilateral proptosis can be the first and only symptom caused by the tumor (Fig. 19–19C). The tumor mass often is not palpable in the young baby, for it is obscured by a greatly enlarged liver, the surface of which is smooth rather than nodular. In older infants, involved liver is nodular and the tumor itself is palpable as a hard, nodular mass in either side of the abdomen and extending across the midline. Less often, chronic diarrhea or milk anemia is the only

symptom to signify the presence of tumor. Rarely, the tumor presents as a brain or a mediastinal tumor. In a few cases, ataxia, myoclonic seizures, and "dancing" eyes or feet precede other symptoms by months or years. In such cases the tumor usually lies outside the abdomen. In one instance, the tumor underwent spontaneous rupture and presented as hemoperitoneum.[39a]

Tumors arising in the lower abdomen or from the pelvic sympathetic ganglia produce local pressure upon the urinary tract and cause an outlet type of urinary obstruction, or upon the rectum to cause difficulties in defecation. The tumor mass is palpable on rectal examination. Renal ganglioneuroblastoma may cause Cushing's syndrome.

Metastatic subcutaneous nodules appear as bluish-pink indurated lesions that blanch on pressure, a phenomenon probably due to the local release of catecholamines (Fig. 19–19B).

Clinically the tumor is named according to the distribution of its metastases: the right or Pepper type metastasizes to the liver, while the left or Hutchinson type metastasizes widely to bone, skull, soft tissue, and lung.

Diagnosis. The tumor must be suspected in any child with abdominal enlargement and hepatomegaly and is of prime consideration in those with unilateral proptosis whether or not an abdominal mass is present. The characteristics of the mass in older children differentiate it from Wilms' tumor, which usually does not extend across the midline. Intravenous pyelography often shows displacement of one of the renal calyces, and bone marrow aspirate may be positive for tumor cells. Some patients have increased catecholamine levels in the urine. (See the next section, Ganglioneuroma.)

Treatment. Once the diagnosis is established, the first line of treatment is surgical removal of the entire tumor or as much of it as is feasible. Irradiation and chemotherapy seem of little help in changing survival rates. Recommended therapy for type IV S disease is removal of the primary tumor and liver biopsy. If there is severe hepatomegaly, then irradiation or cyclophosphamide and vincristine should be given. The majority of studies indicate that irradiation is of import in increasing the cure rate, particularly when it is begun immediately after surgery. Irradiation followed by prolonged chemotherapy seems to produce the best results, with dosage and type of drug determined by tumor chemotherapists. Cyclophosphamide (Cytoxan) and vincristine are alternated weekly over a nine to ten month period or combinations of doxorubicin hydrochloride, dacarbazine, and vincristine are used. One child with metastatic disease refractory to therapy was treated with lethal chemotherapy doses, total body irradiation, and bone marrow transplantation to attain a six-month remission.[307]

Prognosis. The peripheral lymphocyte count seems to be an important indicator of prognosis, for infants under one year of age who survived after treatment for neuroblastoma had higher total lymphocyte counts than those who died. Survival after total excision of the tumor ranges from 36 to 100 per cent; after partial excision, the survival rate is from 18 to 64 per cent, no matter what other modes of treatment are used. It is stated that neuroblastoma in infants has the highest rate of spontaneous regression of any type of human malignant disease; although this is only in the range of 5 to 10 per cent, it is significant. Most series consider two or more years adequate for determining survival from this tumor, but death may occur up to six and a half years after a tumor-free period.

Swank et al. reported the factors they found to indicate a good prognosis as onset in the first year, an extra-abdominal primary site, either no metastases or spread limited to regional nodes, total or subtotal tumor excision, and an elevated peripheral total lymphocyte count.[314a] Poor prognostic signs, on the other hand, are bone or bone marrow metastases, which carry a 94 to 100 per cent mortality, liver metastases, with a 93 per cent mortality, and lung, kidney, or brain metastases, which are universally fatal.[194] Extra-abdominal and pelvic tumors carry a far better prognosis than those within the abdomen, in which the survival rate is 25 per cent. Survival with adrenal tumors is 32 per cent; with thoracic, 43 to 75 per cent;

sacral, 50 to 100 per cent; and cervical, 80 to 100 per cent. Spontaneous maturation-regression recently has been reported in seven of seven patients with pelvic neuroblastoma.

Differentiation of the tumor cell is of some help in determining the eventual outlook, since 31 per cent of those with well-differentiated tumors survive, compared with 9 per cent of those with poorly differentiated ones. Endocrine activity also has some bearing upon prognosis, for those with a relatively low homovanillic acid (HVA) excretion have a more benign course than those who have a considerably increased urinary HVA. Some feel that tumors that secrete norepinephrine and epinephrine metabolites carry a better outlook than those that secrete dopamine. Failure of catabolite excretion to return to normal after surgery is ominous and represents persistent tumor activity. Less than 5 per cent of patients fail to excrete excessive quantities of catecholamines, and their prognosis cannot be determined by biochemical analysis, for their tumors may be either undifferentiated or highly differentiated. Others studied prognostic factors and concluded that prognosis in disseminated disease correlated directly with the vanillylmandelic acid (VMA):HVA ratio but not with absolute levels of HVA. The presence of vanillacetic acid and increased amounts of cystathionine and/or low levels of VMA indicate poor prognosis. Patients with initially high IgG levels and in whom IgG and IgM do not decrease during treatment seem to have a good prognosis. The serum lactic dehydrogenase is elevated in advanced disease (90 per cent type IV) and may serve as an indicator of tumor activity,[271] as may serum immunoglobulin levels.[286]

Ganglioneuroma

Ganglioneuromas arising from neural crest tissue cause diarrhea by way of increased production of catecholamines and their metabolites, prostaglandins, or vasoactive intestinal peptide.[315]

Incidence. Over 500 cases have been reported. The tumor is far less common than is neuroblastoma, with an estimated occurrence of one benign ganglioneuroma to every six neuroblastomas. There is a slight preponderance of females over males (3:2).

Etiology. It is believed that some ganglioneuromas derive from neuroblastomas.

Pathology. Some of these nonfunctioning tumors arise in the intestine, where they act as polypoid lesions and interfere with motility. Most, however, arise from the sympathetic chain extending from the base of the skull to the pelvis, including the adrenal medulla, and originate most often in the posterior mediastinum or in or near the adrenal gland. Less often they arise in the neck and rarely they originate in the breast, joints, maxilla, kidney, peritoneum, or brain. Ganglioneuroma is the most mature, fully differentiated, and benign of all of the neural crest tumors and, since it grows slowly, rarely causes local symptoms unless it is located in the neck or brain. The criterion for diagnosis of benign ganglioneuroma is to find tumor of adult ganglion cells in a matrix of large numbers of neurites with Schwann's sheaths, which are occasionally myelinated and lie within a fibrous framework. One fifth of ganglioneuromas contain some anaplasia, and in some tumors one portion may appear mature and another resemble a malignant neuroblastoma. Sixty-five per cent of this latter type will metastasize. Calcification occurs frequently and is considered by some to represent tumor immaturity and malignancy and by others, a rapid tissue growth beyond the capacity of the blood supply, resulting in necrosis. Differences of opinion exist concerning hormone secretion by the tumor. Some feel that more actively secreting tumors are more immature and malignant, whereas others consider active secretion a sign of better differentiation and therefore of a more benign tumor. Increased catecholamine secretion is found in both benign or metastasizing tumors, however.

Pathophysiology. The synthesis of catecholamines is from the precursors dihydroxyphenylalanine to dopamine. From dopamine are derived 3-methyldopamine, norepinephrine, and epinephrine. The catechols are broken down through O-methylation to yield vanillylmandelic acid (VMA) from the epinephrines and homovanillic acid (HVA) from 3-methyldopamine. Norepinephrine, the major hormone of the sympathetic nervous system, is present in greater quantity than epinephrine, and the urinary excretion of its metabolite, VMA, is 10 to 100 times greater. Only 3 to 6 per cent of norepinephrine is excreted unchanged in the urine, while 20 to 40 per cent is excreted as normetanephrine and over 30 per cent as VMA.

The hypertension often associated with these tumors is probably a direct result of increased norepinephrine and is caused by peripheral vasoconstriction with only a small decrease in cardiac output. This is in contrast to that caused by epinephrine, which is accompanied by vasoconstriction and increase in heart rate and pulse pressure. Other catecholamine-induced symptoms are sweating, flushing, pallor, and polydipsia. The Cushing's syndrome induced by the intermediate ganglioneuroblastoma is probably caused by catecholamine stimulation of the adrenal or pituitary gland.

Although most of these tumors secrete catecholamines, only about 10 per cent are associated with diarrhea, with stool containing massive amounts of water, sodium, and potassium. This impairment of water and electrolyte transport is probably related to vasoconstriction in the blood vessels of the intestinal muscularis and mucosa. Some effect upon the distal small bowel is suggested by impaired vitamin B_{12} absorption. Although some patients have a milky, generalized steatorrhea, other specific absorptive defects have not been demonstrated.

Symptoms. Many of these tumors are asymptomatic, but the most common symptom in the infant is chronic watery diarrhea that is refractory to all methods of dietary and medical management. Abdominal distention is marked, and as the diarrhea progresses extreme muscle wasting develops. Respiratory symptoms or chest pain is sometimes noted in those with thoracic lesions. Water and electrolyte losses result in dehydration, hyponatremia, and hypokalemia. The physical examination reveals only an emaciated infant with a greatly distended abdomen that is extremely tympanitic. The bowel sounds are hyperactive. The presence of hypertension is an extremely important diagnostic clue. It has been associated with heterochromia iridis and Horner's syndrome.

Diagnosis. Early in its course the disease is confused with celiac disease or with enteritis or enterocolitis. As its refractory nature becomes obvious, intensive diagnostic studies for tumor must be undertaken. The radiologic examination begins with examination of the chest, for ganglioneuroma is the most common posterior mediastinal tumor of children. Calcification in the mass will help to differentiate it from a duplication cyst. Flat films of the abdomen or pyelogram will demonstrate displacement of a kidney or the presence of a calcified mass. The only abnormal gastrointestinal manifestation is dilation or hypotonicity of the colon. Computed axial tomography is valuable in identifying paraspinal tumors.

The measurement of urinary catecholamines and particularly their metabolite, VMA, is the most reliable diagnostic test although the levels are not elevated in all patients early in the disease even if symptoms are present. Several patterns are possible, including a normal VMA but increased norepinephrine or a normal VMA with increased dopamine and HVA, and so all the metabolites must be evaluated. Voorhees and Gardner classified their patients into four groups according to the urinary patterns of catechol and catechol metabolites: (1) elevated dopamine, norepinephrine and VMA, (2) elevated dopamine and norepinephrine, (3) elevated metanephrine, normetanephrine and VMA, and (4) normal catechol excretion.[330a] Those with normal VMA but elevated dopamine and norepinephrine had extremely malignant tumors.

The normal total urinary catecholamines range between 30 and 200 μg per 24 hours. Various laboratories report normal values for VMA excretion varying from 405 to 1440 μg per 24 hours; from 1.5 to 3.6 mg per 24 hours with means of 116 μg $\pm$ 5 μg per 5 kg per 24 hours; and 2.3 $\pm$ 2.4 mg per liter in children under two years of age. The values

are lowest during the first week of life, with neonates excreting 0.13 μg per 24 hours, and 5-day-old infants excreting 0.3 μg per 24 hours. Values for norepinephrine vary from 6.4 to 16.4 μg per 24 hours; for epinephrine, 0.5 to 1.2 μg per 24 hours; and for metanephrine and normetanephrine, 20.3 to 198 μg per 24 hours.

Some neural crest tumors also produce prostaglandins, some of which cause diarrhea in human beings.

Treatment. The only definitive treatment is surgical removal of the tumor. At times this is not possible if the tumor has invaded the spine or is intimately wrapped about a major blood vessel Even partial resection in such cases may alleviate the symptoms, although the catecholamine excretion remains elevated. Postoperative irradiation is of no use, for the tumor is resistant to radiation. Regular determinations of urinary catecholamines are necessary to detect any residual or metastatic tumor. Patients who have persistent diarrhea after incomplete tumor excision are sometimes helped by prednisone.

Prognosis. The prognosis is excellent in patients after complete excision of the tumor; it is poor otherwise.

UNUSUAL CHRONIC DIARRHEAL SYNDROMES

An *X-linked syndrome of diarrhea, polyendocrinopathy, and fatal infection* in infancy has been reported in eight boys, six of whom died. In addition to chronic diarrhea, there was eczema, hemolytic anemia, diabetes, or thyroid autoimmunity. Eleven other boys in the kindred had died in infancy. Immunologically, T and B cell function was normal, but one patient had delayed skin anergy and one, decreased lymphocyte stimulation upon exposure to phytohemagluttinin.[269b]

Chronic diarrhea and failure to thrive in association with unusual facies and abnormal scalp hair shafts has been reported in two siblings born at 38 and 39 weeks' gestation, weighing 1680 and 1620 gm. They had low-set ears, prominent eyes, a supraorbital ridge, antimongoloid slant to the eyes, woolly black hair, galactosuria without galactosemia, hepatic cirrhosis, and islet cell hyperplasia. Electron microscopy showed the hair to be kinked, ropelike, and ghostlike, with budding projections. The hair had a decreased cystine content.[308b]

Two first cousins have been reported with the *nephrotic syndrome caused by tubulointerstitial renal disease and diarrhea*, with malabsorption as a result of villous atrophy, associated with tissue autoantibodies.[85b]

The *Polle syndrome*, named after the son of Munchausen, is a phenophthalein laxative–induced diarrhea resulting from maternal administration of medication. The diagnosis may be made by eliciting a pink color after alkalinization of the stool.[1, 267a]

TESTS FOR FAT MALABSORPTION

The serum carotene test is a conventional method of assessing fat absorption, as long as the patient is ingesting carotene (present in yellow vegetables, oranges, and tomatoes). Since carrots seem to be the first vegetable matter identified in diarrheal stools, mothers often attribute the cause of diarrhea to them and delete them from the diet. Some ingested carotene is absorbed unchanged, and some is converted to vitamin A. Since carotene is not stored, its level can be depleted within three to four weeks. Normal carotene levels range between 70 and 120 μg/per dl, but values may fall between 25 and 40 μg per dl in those whose diets are restricted. In malabsorption, levels are 22 μg or less, often in single numbers. A carotene loading test is recommended to differentiate dietary from intestinal etiology. Adults given 15,000 units of carotene three times daily for three days will increase serum carotene by 35 μg per dl or more. Similarly, infants taking one-half jar of carrots daily for one week will increase their serum levels.

Stool fat and nitrogen may be measured in a single stool collection. Although the presence of fat globules in a random stool stained with Sudan III suggests malabsorption, and, similarly, the steatocrit has been cited as a simple method for evaluating stool fat content,[267b] the only true documentation is by a quantitative study. Children should have no enzyme therapy, tolerance tests, or barium studies for at least 48 hours prior to the collection. A daily dietary diary should be maintained for one to two days before and during the collection period. It should be noted that anorectic patients may ingest well below normal levels of fat and total calories.

Method of Collection. The child should take a normal diet for at least three days before the collection begins. A charcoal or red dye marker is given at the beginning of the collection period (usually 8 A.M.) and repeated in 72 hours. The stool with the first marker is noted, and that and subsequent stools are collected. The last stool containing the second marker is discarded. Collections may be carried out at home with the mother collecting all stools between 8 A.M. on day 1 and 8 A.M. 72 hours later. If the stools are semiformed or liquid, they are best collected using a Saran-Wrap liner or revised disposable diapers. Stools are scraped from these into a weighed container that is kept refrigerated during the collection.

Fecal fat is measured as total fecal fatty acids determined according to the method of Van de Kamer or a modification of it. The coefficient of fat absorption represents the per cent of fat absorbed from that which was ingested. Normal infants taking a regular diet for age excrete less than 3.5 gm per day, which represents 5 to 10 per cent of their fat intake. Other workers define the limits more stringently, using 2.3 gm per day as the mean fat excretion for infants under one year of age (upper limit, 4.3 gm per day); and 1.72 gm per day the mean for those over one year of age (upper limit, 3.02 gm per day). In comparison, the normal fecal fat excretion for adolescents and adults is 5 gm per day. In infants with celiac disease, fecal fat ranges from 4 to 26 gm per day, but the highest values are in those with pancreatic insufficiency or intestinal lymphangiectasia. Since fecal fat is derived from ingested fat, bile fats, intestinal secretions, desquamated cells, and bacteria, normal persons taking a fat-free diet will still excrete 0.5 to 1 gm of fat per day. Even increasing dietary fat from 50 to 100 gm per day will not increase fat excretion in the normal person, although it will do so in the malabsorber. Those with malabsorption not only fail to absorb ingested fat but have increased endogenous fecal fat.

Fecal nitrogen is measured from the same 72-hour collection and provides information about protein digestion and loss. Infants under one year of age excrete less than 1 gm per day and older infants no more than 1.2 gm. Endogenous fecal nitrogen is derived from cellular proteins and intestinal secretions.

Other Measures of Fat Absorption

1. Radioiodine-labeled oleic and trioleic tests have been used to differentiate pancreatic from intestinal fat malabsorption. Triolein must be broken down by pancreatic lipase for absorption and the free oleic acid is absorbed by the small intestine. The blood level of radiolabeled iodine in the normal patient rises within two hours of its ingestion and remains high for five hours. If the etiology of the malabsorption is pancreatic, the ^{131}I blood curves are depressed 50 per cent or more after triolein feeding and are normal after oleic acid feeds. In small bowel disease, both levels are low after ingestion. Commercial preparations have given normal results in some patients with steatorrhea and are no longer generally used. It has been suggested that fecal rather than blood radioactivity measurements may be preferable, for triolein may undergo deiodination within the intestinal wall and thoracic duct.

2. ^{14}C-labeled tripalmitate has been used to indicate pancreatic insufficiency by measuring $^{14}CO_2$ in breath, with patients having lower values than controls. A mixed triglyceride breath test is also effective.[105b]

3. Lipiodol, composed of poppyseed oil with hydriodic acid added to contain a total of 40 per cent iodine, is another indicator of fat absorption. Iodine attached to the unsaturated double bonds of fat is split off during transport and assimilation of the fat. Urinary excretion of the iodine, therefore, reflects the per cent absorption of lipiodol. The lipiodol is given in orange juice one hour after breakfast — 5 ml for a child of 10 kg or less; 0.5 ml per kg for those weighing 10 to 20 kg; and 10 ml to those 20 kg or more. A spot urine sample is tested for iodine 12 to 18 hours after the oral load.

4. A *butter fat absorption test*, which also indicates integrity of lymphatic transport as well as fat absorption, measures serum turbidity after the ingestion of cream. A dose of 0.5 gm of butter fat per kg is given as 15 per cent cream to the fasting patient, and capillary blood specimens are taken at 1, 2, 3, and 4 hours. Optimal density (OD) of the serum is read at 620 μg in a Beckman DU spectrophotometer. Maximal turbidity appears at three hours, with a rise of more than 0.170 OD over fasting.

5. *The vitamin A absorption test* measures the blood level after ingestion of a known quantity of the fat-soluble vitamin. However, it does not always correlate well with the degree of steatorrhea. Results vary with age, for the serum vitamin A level increases with age. For the test, the vitamin is omitted from the diet for 24 hours. Oleum percomorph, 0.2 ml (6000 USP units), is administered orally and blood samples obtained at 3, 5, and 7 hours. Tubes must be covered by foil. Normal increases are 360 μg per dl at 5 and 125 μg per dl at 7 hours. Studies in which vitamin A was expressed as micromoles per liter revealed a rise after ingestion of 75,000 units per kg to be 1.9 μmol per liter to one month of age and 7.3 to 7.5 μmol per liter between one month and three years of age. Mean fasting vitamin A levels in infants under one month of age are 0.5 μmol per liter, and in older children, 1.0 μmol per liter.

6. A *25-hydroxyvitamin D (25-OHD)* oral tolerance test may be used to evaluate vitamin D absorption. The fasting patient is given 10 μg per kg of an oily solution of 25-hydroxycalciferol (25-OHD_3), alone or in capsule form in older patients. Blood sam-

ples for 25-OHD are obtained at 0, 2, 4, 8, and 24 hours. Normally, levels peak after 4 to 8 hours and fall slowly, with the 24-hour levels being 84 per cent of the mean peak level (to 450 ng/ml per liter).

Small Bowel Absorption

Folic acid is absorbed through the jejunal mucosa and, if the dietary folate is adequate, serum and red blood cell folate levels mirror jejunal function. Levels may be low, however, in infants taking goat's milk. RBC folate is more accurate than serum levels, which may fluctuate. In general, a serum level over 7 μg per dl is normal; one less than 5 μg per dl is suggestive and less than 3 μg per dl indicates malabsorption. Normal RBC folate is greater than 250, with levels less than 200 indicating malabsorption.

Although the lactose hydrogen breath test is a sensitive means of indicating mucosal damage, it may at times represent a congenital type of lactose intolerance in which the small intestinal mucosa is normal. Other tests of small intestinal function are merited.

The xylose absorption test has been used with varying techniques over the past 40 years to measure intestinal absorption. Although the question has been raised that it may have an element of active transport, it is generally considered to be absorbed from the duodenum and proximal jejunum without energy-dependent transport mechanisms. Of the ingested sugar, 65 per cent is absorbed and 35 per cent excreted by adults in a five-hour urine collection. The test is affected by delayed gastric emptying, poor hydration, renal disease, thyroid disease,

iron deficiency anemia, and pernicious anemia, as well as by adequacy of urine collection. We have noted abnormal xylose tolerance tests in some patients with pancreatic insufficiency.

The test is administered to the infant who has been fasted for at least four hours. A dose of 0.3 to 0.5 gm per kg (we use 0.5 gm per kg) or 14.5 gm per square meter is administered in water. The test may be performed using blood or urine values. Water is offered freely during the five-hour urine collection period to assure adequate urinary output. Blood values at 15 minutes show a rise of 20 to 30 mg per dl and at 30 and 60 minutes normally show a rise of at least 15 mg per dl. A screening test using one blood level at one hour after ingestion of 5 gm of sugar shows a level of 20 or more mg per dl. In suspected celiac disease, specimens should be extended to 90 or even 120 minutes to compensate for delayed motility.

Urine excretion is low in young infants and children, with normal infants under six months of age excreting 8 to 16 per cent, and those 6 to 12 months old excreting 20 to 25 per cent of the sugar.

The dependability of the test in diagnosing celiac disease has been questioned, with false-negative and -positive results noted (Table 19–19).

Bacterial Overgrowth

As noted in an earlier section of the text, several tests are available for the diagnosis of bacterial overgrowth. Use of urinary indican and the Schilling test before and after antibiotics was discussed.

Breath tests have now been utilized to

Table 19–19   Results of Xylose Tolerance Tests in Celiac Disease

NUMBER OF PATIENTS	DOSE	FALSE-NEGATIVE (%)	FALSE-POSITIVE (%)
254	5 gm	2	0
68	0.4 gm/kg	15 (Gr 3–4 mucosal disease) 61 (Gr 2–4 mucosal disease)	66
148	5 gm	2	12
33	5 gm	25	46
435	14.5 gm/m²	4	0
46	0.5 gm/kg	33	22

evaluate small bowel overgrowth, since bacteria catabolize the sugars. The ^{14}C-d-$xylose$ breath test is administered using 1 or 25 gm of xylose plus 10 μC of ^{14}C-D-xylose. Patients excreted 10.1 ± 0.9 per cent versus 7.0 ± 0.7 per cent by controls in 30 minutes. No false-negative results were reported.

A *bile acid breath test* measures excessive breath [13]- or $^{14}CO_2$ after bacterial deconjugation of orally administered cholyl-[13 or 14]C-glycine, but it has been associated with false-negative results in patients with overgrowth and with false-positive results in those with ileal disease or resection.

Although the radiation hazard from ^{14}C is small, we have been hesitant to use such isotopes in infants.

Lactulose, a sugar not metabolized by the human intestine, now is being studied in conjunction with the hydrogen breath test to measure bacterial overgrowth. Normally, as the sugar is metabolized in the colon there is a rise in breath hydrogen. An earlier peak when the sugar is degraded by bacteria in the small bowel suggests overgrowth.

Small Bowel Biopsy

All biopsies are preceded by coagulation studies. Infants are sedated lightly with Vistaril, 2 mg per kg intramuscularly. Small bowel biopsy is performed using the Pediatric Crosby or a variation. The tubing is threaded through a Levine duodenal tube and passed through the mouth into the stomach. The infant is placed in the right decubitus position and the tube is slowly advanced. The pH is monitored by gentle aspiration through the Levine tube. When the aspirate becomes alkaline, the infant is fluoroscoped to check the position of the tube and capsule. When the capsule lies beyond the ligament of Treitz, rapid suction is applied to the capsule tube, which causes firing of a spring-loaded blade. The capsule is withdrawn and the specimen is gently removed and oriented on filter paper under a dissecting microscope.

If a delay is encountered in passage of the capsule from the stomach, its progress may be enhanced by the intravenous administration of metoclopramide in a dosage of 0.2 mg per kg.

Complications. The perforation rate ranges from 1:100 to 1:500 and seems to be at highest risk in the hypoalbuminemic celiac patient. Bleeding or duodenal hematoma is rarely a problem with normal coagulation studies. Failure of the capsule to completely sever the tissue may result in a need to clip the tubing and allow the tissue to slough and the capsule to pass per rectum.

Intestinal Aspiration

During the procedure and before the biopsy, intestinal fluid may be withdrawn for examination for parasites, bacterial culture, immunoglobulins, bile, and pancreatic secretions. A formal secretin test to evaluate pancreatic function is described in Chapter 15.

REFERENCES

1. Ackerman, N., and Strobel, C.: Polle syndrome: Chronic diarrhea in Munchausen's child. Gastroenterology 81:1140, 1981.
1a. Akesode, F., Lifshitz, F., and Hoffman, K.: Transient monosaccharide intolerance in a newborn infant. Pediatrics 51:8911, 1973.
2. Allen, R. H., Seetharam, B., Podell, E., et al.: Effect of proteolytic enzymes on the binding of cobalamin to R protein and intrinsic factor. J. Clin. Invest 61:47, 1978.
3. Alpers, D. H., Grimme, W., Smith R., and Avioli, A.: Dog intestinal mucosa contains two vitamin D–stimulated calcium-binding proteins. Gastroenterology 79:259, 1980.
4. Alpers, D. H., and Seetharam, B.: Pathophysiology of diseases involving brush border proteins. N. Engl. J. Med. 296:1046, 1977.
5. Ament, M., Perera, D., and Esther, L.: Sucrase-isomaltase deficiency — a frequently misdiagnosed disease. J. Pediatr. 83:721, 1973.
6. Ament, M. E., and Rubin, C. E.: Soy protein: Another cause of the flat intestinal lesion. Gastroenterology 62:227, 1972.
7. American Academy of Pediatrics Committee on Nutrition: The practical significance of lactose intolerance in children. Pediatrics 62:240, 1978.
8. Anderson, C. M., Kerry, K. R., and Townley, R. R. W.: An inborn defect of intestinal absorption of certain monosaccharides. Arch. Dis. Child. 40:1, 1965.
9. Anderson, C. M., Messer, M., Townley, R. R., and Freeman, M.: Intestinal sucrase and isomaltase deficiency in 2 siblings. Pediatrics 31:1003, 1963.

9a. Anderson, G., Trojaborg, W., and Lou, H. C.: A clinical and neurophysiological investigation of a Danish kindred with heterozygous familial hypobetalipoproteinemia. Acta Paediatr. Scand. 68:155, 1979.

10. Antonowicz, I., Lloyd-Still, J. D., Khaw, K. T., and Shwachman, H.: Congenital sucrase-isomaltase deficiency. Pediatrics 49:847, 1972.

11. Arand, B. S., Truelove, S. C., and Offord, R. E.: Skin test for celiac disease using a subfraction of gluten. Lancet 1:118, 1977.

12. Arey, L. B.: Developmental Anatomy. Philadelphia, W. B. Saunders Company, 1974.

12a. Arvanitakis, C., and Cooke, A.: Diagnostic tests of exocrine pancreatic function and disease. Gastroenterology 74:932, 1978.

13. Ashkenazi, A., Handzel, Z. T., Idar, D., Offarim, M., and Levin, S.: An in vitro immunological assay for diagnosis of coeliac disease. Lancet 1:627, 1978.

13a. Ashkenazi, A., Levin, S., Idar, D., Or, A., Rosenberg, I., and Handzel, Z. T.: In vitro cell-mediated immunologic assay for cow's milk allergy. Pediatrics 66:399, 1980.

14. Asp, N. G., and Dahlquist, A.: Human small intestinal β-galactosidases. Specific assay of three different enzymes. Anal. Biochem. 47:527, 1972.

15. Astley, R., and French, J. M.: The small intestine pattern in normal children and in coeliac disease. Its relationship to the nature of opaque medium. Br. J. Radiol. 24:321, 1951.

16. Auricchio, S., Buffolano, W., Campiere, M., Ciccimama, F., Follo, D., Lanfranchi, G., and Labo, G.: Skin tests for coeliac disease. Lancet 1:611, 1979.

17. Auricchio, S., Rubino, A., and Murset, E.: Intestinal glycosidase activities in the human embryo, fetus and newborn. Pediatrics 35:944, 1965.

17a. Avery, G. B., Villiavicencio, O., Lilly, J., and Randolph, J.: Intractable diarrhea in early infancy. Pediatrics 41:712, 1968.

18. Awrich, A. E., Stackhouse, W. J., Centrell, J. E., Patterson, J. H., and Rudman, D.: Hyperdibasicaminoaciduria, hyperammonemia and growth retardation. J. Pediatr. 87:731, 1975.

19. Azizi, E., Zaidman, J., Eschar, J., and Szeinberg, A.: Abetalipoproteinemia treated with parenteral and oral vitamins A and E and with medium-chain triglycerides. Acta Paediatr. Scand. 67:797, 1978.

20. Bachman, K. D., and Dees, S. C.: Milk allergy. II. Observations on incidence and symptoms of allergy to milk in allergic infants. Pediatrics 20:400, 1957.

21. Bachna, S., and Heiner, D. C.: Cow's milk allergy. Adv. Pediatr. 25:1, 1978.

21a. Bakkeren, J., Monnens, L., and Van Os, C.: Defect in bile acid concentrating ability of the gallbladder in congenital chloride diarrhea. Acta Paediatr. Scand. 70:43, 1981.

22. Balsan, S., and Garabedian, M.: 25-Hydroxycholecalciferol: A comparative study in deficiency rickets and different types of resistant rickets. J. Clin. Invest. 51:749, 1972.

23. Barr, R. G., Levine, M., and Watkins, J. B.: Recurrent abdominal pain of childhood due to lactose intolerance. N. Engl. J. Med. 300:1449, 1979.

23a. Barr, R. G., Perman, J., Schoeller, D., and Watkins, J.: Breath tests in pediatric gastrointestinal disorders; New diagnostic opportunities. Pediatrics 62:393, 1978.

24. Barry, R. E., and Read, A. E.: Coeliac disease and malignancy. Q. J. Med. 42:665, 1973.

25. Bayless, T. M., and Huang, S. S.: Recurrent abdominal pain due to milk and lactose intolerance in school-aged children. Pediatrics 40:1029, 1971.

26. Bayless, T. M., and Rosensweig, N. S.: A racial difference in the incidence of lactase deficiency. JAMA 197:968, 1966.

27. Bayless, T. M., Kapelowitz, R. F., Shelley, W. M., et al.: Intestinal ulcerations, a complication of celiac disease. N. Engl. J. Med. 276:996, 1967.

27a. Beach, R. C., Menzies, I. S., Clayden, G. S., and Scopes, J. W.: Gastrointestinal permeability changes in the preterm infant. Arch. Dis. Child. 57:141, 1982.

28. Becroft, D. M. O., Costello, J. M., and Scott, P. J.: A-β-lipoproteinemia. Arch. Dis. Child. 40:40, 1965.

28a. Beckwith, J. B., and Perrin, E. V.: In situ neuroblastoma: A contribution to the natural history of neural crest tumors. Am. J. Pathol. 43:1089. 1963.

29. Beratis, N., Price, P., LaBadie, G., and Hirschhorn, K.: Copper metabolism in Menkes' disease. Pediatr. Res. 13:206, 1979.

30. Beratis, N., Price, P., LaBadie, G., and Hirschhorn, K.: Cu metabolism in Menkes' and normal cultured skin fibroblasts. Pediatr. Res. 12:699, 1978.

30a. Berg, N. O., Borulf, S., Jakobsson, I., and Lindberg, T.: How to approach the child suspected of malabsorption. Acta Paediatr. Scand. 67:403, 1978.

31. Berg, N. O., Dahlqvist, A., Lindberg, T., et al.: Severe familial lactose intolerance — a gastrogen disorder? Acta Paediatr. Scand. 58:525, 1969.

32. Berg, N. O., and Dahlqvist, A.: A boy with severe infantile gastrogen lactose intolerance and acquired lactase deficiency. Acta Paediatr. Scand. 68:751, 1979.

33. Berg, N. O., Jakobsson, I., and Lindberg, T.: Do pre- and post-challenge small intestinal biopsies help to diagnose cow's milk protein intolerance? Acta Paediatr. Scand. 68:657, 1979.

34. Bergoz, R.: Trehalose malabsorption causing intolerance to mushrooms. Gastroenterology 60:909, 1971.

35. Bianchi, A., Chipman, D. W., Dreskin, A., and Rosensweig, N. S.: Nutritional folic acid deficiency with megaloblastic changes in the small bowel epithelium. N. Engl J. Med. 282:859, 1970.

36. Bobo, R. C., Partin, J. C., Schubert, W. K., et al.: Abnormal lipid accumulation within the small intestinal mucosa of children with juvenile-onset diabetes. Am. J. Dis. Child. 131:962, 1977.

37. Bock, S. A., Buckley, J., Holst, A., and May, C. D.:

Proper use of skin tests with food extracts in diagnosis of hypersensitivity to food in children. Clin. Allergy 7:375, 1977.

37a. Bloom, S. R., Polak, J. M., and Pearse, A. G. E.: Vasoactive intestinal peptide and watery diarrhea syndrome. Lancet 2:14, 1973.

38. Bolin, T. E., and Davis, A. E.: Asian lactose intolerance and its relationship to intake of lactose. Nature 222:382, 1969.

39. Borgfars, I. V., and Selander, P.: The incidence of coeliac disease in Sweden. Acta Paediatr. (Stockh.) 57:260, 1968.

39a. Brock, C. E., and Ricketts, R. R.: Hemoperitoneum from spontaneous ruptured neonatal neuroblastoma. Am. J. Dis. Child. 136:370, 1982.

40. Brooks, M. H., Bell, N., Love, L., Stern, P., Orfei, E., Queener, S., Hamstra, A., and de Luca, H.: Vitamin D–dependent rickets type II. N. Engl. J. Med. 298:966, 1978.

41. Brown, J. H., Fabre, L. F., and Farrell, G. L.: Hyperlysinuria with hyperammonemia; A new metabolic disorder. Am. J. Dis. Child 124:127, 1972.

41a. Brown, W., Isobe, K., Nakane, P., and Pacini, B.: Studies on translocation of immunoglobulins across the intestinal epithelium. Gastroenterology 73:1333, 1977.

42. Buchanan, G., and Sheehan, R.: Malabsorption and defective utilization of iron in three siblings. Pediatrics 98:723, 1981.

43. Bucknall, W. E., Halsam, R. H., and Holtzman, N.: Kinky hair syndrome. Response to copper therapy. Pediatrics 52:653, 1973.

44. Burke, V., and Danks, D. M.: Monosaccharide malabsorption in young infants. Lancet 1:1177, 1966.

45. Butler, H. L., Byrne, W. J., Marmer, D. J., Euler, A. R., and Steele, R. W.: Depressed neutrophil chemotaxis in infants with cow's milk and/or soy protein intolerance. Pediatrics 67:264, 1981.

46. Buts, J. P., Morin, C. L., Roy, C. C., Weber, A., and Bonin, A.: One hour blood xylose test: A reliable index of small bowel function. J. Pediatr. 90:729, 1978.

47. Carter, C., Sheldon, W., and Walker, C.: The inheritance of coeliac disease. Ann. Human Genet. 23:266, 1959.

48. Christie, D. L.: Use of the 1-hour blood xylose test as an indicator of small bowel mucosal disease. J. Pediatr. 92:725, 1978.

49. Coello-Ramirez, P., Gutierres-Topete, G., and Lifshitz, F.: Pneumatosis intestinalis. Am. J. Dis. Child. 120:3, 1970.

50. Cohen, M., McNamara, H., Blumfeld, D., and Arias, L.: The relationship between glutamyl transpeptidase and the syndrome of celiac sprue, in Booth, C. (ed.): First International Conference on Celiac Disease. Edinburgh, E. and S. Livingstone, 1971, p. 91.

51. Coicadan, L., Heyman, M., Grasset, E., and Desjeux, J. F.: Cystinuria: Reduced lysine permeability at the brush border of intestinal membrane cells. Pediatr. Res. 14:109, 1980.

52. Colle, E., Greenberg, L., and Krivit, W.: Studies of a patient with selective deficiency in

absorption of vitamin B$_{12}$. Blood 18:48, 1961.

53. Collin, P. P., Schmidt, M., Bernsoussan, A., Blanchard, H., and Desjardins, J. G.: Neurogenic tumors and VIP-induced diarrhea. J. Pediatr. Surg. 14:525, 1979.

54. Committee on Nutrition of American Academy of Pediatrics: The practical significance of lactose intolerance in children. Pediatrics 62:240, 1978.

55. Committee on Nutrition of American Academy of Pediatrics: Zinc. Pediatrics 62:408, 1978.

55a. Congdon, P. J., Fiddler, G. I., Littlewood, J. M., and Scott, O.: Coeliac disease associated with congenital heart disease. Arch. Dis. Child. 57:78, 1982.

56. Congdon, P., Mason, M. K., Smith, S., Crollick, A., Steel, A., and Littlewood, J.: Small bowel mucosa in asymptomatic children with celiac disease. Am. J. Dis. Child. 135:118, 1981.

56a. Conklin, K., Yamashiro, K., and Gray, G.: Human intestinal sucrase-isomaltase: Identification of free sucrase and isomaltase and cleavage of the hybrid into active distinct subunits. J. Biol. Chem. 250:5735, 1975.

57. Cooper, G. A., and Castle, W. B.: Sequential mechanisms in the enhanced absorption of vitamin B$_{12}$ by intrinsic factor in the rat. J. Clin. Invest 39:199, 1960.

58. Corradino, R. A., Fullmer, C. S., and Wasserman, R. H.: Calcium transport and calcium-binding protein. Arch. Biochem. Biophys. 174:738, 1976.

58a. Crane, R. K.: Hypothesis for the mechanism of intestinal active transport of sugars. Fed. Proc. 21:891, 1962.

58b. Crane, R. K.: Na$^+$-dependent transport in the intestine and other anal tissues. Fed. Proc. 24:1000, 1965.

59. Cunningham-Rundles, C., Brandeis, W. E., Good, R. A., and Day, N. K.: Milk precipitins, circulating immune complexes and IgA deficiency. Proc. Natl. Acad. Sci. 75:3387, 1978.

60. Dahlqvist, A.: The basic aspects of the chemical background of lactase deficiency. Postgrad. Med. J. 53(Suppl. 2):57, 1977.

61. Daish, P., Wheeler, E. M., Roberts, P. F., and Jones, R.: Menke's syndrome: Report of a patient treated from 21 days of age with parenteral copper. Arch. Dis. Child. 53:956, 1978.

62. Danbolt, N., and Closs, K.: Acrodermatitis enteropathica. Acta Dermatol. Venereol. 23:127, 1942.

63. Danks, D. M., Campbell, P. E., Stevens, B. J., et al.: Menke's kinky hair syndrome: An inherited defect in copper absorption with widespread effects. Pediatrics 50:188, 1972.

64. Danks, D.: Steely hair, mottled mice and copper metabolism. N. Engl. J. Med. 293:1147, 1975.

65. Dannaeus, A., Johansson, S. G. O., Foucard, T., and Ohman, S.: Clinical and immunological aspects of food allergy in childhood. Acta Paediatr. Scand. 66:31, 1977.

66. Darling, S., Mortensen, O., and Sondergaard, G.:

Lactosuria and amino-aciduria in infancy. A new inborn error of metabolism? Acta Paediatr. 49:281, 1960.

67. Davidson, G. P., and Townley, R. R. W.: Structural and functional abnormalities of the small intestine due to nutritional folic acid deficiency in infancy. J. Pediatr. 90:590, 1977.

68. Davis, A., and Pirola, R.: Absorption of phenoxymethylpenicillin in patients with steatorrhea. Aust. Ann. Med. 17:63, 1968.

69. Davis, A. E., and Bolin, T.: Lactose intolerance in Orientals. Gastroenterology 54:225, 1968.

70. Davis, S. D., Bierman, C. W., Pierson, W. E., et al.: Clinical nonspecificity of milk coproantibodies in diarrheal stools. N. Engl. J. Med. 282:612, 1970.

71. Delire, M., Cambiaso, C. L., and Masson, P. L.: Circulating immune complexes in infants fed on cow's milk. Nature 272:632, 1978.

72. Deren, J. J.: Gastrointestinal development, in Barnes, A. C. (ed.): Intrauterine Development. Philadelphia, Lea & Febiger, 1968, pp. 221–232.

73. Desjeux, J., Rajantie, J., Simell, O., Dumontur, A., and Perleenlupa, J.: Lysine fluxes across jejunal epithelium in lysinuric protein intolerance. J. Clin. Invest. 65:1387, 1980.

74. Dicke, W. K.: Celiac disease. A study of the damaging effects of some cereals, especially wheat, caused by a factor outside of their starch, on the fat absorption of children with celiac disease. Zurich, International Congress of Pediatrics, 1950.

75. Dissanayake, A. S., Offord, R. E., Truelove, S. C., and Whitehead, R.: Nature of toxic component of wheat gluten in celiac disease. Lancet 2:709, 1973.

76. Dobbins, W. O., III: Electron microscope study of the intestinal mucosa in intestinal lymphangiectasis. Gastroenterology 51:1004, 1966.

77. Doe, W. F., Henry, K., and Booth, C. C.: Complement in coeliac disease, in Hekkens, W. T. J. M., and Pena, A. S. (eds.): Coeliac Disease. Leiden, Stenfert-Kroese, 1974, p. 189.

78. Douglas, A. P., and Peters, T. J.: Peptide hydrolase activity of the human intestinal mucosa in adult celiac disease. Gut 11:15, 1970.

78a. Douwes, A. C., Fernandes, J., and Degenhart, H. J.: Improved accuracy of lactose tolerance test in children using expired H$_2$ measurement. Arch. Dis. Child. 53:939, 1979.

79. Drummond, K., Michael, A., Ulstrom, R., and Good, R.: The blue diaper syndrome. Am. J. Med. 37:928, 1964.

80. Durand, P.: Intolerance au lactose. Insuffisante hydrolyse intestinale du lactose. Pediatrie 15:407, 1960.

81. Durand, P., and Lamedica, G. M.: Disaccharide intolerance. Helv. Paediatr. Acta 17:395, 1962.

82. Eagan-Mitchell, B., and McNicholl, B.: Constipation in celiac disease. Arch. Dis. Child. 47:238, 1972.

83. Eastham, E. J., Lichauco, T., Grady, M. I., and Walker, W. A.: Antigenicity of infant formulas: Role of immature intestine on protein permeability. J. Pediatr. 93:561, 1978.

84. Eastham, E. J., and Walker, W. A.: Effect of cow's milk on the gastrointestinal tract: A persistent dilemma for the pediatrician. Pediatrics 60:477, 1977.

84a. Eastham, E., Lichanco, T., Pang, K., and Walker, W. A.: Antigenicity of infant formulas and the induction of systemic tolerance by oral feeding: Cow's milk versus soy milk. J. Pediatr. Gastroenterol. Nutr. 1:23, 1982.

85. Eastwood, G. L.: Gastrointestinal epithelial renewal. Gastroenterology 72:962, 1977.

85a. Eil, C., Liberman, U., Rosen, J., and Marx, S.: A cellular defect in hereditary vitamin D–dependent rickets type II: Defective nuclear uptake of 1,25-dihydroxy vitamin D in cultured skin fibroblasts. N. Engl. J. Med. 304:1558, 1981.

85b. Ellis, D., Fischer, S. E., Smith, W. I., and Jaffe, R.: Familial occurrence of renal and intestinal diseases associated with tissue autoantibodies. Am. J. Dis. Child. 136:323, 1982.

86. Elsas, L. J., Hillman, R. E., Patterson, J. H., et al.: Renal and intestinal hexose transport in familial glucose-galactose malabsorption. J. Clin. Invest. 49:576, 1970.

87. Elsas, L. J., and Lambe, D. W.: Familial glucose-galactose malabsorption. Remission of glucose intolerance. J. Pediatr. 83:226, 1973.

88. Erbe, R. W.: Inborn errors of folate metabolism. N. Engl. J. Med. 293:753, 1975.

89. Evans, A., Chatten, J., D'Angio, R., Gerson, J., Robinson, J., and Schnaufer, L.: Review of 17 IV-S neuroblastoma patients at Children's Hospital of Philadelphia. Cancer 45:833, 1980.

90. Evans, G., and Johnson, P.: Characterization of a zinc-binding liquid in human milk. Pediatr. Res. 14:876, 1980.

91. Evans, G. W., and Johnson, P. E.: Zinc-binding factor in acrodermatitis enteropathica. Lancet 1:52, 1977.

92. Evans, G. W., and Johnson, P. E.: Defective prostaglandin synthesis in acrodermatitis enteropathica. Lancet 1:52, 1977.

93. Fairclough, P. D., Clark, M. L., Dawson, A. M., Silk, D., Milla, P. J., and Harries, J. T.: Absorption of glucose and maltose in congenital glucose-galactose malabsorption. Pediatr. Res. 12:1112, 1978.

94. Falchuk, Z. M., Gebhard, R. L., and Sessoms, C.: An *in vitro* model of gluten-sensitive enteropathy. J. Clin. Invest. 53:487, 1974.

95. Falchuk, Z. M., Nelson, D. L., Katz, A., Bernarden, J., and Kasarda, D.: Gluten-sensitive enteropathy — influence of histocompatibility type on gluten sensitivity. J. Clin. Invest. 66:227, 1980.

96. Ferguson, A., and Canswell, F.: Precipitins to dietary proteins in serum and upper intestinal secretions of coeliac children. Br. Med. J. 1:75, 1972.

96a. Florent, C., Aymes, C., and Rambaud, J. C.: Selection of timing of blood-xylose oral test— Correlation between the 30th min. xylosemia and D-xylose gastric emptying. Gastroenterol. Clin. Biol. 6:252, 1982.

97. Ford, J. D., and Haworth, J. C.: The fecal excretion of sugars in children. J. Pediatr. 63:988, 1963.

98. Fordtran, J. S., Rector, F. C., Locklear, T. W., et al.: Water and solute movement in the small intestine of patients with sprue. J. Clin. Invest. 46:287, 1967.

99. Fox, H. J.: Sucrose absorption in sprue. Am. J. Dig. Dis. 2:663, 1957.

99a. Fraterschroeder, M., Hitzig, W. H., and Sacher, M.: Inheritance of transcobalamin II in 2 families with TCII deficiency and related immunodeficiency. J. Inher. Metab. Dis. 4: 165, 1981.

100. Frazer, A. C., Fletcher, R. F., Ross, C. A. C., Shaw, B., Sammons, H. G., and Schneider, R.: Gluten-induced enteropathy — the effect of partially digested gluten. Lancet 2:252, 1959.

101. Frier, S., and Gerger, H.: Disodium cromoglycate in gastrointestinal protein intolerance. Lancet 1:913, 1973.

101a. Fromm, H., and Hofmann, A.: Breath test for altered bile acid metabolism. Lancet 1:621, 1971.

102. Gamble, J. L., Fahey, K. R., Appleton, J., et al.: Congenital alkalosis with diarrhea. J. Pediatr. 26:509, 1945.

103. Garretts, M., and Molokhia, M.: Acrodermatitis enteropathica without hypozincemia. J. Pediatr. 91:492, 1977.

104. Gee, S. J.: On the coeliac affection. St. Bartholomew's Hospital Reports 24:17, 1888.

105. Gerrard, J. W., Mackenzie, J., Goluboff, N., Garson, J., and Maningas, C. S.: Cow's milk allergy prevalence and manifestations in an unselected series of newborns. Acta Paediatr. Scand. (Suppl.) 234:1, 1973.

105a. Gertner, J. M., Lilburn, M., and Domenech, M.: 25-Hydroxycholecalciferol absorption in steatorrhoea and postgastrectomy osteomalacia. Br. Med. J. 1:1310, 1977.

105b. Ghoos, Y. F., Van Trappen, G. R., Rutgurts, P. J., and Schurmans, P. C.: A mixed triglyceride breath test for intraluminal fat digestive activities. Digestion 22:239, 1981.

106. Gilat, T., Benaroya, Y., Gelman-Malachi, E., and Adam, A.: Genetics of primary lactase deficiency. Gastroenterology 64:562, 1973.

107. Giradin, E. P., DeWolfe, M. S., and Crocker, J. F. S.: Treatment of cystinosis with cysteamine. J. Pediatr. 94:838, 1979.

108. Glorieux, F. H., Holick, M. I., Scriver, C. R., et al.: X-linked hypophosphatemic rickets: Inadequate therapeutic response to 1,25-dihydroxycholecalciferol. Lancet 2:287, 1973.

109. Gluckman, R., Green, P., Lees, R., Lux, S., and Kilgore, A.: Immunofluorescence studies of apolipoprotein B in intestinal mucosa. Gastroenterology 76:288, 1979.

110. Goel, K., Lifshitz, F., Kahn, E., and Teichberg, S.: Monosaccharide intolerance and soy protein hypersensitivity in an infant with diarrhea. J. Pediatr. 93:617, 1978.

111. Goka, T. J., Stevenson, R. E., Hefferan, P. M., and Howell, R. R.: Menke's disease: A biochemical abnormality in human fibroblasts. Proc. Natl. Acad. Sci. 73:604, 1976.

112. Goldberg, L. S., Barnett, E. V., and Desai, R.: Effect of transplacental transfer of antibody to intrinsic factor. Pediatrics 40:851, 1967.

113. Goldman, A., Anderson, D., Sellers, W., et al.: Milk allergy. I. Oral challenge with milk and isolated milk proteins in allergic children. Pediatrics 32:425, 1963.

114. Goodman, S. I., McIntyre, C. A., and O'Brien, D.: Impaired intestinal transport of proline in a patient with familial iminoaciduria. J. Pediatr. 71:246, 1967.

115. Gordon, P., and Levitin, H.: Congenital alkalosis with diarrhea. A sequel to Darrow's original description. Ann. Intern. Med. 78:876, 1973.

116. Gotto, A. M., Levy, R. I., John, K., and Frederickson, D. S.: On the protein defect in abetalipoproteinemia. N. Engl. J. Med. 284:813, 1971.

117. Grand, R., Sutphen, J., and Montgomery, R.: The immature intestine: Implications for nutrition of the neonate, in Development of mammalian Absorptive Processes. Amsterdam, Excerpta Medica, 1979, p. 293.

118. Grasbeck, R., Gordin, R., Kantero, I., et al.: Selective vitamin B_{12} malabsorption and proteinuria in young people. A syndrome. Acta Med. Scand. 167:289, 1960.

119. Gray, G. M.: Assimilation of Dietary Carbohydrate: Viewpoints on Digestive Diseases. Vol. 12, no. 3, 1980.

119a. Groll, A., Candy, D. C., Preece, M. A., Tanner, J. M., and Harries, J. T.: Short stature as the primary manifestation of coeliac disease. Lancet 2:1097, 1980.

120. Grover, W. D., and Scrutton, M. C.: Copper infusion therapy in trichopoliodystrophy. J. Pediatr. 86:216, 1975.

121. Gryboski, J. D.: Diarrhea from dietetic candy. N. Engl. J. Med. 275:818, 1966.

122. Gryboski, J. D., Burkle, F., and Hillman, R.: Milk-induced colitis in an infant. Pediatrics 38:299, 1966.

123. Gryboski, J. D.: False security of a gluten-free diet. Am. J. Dis. Child. 135:110, 1981.

124. Gryboski, J. D.: Gastrointestinal Problems in the Infant. Philadelphia, W. B. Saunders Company, 1975.

125. Gryboski, J. D.: Congenital disorders of absorption, in Lebenthal, E. (ed.): Textbook of Gastroenterology and Nutrition. New York, Raven Press, 1981, p. 931.

126. Gryboski, J. D., Zellis, J., and Ma, O. H.: A study of fecal sugars by high voltage electrophoresis. Gastroenterology 47:26, 1964.

127. Gryboski, J. D., and Boehm, J.: Lactulosuria in the neonate. Pediatrics 35:340, 1965.

128. Gunther, M., Aschaffenburg, R., Matthews, R. H., Parish, W., and Coombs, R. R.: The level of antibodies to the proteins of cow's milk in the serum of normal infants. Immunology 3:296, 1960.

129. Hadorn, B.: Diseases of the pancreas in children. Clin. Gastroenterol. 1:125, 1972.

130. Hadorn, B., Tarlow, M., Lloyd, J., and Wolff, O.: Intestinal enterokinase deficiency. Lancet 1:812, 1969.

130a. Haeney, M. R., Culank, L. S., Montgomery, R. D., and Sammons, H. G.: Evaluation of xylose absorption as measured in blood and urine. Gastroenterology 75:393, 1978.

131. Hakami, N., Newman, P. E., Camelles, G. P., et

al.: Neonatal megaloblastic anemia due to inherited transcobalamin II deficiency in two siblings. N. Engl. J. Med. 285:1163, 1971.

132. Hall, C.: Congenital disorders of vitamin B₁₂ transport and their contribution to concepts. Gastroenterology 65:684, 1973.

132a. Hall, C. A.: Congenital disorders of vitamin B₁₂ transport and their contribution to concepts II. Yale J. Biol. Med. 54:485, 1981.

133. Halpin, T. C., Byrne, W. J., and Ament, M. E.: Colitis, persistent diarrhea and soy protein intolerance. J. Pediatr. 91:404, 1977.

134. Hamilton, J. R., Lynch, M. J., and Reilly, B. J.: Active coeliac disease in childhood. Q. J. Med. 38:135, 1969.

135. Hamilton, J. R., and McNeill, L. K.: Childhood celiac disease: Response of treated patients to a small uniform daily dose of wheat gluten. J. Pediatr. 81:885, 1972.

136. Hann, H. L., Evans, A., Cohen, I., and Leitmeyer, J.: Biologic differences between neuroblastoma stages IV-S and IV. N. Engl. J. Med. 305:425, 1981.

137. Hanson, L. A., and Anderson, R. J.: A comparison of the antigenic relationships of human milk and goat's milk to bovine milk. Acta Paediatr. 51:509, 1962.

138. Hara, K., Oohira, A., Nogami, H., Watanabe, K., and Miyazaki, S.: Kinky hair disease. Biochemical, histochemical and ultrastructural studies. Pediatr. Res. 13:1222, 1979.

139. Harris, O. D., Cooke, W. T., Thompson, H., et al.: Malignancy in adult coeliac disease and idopathic steatorrhea. Am. J. Med. 42:899, 1967.

140. Harrison, H. E., and Harrison, H. C.: Disorders of calcium and phosphate metabolism in childhood and adolescence. Philadelphia, W. B. Saunders Company, 1979, p. 141.

140a. Harrison, M., Kilby, A., Walker-Smith, J. A., et al.: Cow's milk protein intolerance: A possible association with gastroenteritis, lactose intolerance and IgA deficiency. Br. Med. J. 1: 1501, 1976.

141. Haurani, F. I., Hall, C. A., and Rubin, R.: Megaloblastic anemia as a result of an abnormal transcobalamin II. J. Clin. Invest. 64:1250, 1979.

142. Haworth, E. M., Hodson, C., Pringle, E., and Young, W.: The value of radiologic investigations of the alimentary tract in children with the coeliac syndrome. Clin. Radiol. 19:65, 1968.

143. Haworth, J. C., Gourley, B., Hadorn, B., and Sumida, C.: Malabsorption and growth failure due to intestinal enterokinase deficiency. J. Pediatr. 78:481, 1971.

144. Heaney, R. P., and Skillman, T. G.: Secretion and excretion of calcium by the human gastrointestinal tract. J. Lab. Clin. Med. 4:29, 1964.

145. Hecht, F., and Karser-McCaw, B.: Chromosomes in familial neuroblastoma. J. Pediatr. 98:334, 1981.

146. Heiner, D. C., and Sears, J. W.: Chronic respiratory disease associated with multiple circulating precipitins to cow's milk. Am. J. Dis. Child. 100:500, 1960.

147. Heiner, D. C., Wilson, J. F., and Lahey, M. E.: Sensitivity to cow's milk. JAMA 189:561, 1964.

148. Heiner, D. C., and Lahey, M. E.: The celiac syndrome. Pediatr. Clin. North Am. 9:975, 1962.

149. Herbert, P. N., Gotto, A. M., and Frederickson, D. S.: Familial lipoprotein deficiency, in Stanbury, J. B., Wyngaarden, J. B., and Frederickson, D. S., (eds.): The Metabolic Basis of Inherited Disease. New York, McGraw-Hill, 1978, Chart 28.

150. Herbert, U., Colman, N., and Jacob, E.: Folic acid and vitamin B₁₂, in Shilo, M. E. (ed.): Modern Nutrition in Health and Disease. Philadelphia, Lea & Febiger, 1980, p. 229.

151. Higginbottom, M. C., Sweetman, L., and Nyhan, W. L.: A syndrome of methylmalonic aciduria, homocystinuria, megaloblastic anemia, and neurologic abnormalities in a vitamin B₁₂–deficient breast-fed infant of a strict vegetarian. N. Engl. J. Med. 299:317, 1978.

151a. Hildebrand, H., Borgstrom, B., Bekassy, A., Erlasonalbertsson, C., and Helen, F.: Isolated co-lipase deficiency in 2 brothers. Gut 23:243, 1982.

152. Hill, D. J., Davidson, G. P., Cameron, D. J. S., and Barnes, G. L.: The spectrum of cow's milk allergy in childhood. Acta Paediatr. Scand. 68:847, 1979.

153. Hitzig, W., Dohmann, U., and Pluss, H. J.: Hereditary transcobalamin II deficiency; New clinical findings in a family. J. Pediatr. 85:622, 1974.

154. Holmberg, C., Perheentupa, J., and Launiala, K.: Colonic electrolyte transport in health and in congenital chloride diarrhea. J. Clin. Invest. 56:302, 1975.

155. Holmberg, C., Perheentupa, J., and Pasternack, A.: The renal lesion in congenital chloride diarrhea. J. Pediatr. 91:738, 1977.

156. Holmberg, C., Perheentupa, J., Launiala, K., and Hallman, N.: Congenital chloride diarrhea. Clinical analysis of 21 Finnish patients. Arch. Dis. Child. 52:255, 1977.

157. Holzel, A.: Sugar malabsorption and sugar intolerance in childhood. Proc. Roy. Soc. Med. 61:1095, 1968.

158. Holzel, A., Mereu, T., and Thomson, M. L.: Severe lactose intolerance in infancy. Lancet 2:1346, 1962.

159. Holzel, A.: Sugar malabsorption due to deficiency of disaccharidase activities and of monosaccharide transport. Arch. Dis. Child. 42:341, 1967.

160. Hooft, C., and Antener, I.: Methionine malabsorption syndrome. Mod. Prob. Pediatr. 11:127, 1968.

161. Hooft, T. C., Devos, E., and van Damme, J.: Coeliac disease in a diabetic child. Lancet 2:161, 1969.

162. Horn, N.: Copper incorporation studies on cultured cells for prenatal diagnosis of Menkes' disease. Lancet 1:1156, 1976.

163. Howat, J. M., and Aaronson, I.: Sugar intolerance in neonatal surgery. J. Pediatr. Surg. 6:719, 1971.

163a. Howdle, P. D., Corazza, G. R., Bullen, A. W., and Losowsky, M. S.: In vitro diagnosis of coeliac diseases. Gut 22:939, 1981.

164. Hurley, L. S., Duncan, J. R., Sloan, M. V., and Eckhert, C. D.: Development of zinc-binding ligands during the post-natal period. Fed. Proc. 35:1667, 1977.

165. Hyams, J. S., Stafford, R. J., Grand, R. J., and Watkins, J.: Correlation of lactose breath hydrogen test, intestinal morphology and lactose activity in young children. J. Pediatr. 97:609, 1980.

166. Hamed, I. A., Czerwinski, A. W., Coats, B., Kaufman, C., and Altmiller, D. H.: Familial absorptive hypercalciuria and renal tubular acidosis. Am. J. Med. 67:385, 1979.

167. Imerslund, O.: Idiopathic chronic megaloblastic anemia in children. Acta Paediatr. 49:suppl. 119, 1964.

168. Inall, J. A., and Burkinshaw, J. H.: Lactosuria and sucrosuria with failure-to-thrive. Proc. Roy. Soc. Med. 53:318, 1960.

169. Isaacson, P., and Wright, D. H.: Intestinal lymphoma associated with malabsorption. Lancet 1:67, 1978.

170. Isaacson, P.: Malignant histiocytosis of the intestine: The early histological lesion. Gut 21:381, 1980.

170a. Iyngkaran, N., Robinson, M. J., Sumithran, E., Lam, S. K., Puthucheary, S. D., and Yadav, M.: Cow's milk protein–sensitive enteropathy. Arch. Dis. Child. 53:150, 1978.

170b. Iyngkaran, N., Robinson, M. J., Prathap, K., Sumithran, E., and Yadav, M.: Cow's milk protein–sensitive enteropathy; Combined clinical and histologic criteria to diagnosis. Arch. Dis. Child. 53:20, 1978.

170c. Iyngkaran, N., Abidin, Z., Meng, L., and Yadav, M.: Egg protein-induced villous atrophy. J. Pediatr. Gastroenterol. Nutr. 1:29, 1982.

171. Jakobsson, I., and Lindberg, T.: A prospective study of cow's milk protein intolerance in Swedish infants. Acta Paediatr. Scand. 68:853, 1979.

171a. Jakobsson, I., Lindberg, T., and Benediktsson, B.: In vitro digestion of cow's milk proteins by duodenal juice from infants with various gastrointestinal disorders. J. Pediatr. Gastroenterol. Nutr. 1:183, 1982.

171b. Jenkins, W. J., Empson, R., Jewell, D. P., and Taylor, K. B.: Subcellular localization of vitamin B_{12} during absorption in the guinea pig. Gut 22:617, 1981.

172. Jones, D. V., and Latham, M. C.: Lactose intolerance in young children and their parents. Am. J. Clin. Nutr. 27:547, 1974.

172a. Jones, J., Mehta, N., and Hamosh, M.: α-Amylase in preterm human milk. J. Pediatr. Gastroenterol. Nutr. 1:43, 1982.

173. Jos, J., and Charbonnier, L.: In vitro toxicity of wheat gluten fractions and subfractions on coeliac intestinal mucosa. Acta Paediatr. Belg. 29:261, 1976.

173a. Kahan, J.: The vitamin A absorption test. Scand. J. Gastroenterol. 4:313, 1969.

174. Kaijser, K., and Ockerman, P. A.: Diagnostic problems in glucose-galactose malabsorption. Acta Paediatr. Scand. 59:214, 1970.

175. Kapadia, C. R., Schafer, D. E., Donaldson, R. M., Jr., and Ebersole, E. R.: Evidence for involvement of cyclic nucleotides in intrinsic factor secretion by isolated rabbit gastric mucosa. J. Clin. Invest. 64:1044, 1979.

176. Kaplan, B., and Vitullo, B.: Acquired chloride diarrhea. J. Pediatr. 99:211, 1981.

177. Kaplan, S., Holbrook, C. T., McDaniel, H., Buntain, W., and Crist, W.: Vasoactive intestinal peptide secreting tumors of childhood. Am. J. Dis. Child. 134:21, 1980.

178. Kasper, H.: The effect of a gluten-free diet on the absorption of foodstuffs in nontropical sprue. Gastroenterologia 108:239, 1967.

179. Katz, A. J., and Falchuk, Z. M.: Definitive diagnosis of gluten-sensitive enteropathy. Gastroenterology 75:695, 1978.

180. Katz, A. J., and Grand, R. J.: All that flattens is not "sprue." Gastroenterology 76:375, 1979.

181. Katz, M., and O'Brien, R.: Vitamin B_{12} absorption studied by vascular perfusion of rat intestine. J. Lab Clin. Med. 94:817, 1979.

182. Kekomaki, M., Visakorpi, J. K., Perhentupa, J., et al.: Familial protein intolerance with deficient transport of basic amino acids. Acta Paediatr. Scand. 56:617, 1967.

182a. Kerry, K. R., and Anderson, C. M.: A ward test for sugar in feces. Lancet 1:980, 1964.

183. Kerry, K. R., and Townley, R. R.: Genetic aspects of intestinal sucrase-isomaltase deficiency. Aust. Paediatr. J. 1:223, 1965.

184. Keuning, J. J., Peña, A. S., van Leeuwen, A., et al.: HLA-DW3 associated with celiac disease. Lancet 1:506, 1976.

184a. Kilby, A., Burgess, E. A., Wigglesworth, S., and Walker-Smith, J. A.: Sucrase-isomaltase de-deficiency; A follow-up report. Arch. Dis. Child. 53:677, 1978.

184b. King, C. E., Toskes, P., Spivey, J. C., Lorenz, E., and Welkos, S.: Detection of small intestinal bacterial overgrowth by means of a ^{14}C-D-xylose breath test. Gastroenterology 77:75, 1979.

185. Kinney, H., Faix, R., and Brazy, J.: The fetal alcohol syndrome and neuroblastoma. Pediatrics 66:131, 1980.

186. Klipstein, F. A., Lipton, S. D., and Schenk, E. A.: Folate deficiency of the intestinal mucosa. Am. J. Clin. Nutr. 26:728, 1973.

187. Kocoshis, S., and Gryboski, J. D.: Combined G. I. allergy and immunoglobulin deficiency: Role of Cromolyn. Pediatr. Res. 12:438, 1978.

187a. Kokonen, J., Similä, S., and Herva, R.: Impaired gastric function in children with cow's milk intolerance. Eur. J. Pediatr. 132:1, 1979.

188. Koldovsky, O.: Development of the Functions of the Small Intestine in Mammals and Man. Ciba Foundation Symposium 70. New York, Excerpta Medica, 1979, p. 147.

189. Kraft, S., Rothberg, R. M., and Kriebel, G.: Non-immunologic precipitin lines between serum and enteric contents giving false-positive evidence of local antibody production. J. Immunol. 104:528, 1970.

189a. Kreiger, I., Evans, G., and Zelkowitz, P.: Zinc dependency as a cause of chronic diarrhea in variant acrodermatitis enteropathica. Pediatrics 69:773, 1982.

190. Kuitunen, P., Visakorpi, J. K., Savilahti, E., and Pelkonen, P.: Malabsorption syndrome with cow's milk intolerance; Clinical findings and cause in 54 cases. Arch. Dis. Child. 50:351, 1975.

191. Kumento, A.: Studies on the serum binding of

vitamin B$_{12}$ in the newborn infant. Acta Paediatr. Scand. (Suppl.)*194*:1, 1969.

192. Kurome, T., Oguri, M., Matsumara, T., Iwasaki, I., Kanabe, Y., Yamada, T., Kawabe, S., and Negisiki, K.: Milk sensitivity and soy bean sensitivity in production of eczematous manifestations in breast-fed infants. Ann. Allergy 37:41, 1976.

192a. Lamabadusuriya, S. P., Packer, S., and Harries, J. T.: Limitations of xylose tolerance test as a screening procedure in childhood coeliac disease. Arch. Dis. Child. 50:34, 1975.

193. Lampkin, B. C., Shore, N. A., and Chadwick, N. A.: Megaloblastic anemia of infancy secondary to maternal pernicious anemia. N. Engl. J. Med. 274:1168, 1966.

194. Lang, W., Siegel, S., Shaw, K., Landing, B., Baptista, J., and Gutenstein, M.: Initial urinary catecholamine metabolite concentrations and prognosis in neuroblastoma. Pediatrics 62:77, 1978.

195. Lankowsky, P.: Congenital malabsorption of folate. Am. J. Med. 48:580, 1970.

196. Lankowsky, P., Erlandson, M. E., and Bezan, A.: Isolated defect of folic acid absorption associated with mental retardation and cerebral calcification. Blood 34:452, 1969.

196a. Lebenthal, E., Hatch, T., and Lee, P. C.: Carbohydrates in pediatric nutrition — consumption, digestibility, and disease, in Barness, L. A. (eds.): Advances in Pediatrics. Chicago, Year Book Medical Publishers, 1981, p 99.

196b. Lebenthal, E., and Rossi, T.: Lactose malabsorption and intolerance, in Lebenthal, E. (ed.): Textbook of Gastroenterology and Nutrition in Infancy. New York, Raven Press, 1981, p. 673.

197. Lebenthal, E., and Lee, P. C.: Glucoamylase and disaccharidase activities in normal subjects and in patients with mucosal injury of the small intestine. J. Pediatr. 97:389, 1980.

198. Lebenthal, E., Hatch, T., and Lee, P. C.: Development of disaccharidase in premature, small-for-gestational age and full-term infants, in Lebenthal, E. (ed.): Textbook of Gastroenterology and Nutrition in Infancy. New York, Raven Press, 1981, p. 413.

199. Lee, M.: Human serum precipitins to goat's milk proteins and to cow's milk proteins. Pediatrics 35:247, 1965.

200. Leichter, J.: Comparison of whole milk and skim milk with aqueous lactose solution in lactose tolerance testing. Am. J. Clin. Nutr. 26:393, 1973.

200a. Lemoh, J. N., and Watt, J.: Lactobezoar and cow's milk protein intolerance. Arch. Dis. Child. 55:128, 1980.

200b. Liebman, W. M.: Xylose test in malabsorption. J. Pediatr. 94:508, 1979.

201. Lifshitz, F.: Congenital lactase deficiency. J. Pediatr. 69:229, 1966.

202. Lifshitz, F., Coello-Ramirez, P., and Contreas-Gutierrez, M.: The response of infants to carbohydrate oral loads after recovery from diarrhea. J. Pediatr. 79:612, 1971.

203. Lifshitz, F., Coello-Ramirez, P., Guiterrez-Topete, G., and Coronado-Cornet, M.: Carbohydrate intolerance in infants with diarrhea. J. Pediatr. 79:760, 1971.

204. Lindquist, B., and Meeuwisse, G. W.: Chronic diarrhea caused by monosaccharide malabsorption. Acta Paediatr. Scand. 51:674, 1962.

205. Lippard, V. W., Schloss, C. M., and Johnson, P. H.: Immune reactions induced in infants by intestinal absorption of incompletely digested cow's milk. Am. J. Dis. Child. 51:562, 1936.

206. Lloyd-Still, J., Grand, R. J., Khaw, K. T., and Schwachman, H.: The use of corticosteroids in celiac crisis. J. Pediatr. 81:104, 1972.

207. Lombeck, I., von Bessewitz, D. B., Becker, K., et al.: Ultrastructural findings in acrodermatitis enteropathica. Pediatr. Res. 8:82, 1974.

208. Lott, I. T., DiPaolo, R., Raghavan, S., Clopath, P., Milunsky, A., Robertson, W. C., Jr., and Kanfer, J.: Abnormal copper metabolism in Menkes' steely hair syndrome. Pediatr. Res. 13:845, 1979.

209. Low-Bear, T. S., Harvey, R. F., Davies, E. R., et al.: Abnormalities of serum cholecystokinin and gallbladder emptying in celiac disease. N. Engl. J. Med. 292:961, 1975.

210. Lowe, C. U., and May, C. D.: Selective pancreatic deficiency: Absent amylase, diminished trypsin and normal lipase. Am. J. Dis. Child. 8:459, 1951.

210a. Lucaya, J., Perez-Candela, V., Aso, C., and Calvo, J.: Mastocytosis with skeletal and gastrointestinal involvement in infancy. Radiology 131:363, 1979.

211. Lucky, A. W., and Hsia, E.: Distribution of ingested and injected radiocopper in two patients with Menkes' kinky hair disease. Pediatr. Res. 13:1280, 1979.

212. Luhby, A. L., Eagle, F. J., Roth, E., and Cooperman, J. M.: Relapsing megaloblastic anemia in an infant due to a specific defect in gastrointestinal absorption of folic acid. Am. J. Dis. Child. 102:482, 1961.

213. MacDonald, W. C., Dobbins, W. O., III, and Rubin, C. E.: Studies of the familial nature of celiac sprue using biopsy of the small intestine. N. Engl. J. Med. 272:448, 1965.

214. Mackenzie, I. L., Donaldson, R. M., Trier, J. S., and Mathan, U. I.: Ileal mucosa in familial selective vitamin B$_{12}$ malabsorption. N. Engl. J. Med. 286:1021, 1972.

215. MacLean, W., and Fink, B.: Lactose malabsorption by premature infants. J. Pediatr. 97:383, 1980.

216. Madzarovana-Nohejlova, J.: Trehalase deficiency in a family. Gastroenterology 65:130, 1973.

217. Magotra, M., Tandon, B., and Saraya, A.: Small bowel in iron-deficiency anaemia. Indian J. Med. Res. 59:1788, 1971.

218. Malmquist, J., and Hetter, B.: Leukocyte glutaminase in familial protein intolerance. Lancet 2:129, 1970.

219. Mann, D. L., Katz, S. I., Nelson, D. L., Abelson, L. D., and Strober, W.: Specific B cell antigens associated with gluten-sensitive enteropathy and dermatitis herpetiformis. Lancet 1:110, 1976.

220. Matsuda, I., Pearson, T., and Holtzman, N. A.: Determination of apoceruloplasmin by radioimmunoassay in nutritional copper deficiency, Menkes' kinky hair syndrome, Wilson's disease, and umbilical cord blood. Pediatr. Res. 8:821, 1974.

221. Matthews, T. S., and Soothill, J. F.: Complement

activation after milk feeding in children with cow's milk allergy. Lancet 2:893, 1970.

222. Maurer, H. M.: Solid tumors in children. N. Engl. J. Med. 299:1345, 1978.

223. May, C. D.: Food allergy: Material and ethereal. N. Engl. J. Med. 302:1142, 1980.

223a. May, C. D., Fomon, S. J., and Remigio, L.: Immunologic consequences of feeding infants with cow's milk and soy products. Acta Paediatr. Scand. 71:43, 1982.

224. McDermott, M. R., and Bienenstock, J.: Evidence for a common mucosal immunologic system. J. Immunol. 122:1892, 1979.

225. McNeish, A. S.: Coeliac disease: Duration of gluten-free diet. Arch. Dis. Child. 55:110, 1980.

226. McNeish, A. S., Harms, H. K., Rey, J., Shmerling, D. H., Visakorpi, J. K., and Walker, Smith, J. A.: The diagnosis of celiac disease. Arch. Dis. Child. 54:783, 1979.

227. McNeish, A. S., and Nelson, R.: Coeliac disease in one of monozygotic twins. Clin. Gastroenterol. 3:143, 1974.

228. McNeish, A. S., Rolles, C. J., and Arthur, L. J. H.: Criteria for diagnosis of temporary gluten intolerance. Arch. Dis. Child. 51:275, 1976.

229. McNeish, A. S., Rolles, C. J., Nelson, R., Kyaw-Myint, T. O., Mackintosh, P., and Williams, A. F.: Factors affecting the differing racial incidence of coeliac disease, in Hekkens, W. T. J. M., and Pena, A. S. (eds.): Coeliac Disease. Leiden, Stenfert-Kroese, 1974, p. 330.

230. McNeish, A. S., Rolles, C. J., and Thompson, R. A.: Complement and its degradation products after challenge with gluten in children with coeliac disease, in Hekkens, W. T. J. M., and Pena, A. S. (eds.): Coeliac Disease. Leiden, Stenfert-Kroese, 1974, p. 197.

231. McRae, D., and Shaw, A.: Ganglioneuroma heterochromia iridis and Horner's syndrome. J. Pediatr. Surg. 14:612, 1979.

232. Meeuwisse, G. W., and Dahlqvist, A.: Glucose-galactose malabsorption. A study with biopsy of the small intestinal mucosa. Acta Paediatr. Scand. 57:273, 1968.

233. Meeuwisse, G. W., and Lindquist, B.: Glucose-galactose malabsorption. Acta Paediatr. Scand. 59:74, 1970.

234. Meeuwisse, G. W., and Melin, K.: Glucose-galactose malabsorption. A clinical study of 6 cases and a genetic study. Acta Paediatr. Scand. 188:(Suppl.) 3, 1969.

235. Melin, K., and Meeuwisse, G. W.: Glucose-galactose malabsorption: A genetic study. Acta Paediatr. Scand. 188:(Suppl.) 19, 1969.

236. Menkes, J. H., Alter, M., Steigleder, G. K., et al.: A sex-linked recessive disorder with retardation of growth, peculiar hair and focal cerebral and cerebellar degeneration. Pediatrics 29:764, 1962.

237. Milla, P., Aggett, P. J., Wolfe, O. H., and Harries, J. J.: Studies in primary hypomagnesemia; Evidence of a defective carrier-mediated small intestinal transport of magnesium. Gut 20:160, 1979.

238. Miller, D. R., Bloom, G. E., Strieff, R. R., LoBuglio, A. F., and Diamond, L. K.: Juvenile congenital pernicious anemia: Clinical and immunologic studies. N. Engl. J. Med. 275:978, 1966.

239. Mills, C. F., and Davies, N. T.: Perinatal changes in the absorption of trace elements. Development of mammalian absorptive process. New York, Excerpta Medica, 1979.

240. Milne, M. D.: Hartnup disease. Biochem. J. 111:3, 1969.

241. Morin, C. L., Thompson, M. W., Sanford, J. H., and Sasskortsak, A.: Biochemical and genetic studies in cystinuria: Observations on double heterozygotes of genotype I/II. J. Clin. Invest. 50:1961, 1971

242. Morris, M. D., and Fisher, D. A.: Trypsinogen deficiency disease. Am. J. Dis. Child. 114:203, 1967.

243. Moynahan, E. J.: Acrodermatitis enteropathica: A lethal inherited human zinc deficiency disorder. Lancet 2:399, 1974.

244. Muller, D. P. R., and Lloyd, J. K.: The long-term management of abetalipoproteinemia: A possible role for vitamin E. Arch Dis. Child. 52:209, 1977.

245. Myllarniemi, S., and Holmberg, C.: Caries resistance in children with congenital chloride diarrhea. Arch. Oral Biol. 20:239, 1975.

246. Mylotte, M., Egan-Mitchell, B., McCarthy, C. F., and McNicholl, B.: Incidence of coeliac disease in the West of Ireland. Br. Med. J. 1:703, 1973.

247. Naiman, J. L., Oski, F., Diamond, L., et al.: The gastrointestinal effects of iron deficiency anemia. Pediatrics 33:83, 1964.

248. Navab, F., and Asatoor, A. M.: Studies on intestinal absorption of amino acids and a dipeptide in a case of Hartnup disease. Gut 11:373, 1970.

249. Neldner, K. H., and Hambidge, K. M.: Zinc therapy of acrodermatitis enteropathica. N. Engl. J. Med. 292:879, 1975.

250. Nelson, R., McNeish, A. S., and Anderson, C. M.: Celiac disease in children of Asian immigrants. Lancet 1:348, 1973.

250a. Newcomer, A., Hofman, A., DiMagno, E., Thomas, P. J., and Carlson, G.: Triolein breath test. Gastroenterology 76:6, 1979.

251. Nordio, S., Donath, A., Macagno, F., and Gatti, R.: Chronic hypomagnesemia with magnesium-dependent hypocalcemia. Acta Paediatr. Scand. 60:441, 1971.

252. Nordio, R., Perteentupa, J., Launiala, K., et al.: Congenital chloride diarrhea, an autosomal recessive disease. Clin. Genet. 2:182, 1971.

253. Norman, M. E., Hansell, J. R., Holtzapple, P. G., Parks, J. S., and Waldmann, T. A.: Malabsorption and protein-losing enteropathy. Clin. Immunol. Immunopathol. 4:157, 1975.

254. Ochs, H. D., and Ament, M. E.: Gastrointestinal tract and immunodeficiency, in Ferguson, A., and MacSween, R. N. M. (eds.): Immunological Aspects of the Liver and Gastrointestinal Tract. Lancaster, England, MTP Press, 1976, p. 83.

255. Ochs, H. D., Ament, M. E., and Davis, S. D.: Giardiasis with malabsorption in X-linked agammaglobulinemia. N. Engl. J. Med. 287:341, 1972.

256. Oleske, J., Westphal, M., Shore, S., Gorden, D., Bogden, J., and Nehmias, A.: Zinc therapy

of depressed cellular immunity in acrodermatitis enteropathica. Am. J. Dis. Child. 133:915, 1979.

256a. Onstad, G. R., and Zieve, L.: Carotene absorption: A screening test for steatorrhea. JAMA 221:677, 1972.

257. Owen, R. L., and Jones, A. L.: Epithelial specialization within human Peyer's patches: An ultrastructural study of intestinal lymphoid follicles. Gastroenterology 66:189, 1974.

258. Oyanagi, K., Miura, R., and Yamanouchi, T.: Congenital lysinuria: A new inherited transport disorder of dibasicamino acids. J. Pediatr. 77:259, 1970.

259. Oyanagi, K., Sogawa, H., Minami, R., Nakao, T., and Chiba, T.: The mechanism of hyperammonemia in congenital lysinuria. J. Pediatr. 94:255, 1979.

260. Paige, D. M., Bayless, T. M., Mellitis, E. D., and Davis, L.: Lactose malabsorption in preschool Black children. Am. J. Clin. Nutr. 30:1018, 1977.

260a. Partin, J., and Schubert, W.: Small intestinal mucosa in cholesterol ester storage disease. Gastroenterology 57:542, 1969.

261. Partin, J., and Schubert, W.: White villus disease: A form of hypobetalipoproteinemia in infancy. (Abstr.) SPR Program, American Pediatric Society, 1970, p. 11.

262. Pasternack, A., Perheentupa, J., Launiala, K., and Hallman, N.: Kidney biopsy findings in familial chloride diarrhoea. Acta Endocrinol. 55:1, 1967.

263. Paunier, L., Radde, I., Kooh, S., et al.: Primary hypomagnesemia with secondary hypocalcemia in an infant. Pediatrics 41:385, 1968.

264. Pearse, A. G. E., Polak, J., and Bloom, S. R.: The newer gut hormones. Gastroenterology 72:746, 1977.

265. Pearson, A. J. G., Sladen, G. E., Edmonds, C. J., et al.: The pathophysiology of congenital chloridorrhoea. Q. J. Med. 42:453, 1973.

266. Perheentupa, J., and Visakorpi, J. K.: Protein intolerance with deficient transport of basic amino acid, another inborn error of metabolism. Lancet 2:813, 1965.

267. Petith, M. M., Wilson, H. D., and Schedl, H. P.: Vitamin D dependence of in vivo calcium transport and mucosal calcium-binding protein in rat large intestine. Gastroenterology 78:99, 1979.

267a. Pickering, L. K., and Kohl, S.: Munchausen syndrome by proxy. Am. J. Dis. Child. 135:288, 1981.

267b. Phuapradit, P., Narang, A., Mendonca, P., Harris, D., and Baum, J. D.: The steatocrit: A simple method for evaluating stool fat content in newborn infants. Arch. Dis. Child. 56:725, 1981.

268. Poley, J. R., Bhatia, M., and Welsh, J. D.: Disaccharidase deficiency in infants with cow's milk protein intolerance; Response to treatment. Digestion 17:97, 1978.

269. Polmar, S. H., Stearn, R. C., Schwartz, A. L., Wetzler, E. M., Chase, P. A., and Hinschhorn, R.: Enzyme replacement therapy for adenosine deaminase deficiency and severe combined immunodeficiency. N. Engl. J. Med. 295:1337, 1976.

269a. Poncz, M., Colman, N., Herbert, V., Schwartz, E.,

and Cohen, A.: Therapy of congenital folate malabsorption. J. Pediatr. 98:76, 1981.

269b. Powell, B., Buist, N. R., and Stenzel, P.: An x-linked polyendocrinopathy and fatal infection in infancy. J. Pediatr. 100:711, 1982.

270. Powell, G. K.: Milk- and soy-induced enterocolitis of infancy. J. Pediatr. 93:552, 1978.

270a. Procopis, C., Camakaris, J., and Danks, D. A.: Mild form of Menkes' steely hair syndrome. J. Pediatr. 98:97, 1981.

271. Quinn, J., Altman, A., and Frantz, C.: Serum lactic dehydrogenase, an indicator of tumor activity in neuroblastoma. J. Pediatr. 97:89, 1980.

272. Rajantie, J., Simell, O., and Perheentupa, J.: Intestinal absorption in lysinuric protein intolerance. Gut, 21:519, 1980.

272a. Rangecroft, L., Lauder, I., and Wagget, J.: Spontaneous maturation of stage IV-S neuroblastoma. Arch. Dis. Child. 53:815, 1978.

273. Rask-Madsen, J., Kamper, J., Oddsson, E., et al.: Congenital chloride diarrhoea. A question of reversed brush border transport processes and varying junctional tightness. Scand. J. Gastroenterol. 11:377, 1976.

274. Raydanzadeh, S., and Dantzig, P.: Acrodermatitis enteropathica with pathologic findings in jejunum and skin. Pediatrics 54:77, 1974.

274a. Rhodes, J. M., Middleton, P., and Jewell, D. P.: The lactulose hydrogen breath test as a diagnostic test for small bowel bacterial overgrowth. Scand. J. Gastroenterol. 14:333, 1979.

274b. Roberts, S. A., and Soothill, J. F.: Provocation of allergic response by supplementary feeds of cow's milk. Arch. Dis. Child. 57:127, 1982.

274c. Rolles, C. J., Anderson, C. M., and McNeish, A. S.: Confirming persistence of gluten intolerance in children diagnosed as having coeliac disease in infancy. Arch. Dis. Child. 50:259, 1975.

275. Rolles, C. J., Nutter, S., Kendall, M. J., and Anderson, C. M.: One hour blood-xylose screening test for coeliac disease. Lancet 2:1044, 1973.

276. Rosen, J., Fleischman, A., Finberg, L., Haustra, A., and DeLuca, H.: Rickets with alopecia: An inborn error of vitamin D metabolism. J. Pediatr. 94:729, 1979.

277. Rosenberg, I. H.: Folate absorption and malabsorption. N. Engl. J. Med. 293:1303, 1975.

278. Rosenberg, J. J.: D-Xylose absorption. J. Allergy Metab. 62:19, 1978.

279. Rosenberg, J. J.: Hypergastrinemia. J. Allergy Metab. 69:327, 1979.

280. Rosenberg, L., Downing, S., Durant, J., and Segal, S.: Cystinuria. J. Clin. Invest. 45:365, 1966.

281. Rossi, T., Lebenthal, E., Nord, K., and Fazilla, R.: Extent and duration of small intestinal mucosal injury in intractible diarrhea of infancy. Pediatrics 66:730, 1980.

282. Rubin, C. E., Brandborg, L., Flick, A., et al.: Studies of celiac sprue. III. The effect of repeated wheat instillation into the proximal ileum of patients on gluten-free diets. Gastroenterology 43:621, 1962.

283. Rubin, W.: Celiac disease. Am. J. Clin. Nutr. 24:91, 1971.

283a. Rudman, D., Dedonis, J., Fountain, M., Chandler, J., Gerron, G., Fleming, G. A., and Kutner, M.: Hypocitraturia in patients with gastrointestinal malabsorption. N. Engl. J. Med. *303*:657, 1980.

284. Sandberg, D. H., Bernstein, C. W., McIntosh, R. M., et al.: Severe steroid-responsive nephrosis associated with hypersensitivity. Lancet *1*:388, 1977.

285. Santiago-Borrero, P., Santini, J. R. R., Perez-Santiago, E., et al.: Congenital isolated defect of folic acid absorption. J. Pediatr. *82*:450, 1973.

286. Sawada, T., Sugimoto, T., Tozawa, M., Takada, H., and Kusunoki, T.: Serum immunoglobulin levels in patients with neuroblastoma and their prognosis. J. Pediatr. Surg. *14*:405, 1979.

287. Scanu, A. M., Aggerbeck, L. P., Kruski, A. W., et al.: A study of the abnormal lipoproteins in abetalipoproteinemia. J. Clin. Invest. *53*:440, 1974.

287a. Schaad, U., Gaza, H., and Hadorn, B.: Value of 1-hour blood xylose in diagnosis of childhood coeliac disease. Arch. Dis. Child. *53*:420, 1978.

288. Schmid, W. C., Phillips, S. F., and Summenskill, W. H. J.: Jejunal secretion of electrolytes and water in nontropical sprue. J. Lab. Clin. Med. *73*:772, 1969.

289. Schneider, A. J., Kinter, W. B., and Stirling, C. E.: Glucose-galactose malabsorption. Report of a case with autoradiographic studies of a mucosal biopsy. N. Engl. J. Med. *274*:305, 1966.

290. Schwartz, J. F., Rowland, L. P., Eder, H., et al.: Bassen-Kornzweig syndrome: Deficiency of serum beta lipoprotein. Arch. Neurol. *8*:438, 1963.

291. Scriver, C. R., and Rosenberg, L. E.: Amino Acid Metabolism and its Disorders. Philadelphia, W. B. Saunders Company, 1973.

292. Scriver, C. R.: Renal transport of proline, hydroxyproline and glycine. J. Clin. Invest. *47*:823, 1968.

293. Segal, S.: Tissue transport defects of dibasic aminoacids. Mod. Probl. Pediatr. *11*:56, 1968.

294. Shaw, J.: Trace elements in the fetus and young infant. I. Zinc. Am. J. Dis. Child. *133*:1260, 1979.

295. Sheehy, T. W., and Anderson, P. R.: Disaccharidase activity in normal and diseased small bowel. Lancet *2*:1, 1965.

296. Sheldon, W.: Congenital lipase deficiency. Arch. Dis. Child. *39*:268, 1964.

297. Shepherd, R. W., Gall, D. G., Butler, D. G., and Hamilton, J. R.: Determinants of diarrhea in viral enteritis. Gastroenterology *76*:20, 1979.

298. Shiner, M.: Jejunal surface epithelium in idiopathic steatorrhea. Br. Med. Bull. *23*:233, 1967.

298a. Shiner, M.: Ultrastructural features of allergic manifestations in the small intestine of children. Scand. J. Gastroenterol. *16*:49, 1981.

299. Shiner, M., Ballard, J., and Smith, M. E.: The small intestinal mucosa in cow's milk allergy. Lancet *1*:136, 1975.

300. Shiner, M., Brook, C. G. D., Ballard, J., and Herman, S.: Intestinal biopsy in the diagnosis of cow's milk protein intolerance without acute symptoms. Lancet *2*:1060, 1975.

300a. Shmerling, D. H., Forrer, J. C., and Prader, A.: Fecal fat and nitrogen in health, malabsorption or maldigestion. Pediatrics *46*:690, 1970.

301. Shmerling, D. H., Leisinger, P., and Prader, A.: On the familial occurrence of coeliac disease. Acta Paediatr. (Stockh.) *61*:501, 1972.

302. Simell, O., and Perheentupa, J.: Defective metabolic clearance of plasma arginine and ornithine in lysinuric protein intolerance. Metabolism *23*:691, 1974.

303. Simell, O., Perheentupa, J., and Visakorpi, J. K.: Leukocyte and liver glutaminase in lysinuric protein intolerance. Pediatr. Res. *6*:797, 1972.

303a. Sloper, K. S., Brook, C. G. D., Kingston, D., Pearson, J. R., and Shiner, M.: Eczema and atopy in early childhood: Low IgA plasma cell counts in the jejunal mucosa. Arch. Dis. Child. *56*:12, 1981.

304. Sockalosky, J. J., Ulstrom, R. A., DeLuca, H. F., and Brown, D. M.: Vitamin D–resistant rickets: End-organ unresponsiveness to $1,25(OH)2D_3$. J. Pediatr. *96*:701, 1980.

305. Socken, D. J., Jeejeebhoy, K. N., Bazin, H., and Underdown, B. J.: Identification of secretory component as an IgA receptor on rat hepatocytes. J. Exp. Med. *50*:1538, 1979.

306. Soothill, J. F.: Immunoglobulins in first degree relatives of patients with hypogammaglobulinemia. Lancet *1*:1001, 1968.

306a. Soter, N., Austen, F., and Wasserman, S.: Oral sodium cromoglycate in the treatment of systemic mastocytosis. N. Engl. J. Med. *301*:465, 1979.

307. Spruce, W., Blume, K., Ellington, O., Schmidt, G., and Zusman, J.: Synergeneic bone marrow transplantation in a patient with metastatic neuroblastoma refractory to conventional therapy. Pediatrics *65*:573, 1980.

308. Stanfield, J. P., Hult, M. S. R., and Tunnichliffe, R.: Intestinal biopsy in kwashiorkor. Lancet *2*:519, 1965.

308a. Stankler, L., Lloyd, D., Pollitt, R., Gray, E. S., Thom, H., and Russell, G.: Unexplained diarrhoea and failure-to-thrive in 2 siblings with unusual facies and abnormal scalp hair shafts. Arch. Dis. Child. *57*:212, 1982.

308b. Strauss, R. G., Ghishan, F., Mitros, F., et al.: Rectosigmoid colitis in common variable immunodeficiency disease. Dig. Dis. Sci. *25*:789, 1980.

309. Strober, W., Krakauer, R., Klaeveman, H. L., Reynolds, H. Y., and Nelson, D. L.: Secretory component deficiency: A disorder of the IgA immune system. N. Engl. J. Med. *294*:351, 1976.

310. Stromme, J. H., Nesbakken, R., Normann, T., Skjorten, F., Skyberg, D., and Johannessen, B.: Familial hypomagnesemia: Biochemical, histological and hereditary aspects; studies in 2 brothers. Acta Paediatr. Scand. *58*:433, 1969.

311. Suh, S. M., Fraser, D., and Kooh, S. W.: Pseudo-hypoparathyroidism: Responsiveness to parathyroid extract induced by vitamin D therapy. J. Clin. Endocrinol. Metab. *30*:609, 1970.

312. Sumithran, E., and Iyngkaran, N.: Is jejunal biop-

sy really necessary in cow's milk protein intolerance? Lancet 2:1122, 1977.

313. Sunshine, P., and Kretchmer, N.: Studies of small intestine during development. II. Infantile diarrhea associated with intolerance to disaccharides. Pediatrics 34:38, 1964.

314. Suricchio, S., and Ciccumarra, F.: Glucoamylolytic digestion of starch in human intestinal mucosa, in Digestion and Intestinal Absorption; Proceedings. International Congress on Clinical Chemistry (Clinical Chemistry Series, Vol. 4). Baltimore, University Park Press, 1971, p. 45.

314a. Swank, R. L., Fetterman, G. H., Seiber, W., and Kieswetter, W. B.: Prognostic factors in neuroblastoma. Ann. Surg. 174:428, 1971.

315. Swift, P. F. G., Bloom, S. R., and Harris, F.: Watery diarrhea and ganglioneuroma with secretion of vasoactive intestinal peptide. Arch. Dis. Child. 50:896, 1975.

316. Taylor, B., Norman, A. P., Orgel, M. A., Stokes, C. R., Turner, M. W., and Soothill, J. F.: Transient IgA deficiency and pathogenesis of infantile atopy. Lancet 2:111, 1973.

317. Taylor, K. B., Truelove, S. C., and Wright, R.: Serologic reactions to gluten and cow's milk proteins in gastrointestinal disease. Gastroenterology 46:99, 1964.

318. Thain, M. E., Hamilton, J. R., and Ehrlich, R. M.: Coexistence of diabetes mellitus and celiac disease. J. Pediatr. 85:527, 1974.

319. Tiller, T. L., and Buckley, R. H.: Transient hypogammaglobulinemia of infancy: Review of the literature, clinical and immunologic features of 11 new cases and long-term follow up. J. Pediatr. 92:347, 1978.

319a. Toskes, P. P., King, C. E., Spivey, J. C., et al.: Xylose catabolism in experimental rat blind loop syndrome. Gastroenterology 74:691, 1978.

320. Townley, R.: Celiac disease; An inborn error of metabolism. Am. J. Dig. Dis. 18:797, 1973.

321. Trier, J. S.: Celiac sprue disease, in Sleisenger, M. H., and Fordtran, J. S. (eds.): Gastrointestinal Disease. Philadelphia, W. B. Saunders Company, 1973, p. 864.

322. Trier, J. S., Falchuk, Z. M., Carey, M. C., and Schreiber, D. S.: Celiac sprue and refractory sprue. Gastroenterology 75:307, 1978.

323. Tsang, R. C.: Neonatal magnesium disturbances. Am. J. Dis. Child. 124:282, 1972.

324. Tull, A. R., Green, P., Glickman, R., and Riley, J. W.: Metabolic rate of chylomicron phospholipids and apoproteins in the rat. J. Clin. Invest. 64:977, 1979.

325. Turnberg, L. A.: Abnormalities in intestinal electrolyte transport in congenital chloridorrhoea. Gut 12:544, 1971.

325a. Udall, J.: Dietary proteins, serum immunoglobulins and antigens. J. Pediatr. Gastroenterol. Nutr. 1:155, 1982.

326. Udall, J., Pang, K., Scrimshaw, N. S., and Walker, W. A.: The effect of early nutrition on intestinal maturation. Pediatr. Res. 13:409, 1979.

326a. Unsworth, D. J., Manuel, P. D., Walker-Smith, J. A., Campbell, C. A., Johnson, G. D., and Holborow, E. J.: New immunofluorescent blood test for gluten sensitivity. Arch. Dis. Child. 56:864, 1981.

326b. Verkasalo, M., Kuitenen, P., and Savilahti, E.: Changing patterns of cow's milk intolerance. Acta Paediatr. Scand. 70:289, 1981.

327. Visakorpi, J. K.: An international inquiry concerning the diagnostic criteria of celiac disease. Acta Paediatr. Scand. 59:463, 1970.

327a. Vitoria, J. C., Camarero, C., Sojo, A., Ruiz, A., and Rodriguez-Soriano, J.: Enteropathy related to fish, rice and chicken. Arch. Dis. Child. 57:44, 1982.

328. Von Sydow, S.: Some cases of cow's milk idiosyncrasy. Acta Paediatr. Scand. 23:383, 1939.

329. Voorhess, M. L.: Disorders of the adrenal medulla and multiple endocrine adenomatoses. Pediatr. Clin. North Am. 26:209, 1979.

330. Voorhess, M. L.: Functioning tumors. Am. J. Dis. Child. 134:15, 1980.

330a. Voorhess, M. L., and Gardner, L.: Studies of catecholamine excretion by children with neural tumors. J. Clin. Endocrinol. 22:126, 1962.

331. Waldmann, T. A.: Protein-losing enteropathy. Gastroenterology 50:422, 1966.

332. Waldmann, T. A., Wochner, R. D., Laster, L., et al.: Allergic gastroenteropathy. N. Engl. J. Med. 276:761, 1967.

333. Waldmann, T. A., Durm, M., Broder, S., Blackman, M., Blaese, R. M., and Strober, W.: Role of suppressor T cells in pathogenesis of common variable hypogammaglobulinemia. Lancet 2:609, 1974.

334. Walker, W. A., and Isselbacher, K. J.: Intestinal antibodies. N. Engl. J. Med. 297:767, 1977.

335. Walker-Smith, J.: Diseases of the Small Intestine in Childhood. 2nd ed. London, Pitman Medical, 1979, p. 113.

335a. Walker-Smith, J., Harrison, M., Kilby, A., Phillips, A., and France, N.: Cow's milk–sensitive enteropathy. Arch. Dis. Child. 53:375, 1978.

335b. Walker-Smith, J. A.: Cow's milk intolerance as a cause of postenteritis diarrhea. J. Pediatr. Gastroenterol. Nutr. 1:163, 1982.

336. Walravens, P. A., Hambidge, K. M., Neldner, K. H., et al.: Zinc metabolism in acrodermatitis enteropathica. J. Pediatr. 93:71, 1978.

337. Wara, D., Brunner, W., and Ammann, A.: Graft versus host disease: Pathogenesis, recognition, prevention, and treatment. Curr. Prob. Pediatr. 8:7, 1978.

338. Wardrop, C. A. J., Lee, F. D., Dyet, J. F., et al.: Immunologic abnormalities in splenic atrophy. Lancet 2:4, 1975.

338a. Watson, J. B. G.: Food allergy: Response to treatment with sodium cromoglycate. Arch. Dis. Child. 54:77, 1979.

339. Watson, W. C., Small, J. A., and Luke, R. G.: Beeturia: its incidence and a clue to its mechanism. Br. Med. J. 5:971, 1963.

340. Weber, F. L., and Fresard, K. M.: Comparative effects of lactulose and magnesium sulfate on urea metabolism and nitrogen excretion in cirrhotic subjects. Gastroenterology 80:994, 1981.

341. Wedgwood, R. J.: X-linked agammaglobulinemia, in Seligson, D. (ed.): CRC Handbook Series in Clinical Laboratory Science. West Palm Beach, Fla., CRC Press, 1978, p. 41.

342. Weiser, M. M., and Douglas, A. P.: An alternative mechanism for gluten toxicity in coeliac disease. Lancet 1:561, 1976.

343. Weston, W. L., Huff, J. C., Humbert, J. R., et al.: Zinc correction of defective chemotaxis in acrodermatitis enteropathica. Arch. Dermatol. *113*:422, 1977.

344. Wheller; E. M., and Roberts, P. F.: Menke's steely hair syndrome. Arch. Dis. Child. *51*:269, 1976.

345. Whitington, P. F., and Gibson, R.: Soy protein intolerance: Four patients with concomitant cow's milk intolerance. Pediatrics *59*:730, 1977.

345a. Whyte, R. K., Homer, R., and Pennock, C. A.: Fecal excretion of oligosaccharides and other carbohydrates in neonates. Arch. Dis. Child. *53*:913, 1978.

346. Wilfert, C. M., Buckley, R. H., Mohanakumar, T., et al.: Persistent and fatal central nervous system ECHO virus infections in patients with agammaglobulinemia. N. Engl. J. Med. *296*:1485, 1977.

347. Williams, D. M., Atkin, C. L., Frens, D. B., and Bray, P. F.: Menke's kinky hair syndrome: Studies of copper metabolism and long-term copper therapy. Pediatr. Res. *11*:823, 1977.

348. Williamson, R. C. N.: Intestinal adaptation. N. Engl. J. Med. *298*:1393, 1978.

348a. Wilson, M. C., Fischer, J. J., and Riordan, M. M.: Isolated IgG hypogammaglobulinemia in acrodermatitis enteropathica–correction with zinc therapy. Ann. Allergy *48*:288, 1982.

349. Wilson, J., Heiner, D., and Lahey, M. E.: Milk-induced gastrointestinal bleeding in infants with hypochromic microcytic anemia. JAMA *189*:122, 1964.

350. Wohlman, M., Sterk, V., Gatt, S., and Frenkel, M.: Primary familial xanthomatosis with involvement of the adrenals. Pediatrics *28*:742, 1961.

351. Woodard, J. C., Webster, P. D., and Carr, A. A.: Primary hypomagnesemia with secondary hypocalcemia, diarrhea and insensitivity to parathyroid hormone. Am. J. Dig. Dis. *17*:612, 1972.

352. Zerwekh, J. E., Glass, K., Jowsey, J., and Pak, C.: A unique form of osteomalacia associated with end-organ refractoriness to 1,25-dihydroxy vitamin D and apparent defective synthesis of 25-hydroxy vitamin D. J. Clin. Endocrinol. Metab. *49*:171, 1979.

353. Zimmerman, A., Hambidge, M., Leporo, M., Greenberg, R., Stover, M., and Casey, C.: Acrodermatitis in breast-fed premature infants: Evidence for a defect of mammary zinc secretion. Pediatrics *69*:176, 1982.

354. Zoppi, G., Gerosa, F., Pezzini, A., Bassani, N., et al.: Immunocompetence and dietary protein intake in early infancy. J. Pediatr. Gastroenterol. Nutr. *1*:175, 1982.

Appendix

Section 3   Formula Composition Tables and Guidelines

Feeding Recommendations for Premature Infants
Quality of Growth: Guidelines for Nutrition and Growth for Premature Infants with
    Appropriate Weight for Gestational Age
Selection of Infant Formulas
Delivery of Infant Formulas
Recommended Feeding Schedule at 0–12 Months
Oral Feeding Alternatives to Breast Feeding in Infancy
Suggested Feedings for Gastrointestinal Problems

Section 4   Human Milk Banking Program

Human Milk Banking
Human Milk Banking Procedures of Massachusetts General Hospital
Nutritional Composition of Milk from Mothers Delivering Preterm (PT) and at Term (T)

Section 5   Special Diets and Carbohydrate Content of Foods

Gluten-Free Diet
Soy-Free Diet
Lactose-Free Diet
Low Sucrose Diet
Adequate Fat Diet
Low Long-Chain Triglyceride, High Medium-Chain Triglyceride Diet
Carbohydrate Content of Common Foods
Less Common Carbohydrates in Foods

SECTION 1
PEDIATRIC PARENTERAL NUTRITION MANUAL

This section on parenteral nutrition discusses specific indications for the use and potential complications of parenteral nutrition in pediatric patients. Suggested protein, glucose, vitamin, mineral, and trace element content of solution is included, as well as allowable electrolyte additives. Laboratory and other indices for monitoring patients on parenteral nutrition are recommended. A suggested protocol for initiating parenteral nutrition in a neonate and advancement of the solution is included. Procedures for line insertion, administration of solutions, dressing changes, and administration of Intralipid are outlined.

675

Indications for Use of Pediatric Parenteral Nutrition Solutions

The following booklet is a result of the combined efforts of members of the Pharmacy Department, Children's Service, Pediatric Nursing Service, Pediatric Surgical Service, Hyperalimentation Unit, Dietary Service and Pediatric Gastrointestinal and Nutrition Unit. It is meant to be a guide to the use of parenteral nutrition in pediatric patients at the Massachusetts General Hospital and to stimulate further reading in more complete textbooks of pediatric parenteral nutrition.

Pediatric parenteral nutrition solutions can be used to provide infants and children all of their nutritional requirements by central or peripheral vein in situations where the enteral route cannot be utilized or is inadequate to perform its normal functions. Examples of such situations include providing nutrition to premature or small for gestational age infants, intractable diarrhea, short-gut syndrome, pre and post gastrointestinal surgery to correct congenital malformations such as esophageal or small bowel atresia, extensive burns, inflammatory bowel disease and the complications of inflammatory bowel disease such as obstruction or fistula, and pancreatitis. Where water tolerance is significantly reduced as in cardiac or renal failure, the provision of adequate calories can be accomplished through the use of the more highly concentrated parenteral nutrition solutions.

The pediatric formulations differ from the standard adult formulations significantly in amino acid, electrolyte, mineral, trace element and vitamin content. An adult parenteral nutrition order sheet is included in this manual so that comparisons can be made and because older children and adolescents may utilize the adult solutions, depending on their needs. All patients on total parenteral nutrition should have a consult from the Pediatric Gastrointestinal and Nutrition Unit to insure that nutrient requirements are met through the proper use of either pediatric or adult formulations.

Because these solutions are formulated to provide complete nutritional support they can be used for short as well as extended periods of time. Amino acid, glucose, electrolyte, mineral, trace element, vitamin, lipid, and fluid requirements can be met parenterally.

Ordering Solutions

The Standard solutions which are listed elsewhere in this booklet may be ordered by the House Officer caring for the patient, before consulting the Pediatric Gastrointestinal Unit Fellow. All other formulations require a consultation before ordering the solution. The pharmacy will make all changes in solutions; **no changes are to be made on the floor.** The pharmacy will also refer any questions concerning the use or formulation of a particular solution to the G.I. Service.

New orders or changes in existing orders are to be phoned into the pharmacy once daily: by 10 a.m. to begin at 12:00 p.m. After 12 p.m. solutions of Dextrose 10% in Water (D10W) with electrolytes will be made available by the pharmacy and should be used to correct acute glucose, fluid or electrolyte imbalances. No medication or blood products, such as albumin, may be added to parenteral nutrition solutions or injected through a parenteral nutrition catheter.

The initial solution for central nutrition, following X-ray confirmation that the line has been correctly placed should be Pediatric 10% Solution containing 10% dextrose and providing 42.5 calories per 100 ml. A volume of 100-150 ml/kg/day should be used for infants and children to start, which will initially provide them with 40-63.5 cals/kg/day. In the presence of renal or cardiac failure smaller volumes and more concentrated solutions should be utilized after consulation with the cardiac or renal service. Adolescents will usually tolerate between 75 and 100 ml/kg to begin and can be advanced to higher volumes as tolerated. In order to achieve higher caloric intakes, the formulations containing higher amounts of dextrose must be used. The dextrose concentration should be increased as tolerated over several days to meet caloric requirements. Premature infants are quite variable in their response to a dextrose load but in general will not tolerate more than 14 g/kg/d.

Ten percent intravenous fat emulsion which provides 1.1 cals/ml can be used to provide essential fatty acids as well as a caloric source. The lipid may be delivered together with the glucose/amino acid solution into both central and peripheral veins. The initial recommended amount is 1 g/kg/d advancing to 4 g/kg/d over several days. It should be utilized and delivered continuously over 16-20 hours. Lipid should not comprise more than 45-55% of total daily calories and should be used cautiously in neonates with hyperbilirubinemia, marked pulmonary compromise or platelet disorders. In the absence of these situations, however, lipid should be used to insure that a proper distribution of calories (15% protein, 50% carbohydrate and 35% fat) is delivered.

Parenteral nutrition solutions cannot be stopped abruptly. If this occurs a D10W solution should be started to avoid hypoglycemia and the volume tapered gradually over 4-12 hours. Under normal circumstances the volume of the parenteral nutrition solution itself should be tapered over 24 hours.

PARENTERAL NUTRITION ORDER SHEET PEDIATRIC FORMULATIONS AND PROTOCOL FOR MONITORING PATIENTS

Keep in D.O.B. for duration of Parenteral Nutrition.

1) Infuse "Central" parenteral nutrition via new, sterile catheter terminating in a central vein. X-ray confirmation mandatory and should be documented in chart. Infuse D5W at a keep-open rate until X-ray confirmation.

2) Written orders are telephoned to the Inpatient Pharmacy once daily: By 10:00 a.m. to begin at noon. Changes in electrolytes in solutions at other times may be made by ordering a dextrose/electrolyte solution in place of the parenteral nutrition solution.

3) No additions may be made to any parenteral nutrition solution except by the pharmacy staff.

4) Any change from the standard parenteral solutions listed below requires a Pediatric G.I. service consult and needs to be arranged with the inpatient pharmacy. (May require a 24 hour interval.)

5) Notify Surgical H.O. in event of clotted line, or leakage from catheter or insertion site and record it in the patient's chart.

6) Test urinary sugar and acetone twice a day for 7 days. For 3+ glycosuria or greater obtain serum glucose and notify MD.

7) Accurate I & O. Daily calorie count and weight. Length and head circumference of child on day 1 and then q 7 days.

8) Care of central line dressing (change q 48h or M,W,F, where indicated) and I.V. administration sets and filters (change q 24h at 10 a.m.)

9) Infusion rate should be constant. Check q 30 min. on neonates and q 60 mins. in older infants and children and reset to rate ordered. DO NOT CATCH UP.

PROTOCOL FOR MONITORING PATIENTS

Name									
Unit –									
Dr/Team									
M/F									
Birthdate									
Gestational Age									
Diagnosis									
Date									
Wt kg/									
Ht cm/									
Hc cm/									
Skin Fold Thickness mm									
Parenteral intake									
Enteral intake									
Total calories									
Cal/kg	/	/	/	/	/	/	/	/	/
Gms protein									
Gms fat									
Gm CHO									
Na/K	/	/	/	/	/	/	/	/	/
C1/HCO3-	/	/	/	/	/	/	/	/	/
Bun/Creat	/	/	/	/	/	/	/	/	/
Ca/Phos	/	/	/	/	/	/	/	/	/
Mg									
Glucose									
SGOT									
5' Nucleotidase									
Bili									
T Protein/Albumin	/	/	/	/	/	/	/	/	/
Protime									
HCT/Platelet Ct.	/	/	/	/	/	/	/	/	/
Arterial NH3									
Vit D/Vit A	/	/	/	/	/	/	/	/	/
Copper									
Folate/B12	/	/	/	/	/	/	/	/	/
Triglycerides									

PARENTERAL NUTRITION SOLUTION
STANDARD PEDIATRIC FORMULAE
CONTENTS PER 100 ml

	Pediatric 5%	Pediatric 10%	Pediatric Central 15%	Pediatric Central 20%	Pediatric Central 25%
Amino Acids	2 g	2 g	2 g	2 g	2 g
Dextrose	5 g	10 g	15 g	20 g	25 g
Sodium	0.25mEq	0.25mEq	0.25 mEq	0.25 mEq	0.25mEq
Potassium	0.5mEq	0.5mEq	1.1-5 mEq	1.8-5mEq	1.8-5mEq
Calcium	2 mEq	2 mEq	0.5 mEq	0.5 mEq	0.5 mEq
Magnesium	2 mEq	1 mEq	0.5 mEq	0.5 mEq	0.5 mEq
Chloride	0.4.8mEq	0.4.8mEq	0.4.8mEq	0.4.8mEq	0.4.8mEq
Acetate	1.6 mEq	1.6 mEq	1.4.9mEq	1.4.2mEq	1.4.2mEq
Phosphorus	0.2 mmoles	0.2 mmoles	1 mmole	1.5 mmoles	1.5 mmoles
Trace Elements**	1 ml	1 ml	1 ml	1 ml	1 ml
Multiple Vitamins***	2 ml	2 ml	2 ml	2 ml	2 ml
Osmolarity	700	825	980	1230	1485
Calories Protein	8.5	8.5	8.5	8.5	8.5
Calories Carbohydrate	17	34	51	68	85

Added in sufficient quantites by Pharmacy in 1 mEq increments as whole integers up to 5 mEq.
Sodium added as Sodium Chloride and Potassium added as Potassium Acetate.

**
TRACE ELEMENTS -- 1 ml/100 ml contains:
Zinc 40 mcg, Copper 20 mcg, Fluoride 1 mcg, Iodide 6 mcg, Manganese 20 mcg.

***

MULTIPLE VITAMINS -- 2 ml added to the first bottle daily contains: Vitamin A 4000 I.U., Vitamin D 400 I.U., Vitamin E 2 I.U., Ascorbic Acid 200 mg, Thiamine (B_1) 20 mg, Riboflavin (B_2) 4 mg, Pyridoxine (B_6) 6 mg, Niacinamide 40 mg, Dexpanthenol 10 mg, Folic Acid 200 mcg. Subsequent bottles do not contain vitamins.

10) If parenteral nutrition solution is not available notify MD for appropriate replacement.

11) Lab Work
   A. For infants under 1 year of age
   1. Obtain before initiating TPN: Na, K, Cl, HCO_3-, BUN, Creat., Ca, Phos., Mg, Glucose, SGOT, 5' Nuc., Bili., T. Protein, Albumin, Protime, CBC and Platelet count, Arterial NH_3.
   2. Obtain during TPN on Mondays: SGOT, T.P., 5' Nuc., Protime, Mg, Triglycerides, CBC with diff., Platelet count, Na, K, Cl, Glucose, HCO_2-, Ca, Phos., and arterial NH_3 (NH_3 should be drawn only for first 2 weeks if value remains normal).
   3. Obtain during TPN on Wed. and Fri: Na, K, Cl, HCO_2-, Glucose, Ca, Phos.
   B. For infants and children over 1 year of age the same lab work is indicated but lab tests under 11 (A.3.) only need to be done Mon. and Thurs. Vit. A, Vit. D, copper/folate and B_{12} levels should be obtained prior to TPN and thereafter once a month in all infants and children.
   C. Daily Lipemia checks should be done 2 hrs. after administration of Intralipid. Withhold administration of Intralipid if serum is lipemic.
   D. Weekly urine analysis.

12) Vit. B_{12} should be given IM 100 mcg q month. Vit. K 5 mg q. 2 wks IM.

ADULT FORMULATIONS

PARENTERAL NUTRITION ORDER SHEET
Amino Acids **CENTRAL** Formulation

Initial Order Sheet: Keep in D.O.B. for duration of Parenteral Nutrition.

Date: _____

1) Infuse via new, sterile subclavian or internal jugular catheter terminating in superior vena cava, innominate, or intrathoracic subclavian vein. X-ray confirmation is mandatory. Infuse D_5W at a keep - open rate until X-ray Confirmation.

2) Notify Hyperalimentation Unit or M.D. in event of clotted line, or leakage from catheter or insertion site.

3) Test urinary sugar and acetone q 6h. For 4 + glycousuria obtain serum glucose and notify M.D.

4) Daily I&O, calorie count, and weight before 8 a.m. (Save all I&O sheets).

5) Care of dressing (change q 48h) and IV tubing and filter (change q 24h at 6 p.m.) via Nursing Procedure and Policy Manual.

6) Infusion rate should be constant. check q 30 min. and reset to rate ordered. DO NOT CATCH UP.

7) If CENTRAL solution is not available, infuse $D_{20}W$ at same rate. N.B.: add same amount of C.Z.I. insulin/liter bottle if patient is receiving insulin in T.P.N. solution.

8) Blood Work: Obtain before initiating T.P.N. and bi-weekly on Monday and Thursday. These are fasting bloods if the patient is not n.p.o. - Na, K, Cl, Co_2, Ca, Mg, PO_4, TP, Alb/glob, osm, BUN/creat, glucose, bili D/T, NH_3, PT, platelets, Hct, Wbc, and diff.

9) Catheter cannot be used for other IV's, medications, blood sampling, or CVP readings.

10) Culture catheter tip when removed. Send in culture tube **stat.** Request smear on plate immediately. Request C&S and "hold for fungal testing".

SIGNATURE _____

MAXIMUM ALLOWABLE ELECTROLYTE ADDITIVES

Electrolyte	Total per 100 ml of Parenteral Solution	Additive	Explanation
Magnesium	1 mEq	Magnesium Sulfate Injection 4 mEq/1 ml	Standard quantities may be omitted or additional quantities may be added up to maximum to the 15, 20 and 25% solution after consultation with Pediatric GI Service and Inpatient Pharmacy
Sodium* Chloride	Patient tolerance and/or need	Sodium Chloride Injection 2.5 mEq/1 ml	0 - 5 mEq may be added without consult. Additional quantities may be ordered after consultation with Pediatric GI Service and Inpatient Pharmacy
Potassium Acetate	Patient tolerance and/or need	Potassium Acetate Injection 2 mEg/ml	0 - 5 mEq may be added without consult. Additional quantities may be ordered after consultation with Pediatric GI Service and Inpatient Pharmacy
Calcium Phosphorus	2 mEq 2 mmoles	Calcium Gluconate Injection 0.4 mEq/q ml Potassium Phosphate 4.4 mEq K+ & 3 mM P/.1 ml	Standard quantities may be omitted from all formulas or additional quantities may be added to maximum to the 15, 20 and 25% solution after consultation with pediatric GI Service and Inpatient Pharmacy. Insoluble calcium phosphate will form if the ratio to these two ions is incorrect. Known soluble ratios per 100 ml:

$$\frac{Ca + + \quad P}{}$$

2.0 mEq 0.5 mmole
1.0 mEq 1.0 mmole
0.5 mEq 2.0 mmole

*Sodium Acetate may be ordered in chloride restricted patients

ALLOWABLE ADDITIVE SUPPLEMENTATION

ADDITIVE	PRODUCT	MAXIMUM ALLOWABLE TOTAL PER LITER BOTTLE
† Calcium	*Calcium Gluceptate Inj. / Calcium Chloride	9 mEq
Magnesium	Magnesium Sulfate Inj.	12 mEq
† Phosphate	*Sodium Phosphate Inj. / Potassium Phosphate Inj.	21 mM
† Potassium	Potassium Acetate Inj. / *Potassium Chloride Inj.	80 mEq
† Sodium	Sodium Acetate / *Sodium Chloride	Patient Tolerance and/or need
Chloride	As calcium, Potassium or Sodium	Limited by amount of cation
	As HCl Inj.	100 mEq
Acetate	As Potassium or Sodium	Limited by amount of cation
Insulin	C.Z.I. (regular insulin)	50 units

****

- Calcium + phosphorus salts cannot be mixed in same bottle of renal, cardiac or peripheral formulation.
- Bicarbonate salts should be avoided since they create a number of incompatibilities in parenteral nutrition solutions.
- Medicinal agents not mentioned (such as all antibiotics, cardioactive agents, colloids and electrolytes not specified as compatible) should not be admixed with these formulations due to resultant incompatibilities.

† With these ions, unless specified, the additive will be the noted (*) salt.

PARENTERAL NUTRITION SOLUTION
AMINO ACIDS CENTRAL FORMULATION

Each 1000 ml contains:

Amino Acids (4.25%)	42.5g
Dextrose (25%)	250 g
Total Calories	1000
Nitrogen	6.25g
Vitamins	B Complex (1 ml) and ascorbic acid equiv. (550 mg) every day (white label); multivitamins (B group, A, D, E) (3.5 ml) and ascorbic acid equiv. (800 mg) every Monday (yellow label).
Osmolarity	1900 mOsm.

	*Na	K	Mg	Ca	P(mM)	Cl	Acetae	Insulin (units)
Standard	12	21	8	4.5	13.4 mM	8	29	0
With Added Sodium	12	51	8	4.5	13.4 mM	24	43	0
With Added Insulin	12	21	8	4.5	13.4 mM	8	29	15
With Added Sodium & Insulin	12	51	8	4.5	13.4 mM	24	43	15
With Added Potassium	40	21	8	4.5	17.3 mM	16	43	0
With Added Potassium & Sodium	40	51	8	4.5	17.3 mM	32	57	0
With Added Potassium & Insulin	40	21	8	4.5	17.3 mM	16	43	15
With Added Potassium, Sodium and Insulin	40	51	8	4.5	17.3 mM	32	57	15

*Values expressed in mEq unless otherwise noted.

N.B. For maximum allowable concentrations of electrolytes please consult allowable additive supplementation sheet.

Suggested Protocol for 3 kg Infant On Central parenteral Nutrition

1. Central catheter is placed in central vein and Dextrose 5% in water is infused pending X-ray confirmation that the catheter is in proper position.

Formulation	Volume	Cals/ 24h.	Cals/ k g / d .
2. Pediatric 10% Solution	100 ml/kg/d	127.5	42.5
3. Pediatric 10% Solution	150 ml/kg/d	191	61
4. Pediatric Solution 15% (Central)	150/ml/kg/d	267	89
5. Pediatric Solution 20% (Central)	150/ml/kg/d	344	114.6
6. Pediatric Solution 25% (Central)	150/ml/kg/d	420	140

If glucose intolerance develops during 1-5:

a. rate of infusion can be lowered and then increased slowly over several hours.

b. Intravenous fat emulsion can be started. This will supply 1.1 cals/ml and will allow the use of lower glucose loads while maintaining adequate fluid volumes. The fat emulsion contains 87% w/v water and this should be counted in the total daily fluid intake.

note: Begin intravenous fat emulsion at 10 ml/kg/d given over 20 hrs. and increase the volume over 96 hours to maximum of 40 ml/kg/d or 45% of total calories, whichever is reached first. Essential fatty acid requirements can be met by 5 ml/kg/d once to twice a week.

c. insulin can be administered either as bolus subcutaneous injections or, after consultation with the gastrointestinal service, as a continuous infusion in the parenteral nutrition solution.

A rapid weight gain of greater than 50 grams per day is more likely edema than cell growth and suggests that a more concentrated solution is required to provide adequate calories while limiting fluid.

COMPLICATIONS OF CENTRAL HYPERALIMENTATION IN INFANTS AND CHILDREN

METABOLIC COMPLICATIONS

1. Glucose Metabolism

A. Hyperglycemia is a particularly common problem in the low birth weight infant but is seen in both infants and children receiving high concentrations of glucose through a central venous catheter. It can cause osmotic diuresis, hyperosmolar dehydration, intracranial hemorrhage, coma and ketoacidosis. These problems can be treated by slowing the rate of administration of the solution, repairing the fluid and electrolyte deficit by peripheral vein and keeping the amount of glucose at 7-10 g/kg/d per day. An alternative is to add insulin to the parenteral nutrition solution as a continuous infusion or to give it on a sliding scale as subcutaneous bolus injections.

B. Hypoglycemia may occur with the inadvertent sudden cessation of the intravenous glucose solution because of infiltration at the intravenous site or malfunction of the pump.

C. Hypokalemia and hypophosphatemia may occur with high glucose infusion rates.

2. Amino Acid Metabloism

A. Abnormal serum amino acid profiles have been reported in association with parenteral nutrition. The consequences of these imbalances are unknown, but the elevations of some amino acids such as glutamine may be harmful to the developing central nervous system. In addition, lethargy and altered central nervous system function is seen in some infants who have marked elevations of serum amino acids due to excessive (greater than 5 gm/kg/d) protein intake.

B. Hyperammonemia has been reported in infants receiving protein hydrolysate and crystalline amino acid solutions by several investigators. This is thought to be due to the high loads of preformed ammonia and low levels of arginine found in the original amino acid solutions. These problems have partially been corrected in the newer solutions by lowering the amount of preformed ammonia and by raising the amount of arginine.

C. Prerenal azotemia may occur, particularly in low birth weight infants when protein intakes in excess of 5 g/kg/d are given.

3. Lipid Metabolism

A. Hypertriglyceridemia and high free fatty acid levels have been reported in association with rapid fat emulsion infusion.

B. Displacement of bilirubin from albumin by free fatty acids has been demonstrated in vitro and, therefore, infants at risk for kernicterus with hyperbilirubinemia should not receive intravenous fat emulsions. It should be noted, however, that animal studies and tissue culture experiments have not substantiated any increased risk of kernicterus with the use of Intralipid. Lipemic serum falsely elevates the spectrophotometric determination of bilirubin.

C. Fat overload syndrome is characterized by hyperlipemia, fever, lethargy, liver damage and coagulation defects. This has only rarely been described in infants and children. All children have had grossly lipemic sera, therefore, lipemia levels should be monitored daily while the patient is receiving intravenous fat emulsion. The Lipemia check is done by centrifuging blood in a hematocrit tube 2 hrs. after stopping intralipid, and checking the serum for opalescence.

D. Platelet dysfunction and thrombocytopenia have been associated with the use of cotton seed oil emulsions. Essential fatty acid deficiency as well as many of the underlying conditions of patients receiving parenteral nutrition are associated with thrombocytopenia. In a large series of patients who had thrombocytopenia prior to beginning Intralipid, platelet counts were not affected by the use of the fat emulsion. In several of the infants in this same series with malignancy and thrombocytopenia, platelet counts **rose** concommitent with recovery from sepsis or the recovery of the bone marrow **while the patient was on Intralipid.**

E. Deposition of fat pigment in reticuloendothelial cells in the liver, lungs, and spleen occurs in patients receiving intravenous fat emulsions. At the present time there does not appear to be any adverse clinical effect associated with this histological finding.

F. Essential fatty acid deficiency occurs commonly in patients on long term parenteral nutrition without lipid supplementation. Requirements can be met by administering 5 ml/kg twice a week. While the cutaneous administration of safflower oil may reverse essential fatty acid deficiency, one should not rely on this method unless serum essential fatty acid levels can be monitored.

4. Fluid, acid base, electrolyte, calcium, phosphorous, trace element and vitamin imbalance have all been seen with parenteral nutrition and close monitoring of these nutrients is important. For a complete review see references at the end of this manual.

5. Hepatic Dysfunction and Hepatic Failure

Elevation of alkaline phosphatase, bilirubin and hepatic transaminases occur in approximately 30% of infants and children on prolonged parenteral nutrition. Hepatomegaly with accumulation of bilirubin in bile ductules as well as in hepatocytes occurs. Though generally a reversible process even with continuation of parenteral nutrition, it may progress to hepatic fibrosis and cirrhosis with concommitant hepatic failure. There is no way to predict which patients will develop these changes or which patients will progress to hepatic failure.

COMPLICATIONS OF CENTRAL VENOUS CATHETERS

1. Malposition of the central venous cateter

Extravasation of the catheter with infusion of hypertonic solutions into the pleural or pericardial space may be life threatening. A rapid fall in serum glucose or the acute onset of circulatory compromise should alert one to this complication. Hemorrhage associated with erosion of central veins or the right atrium has also been reported.

2. Pneumothorax, hemorrhage and brachial plexus injuries are relatively common complications of percutaneous subclavian line insertion, a relatively difficult technique to undertake in the pediatric age group.

3. Placement of central venous catheters in the neonate and small infant is particularly difficult and most commonly is performed by cutdown under general anesthesia. Included in the risks of central line placement in this age group are those associated with transport of a critically ill patient as well as the risks of general endotracheal anesthesia.

4. Air embolus may occur if the proper filters are not in place.

5. Catheter embolus may occur if the tip of the catheter breaks off the main body of the catheter. Very high pressures may rupture silastic catheters or the tip may be sheared off by pulling the catheter back through the hub of the needle used to insert it.

6. Thrombophlebitis of peripheral and central veins and catheter sepsis:

A. Thrombophlebitis is recognized by swelling and erythema of the neck or extremity distal to the cannulated vein as well as reduced flow under gravity of the parenteral nutrition solution.

B. Catheter sepsis is a life threatening complication of parenteral nutrition and must be treated aggressively by discontinuation of the line as well as considering antibiotic theorapy. Signs of sepsis in the neonate include lethargy, hyperbilirubinemia, temperature instability, poor feeding, vomiting and diarrhea, and intolerance to previously tolerated glucose and lipid loads. Whenever a high index of suspicion of catheter sepsis exists, the catheter must be removed immediately. A substitute $D_{10}W$ solution must be started in a different site, and patient, catheter and solutions cultured appropriately. **Central parenteral nutrition catheters are to be considered inviolate.** They should not be used for serum sampling, blood or medication administration, or CVP monitoring.

In small infants and children the risk of complications associated with central parenteral nutrition must be weighed carefully against the risk of replacement of that central catheter. That is to say, before discontinuation of a central line for a break in technique or other minor complications one must consider the risk of transporting the infant back to the operating room and subjecting the patient to general anesthesia for replacement of that central catheter.

If the parenteral nutrition catheter is used to administer lifesaving medication or fluids during an emergency situation, as in the case of circulatory failure without other sites of rapid access, the decision to resume therapy via the same catheter must be made only by the **primary physician and noted in the chart.**

In extraordinary circumstances, the patient's condition may necsssiate the intermittent administration of medication via the parenteral nutrition catheter. This should be done in a manner consistent with the accepted nursing procedures. This decision must be made only by the primary physician and noted in the patient's record. Solution and drug compatibility must be approved by the Pharmacy to prevent chemical complications.

In the event that the external catheter is damaged, the catheter should immediately be clamped at a point between the patient and the damaged catheter area, and the IV infusion apparatus should be turned off. The house officer is to be notified immediately. Repair of the catheter is done as soon as possible by a member of the parenteral nutrition team in an aseptic manner. (See Procedure for Catheter Repair) A damaged or leaking catheter is a disruption of the closed system and makes the catheter highly suspect as a source of sepsis if a future febrile incident occurs. **A clotted catheter must be removed, and not flushed.**

ASSISTING THE PHYSICIAN WITH INSERTION OF CENTRAL INTRAVENOUS LINES FOR HYPERALIMENTATION

Objective: To provide aseptic insertion of a central Hyperalimentation catheter if performed on the patient care unit.

Policy: The physician must order the Hyperalimentation solution from Pharmacy before 10 a.m. on the day of the procedure. Dextrose 5%/Water (D5W) will be infused until X-ray confirmation of catheter tip obtained and if solution is unavailable.

Equipment:

Masks
Gown
Sterile gloves
Sterile drapes
Sterile 4 x 4 gauze sponges
3 cc Syringe
25 g. needle
Xylocaine 1% s epinephrine
Sterile suture material
Sterile scissors
   or Subclavian Replacement Set

Other Equipment

70% Isopropyl Alcohol
1% Iodine tincture or povidone-iodine solution
Intravenous catheter (radiopaque with wire stylet)
Alcohol Swabs
D10W with administration set and filter
Subclavian dressing set
Benzoin

Procedure	Points of Emphasis
1. Obtain equipment. Explain procedure to patient and/or parents.	A complete explanation will alleviate some fears.
2. Prime intravenous tubing with D5W immediately prior to beginning procedure. (see page 248).	See procedure for Administration of Pediatric Central Hyperalimentation Solution and Care of Central Venous Catheter and Line for Hyperalimentation.
3. Physician and assistant must wear mask, gown and gloves. patient must wear a mask.	It is essential for aseptic technique to be maintained.
4. Assist physician as needed.	
5. Position patient on back in Trendelenberg position with arm extended. If neck vein used, turn patient's face away from site.	Alters the negative pressure in the superior vena cava which decreases the chance of air embolus.
6. Have patient perform Valsalva maneuver when catheter is threaded through the needle and when IV tubing is connected to catheter hub.	If child is cooperative have him or her bear down or breathe out forcibly after they have exhaled normally. This is called the Valsalva maneuver. If child is unable to cooperate, perform maneuvers during exhalation. The intubated patient should be ambues and maintained in prolonged inspiration.
7. Apply dressing per Procedure Manual.	
8. Call for X-ray for confirmation of appropriate placement of line.	Central Hyperalimentation solution may only be infused via catheter terminating in a central venous position. Note X-ray report in patient's record.

PROCEDURE FOR CHANGING CENTRAL VENOUS CATHETER DRESSINGS FOR INTRAVENOUS HYPERALIMENTATION IN THE PEDIATRIC PATIENT

Objective: To provide an occlusive and water proof dressing for central venous catheter site to help prevent infection and displacement of the catheter.

Policy:

A. Sterility is essential as intravenous hyperalimentation solution is an excellent culture medium for bacteria and yeast.

B. Procedure is to be done Monday, Wednesday and Friday unless dressing becomes unocclusive. Unocclusive central venous catheter dressing must be changed immediately.

C. Procedure is to be done by a nurse who has been qualified to do the procedure.

Equipment:

"Subclavian Dressing Change Kit" from Central Supply containing:

Sterile Items

1 pair scissors
10 gauze sponges
2 clamps
2 pair gloves
3 cups
1 tray

Unsterile Items (packed in outer plastic bag)

1 roll elastoplast
1 roll 1" adhesive tape
1 package povidone-iodine ointment
2 face masks

Other:

Surgical scrub solution
1 bottle 70% Isoprophyl alcohol
1 bottle acetone (if child older than 1 year of age)
1 bottle 1% tincture of iodine
Sterile Q-tips (for benzoin application)
1 bottle of tincture of benzoin
Steridrape (size 1035)
Blenderm Tape

Procedure	Points of Emphasis
1. Explain procedure to patient and/or parents.	
2. Wash hands.	
3. Close curtain around bed.	This will provide privacy as well as cut down on air turbulence.
4. Position and restrain patient as necessary in bed with the help of a second nurse for positioning and patient reassurance.	Use nursing judgment. Consider the safety and comfort of the patient. Use second nurse to help restrain when necessary.
5. Wash the table to be used with alcohol, then surgical scrub solution and let dry.	This solution is bacteriostatic. Do not wipe or fan dry the table.
6. Wash your hands, apply the surgical scrub solution to hands, and allow hands to air dry. Then open the dressing change kit.	Use the plastic bag for the discarded solutions, sponges and old dressing as well as other discarded items.

Procedure	Points of Emphasis
7. Everyone behind curtain must wear face mask.	This will aid in preventing organisms of the mouth and nose from contaminating the catheter site.
8. Have the patient put on face mask or lay a gauze over nose and mouth area and turn patient's to the side away from the dressing if possible.	This protects the insertion site from the patient's organisms and also protects the patient from unpleasant ordors from the prep solutions. If the patient's breathing is compromised or if he is receiving O₂ therapy, omit mask.
9. Pour off a small amount of each solution into the waterproof plastic bag. Fill the cups in the kit with acetone (if child older than 1 year), iodine and alcohol. **N.B.** Alcohol should be used as a substitute for acetone if the child is 1 year of age or younger or in the event that catheter is silastic.	**ALWAYS** use a new, unopened bottle of each solution to insure sterility of each solution.
10. Squeeze the entire amount of povidone-iodine ointment onto a gauze spong in the tray.	Check the old dressing when you remove it for traces of povidone-iodine ointment. If there are no traces of the ointment present on the old dressing then double the amount of povidone-iodine ointment and note this in the Nursing care plan. Continue to make consistent observations to determine the correct amount of povidone-iodine ointment to be used.
11. Do not cut Steridrape or tape ahead of time.	The tape and Steridrape will become contaminated.
12. Remove old dressing and examine catheter site.	Remove dressing slowly to prevent catheter displacement. It is only necessary to glove for dressing removal if you must touch the area **underneath** the dressing. Notify MD immediately if sutures are not intact, or if you have any questions about catheter sit condition. Culture any drainage from catheter site.
13. Put on sterile gloves. Wash catheter with iodine, hold above skin, then:	
14. Holding sponge with clamp, clean area with acetone beginning at insertion site and moving out to the periphery in a circular motion. Prep out to tape or dressing border and do not return to the center with the same sponge. Repeat until sponge comes off skin area unstained. N.B. For children under 1 year of age for all silastic catheters, omit acetone and use alcohol in the same manner.	Acetone defats the skin, destroys the integrity of the bacterial cell wall and will remove old adhesive tape which could ulcerate the skin if left on. Do not justle catheter in and out during the prep because this could introduce bacteria internally and/or dislodge the catheter. Gentle friction should be used to clean area. Acetone may destroy the integrity of the silastic catheter.

Procedure	Points of Emphasis
15. In the same manner clean the area with iodine solution. Repeat this step with additional sponges for **two minutes** spending most of the time directly on the insertion site.	Use at least two sponges. Let the iodine air dry before you remove it. This will increase the effectiveness. This takes about 30 seconds. Do not jostle the catheter. If patient demonstrates sensitivity or allergic reaction to iodine, povidone-iodine solution may be used. Scrub in similar fashion for two minutes, and allow to air-dry and remain on the skin. Do not remove with alcohol. Note in patient's record.
16. In the same manner clean the area with alcohol until all of the dried iodine tincture is removed from the skin. Allow the alcohol to air dry.	Use at least two sponges. This completes the defatting process and removes iodine. Any remaining iodine tincture under the occlusive seal could cause burning. Alcohol is also an antiseptic. Do not jostle the catheter.
17. With your gloves still on, pick up gauze sponge containing the povidone-iodine ointment. Apply a generous amount of ointment to the insertion site.	If patient has shown sensitivity or allergic reaction to povidone-iodine ointment, use a combination of equal amounts of Neosporin and Nystatin ointments until site is again clear. Requires physician's order. Note in patient's record.
18. Gently curve prepped catheter within area to be covered by gauze sponges.	This reduces tension on light-weight scalp sutures.

Procedure	Points of Emphasis
19. Cover the insertion site with 1 or 2 gauze sponges.	Trim the sponges to the appropriate size for the patient.
20. Remove your gloves	
21. Using sterile Q-tips, apply Benzoin tincture (or use Benzoin aerosol) to skin area around gauze and allow it to air dry.	This will provide a protective coating on the skin as well as increase effectiveness of tape adherence. Benzoin aerosol may cause respiratory distress in neonates.
22. Open and cut Steridrape to size.	Keep it as clean as possible. Do not touch adhesive area.
23. Sterilely peel away part of the paper backing from Steridrape. Beginning 1/2" above sponges, place drape on skin. Slowly pull backing away from adhesive as you lay down the drape.	Do not remove all of paper backing at once as the Steridrape then becomes difficult to handle and could contaminate the dressing cover. This provides an occlusive, waterproof dressing that also provides increased visualization of area.
24. Seal all the edges with Blenderm tape. Place a piece of slit tape under the catheter and over the lower edge of the Steridrape.	This insures a seal around the edges of the Steridrape and around the catheter.
25. Place a strip of Blenderm tape on Steridrape and lengthwise over the catheter to secure catheter to skin. Loop remaining external portion of catheter and secure it to Steridrape with tape.	This will prevent tension on the catheter site.

ADMINISTRATION OF PEDIATRIC CENTRAL HYPERALIMENTATION SOLUTION VIA CENTRAL VENOUS CATHETER (CHANGING TUBING AND SOLUTION)

Objective: To provide aseptic central intravenous administration of supplemental nutrients to children whose caloric intake is not sufficient through intragastric feeding or pediatric peripheral supplemental caloric solutions.

Policy:
1. Hyperalimentation solution to be ordered by physician.

2. Hyperalimentation solution, prepared by Pharmacy is stable for 24 hours. It does not require refrigeration.

3. Bottle, tubing and filter should be changed at 10 a.m.

Equipment
1. Bottle of Hyperalimentation solution
2. Graduated burette
3. Sterile disposable intravenous administration set
4. Intravenous air elimination filter
5. Holter pump and appropriate pump tubing, if applicable or
   I-Med with cassette
6. Tape

Procedure	Points of Emphasis
1. Check solution label with Physician's order.	
2. Check solution expiration date.	
3. Check solution clarity and bottle integrity.	

Procedure	Points of Emphasis
26. Secure catheter-filter junction with tape. Catheter and filter should not interfere with movement of extremity.	This will prevent separation of the filter tubing from the catheter hub which could result in accidental air embolus.
27. Secure filter-IV tubing junction with 1"tape.	Be careful not to occlude air-eliminating vents of filter. This will prevent accidental separation.
28. Date, initial and time dressing.	Label it on a part of the dressing that will remain until the next dressing change. Do not write on a piece of tape that will be removed during intravenous tubing and filter.
29. Write a Progress note when the procedure is completed.	

Procedure	Points of Emphasis
4. Assemble equipment as follows: hyperalimentation fluid to graduated burette, intravenous tubing, pump tubing if applicable and final filter. Sterile gloves should be worn while assembling equipment.	
5. Prime new intravenous tubing with fresh solution from pharmacy making sure all air bubbles are removed.	Refer to package insert for filter priming instructions.
6. Indentify patient and explain procedure to him.	
7. Place patient flat in bed.	Alters the negative pressure in the superior vena cava which decreases the chance of air embolus.
8. Remove tape securing catheter hub to tubing.	
9. Using a clean Kelly clamp for leverage gently grasp catheter hub, rotate old tubing out of hub, quickly attaching new intravenous tubing.	If child is cooperative have him or her bear down or breathe out forcibly after they have exhaled normally. (Valsalva maneuver). If child is unable to cooperate (i.e. neonate) perform tubing change during exhalation. External portion of soft silastic catheter should be pinched off (scalp exit catheter). The intubated patient should be ambued and maintained in prolonged inspiration.
10. Adjust clamps or infusion apparatus to achieve prescribed flow rate	
11. Secure all tubing junctions with tape.	Prevents accidental separation. Be careful not to occlude air-eliminating vents of filter.
12. Do not add any extra connectors unless planning to administer Intralipid.	Decreases possibility of line violation and contamination.

CENTRAL HYPERALIMENTATION WITH SIMULTANEOUS INTRAVENOUS FAT EMULSION INFUSION

Objective: To run Central Venous Hyperalimentation and intravenous fat emulsion through the same line with minimal mixing of solutions where there are no alternative peripheral vein infusion sites for intravenous fat emulsion.

Policy:

1. Intravenous fat emulsion must be ordered by the doctor.

2. Intravenous fat emulsion must be refrigerated until used.

3. tubing should be changed every morning at 10 a.m. with central hyperalimentation tubing.

4. Between daily tubing changes, the only break in the system must be when changing intravenous fat emulsion syringes.

Equipment:

1. Bottle of prescribed sterile intravenous fat emulsion and Hyperalimentation Solution.

3. Harvard pump, Holter pump, or IMED with appropriate tubing

3. Sterile 35cc or 50cc (luer-lock) syringe

4. Sterile T-connector

5. Sterile extension tubing

Procedure

1. FOLLOW procedure for administration of Pediatric Central Hyperalimentation Solution via central venous catheter (changing tubing and solution).

2. Intravenous fat emulsion tubing and T-connector must be changed when changing hyperalimentation tubing and bottle.

3. Connect extension tubing or pump tubing and sterile T-connector.

4. From an unopened bottle of intravenous fat emulsion, draw into 35cc or 50cc (luer-lock) syringe the desired amount of intravenous fat emulsion and connect to tubing. Discard any remaining solution.

5. Prime the tubing with the intravenous fat emulsion.

Points of Emphasis

This minimizes the number of times the system is broken and prevents contamination of Central Venous Line.

Sterile technique is required when removing rubber stopper from T-connector. Extension tubing is used with Harvard pump and appropriate size pump tubing with the Holter pump. Use syringes for smaller volume infusion with the Harvard and Holter pumps.

Inject the intravenous fat emulsion into a burette to use a drip method for larger volumes. If the drip method is used, a macro drip administration set is needed.

Intravenous fat emulsion vials may only be entered once, because of chance of introducing bacteria.

PEDIATRIC PERIPHERAL PARENTERAL NUTRITION SOLUTIONS

Objective:

To provide aseptic peripheral intravenous administration of supplemental nutrients to children whose caloric intake is not sufficient through intragastric feeding.

Equipment:

1. Bottle of sterile prescribed pediatric peripheral caloric solution.
2. Graduated burette
3. Sterile disposable intravenous administration set
4. Intravenous air elimination filter
5. Holter pump or Imed and appropriate pump tubing, if applicable.

Procedure	Points of Emphasis
1. Refer to doctor's order for prescribed solution and infusion rate, and order solution from pharmacy.	Orders must be written by physician on prescribed form (Total Parenteral Nutrition Sheet).
2. Neither physicians nor nurses may add any intravenous additives to prescribed solution received from the pharmacy.	If the electrolyte contents must be altered according to the needs of the child, the solution should be disconnected and $D_{10}W$ plus desired additive should be hung until the new solution can be prepared by the pharmacy.
3. Check the label of the bottle of solution against the physician's order prior to administration of the solution.	

Procedure	Points of Emphasis
6. Connect tubing to desired pump.	
7. Connect female end of filter of the T-connector to the male end of filter and connect male end to central venous catheter so that the intravenous fat emulsion is between the filter and the patient.	See Diagram Page 41
8. Check that intravenous fat emulsion is running through the part closest to the central venous catheter site.	Because of the viscosity of intravenous fat emulsion, it must have the shortest distance to travel.
9. Central venous hyperalimentation may run simultaneously.	Intravenous fat emulsion is the only product that may run simultaneously with central venous hyperalimentation.

PERIPHERAL SOLUTION WITH ANTIBIOTICS OR OTHER ADDITIVES: IN INFANTS AND CHILDREN TO THE AGE OF 5.

Equipment:

1. Bottle of perscribed sterile antibiotic solution
2. Graduated burette
3. Sterile disposable intravenous administration set
4. T-connector (number of T-connectors will vary according to number of antibiotics ordered. One T-connector will be for flushing.)
5. Butterfly clamp
6. Sterile normal saline for injection
7. 2-6cc syringes

Procedure	Points of Emphasis
4. Identify the patient.	
5. Check the site of infusion for proper placement of needle or catheter and check for signs of infiltration.	Watch closely for infiltrates. Increased concentration of dextrose can cause sloughing and necrosis of tissue.
6. Connect bottle of solution to burette, intravenous tubing and final filter.	
7. If pump is necessary for accuracy of infusion, add either Holter pump or Imed cassette, tubing and filter.	
8. Prime solution through tubing and attach to intravenous site.	
9. Solution is good for 24 hours.	
10. Change administration set-up every 24 hours.	Eliminate all air bubbles.

Procedure	Points of Emphasis
1. Connect bottle of antibiotics to intravenous administration set, graduated burette and T-connector.	Use sterile technique. Sterile technique also required when removing rubber stopper from T-connector.
2. Prime solution through tubing.	
3. Connect antibiotic tubing to solution tubing by placing male end of T-connector in female end filter and reconnection with solution tubing.	See Diagram Page 41

PERIPHERAL SOLUTIONS WITH INTRALIPIDS

Equipment:

1. Bottle of prescribed sterile intralipid solution (fat Emulsion)
2. Holter pump, Imed, Harvard pump and appropriate tubing if applicable.
3. Sterile 50 ml syringe (luer lock)
4. Sterile extension tubing
5. Steile T-connector

Procedure	Points of Emphasis
1. Connect extension tubing/pump tubing and sterile T-connector.	Sterile technique required when removing rubber stopper from T-Connector. Extension tubing is used with the Harvard pump and pump tubing with the Holter pump. Use syringe method for smaller volume infusions with the Harvard pump and Holter pump. Inject the intralipids into a burette to use a drip method for larger volumes. If the drip method is used, a macro drip administration set is needed.
2. If less than a whole bottle of Intralipid is to be used: from an unopened bottle, draw into 50 ml luer lock syringe the desired amount of intralipids and connect to tubing. Discard any remaining intralipid solution.	
3. Prime intralipid through tubing.	
4. Connect tubing to Holter pump, Harvard pump or new IMED pump.	

Procedure	Points of Emphasis
4. To administer antibiotics: A. Clamp off solution B. Remove intravenous plug and flush line with 6cc sterile normal saline for injection before antibiotic. Then replace plub. C. Unclamp antibiotic solution tubing and regulate drip as in B.	Parenteral nutrition solution is not administered simultaneously with antibiotics. Normal saline flush will decrease mixing.
5. Keep antibiotics clamped at T-connector when not in use.	Prevents inadvertent administration of intravenous antibiotics.

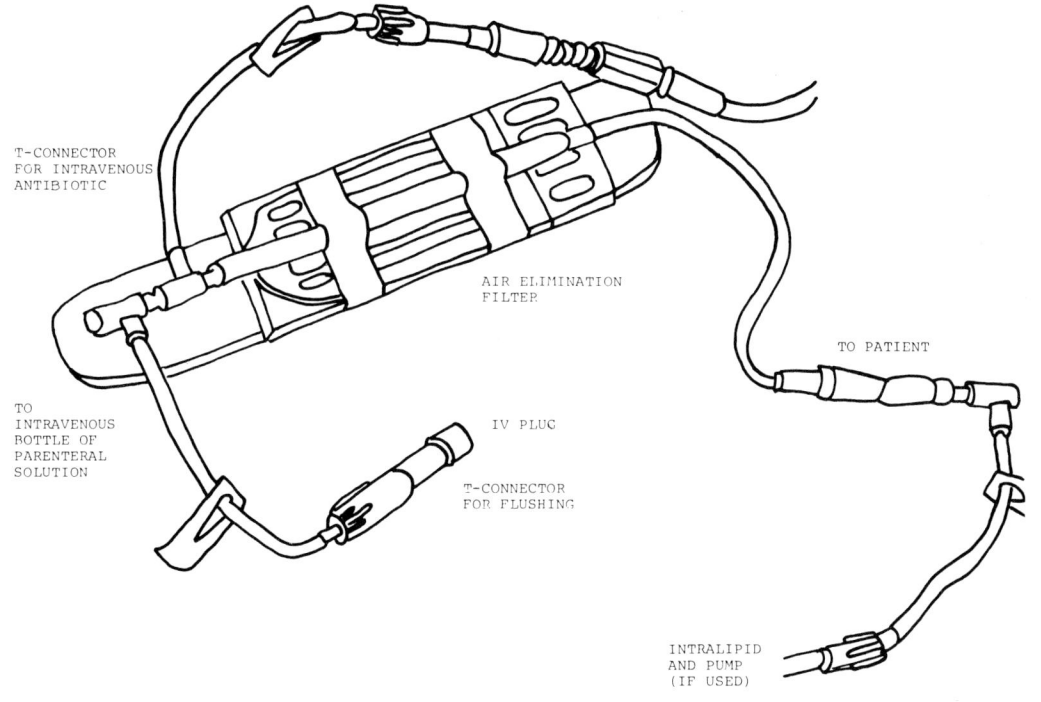

T-CONNECTOR
FOR INTRAVENOUS
ANTIBIOTIC

AIR ELIMINATION
FILTER

TO PATIENT

TO
INTRAVENOUS
BOTTLE OF
PARENTERAL
SOLUTION

IV PLUG

T-CONNECTOR
FOR FLUSHING

INTRALIPID
AND PUMP
(IF USED)

Procedure

5. Place female end of T-connector to male end of filter and connect male end to intravenous catheter so that the intralipid is between the filter and the patient.

6. Check that intralipids are running through the port closest to the intravenous catheter site.

7. Peripheral solution and intralipids may run simultaneously.

Points of Emphasis

See Diagram Page 41

Because of its viscosity intralipids must have the shortest distance to travel.

Intralipid is the only product that may run simultaneously with the solution. This should be done only when there is no alternate line.

PERIPHERAL SOLUTION WITH ANTIBIOTICS AND INTRALIPIDS

Objective:

1. To run the solution, antibiotics and intralipids through the same line when there are no alternative infusion sites, follow procedures for administering the solution (p. 35), antibiotic solutions (p. 37), and intralipids (p. 39). See diagram, p. 41 also.

2. When infusing antibiotics, the solution and intralipids must be clamped off.

3. When patient requires transport the solutions may be removed and intravenous plugs in the T-connectors. Peripheral solution infusion is not a required closed system like central hyperalimentation. Keep all hanging solutions sterile according to policy.

NOTE: If the peripheral solution is administered centrally, another peripheral intravenous should be used for antibiotics.

PROPOSED PROCEDURE FOR REPAIR OF HYPERALIMENTATION CATHETERS

In the event that the external catheter is damaged, the catheter should immediately be clamped at a point between the patient and the damaged area of the catheter to prevent bacterial contamination and potential air embolism. The clamp should be positioned as close as possible to the damaged area of the catheter to prevent bacterial contamination and potential air embolism. The clamp should be positioned as close as possible to the damaged area of the catheter.

Then, obtain the Proposed Pediatric Hyperalimentation Repair Kit.

1. Open plastic bag. Remove and put on mask.
2. Open sterile kit on cleaned work area.
3. Put on sterile gloves and gown.
4. Place sterile towel under catheter. (Assistant should remove IV tubing from catheter hub, attach and prime new sterile filter, and cover luer tip with a sterile needle.)
5. Scrub the area of the catheter to be cut first with alcohol, then with tincture of iodine. Allow to dry approximately 20 seconds; then wipe dry with sterile gauze.
6. Clamp catheter with sterile rubber-shod clamp at a point between first clamp and patient.
7. Cut prepped area of catheter with sterile scissors or blade and allow damaged catheter and distal clamp to fall away from sterile field. The sterile rubber-shod clamp should remain clamped on catheter.
8. Attach a new sterile blunt-needle adaptor.
9. Connect sterile syringe to new catheter hub, release rubber shod clamp, and clamp catheter.
10. Quickly reattach IV tubing to new catheter hub.
11. Remove rubber-shod clamp. Reset infusion rate.
12. Tape all tubing junctions to prevent accidental separations.

SELECTED BIBLIOGRAPHY

Shenkin, Alan and Wretlind, Arvid.
    Parenteral Nutrition World Review of Nutrition and Dietetics 28,
    pp. 1-111, Karger, Basel, 1978.

Ota, D., Imbembo, A., Zuidema, G.
    Total Parenteral Nutrition. Surgery 83 (5): 503-519, 1978.

Heird, W.C., Winters, R.W.
    Total Parenteral Nutrition. Journal of Pediatrics, 86(2): 2-16, 1975.

Quinby, G.E., et. al.
    Parenteral Nutrition in the Neonate. Clinics in Perinatology, 2(1):
    59-81, March 1975.

Seashore, J.H. and Seashore, M.R.
    Protein Requirements of Infants Receiving T.P.N. Journal of
    Pediatric Surgery, 11(5): 645-653, 1976.

Lowry, S.F. et. al.
    Parenteral Vitamin Requirements during intravenous feeding.
    American Journal of Clinical Nutrition, 31: 2149-2158, 1978.

Filler, R.M. and Coran, A.G.:
    Total parenteral nutrition in infants and children: Central and
    Peripheral approaches. Surgical Clinics of North America. 56'
    395-412, 1976.

Keating, J. and Teanberg.
    Amino acid hypertonic glucose treatment for intractable diarrhea
    in infants. American Journal of Disease in Children, 123-336, 1971.

Goodgame, J.T. et. al.
    Essential fatty acid deficiency in total parenteral nutrition: Time
    course of development ? suggestions for therapy. Surgery 84(2),
    271-277, 1978.

Cohen, I.T., et. al.
    Peripheral total parenteral nutrition employing a lipid emulsion
    (Intralipid) Complications encountered in pediatric patients. Jour-
    nal of Pediatric Surgery, 12: 837-845, 1977.

Bryan, H. et al.
    Intralipid - Its rational use in parenteral nutrition of the newborn.
    Pediatrics, 58(no. 6): 787-790, 1976.

Bernstein, J., Chang, C.H., Brough, A.J., Heidelberger, K.P.
    Conjugated hyperbilirubinemia infancy associated wit parenteral
    alimentation. Journal of Pediatrics, 90(3): 361-367, 1977.

Driscoll, R.H., Jr, Rosenberg, I.H.
    Total parenteral nutrition in inflammatory bowel disease. Medical
    Clinics of North America, 62(1): 185-201, 1978.

Dale, G.
    Biochemical consequences of intravenous nutrition in the
    newborn. Advances in Clinical Chem., 19, 207-249.

SECTION 2
NUTRITIONAL ASSESSMENT OF PREMATURE BABY, NEONATE, AND INFANT

Growth Chart for Low Birth Weight Infants
Nutritional Requirements of Low Birth Weight Infants
Neonatal Intensive Care Unit Nutrition Care Plan
Pediatric Nutrition and Metabolic Assessment
Pediatric Charts for Length and Weight
Recommended Daily Dietary Allowances
Mean Heights and Weights and Recommended Energy Intake

Provided in this section on nutritional assessment of the premature baby and newborn infant are recommendations for calorie and nutrient intake as well as standardized growth charts for premature and full-term neonates. Two suggested information sheets to evaluate anthropometric, laboratory, and dietary status of premature and other pediatric patients are included.

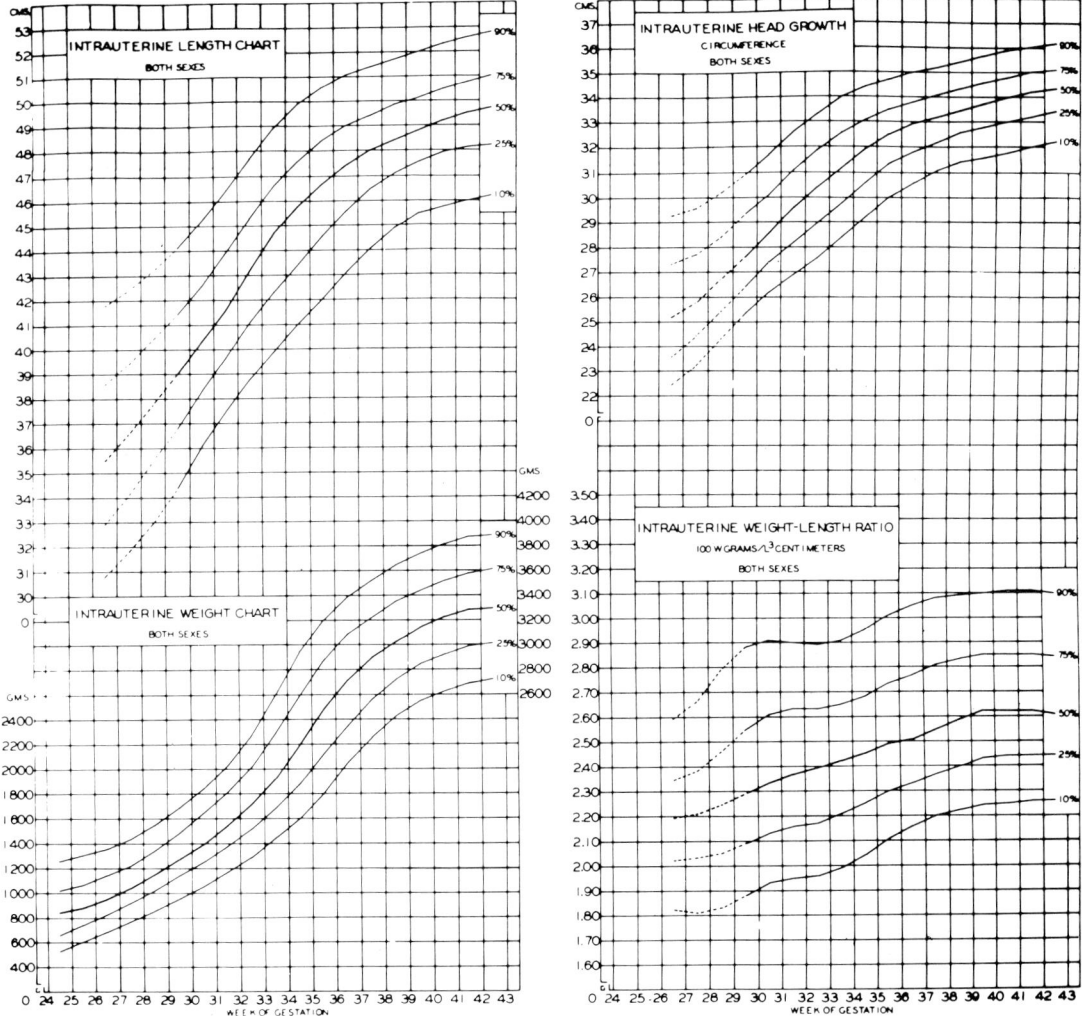

Nutritional Requirements of Low Birth Weight Infants[1-4]

Energy	120 kcal/kg/day
Protein	2.25 to 5.0 gm/kg/day (8–10% of total energy intake)
Carbohydrate	50% of total energy intake
Fat	40–50% of total energy intake (3–5% of total energy intake from linoleic acid)
Fluid	140 to 160 ml/kg
Calcium	160 mg/kg/day
Phosphorus	140 mg/kg/day
Sodium	0.9 mEq per 100 kcalories
Potassium	2.1 mEq per 100 kcalories
Iron	2 mg elemental iron/kg/day by 2 mo of age
Vitamin A	1500 IU
Vitamin D	400 IU
Vitamin C	35 mg
Vitamin E	25 IU α-tocopherol to 6 wk of age
Thiamine	0.5 mg
Niacin	8 mg
Riboflavin	0.6 mg
Vitamin B_6	0.4 mg
Folic acid	50–70 μg/day supplement until 3 mo of age
Vitamin B_{12}	2 μg

1. Sinclair, J. C.: Heat production and thermoregulation in the small-for-date infant. Pediatr. Clin. North Am. 17:147, 1970.

2. Zeigler, E. E., Bigi, R. L., and Fomon, S. J.: Nutritional requirements of the premature infant, in Suskind, R. M. (ed.): Textbook of Pediatric Nutrition. New York, Raven Press, 1980.

3. Committee on Nutrition: Nutritional needs of low-birth-weight infants. Pediatrics 60:519, 1977.

4. Ernest J., Brody, S., Gresborn, E., and Richard, K.: Suggested protocol for vitamin and mineral supplementation. Intensive Care Newborn Unit, James Whitcomb Riley Hospital for Children, Indianapolis, 1978.

NEONATAL INTENSIVE CARE UNIT NUTRITION CARE PLAN

DIAGNOSIS

MD
RN

HX

BW
BL
GA

DATE	HBG HCT	BILI	TP	ALB	BS	BUN/CR	CA	PO$_4$	NA/CL K/CO$_2$	URINE S/A KETONES	OTHER	FDG/ IV AMT RATE SUP	KCAL PRO ML PER KG	WT LT HC	PROGRESS NOTES, PLANS

MASSACHUSETTS GENERAL HOSPITAL PEDIATRIC NUTRITION AND METABOLIC ASSESSMENT

Initial Assessment Date _____

I. ASSESSMENT

Diagnosis _____

A. Anthropometric Data

Height (Ht) _____cm _____percentile   Triceps Skinfold Thickness (TSF)_____mm
(Length)(Lt)_____cm _____percentile   _____percentile
Weight (Wt)_____kg _____percentile   Arm Muscle Circumference (AMC)_____cm
                                                                       _____percentile
Wt for Ht (Wt/Ht)_____percentile   Arm Muscle Area (AMA)_____cm^2
      (Lt) (Wt/Lt) _____percentile
Head Circumference (HC)_____cm
                    _____percentile

B. Laboratory Data

Hematocrit (Hct) _____   White Blood Cell Count (WBC) _____
Mean Corpuscular Volume (MCV) _____   Lymphocyte % (LYM %) _____
Albumin (Alb) _____   Other _____
Total Protein (TP) _____   _____
Transferrin (Trans) _____   _____
Iron-Binding Capacity (IBC) _____   _____

C. Dietary History

Est. KCal Intake: Total KCal/day _____, KCal/kg _____
Pro (gm)_____% KCal_____; Fat_____(gm)_____% KCal CHO (gm)_____%
KCal_____
Unusual Losses: _____
Vitamin/Mineral Supplements (Dosage): _____
Nutrient Deficiencies _____
Nutritional Problems _____

D. Summary/Recommendations

Ideal Body Weight (IBW)_____Kg   Recommended KCal/Day_____ Protein gm/Day_____
   for present heights
Recommendations _____

_____

_____

_____

_____

_____

_____

_____

_____

II. FLOW SHEET

DATE:						
Ht. (cm)/						
Ht. %'tile						
Wt (kg)/						
Wt %'tile						
Ht/Wt %'tile						
HC (cm)						
HC %'tile						
TSF (mm)						
TSF %'tile						
AMC (cm)						
AMC %'tile						
AMA (cm^2)						
Hct/MCV						
Alb/TP						
Trans/IBC						
WBC/LYM%						

(Continued)

II. FLOW SHEET *(Continued)*

KCal/Day						
Pro (gm)						
Fat (gm)						
CHO (gm)						
KCal/kg						
Pro gm/kg						

PEDIATRIC CHARTS FOR LENGTH AND WEIGHT

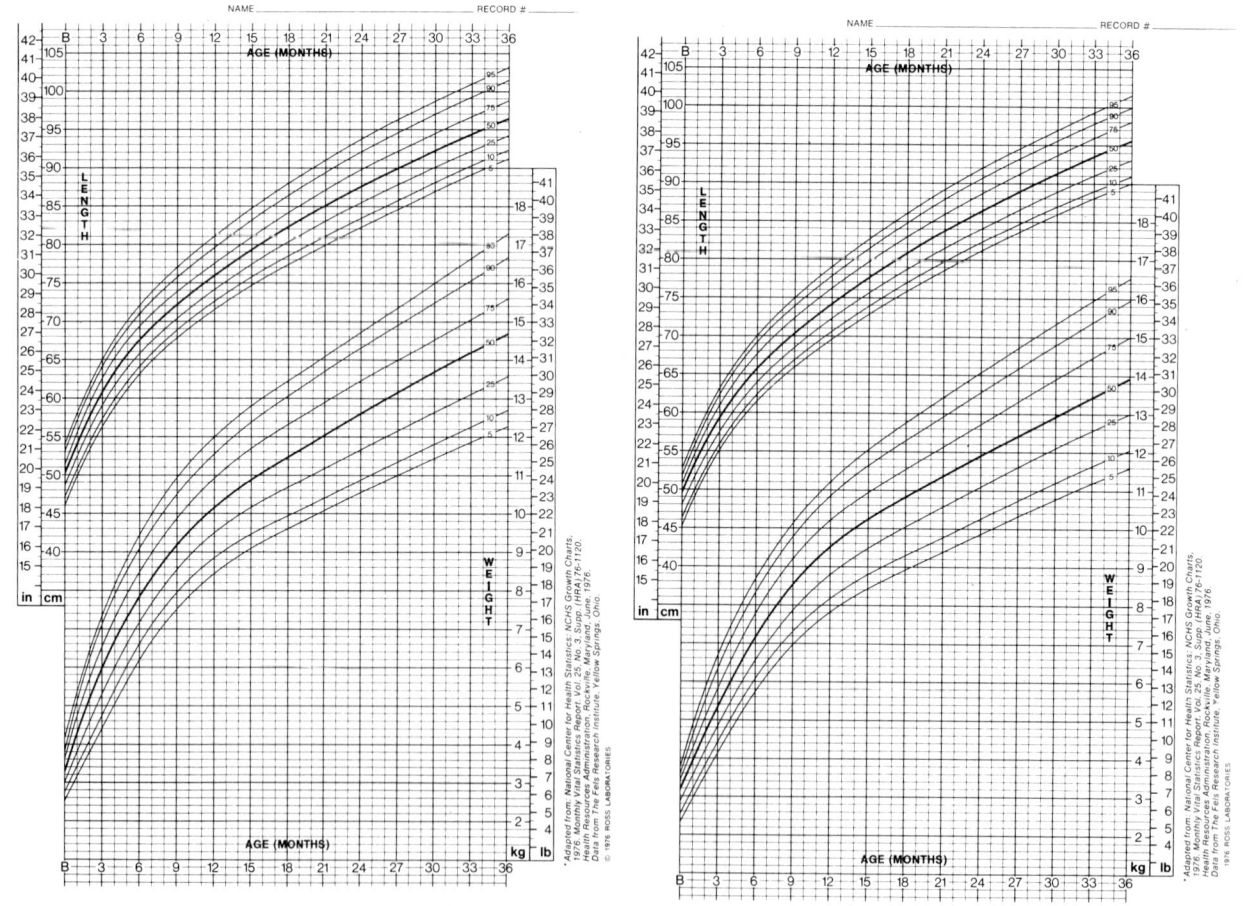

LENGTH AND WEIGHT BY AGE: **BOYS,** 0 to 36 months

LENGTH AND WEIGHT BY AGE: **GIRLS,** 0 to 36 months

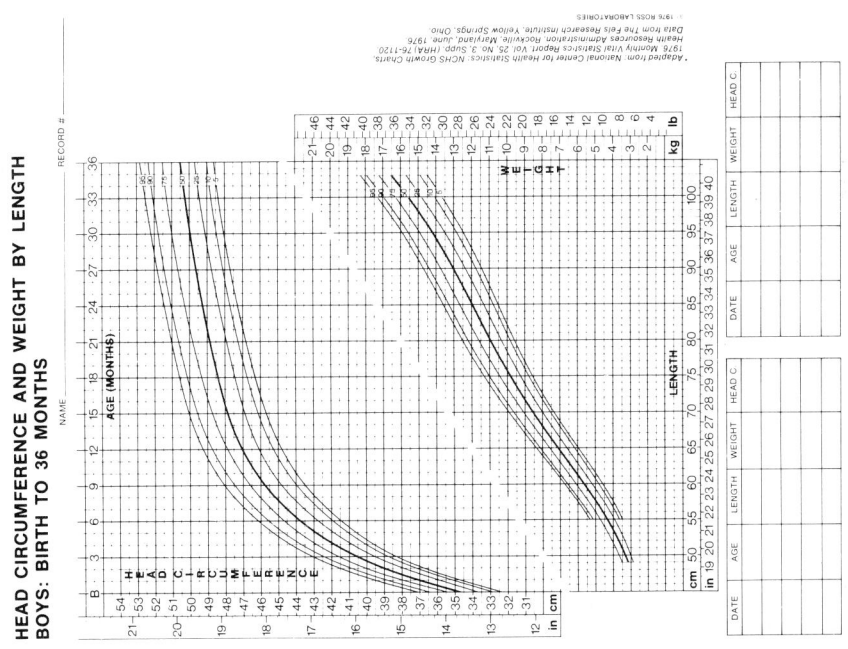

HEAD CIRCUMFERENCE AND WEIGHT BY LENGTH
GIRLS: BIRTH TO 36 MONTHS

HEAD CIRCUMFERENCE AND WEIGHT BY LENGTH
BOYS: BIRTH TO 36 MONTHS

Recommended Daily Dietary Allowances,[1] Food and Nutrition Board,
National Academy of Sciences–National Research Council, Revised 1980
*Designed for the maintenance of good nutrition of
practically all healthy people in the U.S.A.*

	Age (years)	Weight (kg)	Weight (lb)	Height (cm)	Height (in)	Protein (g)	FAT-SOLUBLE VITAMINS Vitamin A (μg RE)[2]	Vitamin D (μg)[3]	Vitamin E (mg α-TE)[4]
Infants	0.0–0.5	6	13	60	24	kg × 2.2	420	10	3
	0.5–1.0	9	20	71	28	kg × 2.0	400	10	4
Children	1–3	13	29	90	35	23	400	10	5
	4–6	20	44	112	44	30	500	10	6
	7–10	28	62	132	52	34	700	10	7
Males	11–14	45	99	157	62	45	1000	10	8
	15–18	66	145	176	69	56	1000	10	10
	19–22	70	154	177	70	56	1000	7.5	10
	23–50	70	154	178	70	56	1000	5	10
	51+	70	154	178	70	56	1000	5	10
Females	11–14	46	101	157	62	46	800	10	8
	15–18	55	120	163	64	46	800	10	8
	19–22	55	120	163	64	44	800	7.5	8
	23–50	55	120	163	64	44	800	5	8
	51+	55	120	163	64	44	800	5	8
Pregnant						+30	+200	+5	+2
Lactating						+20	+400	+5	+3

[1]The allowances are intended to provided for individual variations among most normal persons as they live in the United States under usual environmental stresses. Diets should be based on a variety of common foods in order to provide other nutrients for which human requirements have been less well defined.

[2]Retinol equivalents. 1 retinol equivalent = 1 μg retinol or 6 μg β carotene.

[3]As cholecalciferol. 10 μg cholecalciferol = 400 IU of vitamin D.

[4]α-tocopherol equivalents. 1 mg d-α tocopherol = 1 α-TE.

Recommended Daily Dietary Allowances,[1] Food and Nutrition Board, National Academy
of Sciences–National Research Council, Revised 1980 (Continued)
Designed for the maintenance of good nutrition
of practically all healthy people in the U.S.A.

WATER-SOLUBLE VITAMINS							MINERALS					
Vita- min C (mg)	Thia- min (mg)	Ribo- flavin (mg)	Niacin (mg NE)[5]	Vita- min B-6 (mg)	Fola- cin[6] (µg)	Vitamin B-12 (µg)	Cal- cium (mg)	Phos- phorus (mg)	Mag- nesium (mg)	Iron (mg)	Zinc (mg)	Iodine (mg)
35	0.3	0.4	6	0.3	30	0.5[7]	360	240	50	10	3	40
35	0.5	0.6	8	0.6	45	1.5	540	360	70	15	5	50
45	0.7	0.8	9	0.9	100	2.0	800	800	150	15	10	70
45	0.9	1.0	11	1.3	200	2.5	800	800	200	10	10	90
45	1.2	1.4	16	1.6	300	3.0	800	800	250	10	10	120
50	1.4	1.6	18	1.8	400	3.0	1200	1200	350	18	15	150
60	1.4	1.7	18	2.0	400	3.0	1200	1200	400	18	15	150
60	1.5	1.7	19	2.2	400	3.0	800	800	350	10	15	150
60	1.4	1.6	18	2.2	400	3.0	800	800	350	10	15	150
60	1.2	1.4	16	2.2	400	3.0	800	800	350	10	15	150
50	1.1	1.3	15	1.8	400	3.0	1200	1200	300	18	15	150
60	1.1	1.3	14	2.0	400	3.0	1200	1200	300	18	15	150
60	1.1	1.3	14	2.0	400	3.0	800	800	300	18	15	150
60	1.0	1.2	13	2.0	400	3.0	800	800	300	18	15	150
60	1.0	1.2	13	2.0	400	3.0	800	800	300	10	15	150
+20	+0.4	+0.3	+2	+0.6	+400	+1.0	+400	+400	+150	[8]	+5	+25
+40	+0.5	+0.5	+5	+0.5	+100	+1.0	+400	+400	+150	[8]	+10	+50

[5] 1 NE (niacin equivalent) is equal to 1 mg of niacin or 60 mg of dietary tryptophan.

[6] The folacin allowances refer to dietary sources as determined by Lactobacillus casei assay after treatment with enzymes (conjugases) to make polyglutamyl forms of the vitamin available to the test organism.

[7] The recommended dietary allowance for vitamin B_{12} in infants is based on average concentration of the vitamin in human milk. The allowances after weaning are based on energy intake (as recommended by the American Academy of Pediatrics) and consideration of other factors, such as intestinal absorption.

[8] The increased requirement during pregnancy cannot be met by the iron content of habitual American diets nor by the existing iron stores of many women; therefore the use of 30–60 mg of supplemental iron is recommended. Iron needs during lactation are not substantially different from those of nonpregnant women, but continued supplementation of the mother for two–three months after parturition is advisable in order to replenish stores depleted by pregnancy.

Mean Heights and Weights and Recommended Energy Intake*

CATEGORY	AGE (years)	WEIGHT (kg)	WEIGHT (lb)	HEIGHT (cm)	HEIGHT (in)	ENERGY NEEDS (WITH RANGE) (kcal)		ENERGY NEEDS (WITH RANGE) (Mega Joule)
Infants	0.0–0.5	6	13	60	24	kg × 115	(95–145)	kg × 0.48
	0.5–1.0	9	20	71	28	kg × 105	(80–135)	kg × 0.44
Children	1–3	13	29	90	35	1300	(900–1800)	5.5
	4–6	20	44	112	44	1700	(1300–2300)	7.1
	7–10	28	62	132	52	2400	(1650–3300)	10.1
Males	11–14	45	99	157	62	2700	(2000–3700)	11.3
	15–18	66	145	176	69	2800	(2100–3900)	11.8
	19–22	70	154	177	70	2900	(2500–3300)	12.2
	23–50	70	154	178	70	2700	(2300–3100)	11.3
	51–75	70	154	178	70	2400	(2000–2800)	10.1
	76+	70	154	178	70	2050	(1650–2450)	8.6
Females	11–14	46	101	157	62	2200	(1500–3000)	9.2
	15–18	55	120	163	64	2100	(1200–3000)	8.8
	19–22	55	120	163	64	2100	(1700–2500)	8.8
	23–50	55	120	163	64	2000	(1600–2400)	8.4
	51–75	55	120	163	64	1800	(1400–2200)	7.6
	76+	55	120	163	64	1600	(1200–2000)	6.7
Pregnancy						+300		
Lactation						+500		

*The data in this table have been assembled from the observed median heights and weights of children, together with desirable weights for adults for the mean heights of men (70 in) and women (64 in) between the ages of 18 and 34 years as surveyed in the U.S. population (HEW/NCHS data).

The energy allowances for the young adults are for men and women doing light work. The allowances for the two older age groups represent mean energy needs over these age spans, allowing for a 2 per cent decrease in basal (resting) metabolic rate per decade and a reduction in activity of 200 kcal/day for men and women between 51 and 75 years, 500 kcal for men over 75 years, and 400 kcal for women over 75 years. The customary range of daily energy output is shown in parentheses for adults and is based on a variation in energy needs of ±400 kcal at any one age, emphasizing the wide range of energy intakes appropriate for any group of people.

Energy allowances for children through age 18 are based on median energy intakes of children of these ages followed in longitudinal growth studies. The values in parentheses are 10th and 90th percentiles of energy intake, to indicate the range of energy consumption among children of these ages.

From Food and Nutrition Board, National Research Council, Committee on Dietary Allowances. Recommended Dietary Allowances. Washington, D.C., National Academy of Sciences, 1980.

SECTION 3
FORMULA COMPOSITION TABLES AND
FEEDING GUIDELINES

Feeding Recommendations for Premature Infants
Quality of Growth: Guidelines for Nutrition and Growth for Premature Infants with
   Appropriate Weight for Gestational Age
Selection of Infant Formulas
Delivery of Infant Formulas
Recommended Feeding Schedule at 0-12 Months
Oral Feeding Alternatives to Breast Feeding in Infancy
Suggested Feedings for Gastrointestinal Problems

In addition to comprehensive tables showing the composition of the various formulas available for use, a discussion of those specific needs of the premature infant and what composition would be most appropriate follows. Suggested feeding and advancement, depending on gestational age, and recommended formulas to use in infants with gastrointestinal problems are included. Recommendations for normal infant feeding from birth to age 12 months are given.

Feeding Recommendations for Premature Infants

AGE	CONDITION	FORMULA	METHOD OF DELIVERY
26–34 wks	Without GI complications	1. Own mother's milk 2. Enfamil Premature Formula 3. Central or peripheral parenteral nutrition to achieve 150 kcal/kg 4. Vitamin E	continuous infusion nasogastric or nasojejunal ↓ nasogastric bolus nasogastric bolus and nipple ↓ nipple
	Renal complications	1. Own mother's milk 2. Dilute Enfamil Premature Formula to 20 kcal/oz or PM 60/40 3. Central or peripheral parenteral nutrition to achieve 150 kcal/kg 4. Vitamin E	same as above
34–36 wks	Without GI complications	1. Own mother's milk 2. Enfamil Premature Formula 3. Supplemental peripheral parenteral nutrtion	same as above
36 wks–term	Without GI complications	1. Own mother's milk or banked human milk 2. Proprietary cow's milk formula, i.e., Enfamil	bolus and nipple ↓ nipple
Any age	Maldigestion	1. Pregestimil	same as above, depending on age

QUALITY OF GROWTH: GUIDELINES FOR NUTRITION AND GROWTH FOR PREMATURE INFANTS WITH APPROPRIATE WEIGHT FOR GESTATIONAL AGE*

1. Low weight should be reached between two and eight days of age and should be no more than a 5 to 10 per cent reduction in body weight, depending on gestational age.

2. Birth weight should be regained in one to two weeks. The ideal weight gain of infants weighing 1 to 2 kg is 20 gm per day.

3. Length as measured by a satisfactory method should increase on the average approximately 1 cm per week.

SELECTION OF INFANT FORMULAS

I. Basic Requirements of Normal Nutrition

Calories:	Basal metabolism	50–60	Kcal/kg/day
	Stool losses and activity	15–20	Kcal/kg/day
	Weight gain	4–7	Kcal/kg/day for each gram of daily weight gain

100–120 Kcal/kg/day

Fluid: 130–200 ml/kg/day. (Few infants drink >180 ml/kg/day after age three months)
Protein: 8 per cent of total caloric consumption or approximately 2 gm/kg/day
Fat: 40 per cent if total calories should be supplied as fat
Weight gain: Approximately 20 gm/day

II. Formulas for the Healthy Infant. Infants should be formula fed or breast fed the first 6–12 months. In comparing milks, review caloric density, osmolarity, quality and quantity of proteins, fat, carbohydrate, renal solute load, iron, and vitamin and mineral content.

    A. Breast milk in the term infant. Bacteriologically safe, may confer antibody and other immune protection to the neonate as well.

        1. Protein 1.6 gm/dl (6 per cent of total calories)
            60:40 lactalbumin:casein ratio
            100 per cent biologically available protein (low protein may facilitate Fe absorption)

        2. Osmolarity = 300 mOsm/L   Caloric density = 20 Kcal/oz

        3. Low renal solute load = 81 mOsm/L

        4. Fats = saturated animal fat (50 per cent of total calories). Five per cent of this is linoleic acid (essential fatty acid).

        5. Carbohydrate = lactose

        6. High in taurine (? reason for this)

        7. Vitamins = low in vitamin D. Need to supplement breast-fed babies with 400 IU vitamin D daily. Although A and C are commonly given, they are not necessary.

        8. Iron = 1.0–1.5 mg/liter. Lactoferrin present in large amounts in human milk is largely unsaturated with iron and is believed to compete with microorganisms in the environment for iron, thus inhibiting their growth. The low protein in breast milk may in some way enhance Fe absorption. Fe deficiency is rare in term infants fed human milk. Stores are depleted by the third to

*From Richard, K., and Gresham, E.: Nutritional considerations for the newborn requiring intensive care. J. Am. Dietet. Assoc. 66:592, 1975.

sixth month, however. A good guide is supplementation when birth weight doubles or reticulocyte count starts to rise.

    9. $Ca:PO_4$ = 2:1 ratio to prevent neonatal tetany

B. Milk or soy protein-based formulas. Most are formulated to be as close to human milk as possible. An iron-fortified, commercially prepared formula is a complete food for infants and requires no supplements, vitamins, or minerals.

    Contents: The American Academy of Pediatrics recommends the following for normal infant formulas:

1. Osmolarity = 300 mOsm/L
2. Caloric density = 20 cal/oz (0.67 cal/ml)
3. Protein = 1.5 gm/dl → 3.0 gm/ml maximum.

    Protein quality is compared with casein and must be at least 70 per cent as bioavailable as casein. Soy protein is lower quality than milk protein because it is lower in essential fatty acids, especially methionine, and must be supplemented to meet the Committee's standards. There is no evidence that protein concentrations greater than 1.5 gm/dl (~2.2 gm/kg) are beneficial to the neonate.

4. Fat = A minimum of 30 per cent → maximum 54 per cent of calories should be from fat. 2.7 per cent of these calories from linoleic acid (excess linoleic acid causes excessive peroxidation and can increase vitamin E requirements)
5. Carbohydrates: 40–50 per cent of calories from CHO. Lactose is the milk sugar in most proprietary formulas, as in breast milk. Soy formulas contain sucrose and corn syrup solids.
6. $Ca:PO_4$ ratio = no more than 2:1 and no less than 1.1:1
7. Vitamins: Formulas must be fortified with vitamins, minerals, and electrolytes.
8. Iron: Most iron-supplemented formulas contain 12 mg Fe/liter. The higher the protein content of an unsupplemented formula, the more likely the baby is to develop iron deficiency.

III. Nutrition of the Premature Infant

  A. Weight gain

    Intrauterine (28–32 weeks) 18 gm/day

                  (32–36 weeks) 38 gm/day

    Prematures weighing 1000–1250 gm = 20 gm/day weight gain

                          1250–1500 gm = 25 gm/day

                          >1500 grams = 30 gm/day

  B. Requirements

    Calories: 120–150 Kcal/kg/day

    Fluid: 150–200 ml/kg/day

    Protein: 2.0–4.0 gm/kg/day

    Fat: 4–7 gm/kg/day

    CHO: 10–15 gm/kg/day

  C. Protein. Digestion requires pancreatic enzymes and intestinal peptidases, which are present at 28–30 weeks. Absorption is maximal as di- and oligopeptides.

    Breast milk from mothers of premature babies is approximately 2.3 gm/dl in colostrum, decreasing to 1.1 gm/dl after the second week.

    Cystine, tyrosine, and taurine are probably essential amino acids for the premature infant. Breast milk contains high taurine levels for an unknown reason.

    Breast milk has a 60:40 whey (lactalbumin) to casein ratio. This protein is 100 per cent biologically available. Cysteine is absorbed in adequate amounts from the whey protein in breast milk. LBW babies grow normally on the low concentrations of protein (1.1–1.6 gm/dl) in breast milk.

Intakes of 6–9 gm/kg/day have been associated with irritability, lethargy, hyper-pyrexia, late acidosis of prematurity. One long-term follow-up study suggested that premature infants fed high protein (> 6 gm/kg) had lower IQs in school than a matched group with < 4 gm/kg.

High concentrations of protein also increase the renal solute delivered to the premature infant's kidneys.

D. Fat. Long-chain triglycerides require pancreatic lipase and bile salts for digestion. LBW infants malabsorb about 20 per cent of this fat intake. This may be due to low concentrations of bile salts. Also in the premature infant, bile salts are con-jugated to taurine instead of glycine and suboptimal micelles are formed. Lipase does not reach peak levels for four to nine months. Polyunsaturated fats are better absorbed than butterfat.

MCT oil — medium chain triglycerides (C8–C10) are partially water soluble and do not require micelle formation for absorption. Pancreatic lipase may not be necessary for their digestion. MCT is absorbed directly into the portal circula-tion. MCT has been shown to increase weight gain, calcium absorption, and nitro-gen retention in the premature infant. MCT does not contain essential fatty acids.

Essential fatty acids (EFAs) — linoleic (18:2), linolenic (18:3), and arachidonic (20:4) cannot be made by the infant. A premature infant on MCT who cannot digest EFAs should get Intralipid or cutaneous safflower oil. They are key lipids for CNS and dermal integrity and are essential for growth and the formation of prosta-glandins. 2–3 per cent of the total calories of the LBW infant should be as linoleic acid.

E. Carbohydrate. Forty per cent of the calories in LBW formulas should be as CHO. Lactose and sucrose must be cleared by disaccharidases. These are first present by the tenth week. Sucrose/isomaltase reach mature levels by the sixth to eighth month. Lactase does not reach mature levels until the 38th week. Glucose, dextrose, fructose, and polycose do not require breakdown by disaccharidases. Polycose re-quires pancreatic amylase to break starch linkages. Polysaccharides are well absorbed by the premature infant and have low osmolarity. "Preemies" appear to possess pancreatic amylase.

Disaccharidases are found in the intestinal "brush borders" and may be dimi-nished by shock, ischemia, or diarrhea.

F. Vitamins. The amount of vitamins present in formula, while adequate for full-term infants, is not adequate for premature infants because of the small volumes con-sumed. Rickets and folate and B_{12} deficiencies have been seen in those consuming infant formula without supplementation. One daily oral multivitamin and 50 μg/day of folate should be given to all premature babies.

G. Vitamin E. Antioxidant deficiency presents in the first month with anemia, thrombocytosis or thrombocytopenia, and peripheral edema. Premature infants have decreased absorption of vitamin E.

Infants supplemented with iron and not vitamin E may develop hemolytic anemia. Iron is a cofactor that catalyzes the oxidative breakdown of red cell lipids *in vitro*. This effect may be exacerbated without the antioxidant effect of vitamin E. In addition, there is evidence that the concurrent administration of iron and vitamin E results in decreased absorption of vitamin E.

Dosage: 25–50 IU/day for the first two to three months.

H. Iron. The premature baby is susceptible to development of iron deficiency anemia because of insufficient iron stores. These stores are increased by destruction of "old" RBCs after birth. Active erythropoiesis resumes between one and two months of age. Premature infants should be supplemented at two months or when their birth weight doubles. Dosage: 2 mg Fe/kg/day.

I. Renal solute load. Not > 200 mOsm/L — urine osmolarity should not exceed 400 mOsm/L.

DELIVERY OF INFANT FORMULAS

1. At less than 32–34 weeks, suck/swallow not well developed. Needs gavage feeding.
2. Gastric capacity may be only a few millimeters.
3. Gastric distention may result when baby is fed less than q two to three hours.
4. Aspiration may result from overfeeding. Risk factors:
   a. Relaxed LES
   b. Short esophagus
   c. Recumbent posture
   d. Hyperinflated, stiff lungs with secondary decreased movement of diaphragm

Strategies of Intake

1. On admission, start IV with D10.
2. When baby's condition permits, test patency of GI tract with a sterile H_2O feeding.
3. Over the next one to two weeks, an overlapping regimen will be followed, with decreased IV as oral feedings tolerated. (Obviously the healthy premature infant will be able to bottle or breast feed quickly.)
4. If baby is unable to receive oral feeds, peripheral HAL should be started.

Gavage Feedings — Bolus or Constant Drip

1. Gastric emptying is influenced by volume, duodenal osmoreceptors, and hormonal responses to feeding. Continuous drip gastric feedings are less dependent on osmolarity or volume.
2. With gastric feedings, volume rather than osmolarity is the important determinant of gastric emptying. Therefore, advance concentration first before volume.
3. For continuous gastric feeds, drip in no more than two hours' feeding and then check for gastric aspirates (danger of aspiration).
4. If ≥ one hour's volume is left in the stomach after two hours, decrease the rate of infusion.
5. Once the volume limit has been reached, the formula can be further concentrated in a stepwise manner to 1 cal/ml. If the formula itself is concentrated, the same distribution of fat/CHO/protein is maintained. A LBW baby should not get 4 kg/kg, however. Concentrating can also increase the renal solute load by decreasing the amount of free water the baby is receiving.
   When the protein concentration is maximal, polycose and MCT should be added. Protein intake should not fall to less than 8 per cent of total calories. Polycose = 4 kcal/gm. MCT = 8.3 kcal/gm. MCT oil may delay gastric emptying because of duodenal osmoreceptors.
6. Jejunal feeds can be instituted using a soft, gage 7.3, Silastic keofeed tube with weighted end — very useful for delayed gastric emptying or severe reflux. To pass, use metoclopramide, lay baby on right side, advance volume before concentration of feeds.

Choosing a Formula

For the premature infant we recommend Premature Enfamil, 24 cal/oz, because for protein it has a favorable 60:40 lactalbumin to whey ratio; for fat it contains 40 per cent MCT, 40 per cent corn oil, and 20 per cent coconut oil; carbohydrate consists of 60 per cent polycose and 40 per cent lactose; osmolarity is 300 mOsm/L; and it contains 1.3 mg of iron and has a calcium to phosphorus ratio of 2:1.

This combines several important features for the premature baby:

(1) increased protein content (2.4 gm/dl) and good bioavailability of protein;
(2) decreased polyunsaturates (50 per cent of fat), the rest being from MCT (decreased chance of hemolysis);
(3) polycose is good for infants with decreased lactase levels; and
(4) favorable osmolarity. It is not perfect but recommended.

For babies with fat malabsorption, formulas containing MCT and hydrolyzed casein, that is, Pregestimil, should be used.

RECOMMENDED FEEDING SCHEDULE AT 0–12 MONTHS*

Schedules vary and overlap, as each infant will progress at his or her own rate, generally taking one to one and a half months from starting one food group to the next. In all instances: (1) start with small serving sizes of one to two teaspoons, increasing gradually to three to four tablespoons per feeding; (2) introduce single-ingredient foods one at a time and continue them four to five days before introducing another food; and (3) remember, do not overfeed — quantity counts even though a food is nutritious.

	BIRTH–4 MONTHS	4–6 MONTHS	6–8 MONTHS	8–10 MONTHS	10–12 MONTHS
Milk	Breast milk or formula; 180 ml/ kg provides 120 calories/kg	Breast milk or formula, 160–180 ml/kg	Breast milk or formula — about 32 ounces	Breast milk or formula; encourage use of a cup (may be taking breast milk and formula)	Breast milk or formula (24 oz/day) should be continued until age 12 months. Wait until infant is well established on table food to begin pasteurized whole milk
Fruit and Vegetable Group	None	None	Commercial baby food or mashed or milled table food without added sugar or salt. Work toward 1 source of vitamin C/day and a dark green or yellow fruit or vegetable 3 times a week for vitamin A	Juices may be introduced one at a time, preferably from a cup — more than 3 oz per day may replace other nutritious foods. Be sure to use real juices, not canned fruit drinks	Aim for 3–4 servings per day, including juice (3 oz juice or about 2 tablespoons per serving). Include one good vitamin A source 3 times per week, one vitamin C source daily
Cereal and Bread Group	None	May begin iron-fortified baby rice cereal mixed with formula. Gradually increase amount	Begin one new grain at a time	Good finger foods to try include crackers, bread, pasta, regular cereals. Begin one new grain at a time	Grains provide B vitamins and iron. Try to include 4 servings daily. A serving for this age would be ¼ slice bread, 2 tablespoons cereal or pasta, 2 small crackers. Continue infant cereals
Meat and Other Protein Sources	None	None	None	Commercial baby food or finely milled meat. Casseroles, eggs, fish, poultry, peanut butter, legumes, cheese are all good protein sources to try	Aim for 1–2 ounces per day

*Based on the Recommendations of the Committee on Nutrition of The American Academy of Pediatrics.

Oral Feeding Alternatives to Breast Feeding in Infancy

	MANU-FACTURER	PROTEIN			FAT			CHO		
		Gm/dl	Source	% Cal	Gm/dl	Source	% Cal	Gm/dl	Source	% Cal
Enfamil	Mead Johnson	1.5	Skim milk	9	3.7	80% soy, 20% coconut oil	50	7	Lactose	41
Enfamil Premature Formula*	Mead Johnson	2.4	Skim milk, whey	12	4.1	40% MCT, corn oil, coconut oil	44	8.9	Glucose polymers, lactose	44
Human milk (mature)		1.2	Human	7	4.0	Human	54	6.8	Lactose	41
Isomil	Ross	2.0	Soy protein isolate	12	3.6	Coconut, soy oil	48	6.8	Corn syrup, sucrose	40
Lytren*	Mead Johnson							8.3	Corn syrup solids, dextrose	100
Meat Base Formula	Gerber	2.8	Beef hearts	17	3.3	Sesame	44	6.2	Cane sugar	37
Nutramigen	Mead Johnson	2.6	Hydrolyzed casein	13	2.6	Corn oil	35	8.76	Sucrose	52
Pedialyte*	Ross							5	Dextrose	100
PM 60/40	Ross	1.58	Whey, casein	9	3.76	Coconut, corn oil	50	6.9	Lactose	41
Portagen	Mead Johnson	2.4	Sodium caseinate	14	3.2	MCT 50%, corn 30%, coconut 30%	40	7.8	Corn syrup solids, sucrose	45
Pregestimil	Mead Johnson	1.9	Hydrolyzed casein	11	2.7	Corn oil 60%, MCT 40%	35	9.1	Glucose polymers	54
Prosobee	Mead Johnson	2	Soy protein isolate	12	3.6	80% soy, 20% coconut oil	48	6.9	Corn syrup solids	40
RCF*	Ross	2	Soy protein isolate	21	3.6	Coconut, soy oil	79			
Similac	Ross	1.55	Skim milk	9	3.6	Coconut, soy oil	48	7.2	Lactose	43
Similac LBW*	Ross	2.2	Skim milk	11	4.5	MCT 50%, corn 30%, coconut 20%	47	8.5	Lactose 50%, polycose 50%	42
Similac Special Care*	Ross	2.2	Whey, casein	11	4.4	MCT 50%, corn 30%, coconut 20%	46	8.6	Lactose 50%, polycose 50%	42
SMA	Wyeth	1.5	Skim milk, whey	9	3.6	Coconut, corn, soy oil	48	7.2	Lactose	43
Vivonex (2/3 strength)	Eaton	1.5	L-amino acids	9	0.2	Safflower oil	3	15	Glucose oligosaccharides	89
Whole cow's milk		3.3		20	3.7	Butter fat	50	4.9	Lactose	30

*All values for 0.67 cal/ml or 20 cal/oz concentration unless otherwise noted.

Oral Feeding Alternative to Breast Feeding in Infancy (*Continued*)

	Osmol-ality	Renal Solute Load/L	Na mEq/L	K mEq/L	Ca Mg/L	Phos Mg/L	Ca/Phos Ratio	Indications for Use
Enfamil	278	100	10	16	500	420	1.2:1	Normal infant feeding
Enfamil Premature Formula*	300	220	13	22	900	450	2:1	24 cal/oz; premature infants
Human milk (mature)	300	81	7	13	340	140	2.2:1	Normal infant feeding
Isomil	250	130	13	18	700	500	1.4:1	Milk protein allergy, lactose intolerance, galactosemia
Lytren*	290		30	25	80			9 cal/oz, oral electrolyte solution; rehydration
Meat Base Formula		176	8	10	980	650	1.5:1	
Nutramigen	479	130	13	17	600	450	1.3:1	Hypoallergenicity
Pedialyte*		130	30	20	80	450		6 cal/oz oral electrolyte solution; rehydration
PM 60/40	260	90	7	15	400	200	2:1	Renal conditions
Portagen	158	150	13	21	600	450	1.3:1	Fat malabsorption
Pregestimil	348	130	13	18	600	400	1.5:1	Malabsorption, maldigestion
Prosobee	200	130	9.6	16	500	420	1.2:1	Milk protein allergy, sucrose or lactose intolerance, galactosemia
RCF*		126	13	18	700	500		12 cal/oz without added carbohydrate; carbohydrate intolerance
Similac	290	108	11	20	510	390	1.3:1	Normal infant feeding
Similac LBW*	300	160	16	31	730	560	1.3:1	24 cal/oz; low birth weight infants
Similac Special Care*	300	150	15	26	1440	720	2:1	24 cal/oz; very low birth weight infants
SMA	295	90	6.5	13.6	420	312	1.3:1	Renal or cardiac conditions
Vivonex (2/3 strength)	430		37	30	295	295	1:1	Intractable diarrhea, severe malabsorption
Whole cow's milk	288	226	24	35	1150	920	1.3:1	Normal infant feeding after 12 months of age

SUGGESTED FEEDINGS FOR GASTROINTESTINAL PROBLEMS

COMMON GASTROINTESTINAL PROBLEMS IN INFANCY	SUGGESTED FORMULAS TO USE	RATIONALE
Allergy — cow's milk protein soy protein	Protein hydrolysate (Nutramigen or Pregestimil)	protein sensitivity
Biliary atresia	Portagen	impaired intraluminal digestion/absorption of long-chain fats
Celiac disease	Pregestimil, soy-based formula, cow's milk formula	advance to more complex formula as intestinal epithelium returns to normal
Colic	Lactose-free formula may be helpful (Prosobee, Isomil, etc.)	↑ hydrogen production with disaccharide intolerance
Constipation	Routine formula ↑ sugar	mild laxative effect
Cystic fibrosis	Portagen	impaired intraluminal digestion/absorption of long-chain fats
	Pregestimil	whey protein, disaccharide digestion/absorption impaired
Diarrhea — CNSD intractable	Routine formula, Pregestimil	appropriate distribution of calories — impaired digestion of intact protein, long-chain fats, and disaccharides
Failure to thrive	Pregestimil	advance to more complex formula as intestinal epithelium returns to normal
Gastroesophageal Reflux	Routine formula	thickened, small frequent feeds
GI bleed	Consider cow's milk–free formula — ? soy	milk toxicity in infancy
Hepatitis — without failure with failure	Routine formula, Portagen	impaired intraluminal digestion/absorption of long-chain fats
Jaundice	Routine formula	
Lactose intolerance	Soy-based formula (Isomil, Prosobee, etc.)	impaired digestion or utilization of lactose
Necrotizing enterocolitis	Pregestimil	impaired digestion/absorption
Short bowel syndrome > 100 cm remaining < 100 cm remaining	None Pregestimil	impaired end-stage digestion/absorption
Sucrose intolerance Primary	Cow's milk formula (Enfamil, Similac, etc.)	as intestinal epithelium returns to normal
Secondary (sucrose and lactose)	Pregestimil, RCF, soy or cow's milk	

SECTION 4
HUMAN MILK BANKING PROGRAM

Human Milk Banking
Human Milk Banking Procedures of Massachusetts General Hospital
Nutritional Composition of Milk from Mothers Delivering Preterm (PT) and at Term (T)

The rationale for breast milk banking; procedures to establish such a unit include (1) information for mothers on expression of milk, and medical history and information necessary from donating mothers, (2) procedures for collection, culturing, and storage of milk, (3) a consent form appropriate for use in human infants, and (4) composition of preterm milk.

HUMAN MILK BANKING

Banking of human milk for the purposes of feeding the hospitalized premature or sick infant is widely practiced in Europe. In this country, before the development of ready-to-use, commercially prepared modified milk formulas, human milk banking ended almost completely in the period following World War II.

There has been an increased interest in banking of human milk in the past ten years. Various institutions have developed procedures to suit their needs and to protect the quality of the milk provided to the patient. Many of the modern human milk banks are "donor" banks; that is, human milk is collected from volunteer mothers to feed an infant other than their own.

We have included in this section the protocol used at one hospital for the donation of human milk for the feeding of ill low birth weight infants. References are given on page 000.

HUMAN MILK BANKING PROCEDURES OF
MASSACHUSETTS GENERAL HOSPITAL

PROTOCOL FOR COLLECTION AND STORAGE OF BREAST MILK

I. Collection

A. Sterile water bottles and culture tubes will be provided by the Massachusetts General Hospital.
B. All milk will be immediately frozen and labeled with date of expression, time of expression, code number, and a note whether culture has been sent. Bottles approved for use will be color coded.
C. Milk will be brought to the central depot by designated council members in a plastic ice chest filled with ice in the frozen state, and then transported to Massachusetts General Hospital in the same type of ice chest and still in the frozen state.

II. Storage

A. Bottles should be kept no longer than four weeks at −20°C from the day of expression. All information on the bottles will be kept in a log book, and culture reports will be kept on file. The Dietary Department will supervise these tasks.
B. Dates on bottles will be checked daily by Dietary personnel for expired milk, and bottles will be rotated to use the oldest milk first.
C. A sample of every bottle of milk will be sent for culture and colony counts and the milk will not be used until the culture results are known.

III. Preparation for Use

    A. All personnel handling breast milk will follow standard nursing procedures for hand washing and handling of infants' milk.

    B. The breast milk should be thawed in tepid water just before use and kept in the refrigerator until used but for no longer than 12 hours from the time it is defrosted. Milk defrosted for longer than 12 hours should be discarded by the nurses.

    C. If feeding is to be continuous, syringe and tubing should be changed every eight hours. The syringe should be dated and timed.

HISTORY SHEET AND LABORATORY DATA

History from Mother

1. Are you on any medication?   If so, what?

    Are you taking birth control pills?

2. Do you smoke?   How many packs of cigarettes per day?

3. Do you drink alcohol?   How much per day?

4. Do you drink more than 6 cups of coffee per day?

5. Do you have any major illnesses at the present time?
   Havy you ever had TB?
   Have you ever had hepatitis?
   Have you ever had a blood transfusion?

6. Was your baby jaundiced for more than 10 days?

7. How long have you been nursing continuously?
   What is your nursing history? (Birth date of each child, and length of time nursed and reason for stopping.)

Laboratory Data

Date being examined:

VDRL	positive	negative
Hepatitis B surface antigen	positive	negative
Tine test	positive	negative

INSTRUCTION SHEET FOR MOTHER DONATING BREAST MILK

It is important to maintain as clean a procedure as possible as the milk will not be sterilized before being fed to a small infant.

    1. Wash hands vigorously with soap for two minutes.

    2. Wash nipples well and rinse with the sterile water provided in the sterile water bottles that will be used to collect the breast milk.

3. Discard the first half-ounce of breast milk expressed. Express the remaining breast milk directly into the empty sterile water bottle provided by the Bank. A small amount should be emptied into the culture tube attached to each sterile water bottle.

4. Once the milk is expressed, cap the sterile bottle immediately and place the bottle in the back of your home freezer. The breast milk must be kept frozen at all times. Bottles of milk are not to remain in any home freezer longer than 48 hours prior to transfer to the hospital.

5. The bottle should be labeled with your code number, date of expression, and time of expression of the milk. Please place an asterisk on the label if the milk is being expressed within two weeks following the birth of your last baby. Please do not put more than two ounces in each bottle.

6. If breast milk has started to thaw, it must be discarded.

7. Alcohol, coffee, and other caffeine-containing foods may be taken in only moderate amounts.

8. Do not express milk for the Milk Bank while taking any medication and for at least 48 hours after medication has been discontinued.

9. The following foods should be avoided 18 hours before pumping: cabbage, Brussels sprouts, cauliflower, garlic, and onions.

10. If you or your baby are sick (if you have localized infection of the breast, fissured nipples), you must wait until you have been well for 48 hours before donating your milk.

11. If possible, please inform your child's pediatrician and your obstetrician of your intention to donate your breast milk to the Massachusetts General Hospital Breast Milk Bank. If they have any objections, ask them to please contact the director of the Breast Milk Bank.

PROCEDURE FOR MANUALLY EXPRESSING MILK

Preparation

Place warm towel on breasts for approximately five minutes prior to expressing. Clean hands throughly, using soap and hot running water; scrub nails with brush. Wash breasts with warm water or sterile water from bottles, and pat dry with a clean towel. Remove cap from the bottle without touching the inside of the bottle. Place cap inside up on a clean surface. Avoid touching the top of the bottle or the inside of the cap. Use the four-ounce size bottles of sterile water supplied by the hospital whenever possible (discard extra water).

1. Manual expression is simple and preferred since it eliminates extra equipment that may harbor bacteria. If milk can be expressed only by pump, it is essential that the pump be cleaned well before each use.

To express manually, support the breast with index and middle finger of one hand, placing them on the outside margin of the areola (brown ring) and your thumb on the upper rim of the areola. Use gentle scissor-like motion on your breast, holding bottle to nipple with the other hand.

It may take time for the milk let-down reflex to adjust to manual stimulation; therefore, relax and do not be discouraged. Bacteriologic quality of milk can be improved by discarding the first half-ounce and collecting the remaining milk. Total expression time should not exceed 15 or 20 minutes. After you have worked on one side, start expressing from the other breast, again discarding the first half-ounce. Then do each side once more. This changing back and forth gives the milk a greater chance to come down the ducts. (The first half-ounce from each breast is discarded as it often has the greatest number of bacteria in it.)

2. Since milk at room temperature is an excellent medium for bacterial growth, replace cap firmly when finished. Label and put in back of home freezer at once. Do not reopen bottle — use new a bottle for the next expression. Transfer bottles of milk in a cooler or packed in ice to the hospital as soon as possible, preferably within 48 hours.

3. If you have hepatitis or tuberculosis, you should not breast feed your infant. If you have localized infection of the breast, you must wait until you have been well for 48 hours before expressing your milk.

4. Information provided on the "Instruction Sheet for Mothers Donating Breast Milk" also applies.

Consent Form for Donors

I, _____, have agreed voluntarily to donate my breast milk to the Massachusetts General Hospital Breast Milk Bank. I understand that the milk will be donated anonymously and that I am not responsible for any use to which the milk is put. I understand that this milk will be used to help infants grow and for certain other conditions of infancy that may be helped by breast milk and that I am not responsible for any condition that may arise in the infants from the use of this breast milk.

_____   _____
Date   Signature

_____
Witness

Consent Form for Recipients

I, _____, give permission for my child, _____,
      (name)   (name)
to receive banked breast milk. I am aware that there are several conditions of infancy that may respond favorably to feedings of breast milk, and I am also aware of the risks present in the taking of breast milk. Some of these risks involve the presence of infection or toxic substances in milk which are undetectable by present methods and also the theoretic possibility that because the breast milk contains living tissue much the same as blood that some infants may react immunologically with the living cells in mother's breast milk. However, despite these risks no harm is actually expected to arise from the consumption of donated breast milk, and I agree to allow my child _____to receive this
                                           (name)
breast milk. I also understand that no breast milk will be prescribed for my child unless the benefits are believed to outweigh the theoretic risks.

_____   _____
Date   Signature

_____   _____
Witness   Physician

CULTURING HUMAN MILK FOR THE HUMAN MILK BANK IN THE INFECTION CONTROL LABORATORY

Samples of frozen human milk collected weekly by the Dietary Department for use in the Human Milk Bank are cultured for total colony counts and screened qualitatively for the presence or predominance of potential pathogens.

Total colony counts are determined by the Standard Plate Count Method as described in Chapter 5 of Standard Methods for the Examination of Dairy Products (American Public Health Association, 1978, 14th ed.) and detailed below. At present the Dietary Department considers counts under 100,000 per ml acceptable.

State milk standards: pasteurized milk: 5,000 col per ml tpc, 3 col per ml colif; raw milk: 100,000 tpc.

Screening for potential pathogens is performed by inoculating a TSA with 5 per cent sheep blood plate with 0.1 ml of milk, which is streaked out to obtain isolated colonies. Normally, the growth is a mixture of skin flora (*Staphyloccus* spp., diphtheroids) and sometime some normal mouth flora (alpha-streptococcus). This is easy to determine from colony morphology and a few simple tests (Gram stain, catalase) and is reported as mixed skin (and/or normal mouth) flora. If a potential pathogen, such as *S. aureus*, gram-negative bacillus, or beta-strep, is either predominant or abundant, then that organism is identified by standard bacteriologic techniques and reported.

PLATING PROCEDURE FOR HUMAN MILK OF THE INFECTION CONTROL LABORATORY

Turn on water bath, check temperature (it should be 44–46° C). Melt Standard Methods Agar in autoclave (5 min), cool in cold water, temper to 45° C in water bath. Thaw milk specimens in refrigerator. It may be necessary to thaw large (several ounce) specimens at room temperature. Log specimen identification in book.

Plating cultures: Complete each step for all specimens in series before proceeding.

1. a. *Label* BAP, 9 ml tube of buffered dilution water.
    b. *Label* 2 Petri dishes for SPC — spec ident and dilutions (−1, −2).
2. Using a 1.1 ml pipet, transfer 0.1 ml shaken milk onto BAP, 1 ml into dilution blank (blow out).
3. *Shake* diluted sample (25 movements in 7 seconds), then, using 1.1 ml pipet, transfer 1 and 0.1 ml aliquots to Petri dishes. (Don't blow out.) Transfer a 1 ml aliquot of dilution water for sterility control.
4. *Pour* 10–12 ml melted SMA into the dishes and mix. After *solidification*, invert plates and incubate at 32° C.
5. Streak out the previously inoculated BAPs, invert, and incubate at 35° C.

NUTRITIONAL COMPOSITION OF MILK FROM MOTHERS DELIVERING PRETERM (PT) AND AT TERM (T)*

| NUTRIENT | | DAYS POSTPARTUM | | | | |
		3	7	14	21	28
Lactose (gm/dl)	PT†	5.96 ± 0.20 (26)	6.05 ± 0.18 (29)	6.21 ± 0.18 (22)	6.49 ± 0.21 (15)	6.95 ± 0.27 (13)
	T	6.16 ± 0.10 (10)	6.52 ± 0.20 (13)	6.78 ± 0.19 (13)	7.12 ± 0.19 (12)	7.26 ± 0.17 (11)
Fat (gm/dl)	PT	1.63 ± 0.23 (25)	3.81 ± 0.21 (27)	4.40 ± 0.31 (21)	3.68 ± 0.40 (15)	4.00 ± 0.33 (13)
	T	1.71 ± 0.24 (10)	3.06 ± 0.46 (12)	3.48 ± 0.40 (12)	3.89 ± 0.49 (12)	4.01 ± 0.30 (11)
Protein (gm/dl)	PT‡	3.24 ± 0.31 (26)	2.44 ± 0.15 (29)	2.17 ± 0.12 (22)	1.83 ± 0.14 (15)	1.81 ± 0.11 (13)
	T	2.29 ± 0.07 (12)	1.87 ± 0.08 (14)	1.57 ± 0.05 (13)	1.52 ± 0.06 (12)	1.42 ± 0.05 (11)
Energy (Kcal/dl)	PT	51.4 ± 2.4 (25)	67.4 ± 1.7 (27)	72.3 ± 3.0 (21)	65.6 ± 4.3 (15)	70.1 ± 3.3 (13)
	T	48.7 ± 2.0 (10)	60.6 ± 4.3 (12)	64.2 ± 3.7 (12)	68.6 ± 4.0 (12)	69.7 ± 2.9 (11)
Sodium (mEq/L)	PT†	26.6 ± 3.0 (26)	21.8 ± 2.7 (29)	19.7 ± 2.3 (22)	13.4 ± 1.8 (15)	12.6 ± 2.5 (13)
	T	22.3 ± 2.4 (10)	16.9 ± 2.8 (13)	11.0 ± 1.7 (13)	10.8 ± 1.6 (12)	8.5 ± 1.8 (11)
Chloride (mEq/L)	PT†	31.6 ± 2.4 (26)	25.3 ± 2.2 (29)	22.8 ± 2.2 (22)	17.0 ± 1.7 (15)	16.8 ± 2.8 (13)
	T	26.9 ± 2.4 (10)	21.3 ± 2.7 (13)	14.5 ± 1.5 (13)	15.2 ± 1.9 (12)	13.1 ± 2.3 (11)
Potassium (mEq/L)	PT	17.4 ± 0.7 (26)	17.6 ± 0.5 (29)	16.2 ± 0.5 (22)	16.3 ± 0.9 (15)	15.5 ± 0.6 (13)
	T	18.5 ± 1.0 (10)	16.5 ± 0.5 (13)	15.4 ± 0.8 (13)	15.8 ± 0.6 (12)	15.0 ± 0.7 (11)
Calcium (mg/L)	PT	208 ± 17 (25)	247 ± 16 (27)	219 ± 12 (20)	204 ± 15 (13)	216 ± 15 (11)
	T	214 ± 38 (6)	254 ± 11 (8)	258 ± 17 (9)	266 ± 25 (8)	249 ± 18 (7)
Phosphorus (mg/L)	PT	95 ± 7 (25)	142 ± 10 (27)	144 ± 8 (20)	149 ± 13 (13)	143 ± 11 (11)
	T	110 ± 12 (6)	151 ± 18 (8)	168 ± 6 (9)	153 ± 14 (8)	158 ± 13 (7)
Magnesium (mg/L)	PT	28 ± 1 (25)	31 ± 1 (27)	30 ± 1 (20)	24 ± 1 (13)	25 ± 1 (11)
	T	25 ± 4 (6)	29 ± 2 (8)	26 ± 2 (9)	29 ± 3 (8)	25 ± 2 (7)

*Results are expressed as mean ± SEM with the number of subjects at each period in parentheses.
†$P < 0.05$ for PT milk against T milk.
‡$P < 0.005$ for PT milk against T milk.
  From Gross, S. J., David, R. J.: Bauman, L., and Tomarelli, R. M.: Nutritional composition of milk produced by mothers delivering preterm. J. Pediatr. 96:643, 1980.

REFERENCES

AAP Committee on Nutrition: Human milk banking. Pediatrics 65:854, 1980.
Dauncey, S., Shaw, J. C. L., and Urman, J.: The absorption and retention of magnesium zinc and copper by low-birth-weight infants fed pasteurized human breast milk. Pediatr. Res. 11:991, 1977.
Fomon, S. J.: Human milk in premature infant feeding: Report of a second workshop. Am. J. Public Health 67:361, 1977.
Human milk in premature infant feeding: Summary of a workshop. Pediatrics 57:741, 1976.
Siimes, M., and Hallman, N.: A perspective on human milk banking, 1978. J. Pediatr. 94:173, 1979.

SECTION 5
SPECIAL DIETS AND CARBOHYDRATE CONTENT OF FOODS

Gluten-Free Diet
Soy-Free Diet
Lactose-Free Diet
Sucrose-Free Diet
Low Sucrose Diet
Adequate Fat Diet
Low Long-Chain Triglyceride, High Medium-Chain Triglyceride Diet
Carbohydrate Content of Common Foods
Less Common Carbohydrates in Foods

Multiple pediatric problems require special dietary manipulation. Those therapeutic diets generally seen with gastrointestinal disease and included here are gluten free, adequate fat for treatment of chronic nonspecific diarrhea, lactose free, and recommendations for a low intake of long-chain fats and increased medium-chain triglycerides.

GLUTEN-FREE DIET

At present, the only practical way to control celiac sprue is to remove completely wheat, rye, oats, and barley from the diet. Rice, corn, and soy seem to be safe.

1. In order to eliminate the gluten from the diet, omit wheat, oats, rye, and barley, and foods containing these grains.

2. It is important to be *absolutely sure* of the ingredients used in the preparation of all foods eaten. *Read labels* on foodstuff when shopping and *avoid* any that contain *wheat, wheat flour, flour, oats, rye, barley, malt, gluten, cereal additive, hydrolyzed vegetable protein, starch, emulsifiers,* and *stabilizers.*

If in doubt about specific ingredients in products, write to the manufacturer for additional information.

The labels on some foods do not list their ingredients because of standards of identity set up by the federal government. Locally produced foods not entered into interstate commerce are not required to list ingredients. Standards of identity require that certain basic ingredients must be used, and designate other ingredients that may be used at the packer's option. No other ingredient may be added. A full list of ingredients may not appear on the label of a food for which a definition of standard of identity has been set. For confirmation on current definitions and standards, contact the area office of the Food and Drug Administration.

3. Pure spices and herbs may be used for seasoning.

4. When eating in restaurants, avoid mixed dishes — choose simply prepared, easily identified foods.

5. Periodic review of the diet and nutritional care plan by a registered dietitian is advisable.

REMEMBER: Even a small amount of gluten in the diet may prevent any improvement in the patient's condition.

A gluten-free diet controls, but does not cure, celiac sprue. Lifelong adherence to a gluten-free diet is recommended for the individual who is gluten-sensitive.

Constant and careful adherence to this diet is *essential* at *all times!*

FOODS ALLOWED	FOODS NOT ALLOWED
Milk: Whole, low fat, or skim; fresh, dried, or evaporated. Yogurt — plain or flavored.	Malted milk, Ovaltine. Flavoring syrups of unknown content, or those that contain wheat products or malt.
Beverages: Tea, coffee (decaffeinated, freeze-dried, and other instant varieties that do not contain cereal products). Carbonated beverages. Cocoa and chocolate syrup (read labels to see that no wheat product has been added). Distilled alcoholic beverages and wine as permitted.	Postum and other beverage mixes that contain the prohibited cereals. Beer and ale.
Eggs: As desired.	Egg dishes thickened with prohibited flour or containing bread crumbs.
Cheese: Aged or processed. All kinds of pure cheese — cottage or cream.	Cheese sauce or cheese spread containing prohibited flours.
Meat, Fish, Poultry: Bake, boil, broil, stew, or fry. The allowed special flours (for example, rice, soy, potato, or cornmeal, or potato chips) may be used in "breading" or in preparing stuffing or gravies. Homemade combination dishes, such as meatballs and casseroles of allowed ingredients.	Combination dishes (unless prohibited foods have been omitted), such as meatloaf, croquettes, breaded meat, fish, chicken; canned meat dishes; prepared meats, such as frankfurters and bologna (unless guaranteed pure meat); luncheon meats, scrapple, extenders, sausage and commercial hamburgers that may contain cereal fillers. Sauces and gravies that contain prohibited flours.
Bread and Cereal: Those made from rice, corn, soybean, potato, or arrowroot flour only. Cornmeal, hominy grits, rice, puffed rice, cream of rice, precooked rice cereal prepared for infants. Ready-to-eat cereals made from foods allowed. Do not use wheat starch flour.	Wheat, oats, rye, barley, and any foods containing these grains. Oatmeal, buckwheat, wheat germ, bulgur wheat, crude bran, noodles, macaroni, spaghetti, dumplings, stuffing, kasha. Bakery bread, rolls, cake, crackers, muffins, biscuits, waffles, pancakes, doughnuts, prepared mixes, rusk, zwieback, matzoth, pretzels. Prepared cereals containing malt flavoring, including those made from rice and corn.
Vegetables and Potatoes: All kinds — raw, baked, boiled, or steamed. May be seasoned with salt, pure spices and herbs, and the fats allowed. Sauces may be thickened with cream, cornstarch, or allowed special flour.	Creamed or scalloped vegetables if thickened with wheat flour and/or topped with bread crumbs or matzoth meal. Avoid sauces unless homemade of allowed foods.
Fruits and Juices: Raw, cooked, canned, frozen, dried. Stewed fruits thickened with tapioca, cornstarch, or allowed special flours.	Stewed fruits or combination dishes that are thickened with wheat flour.

FOODS ALLOWED

Desserts: Fruits, fruit-flavored gelatin desserts (plain or with fruit). Sherbet, ices, and vanilla ice cream, homemade custard, rice pudding, junket, cornstarch pudding, tapioca, and similar puddings made without prohibited cereals. Baked desserts made with allowed special flours.

Soups: Clear, unthickened broth. Vegetable soups made with clear stock and without barley, noodles, or macaroni. Cream soups and chowders only if thickened with cream, cornstarch, or allowed special flour.

Fats. Butter, margarine, oil, pure mayonnaise (and other salad dressings that are thickened with egg, cornstarch or allowed special flour), cream, bacon, lard, vegetable shortening, nuts, olives, and peanut butter.

Seasonings and Sweets: Pure spices and herbs. Salt, sugar, molasses, honey, jelly, jam, corn syrup, maple sugar and syrup, marshmallows, and candies made from foods allowed. Pure cocoa and chocolate. Catsup, prepared mustard, pickles, relish, vinegar, monosodium glutamate.

FOODS NOT ALLOWED

Any pudding or frozen dessert that is thickened with wheat flour or with cereals added; commercial ice cream with cereal additives. Bakery products made with prohibited flour, such as cake, pasty, cookies, pie crust, pudding, ice cream cones; prepared mixes.

Ingredients of canned soup other than clear broth must be checked. Soups containing barley, noodles, macaroni. Cream soups, bisques, and chowders, unless made only with ingredients allowed.

Commercial salad dressings that may contain wheat flour. Gravies or sauces thickened with wheat flour.

Candy and other confections that contain prohibited cereals or are of unknown content.

RECIPES FOR THE GLUTEN-FREE DIET

Many favorite recipes can be modified by substituting one of the allowed starches for flour. This is not true of yeast bread, however, since gluten contributes to the characteristic texture of loaf bread.

Recipes for breads, cakes, and cookies using the allowed flours are available from a number of sources. Wheat starch is not recommended even though it is advertised as a "low gluten" or "gluten-free" product. Since the gluten and gliadin fractions are characteristic of wheat protein, it is not considered wise to take the chance on the presence of even traces of these toxic factors in starch from wheat. Hence, patients are urged to use only those flours and starches that are of known derivation and avoid *wheat, rye, oats,* and *barley*. Cornstarch, rice flour, potato flour, arrowroot, and tapioca are widely available and acceptable alternatives.

SOY-FREE COMMERCIAL PRODUCTS*

This list does not include all commercial products that can/cannot be used; many more could be added. It is always wise to check the label for ingredients when purchasing any processed foods, since product content may change periodically. Key words to look for on product labels are soy, soybean oil, sprouts, flour, milk, curd, vegetable protein, protein isolate, and lecithin (a soybean derivative). Soy or soy products are commonly found in bread and pastry products, breaded food, chocolates, cold cuts, ground meat products, and oils and margarines.

CONTAINS SOY	SOY-FREE
Breads	
Pepperidge Farm breads	Rositani Italian Bread (also other Italian breads made with flour, water, yeast, and salt only)
Arnold breads	
Wonder Bread	
English muffins	
Hot dog/hamburger buns	
Dinner rolls	
Cereals	
Nature Valley Granola — all flavors	General Mills: Cheerios, Total, Buck Wheats, Wheaties, 40% Bran, Trix, Lucky Charms
Kellogg's Country Morning	
Quaker 100% Natural	Kellogg's: Raisin Bran, Bran Buds, Product 19, Corn Flakes, Rice Krispies, Special K, Frosted Flakes, Sugar Pops
Nabisco Ready-to-Eat Cream of Wheat	
	Ralston: Rice Chex, Corn Chex, Wheat Chex
	Nabisco: Shredded Wheat
	Quaker: Puffed Rice, Puffed Wheat
	Plain Cream of Wheat
	Wheatena
	Maltex
	Farina
	Cream of Rice
Rice	
Rice-a-Roni	Plain rice — regular or instant
Stroganoff	Rice-a-Roni Risotto Flavored
Beef-Flavored	
Fried Rice with Almonds	
Spanish Rice	
Long Grain and Wild Rice	
Chicken-Flavored	
Minute	
Long Grain and Wild Rice	
Spanish	
Rib Roast	
Fried	
Drumstick	
Uncle Ben's	
Rice and Gravy	
Long Grain and Wild Rice	

*From Yale–New Haven Hospital Department of Food and Nutritional Services.

CONTAINS SOY	SOY-FREE

Rice Pilaf
  Chicken Flavored
  Beef Flavored

Stuffing

Stuff 'n' Such	Bell's Stuffing
Stove Top Stuffing	
Arnold's Great Stuff	
Shake'n Bake — all flavors	
Kellogg's Croutettes Stuffing	
Noodle-Roni	

Potatoes

Idahoan

Au Gratin	Fresh potatoes
Mashed	Fresh frozen potatoes
Scalloped	Idahoan Hashed Browns
	Ore Ida Southern Style Hash Browns
	Ore Ida Small Whole Potatoes

Borden's
  Country Store Mashed
  Potato with Bacon Bits
French'es
  Au Gratin
Most instant mashed potatoes contain vegetable oil — check label
All prepared fried potatoes

Flours

Hungry Jack	All-purpose flour
Complete Pancake Mix	Cake flour
Buttermilk Pancake Mix	Presto Self-Rising Cake Flour
Aunt Jemima	Hungry Jack Extra Light Pancake Mix
Complete Pancake Mix	Aunt Jemima Original Pancake Mix, Butter-
Bisquick Mix	milk Pancake Mix
Jiffy Mix	Baking powder

Beverages

General Foods International Coffee, all flavors	Whole and skim milk
Hills Brothers European Coffee, all flavors	Coffee — regular and instant
Carnation Coffeemate	Fruit juice — fresh or frozen
Coffee Rich	Fruit-flavored drinks
Poly Perx	Soft drinks
Mitchells Perx	Koolaid — all flavors
Carnation Slender — all flavors	Funny Face — all flavors
Carnation Instant Breakfast — all flavors	Tea — regular and instant
Carnation	
Hot Cocoa mix	
Rich Chocolate Flavor	
Milk Chocolate Flavor	
Chocolate and Marshmallow	
Malted Milk	

CONTAINS SOY	SOY-FREE

Beverages (*Continued*)

Nestlé's Quik Cocoa Mix	Nestlé's Strawberry Quik
Ovaltine Cocoa Mix, Chocolate Flavor, Malt Flavor	Bosco
Hershey's Instant Chocolate	
Swiss Miss Cocoa Mix	

Desserts and Sweets/Snacks

All potato chips
Corn chips
Popcorn
Pretzels
Bambeanos Roasted Soybeans
McCormick Party Dip
Frito-Lay Dip Mixes

Cookies

Must look on all labels	Pepperidge Farm Butter Cookies
Estee Dietetic Foods	Cakes made with butter
Cakes and cake mixes	Duncan Hines Angel Food Cake Mix
Pillsbury Figurines	General Foods Cherry Fluff Frosting, Fluffy
Most prepared frostings	White Frosting, Lemon Frosting
Pop Tarts — all types	Gelatin
Doughnuts	D–Zerta Gelatin
Puddings — most chocolate flavors	

Baking Products

Baker's Chocolate Flavored Chips, Semi-Sweet Chocolate	Baker's Cocoa Unsweetened Baking Chocolate
Nestlé's Coconut Morsels, Butterscotch Chips, Semi-Sweet Chocolate Chips, Milk Chocolate Chips	Hershey's Baking Chocolate
	Fruit pie fillings

Syrups

General Foods Log Cabin Buttery Syrup	General Foods Log Cabin Syrup
Vermont Maid Butter-Flavored Syrup	Karo corn syrup — dark or light, pancake and waffle syrup
	Vermont Maid Syrup
	Sugar and sugar substitutes
	Jams and jellies
	Honey

Candy

Cadbury Chocolate Bar — all types	Brachs' Circus Peanuts, Sour balls, Licorice,
Nestlé's Chocolate Bars — all	Good-and-Plenty, Good-and-Fruity,
Hershey's Chocolate Bars — all	Life-Savers
Reese's, Payday, 5th Avenue, Bolster,	
Oh Henry!, No Jelly, Kraft Toffee, Tootsie	
Rolls, Tootsie Pop Drops, Bit-o-Honey,	
M & Ms, Pom Poms, Junior Mints, Pepper-	
mint Patties, Baby Ruth, Butterfingers,	
Mounds, Almond Joy, Caravelle, 3 Mus-	
keteers, Snickers, Mar's Almond, Choco'-	
Lite, $100,000 Bar, Milky Way	

CONTAINS SOY	SOY-FREE

Oils, Butters, Margarine

CONTAINS SOY	SOY-FREE
Most margarines — check label	Fleischman's Liquid Corn Oil
Progresso Oil	Mazola Corn Oil
Wesson Oil	Planters Peanut Oil
Crisco Oil	Olive oil
Sweet Life Oil	Butter
Spry Hydrogenated Oil	Skippy Peanut Butter
Fluffo Hydrogenated Oil	
Crisco Hydrogenated Oil	
Spray-type oils	
Jif Peanut Butter	
Big-Top Peanut Butter	

Meat and Meat Products

CONTAINS SOY	SOY-FREE
Breaded meats, fish, or poultry	All fresh fish, meat, poultry
Tunafish packed in oil	Tunafish packed in water
Salmon packed in oil	Salmon packed in water
Chef-Boy-ar-dee Meatball Stew	Dinty Moore Beef Stew, Meatball Stew
Armour Treet	Armour Chopped Ham, Chili, Beef, Corned
Underwood Chicken Spread, Roast Beef	Beef, Corned Beef Hash
Spread	Spam
Bac-os	Prudence Roast Beef Hash, Corned Beef
Cold cuts	Hash
Hot dogs	Hormel Chili
Swanson Chicken à la King	Underwood Deviled Ham, Corned Beef,
Armour Sloppy Joe	Liverwurst
Most prepared canned spaghetti dinners	Armour Vienna Sausage, Vienna Sausage
Most prepared canned Chinese dinners	Spread, Potted Meat Food Product, Dried
Hamburger Helper — all styles	Beef
Lipton Make a Better Burger	Swanson Boned Chicken, Boned Turkey
Kraft Egg Noodles with Chicken	Hunt's Manwich
Golden Grain Macaroni and Cheese	Sweet Life Dried Beef
Chef-Boy-ar-dee Pizza Mix	Bounty Chili con Carne, Corned Beef Hash,
Appian Way Pizza Mix	Chili Mac, Chicken Stew
Most prepared spaghetti sauces	Campbell's Pork and Beans, Home-Style
Pennsylvania Dutch Egg Noodles Plus,	Beans, Beans and Franks, Beans and Ground
Chicken Sauce, Butter Sauce	Beef, Old-Fashioned Beans
	Sweet Life Boston Baked Beans
	Palmieri Pizza Sauce
	Betty Crocker Noodles Romanoff
	Kraft Macaroni and Cheese
	Pennsylvania Dutch: Egg Noodles Plus,
	Macaroni and Cheese, Beef Sauce, Cheese
	Sauce

Salad Dressings and Sauces

CONTAINS SOY	SOY-FREE
Kraft Salad Dressings — all	Good Season Mild Italian, Italian, Blue
Pfeiffer Salad Dressings — all	Cheese, Cheese Garlic, Garlic
Frenchette Salad Dressings — all	Weight Watchers French Dressing, Blue
Cains — all	Cheese
Ken's Steak House Dressings — all	Saucy Susan Golden Sauce
Wish Bone Salad Dressings — all	Prime Choice Steak Sauce
Sweet Life Salad Dressings — all	A-1 Sauce

CONTAINS SOY	SOY-FREE

Salad Dressings and Sauces *(Continued)*

Good Season Italian with Cheese and
Croutons, Caesar with Croutons, French,
Low-Calorie Italian
Weight Watchers Italian Dressing, Creole
Mix, Brown Gravy Mix
Good Season Open Pit Barbeque Sauce —
all
Heinz Barbeque Sauce — all flavors
Kraft Barbeque Sauce — all flavors
Grandma's Molasses Barbeque Sauce
Heinz 57 Steak Sauce
French's Worcestershire Sauce
Lea & Perrins Worcestershire Sauce
Soy Sauce — all brands
Frenchette Mayonette Gold
Kraft Miracle Whip, Imitation Mayonnaise,
Real Mayonnaise
Bright Day Mayonnaise
Most gravy/sauce mixes — check labels

Miscellaneous

CONTAINS SOY	SOY-FREE
Frozen vegetables in sauces	Eggs, cheese, cream, pure yogurt, fresh fruits, fresh vegetables, fresh-frozen fruits, fresh-frozen vegetables

Soups

CONTAINS SOY	SOY-FREE
Campbell's	Campbell's
Chunky Beef	Chunky Split Pea with Ham
Chunky Vegetable	Chunky Chicken
Chunky Turkey	Chunky Chicken with Rice
Chunky Sirloin Beef	Tomato
Chunky Minestrone	Vegetarian Vegetable
Chunky Clam Chowder	Chili Beef
Vegetable	Pepper Pot
Vegetable with Beef	Turkey Noodle
Old Fashion Vegetable	Chicken Gumbo
Cream of Asparagus	Curly Noodle
Cream of Potato	Chicken Vegetable
Cream of Shrimp	Noodles and Ground Beef
Cream of Onion	Chicken Noodle Os
Cream of Celery	Chicken and Stars
Cream of Mushroom	
Cream of Chicken	
Golden Mushroom	
Cheddar Cheese	
Green Pea	
Split Pea with Ham	
Tomato Rice	
Tomato Bisque	
Old Fashioned Tomato	

Contains Soy	Soy-Free

Contains Soy

Manhattan Clam Chowder
New England Clam Chowder
Oyster Stew
Chicken Noodle
Beef Broth
Chicken Broth
Beef Consomme
Scotch Broth
Minestrone
Noodle Os
Stock Pot
Onion
Beef
Lipton
   Vegetable Beef
   Chicken Rice
   Tomato Vegetable
   Italian Style Vegetable
   Ring-O-Noodle
   Green Pea
   Beef-Flavor Mushroom
   Chicken Noodle
   Noodle
   Onion
Herb-Ox Bouillon Cubes, Beef, Chicken
MBT Instant Broth
Knorr Instant Soups — all types

MILK PROTEIN OR LACTOSE-FREE DIET

This diet is for the patient who must eliminate *all* sources of lactose from the diet. Lactose is the sugar found in milk, so all foods containing milk are to be excluded from the diet.

Read the label carefully. Avoid any food containing *milk, nonfat milk solids, skim milk, butter, cream, lactose, casein, caseinate,* or *sodium caseinate.* Some children sensitive to milk protein may not tolerate beef products.

Foods Allowed	Foods Not Allowed
Milk: None (exception: use of Lactaid additive to predigest lactose).	All milk and milk drinks — including whole, skim, low fat, dried, evaporated, and condensed milk; human breast milk. Yogurt — any type. Cream — sweet or sour. Infant formulas other than those permitted. Ice cream sodas, milk shakes.
Beverages: Powdered, fruit-flavored drinks, ginger ale, tonics. **Eggs:** As desired.	Any made with milk, such as milkshakes, eggnog, hot chocolate. Eggs made with milk — use specific formula. Do not prepare with butter.

FOODS ALLOWED	FOODS NOT ALLOWED
Meats: Any baked, broiled, roasted, or boiled, except those to be avoided.	Creamed or breaded meat, fish, or poultry. Prepared meats that may contain dried milk solids, including bologna and cold cuts, frankfurts, salami, commercially prepared fish sticks, and some sausage.
Cheese: Although made from milk, some cheeses are lactose-free and may be permitted. These are Camembert, brick, cheddar, Edam, Provolone, Swiss, pasteurized processed American.	All types of cheese and cheese dishes not listed as allowed.
Breads: Breads made without milk only, such as French bread, Italian bread, water bagels, or 'parva' breads.	Made with any form of milk. Any baked product made with milk. Muffins, biscuits, waffles, pancakes, doughnuts, sweet rolls, commercial mixes.
Cereal: Any made without milk, cooked or ready to eat. Macaroni, spaghetti, pasta, rice — all prepared without milk or cheese.	Any prepared cereal that contains dry milk solids.
Vegetables and Potatoes: All — cooked, canned, frozen, or fresh.	Any vegetable prepared with milk, butter, milk solids, bread, or bread crumbs. No cheese or cream sauces.
Fruits: All.	All are allowed.
Desserts: Any made without milk or milk products, such as gelatin desserts, fruit crisp, snow puddings, fruit and water sherbets, pie with fruit filling, angel cake.	All commercial cake and cookie mixes, ice cream, custard puddings, junket, ice milk, or sherbets that contain milk. Frosting made with milk or butter, dessert sauces, cheese cakes.
Soup: Any prepared without milk or milk products. Homemade or canned, e.g., chicken rice.	All creamed soups, chowders.
Fats: Milk-free margarine or 'parva' margarine. Oils, nuts, peanut butter.	Butter, margarine, some commercial salad dressings (check labels).
Sugar and Seasonings: Sugar, honey, molasses, maple syrup, corn syrup, jelly and jam, hard candy, gum drops, marshmallows, hard peppermints, fondant. Salt, pepper, spices, herbs, condiments, vinegar, catsup, relish, pickles, olives, tomato sauce, coconut, wheat germ. Artificial flavoring and extracts.	Any product made from milk, butter, cream, chocolate, toffee, cream mints, caramel candy, candy with cream centers.
Miscellaneous:	Medications that may contain lactose as filler or bulk agents; party dips; nonprescription vitamins; spice blends; Easter egg dyes. Dietetic foods and foods advertised as "high protein" sometimes contain lactose or dry milk solids. *Check all labels carefully.*

SUCROSE-FREE DIET

FOODS ALLOWED	FOODS NOT ALLOWED
Meat and Meat Substitutes: Beef, pork, lamb, veal, chicken, turkey, and other meats and poultry prepared without the addition of sugar such as sucrose or corn syrup, etc.; eggs; cream cheese, cottage cheese, other plain cheeses unprocessed; fish.	Frankfurter, cold cuts to which sucrose may be added as a filler, commercially prepared infant meat and vegetable dinners to which sucrose may be added; some processed cheese spreads.
Beverages: CHO-Free infant formula (Borden's), whole milk, skimmed milk, evaporated milk, buttermilk, plain yogurt; diet sodas not sweetened with sucrose.	Chocolate milk and drink, condensed milk, flavored yogurt or any made with sweetened fruit, milk shakes, ice cream, sherbet, regularly sweetened carbonated beverages.
Vegetables: None.	All
Fruits: None.	All
Fats: Butter, margarine, vegetable oils, sour cream, cream cheese, cream.	Mayonnaise, salad dressings, peanut butter.
Desserts: Custard and vanilla pudding made with allowed ingredients without sugar or sucrose-containing beverages.	Commercially prepared gelatin desserts sweetened with sucrose; cakes, cookies, pies, pastries containing sucrose or wheat germ.
Miscellaneous: Saccharin, sugars, and artificial sweeteners that are free of sucrose such as Sweet 'n' Low, Sugar Twin, Sucaryl, pure spices, and herbs.	Allspice; cane sugar, molasses, honey; most pickles, ketchup, carob powder; almonds, chestnuts, coconut and coconut milk, macadamia nuts, pecans; jams, jellies, preserves made with sucrose, corn syrup, invert sugar.

SUCROSE-RESTRICTED DIET

In addition to all foods permitted on the sucrose-free diet, the following foods should be added to the diet:

Fruits and Fruit Juices Containing 1% or Less Sucrose
Gooseberries, loganberries, blackberries, cranberries, currants, lemons, rhubarb, pomegranates.

Limit to three to four half cup servings daily.

Fruits and Fruit Juices Containing More Than 1% but Less Than 2% Sucrose
Boysenberries, Bing cherries, figs, Tokay or Thompson seedless grapes, guava, lime juice, pears, raspberries, strawberries.

Limit to one-half cup serving only.

Vegetables Containing 1% or Less Sucrose
Snap, string or green beans, cabbage, cauliflower, celery, corn, eggplant, lettuce, white potato, pumpkin, radishes, Hubbard, butternut, or crookneck squash, tomatoes, tomato juice.

Limit to three to four half cup servings daily.

---

*From ADA Manual of Applied Nutriton.
†Adapted from Sucrase-isomaltase deficiency — a frequently misdiagnosed disease (1).

Grains, Cereals, Nuts, Miscellaneous
Containing 1% or Less Sucrose
Cornmeal, puffed rice, whole wheat cereals   As desired.
and crackers, patent wheat flour, brown or
white rice, macaroni, spaghetti; Kraft
mayonnaise, Kraft Salad Bowl Mayonnaise,
commercial salad dressings, pecans, honey.

SAMPLE MENU*

Breakfast
4 oz cranberry juice
1 cup milk
scrambled egg in butter
puffed rice, ½ cup with 2 teaspoons fructose
toast, butter

Lunch
hamburger on a bun with 1 sliced tomato
French fried potatoes
½ cup corn
½ cup fresh or frozen unsweetened strawberries with 1 teaspoon fructose
1 cup milk
1 teaspoon butter

Dinner
3 oz rib eye steak
½ cup mashed potato
½ cup butternut squash
bread — 1 slice
butter — 2 teaspoons
milk — 1 cup
Bing cherries — ½ cup

Bedtime Snack
custard, made with fructose

ADEQUATE FAT DIET

1. To achieve an adequate intake of fat, the patient's diet should contain 35 per cent of total kilocalories as dietary fats. The level of fat is derived from the estimated energy needs (Kilocalories) for patient age and size.

2. The diet is planned to provide the recommended fat level from formula, milk, or commonly available foods (see following list). When the child is unable to take adequate fat in the diet, it may be given in the liquid form (oil).

3. When an adequate fat diet is to be given for quantitative analysis of fat in stool, the diet adequate in fat should be instituted 24 hours prior to the start of the stool collection. A careful food record should be kept during the collection period and analyzed by a registered dietitian for adequacy. A list of the fat content of common foods is helpful to families in maintaining adequate levels in the diet.

4. When an adequate fat diet is presented on a long-term basis, counseling by a registered dietitian is helpful to the family in planning menus to suit the patient's particular needs.

FOOD	AMOUNT (Level Household Measure)	FAT VALUE (Grams)
Whole milk	4 ounces	5
Cheese	1 slice or 1 ounce	6
Custard	½ cup	9
Yogurt, low fat milk–based	½ cup	4
Ice cream	½ cup	10
Pudding	½ cup	5
Cottage cheese	½ cup	5
Sour cream	1 tablespoon	3
Cream cheese	1 tablespoon	5
Mayonnaise	1 tablespoon	10
Imitation mayonnaise	1 tablespoon	5
Salad dressing	1 tablespoon	5
Margarine or butter	1 teaspoon	5
Cooking oil	1 teaspoon	5
Meat	1 ounce	5
Egg	1 (whole, medium)	5
Luncheon meat	1 slice	7
Hot dog	1 (8 per pound)	10
Bacon	1 slice	5
Nuts	8 small	5
Peanut butter	1 level tablespoon	7
French fries, frozen	10 pieces	5
Potato chips	7 average (½ ounce)	5
Cookie	1 average	2
Milk chocolate	1 ounce	10

LOW LONG-CHAIN TRIGLYCERIDE, HIGH MEDIUM-CHAIN TRIGLYCERIDE DIET

The fat content of this diet is altered to decrease the long-chain triglyceride (LCT) fat content and to replace this with medium-chain triglyceride–containing fats (MCT). MCT is provided as an oil or as part of a special formula. It is a form of fat that is more easily absorbed and digested than fat found in conventional food.

The diet should be planned with the assistance of a registered dietitian to meet the energy, protein, and nutrient needs of the patient while limiting the LCT fats and incorporating the desired level of MCT oil.* Specific amounts of MCT oil and/or MCT-containing formula (Portogen and Pregestimil) should be identified in a meal plan to help assure adequacy of the diet.

Foods Allowed	Foods Not Allowed
Milk: Skim milk, skim milk–based beverages.	Whole milk, low-fat milk, buttermilk, cream in any form.
Beverages: Powdered fruit-flavored drinks, ginger ale, soda.	Any beverage made with whole or low-fat milk, milkshakes, ice cream soda.
Eggs: Egg whites, egg yolks, and whole eggs only when calculated into diet.	Whole eggs, egg yolks, egg substitutes unless calculated into diet.
Cheese: Skim milk cottage cheese, skim milk mozzarella cheese.	Any cheese made from whole or low-fat milk.
Meat, Fish, Poultry: Only in amount calculated: lean meat (well trimmed of fat), fish, poultry, tuna in water.	Fatty meats, fish, tuna in oil, poultry. Any fried meats. Cold cuts, frankfurts, salami, sausages.
Bread and Cereal: Bread — whole wheat, white enriched, rye, pumpernickel; hard rolls, hamburger type rolls, English muffins, most cooked and dry cereals, rice, pasta. Plain crackers such as soda crackers or saltines.	Commercial or homemade biscuits, muffins, cornbread, commercial crackers containing fat or butter. Doughnuts.
Vegetables and Potatoes: All are permitted provided they are prepared without fat, sauces, or frying.	All fried foods including French fried potatoes, sautéed vegetables, potato chips. No sauces. Avocadoes.
Fruit and Juices: All.	Avocadoes.
Desserts: Angel food cake, meringue, gelatin, water ice. Desserts made with skim milk and MCT oil may be permitted.	Ice cream, sherbet, pudding, custard, cake, coffeecake, Danish pastries, pies, cookies, commercial mixes.
Soups: Fat-free bouillon, consomme, and broth. Soups made from these and no other fat added.	Chowders, cream soups.
Fats: None except MCT oil, which may be used in preparation of some items.	Sauces, gravies, nuts, chocolate, and olives.
Seasonings: Sugar, salt, pepper, spices, and herbs.	Any seasoning containing fat.
Miscellaneous: Hard candy containing no fat. Plain popcorn.	Most convenience foods; snack foods such as corn chips, cheese-flavored snacks, etc. Candy made with chocolate, cream, butter, or coconut. Chocolate fudge. Commercial popcorn.

---

*MCT oil is available from Mead Johnson.

Carbohydrate Content of Common Foods (per 100 gm edible portion)

	Mono-saccharides		Reducing	Disaccharides			Polysaccharides					
Food	Fructose (gm)	Glucose (gm)	Sugars* (gm)	Lactose (gm)	Maltose (gm)	Sucrose (gm)	Cellulose (gm)	Dextrins (gm)	Hemi-cellulose (gm)	Pectin (gm)	Pento-sans (gm)	Starch (gm)
Fruits												
Agave juice	17.0		19.0	†		3.1						0.6
Apple	5.0	1.7	8.3			4.2	0.4		0.7	0.6		
Apple juice		1.9	8.0									
Apricots	0.4					5.5	0.8		1.2	1.0		
Banana												
Yellow green			5.0			5.1						8.8
Yellow	3.5	4.5	8.4			8.9						1.9
Flecked						11.9						1.2
Powder			32.6			33.2		9.6				7.8
Blackberries	2.9	3.2				0.2						
Blueberry juice, commercial			9.6			0.2						
Boysenberries			5.3			1.1				0.3		
Breadfruit												
Hawaiian			1.8			7.7						
Samoan			4.9			9.7						
Cherries												
Eating	7.2	4.7	12.5			0.1				0.3		
Cooking	6.1	5.5	11.6			0.1						
Cranberries	0.7	2.7				0.1						
Currants												
Black	3.7	2.4				0.6						
Red	1.9	2.3				0.2						
White	2.6	3.0										
Dates												
Invert sugar, seedling type	23.9	24.9				0.3						
Deglet Noor			16.2			45.4						
Egyptian			35.8			48.5						3.0
Figs, Kadota												
Fresh	8.2	9.6				0.9						0.1
Dried	30.9	42.0				0.1						0.3
Gooseberries	4.1	4.4				0.7						

(Continued)

Carbohydrate Content of Common Foods (per 100 gm edible portion) (Continued)

FOOD	MONO-SACCHARIDES		REDUCING SUGARS* (gm)	DISACCHARIDES			POLYSACCHARIDES					
	Fructose (gm)	Glucose (gm)		Lactose (gm)	Maltose (gm)	Sucrose (gm)	Cellulose (gm)	Dextrins (gm)	Hemi-cellulose (gm)	Pectin (gm)	Pento-sans (gm)	Starch (gm)
Fruits, *continued*												
Grapes												
Black	7.3	8.2										
Concord	4.3	4.8	9.5			0.2						
Malaga			22.2			0.2						
White	8.0	8.1										
Grapefruit	1.2	2.0	4.4			2.9					1.3	
Guava						1.9						
Lemon												
Edible portion			1.3			0.2				3.0		
Whole	1.4	1.4				0.4					0.7	
Juice	0.9	0.5				0.1						
Peel			3.4			0.1						
Loganberries	1.3	1.9				0.2						
Loquat												
Champagne	12.0					0.8						
Thales		9.0				0.9						
Mango			3.4			11.6						0.3
Melon												
Cantaloupe	0.9	1.2	2.3			4.4				0.3		
Cassaba												
Vine ripened			2.8			6.2						
Picked green			3.2			3.9						
Honeydew												
Vine ripened			3.3			7.4						
Picked green			3.6			3.3						
Yellow	1.5	2.1				1.4						
Mulberries	3.6	4.4										
Orange												
Valencia (Calif.)	2.3	2.4	4.7			4.2						
Composite values	1.8	2.5	5.0			4.6	0.3		0.3	1.3	0.3	
Juice												
Fresh	2.4	2.4	5.1			4.7						
Frozen, reconstituted			4.6			3.2						
Palmyra palm, tender kernel	1.5	3.2				0.4						

Papaw (Asimina triloba) (North America)	3.6		5.9		2.7		
Papaya (Carica papaya)							
(tropics)	1.6		9.0		0.5		1.8
Passion fruit juice		3.6	3.1		3.8	0.7	
Peaches		1.5			6.6		0.7
Pears							
Anjou	5.0	2.5	7.6		1.9		0.7
Bartlett	6.5	2.6	8.0		1.5		0.6
Bosc					1.7		0.6
Persimmon			17.7				
Pineapple							
Ripened on plant	1.4	2.3	4.2		7.9		
Picked green			1.3		2.4		
Plums							
Damson	3.4		8.4		1.0		
Greengage	4.0	5.2			2.9		
Italian prunes	2.9	5.5	4.6		5.4	0.5	0.9
Sweet	1.3	4.5	7.4		4.4		1.0
Sour		3.5			1.5		1.0
Pomegranate	15.0		12.0	2.8	0.6		0.9
Prunes, uncooked		30.0	47.0		2.0		1.0
Raisins, Thompson seedless			70.0			2.0	0.8
Raspberries	2.4	2.3	5.0				
Sapote	3.8	4.2			0.7		0.7
Strawberries							
Ripe	2.3		3.8		1.4		
Medium ripe		2.6	4.8		0.3		
Tangerine	1.2	1.6	3.4		9.0	0.3	0.3
Tomatoes							
Canned			3.0	0.2	0.3		
Seedless pulp			6.5	0.4	0.4	0.5	0.5
Watermelon							
Flesh red and firm, ripe			3.8		4.0	0.1	0.1
Red, mealy, overripe			3.0		4.9	0.1	0.1

Vegetables

Asparagus, raw	1.2				0.2		0.3
Bamboo shoots	0.5				1.2		
Beans							
Lima							
Canned					1.4		
Fresh					1.4		
Fresh	1.7				0.5	0.3	1.0
Snap, fresh			1.0	0.9	12.9	0.5	0.8
Beets, sugar			0.8		0.9	0.9	1.2
Broccoli			0.9		12.9	0.9	2.0

(Continued)

Carbohydrate Content of Common Foods (per 100 gm edible portion) (Continued)

FOOD	MONOSACCHARIDES		REDUCING SUGARS* (gm)	DISACCHARIDES			POLYSACCHARIDES					
	Fructose (gm)	Glucose (gm)		Lactose (gm)	Maltose (gm)	Sucrose (gm)	Cellulose (gm)	Dextrins (gm)	Hemicellulose (gm)	Pectin (gm)	Pentosans (gm)	Starch (gm)
Vegetables, continued												
Brussels sprouts							1.1		1.5			
Cabbage, raw			3.4			0.3	0.8		1.0			
Carrots, raw			5.8			1.7	1.0		1.7			
Cauliflower		2.8				0.3	0.7		0.6	0.9		
Celery												
Fresh			0.3			0.3						
Hearts			1.7			0.2						
Corn												
Fresh									0.9		1.3	
Bran		0.5				0.3	0.6	0.1	77.1		4.0	14.5
Cucumber			2.5			0.1						
Eggplant			2.1			0.6			0.5			
Lettuce			1.4			0.2	0.4		0.6			
Licorice root		1.4				3.2						22.0
Mushrooms, fresh			0.1			2.9			0.7			2.5
Onions, raw			5.4			3.5	0.9		0.3			
Parsnips, fresh						5.5				0.6		7.0
Peas, green	0.1					0.1	1.1		2.2			4.1
Potatoes, white	0.1	0.1	0.8			0.6	0.4		0.3			17.0
Pumpkin			2.2			0.3			0.5			0.1
Radishes			3.1			1.3			0.3			
Rutabagas		5.0								0.4		
Spinach			0.2				0.4		0.8		0.8	
Squash												
Butternut	0.2	0.1				0.4						2.6
Blue Hubbard	1.2	1.1				0.4	0.7					4.8
Golden crookneck			2.8			1.0						
Sweet potato												
Raw	0.3	0.4	0.8		1.6	4.1	0.6		1.4	2.2		16.5
Baked			14.5			7.2						4.0

Mature Dry Legumes

Beans							
Mung	1.6						
Black gram	1.8						
Green gram							
Navy	7.2		3.1	3.7	6.4	8.2	35.2
Soy	1.5		2.6	1.4	6.6	4.0	1.9
Cow pea	2.4	1.6	5.4		4.8		
Garbanzo (chickpeas)							
Garden pea (*Pisum sativum*)‡	6.7		5.0		5.1		38.0
Horse gram (*Dolichos biplorus*)	2.7						
Lentils	2.1						
Pigeon pea (red gram)	1.6						28.5
Soybean							
Flour	6.8						
Meal	6.8						

Milk and Milk Products

Buttermilk				
Dry			39.9	
Fluid, genuine and cultured			5.0	
Casein	0.1	16.6	4.9	
Ice cream (14.5% cream)			3.6	
Milk				
Ass			6.0	
Cow			4.9	
Dried				
Skim			52.0	
Whole			38.1	
Fluid				
Skim			5.0	
Whole			4.9	
Sweetened, condensed			14.1	43.5
Ewe			4.9	
Goat			4.7	
Human				
Colostrum			5.3	
Mature			6.9	
Whey			4.9	
Yogurt			3.8	

(Continued)

Carbohydrate Content of Common Foods (per 100 gm edible portion) (Continued)

FOOD	MONO-SACCHARIDES		REDUC-ING SUGARS* (gm)	DISACCHARIDES			POLYSACCHARIDES					
	Fructose (gm)	Glucose (gm)		Lactose (gm)	Maltose (gm)	Sucrose (gm)	Cellulose (gm)	Dextrins (gm)	Hemicellulose (gm)	Pectin (gm)	Pentosans (gm)	Starch (gm)
Nuts and Nut Products												
Almonds, blanched						2.3					2.1	
Chestnuts			0.2			3.6					1.2	18.0
Virginia			2.2			8.1					2.8	18.6
French			3.3			3.6					2.5	33.1
Coconut milk, ripe						2.6		0.3				
Copra meal, dried	1.2	1.2				14.3	15.6	0.6			2.2	0.9
Macadamia nut			0.3			5.5						
Peanuts			0.2			4.5	2.4					
Peanut butter			0.9					2.5	3.8			4.0
Pecans						1.1					0.2	5.9
Cereals and Cereal Products												
Barley												
Grain, hulled							2.6		6.0		8.5	62.0
Flour											1.2	69.0
Corn, yellow						3.1					6.2	62.0
Flaxseed							4.5		4.9			
Millet grain							1.8		5.2		6.5	56.0
Oats, hulled									0.9		6.4	56.4
Rice												
Bran			1.4			10.6	11.4		7.0		7.4	
Brown, raw			0.1			0.8		2.1			2.1	69.7
Polished, raw		2.0	trace#			0.4	0.3	0.9			1.8	72.9
Polished			0.7								3.8	
Rye												
Grain											6.8	57.0
Flour											4.1	71.4
Sorghum grain							3.8		5.6		2.5	70.2
Soya-wheat (cereal)											3.3	46.4
Wheat												
Germ, defatted			2.0			8.3					6.2	
Grain			2.0			1.5	2.0	2.5	5.8		6.6	59.0
Flour, patent					0.1	0.2		5.5			2.1	68.8

Spices and Condiments

Allspice (pimenta)			18.0			3.0			
Cassia			23.3						
Cinnamon			19.3						2.7
Cloves			9.0						
Nutmeg			17.2						14.6
Pepper, black			38.6						34.2

Syrups and Other Sweets

Corn syrup	21.2				26.4	56.4	34.7		
High conversion	33.0				23.0	31.0	19.0		
Medium conversion	26.0				21.0		23.0		
Corn sugar	87.5				3.5		0.5		
Chocolate, sweet dry			37.5						
Golden syrup	34.2						1.5		
Honey		40.5				1.9			
Invert sugar			74.0			6.0			
Jellies, pectin		11.3				40–65			
Royal jelly	9.8					0.9			7–12
Jellies, starch						25–60			
Maple syrup			1.5			62.9			
Milk chocolate				8.1		43.0			
Molasses	8.8	8.0	26.9			53.6			
Blackstrap	6.8	6.8				36.9			
Sorghum syrup			27.0			36.0			

Miscellaneous

Beer			1.5			1.9	0.3		
Cacao beans, raw, Arriba	0.6	0.5	1.1						
Carbo bean								1.4	
Pod			11.2			23.2			
Pod and seeds			11.1			19.4			
Soy sauce	0.9								

*Mainly monosaccharides plus the disaccharides, maltose and lactose.
‡Blanks indicate lack of acceptable data.
‡Also known as Alaska pea, field pea, and common pea.
#Trace = less than 0.05 gm.
From Hardinge, M. G., Swarner, J. B., and Crooks, H.: Carbohydrates in foods. J. Am. Dietet. Assoc. 46:197, 1965.

Less Common Carbohydrates in Foods, Per 100 Gm. Edible Portion

FOOD	CARBOHYDRATES (gm)		
	Arabinose	*Araban*	
Beet sugar	0.6	—	
Soybean meal	—	4.7	
Soybean flour	—	3.6	
Soy sauce	0.3	—	
	Galactose	*Galactans*	
Peach	0.2	—	
Sapote	0.6	—	
Beet sugar	0.3	—	
Rutabagas	—	0.3	
Navy bean	—	1.3	
Soybean	—	2.3	
Soybean flour	—	4.2	
Soybean meal	—	4.1	
Soybean sauce	0.4	—	
Casein	0.2	—	
Pear	0.2	—	
Apple	0.2	—	
	Glycogen (Phytoglycogen)		
Corn, fresh	4.4		
Mushrooms, fresh	0.6		
	Mannose	*Mannans*	
Egg albumin	0.3	—	
Casein	0.1	—	
Brewer's yeast	—	14.0	
	Pentose		
Copra meal	2.4		
Corn kernel	0.2		
	Raffinose	*Stachyose*	*Verbascose*
Beans, black mung, dry	0.5	1.8	3.7
Beans, green mung, dry	0.8	2.5	3.8
Beans, soy, dry	1.9	5.2	—
Cacao seeds, raw	—	1.9	—
Copra meal	2.4	—	—
Cow pea	0.4	2.0	3.1
Field bean (*Dolichos lablab*)	0.5	2.1	3.6
Garbanzo (chickpea)	1.0	2.5	4.2
Horse gram	0.7	2.0	3.1
Lentils	0.6	2.2	3.0
Lima beans, canned	—	0.2	—
Molasses, beet	1.8	—	—
Pigeon pea	1.1	2.7	4.1
Wheat germ, defatted	6.6	—	—
	Sorbitol		
Apple	1.0		
Apple juice	0.3		
Apricot	1.0		
Hawthorn	4.7		
Hawthorn, English	7.6		
Loquat	0.2		
Pear, small green	2.4		
Pear, large green	1.9		
Pear, ripe	2.3		
Pear, Bose	3.5		
Peach	0.2		
Plum, Kelsey	2.8		
Pyracantha berry	4.0		
Rowan berries (mountain ash)	8.7		
Toyon berry, green	2.5		

From Hardinge, M. G., Swarner, J. B., and Crooks, H.: Carbohydrates in foods. J. Am. Dietet. Assoc. *46*:197, 1965.

Index

Page numbers in *italics* denote illustrations; (t) indicates tabular material.

747